NURSING DIAGNOSIS HANDBOOK

*An Evidence-Based
Guide to Planning Care*

NURSING DIAGNOSIS HANDBOOK

An Evidence-Based
Guide to Planning Care

Betty J. Ackley, MSN, EdS, RN

Gail B. Ladwig, MSN, RN, CHTP

Eighth Edition

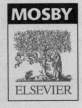

MOSBY

ELSEVIER

MOSBY
ELSEVIER

11830 Westline Industrial Drive
St. Louis, Missouri 63146

NURSING DIAGNOSIS HANDBOOK: AN EVIDENCE-BASED GUIDE TO
PLANNING CARE, EIGHTH EDITION

ISBN: 978-0-323-04826-2

Notice

Knowledge and best practice in this field are constantly changing. As new research and experience
broaden our knowledge, changes in practice, treatment and drug therapy may become necessary or
appropriate. Readers are advised to check the most current information provided (i) on procedures
featured or (ii) by the manufacturer of each product to be administered, to verify the recommended dose
or formula, the method and duration of administration, and contraindications. It is the responsibility of
the practitioner, relying on their own experience and knowledge of the patient, to make diagnoses, to
determine dosages and the best treatment for each individual patient, and to take all appropriate safety
precautions. To the fullest extent of the law, neither the Publisher nor the Authors assume any liability
for any injury and/or damage to persons or property arising out or related to any use of the material
contained in this book.

The Publisher

Library of Congress Control Number 2007928537

Senior Acquisitions Editor: Sandra Clark Brown
Senior Developmental Editor: Cindi Anderson
Publishing Services Manager: Deborah L. Vogel
Senior Project Manager: Steve Ramay
Design Direction: Julia Dummitt

Printed in the United States of America

Working together to grow
libraries in developing countries

www.elsevier.com | www.bookaid.org | www.sabre.org

ELSEVIER **BOOK AID International** **Sabre Foundation**

Last digit is the print number: 9 8 7 6 5 4 3 2 1

To:

Dale Ackley, the greatest guy in the world, without whose support this book would have
never happened, and my daughter, Dr. Dawn and her husband Cameron Goulding.
And the absolute joy of my life, granddaughter Althea Rose Goulding.

Jerry Ladwig, my wonderful husband, who after 43 years is still supportive and helpful—
he is "my right hand man" in revising this book every two years.
Also to my very special children, their spouses and all of my grandchildren;
Jerry, Kathy, Alexandra, Elizabeth, and Benjamin Ladwig; Christine, John, Sean, Ciara and
Bridget McMahon; Jennifer, Jim, Abby, Katelyn, Blake and Connor Martin;
Amy, Scott, Ford and Vaughn Bertram—the greatest family anyone could ever hope for.

A special thank you to Cindi Anderson, Senior Developmental Editor for Elsevier.
She has worked tirelessly on this project for many editions.
She is not only a colleague but has become a treasured and very special friend.

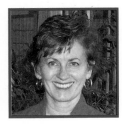

Betty Ackley has worked in nursing for more than 37 years in many capacities. She has been a staff nurse on a CCU unit, medical ICU unit, respiratory ICU unit, intensive care unit, and step-down unit. She has worked on a gynecological surgery floor, and an orthopedic floor, and she has spent many years working in oncology. She also has been in management, has been in nursing education in a hospital, and spent 31 years as a professor of nursing at Jackson Community College. In 1996, she began the online learning program at Jackson Community College, offering a course in nutrition online. In 2000 Betty was named Faculty of the Year at her college.

Betty has presented conferences nationally and internationally in the areas of nursing diagnosis, nursing process and online learning. She has written NCLEX-RN questions for the national licensure examination four times and is an expert in the area of testing and NCLEX preparation.

Betty obtained her BSN from Michigan State University, MS in nursing from the University of Michigan, and education specialist degree from Michigan State University.

Presently Betty has her own company and serves as a nursing consultant for the Research Committee at W.A. Foote Memorial Hospital. In addition she has written/edited another text entitled *Evidence-based Nursing Care Guidelines: Medical-Surgical Interventions.* This text will be available in November of 2007, and will help nurses utilize evidence to provide excellent nursing care.

Her free time is spent exercising, especially spinning and Pilates. She is certified in both and teaches Pilates. In addition, she loves to travel, read, garden, spend time with her granddaughter, and learn anything new!

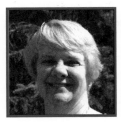

Gail Ladwig is a professor Emeritus of Jackson Community college. During her tenure there she served four years as the Department Chairperson of Nursing and as a nurse consultant for Continuing education. She was instrumental in starting a BSN transfer program with the University of Michigan.

Gail has taught classroom and clinical at JCC in Fundamentals, Med-Surg, and Mental Health; as well as transfer course for BSN students. In addition she has taught online courses in pharmacology and a hybrid course (partially online) for BSN transfer students. She has also taught a course in pathophysiology online for the Medical University of South Carolina.

She worked as a staff nurse in medical-surgical nursing and intensive care for over 20 years prior to beginning her teaching career. She was a Certified Critical Care Nurse for several years. She has a Masters Degree in Psychiatric Mental Health Nursing from Wayne State University. Her Masters research was published in the *International Journal of Addictions.*

She has presented nationally and internationally, in Paris, Japan, and Puerto Rico. She has presented on many topics including nursing diagnosis, computerized care planning, and holistic nursing topics.

In addition to co-authoring this text, Gail is also a coauthor/editor of a new text entitled *Evidence-based Nursing Care Guidelines: Medical-Surgical Interventions.* This text will be available in November of 2007, and will help nurses utilize evidence to provide excellent nursing care. Gail also is a reviewer for *WORLDviews on EVIDENCE-BASED NURSING.* She published an article in *always a nurse,* Sigma Theta Tau's online newsletter, "Joys of Retirement," Summer 2006.

She is certified as a Healing Touch practitioner and is co-owner and founder of Holistic Choices, specializing in Alternative presentations and Healing Touch and Guided Imagery treatments. She helped to start the first "Healthy Living Day" in Jackson, Michigan.

Gail volunteers at Saint Luke's clinic in Jackson, Michigan. She has also volunteered at Volunteers in Medicine on Hilton Head Island. Both of these clinics serve the underserved and uninsured populations, the working poor. Gail gets a great deal of satisfaction working at both of these clinics.

Gail is the mother of four children and grandmother of twelve. She loves to spend time with her grandchildren. She has been married to Jerry for almost 43 years. She is passionate about her family and the profession of nursing.

CONTRIBUTORS

Betty Ackley, MSN, EdS, RN
President and Owner
The Betty Ackley, LLC
Consultant in Nursing Process, Evidence-based Nursing
    and Pilates
Jackson, Michigan
*Activity Intolerance; Risk for Aspiration; Acute Confusion;
    Impaired Dentition; Diarrhea; Deficient Diversional Activity;
    Readiness for enhanced Fluid Balance; Deficient Fluid balance;
    Excess Fluid volume; Risk for deficient Fluid volume; Risk for
    enhanced Fluid volume; Hyperthermia; Hypothermia; Risk
    for Injury; Sedentary Lifestyle; Impaired physical Mobility;
    Nausea; Noncompliance; Imbalanced Nutrition: less than
    body requirements; Imbalanced Nutrition: more than body
    requirements; Readiness for enhanced Nutrition; Risk for
    imbalanced Nutrition: more than body requirements; Impaired
    Oral mucous membrane; Risk for Peripheral neurovascular
    dysfunction; Pruritus; Disturbed Sensory perception; Chronic
    Sorrow; Impaired Swallowing; Ineffective Thermoregulation*

Nadine M. Aktan, MS, RN, APN-C, PhD(c)
Instructor
Nursing Department
William Paterson University
Wayne, New Jersey
*Risk for Suffocation, Consultant in Pediatric Diagnoses and
    Interventions, Sections II and III*

Donna L. Algase, PhD, RN, FAAN, FGSA
Professor and Faculty Associate, Institute of Gerontology
Director, Center on Frail and Vulnerable Elders
University of Michigan
Ann Arbor, Michigan
Wandering

Keith A. Anderson, PhD
Assistant Professor
College of Social Work
The Ohio State University
Columbus, Ohio
Readiness for enhanced family Coping

Sharon Baranoski, MSN, RN, CWOCN, APN, FAAN
Director of Medical Surgical Nursing
Provena Saint Joseph Medical Center
Joliet, Illinois
*Impaired Skin integrity; Risk for impaired Skin integrity; Impaired
    Tissue integrity*

Nancy Albright Beyer, RN, MSN, CEN
Teaching Specialist
School of Nursing
University of Minnesota
Minneapolis, Minnesota
Risk for impaired Liver function

Kathaleen C. Bloom, PhD, CNM
Professor and Undergraduate Coordinator
School of Nursing
University of North Florida
Jacksonville, Florida
*Ineffective Health maintenance; Health-seeking behaviors; Deficient
    Knowledge; Readiness for enhanced Knowledge*

Lisa Burkhart, PhD, RN
Assistant Professor
Marcella Niehoff School of Nursing
Loyola University
Chicago, Illinois
*Decisional Conflict; Moral distress; Spiritual distress; Risk for
    Spiritual distress; Readiness for enhanced Spiritual well-being*

Stacey M. Carroll, PhD, APRN, BC
Associate Professor
School of Nursing
University of Massachusetts at Amherst
Amherst, Massachusetts
*Readiness for enhanced Communication; Impaired verbal
    Communication*

Susan Mee Coleman, RN, PhD(c), CPNP
Assistant Professor
Department of Nursing
College of Staten Island
The City University of New York
Staten Island, New York
Readiness for enhanced Immunization

June M. Como, RN, MSA, MS, CCRN, CCNS
Faculty
Department of Nursing
College of Staten Island
The City University of New York
Staten Island, New York
Stress Overload

Elizabeth Crago, RN, MSN
Research Associate
School of Nursing
University of Pittsburgh
Pittsburgh, Pennsylvania
Autonomic dysreflexia

Maryanne Crowther, MSN, RN, APNC, CCRN
CHF Coordinator; Nurse Practitioner
Jersey Shore University Medical Center
Neptune, New Jersey
Ineffective Tissue perfusion; Decreased Cardiac output

Ruth Davidhizar, RN, DNS, ARNP, BC, FAAN
Dean
School of Nursing
Bethel College
Mishawaka, Indiana
Consultant in Culturally Competent Nursing Care

Rebecca L. Davis, RN, PhD
Kirkhoff School of Nursing
Grand Valley State University
Grand Rapids, Michigan
Chronic Confusion

Mary DeWys, BS, RN
Infant and Feeding Developmental Specialist
Spectrum Health Healthier Communities
Grand Rapids, Michigan
*Disorganized Infant behavior; Risk for disorganized Infant
    behavior; Readiness for enhanced organized Infant behavior;
    Ineffective Infant feeding pattern; Risk for impaired parent/child
    attachment*

Brenda Emick-Herring, RN, MSN, CRRN
Rehabilitation Clinical Nurse
St. Lukes Hospital
Cedar Rapids, Iowa
*Impaired bed Mobility; Impaired wheelchair Mobility; Impaired
    transfer Ability; Impaired Walking*

Dawn Fairlie, MS, ANP, FNP, GNP
Faculty
College of Staten Island
The City University of New York
Staten Island, New York
*Ineffective community Coping; Readiness for enhanced community
    Coping; Effective Therapeutic regimen management; Ineffective
    family Therapeutic regimen management; Ineffective
    Therapeutic regimen management; Readiness for enhanced
    Therapeutic regimen management*

Arlene T. Farren, RN, PhD, AOCN
Assistant Professor
College of Staten Island
The City University of New York
Staten Island, New York
Ineffective Coping; Defensive Coping; Hopelessness

Terri A. Foster, RN, BSN, CNOR
Surgical Services Educator
Surgery Department
Foote Hospital
Jackson, Michigan
*Risk for imbalanced Fluid volume; Risk for perioperative
    positioning Injury*

Judith A. Floyd, PhD, RN, FAAN
Associate Dean for Research
College of Nursing
Wayne State University
Detroit, Michigan
Insomnia; Readiness for enhanced Sleep; Sleep Deprivation

Joseph E. Gaugler, PhD
Assistant Professor
Center on Aging
Center for Gerontological Nursing
School of Nursing
The University of Minnesota
Minneapolis, Minnesota
Readiness for enhanced family Coping; Compromised family Coping

Judith R. Gentz, APRN-BC
President
Nurse Practitioner Care, Inc.
Grass Lake, Michigan
*Chronic low Self-esteem; Situational low Self-esteem; Risk for
    situational low Self-esteem; Disturbed Thought processes*

Joyce Newman Giger, EdD, APRN, BC, FAAN
Professor and Lulu Wolff Hassenplug Endowed Chair
School of Nursing
University of California Los Angeles
Los Angeles, California
Consultant in Culturally Competent Nursing Care

Marie Giordano, RN, MS
Instructor
Department of Nursing
College of Staten Island
The City University of New York
Staten Island, New York
*Readiness for enhanced Power; Readiness for enhanced Hope;
    Readiness for enhanced Decision-making*

Barbara Given, RN, PhD, FAAN
University Distinguished Professor
College of Nursing
Michigan State University
East Lansing, Michigan
Fatigue; Caregiver role strain

Mikel Gray PhD, FNP, PNP, CUNP, CCCN, FAANP, FAAN
Professor and Nurse Practitioner
School of Nursing
Department of Urology
University of Virginia
Charlottesville, Virginia
Bowel Incontinence; Functional urinary Incontinence; Reflex urinary Incontinence; Stress urinary Incontinence; Total urinary Incontinence; Urge urinary Incontinence; Overflow urinary Incontinence; Impaired Urinary elimination; Urinary retention; Risk for urge urinary Incontinence; Readiness for enhanced Urinary elimination

Pauline McKinney Green, PhD, RN
Professor
Division of Nursing
Howard University
Washington, DC
Contamination; Risk for Contamination

Sherry A. Greenberg, MSN, APRN, BC, GNP
Consultant
Hartford Institute for Geriatric Nursing
New York University College of Nursing
New York, New York
Risk for Falls

Elizabeth A. Henneman, RN, PhD, CCNS
Assistant Professor
School of Nursing
University of Massachusetts Amherst
Amherst, Massachusetts
Dysfunctional Ventilatory weaning response; Impaired spontaneous Ventilation

T. Heather Herdman, RN, PhD
Executive Vice President
Matousek & Associates Inc., medFOCUS Research
Green Bay, Wisconsin
Readiness for enhanced Parenting; Impaired Parenting; Risk for impaired Parenting; Grieving; Complicated Grieving; Risk for complicated Grieving

Paula D. Hopper, MSN, RN
Professor of Nursing
Jackson Community College
Jackson, Michigan
Risk for unstable blood Glucose

Teresa Howell, MSN, RN
Associate Professor of Nursing
Morehead State University
Morehead, Kentucky
Section II, Maternal Child; Effective Breastfeeding; Ineffective Breastfeeding; Interrupted Breastfeeding

Jean D. Humphries, MSN, RN
Doctoral Student
Wayne State University
Detroit, Michigan
Insomnia; Readiness for enhanced Sleep; Sleep deprivation

Mike Jacobs, RN, DNS
Chair and Associate Professor
Department of Adult Health Nursing
College of Nursing
University of South Alabama
Mobile, Alabama
Impaired Gas exchange; Ineffective Breathing pattern; Ineffective Airway clearance

Rebecca A. Johnson, PhD, RN
Millsap Professor of Gerontologic Nursing
Sinclair School of Nursing
Director, Research Center for Human Animal Interaction (ReCHAI)
College of Veterinary Medicine
University of Missouri—Columbia
Columbia, Missouri
Relocation stress syndrome

Beverly Kopala, PhD, RN
Associate Professor
Marcella Niehoff School of Nursing
Loyola University
Chicago, Illinois
Moral distress; Decisional conflict

Gail B. Ladwig, MSN, RN, CHTP
Co-Owner Holistic Choices
Consultant: Guided Imagery, Healing Touch, Holistic Nursing, Nursing Diagnosis
Jackson, Michigan,
Hilton Head, South Carolina
Parental role Conflict; Readiness for enhanced Coping; Defensive Coping; Disabled family Coping; Risk for delayed Development; Disturbed Energy field; Adult Failure to thrive; Dysfunctional Family processes: alcoholism; Readiness for enhanced Family processes; Interrupted Family processes; Delayed Growth and development; Risk for disproportionate Growth; Risk-prone health Behavior; Impaired Home maintenance; Hopelessness; Disturbed personal Identity; Risk for Infection; Ineffective Protection; Ineffective Role performance; Readiness for Enhanced Self-Concept; Impaired Social interaction; Social isolation; Delayed Surgical recovery

Barbara Kraynyak Luise, RN, EdD
Associate Professor
Department of Nursing
College of Staten Island
The City University of New York
Staten Island, New York
Readiness for enhanced Comfort; Readiness for enhanced Self-Care

Margaret Lunney, RN, PhD
Professor
Department of Nursing
College of Staten Island
The City University of New York
Staten Island, New York
Readiness for enhanced community Coping; Ineffective community Coping; Ineffective community Therapeutic regimen management; Ineffective family Therapeutic regimen management; Readiness for enhanced Therapeutic regimen management; Ineffective Therapeutic regimen management; Effective Therapeutic regimen management; Stress Overload; Readiness for enhanced Power; Readiness for enhanced Hope; Readiness for enhanced Decision-making

Margo McCaffery, MS, RN-BC, FAAN
Consultant in the Nursing Care of Patients with Pain
Los Angeles, California
Acute Pain; Chronic Pain

Ruth McCaffrey, DNP, ARNP-BC
Associate Professor
Christine E. Lynn College of Nursing
Florida Atlantic University
Boca Raton, Florida
Anxiety; Death Anxiety

Graham J McDougall, Jr., PhD, APRN-BC, FAAN
Professor
School of Nursing
University of Texas—Austin
Austin, Texas
Impaired Memory

Laura H. Mcilvoy, PhD, RN, CCRN, CNRN
Assistant Professor
Indiana University Southeast
New Albany, Indiana
Decreased Intracranial adaptive capacity

Dale A. Nasby, MA, MS, RN, CNS
Certified Clinical Nurse Specialist
Adult Psychiatric and Mental Health Nursing
Administrative Specialist
Division of Nursing Research
Mayo Clinic
Rochester, Minnesota
Disturbed Body image

DeLancey Nicoll, SN
Nursing Student
Hartwick College
Oneonta, New York
Latex Allergy response; Risk for latex Allergy response

Leslie H. Nicoll, PhD, MBA, RN, BC
President and Owner
Maine Desk, LLC
Portland, Maine
Latex Allergy response; Risk for latex Allergy response

Katherina A. Nikzad, MSW
Hartford Doctoral Fellow
Graduate Center for Gerontology
University of Kentucky
Lexington, Kentucky
Compromised family Coping

Lisa Oldham, PhD, MSN, RN, BC, CNA, FABC, GCM
Professor
William Patterson University
Wayne, New Jersey
Consultant in Geriatric Diagnoses and Interventions, Sections II and III

Barbara J. Olinzock, MSN, EdD, RN
Assistant Professor in Nursing
School of Nursing
Brooks College of Health
University of North Florida
Jacksonville, Florida
Ineffective Health maintenance; Health-seeking behaviors; Deficient Knowledge; Readiness for enhanced Knowledge

Peg Padnos, AB, BSN, RN
Nursing Consultant
NICU Transition Services
Spectrum Health System
Grand Rapids, Michigan
Disorganized Infant behavior; Risk for disorganized Infant behavior; Readiness for enhanced organized Infant behavior; Ineffective Infant feeding pattern; Risk for impaired parent/child Attachment

Chris Pasero, MS, RN-BC, FAAN
Pain Management Educator and Clinical Consultant
El Dorado, California
Acute Pain; Chronic Pain

Kathleen L. Patusky, PhD, APRN-BC
Assistant Professor
School of Nursing
University of Medicine and Dentistry of New Jersey
Newark, New Jersey
Powerlessness; Risk for Powerlessness; Self-mutilation; Risk for Self-mutilation; Risk for Suicide; Risk for other-directed Violence; Risk for self-directed Violence

Laura V. Polk, DNSc, RN
Associate Professor
College of Southern Maryland
La Plata, Maryland
Contamination; Risk for Contamination

Lori M. Rhudy, RN, PhDc
Nursing Research Specialist
Department of Nursing
Mayo Clinic College of Medicine
Rochester, Minnesota
Unilateral Neglect

Susan M. Rosenberg, RN, MSN, CNRN, CHI
Clinical Consultant
McKesson Corporation
Adjunct Faculty
Lewis University
Bloomingdale, Illinois
Risk for compromised Human Dignity

Julie T. Sanford, DNS, RN
Associate Professor
College of Nursing
University of South Alabama
Mobile, Alabama
Impaired Gas exchange; Ineffective Airway clearance; Ineffective Breathing pattern

Marilee Schmelzer, PhD, RN
Associate Professor
School of Nursing
The University of Texas at Arlington
Arlington, Texas
Constipation; Perceived Constipation

Paula R. Sherwood, RN, PhD, CNRN
Assistant Professor
School of Nursing
Assistant Professor
Department of Neurosurgery
University of Pittsburgh
Pittsburgh, Pennsylvania
Fatigue; Caregiver role strain; Autonomic dysreflexia

Mary T. Shoemaker, RN, MSN, SANE
Assistant Professor of Nursing
Morehead State University
Morehead, Kentucky
Rape-trauma syndrome; Rape-trauma syndrome compound reaction; Rape-trauma syndrome silent reaction

Sheryl K. Sommer, PhD, RN
Associate Professor and Program Chair
School of Nursing
Creighton University
Omaha, Nebraska
Disturbed Sensory perception: auditory

Mary Stahl, RN, CEN, MSN-NEdu
Clinical Faculty Specialist
Bronson School of Nursing
Western Michigan University
Kalamazoo, Michigan
Risk for Poisoning; Risk for sudden infant Death syndrome

Elaine E. Steinke, PhD, RN
Professor of Nursing
School of Nursing
Wichita State University
Fairmount, Wichita
Sexual dysfunction; Ineffective Sexuality pattern

Michele Walters, MSN, ARNP
Assistant Professor of Nursing
Morehead State University
Morehead, Kentucky
Fear; Risk for Trauma; Post-trauma syndrome; Risk for Post-trauma syndrome

Linda S. Williams, MSN, RNBC
Professor of Nursing
Jackson Community College
Jackson, Michigan
Bathing/hygiene Self-care deficit; Dressing/grooming Self-care deficit; Feeding Self-care deficit; Toileting Self-care deficit

Diane Wind Wardell, PhD, RNC
Associate Professor
School of Nursing
The University of Texas Health Science Center at Houston
Houston, Texas
Disturbed Energy field

PREFACE

Nursing Diagnosis Handbook: An Evidence-Based Guide to Planning Care is a convenient reference to help the practicing nurse or nursing student make a nursing diagnosis and write a care plan with ease and confidence. This handbook helps nurses correlate nursing diagnoses with known information about clients on the basis of assessment findings; established medical, surgical, or psychiatric diagnoses; and the current treatment plan.

Making a nursing diagnosis and planning care are complex processes that involve diagnostic reasoning and critical thinking skills. Nursing students and practicing nurses cannot possibly memorize the extensive list of defining characteristics, related factors, and risk factors for the 188 diagnoses approved by NANDA-International. This book correlates suggested nursing diagnoses with what nurses know about clients and offers a care plan for each nursing diagnosis.

Section I, Nursing Diagnosis, the Nursing Process, and Evidence-Based Nursing, explains how the nurse formulates a nursing diagnosis using assessment findings, determines outcomes, writes appropriate interventions, and evaluates the plan of care.

In **Section II, Guide to Nursing Diagnoses,** the nurse can look up symptoms and problems and their suggested nursing diagnoses for more than 1400 client symptoms; medical, surgical and psychiatric diagnoses; diagnostic procedures; surgical interventions; and clinical states.

In **Section III, Guide to Planning Care,** the nurse can find care plans for all nursing diagnoses suggested in Section II. We have included the suggested nursing outcomes from the Nursing Outcomes Classification (NOC) and interventions from the Nursing Interventions Classification (NIC) by the Iowa Intervention Project. We are excited about this work and believe it is a significant addition to the nursing process to further define nursing practice.

Rationales based on research are included for many of the interventions. This is done to make the research base of nursing practice very apparent to the nursing student and practicing nurse.

New special features of the eighth edition of *Nursing Diagnosis Handbook: An Evidence-Based Guide to Planning Care* include the following:
- **Fifteen** new nursing diagnoses recently approved by NANDA-I
- **Twenty-five** revisions made by NANDA-I in existing nursing diagnoses
- Revised NOC outcomes for each nursing diagnosis, including the rating scale as appropriate
- Revised NIC interventions for each nursing diagnosis as appropriate
- Addition of pediatric interventions to appropriate care plans

- Even more culturally appropriate interventions added to care plans as relevant by nationally known experts on multicultural nursing care: Dr. Joyce Giger and Dr. Ruth Davidhizar.
- An associated EVOLVE Course Management System that includes additional critical thinking case studies; worksheets; and the ability to post a class syllabus, outline, and lecture notes, share e-mail, and encourage student participation through chat rooms and discussion boards
- An Instructor's Electronic Resource and additional PowerPoint lecture slides

The following features of *Nursing Diagnosis Handbook: An Evidence-Based Guide to Planning Care* are also included:
- Suggested nursing diagnoses for more than 1400 clinical entities including signs and symptoms, medical diagnoses, surgeries, maternal-child disorders, mental health disorders, and geriatric disorders
- Labeling of nursing research as **EBN** (Evidence-Based Nursing) and clinical research as **EB** (Evidence-Based) to identify the source of evidence-based rationales
- An EVOLVE Courseware System with the Ackley Ladwig Care Plan Constructor that helps the student or nurse write a nursing care plan, including links to websites for client education
- Rationales for nursing interventions that are based on nursing research and literature
- Comprehensive nursing references identified for each care plan
- A complete list of NOC outcomes on the EVOLVE website
- A complete list of NIC interventions on the EVOLVE website
- Nursing care plans that contain many holistic interventions
- Care plans for **Caregiver role strain** and **Fatigue** written by two national experts, Dr. Barbara Given and Dr. Paula Sherwood
- Care plans for **Constipation** written by Dr. Merilee Schmelzer
- Care plans for **Contamination** and **Risk for Contamination** written by Dr. Laura Polk
- Care plans for **Pain** written by two national experts on pain, Margo McCaffery and Christine Pasero
- Care plans for **Spirituality** written by national experts Ann Solari-Twadell and Dr. Lisa Burkhart
- Care Plans for **Religiosity** written by national expert Dr. Lisa Burkhart
- Care plans for **Skin integrity** written by national expert Dr. Sharon Baranoski

- Care plans for **Community** written by national expert Dr. Margaret Lunney
- Care plan for **Impaired Memory** written by national expert Dr. Graham McDougall
- Care plans for **Incontinence** written by national expert Dr. Mikel Gray
- Care Plans for **Insomnia** and **Sleep deprivation** written by national expert Dr. Judith Floyd
- Care plan for **Decreased Intracranial adaptive capacity** written by national expert Dr. Laura Mcilvoy
- Care plan for **Latex Allergy response** written by national expert Dr. Leslie Nicoll
- Care plans for **Sexual dysfunction** and **Ineffective Sexual pattern** written by Dr. Elaine Steinke
- Care plan for **Unilateral Neglect** written by national expert Dr. Lori Rhudy
- Care plan for **Wandering** written by national expert Dr. Donna Algase
- Care plan for **Impaired spontaneous Ventilation** and **Dysfunctional Ventilatory weaning response** written by national expert Dr. Beth Ann Henneman
- A format that facilitates analyzing signs and symptoms by the process already known by nurses, which involves using defining characteristics of nursing diagnoses to make a diagnosis
- Use of 2007-2008 NANDA-I terminology and approved diagnoses
- An alphabetical format for Sections II and III, which allows rapid access to information
- Nursing care plans for all nursing diagnoses listed in Section II
- Specific geriatric interventions in appropriate plans of care updated by Dr. Lisa Oldham
- Specific client/family teaching interventions in each plan of care
- Inclusion of commonly used abbreviations (e.g., AIDS, MI, CHF) and cross-references to the complete term in Section II
- Contributions by leading nurse experts from throughout the United States, who together represent all of the major nursing specialties and have extensive experience with nursing diagnoses and the nursing process

We acknowledge the work of NANDA-I, which is used extensively throughout this text. In some cases the authors and contributors have modified the NANDA-I work to increase ease of use. The original NANDA-I work can be found in *NANDA-I Nursing Diagnoses: Definitions & Classification 2007-2008*. Several contributors are the original authors of the nursing diagnoses established by NANDA-I. These contributors include the following:

Margaret Lunney, RN, PhD
Ineffective community Coping; Readiness for enhanced community Coping; Effective Therapeutic regimen management; Ineffective Therapeutic regimen management; Ineffective community Therapeutic regimen management; Ineffective family Therapeutic regimen management; Stress Overload (Co-Contributor); Readiness for enhanced Self-Care; Readiness for enhanced Comfort; Readiness for enhanced Decision-making; Readiness for enhanced Hope; Readiness for enhanced Immunization status; Readiness for enhanced Power

Barbara Kraynyak Luise, RN, EdD
Readiness for enhanced Self-Care

Lisa Burkhart, PhD, RN
Spiritual distress; Readiness for enhanced Spiritual well-being; Impaired Religiosity; Risk for impaired Religiosity; Readiness for enhanced Religiosity

Lisa Burkhart, MPH, PhD, RN & Beverly Kopala, PhD, RN
Moral Distress

Brenda Emick-Herring, RN, MSN, CRRN
Impaired bed Mobility; Impaired Transfer ability; Impaired Walking; Impaired wheelchair Mobility

Susan M. Rosenberg, RN, MSN, CNRN, CHI
Risk for compromised human Dignity

Laura V. Polk, DNSc, RN
Contamination and Risk for Contamination

We and the consultants and contributors trust that nurses will find this eighth edition of *Nursing Diagnosis Handbook: An Evidence-Based Guide to Planning Care* a valuable tool that simplifies the process of diagnosing clients and planning for their care, thus allowing nurses more time to provide evidence-based care that speeds each client's recovery.

Betty J. Ackley
Gail B. Ladwig

ACKNOWLEDGMENTS

We would like to thank the following people at Elsevier: Sandra Brown, Senior Acquisition Editor, who supported us with this eighth edition of the text with intelligence and kindness; Cindi Anderson, Senior Developmental Editor, who was a continual support and constant source of wise advice and who is frankly wonderful; and a special thank-you to Steve Ramay for project management of this edition, and Brooke Bagwill, Editorial Assistant, for her ongoing support and hard work.

We acknowledge with gratitude nurses and student nurses who are always an inspiration for us to provide fresh and accurate material. We are honored that they continue to value this text and to use it in their studies and practice.

Care has been taken to confirm the accuracy of information presented in this book. However, the authors, editors, and publisher cannot accept any responsibility for consequences resulting from errors or omissions of the information in this book and make no warranty, express or implied, with respect to its contents. The reader should use practices suggested in this book in accordance with agency policies and professional standards. Every effort has been made to ensure the accuracy of the information presented in this text.

We hope you find this text useful in your nursing practice.

Betty J. Ackley
Gail B. Ladwig

HOW TO USE NURSING DIAGNOSIS HANDBOOK: AN EVIDENCE-BASED GUIDE TO PLANNING CARE

ASSESS

Assess the client using the format provided by the clinical setting. Collect data including client's symptoms, clinical state, and known medical or psychiatric diagnoses.

DIAGNOSIS

Turn to Section II, Guide to Nursing Diagnoses, and locate the client's symptoms, clinical state, medical or psychiatric diagnoses, and anticipated or prescribed diagnostic studies or surgical interventions (listed in alphabetical order). Note suggestions for appropriate nursing diagnoses.

Use Section III, Guide to Planning Care, to evaluate each suggested nursing diagnosis and "related to" etiology statement. Section III is a listing of care plans according to NANDA-I, arranged alphabetically by diagnostic concept, for each nursing diagnosis referred to in Section II. Determine the appropriateness of each nursing diagnosis by comparing the Defining Characteristics and Risk Factors to the client data collected.

DETERMINE OUTCOMES

Use Section III, Guide to Planning Care, to find appropriate outcomes for the client. Use either the NOC outcomes with the associated rating scales, or Client Outcomes as desired.

PLAN INTERVENTIONS

Use Section III, Guide to Planning Care, to find appropriate interventions for the client. Use either the NIC interventions or Nursing Interventions as found in that section.

GIVE NURSING CARE

Administer nursing care following the plan of care based on the interventions.

EVALUATE NURSING CARE

Evaluate nursing care administered using either the NOC outcomes or Client Outcomes. If the outcomes were not met, and the nursing interventions were not effective, reassess the client and determine if the appropriate nursing diagnoses were made.

DOCUMENT

Document all of the previous steps using the format provided in the clinical setting.

CONTENTS

NURSING DIAGNOSIS HANDBOOK

*An Evidence-Based
Guide to Planning Care*

Nursing Process, Nursing Diagnosis, and Evidence-Based Nursing

Section I is an overview of the nursing process and evidence-based nursing. It includes how to make a nursing diagnosis and how to plan nursing care.

Components of the five key steps in the Nursing Process include:

1. **Assessing:** performing a nursing assessment
2. **Diagnosing:** making nursing diagnoses
3. **Planning:** formulating and writing outcome/goal statements and determining appropriate nursing interventions
4. **Implementing care**
5. **Evaluating** the nursing care that has been given (making necessary revisions)

The nursing process is an organizing framework for professional nursing practice. It is very similar to the steps used in scientific reasoning and problem solving. Critical thinking is used as part of the process.

Components of the five key steps in the Nursing Process include:

1. **A**ssessing: performing a nursing **A**ssessment
2. **D**iagnosing: making nursing **D**iagnoses
3. **P**lanning: formulating and writing outcome/goal statements and determining appropriate nursing interventions
4. **I**mplementing care
5. **E**valuating the nursing care that has been given (making necessary revisions)

An easy way to remember the steps of the Nursing Process is to use an acronym: **ADPIE.** ADPIE stands for **A**ssessment, **D**iagnosis, **P**lanning, **I**mplementation, and **E**valuation. The process can be visualized as a circular, continuous process (Figure I-1).

A concept that has been added to the nursing process is basing nursing practice on evidence or research. This concept is called *evidence-based nursing* (EBN). Evidence-based nursing is a systematic process that utilizes current evidence in making decisions about the care of clients, including evaluation of quality and applicability of existing research, client preferences, costs, clinical expertise, and clinical settings (Fineout-Overholt & Johnston, 2005).

It is a problem-solving approach designed to enhance the profession of nursing and to promote quality client care (Spear, 2006). EBN is very much like the nursing process (see Table I-1).

Evidence-based nursing emphasizes asking searchable, answerable, clinical questions (Fineout-Overholt & Johnston, 2005). In this text, the abbreviation **EBN** is used when interventions have rationale supported by nursing research. The abbreviation **EB** is used when interventions have rationale for research that has been obtained from other disciplines.

A barrier to implementing EBN has been a lack of understanding of the process and limited knowledge of the research process (Hockenberry, Wilson, & Barrera, 2006). This text utilizes both research and the nursing process and assists the nurse in increasing use of evidence-based interventions in the clinical setting.

This book first focuses on an essential part of the nursing process: how to make and use a nursing diagnosis. A nursing diagnosis is a clinical judgment about individual, family, or community responses to actual or potential health problems or life processes. Nursing diagnoses provide the basis for selection of nursing interventions to achieve outcomes for which the nurse is accountable (NANDA-I, 2007).

The nursing diagnoses that are used throughout this book are taken from NANDA-International (NANDA-I, 2007). The complete nursing diagnosis list by the NNN (Taxonomy of Nursing practice by domains, classes, diagnosis, outcomes, interventions, and NANDA) can be found on the EVOLVE website.

The diagnoses used throughout this text are listed in alphabetical order by the **diagnostic concept.** If you were looking for *impaired wheel chair mobility, you would find it under "mobility" not under "wheelchair" or "impaired" (NANDA- I, 2007).*

The following is an overview and practical application of the steps of the nursing process. The steps are listed in the usual order in which they are performed.

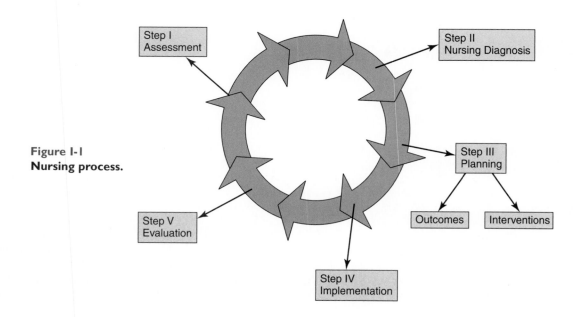

Figure I-1
Nursing process.

TABLE 1-1

Implementing the Nursing Process and Evidence-Based Nursing

Nursing Process	Implementing	Evidence-Based Nursing	Implementing
Assessment	Collecting data about the client using physical assessment and interviewing techniques	Ask the clinical question	Identifying the problem and clinical question
Nursing Diagnosis	Using client data and critical thinking skills to identify and validate an appropriate nursing diagnosis	Searching for and critically appraising the evidence	Searching for evidence (research) applicable to the clinical question. Using critical thinking to appraise the evidence for validity, reliability, generalizability, and appropriateness for the question.
Planning	This phase consists of writing **measurable client outcomes and nursing interventions** to accomplish the outcomes.	Determining the outcome(s) and evidence-based interventions	Writing appropriate measurable outcome(s) and evidence-based interventions to accomplish the outcomes.
Implementing Care	Initiating the care plan and performing the interventions	Apply the evidence to nursing practice	Initiating the care and performing the evidence-based interventions
Evaluate the nursing care	Evaluating if met the outcome(s) and appropriateness of the interventions to meet the needs of the client.	Evaluate the evidence-based nursing care	Evaluating if met the outcome(s) and appropriateness of the interventions to meet the needs of the client.

Adapted from Hockenberry M, Wilson D, Barrera P: Implementing evidence-based nursing practice in a pediatric hospital, *Pediatr Nurs* 32(4):371, 2006.

STEP 1: ASSESSMENT (ADPIE)

Assessment is the data collection step. It involves performing a thorough holistic nursing assessment of the client. This is the first step needed to make an appropriate nursing diagnosis. This is done using the assessment format adopted by the facility or educational institution in which the practice is situated. Several organizational approaches to assessment are available, including Gordon's Functional Health Patterns (see Appendix B) and head-to-toe and body systems approaches. Regardless of the approach used, the nurse assesses the client, being alert for symptoms that will help formulate a nursing diagnosis.

Assessment information is obtained first by doing a thorough health and medical history, and listening to and observing the client. To elicit as much information as possible, the nurse should use open-ended questions rather than questions that can be answered by a simple yes or no

(Dreyer, 2006). The client should be asked questions such as the following:

"Describe what you are feeling."
"How long have you been feeling this way?"
"How did the symptoms start?"
"Describe the symptoms."

These types of questions will encourage the client to give more information about his or her situation. Listen carefully for cues and record relevant information that the client shares.

Information is also obtained by performing a physical assessment, taking vital signs, and noting diagnostic test results. If the client is critically ill or unable to respond verbally, much of the information will be gathered from the physical assessment and diagnostic test results, and possibly from the client's significant others. The information from each of these sources is used to formulate a nursing diagnosis. All of this information needs to be carefully documented on the forms provided by the agency or school of nursing. HIPAA (Health Insurance Portability & Accountability Act) (Brown, 2007) regulations need to be followed. The client's name should NOT be used on the student care plan to protect client confidentiality. When the assessment is complete, proceed to the next step.

STEP 2: NURSING DIAGNOSIS (ADPIE)

Formulating a Nursing Diagnosis with Related Factors and Defining Characteristics

A working nursing diagnosis may have two or three parts. The two-part system consists of the nursing diagnosis and the "related to" statement. "Related factors are factors that appear to show some type of patterned relationship with the nursing diagnosis: such factors may be described as antecedent to, associated with, relating to, contributing to, or abetting" (NANDA-I, 2007). The three-part system consists of the nursing diagnosis, the "related to" statement, and the defining characteristics, which are "observable cues/inferences that cluster as manifestations of an actual or wellness nursing diagnosis" (NANDA-I, 2007).

Some nurses refer to the three-part diagnostic statement as the **PES system:**

P (problem)—The nursing diagnosis label; a concise term or phrase that represents a pattern of related cues. The nursing diagnosis is taken from the official NANDA-I list.

E (etiology)—"Related to" (r/t) phrase or etiology; related cause or contributor to the problem

S (symptoms)—Defining characteristics phrase; symptoms that the nurse identified in the assessment

Application and Examples of Making a Nursing Diagnosis

When the assessment is complete, identify common patterns/symptoms of response *to actual or potential health problems from the assessment* and select an appropriate nursing diagnosis label using critical thinking skills. Use the steps below with Case Study 1. (The same steps can be followed using an actual client assessment in the clinical setting or from a student assessment.)

A. Highlight or underline the relevant symptoms (defining characteristics).
B. Make a short list of the symptoms.
C. Cluster similar symptoms.
D. Analyze/interpret the symptoms.
E. Select a nursing diagnosis label that fits with the appropriate related factors and defining characteristics.

Case Study 1—An Elderly Man With Breathing Problems

A. Underline the Symptoms (Defining Characteristics)

A 73-year-old man has been admitted to the unit with a diagnosis of <u>chronic obstructive pulmonary disease (COPD)</u>. He states that he has "<u>difficulty breathing when walking short distances</u>." He also states that his "<u>heart feels like it is racing</u>" at the same time. He states that he is "<u>tired all the time</u>," and while talking to you, he is continually <u>wringing his hands</u> and <u>looking out the window</u>.

B. List the Symptoms

Chronic obstructive pulmonary disease (COPD); "difficulty breathing when walking short distances"; "heart feels like it is racing"; "tired all the time"; continually wringing his hands and looking out the window.

C. Cluster Symptoms

Chronic obstructive pulmonary disease (COPD)
"Difficulty breathing when walking short distances"
"Heart feels like it is racing"
"Tired all the time"

Continually wringing his hands
Looking out the window

D. Analyze
Interpret the "Subjective Symptoms" (What the Client Has Stated)

• "difficulty breathing when walking short distances" = exertional dyspnea
• "heart feels like it is racing" = abnormal heart rate response to activity
• "tired all the time" = verbal report of weakness

Interpret the "Objective Symptoms" (Observable Information)

• continually wringing his hands = (extraneous movement, hand/arm movements; defining characteristics of Anxiety)
• looking out the window = (poor eye contact, glancing about; defining characteristics of **Anxiety**)

E. Select the Nursing Diagnosis Label

In Section II, look up *dyspnea* or *dysrhythmia (abnormal heart rate or rhythm)*, (these are chosen because they are high priority) and you will find the nursing diagnosis **Activity intolerance** listed with these symptoms. Is this diagnosis appropriate for this client?

In order to validate the **Activity intolerance** nursing diagnosis as appropriate for the client, turn to Section III, and read its NANDA-I definition. **Activity intolerance** is defined as "Insufficient physiological or psychological energy to endure or complete required or desired daily activities." When reading the definition, ask, "Does this definition describe the symptoms demonstrated by the client?" If the appropriate nursing diagnosis has been selected, the definition should describe the condition that has been observed.

The client should also have defining characteristics for this particular diagnosis. Are the client symptoms that you identified in the list of defining characteristics (verbal report of fatigue, abnormal heart rate response to activity, exertional dyspnea)?

Another way to use this text and to help validate the diagnosis is to look up the client's medical diagnosis in Section II. This client had a medical diagnosis of COPD. Is **Activity intolerance** listed with this medical diagnosis?

The process of identifying significant symptoms, clustering or grouping them into logical patterns, and then choosing an appropriate nursing diagnosis involves diagnostic reasoning (critical thinking) skills that must be learned in the process of becoming a nurse. This text serves as a tool to help the learner in this process.

A concept map may also be used to identify the nursing diagnosis. See Figure I-2 for an example.

Concept mapping diagrams the critical thinking strategy involved in using the nursing process (Abel & Freeze, 2006). To create a concept map, start with a blank sheet of paper. Write a client descriptor at the center of the paper. The next steps involve linking the client via arrows to the symptoms (defining characteristics) from the assessment. After the symptoms are visualized, similar ones can be put together to formulate a nursing diagnosis using another concept map (see Figure I-3).

The central theme in this concept map is "I can only walk short distances"; the defining characteristics/client symptoms support the nursing diagnosis **Activity intolerance.**

"Related to" Phrase or Etiology

The second part of the nursing diagnosis is the "related to" (r/t) phrase. Related factors are factors that appear to show some type of patterned relationship with the nursing diagnosis. Such factors may be described as antecedent to, associated with, related to, contributing to, or abetting. Only actual nursing diagnoses have related factors (NANDA-I, 2007). Pathophysiological and psychosocial changes, such as developmental age and cultural and environmental situations, may be causative or contributing factors. Exceptions to including a "related to" statement occur when the client has a "risk" or "readiness" for diagnosis. The risk diagnoses will have risk factors, and the readiness diagnoses will have defining characteristics. This information can be found in Section III, which contains all 188 nursing diagnoses with definitions, defining characteristics, related factors, or risk factors.

Ideally the etiology, or cause, of the nursing diagnosis is something that can be treated by a nurse. When this is the case, the diagnosis is identified as an independent nursing diagnosis. If medical intervention is also necessary, it might be identified as a collaborative diagnosis. A carefully written, individualized r/t statement enables the nurse to plan nursing interventions that will assist the client in accomplishing goals and returning to a state of optimum health.

For each suggested nursing diagnosis, the nurse should refer to the statements listed under the heading "Related Factors (r/t)" in Section III. These r/t factors may or may not be appropriate for the individual client. If they are not appropriate, the nurse should develop and write an r/t statement that is appropriate for the client. For the client from Case Study I a two-part statement could be made here:

Problem = Activity intolerance
Etiology = r/t Imbalance between oxygen supply and demand

It was already determined that the elderly man had **Activity intolerance.** With the respiratory symptoms identified from the assessment, imbalance between oxygen supply and demand is appropriate.

Defining Characteristics Phrase

The defining characteristics phrase is the third part of the three-part diagnostic system, and it consists of the signs and symptoms that have been gathered during the assessment phase. The phrase "as evidenced by" (aeb) may be used to connect the etiology (r/t) with the defining characteristics. The use of identifying defining characteristics is similar to the process the physician uses when making a medical diag-

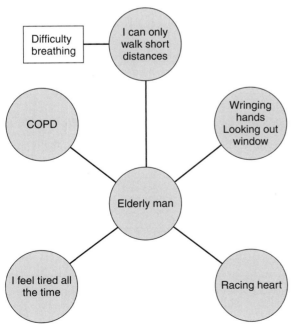

Figure I-2
Example of a concept map.

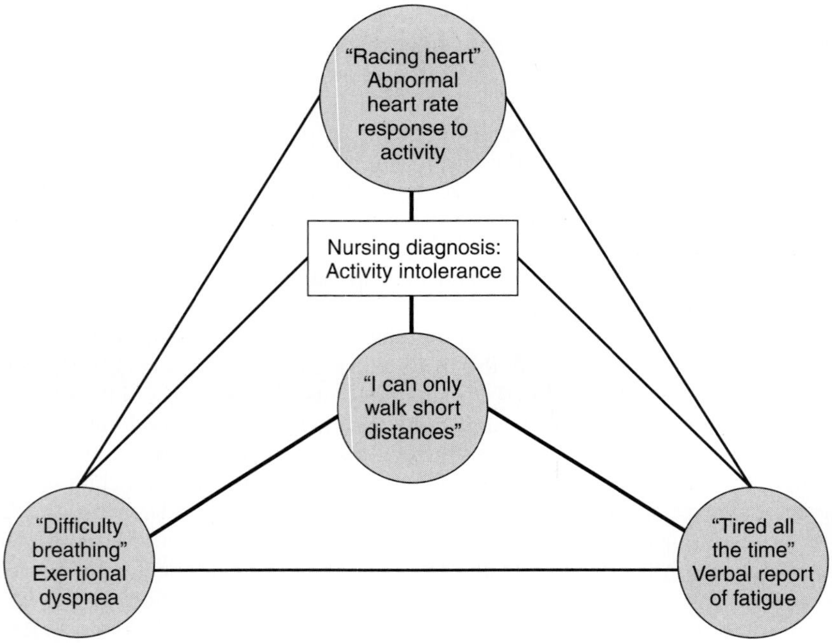

Figure I-3
Formulating a nursing diagnosis using a concept map.

nosis. For example, the physician who observes the following signs and symptoms—diminished inspiratory and expiratory capacity of the lungs, complaints of dyspnea on exertion, difficulty in inhaling and exhaling deeply, and sometimes chronic cough—may make the medical diagnosis of COPD. This same process is used to identify the nursing diagnosis of **Activity intolerance.**

Put It All Together: Writing the Three-Part Nursing Diagnosis Statement

Problem—Choose the label (nursing diagnosis) using the guidelines explained previously. A list of nursing diagnosis labels (arranged alphabetically by diagnostic concept) can be found in Section II and Section III.

Etiology—Write an r/t phrase (etiology). These can be found in Section II.

Symptoms—Write the defining characteristics (signs and symptoms). A list of the signs and symptoms associated with each nursing diagnosis can be found in Section III.

Case Study I—Elderly Man with COPD (cont'd)

Using the information from the above case study/example, the nursing diagnostic statement would be as follows:

Problem—Activity intolerance
Etiology—r/t Imbalance between oxygen supply and demand
Symptoms—Verbal reports of fatigue, exertional dyspnea ("difficulty breathing when walking"), and abnormal heart rate response to activity ("racing heart")

Consider a second case study:

Case Study 2—Woman with Insomnia

As before, the nurse always begins with an assessment. To make the nursing diagnosis, the nurse follows the steps below.

A. Underline the Symptoms

A 45-year-old woman comes to the clinic and asks for medication to help her sleep. She states she is worrying about too much and states, "It takes me about an hour to get to sleep, and it is very hard to fall asleep. I feel like I can't do anything because I am so tired. My husband passed away recently."

B. Make a Short List of the Symptoms

Asks for medication to help her sleep; states she is worrying about too much; "It takes me about an hour to get to sleep; it is very hard to fall asleep; I feel like I can't do anything because I am so tired; My husband passed away recently."

C. Cluster Similar Symptoms

Asks for medication to help her sleep
"It takes me about an hour to get to sleep."
"It is very hard to fall asleep."
"I feel like I can't do anything because I am so tired."

States she is worrying about too much
"My husband passed away recently."

D. Analyze/Interpret the Symptoms
Subjective Symptoms

- Asks for medication to help her sleep, "It takes me about an hour to get to sleep; it is very hard to fall asleep. I feel like I can't do anything because I am so tired." (all defining characteristics = verbal complaints of difficulty with sleeping)
- States she is worrying about too much (anxiety)
- "My husband passed away recently." **(Grieving)**

E. Select a Nursing Diagnosis with Related Factors and Defining Characteristics

Look up *sleep* in Section II. Listed under the heading "Sleep Pattern Disorders" is the following information:

> **Insomnia** r/t anxiety, depression grief
> This client states that she is worrying too much, which may indicate anxiety; she also recently lost her husband (grief).
> Look up **Insomnia** in Section III.
> Check the definition: A disruption in amount and quality of sleep that impairs functioning
> Does this describe the client in the case study? What are the related factors? What are the symptoms? Write the diagnostic statement:

Problem—Insomnia
Etiology—r/t Anxiety, grief
Symptoms—Difficulty falling asleep, "I am so tired, I can't do anything"

After the diagnostic statement is written, proceed to the next step: planning.

STEP 3: PLANNING (AD**P**IE)

This phase consists of writing **measurable client outcomes and nursing interventions** to accomplish the outcomes. Before this can be done, if the client has more than one diagnosis, the priority of the nursing diagnoses must be determined. The highest priority nursing diagnoses can be determined by using Maslow's hierarchy of needs. In this hierarchy, priority is generally given to immediate problems that may be life threatening. For example, **Activity intolerance,** a physiological need, may be a higher priority than **Grieving,** a love and belonging need. Refer to Appendix A, Nursing Diagnoses Arranged by Maslow's Hierarchy of Needs, for assistance in prioritizing nursing diagnoses.

Outcomes

After the appropriate priority of the nursing diagnoses is determined, outcomes are developed. This text includes standardized outcomes written by a large team of University of Iowa College of Nursing faculty and students in conjunction with clinicians from a variety of settings: "Nursing-sensitive

outcome (NOC) is an individual, family, or community state, behavior, or perception that is measured along a continuum in response to nursing interventions. The outcomes are variable concepts that can be measured along a continuum, which means the outcomes are stated as concepts that reflect a client, family caregiver, family, or community actual state rather than expected goals. It also means that the outcomes are neutral; that is, they don't specify the desired state, although they can be used to set goals. This retains the variability of the outcome and allows measurement of the client condition at any point in time." (Moorhead, Johnson & Maas, 2004).

If at all possible, the nurse *involves* the client in determining appropriate outcomes. The use of outcomes information creates a continuous feedback loop that is essential to ensuring evidence-based care and the best possible client outcomes, not only for individuals, but also for families, communities, and populations (Orchard et al, 2006). The minimum requirements that an outcome is rated is when the outcome is selected (i.e., the baseline measure) and when care is completed (i.e., the discharge summary). This may be sufficient in short stay acute care settings. Depending on how rapid client condition changes are anticipated, some settings may evaluate once a day or once a shift. Community agencies may evaluate every visit, every other visit, and so on. Since measurement times are not standardized, they can be individualized for the client and the setting (Moorhead, Johnson & Maas, 2004).

Development of appropriate outcomes can be done one of two ways: using the Nursing Outcomes Classification (NOC) list or developing an appropriate outcome statement, both of which are included in this book in Section III. There are suggested outcome statements for each nursing diagnosis in this text that can be used as written or modified as necessary to meet the needs of the client.

The EVOLVE website includes a listing of additional NOC outcomes. "Each outcome has a group of indicators that are used to determine client status in relation to the outcome. A *nursing-sensitive client outcome indicator* is defined *as* a more concrete individual, family, or community state, behavior, or perception that serves as a cue for measuring an outcome" (Moorhead, Johnson & Maas, 2004). The use of NOC outcomes can be very helpful to the nurse because they contain a five-point Likert-type rating scale that can be used to evaluate progress toward achieving the outcome. In this text the rating scale is listed, along with some of the more common indicators. As an example, the rating scale for the outcome **Sleep** is shown in Table I-2.

Because the NOC outcomes are very specific, they enhance the nursing process by helping the nurse record change after interventions have been performed. The nurse can choose to have clients rate their own progress using the Likert-type rating scale. This involvement can help increase client motivation to progress *toward* outcomes change or resolution.

TABLE I-2

NOC Outcome—Sleep
Definition: Natural periodic suspension of consciousness during which the body is restored

Sleep	Severely Compromised 1	Substantially Compromised 2	Moderately Compromised 3	Mildly Compromised 4	Not Compromised 5	
Hours of sleep (at least 5 hr/24 hr)*	1	2	3	4	5	
Observed hours of sleep	1	2	3	4	5	
Sleep pattern	1	2	3	4	5	
Sleep quality	1	2	3	4	5	
Sleep quantity	1	2	3	4	5	
Sleep efficiency (ratio of sleep time/total time trying)	1	2	3	4	5	
Sleep routine	1	2	3	4	5	
Sleeps through the night consistently	1	2	3	4	5	
Feels rejuvenated after sleep	1	2	3	4	5	
Wakeful at appropriate times	1	2	3	4	5	
EEG	1	2	3	4	5	
EMG	1	2	3	4	5	
EOG	1	2	3	4	5	
	Severe	Substantial	Moderate	Mild	None	NA
Interrupted sleep	1	2	3	4	5	
Inappropriate napping	1	2	3	4	5	
Sleep apnea	1	2	3	4	5	
Dependence on sleep aids	1	2	3	4	5	

EEG, Electroencephalogram; *EMG,* electromyogram; *EOG,* electro-oculogram.
From Moorhead S, Johnson M, Maas M: *Nursing outcomes classification (NOC),* ed 3, St Louis, 2004, Mosby.
*Appropriate for adults.

After client outcomes are selected and *discussed* with a client, the nurse plans nursing care and establishes a means that will help the client achieve the selected outcomes. The usual means are nursing interventions.

Interventions

Interventions are like road maps directing the best ways to provide nursing care. The more clearly a nurse writes an intervention, the easier it will be to complete the journey and arrive at the destination of successful client outcomes.

Section III supplies choices of interventions for each nursing diagnosis. The interventions are identified as independent (autonomous actions that are initiated by the nurse in response to a nursing diagnosis) or collaborative (actions that the nurse performs in collaboration with other health care professionals and that may require a physician's order and may be in response to both medical and nursing diagnoses). The nurse may choose the interventions appropriate for the client and individualize them accordingly or determine additional interventions. This text also contains several suggested Nursing Interventions Classification (NIC) interventions for each nursing diagnosis to help the reader see how NIC is used along with NOC and nursing diagnoses. The NIC interventions are a comprehensive, standardized classification of treatments that nurses perform. The classification includes both physiological and psychosocial interventions and covers all nursing specialties. A listing of NIC interventions is included on the EVOLVE website. For more information about NIC interventions, the reader is referred to the NIC text, which is identified in the reference list (McCloskey Dochterman & Bulechek, 2004).

Many of the nursing interventions in this text involve assessment, initial and ongoing, versus action type nursing interventions. These interventions are an important component of caring for clients. NIC has identified many activities under the NIC label surveillance. Examples include monitoring of neurological status, vital signs, coping, and so on. Surveillance is defined as "purposeful and ongoing acquisition, interpretation, and synthesis of client data for clinical decision making" (McCloskey Dochterman & Bulechek, 2004).

It is here, while determining interventions, that you might pose a "clinical question" to incorporate the concept of EBN. *What are some of the most effective ways to help a client who has difficulty sleeping? Has intolerance to activity? What does the research say? What has helped this person in the past?* Development of EBN is an ongoing process that should involve all nurses to determine the best nursing interventions to provide nursing care. To implement EBN, nurses must work together to develop practice guidelines that ensure the care is excellent and supported by a research base.

This text includes research-based rationales whenever possible, which are labeled EBN for nursing research or EB for multidisciplinary research. The research ranges along a continuum from a case study about a single client to a systematic review performed by experts that gives quality information to guide nursing care.

Every attempt has been made to supply the most current research for the nursing interventions. Some references may have earlier dates because they are classic studies that have not been replicated. For example, in the Spiritual care plans, the work by Koenig, Pargament, Fry, Reed, Engebretson, and Dossey is considered seminal work.

"Theoretical perspectives may be used as a source of evidence. Many theories and models are based on past research and have strong consensus among people in the field (also evidence). Sometimes this type of evidence is better than one small research study with the inherent biases that are present in small research studies" (Lunney, 2005).

If you are aware of or have information on more current research, we encourage you to submit the information to customer.support@elsevier.com. We appreciate your interest in keeping this text up-to-date and current and your support of providing the best "evidence" for state-of-the-art nursing practice.

Nurses in all clinical settings make hundreds of clinical decisions every day. Accurate diagnosis and selection of interventions based on searching and evaluating evidence at the point of care is essential (Swan & Boruch, 2004; Swan, Lang, & McGinley, 2004). Nurses can find evidence to guide their practice in many places. The Agency for Healthcare Research and Quality (AHRQ), formerly the Agency for Health Care Policy and Research (AHCPR), began producing clinical practice guidelines in 1989. Clinical practice guidelines are defined as "systematically developed statements to assist practitioners and client decisions about appropriate health care for specific clinical circumstances" (IOM, p.38). Although AHRQ no longer develops guidelines, it supports the National Guidelines Clearinghouse (NGC). The NGC is a comprehensive database of evidence-based clinical practice guidelines and related documents produced by the AHRQ in partnership with the American Medical Association (AMA) and the American Association of Health Plans (AAHP).

The NGC mission is to provide physicians, nurses, and other health professionals, health care providers, health plans, integrated delivery systems, purchasers, and others an accessible mechanism for obtaining objective, detailed information on clinical practice guidelines and to further their dissemination, implementation, and use. There are currently over 13,000 guidelines in the clearinghouse with new and frequent additions. The guidelines are easily accessed at www.guideline.gov. Both professionals and consumers use this resource to access the guidelines and information for specific health problems.

The journal *Evidence-Based Nursing* is another rich and useful resource. This journal is devoted to helping nurses identify and appraise high-quality, clinically relevant research. The journal selects from the health-related literature articles reporting studies and reviews that warrant immediate attention by nurses attempting to keep pace with their practice and delivering quality care (www.evidencebased-nursing. com). *The Annual Review of Nursing Research* is very useful. Many nursing journals now publish practice guidelines based on reviews of nursing research that are helpful to the nurse heading in the direction of EBN.

In an effort to support nursing knowledge worldwide, Sigma Theta Tau International (STTI) (www.stti.iupui.edu/library), through the Virginia Henderson International Library, provides the *Registry of Nursing Research* (RNR) as a resource to its members. The RNR is an electronic research resource that contains information and abstracts from more than 13,000 studies. As part of an evidence-based practice initiative, the *Online Journal of Knowledge Synthesis for Nursing* (OJKSN) has added a new clinical column. This column includes exemplars of EBN practice (Capasso et al, 2002). In March 2004, STTI introduced its new journal, *WORLDviews on Evidence-Based Nursing*, an international source of information for using EBN practice to improve client care.

Websites for Evidence-Based Care

Some of the multiple helpful websites for evidence-based care include:

- *Pubmed.* This site offers *free* searching of the medical and some of the nursing literature. It is provided by the National Library of Medicine and the National Institute of Health. Information on more than 33,000 journals is found here. Website: www.ncbi.nlm.nih.gov/entrez/query.fcgi?DB=pubmed
- *CINAHL The Cumulative Index to Nursing and Allied Health Literature.* This is the best site to search the nursing literature. There is a cost to utilize this database. It is available in most school and medical/nursing libraries. Website: http://www.cinahl.com
- *The Joanna Briggs Institute for Evidence-Based Nursing and Midwifery.* On this site nurses can find summarized research evidence on which to base their practice. The site provides systematic reviews of international research, undertakes multisite, randomized, controlled clinical trials in areas in which research is needed, and prepares easy-to-read summaries of best practice in the form of Practice Information Sheets based on the results of systematic reviews. Website: www.joannabriggs.edu.au
- *The Cochrane Collaboration.* This international collaboration facilitates the creation, maintenance, and dissemination of more than 1000 systematic reviews of the effects of health care interventions in multiple conditions. More than 60 interdisciplinary working groups and collaborative review groups are composed of people from around the world who share an interest in developing and maintaining systematic reviews relevant to a particular health area. Website: www.cochrane.org

When using EBN, it is vitally important that the clients' concerns and individual situations be taken under consideration (website: www.ahcpr.gov). The nurse must always use critical thinking when applying EBN guidelines to any particular nursing situation. Each client is unique in his or her needs and capabilities. Prescriptive guidelines can be applied inappropriately, resulting in increased problems for the client (Thompson, 2004). The goal is to provide the best care based on input from researchers, practitioners, and the recipients of care.

Putting It All Together—Documenting the Care Plan

The final planning phase is documenting the actual care plan, including prioritized nursing diagnostic statements, outcomes, and interventions. This may be done electronically or by actual writing. To ensure continuity of care, the plan must be documented and shared with all health care personnel caring for the client. This text provides rationales, most of which are research based, to validate that the interventions are appropriate and workable. Because it usually takes at least 1 year from the time a manuscript is accepted for publication for it to appear in print, we have provided many websites as references for rationales and client/family teaching. In this time of rapid change in health care, we cannot wait a year for access to vital information. Today some material appears only in electronic form (Sparks & Rizzolo, 1998). Websites for client/family teaching are available at the EVOLVE website. A sample care plan is illustrated in Figure I-4.

The EVOLVE website includes resources to develop an electronic care plan that can be easily accessed, updated, and individualized. Many agencies are using electronic records, and this is an ideal resource.

STEP 4: IMPLEMENTATION (ADPIE)

The implementation phase of the nursing process is the actual initiation of the nursing care plan. Client outcomes are achieved by the performance of the nursing interventions. During this phase the nurse continues to assess the client to determine whether the interventions are effective and the desired outcomes are met. An important part of this phase is documentation. The nurse should use the facility's tool for documentation and record the results of implementing nursing interventions. Documentation is also necessary for legal reasons because in a legal dispute, *if it wasn't charted/recorded, it wasn't done.*

STEP 5: EVALUATION (ADPIE)

Although evaluation is listed as the last phase of the nursing process, it is actually an integral part of each phase and something the nurse does continually. When evaluation is performed as the last phase, the nurse refers to the client's outcomes and determines whether they were met. If the outcomes were not met, the nurse begins again with assessment and determines the reason they were not met. Were the outcomes attainable? Was the wrong nursing diagnosis made? Should the interventions be changed? At this point the nurse can look up any new symptoms or conditions that have been identified and adjust the care plan as needed. When using EBN, it is at this point the nurse determines whether the practice that was followed was effective. Necessary revisions may be made at this time.

Many health care providers are using critical pathways to plan nursing care. The use of nursing diagnoses should be an integral part of any critical pathway to ensure that nursing care needs are being assessed and appropriate nursing interventions are planned and implemented.

The use of nursing diagnoses, NOC outcomes, and NIC interventions ensures that nurses are speaking a common language when providing nursing care. This system also is easily computerized for simplified documentation and analysis of patterns of care. Nursing diagnosis is the essence of nursing, used to ensure that clients receive excellent, holistic nursing care.

Just as nurses continually evaluate the interventions and outcomes of care delivered, so too must they continually evaluate the research supporting the interventions, to provide state-of-the-art evidence-based care. The nursing process is continually evolving. In this text, our goal is to present state-of-the-art information to assist the nurse and nursing student to provide the best nursing care possible.

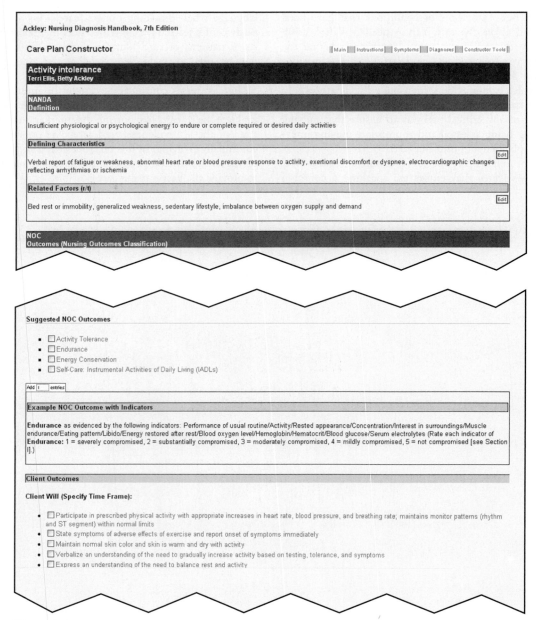

Figure I-4

Activity intolerance care plan from the EVOLVE website.   *Continued*

- ☐ Maintain normal skin color and skin is warm and dry with activity
- ☐ Verbalize an understanding of the need to gradually increase activity based on testing, tolerance, and symptoms
- ☐ Express an understanding of the need to balance rest and activity
- ☐ Demonstrate increased activity tolerance

`Add [1] entries`

NIC
Interventions (Nursing Interventions Classification)

Suggested NIC Interventions

- ☐ Activity Therapy
- ☐ Energy Management

`Add [1] entries`

Example NIC Activities—Energy Management

Monitor cardiorespiratory response to activity; monitor location and nature of discomfort or pain during movement/activity

Nursing Interventions and Rationales

- ☐ Determine cause of activity intolerance (see Related Factors) and determine whether cause is physical, psychological, or motivational. *Determining the cause of a disease can help direct appropriate interventions.*
- ☐ Assess the client daily for appropriateness of activity and bed rest orders. *Inappropriate prolonged bed rest orders may contribute to activity intolerance (Kasper, Braunwald, & Fauci, 2005).* EB: *A review of 39 studies on bed rest resulting from 15 disorders demonstrated that bed rest for treatment of medical*

`Add [1] entries`

Client/Family Teaching

- ☐ Instruct the client on rationale and techniques for avoiding activity intolerance.
- ☐ Teach the client to use controlled breathing techniques with activity.
- ☐ Teach the client the importance and method of coughing, clearing secretions.
- ☐ Instruct the client in the use of relaxation techniques during activity.
- ☐ Help client with energy conservation and work simplification techniques in ADLs.
- ☐ Teach the client the importance of proper nutrition.
- ☐ Describe to the client the symptoms of activity intolerance, including which symptoms to report to the physician.
- ☐ Explain to the client how to use assistive devices or medications before or during activity.
- ☐ Help client set up an activity log to record exercise and exercise tolerance.

`Add [1] entries`

References

1. Allen C, Glasziou P, Del Mar C: Bed rest: a potentially harmful treatment needing more careful evaluation, *Lancet* 354(9186):1229, 1999.
2. Asbring P, Narvanen A: Patient power and control: a study of women with uncertain illness trajectories, *Qual Health Res* 14(2):226, 2004.
3. Belza B, Steele BG, Hunziker J et al: Correlates of physical activity in chronic obstructive pulmonary disease, *Nurs Res* 50(4):195, 2001.
4. Bianchi R, Gigliotti F, Romagnoli I et al: Chest wall kinematics and breathlessness during pursed-lip breathing in patients with COPD, *Chest* 125(2):459, 2004.
5. Bloomfield SA: Changes in musculoskeletal structure and function with prolonged bed rest, *Med Sci Sports Exerc* 29(2):197, 1997.
6. Bradley JG, Davis KA: Orthostatic hypotension, *Am Fam Physician* 68(12):2393, 2003.
7. California Pulmonary Rehabilitation Collaborative Group: Effects of pulmonary rehabilitation on dyspnea, quality of life and healthcare costs in California, *J Cardiopulm Rehabil* 24(1):52, 2004.
8. Demers C, McKelvie RS, Negassa A et al: Reliability, validity, and responsiveness of the six-minute walk test in patients with heart failure, *Am Heart J* 142.

Figure I-4, cont'd.

REFERENCES

Abel W, Freeze M: Evaluation of concept mapping in an associate degree nursing program, *J Nurs Educ* 45(9):356-364, 2006.

Agency for Healthcare Research and Quality (AHRQ): *Evidence-based practice outcomes and effectiveness,* retrieved from the World Wide Web March 16, 2003, available online at: www.ahcpr.gov/clinic/outcomix.htm.

Agency for Healthcare Research and Quality (AHRQ): Systems to rate the strength of scientific evidence, *Evid Rep/Technol Assess* 47, 2002.

Brown B: Top 10 HIPAA misconceptions, *J Health Care Compliance* 9(1):41-44, 2007.

Capasso V, Burke D, Stanley D et al: Unit-based specialty vascular transitional home care program: an example of evidence-based nursing practice, *Online J Knowl Synth Nurs* 9:3C, 2002.

Dreyer L: The patient interview: learn to communicate, *RDH* 26(2):46, 2006.

Fineout-Overholt E, Johnston L: Teaching EBP: asking searchable, answerable clinical questions, *Worldviews Evid Based Nurs* 2(3):157-160, 2005.

Hockenberry M, Wilson D, Barrera P: Implementing evidence-based nursing practice in a pediatric hospital, *Pediatr Nurs* 32(4):371-377, 2006.

Lunney M: Personal communication, March 15, 2005.

McCloskey Dochterman JC, Bulechek GM: *Nursing interventions classification (NIC),* ed 4, St Louis, 2004, Mosby.

Moorhead S, Johnson M, Maas M: *Nursing outcomes classification (NOC),* ed 3, St Louis, 2004, Mosby.

(NANDA-I): *Nursing diagnoses: definitions and classification, 2007-2008,* Philadelphia, 2007, Author.

Orchard C, Reid-Haughian C, Vanderlee R: Health Outcomes for Better Information and Care (HOBIC): integrating patient outcome information into nursing undergraduate curricula. *Can J Nurs Leadersh* 19(3):28-33, 2006.

Sparks SM, Rizzolo MA: World Wide Web search tools, *Image J Nurs Sch* 30(2):167-171, 1998.

Spear HJ: Evidence-based nursing practice: making progress and making a difference, *Worldviews Evid Based Nurs* 3(2):52-54, 2006.

Swan BA, Boruch RF: Quality of evidence: usefulness in measuring the quality of health care, *Medical Care* 42(suppl 2):II-12-II-20, 2004.

Swan BA, Lang NM, McGinley AM: Access to quality health care: links between evidence, nursing language, and informatics, *Nurs Econ* 22(6):325-332, 2004.

Thompson C: Fortuitous phenomena: on complexity, pragmatic randomized controlled trials, and knowledge for evidence-based practice, *Worldviews Evid Based Nurs* 1(1):9-17, 2004.

SECTION

II

Guide to Nursing Diagnoses

Section II is an alphabetical listing of client symptoms, client problems, medical diagnoses, psychiatric diagnoses, and clinical states. Use this section to find suggestions for nursing diagnoses for your client.

First assess the client using the format provided by the clinical setting. Then use this section to locate the client's symptoms, problems, clinical state, diagnoses, surgeries, and diagnostic testing. Note suggestions given for appropriate nursing diagnoses.

Using information found in Section III, evaluate each suggested nursing diagnosis to determine if it is appropriate for the client.

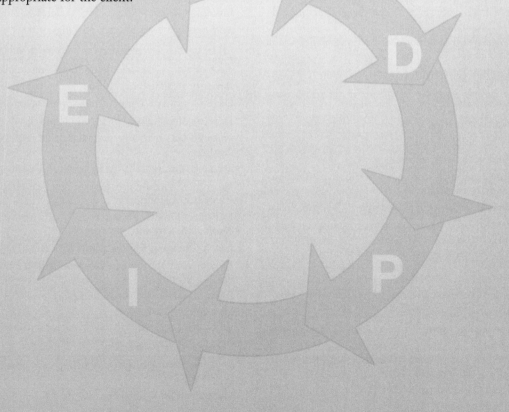

A

A

Abdominal Distention

Acute **Pain** r/t retention of air, gastrointestinal secretions

Constipation r/t decreased activity, decreased fluid intake, decreased fiber intake, pathological process

Delayed **Surgical** recovery r/t retention of gas, secretions

Imbalanced **Nutrition**: less than body requirements r/t nausea, vomiting

Nausea r/t irritation of gastrointestinal tract

Abdominal Hysterectomy

See Hysterectomy

Abdominal Pain

Acute **Pain** r/t injury, pathological process

Imbalanced **Nutrition**: less than body requirements r/t unresolved pain

See cause of Abdominal Pain

Abdominal Surgery

Acute **Pain** r/t surgical procedure

Constipation r/t decreased activity, decreased fluid intake, anesthesia, narcotics

Imbalanced **Nutrition**: less than body requirements r/t high metabolic needs, decreased ability to ingest or digest food

Ineffective **Health** maintenance r/t knowledge deficit regarding self-care after surgery

Ineffective **Tissue** perfusion: peripheral r/t immobility, abdominal surgery

Risk for **Infection**: Risk factor: invasive procedure

See Surgery, Perioperative Care; Surgery, Postoperative Care; Surgery, Preoperative Care

Abdominal Trauma

Acute **Pain** r/t abdominal trauma

Deficient **Fluid** volume r/t hemorrhage

Disturbed **Body** image r/t scarring, change in body function, need for temporary colostomy

Ineffective **Breathing** pattern r/t abdominal distention, pain

Risk for **Infection**: Risk factor: possible perforation of abdominal structures

Abortion, Induced

Acute **Pain** r/t surgical intervention

Chronic low **Self-esteem** disturbance r/t feelings of guilt

Chronic **Sorrow** r/t loss of potential child

Compromised family **Coping** r/t unresolved feelings about decision

Ineffective **Health** maintenance r/t deficient knowledge regarding self-care after abortion

Risk for delayed **Development**: Risk factors: unplanned or unwanted pregnancy

Risk for imbalanced **Fluid** volume: Risk factor: possible hemorrhage

Risk for **Infection**: Risk factors: open uterine blood vessels, dilated cervix

Risk for **Post-trauma** syndrome: Risk factor: psychological trauma of abortion

Risk for **Spiritual** distress: Risk factor: perceived moral implications of decision

Abortion, Spontaneous

Acute **Pain** r/t uterine contractions, surgical intervention

Chronic **Sorrow** r/t loss of potential child

Disabled family **Coping** r/t unresolved feelings about loss

Disturbed **Body** image r/t perceived inability to carry pregnancy, produce child

Fear r/t implications for future pregnancies

Grieving r/t loss of fetus

Ineffective **Coping** r/t personal vulnerability

Ineffective **Health** maintenance r/t deficient knowledge regarding self-care after abortion

Interrupted **Family** processes r/t unmet expectations for pregnancy and childbirth

Risk for deficient **Fluid** volume: Risk factors: hemorrhage

Risk for **Infection**: Risk factors: septic or incomplete abortion of products of conception, open uterine blood vessels, dilated cervix

Risk for **Post-trauma** syndrome: Risk factor: psychological trauma of abortion

Risk for **Spiritual** distress: Risk factor: loss of fetus

Self-esteem disturbance r/t feelings of fetus

Abruptio Placentae <36 Weeks

Acute **Pain** r/t irritable uterus, hypertonic uterus

Anxiety r/t unknown outcome, change in birth plans

Death **Anxiety** r/t unknown outcome, hemorrhage, or pain

Fear r/t threat to well-being of self and fetus

Impaired **Gas** exchange: placental r/t decreased uteroplacental area

Impaired **Tissue** integrity: maternal r/t possible uterine rupture

Interrupted **Family** process r/t unmet expectations for pregnancy and childbirth

Ineffective **Health** maintenance r/t deficient knowledge regarding self-care with disorder

Risk for deficient **Fluid** volume: Risk factor: hemorrhage

Risk for disproportionate **Growth**: Risk factor: uteroplacental insufficiency

Risk for ineffective **Tissue** perfusion: fetal: Risk factor: uteroplacental insufficiency

Risk for **Infection**: Risk factor: partial separation of placenta

Abscess Formation

Impaired **Tissue** integrity r/t altered circulation, nutritional deficit or excess

Ineffective **Health** maintenance r/t deficient knowledge regarding self-care with abscess

Ineffective **Protection** r/t inadequate nutrition, abnormal blood profile, drug therapy, depressed immune function

Abuse, Child

See Child Abuse

Abuse, Spouse, Parent, or Significant Other

Anxiety r/t threat to self-concept, situational crisis of abuse

Caregiver role strain r/t chronic illness, self-care deficits, lack of respite care, extent of caregiving required

Compromised family **Coping** r/t abusive patterns

Defensive **Coping** r/t low self-esteem

Impaired verbal **Communication** r/t psychological barriers of fear

Insomnia r/t psychological stress

Interrupted **Family** process: alcoholism r/t inadequate coping skills

Post-trauma syndrome r/t history of abuse

Powerlessness r/t lifestyle of helplessness

Risk for self-directed **Violence**: Risk factor: history of abuse

Self-esteem disturbance r/t negative family interactions

Accessory Muscle Use (to Breathe)

Ineffective **Breathing** pattern (See **Breathing** pattern, ineffective, Section III)

See Asthma; Bronchitis; COPD (Chronic Obstructive Pulmonary Disease); Respiratory Infections, Acute Childhood

Accident Prone

Acute **Confusion** r/t altered level of consciousness

Adult **Failure** to thrive r/t fatigue

Ineffective **Coping** r/t personal vulnerability, situational crises

Risk for **Injury**: Risk factor: history of accidents

Achalasia

Acute **Pain** r/t stasis of food in esophagus

Impaired **Swallowing** r/t neuromuscular impairment

Ineffective **Coping** r/t chronic disease

Risk for **Aspiration**: Risk factor: nocturnal regurgitation

Acidosis, Metabolic

Acute **Pain**: headache r/t neuromuscular irritability

Decreased **Cardiac** output r/t dysrhythmias from hyperkalemia

Disturbed **Thought** processes r/t central nervous system depression

Imbalanced **Nutrition**: less than body requirements r/t inability to ingest, absorb nutrients

Impaired **Memory** r/t electrolyte imbalance

Ineffective **Tissue** perfusion: cardiopulmonary r/t progressive shock

Risk for **Injury**: Risk factors: disorientation, weakness, stupor

Acidosis, Respiratory

Activity intolerance r/t imbalance between oxygen supply and demand

Decreased **Cardiac** output r/t dysrhythmias associated with respiratory acidosis

Disturbed **Thought** processes r/t central nervous system depression

Impaired **Gas** exchange r/t ventilation perfusion imbalance

Impaired **Memory** r/t hypoxia

ACS (Acute Coronary Syndrome)

See Myocardial Infarction

Acne

Disturbed **Body** image r/t biophysical changes associated with skin disorder

Impaired **Skin** integrity r/t hormonal changes (adolescence, menstrual cycle)

Ineffective management of **Therapeutic** regimen r/t deficient knowledge (medications, personal care, cause)

Acquired Immunodeficiency Syndrome

See AIDS (Acquired Immunodeficiency Syndrome)

Acromegaly

Disturbed **Body** image r/t changes in body function and appearance

Impaired physical **Mobility** r/t joint pain

Ineffective **Airway** clearance r/t airway obstruction by enlarged tongue

Sexual dysfunction r/t changes in hormonal secretions

Activity Intolerance

Activity intolerance (See **Activity** intolerance, Section III)

Activity Intolerance, Potential to Develop

Risk for **Activity** intolerance (See **Activity** intolerance, risk for, Section III)

Acute Abdomen

Acute **Pain** r/t pathological process

Deficient **Fluid** volume r/t air and fluids trapped in bowel, inability to drink

See cause of Acute Abdomen

Acute Alcohol Intoxication

Disturbed **Thought** processes r/t central nervous system depression

Dysfunctional **Family** processes: alcoholism r/t abuse of alcohol

Ineffective **Breathing** pattern r/t depression of the respiratory center

Risk for **Aspiration**: Risk factor: depressed reflexes with acute vomiting

Risk for **Infection**: Risk factor: impaired immune system from altered nutrition

Acute Back

Acute **Pain** r/t back injury

Anxiety r/t situational crisis, back injury

Constipation r/t decreased activity, effect of pain medication

Impaired physical **Mobility** r/t pain

Ineffective **Coping** r/t situational crisis, back injury

Ineffective **Health** maintenance r/t deficient knowledge regarding self-care with painful back

Acute Confusion

See Confusion, Acute

Acute Respiratory Distress Syndrome

See ARDS (Acute Respiratory Distress Syndrome)

Adams-Stokes Syndrome

See Dysrhythmia

Addiction

See Alcoholism; Drug Abuse

Addison's Disease

Activity intolerance r/t weakness, fatigue

Deficient **Fluid** volume r/t failure of regulatory mechanisms

Disturbed **Body** image r/t increased skin pigmentation

Imbalanced **Nutrition**: less than body requirements r/t chronic illness

Ineffective **Health** maintenance r/t deficient knowledge

Risk for **Injury**: Risk factors: weakness

Adenoidectomy

Acute **Pain** r/t surgical incision

Ineffective **Airway** clearance r/t hesitation or reluctance to cough as a result of pain, fear

Ineffective **Health** maintenance r/t deficient knowledge of postoperative care

Nausea r/t anesthesia effects, drainage from surgery

Risk for **Aspiration**: Risk factors: postoperative drainage, impaired swallowing

Risk for deficient **Fluid** volume: Risk factors: decreased intake as a result of painful swallowing, effects of anesthesia

Risk for imbalanced **Nutrition**: less than body requirements: Risk factors: hesitation or reluctance to swallow

Adhesions, Lysis of

See Abdominal Surgery

Adjustment Disorder

Anxiety r/t inability to cope with psychosocial stressor

Disturbed personal **Identity** r/t psychosocial stressor (specific to individual)

Risk-prone health **Behavior** r/t assault to self-esteem

Impaired **Social** interaction r/t absence of significant others or peers

Situational low **Self-esteem** r/t change in role function

Adjustment Impairment

Risk-prone health **Behavior** (See health **Behavior**, risk-prone, Section III)

Adolescent, Pregnant

Anxiety r/t situational and maturational crisis, pregnancy

Decisional **Conflict**: keeping child versus giving up child versus abortion r/t lack of experience with decision making, interference with decision making, multiple or divergent sources of information, lack of support system

Deficient **Knowledge** r/t pregnancy, infant growth and development, parenting

Delayed **Growth** and development r/t pregnancy

Disabled family **Coping** r/t highly ambivalent family relationships, chronically unresolved feelings of guilt, anger, despair

Disturbed **Body** image r/t pregnancy superimposed on developing body

Fear r/t labor and delivery

Health-seeking behaviors r/t desire for optimal maternal and fetal outcome

Imbalanced **Nutrition**: less than body requirements r/t lack of knowledge of nutritional needs during pregnancy and as growing adolescent

Impaired **Social** interaction r/t self-concept disturbance

Ineffective **Coping** r/t situational and maturational crisis, personal vulnerability

Ineffective **Denial** r/t fear of consequences of pregnancy becoming known

Ineffective **Health** maintenance r/t deficient knowledge with denial of pregnancy, desire to keep pregnancy secret, fear

Ineffective **Role** performance r/t pregnancy

Interrupted **Family** processes r/t unmet expectations for adolescent, situational crisis

Noncompliance r/t denial of pregnancy

Risk for **Constipation**: Risk factors: hormonal effects, inadequate fiber in diet, inadequate fluid in diet

Risk for delayed **Development**: Risk factor: unplanned or unwanted pregnancy

Risk for impaired parent/child **Attachment**: Risk factors: anxiety associated with the parent role

Risk for impaired **Parenting**: Risk factors: adolescent parent, unplanned or unwanted pregnancy, single parent

Risk for urge urinary **Incontinence**: Risk factor: pressure on bladder by growing uterus

Situational low **Self-esteem** r/t feelings of shame and guilt about becoming or being pregnant

Social isolation r/t absence of supportive significant others

Adoption, Giving Child Up for

Chronic **Sorrow** r/t loss of relationship with child

Decisional **Conflict** r/t unclear personal values or beliefs, perceived threat to value system, support system deficit

Ineffective **Coping** r/t final decision

Insomnia r/t depression or trauma of relinquishment of child

Interrupted **Family** processes r/t conflict within family regarding relinquishment of child

Grieving r/t loss of child, loss of role of parent

Readiness for enhanced **Spiritual** well-being: harmony with self regarding final decision

Risk for **Post-trauma** syndrome: Risk factor: psychological trauma of relinquishment of child

Risk for **Spiritual** distress: Risk factor: perceived moral implications of decision

Social isolation r/t making choice that goes against values of significant others

Adrenal Crisis

Deficient **Fluid** volume r/t insufficient ability to reabsorb water

Delayed **Surgical** recovery r/t inability to respond to stress

Ineffective **Protection** r/t inability to tolerate stress

See Addison's Disease; Shock

Advance Directives

Death **Anxiety** r/t planning for end-of-life health decisions

Decisional **Conflict** r/t unclear personal values or beliefs, perceived threat to value system, support system deficit

Grieving r/t possible loss of self, significant other

Readiness for enhanced **Spiritual** well-being: harmonious interconnectedness with self, others, higher power, God

Affective Disorders

Adult **Failure** to thrive r/t altered mood state

Chronic low **Self-esteem** r/t repeated unmet expectations

Chronic **Sorrow** r/t chronic mental illness

Constipation r/t inactivity, decreased fluid intake

Insomnia r/t inactivity

Fatigue r/t psychological demands

Hopelessness r/t feeling of abandonment, long-term stress

Ineffective **Coping** r/t complicated grieving

Ineffective **Health** maintenance r/t lack of ability to make good judgments regarding ways to obtain help

Risk for complicated **Grief**: Risk factors: lack of previous resolution of former grieving response

Risk for **Loneliness**: Risk factors: pattern of social isolation, feelings of low self-esteem

Risk for **Suicide**: Risk factor: panic state

Self-care deficit: specify r/t depression, cognitive impairment

Sexual dysfunction r/t loss of sexual desire

Social isolation r/t ineffective coping

See specific disorder: Depression; Dysthymic Disorder; Manic Disorder, Bipolar I

Age-Related Macular Degeneration

See Macular Degeneration

Aggressive Behavior

Fear r/t real or imagined threat to own well-being

Risk for other-directed **Violence** (See **Violence**, other-directed, risk for, Section III)

Risk for self-directed **Violence**
*See **Violence**, self-directed, risk for, Section III*

Aging

Adult **Failure** to thrive r/t depression, apathy, fatigue

Chronic **Sorrow** r/t multiple losses

Death **Anxiety** r/t fear of unknown, loss of self, impact on significant others

Disturbed **Sensory** perception: visual or auditory r/t aging process

Functional urinary **Incontinence** r/t impaired vision, impaired cognition, neuromuscular limitations, altered environmental factors

Grieving r/t multiple losses, impending death

Health-seeking behaviors r/t knowledge about medication, nutrition, exercise, coping strategies

Impaired **Dentition** r/t ineffective oral hygiene

Ineffective management of **Therapeutic** regimen r/t deficient knowledge: medication, nutrition, exercise, coping strategies

Ineffective **Thermoregulation** r/t aging

Readiness for enhanced community **Coping** r/t providing social support and other resources identified as needed for elderly client

Readiness for enhanced family **Coping** r/t ability to gratify needs, address adaptive tasks

Readiness for enhanced **Knowledge**: specify: need to improve health

Readiness for enhanced **Nutrition**: need to improve health

Readiness for enhanced **Sleep**: need to improve sleep

Readiness for enhanced **Spiritual** well-being: one's experience of life's meaning, harmony with self, others, higher power, God, environment

Readiness for enhanced **Urinary** elimination: need to improve health

Risk for **Caregiver** role strain: Risk factor: inability to handle increasing needs of significant other

Risk for **Injury**: Risk factor: disturbed sensory perception

Risk for **Loneliness**: Risk factors: inadequate support system, role transition, health alterations, depression, fatigue

Sleep deprivation r/t aging-related sleep stage shifts

Agitation

Acute **Confusion** r/t side effects of medication, hypoxia, decreased cerebral perfusion, alcohol abuse or withdrawal, substance abuse or withdrawal, sensory deprivation or overload

Sleep deprivation r/t sundown syndrome

Agoraphobia

Anxiety r/t real or perceived threat to physical integrity

Fear r/t leaving home, going out in public places

Impaired **Social** interaction r/t disturbance in self-concept

Ineffective **Coping** r/t inadequate support systems

Social isolation r/t altered thought process

A

Agranulocytosis

Delayed **Surgical** recovery r/t abnormal blood profile

Ineffective **Health** maintenance r/t deficient knowledge of protective measures to prevent infection

Ineffective **Protection** r/t abnormal blood profile

AIDS (Acquired Immunodeficiency Syndrome)

Disturbed **Body** image r/t chronic contagious illness, cachexia

Caregiver role strain r/t unpredictable illness course, presence of situation stressors

Chronic **Pain** r/t tissue inflammation and destruction

Chronic **Sorrow** r/t living with long-term chronic illness

Death **Anxiety** r/t fear of premature death

Diarrhea r/t inflammatory bowel changes

Disturbed **Energy** field r/t chronic illness

Fatigue r/t disease process, stress, poor nutritional intake

Fear r/t powerlessness, threat to well-being

Grieving: family/parental r/t potential or impending death of loved one

Grieving: individual r/t loss of physio-psychosocial well-being

Hopelessness r/t deteriorating physical condition

Imbalanced **Nutrition**: less than body requirements r/t decreased ability to eat and absorb nutrients as a result of anorexia, nausea, diarrhea; oral candidiasis pathology in gastrointestinal tract

Ineffective **Health** maintenance r/t deficient knowledge regarding transmission of infection, lack of exposure to information, misinterpretation of information

Ineffective **Protection** r/t risk for infection secondary to inadequate immune system

Ineffective **Sexuality** pattern r/t possible transmission of disease

Interrupted **Family** processes r/t distress about diagnosis of human immunodeficiency virus (HIV) infection

Risk for deficient **Fluid** volume: Risk factors: diarrhea, vomiting, fever, bleeding

Risk for impaired **Oral** mucous membranes: Risk factor: immunological deficit

Risk for impaired **Skin** integrity: Risk factors: immunological deficit, diarrhea

Risk for **Infection**: Risk factor: inadequate immune system

Risk for **Loneliness**: Risk factor: social isolation

Risk for **Spiritual** distress: Risk factor: physical illness

Situational low **Self-esteem** r/t crisis of chronic contagious illness

Social isolation r/t self-concept disturbance, therapeutic isolation

Spiritual distress r/t challenged beliefs or moral system

See AIDS, Child; Cancer; Pneumonia

AIDS Dementia

Chronic **Confusion** r/t viral invasion of nervous system

Disturbed **Thought** processes r/t viral infection in the brain

See Dementia

AIDS, Child

Impaired **Parenting** r/t congenital acquisition of infection secondary to intravenous (IV) drug use, multiple sexual partners, history of contaminated blood transfusion

Parental role conflict r/t intimidation with invasive or restrictive modalities

See AIDS (Acquired Immunodeficiency Syndrome); Child with Chronic Condition; Hospitalized Child; Terminally Ill Child, Adolescent; Terminally Ill Child, Infant/Toddler; Terminally Ill Child, Preschool Child; Terminally Ill Child, School-Age Child/ Preadolescent; Terminally Ill Child/Death of Child, Parent

Airway Obstruction/Secretions

Ineffective **Airway** clearance (See **Airway** clearance, ineffective, Section III)

Alcohol Withdrawal

Acute **Confusion** r/t effects of alcohol withdrawal

Anxiety r/t situational crisis, withdrawal

Chronic low **Self-esteem** r/t repeated unmet expectations

Disturbed **Sensory** perception: visual, auditory, kinesthetic, tactile, olfactory r/t neurochemical imbalance in brain

Disturbed **Thought** processes r/t potential delirium tremors

Dysfunctional **Family** processes: alcoholism r/t abuse of alcohol

Imbalanced **Nutrition**: less than body requirements r/t poor dietary habits

Ineffective **Coping** r/t personal vulnerability

Ineffective **Health** maintenance r/t deficient knowledge regarding chronic illness or effects of alcohol consumption

Insomnia r/t effect of depressants, alcohol withdrawal, anxiety

Risk for deficient **Fluid** volume: Risk factors: excessive diaphoresis, agitation, decreased fluid intake

Risk for other-directed **Violence**: Risk factor: substance withdrawal

Risk for self-directed **Violence**: Risk factor: substance withdrawal

Alcoholism

Acute **Confusion** r/t alcohol abuse

Anxiety r/t loss of control

Chronic **Confusion** r/t neurological effects of chronic alcohol intake

Defensive **Coping** r/t alcoholism

Ineffective **Denial** r/t refusal to acknowledge alcoholism

Insomnia r/t irritability, nightmares, tremors

Disabled family **Coping**: alcoholism r/t codependency issues

Imbalanced **Nutrition**: less than body requirements r/t anorexia

Impaired **Home** maintenance r/t memory deficits, fatigue

Impaired **Memory** r/t alcohol abuse

Ineffective **Coping** r/t use of alcohol to cope with life events

Ineffective **Protection** r/t malnutrition, sleep deprivation

Interrupted **Family** process: alcoholism r/t alcohol abuse

Powerlessness r/t alcohol addiction

Risk for **Injury**: Risk factor: alteration in sensory or perceptual function

Risk for **Loneliness**: Risk factor: unacceptable social behavior

Risk for other-directed **Violence**: Risk factors: reactions to substances used, impulsive behavior, disorientation, impaired judgment

Risk for self-directed **Violence**: Risk factors: reactions to substances used, impulsive behavior, disorientation, impaired judgment

Risk-prone health **Behavior** r/t lack of motivation to change behaviors

Self-esteem disturbance r/t failure at life events

Social isolation r/t unacceptable social behavior, values

Alcoholism, Dysfunctional Family Processes

Dysfunctional **Family** processes: alcoholism (See **Family** processes, dysfunctional: alcoholism, Section III)

Alkalosis

See Metabolic Alkalosis

Allergies

Ineffective **Health** maintenance r/t deficient knowledge regarding allergies

Latex **Allergy** response r/t hypersensitivity to natural rubber latex

Risk for latex **Allergy** response: Risk factor: repeated exposure to products containing latex

Alopecia

Deficient **Knowledge** r/t self-care needed to promote hair growth

Disturbed **Body** image r/t loss of hair, change in appearance

Altered Mental Status

See Confusion, Acute; Confusion, Chronic; Memory Deficit

ALS (Amyotrophic Lateral Sclerosis)

See Amyotrophic Lateral Sclerosis (ALS)

Alzheimer's Type Dementia

Adult **Failure** to thrive r/t difficulty in reasoning, judgment, memory, concentration

Disturbed **Thought** processes r/t chronic organic disorder

Caregiver role strain r/t duration and extent of caregiving required

Chronic **Confusion** r/t Alzheimer's disease

Compromised family **Coping** r/t interrupted family processes

Fear r/t loss of self

Hopelessness r/t deteriorating condition

Impaired **Environmental** interpretation syndrome r/t Alzheimer's disease

Impaired **Home** maintenance r/t impaired cognitive function, inadequate support systems

Impaired **Memory** r/t neurological disturbance

Impaired physical **Mobility** r/t severe neurological dysfunction

Ineffective **Health** maintenance r/t deficient knowledge of caregiver regarding appropriate care

Insomnia r/t neurological impairment, daytime naps

Powerlessness r/t deteriorating condition

Risk for **Injury**: Risk factor: confusion

Risk for **Loneliness**: Risk factor: potential social isolation

Risk for other-directed **Violence**: Risk factors: frustration, fear, anger

Risk for **Relocation** stress syndrome: Risk factors: impaired psychosocial health, decreased health status

Self-care deficit: specify r/t psychological or physiological impairment

Social isolation r/t fear of disclosure of memory loss

Wandering r/t cognitive impairment, frustration, physiological state

See Dementia

AMD (Age-Related Macular Degeneration)

See Macular Degeneration

Amenorrhea

Imbalanced **Nutrition**: less than body requirements r/t inadequate food intake

Risk for **Sexual** dysfunction: Risk factor: altered body function

See Sexuality, Adolescent

AMI (Acute Myocardial Infarction)

See MI (Myocardial Infarction)

Amnesia

Acute **Confusion** r/t alcohol abuse, delirium, dementia, drug abuse

Dysfunctional **Family** processes: alcoholism r/t alcohol abuse, inadequate coping skills

Impaired **Memory** r/t excessive environmental disturbance, neurological disturbance

Post-trauma syndrome r/t history of abuse, catastrophic illness, disaster, accident

Amniocentesis

Anxiety r/t threat to self and fetus, unknown future

Decisional **Conflict** r/t choice of treatment pending results of test

Risk for **Infection**: Risk factor: invasive procedure

Amnionitis

See Chorioamnionitis

A

Amniotic Membrane Rupture

See Premature Rupture of Membranes

Amputation

Acute **Pain** r/t surgery, phantom limb sensation

Chronic **Pain** r/t surgery, phantom limb sensation

Chronic **Sorrow** r/t grief associated with loss of body part

Disturbed **Body** image r/t negative effects of amputation, response from others

Grieving r/t loss of body part, future lifestyle changes

Impaired physical **Mobility** r/t musculoskeletal impairment, limited movement

Impaired **Skin** integrity r/t poor healing, prosthesis rubbing

Ineffective **Health** maintenance r/t deficient knowledge of care of stump, rehabilitation

Ineffective **Tissue** perfusion: peripheral r/t impaired arterial circulation

Risk for deficient **Fluid** volume: Risk factors: hemorrhage, vulnerable surgical site

Amyotrophic Lateral Sclerosis (ALS)

Chronic **Sorrow** r/t chronic illness

Death **Anxiety** r/t impending progressive loss of function leading to death

Decisional **Conflict**: ventilator therapy r/t unclear personal values or beliefs, lack of relevant information

Impaired spontaneous **Ventilation** r/t weakness of muscles of respiration

Impaired **Swallowing** r/t weakness of muscles involved in swallowing

Impaired verbal **Communication** r/t weakness of muscles of speech, deficient knowledge of ways to compensate and alternative communication devices

Ineffective **Breathing** pattern r/t compromised muscles of respiration

Risk for **Aspiration**: Risk factor: impaired swallowing

Risk for **Spiritual** distress: Risk factor: chronic debilitating condition

See Neurological Disorders

Anal Fistula

See Hemorrhoidectomy

Anaphylactic Shock

Impaired spontaneous **Ventilation** r/t acute airway obstruction

Ineffective **Airway** clearance r/t laryngeal edema, bronchospasm

Latex **Allergy** response r/t abnormal immune mechanism response

See Shock

Anasarca

Excess **Fluid** volume r/t excessive fluid intake, cardiac/renal dysfunction, loss of plasma proteins

Risk for impaired **Skin** integrity: Risk factor: impaired circulation to skin

See cause of Anasarca

Anemia

Anxiety r/t cause of disease

Delayed **Surgical** recovery r/t decreased oxygen supply to body, increased cardiac workload

Fatigue r/t decreased oxygen supply to the body, increased cardiac workload

Impaired **Memory** r/t anemia

Ineffective **Health** maintenance r/t deficient knowledge regarding nutritional and medical treatment of anemia

Ineffective **Protection** r/t bleeding disorder

Risk for **Injury** r/t alteration in peripheral sensory perception

Anemia, in Pregnancy

Anxiety r/t concerns about health of self and fetus

Fatigue r/t decreased oxygen supply to the body, increased cardiac workload

Ineffective **Health** maintenance r/t deficient knowledge regarding nutrition in pregnancy

Risk for delayed **Development**: Risk factor: reduction in the oxygen-carrying capacity of blood

Risk for **Infection**: Risk factor: reduction in oxygen-carrying capacity of blood

Anemia, Sickle Cell

See Anemia; Sickle Cell Anemia/Crisis

Anencephaly

See Neural Tube Defects

Aneurysm, Abdominal Surgery

Risk for deficient **Fluid** volume: Risk factor: hemorrhage r/t potential abnormal blood loss

Risk for ineffective **Tissue** perfusion: peripheral or renal Risk factor: impaired arterial circulation

Risk for **Infection**: Risk factor: invasive procedure

See Abdominal Surgery

Aneurysm, Cerebral

See Craniectomy/Craniotomy; Subarachnoid Hemorrhage (if aneurysm has ruptured)

Anger

Anxiety r/t situational crisis

Defensive **Coping** r/t inability to acknowledge responsibility for actions and results of actions

Fear r/t environmental stressor, hospitalization

Grieving r/t significant loss

Powerlessness r/t health care environment

Risk for compromised human **Dignity**: Risk factors: inadequate participation in decision making, perceived dehumanizing treatment, perceived humiliation, exposure of the body, cultural incongruity

Risk for other-directed **Violence**: Risk factors: history of violence, rage reaction

Risk for **Post-trauma** syndrome: Risk factor: inadequate social support

Risk for self-directed **Violence**: Risk factors: history of violence, history of abuse, rage reaction

Risk-prone health **Behavior** r/t assault to self-esteem, disability requiring change in lifestyle, inadequate support system

Angina Pectoris

Activity intolerance r/t acute pain, dysrhythmias

Acute **Pain** r/t myocardial ischemia

Anxiety r/t situational crisis

Decreased **Cardiac** output r/t myocardial ischemia, medication effect, dysrhythmia

Grieving r/t pain, lifestyle changes

Ineffective **Coping** r/t personal vulnerability to situational crisis of new diagnosis, deteriorating health

Ineffective **Denial** r/t deficient knowledge of need to seek help with symptoms

Ineffective **Health** maintenance r/t deficient knowledge of care of angina condition

Ineffective **Sexuality** pattern r/t disease process, medications, loss of libido

Angiocardiography (Cardiac Catheterization)

See Cardiac Catheterization

Angioplasty, Coronary

Decreased **Cardiac** output r/t ventricular ischemia, dysrhythmias

Fear r/t possible outcome of interventional procedure

Ineffective **Health** maintenance r/t deficient knowledge regarding care after procedures, measures to limit coronary artery disease

Risk for deficient **Fluid** volume: Risk factors: possible damage to coronary artery, hematoma formation, hemorrhage

Risk for ineffective **Tissue** perfusion: peripheral/cardiopulmonary: Risk factors: vasospasm, hematoma formation

Anomaly, Fetal/Newborn (Parent Dealing with)

Anxiety r/t threat to role functioning, situational crisis

Chronic **Sorrow** r/t loss of ideal child, inadequate bereavement support

Decisional **Conflict**: interventions for fetus or newborn r/t lack of relevant information, spiritual distress, threat to value system

Deficient **Knowledge** r/t limited exposure to situation

Effective **Therapeutic** regimen management r/t verbalized intent to reduce risk factors for progression of illness and sequelae associated with anomaly

Fear r/t real or imagined threat to baby, implications for future pregnancies, powerlessness

Hopelessness r/t long-term stress, deteriorating physical condition of child, lost spiritual belief

Disabled family **Coping** r/t chronically unresolved feelings about loss of perfect baby

Impaired **Parenting** r/t interruption of bonding process

Ineffective **Coping** r/t personal vulnerability in situational crisis

Interrupted **Family** processes r/t unmet expectations for perfect baby, lack of adequate support systems

Parental role **Conflict** r/t separation from newborn, intimidation with invasive or restrictive modalities, specialized care center policies

Powerlessness r/t complication threatening fetus or newborn

Risk for disorganized **Infant** behavior: Risk factor: congenital disorder

Risk for complicated **Grief**: Risk factor: loss of perfect child

Risk for impaired parent/child **Attachment**: Risk factor: ill infant unable to effectively initiate parental contact as result of altered behavioral organization

Risk for impaired **Parenting**: Risk factors: interruption of bonding process; unrealistic expectations for self, infant, or partner; perceived threat to own emotional survival; severe stress; lack of knowledge

Risk for **Spiritual** distress: Risk factor: lack of normal child to raise and carry on family name

Situational low **Self-esteem** r/t perceived inability to produce a perfect child

Social isolation r/t alterations in child's physical appearance, altered state of wellness

Spiritual distress r/t test of spiritual beliefs

Anorectal Abscess

Acute **Pain** r/t inflammation of perirectal area

Disturbed **Body** image r/t odor and drainage from rectal area

Risk for **Constipation**: Risk factor: fear of painful elimination

Anorexia

Deficient **Fluid** volume r/t inability to drink

Delayed **Surgical** recovery r/t inadequate nutritional intake

Imbalanced **Nutrition**: less than body requirements r/t loss of appetite, nausea, vomiting

Anorexia Nervosa

Activity intolerance r/t fatigue, weakness

Chronic low **Self-esteem** r/t repeated unmet expectations

Constipation r/t lack of adequate food, fiber, and fluid intake

Defensive **Coping** r/t psychological impairment, eating disorder

Diarrhea r/t laxative abuse

Disabled family **Coping** r/t highly ambivalent family relationships

Disturbed **Body** image r/t misconception of actual body appearance

Disturbed **Thought** processes r/t anorexia, impaired nutrition

A

Imbalanced **Nutrition**: less than body requirements r/t inadequate food intake, excessive exercise

Ineffective **Denial** r/t fear of consequences of therapy, possible weight gain

Ineffective family **Therapeutic** regimen management r/t family conflict, excessive demands on family associated with complexity of condition and treatment

Ineffective **Sexuality** pattern r/t loss of libido from malnutrition

Interrupted **Family** processes r/t situational crisis

Risk for **Infection**: Risk factor: malnutrition resulting in depressed immune system

Risk for **Spiritual** distress: Risk factor: low self-esteem

See Maturational Issues, Adolescent

Anosmia (Smell, Loss of Ability to)

Disturbed **Sensory** perception: olfactory r/t altered sensory reception, transmission, integration

Imbalanced **Nutrition**: less than body requirements r/t loss of appetite associated with loss of smell

Antepartum Period

See Pregnancy, Normal; Prenatal Care, Normal

Anterior Repair, Anterior Colporrhaphy

Risk for urge urinary **Incontinence**: Risk factor: trauma to bladder

Urinary retention r/t edema of urinary structures

See Vaginal Hysterectomy

Anticoagulant Therapy

Ineffective **Health** maintenance r/t deficient knowledge regarding precautions to take with anticoagulant therapy

Ineffective **Protection** r/t altered clotting function from anticoagulant

Risk for deficient **Fluid** volume: hemorrhage: Risk factor: altered clotting mechanism

Antisocial Personality Disorder

Defensive **Coping** r/t excessive use of projection

Disturbed **Thought** processes r/t internal turmoil and conflict (intrusive thinking)

Hopelessness r/t abandonment

Impaired **Social** interaction r/t sociocultural conflict, chemical dependence, inability to form relationships

Ineffective **Coping** r/t frequently violating the norms and rules of society

Ineffective family **Therapeutic** regimen management r/t excessive demands on family

Risk for impaired **Parenting**: Risk factors: inability to function as parent or guardian, emotional instability

Risk for **Loneliness**: Risk factor: inability to interact appropriately with others

Risk for other-directed **Violence**: Risk factor: history of violence

Risk for **Self-mutilation**: Risk factors: self-hatred, depersonalization

Spiritual distress r/t separation from religious or cultural ties

Anuria

See Renal Failure

Anxiety

Anxiety (See **Anxiety**, Section III)

Anxiety Disorder

Anxiety r/t unmet security and safety needs

Death **Anxiety** r/t fears of unknown, powerlessness

Decisional **Conflict** r/t low self-esteem, fear of making a mistake

Defensive **Coping** r/t overwhelming feelings of dread

Disabled family **Coping** r/t ritualistic behavior, actions

Disturbed **Energy** field r/t hopelessness, helplessness

Disturbed **Thought** processes r/t anxiety

Ineffective **Coping** r/t inability to express feelings appropriately

Ineffective **Denial** r/t overwhelming feelings of hopelessness, fear, threat to self

Insomnia r/t psychological impairment, emotional instability

Powerlessness r/t lifestyle of helplessness

Risk for **Spiritual** distress: Risk factor: psychological distress

Self-care deficit r/t ritualistic behavior, activities

Sleep deprivation r/t prolonged psychological discomfort

Aortic Aneurysm Repair (Abdominal Surgery)

See Abdominal Surgery; Aneurysm, Abdominal Surgery

Aortic Valvular Stenosis

See Congenital Heart Disease/Cardiac Anomalies

Aphasia

Anxiety r/t situational crisis of aphasia

Impaired verbal **Communication** r/t decrease in circulation to brain

Ineffective **Coping** r/t loss of speech

Ineffective **Health** maintenance r/t deficient knowledge regarding information on aphasia and alternative communication techniques

Aplastic Anemia

Activity intolerance r/t imbalance between oxygen supply and demand

Anxiety r/t deficient knowledge of disease process and treatment

Delayed **Surgical** recovery r/t risk for infection

Impaired **Protection** r/t inadequate immune function

Risk for **Infection**: Risk factor: inadequate immune function

Apnea in Infancy

See Premature Infant (Child); Premature Infant (Parent); SIDS (Sudden Infant Death Syndrome)

Apneustic Respirations

Impaired **Breathing** pattern r/t perception or cognitive impairment, neurological impairment

See cause of Apneustic Respirations

Appendectomy

Acute **Pain** r/t surgical incision

Deficient **Fluid** volume r/t fluid restriction, hypermetabolic state, nausea, vomiting

Ineffective **Health** maintenance r/t deficient knowledge regarding self-care after appendectomy

Risk for **Infection**: Risk factors: perforation or rupture of appendix, surgical incision, peritonitis

See Hospitalized Child; Surgery, Postoperative

Appendicitis

Acute **Pain** r/t inflammation

Deficient **Fluid** volume r/t anorexia, nausea, vomiting

Delayed **Surgical** recovery r/t risk for infection

Risk for **Infection**: Risk factor: possible perforation of appendix

Apprehension

Anxiety r/t threat to self-concept, threat to health status, situational crisis

Death **Anxiety** r/t apprehension over loss of self, consequences to significant others

AMD (Age-Related Macular Degeneration)

See Macular Degeneration

ARDS (Acute Respiratory Distress Syndrome)

Death **Anxiety** r/t seriousness of physical disease

Delayed **Surgical** recovery r/t complications associated with respiratory pathology

Impaired **Gas** exchange r/t damage to alveolar-capillary membrane, change in lung compliance

Impaired spontaneous **Ventilation** r/t damage to alveolar capillary membrane

Ineffective **Airway** clearance r/t excessive tracheobronchial secretions

See Child with Chronic Condition; Ventilator Client

Arrhythmia

See Dysrhythmia

Arterial Insufficiency

Delayed **Surgical** recovery r/t ineffective tissue perfusion

Ineffective **Tissue** perfusion: peripheral r/t interruption of arterial flow

Arthritis

Activity intolerance r/t chronic pain, fatigue, weakness

Chronic **Pain** r/t progression of joint deterioration

Disturbed **Body** image r/t ineffective coping with joint abnormalities

Impaired physical **Mobility** r/t musculoskeletal impairment

Ineffective **Health** maintenance r/t deficient knowledge regarding care of arthritis

Self-care deficit: specify r/t pain, musculoskeletal impairment

See JRA (Juvenile Rheumatoid Arthritis)

Arthrocentesis

Acute **Pain** r/t invasive procedure

Arthroplasty (Total Hip Replacement)

Acute **Pain** r/t tissue trauma associated with surgery

Constipation r/t immobility

Impaired physical **Mobility** r/t decreased muscle strength, surgery

Impaired **Walking** r/t decreased muscle strength, surgery

Risk for **Infection**: Risk factors: invasive surgery, foreign object in body, anesthesia, immobility with stasis of respiratory secretions

Risk for **Injury**: Risk factors: interruption of arterial blood flow, dislocation of prosthesis

Risk for perioperative positioning **Injury**: Risk factors: immobilization, muscle weakness

Risk for **Peripheral** neurovascular dysfunction: Risk factor: orthopedic surgery

See Surgery, Perioperative; Surgery, Postoperative; Surgery, Preoperative

Arthroscopy

Ineffective **Health** maintenance r/t deficient knowledge regarding procedure, postoperative restrictions

Ascites

Chronic **Pain** r/t altered body function

Imbalanced **Nutrition**: less than body requirements r/t loss of appetite

Ineffective **Breathing** pattern r/t increased abdominal girth

Ineffective **Health** maintenance r/t deficient knowledge of care with condition of ascites

See cause of Ascites; Cancer; Cirrhosis

Asphyxia, Birth

Fear (parental) r/t concern over safety of infant

Grieving r/t loss of "perfect" child, concern of loss of future abilities

Impaired **Gas** exchange r/t poor placental perfusion, lack of initiation of breathing by newborn

Impaired spontaneous **Ventilation** r/t brain injury

Ineffective **Breathing** pattern r/t depression of breathing reflex secondary to anoxia

Ineffective **Coping** r/t uncertainty of child outcome

Ineffective **Tissue** perfusion: cerebral r/t poor placental perfusion or cord compression resulting in lack of oxygen to brain

Risk for delayed **Development**: Risk factor: lack of oxygen to brain

Risk for disorganized **Infant** behavior: Risk factor: lack of oxygen to brain

A

Risk for disproportionate **Growth**: Risk factor: lack of oxygen to brain

Risk for impaired parent/child **Attachment**: Risk factors: ill infant who is unable to initiate parental contact, hospitalization in critical care environment

Risk for **Injury**: Risk factor: lack of oxygen to brain

Risk for **Post-trauma** syndrome: parental: Risk factor: psychological trauma of sudden potential for loss of newborn

Aspiration, Danger of

Risk for **Aspiration** (See **Aspiration**, risk for, Section III)

Assault Victim

Post-trauma syndrome r/t assault

Rape-trauma syndrome r/t rape

Risk for **Post-trauma** syndrome: Risk factors: perception of event, inadequate social support, unsupportive environment, diminished ego strength, duration of event

Risk for **Spiritual** distress: Risk factors: physical, psychological stress

Assaultive Client

Disturbed **Thought** process r/t use of hallucinogenic substance, psychological disorder

Ineffective **Coping** r/t lack of control of impulsive actions

Risk for **Injury**: Risk factors: confused thought process, impaired judgment

Risk for other-directed **Violence**: Risk factors: paranoid ideation, anger

Asthma

Activity intolerance r/t fatigue, energy shift to meet muscle needs for breathing to overcome airway obstruction

Anxiety r/t inability to breathe effectively, fear of suffocation

Disturbed **Body** image r/t decreased participation in physical activities

Impaired **Home** maintenance r/t deficient knowledge regarding control of environmental triggers

Ineffective **Airway** clearance r/t tracheobronchial narrowing, excessive secretions

Ineffective **Breathing** pattern r/t anxiety

Ineffective **Coping** r/t personal vulnerability to situational crisis

Ineffective **Health** maintenance r/t deficient knowledge regarding physical triggers, medications, treatment of early warning signs

Sleep deprivation r/t ineffective breathing pattern, cough

See Child with Chronic Condition; Hospitalized Child

Ataxia

Anxiety r/t change in health status

Disturbed **Body** image r/t staggering gait

Impaired physical **Mobility** r/t neuromuscular impairment

Risk for **Falls**: Risk factors: gait alteration, instability

Atelectasis

Impaired **Gas** exchange r/t decreased alveolar-capillary surface

Ineffective **Breathing** pattern r/t loss of functional lung tissue, depression of respiratory function or hypoventilation because of pain

Atherosclerosis

See MI (Myocardial Infarction), CVA (Cerebrovascular Accident), Peripheral Vascular Disease

Athlete's Foot

Impaired **Skin** integrity r/t effects of fungal agent

Ineffective **Health** maintenance r/t deficient knowledge regarding treatment and prevention of athlete's foot

See Itching; Pruritus

ATN (Acute Tubular Necrosis)

See Renal Failure

Atrial Fibrillation

See Dysrhythmia

Atrial Septal Defect

See Congenital Heart Disease/Cardiac Anomalies

Attention Deficit Disorder

Disabled family **Coping** r/t significant person with chronically unexpressed feelings of guilt, anxiety, hostility, and despair

Risk for delayed **Development**: Risk factor: behavior disorders

Risk for impaired **Parenting**: Risk factor: lack of knowledge of factors contributing to child's behavior

Risk for **Loneliness**: Risk factor: social isolation

Risk for **Spiritual** distress: Risk factor: poor relationships

Risk-prone health **Behavior** r/t intense emotional state

Self-esteem disturbance r/t difficulty in participating in expected activities, poor school performance

Social isolation r/t unacceptable social behavior

Autism

Compromised family **Coping** r/t parental guilt over etiology of disease, inability to accept or adapt to child's condition, inability to help child and other family members seek treatment

Delayed **Growth** and development r/t inability to develop relations with other human beings, inability to identify own body as separate from those of other people, inability to integrate concept of self

Disturbed personal **Identity** r/t inability to distinguish between self and environment, inability to identify own body as separate from those of other people, inability to integrate concept of self

Disturbed **Thought** processes r/t inability to perceive self or others, cognitive dissonance, perceptual dysfunction

Impaired **Social** interaction r/t communication barriers, inability to relate to others, failure to develop peer relationships

Impaired verbal **Communication** r/t speech and language delays

Risk for delayed **Development**: Risk factor: autism

Risk for **Loneliness**: Risk factors: health alterations, change in cognition

Risk for other-directed **Violence**: Risk factors: frequent destructive rages toward others secondary to extreme response to changes in routine, fear of harmless things

Risk for self-directed **Violence**: Risk factors: frequent destructive rages toward self, secondary to extreme response to changes in routine, fear of harmless things

Risk for **Self-mutilation**: Risk factor: autistic state

See Child with Chronic Condition; Mental Retardation

Autonomic Dysreflexia

Autonomic dysreflexia r/t bladder distention, bowel distention, noxious stimuli

Risk for **Autonomic** dysreflexia: Risk factors: bladder distention, bowel distention, noxious stimuli

Autonomic Hyperreflexia

See Autonomic Dysreflexia

B

Back Pain

Acute **Pain** r/t back injury

Anxiety r/t situational crisis, back injury

Chronic **Pain** r/t back injury

Disturbed **Energy** field r/t chronic pain

Impaired physical **Mobility** r/t pain

Ineffective **Coping** r/t situational crisis, back injury

Ineffective **Health** maintenance r/t deficient knowledge regarding prevention of further injury, proper body mechanics

Risk for **Constipation**: Risk factors: decreased activity, side effect of pain medication

Risk for **Disuse** syndrome: Risk factor: severe pain

Bacteremia

Ineffective **Protection** r/t compromised immune system

See Infection; Infection, Potential for

Barrel Chest

See Aging (if appropriate); COPD (Chronic Obstructive Pulmonary Disease)

Bathing/Hygiene Problems

Bathing/hygiene **Self-care** deficit (See **Self-care** deficit, bathing/hygiene, Section III)

Impaired bed **Mobility** r/t chronic physically limiting condition

Battered Child Syndrome

Chronic **Sorrow** r/t situational crises

Dysfunctional **Family** processes: alcoholism r/t inadequate coping skills

Risk for **Aspiration**: Risk factor: propped bottle

Risk for **Post-trauma** syndrome: Risk factors: physical abuse, incest, rape, molestation

Risk for **Self-mutilation**: Risk factors: feelings of rejection, dysfunctional family

Sleep deprivation r/t prolonged psychological discomfort

See Child Abuse

Battered Person

See Abuse, Spouse, Parent, or Significant Other

Bed Mobility, Impaired

Impaired bed **Mobility** (See **Mobility**, impaired bed, Section III)

Bedbugs, Infestation

Impaired **Home** maintenance r/t deficient knowledge regarding prevention of bedbug infestation

Impaired **Skin** integrity r/t bites of bedbugs

See Itching; Pruritus

Bedrest, Prolonged

Deficient **Diversional** activity r/t prolonged bedrest

Impaired bed **Mobility** r/t neuromuscular impairment

Risk for **Disuse** syndrome: Risk factor: prolonged immobility

Risk for **Loneliness**: Risk factor: prolonged bedrest

Social isolation r/t prolonged bedrest

Bedsores

See Pressure Ulcer

Bedwetting

See Enuresis; Toilet Training

Bell's Palsy

Acute **Pain** r/t inflammation of facial nerve

Disturbed **Body** image r/t loss of motor control on one side of face

Imbalanced **Nutrition**: less than body requirements r/t difficulty with chewing

Risk for **Injury** (eye): Risk factor: dysfunction of facial nerve

Benign Prostatic Hypertrophy

See BPH (Benign Prostatic Hypertrophy); Prostatic Hypertrophy

Bereavement

Chronic **Sorrow** r/t death of loved one, chronic illness, disability

Grieving r/t loss of significant person

Risk for complicated **Grief**: Risk factor: death of a loved one

Insomnia r/t grief

Risk for **Spiritual** distress: Risk factor: death of a loved one

Biliary Atresia

Anxiety r/t surgical intervention, possible liver transplantation

Imbalanced **Nutrition**: less than body requirements r/t decreased absorption of fat and fat-soluble vitamins, poor feeding

Pruritus r/t inflammation of skin

B

Risk for impaired **Skin** integrity: Risk factor: pruritus

Risk for ineffective **Breathing** pattern: Risk factors: enlarged liver, development of ascites

Risk for **Injury**: bleeding Risk factors: vitamin K deficiency, altered clotting mechanisms

See Child with Chronic Condition; Cirrhosis (as complication); Hospitalized Child; Terminally Ill Child, Adolescent; Terminally Ill Child, Infant/Toddler; Terminally Ill Child, Preschool Child; Terminally Ill Child, School-Age-Child/Preadolescent; Terminally Ill Child/Death of Child, Parent

Biliary Calculus

See Cholelithiasis

Biliary Obstruction

See Jaundice

Biopsy

Fear r/t outcome of biopsy

Ineffective **Health** maintenance r/t deficient knowledge regarding biopsy site, further needed health care

Bioterrorism

Contamination r/t exposure to bioterrorism

Risk for **Infection**: Risk factor: exposure to harmful biological agent

Risk for **Post-trauma** syndrome: Risk factor: perception of event of bioterrorism

Bipolar Disorder I (Most Recent Episode, Depressed or Manic)

Chronic low **Self-esteem** r/t repeated unmet expectations

Disturbed **Energy** field r/t disharmony of mind, body, spirit

Fatigue r/t psychological demands

Ineffective **Coping** r/t complicated grieving

Ineffective **Health** maintenance r/t lack of ability to make good judgments regarding ways to obtain help

Risk for complicated **Grief**: Risk factor: lack of previous resolution of former grieving response

Risk for **Loneliness**: Risk factors: stress, conflict

Risk for **Spiritual** distress: Risk factor: mental illness

Risk-prone health **Behavior** r/t low state of optimism

Self-care deficit: specify r/t depression, cognitive impairment

Social isolation r/t ineffective coping

See Depression (Major Depressive Disorder); Manic Disorder, Bipolar I

Birth Asphyxia

See Asphyxia, Birth

Birth Control

See Contraceptive Method

Bladder Cancer

Urinary retention r/t clots obstructing urethra

See Cancer; TURP (Transurethral Resection of the Prostate)

Bladder Distention

Urinary retention r/t high urethral pressure caused by weak detrusor, inhibition of reflex arc, blockage, strong sphincter

Bladder Training

Disturbed **Body** image r/t difficulty maintaining control of urinary elimination

Functional urinary **Incontinence** r/t altered environment; sensory, cognitive, mobility deficit

Ineffective **Health** maintenance r/t deficient knowledge regarding incontinence self-care

Stress urinary **Incontinence** r/t degenerative change in pelvic muscles and structural supports

Urge urinary **Incontinence** r/t decreased bladder capacity, increased urine concentration, overdistention of bladder

Bladder Training, Child

See Toilet Training

Bleeding Tendency

Ineffective **Protection** r/t abnormal blood profile, drug therapies

Risk for delayed **Surgical** recovery: Risk factor: bleeding tendency

Blepharoplasty

Disturbed **Body** image r/t effects of surgery

Ineffective **Health** maintenance r/t deficient knowledge regarding postoperative care of surgical area

Blindness

Disturbed **Sensory** perception: visual r/t altered sensory reception, transmission, integration

Impaired **Home** maintenance r/t decreased vision

Ineffective **Role** performance r/t alteration in health status (change in visual acuity)

Interrupted **Family** processes r/t shift in health status of family member (change in visual acuity)

Risk for delayed **Development**: Risk factor: vision impairment

Risk for **Injury**: Risk factor: sensory dysfunction

Self-care deficit r/t inability to see to be able to perform activities of daily living

See Vision Impairment

Blood Disorder

Ineffective **Protection** r/t abnormal blood profile

See cause of Blood Disorder

Blood Pressure Alteration

See Hypertension; Hypotension; HTN (Hypertension)

Blood Sugar Control

Risk for unstable blood **Glucose** (See **Glucose**, unstable blood, risk for, Section III)

Blood Transfusion

Anxiety r/t possibility of harm from transfusion

See Anemia

Body Dysmorphic Disorder

Disturbed **Body** image r/t overinvolvement in physical appearance

Body Image Change

Disturbed **Body** image (See **Body** image, disturbed, Section III)

Body Temperature, Altered

Imbalanced **Thermoregulation** (See **Thermoregulation**, imbalanced, Section III)

Bone Marrow Biopsy

Acute **Pain** r/t bone marrow aspiration

Fear r/t unknown outcome of results of biopsy

Ineffective **Health** maintenance r/t deficient knowledge of expectations after procedure, disease treatment after biopsy

See disease necessitating bone marrow biopsy (e.g., Leukemia)

Borderline Personality Disorder

Anxiety r/t perceived threat to self-concept

Defensive **Coping** r/t difficulty with relationships, inability to accept blame for own behavior

Disturbed **Thought** processes r/t poor reality testing

Ineffective **Coping** r/t use of maladjusted defense mechanisms (e.g., projection, denial)

Ineffective family **Therapeutic** regimen management r/t manipulative behavior of client

Powerlessness r/t lifestyle of helplessness

Risk for **Caregiver** role strain: Risk factors: inability of care receiver to accept criticism, care receiver taking advantage of others to meet own needs or having unreasonable expectations

Risk for self-directed **Violence**: Risk factors: feelings of need to punish self, manipulative behavior

Risk for **Self-mutilation**: Risk factors: ineffective coping, feelings of self-hatred

Risk for **Spiritual** distress: Risk factor: poor relationships associated with behaviors attributed to borderline personality disorder

Social isolation r/t immature interests

Boredom

Deficient **Diversional** activity r/t environmental lack of diversional activity

Social isolation r/t altered state of wellness

Botulism

Deficient **Fluid** volume r/t profuse diarrhea

Ineffective **Health** maintenance r/t deficient knowledge regarding prevention of botulism, care after episode

Bowel Incontinence

Bowel incontinence r/t decreased awareness of need to defecate, loss of sphincter control, fecal impaction

Bowel Obstruction

Acute **Pain** r/t pressure from distended abdomen

Constipation r/t decreased motility, intestinal obstruction

Deficient **Fluid** volume r/t inadequate fluid volume intake, fluid loss in bowel

Imbalanced **Nutrition**: less than body requirements r/t nausea, vomiting

Bowel Resection

See Abdominal Surgery

Bowel Sounds, Absent or Diminished

Constipation r/t decreased or absent peristalsis

Deficient **Fluid** volume r/t inability to ingest fluids, loss of fluids in bowel

Delayed **Surgical** recovery r/t inability to obtain adequate nutritional status

Bowel Sounds, Hyperactive

Diarrhea r/t increased gastrointestinal motility

Bowel Training

Bowel incontinence r/t loss of control of rectal sphincter

Ineffective **Health** maintenance r/t deficient knowledge regarding treatment of bowel incontinence

Bowel Training, Child

See Toilet Training

BPH (Benign Prostatic Hypertrophy)

Ineffective **Health** maintenance r/t deficient knowledge regarding self-care with prostatic hypertrophy

Insomnia r/t nocturia

Risk for **Infection**: Risk factors: urinary residual after voiding, bacterial invasion of bladder

Risk for urge urinary **Incontinence**: Risk factors: detrusor muscle instability with impaired contractility, involuntary sphincter relaxation

Urinary retention r/t obstruction

See Prostatic Hypertrophy

Bradycardia

Decreased **Cardiac** output r/t slow heart rate supplying inadequate amount of blood for body function

Ineffective **Health** maintenance r/t deficient knowledge of condition, effects of cardiac medications

Ineffective **Tissue** perfusion: cerebral r/t decreased cardiac output secondary to bradycardia, vagal response

Risk for **Injury**: Risk factor: decreased cerebral tissue perfusion

Bradypnea

Ineffective **Breathing** pattern r/t neuromuscular impairment, pain, musculoskeletal impairment, perception or cognitive impairment, anxiety, fatigue or decreased energy, effects of drugs

See cause of Bradypnea

Brain Injury

See Intracranial Pressure, Increased

Brain Surgery

See Craniectomy/Craniotomy

Brain Tumor

Acute **Pain** r/t pressure from tumor

Decreased **Intracranial** adaptive capacity r/t presence of brain tumor

Disturbed **Sensory** perception: specify r/t tumor growth compressing brain tissue

Disturbed **Thought** processes r/t altered circulation, destruction of brain tissue

Fear r/t threat to well-being

Grieving r/t potential loss of physiosocial-psychosocial well-being

Risk for **Injury**: Risk factors: sensory-perceptual alterations, weakness

See Cancer; Chemotherapy; Child with Chronic Condition; Craniectomy/Craniotomy; Hospitalized Child; Radiation Therapy; Terminally Ill Child, Adolescent; Terminally Ill Child, Infant/ Toddler; Terminally Ill Child, Preschool Child; Terminally Ill Child, School-Age Child/Preadolescent; Terminally Ill Child/Death of Child, Parent

Braxton Hicks Contractions

Activity intolerance r/t increased perception of contractions with increased gestation

Anxiety r/t uncertainty about beginning labor

Fatigue r/t lack of sleep

Ineffective **Sexuality** pattern r/t fear of contractions

Insomnia r/t contractions when lying down

Stress urinary **Incontinence** r/t increased pressure on bladder with contractions

Breast Biopsy

Fear r/t potential for diagnosis of cancer

Ineffective **Health** maintenance r/t deficient knowledge regarding appropriate postoperative care of breasts

Risk for **Spiritual** distress: Risk factor: fear of diagnosis of cancer

Breast Cancer

Chronic **Sorrow** r/t diagnosis of cancer, loss of body integrity

Death **Anxiety** r/t diagnosis of cancer

Fear r/t diagnosis of cancer

Ineffective **Coping** r/t treatment, prognosis

Risk for **Spiritual** distress: Risk factor: fear of diagnosis of cancer

Sexual dysfunction r/t loss of body part, partner's reaction to loss

See Cancer; Chemotherapy; Mastectomy; Radiation Therapy

Breast Lumps

Fear r/t potential for diagnosis of cancer

Ineffective **Health** maintenance r/t deficient knowledge regarding appropriate care of breasts

Breast Pumping

Ineffective **Health** maintenance r/t deficient knowledge regarding breast milk expression and storage

Risk for impaired **Skin** integrity: Risk factor: high suction

Risk for **Infection**: Risk factors: contaminated breast pump parts, incomplete emptying of breast

Breastfeeding, Effective

Effective **Breastfeeding** (See **Breastfeeding**, effective, Section III)

Breastfeeding, Ineffective

Ineffective **Breastfeeding** (See **Breastfeeding**, ineffective, Section III)

See Painful Breasts, Sore Nipples; Painful Breasts, Engorgement, Infant Feeding Pattern, Ineffective

Breastfeeding, Interrupted

Interrupted **Breastfeeding** (See **Breastfeeding**, interrupted, Section III)

Breath Sounds, Decreased or Absent

See Atelectasis; Pneumothorax

Breathing Pattern Alteration

Ineffective **Breathing** pattern r/t neuromuscular impairment, pain, musculoskeletal impairment, perception or cognitive impairment, anxiety, decreased energy or fatigue

Breech Birth

Anxiety: maternal r/t threat to self, infant

Fear: maternal r/t danger to infant, self

Impaired **Gas** exchange: fetal r/t compressed umbilical cord

Ineffective **Tissue** perfusion r/t compressed umbilical cord

Risk for **Aspiration**: fetal Risk factor: birth of body before head

Risk for delayed **Development**: Risk factor: compressed umbilical cord

Risk for impaired **Tissue** integrity: fetal Risk factor: difficult birth

Risk for impaired **Tissue** integrity: maternal: Risk factor: difficult birth

Bronchitis

Anxiety r/t potential chronic condition

Health-seeking behavior r/t wish to stop smoking

Ineffective **Airway** clearance r/t excessive thickened mucus secretion

Ineffective **Health** maintenance r/t deficient knowledge regarding care of condition

Bronchopulmonary Dysplasia

Activity intolerance r/t imbalance between oxygen supply and demand

Excess **Fluid** volume r/t sodium and water retention

Imbalanced **Nutrition**: less than body requirements r/t poor feeding, increased caloric needs as a result of increased work of breathing

See Child with Chronic Condition; Hospitalized Child; Respiratory Conditions of the Neonate

Bronchoscopy

Risk for **Aspiration**: Risk factor: temporary loss of gag reflex

Risk for **Injury**: Risk factors: complication of pneumothorax, laryngeal edema, hemorrhage (if biopsy done)

Bruits, Carotid

Ineffective **Tissue** perfusion: cerebral r/t interruption of carotid blood flow

Risk for **Injury**: Risk factors: loss of motor, sensory, visual function

Bryant's Traction

See Traction and Casts

Buck's Traction

See Traction and Casts

Buerger's Disease

See Peripheral Vascular Disease

Bulimia

Chronic low **Self-esteem** r/t lack of positive feedback

Defensive **Coping** r/t eating disorder

Diarrhea r/t laxative abuse

Disturbed **Body** image r/t misperception about actual appearance, body weight

Fear r/t food ingestion, weight gain

Imbalanced **Nutrition**: less than body requirements r/t induced vomiting, excessive exercise

Compromised family **Coping** r/t chronically unresolved feelings of guilt, anger, hostility

Noncompliance r/t negative feelings toward treatment regimen

Powerlessness r/t urge to purge self after eating

See Maturational Issues, Adolescent

Bunion

Ineffective **Health** maintenance r/t deficient knowledge regarding appropriate care of feet

Bunionectomy

Impaired physical **Mobility** r/t sore foot

Impaired **Walking** r/t pain associated with surgery

Ineffective **Health** maintenance r/t deficient knowledge regarding postoperative care of feet

Risk for **Infection**: Risk factors: surgical incision, advanced age

Burns

Acute **Pain** r/t burn injury, treatments

Grieving r/t loss of bodily function, loss of future hopes and plans

Deficient **Diversional** activity r/t long-term hospitalization

Delayed **Surgical** recovery r/t ineffective tissue perfusion

Disturbed **Body** image r/t altered physical appearance

Fear r/t pain from treatments, possible permanent disfigurement

Hypothermia r/t impaired skin integrity

Imbalanced **Nutrition**: less than body requirements r/t increased metabolic needs, anorexia, protein and fluid loss

Impaired physical **Mobility** r/t pain, musculoskeletal impairment, contracture formation

Impaired **Skin** integrity r/t injury of skin

Ineffective **Tissue** perfusion: peripheral r/t circumferential burns, impaired arterial/venous circulation

Post-trauma syndrome r/t life-threatening event

Risk for deficient **Fluid** volume: Risk factors: loss from skin surface, fluid shift

Risk for ineffective **Airway** clearance: Risk factors: potential tracheobronchial obstruction, edema

Risk for **Infection**: Risk factors: loss of intact skin, trauma, invasive sites

Risk for **Peripheral** neurovascular dysfunction: Risk factor: eschar formation with circumferential burn

Risk for **Post-trauma** syndrome: Risk factors: perception, duration of event that caused burns

See Hospitalized Child; Safety, Childhood

Bursitis

Acute **Pain** r/t inflammation in joint

Impaired physical **Mobility** r/t inflammation in joint

Bypass Graft

See Coronary Artery Bypass Grafting

C

Cachexia

Adult **Failure** to thrive r/t imbalanced nutrition: less than body requirements

Imbalanced **Nutrition**: less than body requirements r/t inability to ingest food because of biological factors

Ineffective **Protection** r/t inadequate nutrition

Calcium Alteration

See Hypercalcemia; Hypocalcemia

Cancer

Activity intolerance r/t side effects of treatment, weakness from cancer

Chronic **Pain** r/t metastatic cancer

Chronic **Sorrow** r/t chronic illness of cancer

Compromised family **Coping** r/t prolonged disease or disability progression that exhausts supportive ability of significant others

C

Constipation r/t side effects of medication, altered nutrition, decreased activity

Death Anxiety r/t unresolved issues regarding dying

Decisional Conflict r/t selection of treatment choices, continuation or discontinuation of treatment, "do not resuscitate" decision

Disturbed Body image r/t side effects of treatment, cachexia

Fear r/t serious threat to well-being

Grieving r/t potential loss of significant others, high risk for infertility

Hopelessness r/t loss of control, terminal illness

Imbalanced Nutrition: less than body requirements r/t loss of appetite, difficulty swallowing, side effects of chemotherapy, obstruction by tumor

Impaired Oral mucous membranes r/t chemotherapy, effects of radiation, oral pH changes, decreased oral secretions

Impaired physical Mobility r/t weakness, neuromusculoskeletal impairment, pain

Impaired Skin integrity r/t immunological deficit, immobility

Ineffective Coping r/t personal vulnerability in situational crisis, terminal illness

Ineffective Denial r/t complicated grieving process

Ineffective Health maintenance r/t deficient knowledge regarding prescribed treatment

Ineffective Protection r/t cancer suppressing immune system

Ineffective Role performance r/t change in physical capacity, inability to resume prior role

Insomnia r/t anxiety, pain

Powerlessness r/t treatment, progression of disease

Readiness for enhanced Spiritual well-being: desire for harmony with self, others, higher power, God when faced with serious illness

Risk for Disuse syndrome: Risk factors: immobility, fatigue

Risk for impaired Home maintenance: Risk factor: lack of familiarity with community resources

Risk for Infection: Risk factor: inadequate immune system

Risk for Injury: Risk factor: bleeding secondary to bone marrow depression

Risk for Spiritual distress: Risk factor: physical illness of cancer

Self-care deficit: specify r/t pain, intolerance to activity, decreased strength

Social isolation r/t hospitalization, lifestyle changes

Spiritual distress r/t test of spiritual beliefs

See Chemotherapy; Child with Chronic Condition; Hospitalized Child; Radiation Therapy; Terminally Ill Child, Adolescent; Terminally Ill Child, Infant/Toddler; Terminally Ill Child, Preschool Child; Terminally Ill Child, School-Age Child/ Preadolescent; Terminally Ill Child/Death of Child, Parent

Candidiasis, Oral

Impaired Oral mucous membranes r/t overgrowth of infectious agent, depressed immune function

Ineffective Health maintenance r/t deficient knowledge regarding care of infected mouth

Capillary Refill Time, Prolonged

Impaired Gas exchange r/t ventilation perfusion imbalance

Ineffective Tissue perfusion: peripheral r/t interruption of arterial or venous flow

See Shock

Carbon Monoxide Poisoning

See Smoke Inhalation

Cardiac Arrest

Post-trauma syndrome r/t sustaining serious life event

See cause of Cardiac Arrest

Cardiac Catheterization

Anxiety r/t invasive procedure, uncertainty of outcome of procedure

Decreased Cardiac output r/t ventricular ischemia, dysrhythmia

Ineffective Health maintenance r/t deficient knowledge regarding procedure, postprocedure care, treatment and prevention of coronary artery disease

Risk for ineffective Tissue perfusion: Risk factors: impaired arterial or venous circulation

Risk for Injury: hematoma: Risk factor: invasive procedure

Risk for Peripheral neurovascular dysfunction: Risk factor: vascular obstruction

Cardiac Disorders

Decreased Cardiac output r/t cardiac disorder

See specific cardiac disorder

Cardiac Disorders in Pregnancy

Activity intolerance r/t cardiac pathophysiology, increased demand because of pregnancy, weakness, fatigue

Anxiety r/t unknown outcomes of pregnancy, family well-being

Compromised family Coping r/t prolonged hospitalization or maternal incapacitation that exhausts supportive capacity of significant others

Death Anxiety r/t potential danger of condition

Fatigue r/t metabolic, psychological, and emotional demands

Fear r/t potential maternal effects, potential poor fetal or maternal outcome

Ineffective Coping r/t personal vulnerability

Ineffective Health maintenance r/t deficient knowledge regarding treatment, restrictions with cardiac disorder

Ineffective Role performance r/t changes in lifestyle, expectations from disease process with superimposed pregnancy

Interrupted Family processes r/t hospitalization, maternal incapacitation, changes in roles

Powerlessness r/t illness-related regimen

Risk for delayed Development: Risk factor: poor maternal oxygenation

Risk for disproportionate **Growth**: Risk factor: poor maternal oxygenation

Risk for excess **Fluid** volume: Risk factors: compromised regulatory mechanism with increased afterload, preload, circulating blood volume

Risk for imbalanced **Fluid** volume: Risk factor: sudden changes in circulation after delivery of placenta

Risk for impaired **Gas** exchange: Risk factor: pulmonary edema

Risk for ineffective **Tissue** perfusion: fetal: Risk factor: poor maternal oxygenation

Risk for **Spiritual** distress: Risk factor: fear of diagnosis for self and infant

Situational low **Self-esteem** r/t situational crisis, pregnancy

Social isolation r/t limitations of activity, bed rest or hospitalization, separation from family and friends

Cardiac Dysrhythmia

See Dysrhythmia

Cardiac Output Decrease

Decreased **Cardiac** output r/t cardiac dysfunction

Cardiac Tamponade

Decreased **Cardiac** output r/t fluid in pericardial sac

See Pericarditis

Cardiogenic Shock

Decreased **Cardiac** output r/t decreased myocardial contractility, dysrhythmia

See Shock

Caregiver Role Strain

Caregiver role strain (See **Caregiver** role strain, Section III)

Carious Teeth

See Cavities in Teeth

Carotid Endarterectomy

Fear r/t surgery in vital area

Ineffective **Health** maintenance r/t deficient knowledge regarding postoperative care

Risk for ineffective **Airway** clearance: Risk factor: hematoma compressing trachea

Risk for ineffective **Tissue** perfusion: cerebral: Risk factors: hemorrhage, clot formation

Risk for **Injury**: Risk factor: possible hematoma formation

Carpal Tunnel Syndrome

Chronic **Pain** r/t unrelieved pressure on median nerve

Impaired physical **Mobility** r/t neuromuscular impairment

Self-care deficit: bathing, hygiene, dressing, grooming, feeding r/t pain

Carpopedal Spasm

See Hypocalcemia

Casts

Deficient **Diversional** activity r/t physical limitations from cast

Ineffective **Health** maintenance r/t deficient knowledge regarding cast care, personal care with cast

Impaired physical **Mobility** r/t limb immobilization

Impaired **Walking** r/t cast(s) on lower extremities, fracture of bones

Risk for impaired **Skin** integrity: Risk factor: unrelieved pressure on skin

Risk for **Peripheral** neurovascular dysfunction: Risk factor: mechanical compression from cast

Self-care deficit: bathing, hygiene, dressing, grooming, feeding r/t presence of cast(s) on upper extremities

Self-care deficit: toileting r/t presence of cast(s) on lower extremities

Cataract Extraction

Anxiety r/t threat of permanent vision loss, surgical procedure

Disturbed **Sensory** perception: vision r/t edema from surgery

Ineffective **Health** maintenance r/t deficient knowledge regarding postoperative restrictions

Risk for **Injury**: Risk factors: increased intraocular pressure, accommodation to new visual field

See Vision Impairment

Cataracts

Disturbed **Sensory** perception: vision r/t altered sensory input

See Vision Impairment

Catatonic Schizophrenia

Imbalanced **Nutrition**: less than body requirements r/t decrease in outside stimulation, loss of perception of hunger, resistance to instructions to eat

Impaired **Memory** r/t cognitive impairment

Impaired physical **Mobility** r/t cognitive impairment, maintenance of rigid posture, inappropriate or bizarre postures

Impaired verbal **Communication** r/t muteness

Social isolation r/t inability to communicate, immobility

See Schizophrenia

Catheterization, Urinary

Ineffective **Health** maintenance r/t deficient knowledge of normal sensation of catheter in place, care of catheter

Risk for **Infection**: Risk factor: invasive procedure

Cavities in Teeth

Impaired **Dentition** r/t ineffective oral hygiene, barriers to self-care, economic barriers to professional care, nutritional deficits, dietary habits

Cellulitis

Acute **Pain** r/t inflammatory changes in tissues from infection

Impaired **Skin** integrity r/t inflammatory process damaging skin

Ineffective **Health** maintenance r/t lack of knowledge regarding prevention of further incidences of infection

Ineffective **Tissue** perfusion: peripheral r/t edema

Cellulitis, Periorbital

Acute **Pain** r/t edema and inflammation of skin/tissues

Disturbed **Sensory** perception: visual r/t decreased visual fields secondary to edema of eyelids

Hyperthermia r/t infectious process

Impaired **Skin** integrity r/t inflammation or infection of skin, tissues

See Hospitalized Child

Central Line Insertion

Ineffective **Health** maintenance r/t deficient knowledge regarding precautions to take when central line is in place

Risk for **Infection**: Risk factor: invasive procedure

Cerebral Aneurysm

See Craniectomy/Craniotomy; Intracranial Pressure, Increased; Subarachnoid Hemorrhage

Cerebral Palsy

Chronic **Sorrow** r/t presence of chronic disability

Deficient **Diversional** activity r/t physical impairments, limitations on ability to participate in recreational activities

Imbalanced **Nutrition**: less than body requirements r/t spasticity, feeding or swallowing difficulties

Impaired physical **Mobility** r/t spasticity, neuromuscular impairment or weakness

Impaired **Social** interaction r/t impaired communication skills, limited physical activity, perceived differences from peers

Impaired verbal **Communication** r/t impaired ability to articulate or speak words because of facial muscle involvement

Risk for **Falls**: Risk factor: impaired physical mobility

Risk for impaired **Parenting**: Risk factor: caring for child with overwhelming needs resulting from chronic change in health status

Risk for **Injury**: Risk factors: muscle weakness, inability to control spasticity

Risk for **Spiritual** distress: Risk factors: psychological stress associated with chronic illness

Self-care deficit: specify r/t neuromuscular impairments, sensory deficits

See Child with Chronic Condition

Cerebrovascular Accident

See CVA (Cerebrovascular Accident)

Cervicitis

Ineffective **Health** maintenance r/t deficient knowledge regarding care and prevention of condition

Ineffective **Sexuality** pattern r/t abstinence during acute stage

Risk for **Infection**: Risk factors: spread of infection, recurrence of infection

Cesarean Delivery

Acute **Pain** r/t surgical incision

Anxiety r/t unmet expectations for childbirth, unknown outcome of surgery

Disturbed **Body** image r/t surgery, unmet expectations for childbirth

Fear r/t perceived threat to own well-being

Impaired physical **Mobility** r/t pain

Ineffective **Health** maintenance r/t deficient knowledge regarding postoperative care

Ineffective **Role** performance r/t unmet expectations for childbirth

Interrupted **Family** processes r/t unmet expectations for childbirth

Risk for deficient **Fluid** volume: Risk factor: increased blood loss from surgery

Risk for imbalanced **Fluid** volume: Risk factor: loss of blood

Risk for **Infection**: Risk factors: surgical incision, stasis of respiratory secretions as a result of general anesthesia

Risk for **Urinary** retention: Risk factor: regional anesthesia

Situational low **Self-esteem** r/t inability to deliver child vaginally

Chemical Dependence

See Alcoholism; Drug Abuse

Chemotherapy

Death **Anxiety** r/t chemotherapy not accomplishing desired results

Delayed **Surgical** recovery r/t compromised immune system

Disturbed **Body** image r/t loss of weight, loss of hair

Fatigue r/t disease process, anemia, drug effects

Imbalanced **Nutrition**: less than body requirements r/t side effects of chemotherapy

Impaired **Oral** mucous membranes r/t effects of chemotherapy

Ineffective **Health** maintenance r/t deficient knowledge regarding action, side effects, way to integrate chemotherapy into lifestyle

Ineffective **Protection** r/t suppressed immune system, decreased platelets

Nausea r/t effects of chemotherapy

Risk for deficient **Fluid** volume: Risk factors: vomiting, diarrhea

Risk for ineffective **Tissue** perfusion: Risk factor: anemia

Risk for **Infection**: Risk factor: immunosuppression

See Cancer

Chest Pain

Acute **Pain** r/t myocardial injury, ischemia

Decreased **Cardiac** output r/t ventricular ischemia

Fear r/t potential threat of death

See Angina Pectoris; MI (Myocardial Infarction)

Chest Tubes

Acute **Pain** r/t presence of chest tubes, injury

Impaired **Gas** exchange r/t decreased functional lung tissue

Ineffective **Breathing** pattern r/t asymmetrical lung expansion secondary to pain

Risk for **Injury**: Risk factor: presence of invasive chest tube

Cheyne-Stokes Respiration

Ineffective **Breathing** pattern r/t critical illness

See cause of Cheyne-Stokes Respiration

CHF (Congestive Heart Failure)

Activity intolerance r/t weakness, fatigue

Constipation r/t activity intolerance

Decreased **Cardiac** output r/t impaired cardiac function

Excess **Fluid** volume r/t impaired excretion of sodium and water

Fatigue r/t disease process

Fear r/t threat to one's own well-being

Impaired **Gas** exchange r/t excessive fluid in interstitial space of lungs, alveoli

Ineffective **Health** maintenance r/t deficient knowledge regarding care of disease

Powerlessness r/t illness-related regimen

See Child with Chronic Condition; Congenital Heart Disease/ Cardiac Anomalies; Hospitalized Child

Chickenpox

See Communicable Diseases, Childhood

Child Abuse

Acute **Pain** r/t physical injuries

Chronic low **Self-esteem** r/t lack of positive feedback, excessive negative feedback

Deficient **Diversional** activity r/t diminished or absent environmental or personal stimuli

Delayed **Growth** and development: regression versus delayed r/t diminished or absent environmental stimuli, inadequate caretaking, inconsistent responsiveness by caretaker

Fear r/t threat of punishment for perceived wrongdoing

Imbalanced **Nutrition**: less than body requirements r/t inadequate caretaking

Impaired **Parenting** r/t psychological impairment, physical or emotional abuse of parent, substance abuse, unrealistic expectations of child

Impaired **Skin** integrity r/t altered nutritional state, physical abuse

Ineffective community **Therapeutic** regimen management r/t deficits in community regarding prevention of child abuse

Insomnia r/t hypervigilance, anxiety

Interrupted **Family** process: alcoholism r/t inadequate coping skills

Post-trauma syndrome r/t physical abuse, incest, rape, molestation

Risk for delayed **Development**: Risk factors: shaken baby syndrome, abuse

Risk for disproportionate **Growth**: Risk factor: abuse

Risk for **Poisoning**: Risk factors: inadequate safeguards, lack of proper safety precautions, accessibility of illicit substances because of impaired home maintenance

Risk for **Suffocation**: Risk factors: unattended child, unsafe environment

Risk for **Trauma**: Risk factors: inadequate precautions, cognitive or emotional difficulties

Social isolation: family imposed r/t fear of disclosure of family dysfunction and abuse

Child Neglect

See Child Abuse; Failure to Thrive, Nonorganic

Child with Chronic Condition

Activity intolerance r/t fatigue associated with chronic illness

Chronic low **Self-esteem** r/t actual or perceived differences; peer acceptance; decreased ability to participate in physical, school, and social activities

Chronic **Pain** r/t physical, biological, chemical, or psychological factors

Chronic **Sorrow** r/t developmental stages and missed opportunities or milestones that bring comparisons with social or personal norms, unending caregiving as reminder of loss

Compromised family **Coping** r/t prolonged overconcern for child; distortion of reality regarding child's health problem, including extreme denial about its existence or severity

Decisional **Conflict** r/t treatment options, conflicting values

Deficient **Diversional** activity r/t immobility, monotonous environment, frequent or lengthy treatments, reluctance to participate, self-imposed social isolation

Deficient **Knowledge** r/t knowledge or skill acquisition regarding health practices, acceptance of limitations, promotion of maximal potential of child, self-actualization of rest of family

Delayed **Growth** and development r/t regression or lack of progression toward developmental milestones as a result of frequent or prolonged hospitalization, inadequate or inappropriate stimulation, cerebral insult, chronic illness, effects of physical disability, prescribed dependence

Disabled family **Coping** r/t prolonged disease or disability progression that exhausts supportive capacity of significant others

Hopelessness: child r/t prolonged activity restriction, long-term stress, lack of involvement in or passively allowing care as a result of parental overprotection

Imbalanced **Nutrition**: less than body requirements r/t anorexia, fatigue from physical exertion

Imbalanced **Nutrition**: more than body requirements r/t effects of steroid medications on appetite

Impaired **Home** maintenance r/t overtaxed family members (e.g., exhausted, anxious)

Impaired **Social** interaction r/t developmental lag or delay, perceived differences

Ineffective **Coping**: child r/t situational or maturational crises

C

C

Ineffective **Health** maintenance r/t exhausting family resources (finances, physical energy, support systems)

Ineffective **Sexuality** pattern: parental r/t disrupted relationship with sexual partner

Insomnia: child or parent r/t time-intensive treatments, exacerbation of condition, 24-hour care needs

Interrupted **Family** processes r/t intermittent situational crisis of illness, disease, hospitalization

Parental role **Conflict** r/t separation from child as a result of chronic illness, home care of child with special needs, interruptions of family life resulting from home care regimen

Powerlessness: child r/t health care environment, illness-related regimen, lifestyle of learned helplessness

Readiness for enhanced family **Coping** r/t impact of crisis on family values, priorities, goals, or relationships; changes in family choices to optimize wellness

Risk for delayed **Development**: Risk factor: chronic illness

Risk for disproportionate **Growth**: Risk factor: chronic illness

Risk for impaired **Parenting**: Risk factors: impaired or disrupted bonding, caring for child with perceived overwhelming care needs

Risk for **Infection**: Risk factor: debilitating physical condition

Social isolation: family r/t actual or perceived social stigmatization, complex care requirements

Childbirth

See Labor, Normal; Postpartum, Normal Care

Chills

Hyperthermia r/t infectious process

Chlamydia Infection

See STD (Sexually Transmitted Disease)

Chloasma

Disturbed **Body** image r/t change in skin color

Choking or Coughing with Feeding

Impaired **Swallowing** r/t neuromuscular impairment

Risk for **Aspiration**: Risk factors: depressed cough and gag reflexes

Cholecystectomy

Acute **Pain** r/t trauma from surgery

Imbalanced **Nutrition**: less than body requirements r/t high metabolic needs, decreased ability to digest fatty foods

Ineffective **Health** maintenance r/t deficient knowledge regarding postoperative care

Risk for deficient **Fluid** volume: Risk factors: restricted intake, nausea, vomiting

Risk for ineffective **Breathing** pattern: Risk factor: proximity of incision to lungs, resulting in pain with deep breathing

See Abdominal Surgery

Cholelithiasis

Acute **Pain** r/t obstruction of bile flow, inflammation in gallbladder

Imbalanced **Nutrition**: less than body requirements r/t anorexia, nausea, vomiting

Ineffective **Health** maintenance r/t deficient knowledge regarding care of disease

Chorioamnionitis

Anxiety r/t threat to self and infant

Grieving r/t guilt about potential loss of ideal pregnancy and birth

Hyperthermia r/t infectious process

Risk for delayed **Growth** and development: Risk factor: risk of preterm birth

Risk for **Infection** transmission from mother to fetus: Risk factor: infection in fetal environment

Situational low **Self-esteem** r/t guilt about threat to infant's health

Chronic Confusion

See Confusion, Chronic

Chronic Lymphocytic Leukemia

See Cancer; Chemotherapy; Leukemia

Chronic Obstructive Pulmonary Disease

See COPD (Chronic Obstructive Pulmonary Disease)

Chronic Pain

See Pain, Chronic

Chronic Renal Failure

See Renal Failure

Chvostek's Sign

See Hypocalcemia

Circumcision

Acute **Pain** r/t surgical intervention

Ineffective **Health** maintenance r/t deficient knowledge (parental) regarding care of surgical area

Risk for deficient **Fluid** volume: Risk factor: hemorrhage

Risk for **Infection**: Risk factor: surgical wound

Cirrhosis

Chronic low **Self-esteem** r/t chronic illness

Chronic **Pain** r/t liver enlargement

Chronic **Sorrow** r/t presence of chronic illness

Diarrhea r/t dietary changes, medications

Disturbed **Thought** processes r/t chronic organic disorder with increased ammonia levels, substance abuse

Fatigue r/t malnutrition

Imbalanced **Nutrition**: less than body requirements r/t loss of appetite, nausea, vomiting

Ineffective **Health** maintenance r/t deficient knowledge regarding correlation between lifestyle habits and disease process

Ineffective management of **Therapeutic** regimen r/t denial of severity of illness

Ineffective **Protection** r/t risk of impaired blood coagulation, bleeding from portal hypertension

Nausea r/t irritation to gastrointestinal system

Risk for deficient **Fluid** volume: hemorrhage: Risk factor: abnormal bleeding from esophagus

Risk for impaired **Oral** mucous membranes: Risk factors: altered nutrition, inadequate oral care

Risk for impaired **Skin** integrity: Risk factors: altered nutritional state, altered metabolic state

Risk for **Injury**: Risk factors: substance intoxication, potential delirium tremens

Cleft Lip/Cleft Palate

Acute **Pain** r/t surgical correction, elbow restraints

Chronic **Sorrow** r/t birth of child with congenital defect

Fear: parental r/t special care needs, surgery

Grieving r/t loss of perfect child

Impaired **Oral** mucous membranes r/t surgical correction

Impaired physical **Mobility** r/t imposed restricted activity, use of elbow restraints

Impaired **Skin** integrity r/t incomplete joining of lip, palate ridges

Impaired verbal **Communication** r/t inadequate palate function, possible hearing loss from infected eustachian tubes

Ineffective **Airway** clearance r/t common feeding and breathing passage, postoperative laryngeal, incisional edema

Ineffective **Breastfeeding** r/t infant anomaly

Ineffective **Health** maintenance r/t lack of parental knowledge regarding feeding techniques, wound care, use of elbow restraints

Ineffective **Infant** feeding pattern r/t cleft lip, cleft palate

Risk for **Aspiration**: Risk factor: common feeding and breathing passage

Risk for deficient **Fluid** volume: Risk factor: inability to take liquids in usual manner

Risk for delayed **Development**: Risk factor: inadequate nutrition resulting from difficulty feeding

Risk for disproportionate **Growth**: Risk factor: inability to feed with normal techniques

Risk for disturbed **Body** image: Risk factors: disfigurement, speech impediment

Risk for **Infection**: Risk factors: invasive procedure, disruption of eustachian tube development, aspiration

Clotting Disorder

Fear r/t threat to well-being

Ineffective **Health** maintenance r/t deficient knowledge regarding treatment of disorder

Ineffective **Protection** r/t clotting disorder

Risk for deficient **Fluid** volume: Risk factor: uncontrolled bleeding

See Anticoagulant Therapy; DIC (Disseminated Intravascular Coagulation); Hemophilia

Cocaine Abuse

Disturbed **Thought** processes r/t excessive stimulation of nervous system by cocaine

Ineffective **Breathing** pattern r/t drug effect on respiratory center

Ineffective **Coping** r/t inability to deal with life stresses

See Drug Abuse; Substance Abuse

Cocaine Baby

See Crack Baby; Infant of Substance-Abusing Mother

Codependency

Caregiver role strain r/t codependency

Decisional **Conflict** r/t support system deficit

Ineffective **Coping** r/t inadequate support systems

Ineffective **Denial** r/t unmet self-needs

Impaired verbal **Communication** r/t psychological barriers

Powerlessness r/t lifestyle of helplessness

Cognitive Deficit

Disturbed **Thought** processes r/t neurological impairment

Cold, Viral

Readiness for enhanced **Comfort**: verbalizes desire to enhance comfort (See **Comfort**, readiness for enhanced in Section III)

Ineffective **Health** maintenance r/t deficient knowledge regarding care of viral condition, prevention of further infections

Colectomy

Acute **Pain** r/t recent surgery

Constipation r/t decreased activity, decreased fluid intake

Imbalanced **Nutrition**: less than body requirements r/t high metabolic needs, decreased ability to ingest or digest food

Ineffective **Health** maintenance r/t deficient knowledge regarding procedure, postoperative care

Risk for **Infection**: Risk factor: invasive procedure

See Abdominal Surgery

Colitis

Acute **Pain** r/t inflammation in colon

Deficient **Fluid** volume r/t frequent stools

Diarrhea r/t inflammation in colon

See Crohn's Disease; Inflammatory Bowel Disease

Collagen Disease

See specific disease (e.g., Lupus Erythematosus; JRA [Juvenile Rheumatoid Arthritis]); Congenital Heart Disease/Cardiac Anomalies

Colostomy

Disturbed **Body** image r/t presence of stoma, daily care of fecal material

Ineffective **Health** maintenance r/t deficient knowledge regarding care of stoma, integrating colostomy care into lifestyle

Ineffective **Sexuality** pattern r/t altered body image, self-concept

Risk for **Constipation**: Risk factor: inappropriate diet

Risk for **Diarrhea**: Risk factor: inappropriate diet

Risk for impaired **Skin** integrity: Risk factor: irritation from bowel contents

Risk for **Social** isolation: Risk factor: anxiety about appearance of stoma and possible leakage

Colporrhaphy, Anterior

See Vaginal Hysterectomy

Coma

Death **Anxiety**: significant others r/t unknown outcome of coma state

Disturbed **Thought** processes r/t neurological changes

Ineffective family **Therapeutic** regimen management r/t complexity of therapeutic regimen

Interrupted **Family** processes r/t illness or disability of family member

Risk for **Aspiration**: Risk factors: impaired swallowing, loss of cough or gag reflex

Risk for **Disuse** syndrome: Risk factor: altered level of consciousness impairing mobility

Risk for impaired **Oral** mucous membranes: Risk factor: dry mouth

Risk for impaired **Skin** integrity: Risk factor: immobility

Risk for **Injury**: Risk factor: potential seizure activity

Risk for **Spiritual** distress: significant others: Risk factors: loss of ability to relate to loved one, unknown outcome of coma

Self-care deficit: specify r/t neuromuscular impairment

Total urinary **Incontinence** r/t neurological dysfunction

See cause of Coma

Comfort, Loss of

Readiness for enhanced **Comfort** (See **Comfort**, readiness for enhanced, Section III)

Pruritus r/t dry skin, inflammation of skin

Communicable Diseases, Childhood (e.g., Measles, Mumps, Rubella, Chickenpox, Scabies, Lice, Impetigo)

Acute **Pain** r/t impaired skin integrity, edema

Deficient **Diversional** activity r/t imposed isolation from peers, disruption in usual play activities, fatigue, activity intolerance

Ineffective **Health** maintenance r/t nonadherence to appropriate immunization schedules, lack of prevention of transmission of infection

Pruritus r/t inflammation or infection of skin, subdermal organisms

Risk for **Infection**: transmission to others: Risk factor: contagious organisms

See Meningitis/Encephalitis; Respiratory Infections, Acute Childhood; Reye's Syndrome

Communication

Readiness for enhanced **Communication** (See **Communication**, readiness for enhanced, Section III)

Communication Problems

Impaired verbal **Communication** (See **Communication**, impaired verbal, Section III)

Community Coping

Ineffective community **Coping** (See **Coping**, ineffective community, Section III)

Readiness for enhanced community **Coping** r/t community sense of power to manage stressors, social supports available, resources available for problem solving

Community Management of Therapeutic Regimen

Ineffective community **Therapeutic** regimen management r/t inadequate community resources

Compartment Syndrome

Acute **Pain** r/t pressure in compromised body part

Fear r/t possible loss of limb, damage to limb

Ineffective **Tissue** perfusion: peripheral r/t increased pressure within compartment

Compulsion

See Obsessive-Compulsive Disorder

Conduction Disorders (Cardiac)

See Dysrhythmia

Confusion, Acute

Acute **Confusion** r/t older than 70 years of age with hospitalization, alcohol abuse, delirium, dementia, drug abuse

Adult **Failure** to thrive r/t confusion

Confusion, Chronic

Adult **Failure** to thrive r/t confusion

Chronic **Confusion** r/t Alzheimer's disease, Korsakoff's psychosis, multiinfarct dementia, cerebrovascular accident, head injury

Disturbed **Thought** processes r/t organic mental disorder, disruption of cerebral arterial blood flow, chemical imbalance, intoxication

Impaired **Memory** r/t fluid and electrolyte imbalance, neurological disturbances, excessive environmental disturbances, anemia, acute or chronic hypoxia, decreased cardiac output

Confusion, Possible

Risk for acute **Confusion** (See **Confusion**, acute, risk for, Section III)

Congenital Heart Disease/Cardiac Anomalies

ACYANOTIC

Patent ductus arteriosus, atrial/ventricular septal defect, pulmonary stenosis, endocardial cushion defect, aortic valvular stenosis, coarctation of aorta

CYANOTIC

Tetralogy of Fallot, tricuspid atresia, transposition of great vessels, truncus arteriosus, total anomalous pulmonary venous return, hypoplastic left lung

Activity intolerance r/t fatigue, generalized weakness, lack of adequate oxygenation

Decreased **Cardiac** output r/t cardiac dysfunction

Delayed **Growth** and development r/t inadequate oxygen and nutrients to tissues

Excess **Fluid** volume r/t cardiac defect, side effects of medication

Imbalanced **Nutrition**: less than body requirements r/t fatigue, generalized weakness, inability of infant to suck and feed, increased caloric requirements

Impaired **Gas** exchange r/t cardiac defect, pulmonary congestion

Ineffective **Breathing** pattern r/t pulmonary vascular disease

Risk for deficient **Fluid** volume: Risk factor: side effects of diuretics

Risk for delayed **Development**: Risk factor: inadequate oxygen and nutrients to tissues

Risk for disorganized **Infant** behavior: Risk factor: invasive procedures

Risk for disproportionate **Growth**: Risk factor: inadequate oxygen and nutrients to tissues

Risk for ineffective **Thermoregulation**: Risk factor: neonatal age

Risk for **Poisoning**: Risk factor: potential toxicity of cardiac medications

See Child with Chronic Condition; Hospitalized Child

Congestive Heart Failure

See CHF (Congestive Heart Failure)

Conjunctivitis

Acute **Pain** r/t inflammatory process

Disturbed **Sensory** perception r/t change in visual acuity resulting from inflammation

Consciousness, Altered Level of

Acute **Confusion** r/t alcohol abuse, delirium, dementia, drug abuse

Adult **Failure** to thrive r/t altered level of consciousness

Chronic **Confusion** r/t multiinfarct dementia, Korsakoff's psychosis, head injury, Alzheimer's disease, cerebrovascular accident

Decreased **Intracranial** adaptive capacity r/t brain injury

Disturbed **Thought** processes r/t neurological changes

Impaired **Memory** r/t neurological disturbances

Ineffective **Tissue** perfusion: cerebral r/t increased intracranial pressure, decreased cerebral perfusion

Risk for **Aspiration**: Risk factors: impaired swallowing, loss of cough or gag reflex

Risk for **Disuse** syndrome: Risk factors: impaired mobility resulting from altered level of consciousness

Risk for impaired **Oral** mucous membranes: Risk factor: dry mouth

Risk for impaired **Skin** integrity: Risk factor: immobility

Self-care deficit: specify r/t neuromuscular impairment

Total urinary **Incontinence** r/t neurological dysfunction

See cause of Altered Level of Consciousness

Constipation

Constipation (See **Constipation**, Section III)

Constipation, Perceived

Perceived **Constipation** (See **Constipation**, perceived, Section III)

Constipation, Risk for

Risk for **Constipation** (See **Constipation**, risk for, Section III)

Contamination

Contamination (See **Contamination**, Section III)

Risk for **Contamination** (See **Contamination**, risk for, Section III)

Continent Ileostomy (Kock Pouch)

Imbalanced **Nutrition**: less than body requirements r/t malabsorption

Ineffective **Coping** r/t stress of disease, exacerbations caused by stress

Ineffective **Health** maintenance r/t deficient knowledge regarding postoperative care

Risk for **Injury**: Risk factors: failure of valve, stomal cyanosis, intestinal obstruction

See Abdominal Surgery

Contraceptive Method

Decisional **Conflict**: method of contraception r/t unclear personal values or beliefs, lack of experience or interference with decision making, lack of relevant information, support system deficit

Health-seeking behaviors r/t requesting information about available and appropriate birth control methods

Ineffective **Sexuality** pattern r/t fear of pregnancy

Conversion Disorder

Anxiety r/t unresolved conflict

Disturbed personal **Identity** r/t overwhelming stress

Hopelessness r/t long-term stress

Risk-prone health **Behavior** r/t multiple stressors

Impaired physical **Mobility** r/t physical conversion symptom

Impaired **Social** interaction r/t altered thought process

Ineffective **Coping** r/t personal vulnerability

Ineffective **Role** performance r/t physical conversion system

Powerlessness r/t lifestyle of helplessness

Risk for **Injury**: Risk factors: physical conversion symptom

Self-esteem disturbance r/t unsatisfactory or inadequate interpersonal relationships

C

Convulsions

Anxiety r/t concern over controlling convulsions

Impaired **Memory** r/t neurological disturbance

Ineffective **Health** maintenance r/t deficient knowledge regarding need for medication and care during seizure activity

Risk for **Aspiration**: Risk factor: impaired swallowing

Risk for delayed **Development**: Risk factor: seizures

Risk for **Injury**: Risk factor: seizure activity

See Seizure Disorders, Adult; Seizure Disorders, Childhood

COPD (Chronic Obstructive Pulmonary Disease)

Activity intolerance r/t imbalance between oxygen supply and demand

Interrupted **Family** processes r/t role changes

Anxiety r/t breathlessness, change in health status

Chronic low **Self-esteem** r/t chronic illness

Chronic **Sorrow** r/t presence of chronic illness

Death **Anxiety** r/t seriousness of medical condition, difficulty being able to "catch breath," feeling of suffocation

Health-seeking behaviors r/t wishes to stop smoking

Imbalanced **Nutrition**: less than body requirements r/t decreased intake because of dyspnea, unpleasant taste in mouth left by medications

Impaired **Gas** exchange r/t ventilation-perfusion inequality

Impaired **Social** interaction r/t social isolation because of oxygen use, activity intolerance

Ineffective **Airway** clearance r/t bronchoconstriction, increased mucus, ineffective cough, infection

Ineffective **Health** maintenance r/t deficient knowledge regarding care of disease

Noncompliance r/t reluctance to accept responsibility for changing detrimental health practices

Powerlessness r/t progressive nature of disease

Risk for **Infection**: Risk factor: stasis of respiratory secretions

Self-care deficit: specify: r/t fatigue from the increased work of breathing

Sleep deprivation r/t breathing difficulties when lying down

Coping

Readiness for enhanced **Coping** (See **Coping**, readiness for enhanced, Section III)

Coping Problems

Defensive **Coping** (See **Coping**, defensive, Section III)

Ineffective **Coping** (See **Coping**, ineffective, Section III)

See Community Coping; Family Problems

Corneal Reflex, Absent

Risk for **Injury**: Risk factors: accidental corneal abrasion, drying of cornea

Corneal Transplant

Risk for **Infection**: Risk factors: invasive procedure, surgery

Readiness for enhanced **Therapeutic** regimen management: describes need to rest and avoid strenuous activities during healing phase

Coronary Artery Bypass Grafting

Acute **Pain** r/t traumatic surgery

Decreased **Cardiac** output r/t dysrhythmia, depressed cardiac function, increased systemic vascular resistance

Deficient **Fluid** volume r/t intraoperative fluid loss, use of diuretics in surgery

Fear r/t outcome of surgical procedure

Ineffective **Health** maintenance r/t deficient knowledge regarding postprocedure care, lifestyle adjustment after surgery

Risk for perioperative positioning **Injury**: Risk factors: hypothermia, extended supine position

Costovertebral Angle Tenderness

See Kidney Stone; Pyelonephritis

Cough, Effective/Ineffective

Ineffective **Airway** clearance r/t decreased energy, fatigue, normal aging changes

See Bronchitis; COPD (Chronic Obstructive Pulmonary Disease); Pulmonary Edema

Crack Abuse

See Cocaine Abuse; Drug Abuse; Substance Abuse

Crack Baby

Disorganized **Infant** behavior r/t prematurity, pain, lack of attachment

Risk for impaired parent/child **Attachment**: Risk factors: parent's inability to meet infant's needs, substance abuse

See Infant of Substance-Abusing Mother

Crackles in Lungs, Coarse

Ineffective **Airway** clearance r/t excessive secretions in airways, ineffective cough

See cause of Coarse Crackles

Crackles in Lungs, Fine

Ineffective **Breathing** pattern r/t fatigue, surgery, decreased energy

See Bronchitis or Pneumonia (if from pulmonary infection); CHF (Congestive Heart Failure) (if cardiac in origin); Infection

Craniectomy/Craniotomy

Acute **Pain** r/t recent surgery, headache

Adult **Failure** to thrive r/t altered cerebral tissue perfusion

Decreased **Intracranial** adaptive capacity r/t brain injury, intracranial hypertension

Fear r/t threat to well-being

Impaired **Memory** r/t neurological surgery

Ineffective **Tissue** perfusion: cerebral r/t cerebral edema, decreased cerebral perfusion, increased intracranial pressure

Risk for disturbed **Thought** processes: Risk factor: neurophysiological changes

Risk for **Injury**: Risk factor: potential confusion

See Coma (if relevant)

Crepitation, Subcutaneous

See Pneumothorax

Crisis

Anxiety r/t threat to or change in environment, health status, interaction patterns, situation, self-concept, or role functioning; threat of death of self or significant other

Compromised family **Coping** r/t situational or developmental crisis

Death **Anxiety** r/t feelings of hopelessness associated with crisis

Disturbed **Energy** field r/t disharmony caused by crisis

Fear r/t crisis situation

Grieving r/t potential significant loss

Ineffective **Coping** r/t situational or maturational crisis

Risk for **Spiritual** distress: Risk factors: physical or psychological stress, natural disasters, situational losses, maturational losses

Situational low **Self-esteem** r/t perception of inability to handle crisis

Spiritual distress r/t intense suffering

Crohn's Disease

Acute **Pain** r/t increased peristalsis

Anxiety r/t change in health status

Diarrhea r/t inflammatory process

Imbalanced **Nutrition**: less than body requirements r/t diarrhea, altered ability to digest and absorb food

Ineffective **Coping** r/t repeated episodes of diarrhea

Ineffective **Health** maintenance r/t deficient knowledge regarding management of disease

Powerlessness r/t chronic disease

Risk for deficient **Fluid** volume: Risk factor: abnormal fluid loss with diarrhea

Croup

See Respiratory Infections, Acute Childhood

Cryosurgery for Retinal Detachment

See Retinal Detachment

Cushing's Syndrome

Activity intolerance r/t fatigue, weakness

Disturbed **Body** image r/t change in appearance from disease process

Excess **Fluid** volume r/t failure of regulatory mechanisms

Ineffective **Health** maintenance r/t deficient knowledge regarding needed care

Risk for **Infection**: Risk factors: suppression of immune system caused by increased cortisol levels

Risk for **Injury**: Risk factors: decreased muscle strength, osteoporosis

Sexual dysfunction r/t loss of libido

CVA (Cerebrovascular Accident)

Adult **Failure** to thrive r/t neurophysiological changes

Anxiety r/t situational crisis, change in physical or emotional condition

Caregiver role strain r/t cognitive problems of care receiver, need for significant home care

Chronic **Confusion** r/t neurological changes

Constipation r/t decreased activity

Disturbed **Body** image r/t chronic illness, paralysis

Disturbed **Sensory** perception: visual, tactile, kinesthetic r/t neurological deficit

Disturbed **Thought** processes r/t neurophysiological changes

Grieving r/t loss of health

Impaired **Home** maintenance r/t neurological disease affecting ability to perform activities of daily living

Impaired **Memory** r/t neurological disturbances

Impaired physical **Mobility** r/t loss of balance and coordination

Impaired **Social** interaction r/t limited physical mobility, limited ability to communicate

Impaired **Swallowing** r/t neuromuscular dysfunction

Impaired **Transfer** ability r/t limited physical mobility

Impaired verbal **Communication** r/t pressure damage, decreased circulation to brain in speech center informational sources

Impaired **Walking** r/t loss of balance and coordination

Ineffective **Coping** r/t disability

Ineffective **Health** maintenance r/t deficient knowledge regarding self-care after CVA

Interrupted **Family** process r/t illness, disability of family member

Reflex **Incontinence** r/t loss of feeling to void

Risk for **Aspiration**: Risk factors: impaired swallowing, loss of gag reflex

Risk for **Disuse** syndrome: Risk factor: paralysis

Risk for impaired **Skin** integrity: Risk factor: immobility

Risk for **Injury**: Risk factor: disturbed sensory perception

Self-care deficit: specify r/t decreased strength and endurance, paralysis

Total urinary **Incontinence** r/t neurological dysfunction

Unilateral **Neglect** r/t disturbed perception from neurological damage

Cyanosis, Central with Cyanosis of Oral Mucous Membranes

Impaired **Gas** exchange r/t alveolar-capillary membrane changes

Cyanosis, Peripheral with Cyanosis of Nail Beds

Ineffective **Tissue** perfusion r/t interruption of arterial flow, severe vasoconstriction, cold temperatures

Risk for **Peripheral** neurovascular dysfunction: Risk factor: condition causing disruption in circulation

Cystic Fibrosis

Activity intolerance r/t imbalance between oxygen supply and demand

Anxiety r/t dyspnea, oxygen deprivation

Chronic **Sorrow** r/t presence of chronic disease

Disturbed **Body** image r/t changes in physical appearance, treatment of chronic lung disease (clubbing, barrel chest, home oxygen therapy)

Imbalanced **Nutrition**: less than body requirements r/t anorexia; decreased absorption of nutrients, fat; increased work of breathing

Impaired **Gas** exchange r/t ventilation-perfusion imbalance

Impaired **Home** maintenance r/t extensive daily treatment, medications necessary for health, mist or oxygen tents

Ineffective **Airway** clearance r/t increased production of thick mucus

Risk for **Caregiver** role strain: Risk factors: illness severity of care receiver, unpredictable course of illness

Risk for deficient **Fluid** volume: Risk factors: decreased fluid intake, increased work of breathing

Risk for **Infection**: Risk factors: thick, tenacious mucus; harboring of bacterial organisms; immunocompromised state

Risk for **Spiritual** distress: Risk factor: presence of chronic disease

See Child with Chronic Condition; Hospitalized Child; Terminally Ill Child, Adolescent; Terminally Ill Child, Infant/Toddler; Terminally Ill Child, Preschool Child; Terminally Ill Child, School-Age Child/Preadolescent; Terminally Ill Child/Death of Child, Parent

Cystitis

Acute **Pain**: dysuria r/t inflammatory process in bladder

Impaired **Urinary** elimination: frequency r/t urinary tract infection

Ineffective **Health** maintenance r/t deficient knowledge regarding methods to treat and prevent urinary tract infections

Risk for urge urinary **Incontinence**: Risk factor: infection in bladder

Cystocele

Ineffective **Health** maintenance r/t deficient knowledge regarding personal care, Kegel exercises to strengthen perineal muscles

Stress urinary **Incontinence** r/t prolapsed bladder

Urge urinary **Incontinence** r/t prolapsed bladder

Cystoscopy

Ineffective **Health** maintenance r/t deficient knowledge regarding postoperative care

Risk for **Infection**: Risk factor: invasive procedure

Urinary retention r/t edema in urethra obstructing flow of urine

Deafness

Disturbed **Sensory** perception: auditory r/t alteration in sensory reception, transmission, integration

Impaired verbal **Communication** r/t impaired hearing

Risk for delayed **Development** r/t impaired hearing

Risk for **Injury** r/t alteration in sensory perception

Death

Risk for sudden infant **Death** syndrome (SIDS) (See **Death** syndrome, sudden infant, risk for, Section III)

Death, Oncoming

Grieving r/t loss of significant other

Compromised family **Coping** r/t client's inability to provide support to family

Death **Anxiety** r/t unresolved issues surrounding dying

Fear r/t threat of death

Ineffective **Coping** r/t personal vulnerability

Powerlessness r/t effects of illness, oncoming death

Readiness for enhanced **Spiritual** well-being: desire of client and family to be in harmony with each other and higher power, God

Social isolation r/t altered state of wellness

Spiritual distress r/t intense suffering

See Terminally Ill Child, Adolescent; Terminally Ill Child, Infant/Toddler; Terminally Ill Child, Preschool Child; Terminally Ill Child, School-Age Child/Preadolescent; Terminally Ill Child/Death of Child, Parent

Decisions, Difficulty Making

Decisional **Conflict** r/t support system deficit, perceived threat to value system, multiple or divergent sources of information, lack of relevant information, unclear personal values or beliefs

Readiness for enhanced **Decision** making (See **Decision** making, readiness for enhanced, Section III)

Decubitus Ulcer

See Pressure Ulcer

Deep Vein Thrombosis

See DVT (Deep Vein Thrombosis)

Defensive Behavior

Defensive **Coping** r/t nonacceptance of blame, denial of problems or weakness

Ineffective **Denial** r/t inability to face situation realistically

Dehiscence, Abdominal

Acute **Pain** r/t stretching of abdominal wall

Delayed **Surgical** recovery r/t altered circulation, malnutrition, opening in incision

Fear r/t threat of death, severe dysfunction

Impaired **Skin** integrity r/t altered circulation, malnutrition, opening in incision

Impaired **Tissue** integrity r/t exposure of abdominal contents to external environment

Risk for imbalanced **Fluid** volume: Risk factor: altered circulation associated with opening of wound and exposure of abdominal contents

Risk for **Infection**: Risk factor: loss of skin integrity

Dehydration

Deficient **Fluid** volume r/t active fluid volume loss

Impaired **Oral** mucous membranes r/t decreased salivation, fluid deficit

Ineffective **Health** maintenance r/t deficient knowledge regarding treatment and prevention of dehydration

See cause of Dehydration

Delirium

Acute **Confusion** r/t effects of medication, response to hospitalization, alcohol abuse, substance abuse, sensory deprivation or overload

Adult **Failure** to thrive r/t delirium

Disturbed **Thought** processes r/t head trauma, altered metabolic state, substance abuse, sleep deprivation, sensory deprivation or overload

Impaired **Memory** r/t delirium

Risk for **Injury**: Risk factor: altered level of consciousness

Sleep deprivation r/t nightmares

Delirium Tremens (DT)

See Alcohol Withdrawal

Delivery

See Labor, Normal

Delusions

Acute **Confusion** r/t alcohol abuse, delirium, dementia, drug abuse

Adult **Failure** to thrive r/t delusional state

Anxiety r/t content of intrusive thoughts

Disturbed **Thought** processes r/t mental disorder

Impaired verbal **Communication** r/t psychological impairment, delusional thinking

Ineffective **Coping** r/t distortion and insecurity of life events

Risk for other-directed **Violence**: Risk factor: delusional thinking

Risk for self-directed **Violence**: Risk factor: delusional thinking

Dementia

Adult **Failure** to thrive r/t depression, apathy

Chronic **Confusion** r/t neurological dysfunction

Chronic **Sorrow** r/t chronic mental illness

Imbalanced **Nutrition**: less than body requirements r/t psychological impairment

Impaired **Environmental** interpretation syndrome r/t dementia

Impaired **Home** maintenance r/t inadequate support system

Impaired physical **Mobility** r/t neuromuscular impairment

Insomnia r/t neurological impairment, naps during the day

Interrupted **Family** process r/t disability of family member

Risk for **Caregiver** role strain: Risk factors: number of caregiving tasks, duration of caregiving required

Risk for **Falls**: Risk factor: diminished mental status

Risk for impaired **Skin** integrity: Risk factors: altered nutritional status, immobility

Risk for **Injury**: Risk factors: confusion, decreased muscle coordination

Self-care deficit: specify r/t psychological or neuromuscular impairment

Total urinary **Incontinence** r/t neuromuscular impairment

Denial of Health Status

Ineffective **Denial** r/t lack of perception about health status effects of illness

Ineffective management of **Therapeutic** regimen r/t denial of seriousness of health situation

Dental Caries

Impaired **Dentition** r/t ineffective oral hygiene, barriers to self-care, economic barriers to professional care, nutritional deficits, dietary habits

Ineffective **Health** maintenance r/t lack of knowledge regarding prevention of dental disease

Dentition Problems

See Dental Caries

Depression (Major Depressive Disorder)

Adult **Failure** to thrive r/t depression

Chronic low **Self-esteem** r/t repeated unmet expectations

Chronic **Sorrow** r/t unresolved grief

Constipation r/t inactivity, decreased fluid intake

Death **Anxiety** r/t feelings of lack of self-worth

Disturbed **Energy** field r/t disharmony

Insomnia r/t inactivity

Risk for complicated **Grieving**: Risk factor: lack of previous resolution of former grieving response

Fatigue r/t psychological demands

Hopelessness r/t feeling of abandonment, long-term stress

Impaired **Environmental** interpretation syndrome r/t severe mental functional impairment

Ineffective **Coping** r/t grieving

Ineffective **Health** maintenance r/t lack of ability to make good judgments regarding ways to obtain help

D

D

Powerlessness r/t pattern of helplessness

Risk for **Suicide**: Risk factor: panic state

Self-care deficit: specify r/t depression, cognitive impairment

Sexual dysfunction r/t loss of sexual desire

Social isolation r/t ineffective coping

Dermatitis

Anxiety r/t situational crisis imposed by illness

Impaired **Skin** integrity r/t side effect of medication, allergic reaction

Ineffective **Health** maintenance r/t deficient knowledge regarding methods to decrease inflammation

Pruritus r/t inflammation of skin

See Itching

Despondency

Hopelessness r/t long-term stress

See Depression

Destructive Behavior Toward Others

Risk-prone health **Behavior** r/t intense emotional state

Ineffective **Coping** r/t situational crises, maturational crises, personal vulnerability

Risk for other-directed **Violence** (See **Violence**, other-directed, risk for, Section III)

Developmental Concerns

Delayed **Growth** and development (See **Growth** and development, delayed, Section III)

INDIVIDUAL/ENVIRONMENTAL/CAREGIVER

Risk for delayed **Development** (See **Development**, delayed, risk for, Section III)

See Growth and Development Lag

Diabetes in Pregnancy

See Gestational Diabetes (Diabetes in Pregnancy)

Diabetes Insipidus

Deficient **Fluid** volume r/t inability to conserve fluid

Ineffective **Health** maintenance r/t deficient knowledge regarding care of disease, importance of medications

Diabetes Mellitus

Adult **Failure** to thrive r/t undetected disease process

Disturbed **Sensory** perception r/t ineffective tissue perfusion

Imbalanced **Nutrition**: less than body requirements r/t inability to use glucose (type 1 [insulin-dependent] diabetes)

Imbalanced **Nutrition**: more than body requirements r/t excessive intake of nutrients (type 2 diabetes)

Ineffective **Health** maintenance r/t deficient knowledge regarding care of diabetic condition

Ineffective management of **Therapeutic** regimen r/t complexity of therapeutic regimen

Ineffective **Tissue** perfusion: peripheral r/t impaired arterial circulation

Noncompliance r/t restrictive lifestyle; changes in diet, medication, exercise

Powerlessness r/t perceived lack of personal control

Risk for disturbed **Thought** processes: Risk factors: hypoglycemia, hyperglycemia

Risk for impaired **Skin** integrity: Risk factor: loss of pain perception in extremities

Risk for **Infection**: Risk factors: hyperglycemia, impaired healing, circulatory changes

Risk for **Injury**: Risk factors: hypoglycemia or hyperglycemia from failure to consume adequate calories, failure to take insulin

Risk for unstable blood **Glucose** (See **Glucose**, unstable blood, risk for, Section III)

Sexual dysfunction r/t neuropathy associated with disease

Diabetes Mellitus, Juvenile (IDDM Type 1)

Acute **Pain** r/t insulin injections, peripheral blood glucose testing

Disturbed **Body** image r/t imposed deviations from biophysical and psychosocial norm, perceived differences from peers

Imbalanced **Nutrition**: less than body requirements r/t inability of body to adequately metabolize and use glucose and nutrients, increased caloric needs of child to promote growth and physical activity participation with peers

Impaired **Adjustment** r/t inability to participate in normal childhood activities

Ineffective **Health** maintenance r/t parental/child deficient knowledge regarding dietary management, medication administration, physical activity, and interaction between the three; daily changes in diet, medications, illness, stress, activity associated with child's growth spurts and needs; need to instruct other caregivers and teachers regarding signs and symptoms of hypoglycemia or hyperglycemia and treatment

Noncompliance r/t disturbed body image, impaired adjustment attributable to adolescent maturational crises

See Diabetes Mellitus; Child with Chronic Condition; Hospitalized Child

Diabetic Coma

Deficient **Fluid** volume r/t hyperglycemia resulting in polyuria

Disturbed **Thought** processes r/t hyperglycemia, presence of excessive metabolic acids

Ineffective management of **Therapeutic** regimen r/t lack of understanding of preventive measures, adequate blood sugar control

Risk for **Infection**: Risk factors: hyperglycemia, changes in vascular system

Risk for unstable blood **Glucose** (See **Glucose**, unstable blood, risk for, Section III)

See Diabetes Mellitus

Diabetic Ketoacidosis

See Ketoacidosis, Diabetic

Diabetic Retinopathy

Disturbed **Sensory** perception r/t change in sensory reception

Grieving r/t loss of vision

Ineffective **Health** maintenance r/t deficient knowledge regarding preserving vision with treatment if possible, use of low-vision aids

See Vision Impairment

Dialysis

See Hemodialysis; Peritoneal Dialysis

Diaphragmatic Hernia

See Hiatal Hernia

Diarrhea

Diarrhea r/t infection, change in diet, gastrointestinal disorders, stress, medication effect, impaction

DIC (Disseminated Intravascular Coagulation)

Deficient **Fluid** volume: hemorrhage r/t depletion of clotting factors

Fear r/t threat to well-being

Ineffective **Protection** r/t abnormal clotting mechanism

Risk for ineffective **Tissue** perfusion: peripheral: Risk factors: hypovolemia from profuse bleeding, formation of microemboli in vascular system

Digitalis Toxicity

Decreased **Cardiac** output r/t drug toxicity affecting cardiac rhythm, rate

Ineffective management of **Therapeutic** regimen r/t deficient knowledge regarding action, appropriate method of administration of digitalis

Dignity, Loss of

Risk for compromised human **Dignity** (See **Dignity**, compromised human, risk for, Section III)

Dilation and Curettage (D&C)

Acute **Pain** r/t uterine contractions

Ineffective **Health** maintenance r/t deficient knowledge regarding postoperative self-care

Risk for deficient **Fluid** volume: hemorrhage: Risk factor: excessive blood loss during or after procedure

Risk for ineffective **Sexuality** pattern: Risk factors: painful coitus, fear associated with surgery on genital area

Risk for **Infection**: Risk factor: surgical procedure

Discharge Planning

Deficient **Knowledge**: Risk factor: lack of exposure to information for home care

Impaired **Home** maintenance r/t family member's disease or injury interfering with home maintenance

Ineffective **Health** maintenance r/t lack of material sources

Discomforts of Pregnancy

Acute **Pain**: headache r/t hormonal changes of pregnancy

Acute **Pain**: leg cramps r/t nerve compression, calcium/phosphorus/potassium imbalance

Constipation r/t decreased gastrointestinal tract motility, pressure from enlarged uterus, supplementary iron

Disturbed **Body** image r/t pregnancy-induced body changes

Fatigue r/t hormonal, metabolic, body changes

Insomnia r/t psychological stress, fetal movement, muscular cramping, urinary frequency, shortness of breath

Nausea r/t hormone effect

Readiness for enhanced **Comfort**: Headache: hormonal changes of pregnancy

Risk for **Constipation**: Risk factors: decreased intestinal motility, inadequate fiber in diet

Risk for **Injury**: Risk factors: faintness and/or syncope caused by vasomotor lability or postural hypotension, venous stasis in lower extremities

Risk for urge urinary **Incontinence**: Risk factors: hormone effect, pressure on bladder from growing uterus

Stress urinary **Incontinence**: Risk factors: enlarged uterus, fetal movement

Dislocation

Acute **Pain** r/t dislocation of a joint

Risk for **Injury**: Risk factor: unstable joint

Self-care deficit: specify r/t inability to use a joint

Dissecting Aneurysm

Fear r/t threat to well-being

See Abdominal Surgery; Aneurysm, Abdominal Surgery

Disseminated Intravascular Coagulation

See DIC (Disseminated Intravascular Coagulation)

Dissociative Identity Disorder (Not Otherwise Specified)

Anxiety r/t psychosocial stress

Disturbed personal **Identity** r/t inability to distinguish self caused by multiple personality disorder, depersonalization, disturbance in memory

Disturbed **Sensory** perception: kinesthetic r/t underdeveloped ego

Disturbed **Thought** processes r/t repressed anxiety

Impaired **Memory** r/t altered state of consciousness

Ineffective **Coping** r/t personal vulnerability in crisis of accurate self-perception

See Multiple Personality Disorder (Dissociative Identity Disorder)

Distress

Anxiety r/t situational crises, maturational crises

Death **Anxiety** r/t denial of one's own mortality or impending death

Disturbed **Energy** field r/t disruption in flow of energy as result of pain, depression, fatigue, anxiety, stress

D

Disuse Syndrome, Potential to Develop

Risk for **Disuse** syndrome: Risk factors: paralysis, mechanical immobilization, prescribed immobilization, severe pain, altered level of consciousness

Diversional Activity, Lack of

Deficient **Diversional** activity r/t environmental lack of diversional activity as in frequent hospitalizations, lengthy treatments

Diverticulitis

Acute **Pain** r/t inflammation of bowel

Constipation r/t dietary deficiency of fiber and roughage

Deficient **Knowledge** r/t diet needed to control disease, medication regimen

Diarrhea r/t increased intestinal motility caused by inflammation

Imbalanced **Nutrition**: less than body requirements r/t loss of appetite

Risk for deficient **Fluid** volume: Risk factor: diarrhea

Dizziness

Decreased **Cardiac** output r/t dysfunctional electrical conduction

Impaired physical **Mobility** r/t dizziness

Ineffective **Tissue** perfusion: cerebral r/t interruption of cerebral arterial blood flow

Risk for **Falls**: Risk factor: difficulty maintaining balance

Domestic Violence

Anxiety r/t threat to self-concept, situational crisis of abuse

Caregiver role strain r/t chronic illness, self-care deficits, lack of respite care, extent of caregiving required

Compromised family **Coping** r/t abusive patterns

Defensive **Coping** r/t low self-esteem

Impaired verbal **Communication** r/t psychological barriers of fear

Insomnia r/t psychological stress

Interrupted **Family** processes: alcoholism r/t inadequate coping skills

Post-trauma syndrome r/t history of abuse

Powerlessness r/t lifestyle of helplessness

Risk for **Post-trauma** syndrome r/t inadequate social support

Risk for self-directed **Violence** r/t history of abuse

Self-esteem disturbance r/t negative family interactions

Down Syndrome

See Child with Chronic Condition; Mental Retardation

Dress Self (Inability to)

Dressing or grooming **Self-care** deficit r/t intolerance to activity, decreased strength and endurance, pain, discomfort, perceptual or cognitive impairment, neuromuscular impairment, musculoskeletal impairment, depression, severe anxiety

Dribbling of Urine

Overflow urinary **Incontinence** r/t degenerative changes in pelvic muscles and urinary structures

Stress urinary **Incontinence** r/t degenerative changes in pelvic muscles and urinary structures

Drooling

Impaired **Swallowing** r/t neuromuscular impairment, mechanical obstruction

Risk for **Aspiration** r/t impaired swallowing

Drug Abuse

Anxiety r/t threat to self-concept, lack of control of drug use

Disturbed **Sensory** perception: specify r/t substance intoxication

Disturbed **Thought** processes r/t mind-altering effects of drugs

Imbalanced **Nutrition**: less than body requirements r/t poor eating habits

Impaired **Social** interaction r/t disturbed thought processes from drug abuse

Ineffective **Coping** r/t situational crisis

Insomnia r/t effects of medications

Noncompliance r/t denial of illness

Powerlessness r/t feeling unable to change patterns of abuse

Risk for **Injury**: Risk factors: hallucinations, drug effects

Risk for **Violence**: Risk factor: poor impulse control

Risk-prone health **Behavior**: r/t failure to change destructive behavior

Sexual dysfunction r/t actions and side effects of drug abuse

Sleep deprivation r/t prolonged psychological discomfort

Spiritual distress r/t separation from religious, cultural ties

See Cocaine Abuse; Substance Abuse

Drug Withdrawal

Acute **Confusion** r/t effects of substance withdrawal

Anxiety r/t physiological withdrawal

Disturbed **Sensory** perception: specify r/t substance intoxication

Imbalanced **Nutrition**: less than body requirements r/t poor eating habits

Ineffective **Coping** r/t situational crisis, withdrawal

Insomnia r/t effects of medications

Noncompliance r/t denial of illness

Risk for **Injury**: Risk factor: hallucinations

Risk for **Violence**: Risk factor: poor impulse control

See Drug Abuse

Dry Eye

See Conjunctivitis; Keratoconjunctivitis Sicca

DT (Delirium Tremens)

See Alcohol Withdrawal

DVT (Deep Vein Thrombosis)

Acute **Pain** r/t vascular inflammation, edema

Constipation r/t inactivity, bedrest

Delayed **Surgical** recovery r/t impaired physical mobility

Impaired physical **Mobility** r/t pain in extremity, forced bed rest

Ineffective **Health** maintenance r/t deficient knowledge regarding self-care needs, treatment regimen, outcome

Ineffective **Tissue** perfusion: peripheral r/t interruption of venous blood flow

See Anticoagulant Therapy

Dying Client

See Terminally Ill Adult, Terminally Ill Adolescent; Terminally Ill Child, Infant/Toddler; Terminally Ill Child, Preschool Child; Terminally Ill Child, School-Age Child/Preadolescent; Terminally Ill Child/Death of Child, Parent

Dysfunctional Eating Pattern

Imbalanced **Nutrition**: less than body requirements r/t psychological factors

Risk for imbalanced **Nutrition**: more than body requirements: Risk factor: observed use of food as reward or comfort measure

See Anorexia Nervosa; Bulimia; Maturational Issues, Adolescent

Dysfunctional Family Unit

See Family Problems

Dysfunctional Ventilatory Weaning

Dysfunctional **Ventilatory** weaning response r/t physical, psychological, situational factors

Dysmenorrhea

Ineffective **Health** maintenance r/t deficient knowledge regarding prevention and treatment of painful menstruation

Nausea r/t prostaglandin effect

Acute **Pain** r/t cramping from hormonal effects

Dyspareunia

Sexual dysfunction r/t lack of lubrication during intercourse, alteration in reproductive organ function

Dyspepsia

Acute **Pain** r/t gastrointestinal disease, consumption of irritating foods

Anxiety r/t pressures of personal role

Ineffective **Health** maintenance r/t deficient knowledge regarding treatment of disease

Dysphagia

Impaired **Swallowing** r/t neuromuscular impairment

Risk for **Aspiration**: Risk factor: loss of gag or cough reflex

Dysphasia

Impaired **Social** interaction r/t difficulty in communicating

Impaired verbal **Communication** r/t decrease in circulation to brain

Dyspnea

Activity intolerance r/t imbalance between oxygen supply and demand

Anxiety r/t ineffective breathing pattern

Fear r/t threat to state of well-being, potential death

Impaired **Gas** exchange r/t alveolar-capillary damage

Ineffective **Breathing** pattern r/t compromised cardiac or pulmonary function, decreased lung expansion, neurological impairment affecting respiratory center, extreme anxiety

Insomnia r/t difficulty breathing, positioning required for effective breathing

Sleep deprivation r/t ineffective breathing pattern

Dysrhythmia

Activity intolerance r/t decreased cardiac output

Anxiety/Fear r/t threat of death, change in health status

Decreased **Cardiac** output r/t altered electrical conduction

Ineffective **Health** maintenance r/t deficient knowledge regarding self-care with disease

Ineffective **Tissue** perfusion: cerebral r/t interruption of cerebral arterial flow as a result of decreased cardiac output

Dysthymic Disorder

Chronic low **Self-esteem** r/t repeated unmet expectations

Ineffective **Coping** r/t impaired social interaction

Ineffective **Health** maintenance r/t inability to make good judgments regarding ways to obtain help

Ineffective **Sexuality** pattern r/t loss of sexual desire

Insomnia r/t anxious thoughts

Social isolation r/t ineffective coping

See Depression (Major Depressive Disorder)

Dystocia

Acute **Pain** r/t difficult labor, medical interventions

Anxiety r/t difficult labor, deficient knowledge regarding normal labor pattern

Fatigue r/t prolonged labor

Grieving r/t loss of ideal labor experience

Ineffective **Coping** r/t situational crisis

Powerlessness r/t perceived inability to control outcome of labor

Risk for deficient **Fluid** volume: Risk factor: hemorrhage secondary to uterine atony

Risk for delayed **Development**: Risk factor: difficult labor and birth

Risk for disproportionate **Growth**: Risk factor: difficult labor and birth

Risk for impaired **Tissue** integrity: maternal and fetal: Risk factor: difficult labor

Risk for ineffective **Tissue** perfusion: cerebral (fetal): Risk factor: difficult labor and birth

Risk for **Infection**: Risk factor: prolonged rupture of membranes

D

Risk for **Post-trauma** syndrome: Risk factor: sudden emergency during delivery of infant

Situational low **Self-esteem** r/t perceived inability to have normal labor and delivery

Dysuria

Impaired **Urinary** elimination r/t urinary tract infection

Risk for urge urinary **Incontinence**: Risk factors: detrusor hyperreflexia from cystitis, urethritis

E

E. Coli Infection

Deficient **Knowledge** r/t how to prevent disease; care of self with serious illness

Fear r/t serious illness, unknown outcome

See Gastroenteritis; Gastroenteritis, Child; Hospitalized Child

Ear Surgery

Acute **Pain** r/t edema in ears from surgery

Disturbed **Sensory** perception: hearing r/t invasive surgery of ears, dressings

Ineffective **Health** maintenance r/t deficient knowledge regarding postoperative restrictions, expectations, care

Risk for delayed **Development**: Risk factor: hearing impairment

Risk for **Falls**: Risk factor: dizziness from excessive stimuli to vestibular apparatus

See Hospitalized Child

Earache

Acute **Pain** r/t trauma, edema, infection

Disturbed **Sensory** perception: auditory r/t altered sensory reception, transmission, integration

Eclampsia

Fear r/t threat of well-being to self and fetus

Interrupted **Family** processes r/t unmet expectations for pregnancy and childbirth

Risk for **Aspiration**: Risk factor: seizure activity

Risk for delayed **Development**: Risk factor: uteroplacental insufficiency

Risk for disproportionate **Growth**: Risk factor: uteroplacental insufficiency

Risk for excess **Fluid** volume: Risk factor: decreased urine output as a result of renal dysfunction

Risk for imbalanced **Fluid** volume: Risk factors: retained fluid, decreased renal activity

Risk for ineffective **Tissue** perfusion: fetal: Risk factor: uteroplacental insufficiency

Risk for **Injury**: maternal: Risk factor: seizure activity

ECT (Electroconvulsive Therapy)

Decisional **Conflict** r/t lack of relevant information

Fear r/t real or imagined threat to well-being

Impaired **Memory** r/t effects of treatment

See Depression (Major Depressive Disorder)

Ectopic Pregnancy

Acute **Pain** r/t stretching or rupture of implantation site

Chronic **Sorrow** r/t loss of pregnancy, potential loss of fertility

Death Anxiety r/t emergency condition, hemorrhage

Deficient **Fluid** volume r/t loss of blood

Disturbed **Body** image r/t negative feelings about body and reproductive functioning

Fear r/t threat to self, surgery, implications for future pregnancy

Ineffective **Role** performance r/t loss of pregnancy

Risk for ineffective **Coping**: Risk factor: loss of pregnancy

Risk for **Infection**: Risk factor: traumatized tissue, blood loss

Risk for interrupted **Family** processes: Risk factor: situational crisis

Risk for **Spiritual** distress: Risk factor: grief process

Situational low **Self-esteem** r/t loss of pregnancy, inability to carry pregnancy to term

Eczema

Acute **Pain**: pruritus r/t inflammation of skin

Disturbed **Body** image r/t change in appearance from inflamed skin

Impaired **Skin** integrity r/t side effect of medication, allergic reaction

Ineffective **Health** maintenance r/t deficient knowledge regarding how to decrease inflammation and prevent further outbreaks

ED (Erectile Dysfunction)

See Erectile Dysfunction (ED); Impotence

Edema

Excess **Fluid** volume r/t excessive fluid intake, cardiac dysfunction, renal dysfunction, loss of plasma proteins

Ineffective **Health** maintenance r/t deficient knowledge regarding treatment of edema

Risk for impaired **Skin** integrity: Risk factors: impaired circulation, fragility of skin

See cause of Edema

Elder Abuse

See Abuse, Spouse, Parent, or Significant Other

Elderly

See Aging

Electroconvulsive Therapy

See ECT (Electroconvulsive Therapy)

Emaciated Person

Adult **Failure** to thrive r/t imbalanced nutrition: less than body requirements

Imbalanced **Nutrition**: less than body requirements r/t inability to ingest food, digest food, absorb nutrients because of biological, psychological, economic factors

Embolectomy

Fear r/t threat of great bodily harm from embolus

Ineffective **Tissue** perfusion: specify r/t presence of embolus

Risk for deficient **Fluid** volume: hemorrhage: Risk factors: postoperative complication, surgical area

See Surgery, Postoperative Care

Emboli

See Pulmonary Embolism

Emesis

Nausea (See **Nausea**, Section III)

See Vomiting

Emotional Problems

See Coping Problems

Empathy

Health-seeking behaviors r/t desire to attain maximal level of health

Readiness for enhanced community **Coping** r/t social supports, being available for problem solving

Readiness for enhanced family **Coping** r/t basic needs met, desire to move to higher level of health

Readiness for enhanced **Spiritual** well-being: desire to establish interconnectedness through spirituality

Emphysema

See COPD (Chronic Obstructive Pulmonary Disease)

Emptiness

Chronic **Sorrow** r/t unresolved grief

Social isolation r/t inability to engage in satisfying personal relationships

Spiritual distress r/t separation from religious or cultural ties

Encephalitis

See Meningitis/Encephalitis

Endocardial Cushion Defect

See Congenital Heart Disease/Cardiac Anomalies

Endocarditis

Activity intolerance r/t reduced cardiac reserve, prescribed bedrest

Acute **Pain** r/t biological injury, inflammation

Decreased **Cardiac** output r/t inflammation of lining of heart and change in structure of valve leaflets, increased myocardial workload

Ineffective **Health** maintenance r/t deficient knowledge regarding treatment of disease, preventive measures against further incidence of disease

Ineffective **Tissue** perfusion: cardiopulmonary, peripheral r/t high risk for development of emboli

Risk for imbalanced **Nutrition**: less than body requirements: Risk factors: fever, hypermetabolic state associated with fever

Endometriosis

Acute **Pain** r/t onset of menses with distention of endometrial tissue

Grieving r/t possible infertility

Ineffective **Health** maintenance r/t deficient knowledge about disease condition, medications, other treatments

Nausea r/t prostaglandin effect

Sexual dysfunction r/t painful coitus

Endometritis

Acute **Pain** r/t infectious process in reproductive tract

Anxiety r/t prolonged hospitalization, fear of unknown

Hyperthermia r/t infectious process

Ineffective **Health** maintenance r/t deficient knowledge regarding condition, treatment, antibiotic regimen

Enuresis

Ineffective **Health** maintenance r/t unachieved developmental task, neuromuscular immaturity, diseases of urinary system

See Toilet Training

Environmental Interpretation Problems

Adult **Failure** to thrive r/t impaired environmental interpretation syndrome

Chronic **Confusion** r/t impaired environmental interpretation syndrome

Disturbed **Thought** processes r/t lack of orientation to person, place, time, circumstances

Impaired **Environmental** interpretation syndrome r/t dementia, Parkinson's disease, Huntington's disease, depression, alcoholism

Impaired **Memory** r/t environmental disturbances

Risk for **Injury**: Risk factor: lack of orientation to person, place, time, circumstances

Epididymitis

Acute **Pain** r/t inflammation in scrotal sac

Anxiety r/t situational crisis, pain, threat to future fertility

Ineffective **Health** maintenance r/t deficient knowledge regarding treatment for pain and infection

Ineffective **Sexuality** pattern r/t edema of epididymis and testes

Epiglottitis

See Respiratory Infections, Acute Childhood (Croup, Epiglottis, Pertussis, Pneumonia, Respiratory Syncytial Virus)

E

F

Epilepsy

Anxiety r/t threat to role functioning

Impaired **Memory** r/t seizure activity

Ineffective **Health** maintenance r/t deficient knowledge regarding seizures and seizure control

Ineffective **Therapeutic** regimen management r/t deficient knowledge regarding seizure control

Risk for **Aspiration**: Risk factors: impaired swallowing, excessive secretions

Risk for delayed **Development**: Risk factor: seizure disorder

Risk for disturbed **Thought** processes: Risk factor: excessive, uncontrolled neurological stimuli

Risk for **Injury**: Risk factor: environmental factors during seizure

See Seizure Disorders, Adult; Seizure Disorders, Childhood

Episiotomy

Acute **Pain** r/t tissue trauma

Anxiety r/t fear of pain

Disturbed **Body** image r/t fear of resuming sexual relations

Impaired physical **Mobility** r/t pain, swelling, tissue trauma

Impaired **Skin** integrity r/t perineal incision

Risk for **Infection**: Risk factor: tissue trauma

Sexual dysfunction r/t altered body structure, tissue trauma

Epistaxis

Fear r/t large amount of blood loss

Risk for deficient **Fluid** volume: Risk factor: excessive fluid loss

Epstein-Barr Virus

See Mononucleosis

Erectile Dysfunction (ED)

Readiness for enhanced **Knowledge** of treatment information for erectile dysfunction

Self-esteem disturbance r/t physiological crisis, inability to practice usual sexual activity

Sexual dysfunction r/t altered body function

See Impotence

Esophageal Varices

Deficient **Fluid** volume: hemorrhage r/t portal hypertension, distended variceal vessels that can easily rupture

Fear r/t threat of death

See Cirrhosis

Esophagitis

Acute **Pain** r/t inflammation of esophagus

Ineffective **Health** maintenance r/t deficient knowledge regarding treatment of disease

ETOH Withdrawal

See Alcohol Withdrawal

Evisceration

See Dehiscence, Abdominal

Exposure to Hot or Cold Environment

Risk for imbalanced **Body** temperature: Risk factor: exposure

External Fixation

Disturbed **Body** image r/t trauma, change to affected part

Risk for **Infection**: Risk factor: pressure of pins on skin surface

See Fracture

Eye Surgery

Anxiety r/t possible loss of vision

Disturbed **Sensory** perception: visual r/t surgical procedure

Ineffective **Health** maintenance r/t deficient knowledge regarding postoperative activity, medications, eye care

Risk for **Injury**: Risk factor: impaired vision

Self-care deficit r/t impaired vision

See Hospitalized Child; Vision Impairment

F

Failure to Thrive, Adult

Adult **Failure** to thrive r/t depression, apathy, fatigue

Failure to Thrive, Nonorganic

Chronic low **Self-esteem**: parental r/t feelings of inadequacy, support system deficiencies, inadequate role model

Delayed **Growth** and development r/t parental deficient knowledge, lack of stimulation, nutritional deficit, long-term hospitalization

Disorganized **Infant** behavior r/t lack of boundaries

Imbalanced **Nutrition**: less than body requirements r/t inadequate type or amounts of food for infant, inappropriate feeding techniques

Impaired **Parenting** r/t lack of parenting skills, inadequate role modeling

Insomnia r/t inconsistency of caretaker; lack of quiet, consistent environment

Risk for delayed **Development**: Risk factor: failure to thrive

Risk for disproportionate **Growth**: Risk factor: failure to thrive

Risk for impaired parent/child **Attachment**: Risk factor: inability of parents to meet infant's needs

Social isolation r/t limited support systems, self-imposed situation

Falls, Risk for

Risk for **Falls** (See **Falls**, risk for, Section III)

Family Problems

Compromised family **Coping** (See **Coping**, compromised family, Section III)

Disabled family **Coping** (See **Coping**, disabled family, Section III)

Ineffective family **Therapeutic** regimen management r/t complexity of health care system, complexity of therapeutic regimen, decisional conflicts, economic difficulties, excessive demands made on individual or family, family conflict

Interrupted **Family** processes r/t situation transition and/or crises, developmental transition and/or crises

Readiness for enhanced family **Coping** r/t needs sufficiently gratified, adaptive tasks effectively addressed to enable goals of self-actualization to surface

Family Process

Readiness for enhanced **Family** processes (See **Family** processes, readiness for enhanced, Section III)

Fatigue

Disturbed **Energy** field r/t disharmony

Fatigue (See **Fatigue**, Section III)

Fear

Death Anxiety r/t fear of death

Fear r/t identifiable physical or psychological threat to person

Febrile Seizures

See Seizure Disorders, Childhood

Fecal Impaction

See Impaction of Stool

Fecal Incontinence

Bowel incontinence r/t neurological impairment, gastrointestinal disorders, anorectal trauma

Feeding Problems, Newborn

Disorganized **Infant** behavior r/t prematurity, immature neurological system

Impaired **Swallowing** r/t prematurity

Ineffective **Breastfeeding** r/t prematurity, infant anomaly, maternal breast anomaly, previous breast surgery, previous history of breastfeeding failure, infant receiving supplemental feedings with artificial nipple, poor infant sucking reflex, nonsupportive partner and family, deficient knowledge, maternal anxiety or ambivalence

Ineffective **Infant** feeding pattern r/t prematurity, neurological impairment or delay, oral hypersensitivity, prolonged nothing-by-mouth status

Interrupted **Breastfeeding** r/t maternal or infant illness, prematurity, maternal employment, contraindications to breastfeeding, need to abruptly wean infant

Risk for delayed **Development**: Risk factor: inadequate nutrition

Risk for disproportionate **Growth**: Risk factor: feeding problems

Risk for imbalanced **Fluid** volume: Risk factor: inability to take in adequate amount of fluids

Femoral Popliteal Bypass

Acute **Pain** r/t surgical trauma, edema in surgical area

Anxiety r/t threat to or change in health status

Ineffective **Tissue** perfusion: peripheral r/t impaired arterial circulation

Risk for deficient **Fluid** volume: hemorrhage: Risk factor: abnormal blood loss

Risk for **Infection**: Risk factor: invasive procedure

Risk for **Peripheral** neurovascular dysfunction: Risk factor: vascular surgery, emboli

Fetal Alcohol Syndrome

See Infant of Substance-Abusing Mother

Fetal Distress/Nonreassuring Fetal Heart Rate Pattern

Fear r/t threat to fetus

Ineffective **Tissue** perfusion: fetal r/t interruption of umbilical cord blood flow

Ineffective **Tissue** perfusion: placental r/t small or old placenta, interference with gas exchange transplacentally

Fever

Hyperthermia r/t infectious process, damage to hypothalamus, exposure to hot environment, medications, anesthesia, inability or decreased ability to perspire

Fibrocystic Breast Disease

See Breast Lumps

Filthy Home Environment

Impaired **Home** maintenance (See **Home** maintenance, impaired, Section III)

Financial Crisis in the Home Environment

Impaired **Home** maintenance r/t insufficient finances

Fistulectomy

See Hemorrhoidectomy (same nursing care)

Flail Chest

Anxiety r/t difficulty breathing

Impaired spontaneous **Ventilation** r/t paradoxical respirations

Ineffective **Breathing** pattern r/t chest trauma

Flashbacks

Post-trauma syndrome r/t catastrophic event

Flat Affect

Adult **Failure** to thrive r/t apathy

Hopelessness r/t prolonged activity restriction creating isolation, failing or deteriorating physiological condition, long-term stress, abandonment, lost belief in transcendent values or higher power or God

Risk for **Loneliness**: Risk factors: social isolation, lack of interest in surroundings

See Depression (Major Depressive Disorder); Dysthymic Disorder

Flesh-Eating Bacteria

See Necrotizing Fasciitis

Fluid Balance

Readiness for enhanced **Fluid** balance (See **Fluid** balance, readiness for enhanced, Section III)

Fluid Volume Deficit

Deficient **Fluid** volume r/t active fluid loss, failure of regulatory mechanisms

Fluid Volume Excess

Excess **Fluid** volume r/t compromised regulatory mechanism, excess sodium intake

Fluid Volume Imbalance, Risk for

Risk for imbalanced **Fluid** volume: Risk factor: major invasive surgeries

Foodborne Illness

Deficient **Fluid** volume r/t active fluid loss

Deficient **Knowledge** r/t care of self with serious illness, prevention of further incidences of foodborne illness

Diarrhea r/t infectious material in gastrointestinal tract

Nausea r/t contamination irritating stomach

See Gastroenteritis; Gastroenteritis, Child; Hospitalized Child; E. coli Infection

Foreign Body Aspiration

Impaired **Home** maintenance r/t inability to maintain orderly and clean surroundings

Ineffective **Airway** clearance r/t obstruction of airway

Ineffective **Health** maintenance r/t parental deficient knowledge regarding high-risk items

Risk for **Suffocation**: Risk factor: inhalation of small object

See Safety, Childhood

Formula Feeding

Grieving: maternal r/t loss of desired breastfeeding experience

Ineffective **Health** maintenance r/t maternal deficient knowledge regarding formula feeding

Risk for **Constipation**: infant: Risk factor: iron-fortified formula

Risk for **Infection**: infant: Risk factors: lack of passive maternal immunity, supine feeding position

Fracture

Acute **Pain** r/t muscle spasm, edema, trauma

Deficient **Diversional** activity r/t immobility

Impaired physical **Mobility** r/t limb immobilization

Impaired **Walking** r/t limb immobility

Ineffective **Health** maintenance r/t deficient knowledge regarding care of fracture

Risk for impaired **Skin** integrity: Risk factors: immobility, presence of cast

Risk for ineffective **Tissue** perfusion: Risk factors: immobility, presence of cast

Risk for **Peripheral** neurovascular dysfunction: Risk factors: mechanical compression, treatment of fracture

Fractured Hip

See Hip Fracture

Frequency of Urination

Impaired **Urinary** elimination r/t anatomical obstruction, sensory-motor impairment, urinary tract infection

Stress urinary **Incontinence** r/t degenerative change in pelvic muscles and structural support

Urge urinary **Incontinence** r/t decreased bladder capacity, irritation of bladder stretch receptors causing spasm, alcohol, caffeine, increased fluids, increased urine concentration, overdistended bladder

Urinary retention r/t high urethral pressure caused by weak detrusor, inhibition of reflex arc, strong sphincter, blockage

Frostbite

Acute **Pain** r/t decreased circulation from prolonged exposure to cold

Impaired **Skin** integrity r/t freezing of skin

Impaired **Tissue** integrity r/t freezing of skin

Ineffective **Tissue** perfusion r/t damage to extremities from prolonged exposure to cold

See Hypothermia

Frothy Sputum

See CHF (Congestive Heart Failure); Pulmonary Edema; Seizure Disorders, Adult; Seizure Disorders, Childhood

Fusion, Lumbar

Acute **Pain** r/t discomfort at bone donor site, surgical operation

Anxiety r/t fear of surgical procedure, possible recurring problems

Impaired physical **Mobility** r/t limitations from surgical procedure, presence of brace

Ineffective **Health** maintenance r/t deficient knowledge regarding postoperative mobility restrictions, body mechanics

Risk for **Injury**: Risk factor: improper body mechanics

Risk for perioperative positioning **Injury**: Risk factor: immobilization

G

Gag Reflex, Depressed or Absent

Impaired **Swallowing** r/t neuromuscular impairment

Risk for **Aspiration**: Risk factors: depressed cough or gag reflex

Gallop Rhythm

Decreased **Cardiac** output r/t decreased contractility of heart

Gallstones

See Cholelithiasis

Gangrene

Delayed **Surgical** recovery r/t obstruction of arterial flow

Fear r/t possible loss of extremity

Ineffective **Tissue** perfusion: peripheral r/t obstruction of arterial flow

Gas Exchange, Impaired

Impaired **Gas** exchange r/t ventilation-perfusion imbalance

Gastric Surgery

Risk for **Injury**: Risk factor: inadvertent insertion of nasogastric tube through gastric incision line

See Abdominal Surgery

Gastric Ulcer

See GI Bleed (Gastrointestinal Bleeding); Ulcer, Peptic

Gastritis

Acute **Pain** r/t inflammation of gastric mucosa

Imbalanced **Nutrition**: less than body requirements r/t vomiting, inadequate intestinal absorption of nutrients, restricted dietary regimen

Risk for deficient **Fluid** volume: Risk factors: excessive loss from gastrointestinal tract as a result of vomiting, decreased intake

Gastroenteritis

Acute **Pain** r/t increased peristalsis causing cramping

Deficient **Fluid** volume r/t excessive loss from gastrointestinal tract from diarrhea, vomiting

Diarrhea r/t infectious process involving intestinal tract

Imbalanced **Nutrition**: less than body requirements r/t vomiting, inadequate intestinal absorption of nutrients, restricted dietary intake

Ineffective **Health** maintenance r/t deficient knowledge regarding treatment of disease

Nausea r/t irritation to gastrointestinal system

See Gastroenteritis, Child

Gastroenteritis, Child

Impaired **Skin** integrity: diaper rash r/t acidic excretions on perineal tissues

Ineffective **Health** maintenance r/t lack of parental knowledge regarding fluid and dietary changes

See Gastroenteritis; Hospitalized Child

Gastroesophageal Reflux: Child

Acute **Pain** r/t irritation of esophagus from gastric acids

Anxiety: parental r/t possible need for surgical intervention (Nissen fundoplication, gastrostomy tube)

Deficient **Fluid** volume r/t persistent vomiting

Imbalanced **Nutrition**: less than body requirements r/t poor feeding, vomiting

Ineffective **Airway** clearance r/t reflux of gastric contents into esophagus and tracheal or bronchial tree

Ineffective **Health** maintenance r/t deficient knowledge regarding antireflux regimen (e.g., positioning, oral or enteral feeding techniques, medications), possible home apnea monitoring

Risk for **Aspiration**: Risk factor: entry of gastric contents in tracheal or bronchial tree

Risk for impaired **Parenting**: Risk factors: disruption in bonding as a result of irritable or inconsolable infant

See Child with Chronic Condition; Hospitalized Child

Gastrointestinal Hemorrhage

See GI Bleed (Gastrointestinal Bleeding)

Gastroschisis/Omphalocele

Grieving r/t threatened loss of infant, loss of perfect birth or infant because of serious medical condition

Impaired **Gas** exchange r/t effects of anesthesia, subsequent atelectasis

Ineffective **Airway** clearance r/t complications of anesthetic effects

Risk for deficient **Fluid** volume: Risk factors: inability to feed because of condition, subsequent electrolyte imbalance

Risk for **Infection**: Risk factor: disrupted skin integrity with exposure of abdominal contents

Risk for **Injury**: Risk factors: disrupted skin integrity, ineffective protection

Gastrostomy

Risk for impaired **Skin** integrity: Risk factor: presence of gastric contents on skin

See Tube Feeding

Genital Herpes

See Herpes Simplex II

Genital Warts

See STD (Sexually Transmitted Disease)

Gestational Diabetes (Diabetes in Pregnancy)

Anxiety r/t threat to self and/or fetus

Impaired fetal **Nutrition**: more than body requirements r/t excessive glucose uptake

Impaired **Nutrition**: less than body requirements r/t decreased insulin production and glucose uptake in cells

Ineffective **Health** maintenance: maternal r/t deficient knowledge regarding care of diabetic condition in pregnancy

Powerlessness r/t lack of control over outcome of pregnancy

Risk for delayed **Development**: fetal: Risk factor: endocrine disorder of mother

Risk for disproportionate **Growth**: fetal: Risk factor: endocrine disorder of mother

Risk for impaired **Tissue** integrity: fetal: Risk factors: macrosomia, congenital defects, birth injury

Risk for impaired **Tissue** integrity: maternal: Risk factor: delivery of large infant

See Diabetes Mellitus

GI Bleed (Gastrointestinal Bleeding)

Acute **Pain** r/t irritated mucosa from acid secretion

Deficient **Fluid** volume r/t gastrointestinal bleeding

Fatigue r/t loss of circulating blood volume, decreased ability to transport oxygen

H

Fear r/t threat to well-being, potential death

Imbalanced **Nutrition**: less than body requirements r/t nausea, vomiting

Risk for ineffective **Coping**: Risk factors: personal vulnerability in crisis, bleeding, hospitalization

Gingivitis

Impaired **Dentition** r/t ineffective oral hygiene, barriers to self-care

Impaired **Oral** mucous membrane r/t ineffective oral hygiene

Glaucoma

Deficient **Knowledge** r/t treatment and self-care for disease

Disturbed **Sensory** perception: visual r/t increased intraocular pressure

See Vision Impairment

Glomerulonephritis

Acute **Pain** r/t edema of kidney

Excess **Fluid** volume r/t renal impairment

Imbalanced **Nutrition**: less than body requirements r/t anorexia, restrictive diet

Ineffective **Health** maintenance r/t deficient knowledge regarding care of disease

Gonorrhea

Acute **Pain** r/t inflammation of reproductive organs

Ineffective **Health** maintenance r/t deficient knowledge regarding treatment and prevention of disease

Risk for **Infection**: Risk factor: spread of organism throughout reproductive organs

See STD (Sexually Transmitted Disease)

Gout

Chronic **Pain** r/t inflammation of affected joint

Impaired physical **Mobility** r/t musculoskeletal impairment

Ineffective **Health** maintenance r/t deficient knowledge regarding medications and home care

Grand Mal Seizure

See Seizure Disorders, Adult; Seizure Disorders, Childhood

Grandiosity

Defensive **Coping** r/t inaccurate perception of self and abilities

Grandparents Raising Grandchildren

Anxiety r/t change in role status

Compromised family **Coping** r/t family role changes

Decisional **Conflict** r/t support system deficit

Ineffective family **Therapeutic** regimen management r/t excessive demands on individual or family

Ineffective **Role** performance r/t role transition

Interrupted **Family** processes r/t family roles shift

Parental role **Conflict** r/t change in parental role

Readiness for enhanced **Parenting**: physical and emotional needs of children are met

Risk for impaired **Parenting**: Risk factor: role strain

Risk for **Powerlessness**: Risk factors: role strain, situational crisis, aging

Risk for **Spiritual** distress: Risk factor: life change

Graves' Disease

See Hyperthyroidism

Grieving

Grieving r/t anticipated or actual significant loss, change in life status, style, or function

Grieving, Complicated

Complicated **Grieving** r/t expected or sudden death of a significant other, emotional instability, lack of social support

Risk for complicated **Grieving**: Risk factors: death of a significant other, emotional instability, lack of social support

Groom Self (Inability to)

Dressing/grooming **Self-care** deficit (See **Self-care** deficit, dressing/grooming, Section III)

Growth and Development Lag

Delayed **Growth** and development (See **Growth** and development, delayed, Section III)

PRENATAL/INDIVIDUAL/ENVIRONMENTAL

Risk for disproportionate **Growth** (See disproportionate **Growth**, risk for, Section III)

See Developmental Concerns

Guillain-Barré Syndrome

Impaired spontaneous **Ventilation** r/t weak respiratory muscles

See Neurological Disorders

Guilt

Chronic **Sorrow** r/t unresolved grieving

Grieving r/t potential loss of significant person, animal, prized material possession

Risk for complicated **Grief**: Risk factors: actual loss of significant person, animal, prized material possession

Readiness for enhanced **Spiritual** well-being: desire to be in harmony with self, others, higher power or God

Risk for **Post-trauma** syndrome: Risk factor: exaggerated sense of responsibility for traumatic event

Self-esteem disturbance r/t unmet expectations of self

H

Hair Loss

Disturbed **Body** image r/t psychological reaction to loss of hair

Imbalanced **Nutrition**: less than body requirements r/t inability to ingest food because of biological, psychological, economic factors

Halitosis

Impaired **Dentition** r/t ineffective oral hygiene

Impaired **Oral** mucous membranes r/t ineffective oral hygiene

Hallucinations

Acute **Confusion** r/t alcohol abuse, delirium, dementia, mental illness, drug abuse

Adult **Failure** to thrive r/t altered mental status

Anxiety r/t threat to self-concept

Disturbed **Thought** processes r/t inability to control bizarre thoughts

Ineffective **Coping** r/t distortion and insecurity of life events

Risk for other-directed **Violence**: Risk factors: catatonic excitement, manic excitement, rage or panic reactions, response to violent internal stimuli

Risk for self-directed **Violence**: Risk factors: catatonic excitement, manic excitement, rage or panic reactions, response to violent internal stimuli

Risk for **Self-mutilation**: Risk factor: command hallucinations

Head Injury

Acute **Confusion** r/t brain injury

Decreased **Intracranial** adaptive capacity r/t brain injury

Disturbed **Sensory** perception r/t pressure damage to sensory centers in brain

Disturbed **Thought** processes r/t pressure damage to brain

Ineffective **Breathing** pattern r/t pressure damage to breathing center in brainstem

Ineffective **Tissue** perfusion: cerebral r/t effects of increased intracranial pressure

See Neurological Disorders

Headache

Acute **Pain** r/t lack of knowledge of pain control techniques or methods to prevent headaches

Disturbed **Energy** field r/t disharmony

Ineffective management of **Therapeutic** regimen r/t lack of knowledge, identification, elimination of aggravating factors

Health Maintenance Problems

Ineffective **Health** maintenance (See **Health** maintenance, ineffective, Section III)

Health-Seeking Person

Health-seeking behaviors r/t expressed desire for increased control of own personal health

Hearing Impairment

Disturbed **Sensory** perception: auditory r/t altered state of auditory system

Impaired verbal **Communication** r/t inability to hear own voice

Social isolation r/t difficulty with communication

Heart Failure

See CHF (Congestive Heart Failure)

Heart Surgery

See Coronary Artery Bypass Grafting

Heartburn

Acute **Pain**: heartburn r/t gastroesophageal reflux

Ineffective **Health** maintenance r/t deficient knowledge regarding information about factors that cause esophageal reflex

Nausea r/t gastrointestinal irritation

Risk for imbalanced **Nutrition**: less than body requirements: Risk factor: pain after eating

Heat Stroke

Deficient **Fluid** volume r/t profuse diaphoresis

Disturbed **Thought** processes r/t hyperthermia, increased oxygen needs

Hyperthermia r/t vigorous activity, hot environment

Hematemesis

See GI Bleed (Gastrointestinal Bleeding)

Hematological Disorder

Ineffective **Protection** r/t abnormal blood profile

See cause of Hematological Disorder

Hematuria

See UTI (Urinary Tract Infection); Kidney Stone

Hemianopia

Anxiety r/t change in vision

Disturbed **Sensory** perception r/t altered sensory reception, transmission, integration

Risk for **Injury**: Risk factor: disturbed sensory perception

Unilateral **Neglect** r/t effects of disturbed perceptual abilities

Hemiplegia

Anxiety r/t change in health status

Disturbed **Body** image r/t functional loss of one side of body

Impaired physical **Mobility** r/t loss of neurological control of involved extremities

Impaired **Transfer** ability r/t partial paralysis

Impaired **Walking** r/t loss of neurological control of involved extremities

Risk for impaired **Skin** integrity: Risk factors: alteration in sensation, immobility

Risk for **Injury**: Risk factor: impaired mobility

Self-care deficit: specify: r/t neuromuscular impairment

Unilateral **Neglect** r/t effects of disturbed perceptual abilities

See CVA (Cerebrovascular Accident)

Hemodialysis

Excess **Fluid** volume r/t renal disease with minimal urine output

Ineffective **Coping** r/t situational crisis

Ineffective **Health** maintenance r/t deficient knowledge regarding hemodialysis procedure, restrictions, blood access care

Interrupted **Family** processes r/t changes in role responsibilities as a result of therapy regimen

Noncompliance: dietary restrictions r/t denial of chronic illness

Powerlessness r/t treatment regimen

Risk for **Caregiver** role strain: Risk factor: complexity of care receiver treatment

Risk for deficient **Fluid** volume: Risk factor: excessive removal of fluid during dialysis

Risk for **Infection**: Risk factors: exposure to blood products, risk for developing hepatitis B or C

Risk for **Injury**: clotting of blood access: Risk factor: abnormal surface for blood flow

See Renal Failure; Renal Failure, Acute/Chronic, Child

Hemodynamic Monitoring

Risk for **Infection**: Risk factor: invasive procedure

Risk for **Injury**: Risk factors: inadvertent wedging of catheter, dislodgement of catheter, disconnection of catheter with embolism

Hemolytic Uremic Syndrome

Deficient **Fluid** volume r/t vomiting, diarrhea

Nausea r/t effects of uremia

Risk for impaired **Skin** integrity: Risk factor: diarrhea

Risk for **Injury**: Risk factors: decreased platelet count, seizure activity

See Hospitalized Child; Renal Failure, Acute/Chronic, Child

Hemophilia

Acute **Pain** r/t bleeding into body tissues

Fear r/t high risk for AIDS infection from contaminated blood products

Impaired physical **Mobility** r/t pain from acute bleeds, imposed activity restrictions

Ineffective **Health** maintenance r/t knowledge and skill acquisition regarding home administration of intravenous clotting factors, protection from injury

Ineffective **Protection** r/t deficient clotting factors

Risk for **Injury**: Risk factors: deficient clotting factors, child's developmental level, age-appropriate play, inappropriate use of toys or sports equipment

See Child with Chronic Condition; Hospitalized Child; Maturational Issues, Adolescent

Hemoptysis

Fear r/t serious threat to well-being

Risk for deficient **Fluid** volume: Risk factor: excessive loss of blood

Risk for ineffective **Airway** clearance: Risk factor: obstruction of airway with blood and mucus

Hemorrhage

Deficient **Fluid** volume r/t massive blood loss

Fear r/t threat to well-being

See cause of Hemorrhage; Hypovolemic Shock

Hemorrhoidectomy

Acute **Pain** r/t surgical procedure

Anxiety r/t embarrassment, need for privacy

Constipation r/t fear of pain with defecation

Ineffective **Health** maintenance r/t deficient knowledge regarding pain relief, use of stool softeners, dietary changes

Risk for deficient **Fluid** volume: hemorrhage: Risk factor: inadequate clotting

Urinary retention r/t pain, anesthetic effect

Hemorrhoids

Constipation r/t painful defecation, poor bowel habits

Ineffective **Health** maintenance r/t deficient knowledge regarding care of condition

Pruritus r/t inflammation of skin and tissues with hemorrhoids

Hemothorax

Deficient **Fluid** volume r/t blood in pleural space

See Pneumothorax

Hepatitis

Activity intolerance r/t weakness or fatigue caused by infection

Acute **Pain** r/t edema of liver, bile irritating skin

Deficient **Diversional** activity r/t isolation

Fatigue r/t infectious process, altered body chemistry

Imbalanced **Nutrition**: less than body requirements r/t anorexia, impaired use of proteins and carbohydrates

Ineffective **Health** maintenance r/t deficient knowledge regarding disease process and home management

Risk for deficient **Fluid** volume: Risk factor: excessive loss of fluids from vomiting and diarrhea

Social isolation r/t treatment-imposed isolation

Hernia

See Hiatal Hernia; Inguinal Hernia Repair

Herniated Disk

See Low Back Pain

Herniorrhaphy

See Inguinal Hernia Repair

Herpes in Pregnancy

Acute **Pain** r/t active herpes lesion

Fear r/t threat to fetus, impending surgery

Impaired **Tissue** integrity r/t active herpes lesion

Impaired **Urinary** elimination r/t pain with urination

Ineffective **Health** maintenance r/t deficient knowledge regarding treatment of disease, protection of fetus

Risk for **Infection** transmission: Risk factors: transplacental transfer during primary herpes, exposure to active herpes during birth process

Situational low **Self-esteem** r/t threat to fetus as a result of disease process

Herpes Simplex I

Impaired **Oral** mucous membranes r/t inflammatory changes in mouth

Herpes Simplex II

Acute **Pain** r/t active herpes lesion

Impaired **Tissue** integrity r/t active herpes lesion

Impaired **Urinary** elimination r/t pain with urination

Ineffective **Health** maintenance r/t deficient knowledge regarding treatment, prevention, spread of disease

Sexual dysfunction r/t disease process

Situational low **Self-esteem** r/t expressions of shame or guilt

Herpes Zoster

See Shingles

HHNC (Hyperosmolar Hyperglycemic Nonketotic Coma)

See Hyperosmolar Hyperglycemic Nonketotic Coma (HHNC)

Hiatal Hernia

Acute **Pain** r/t gastroesophageal reflux

Imbalanced **Nutrition**: less than body requirements r/t pain after eating

Ineffective **Health** maintenance r/t deficient knowledge regarding care of disease

Nausea r/t effects of gastric contents in esophagus

Hip Fracture

Acute **Confusion** r/t sensory overload, sensory deprivation, medication side effects

Acute **Pain** r/t injury, surgical procedure

Constipation r/t immobility, narcotics, anesthesia

Fear r/t outcome of treatment, future mobility, present helplessness

Impaired physical **Mobility** r/t surgical incision, temporary absence of weight bearing

Impaired **Transfer** ability r/t immobilization of hip

Impaired **Walking** r/t temporary absence of weight bearing

Powerlessness r/t health care environment

Risk for deficient **Fluid** volume: hemorrhage: Risk factors: postoperative complication, surgical blood loss

Risk for impaired **Skin** integrity: Risk factor: immobility

Risk for **Infection**: Risk factor: invasive procedure

Risk for **Injury**: Risk factors: dislodged prosthesis, unsteadiness when ambulating

Risk for perioperative positioning **Injury**: Risk factors: immobilization, muscle weakness, emaciation

Self-care deficit: specify r/t musculoskeletal impairment

Hip Replacement

See Total Joint Replacement

Hirschsprung's Disease

Acute **Pain** r/t distended colon, incisional postoperative pain

Constipation: bowel obstruction r/t inhibited peristalsis as a result of congenital absence of parasympathetic ganglion cells in distal colon

Grieving r/t loss of perfect child, birth of child with congenital defect even though child expected to be normal within 2 years

Imbalanced **Nutrition**: less than body requirements r/t anorexia, pain from distended colon

Impaired **Skin** integrity r/t stoma, potential skin care problems associated with stoma

Ineffective **Health** maintenance r/t parental deficient knowledge regarding temporary stoma care, dietary management, treatment for constipation or diarrhea

See Hospitalized Child

Hirsutism

Disturbed **Body** image r/t excessive hair

Hitting Behavior

Acute **Confusion** r/t dementia, alcohol abuse, drug abuse, delirium

Risk for other-directed **Violence** (See **Violence**, other-directed, risk for, Section III)

HIV (Human Immunodeficiency Virus)

Fear r/t possible death

Ineffective **Protection** r/t depressed immune system

See AIDS (Acquired Immune Deficiency Syndrome)

Hodgkin's Disease

See Anemia; Cancer; Chemotherapy

Home Maintenance Problems

Impaired **Home** maintenance (See **Home** maintenance, impaired, Section III)

Homelessness

Impaired **Home** maintenance r/t impaired cognitive or emotional functioning, inadequate support system, insufficient finances

Powerlessness r/t interpersonal interactions

Risk for **Trauma**: Risk factor: being in high-crime neighborhood

Hope

Readiness for enhanced **Hope** (See **Hope**, readiness for enhanced, Section III)

Hopelessness

Hopelessness (See **Hopelessness**, Section III)

Hospitalized Child

Activity intolerance r/t fatigue associated with acute illness

Acute **Pain** r/t treatments, diagnostic or therapeutic procedures

Anxiety: separation (child) r/t familiar surroundings and separation from family and friends

H

Compromised family **Coping** r/t possible prolonged hospitalization that exhausts supportive capacity of significant people

Deficient **Diversional** activity r/t immobility, monotonous environment, frequent or lengthy treatments, reluctance to participate, therapeutic isolation, separation from peers

Delayed **Growth** and development r/t regression or lack of progression toward developmental milestones as a result of frequent or prolonged hospitalization, inadequate or inappropriate stimulation, cerebral insult, chronic illness, effects of physical disability, prescribed dependence

Fear r/t deficient knowledge or maturational level with fear of unknown, mutilation, painful procedures, surgery

Hopelessness: child r/t prolonged activity restriction, uncertain prognosis

Ineffective **Coping**: parent r/t possible guilt regarding hospitalization of child, parental inadequacies

Insomnia: child or parent r/t 24-hour care needs of hospitalization

Interrupted **Family** processes r/t situational crisis of illness, disease, hospitalization

Powerlessness: child r/t health care environment, illness-related regimen

Readiness for enhanced family **Coping** r/t impact of crisis on family values, priorities, goals, relationships in family

Risk for impaired parent/child **Attachment**: Risk factor: separation

Risk for delayed **Growth** and development: regression: Risk factors: disruption of normal routine, unfamiliar environment or caregivers, developmental vulnerability of young children

Risk for imbalanced **Nutrition**: less than body requirements: Risk factors: anorexia, absence of familiar foods, cultural preferences

Risk for **Injury**: Risk factors: unfamiliar environment, developmental age, lack of parental knowledge regarding safety (e.g., side rails, IV site/pole)

See Child with Chronic Condition

Hostile Behavior

Risk for other-directed **Violence**: Risk factor: antisocial personality disorder

HTN (Hypertension)

Disturbed **Energy** field r/t pain, discomfort

Imbalanced **Nutrition**: more than body requirements r/t lack of knowledge of relationship between diet and disease process

Ineffective **Health** maintenance r/t deficient knowledge regarding treatment and control of disease process

Noncompliance r/t side effects of treatments, lack of understanding regarding importance of controlling hypertension

Human Immunodeficiency Virus (HIV)

See AIDS (Acquired Immune Deficiency Syndrome); HIV (Human Immunodeficiency Virus)

Humiliating Experience

Risk for compromised human **Dignity** (See **Dignity**, compromised human, risk for, Section III)

Huntington's Disease

Decisional **Conflict** r/t whether to have children

See Neurological Disorders

Hydrocele

Acute **Pain** r/t severely enlarged hydrocele

Ineffective **Sexuality** pattern r/t recent surgery on area of scrotum

Hydrocephalus

Decisional **Conflict** r/t unclear or conflicting values regarding selection of treatment modality

Delayed **Growth** and development r/t sequelae of increased intracranial pressure

Imbalanced **Nutrition**: less than body requirements r/t inadequate intake as a result of anorexia, nausea, vomiting, feeding difficulties

Impaired **Skin** integrity r/t impaired physical mobility, mechanical irritation

Ineffective **Tissue** perfusion: cerebral r/t interrupted flow, hypervolemia of cerebral ventricles

Interrupted **Family** processes r/t situational crisis

Risk for delayed **Development**: Risk factor: sequelae of increased intracranial pressure

Risk for disproportionate **Growth**: Risk factor: sequelae of increased intracranial pressure

Risk for **Infection**: Risk factor: sequelae of invasive procedure (shunt placement)

See Normal Pressure Hydrocephalous (NPH); Child with Chronic Condition; Hospitalized Child; Mental Retardation (if appropriate); Premature Infant (Child); Premature Infant (Parent)

Hygiene, Inability to Provide Own

Adult **Failure** to thrive r/t depression, apathy as evidenced by inability to perform self-care

Self-care deficit: bathing/hygiene (See **Self-care** deficit, bathing/hygiene, Section III)

Hyperactive Syndrome

Compromised family **Coping** r/t unsuccessful strategies to control excessive activity, behaviors, frustration, anger

Decisional **Conflict** r/t multiple or divergent sources of information regarding education, nutrition, medication regimens; willingness to change own food habits; limited resources

Impaired **Social** interaction r/t impulsive and overactive behaviors, concomitant emotional difficulties, distractibility and excitability

Ineffective **Role** performance: parent r/t stressors associated with dealing with hyperactive child, perceived or projected blame for causes of child's behavior, unmet needs for support or care, lack of energy to provide for those needs

Parental role **Conflict**: when siblings present r/t increased attention toward hyperactive child

Risk for delayed **Development**: Risk factor: behavior disorders

Risk for impaired **Parenting**: Risk factor: disruptive or uncontrollable behaviors of child

Risk for other-directed **Violence**: parent or child: Risk factors: frustration with disruptive behavior, anger, unsuccessful relationships

Self-esteem disturbance r/t inability to achieve socially acceptable behaviors; frustration; frequent reprimands, punishment, or scolding for uncontrolled activity and behaviors; mood fluctuations and restlessness; inability to succeed academically; lack of peer support

Hyperalimentation

See TPN (Total Parenteral Nutrition)

Hyperbilirubinemia

Anxiety: parent r/t threat to infant, unknown future

Disturbed **Sensory** perception: visual (infant) r/t use of eye patches for protection of eyes during phototherapy

Imbalanced **Nutrition**: less than body requirements (infant) r/t disinterest in feeding because of jaundice-related lethargy

Parental role **Conflict** r/t interruption of family life because of care regimen

Risk for disproportionate **Growth**: infant: Risk factor: disinterest in feeding because of jaundice-related lethargy

Risk for **Imbalanced** body temperature: infant: Risk factor: phototherapy

Risk for **Injury**: infant: Risk factors: kernicterus, phototherapy lights

Hypercalcemia

Decreased **Cardiac** output r/t bradydysrhythmia

Disturbed **Thought** processes r/t elevated calcium levels that cause paranoia, decreased level of consciousness

Imbalanced **Nutrition**: less than body requirements r/t gastrointestinal manifestations of hypercalcemia (nausea, anorexia, ileus)

Impaired physical **Mobility** r/t decreased tone in smooth and striated muscle

Risk for **Trauma**: Risk factors: risk for fractures

Hypercapnia

Fear r/t difficulty breathing

Impaired **Gas** exchange r/t ventilation perfusion imbalance

Hyperemesis Gravidarum

Anxiety r/t threat to self and infant, hospitalization

Deficient **Fluid** volume r/t vomiting

Imbalanced **Nutrition**: less than body requirements r/t vomiting

Impaired **Home** maintenance r/t chronic nausea, inability to function

Nausea r/t hormonal changes of pregnancy

Powerlessness r/t health care regimen

Social isolation r/t hospitalization

Hyperglycemia

Ineffective management of **Therapeutic** regimen r/t complexity of therapeutic regimen, decisional conflicts, economic difficulties, unsupportive family, insufficient cues to action, deficient

knowledge, mistrust, lack of acknowledgment of seriousness of condition

Risk for unstable blood **Glucose** (See **Glucose**, unstable blood, risk for, Section III)

See Diabetes Mellitus

Hyperkalemia

Decreased **Cardiac** output r/t possible dysrhythmia

Risk for **Activity** intolerance: Risk factor: muscle weakness

Risk for excess **Fluid** volume: Risk factor: untreated renal failure

Hypernatremia

Risk for deficient **Fluid** volume: Risk factors: abnormal water loss, inadequate water intake

Hyperosmolar Hyperglycemic Nonketotic Coma (HHNC)

Deficient **Fluid** volume r/t polyuria, inadequate fluid intake

Disturbed **Thought** processes r/t dehydration, electrolyte imbalance

Risk for **Injury**: seizures: Risk factors: hyperosmolar state, electrolyte imbalance

See Diabetes Mellitus; Diabetes Mellitus, Juvenile

Hyperphosphatemia

Deficient **Knowledge** r/t dietary changes needed to control phosphate levels

See Renal Failure

Hypersensitivity to Slight Criticism

Defensive **Coping** r/t situational crisis, psychological impairment, substance abuse

Hypertension

Imbalanced **Nutrition**: more than body requirements r/t lack of knowledge of relation between diet and disease process

Ineffective **Health** maintenance r/t deficient knowledge regarding treatment and control of disease process

Noncompliance r/t side effects of treatment

Hyperthermia

Hyperthermia (See **Hyperthermia**, Section III)

Hyperthyroidism

Activity intolerance r/t increased oxygen demands from increased metabolic rate

Anxiety r/t increased stimulation, loss of control

Diarrhea r/t increased gastric motility

Imbalanced **Nutrition**: less than body requirements r/t increased metabolic rate, increased gastrointestinal activity

Ineffective **Health** maintenance r/t deficient knowledge regarding medications, methods of coping with stress

Insomnia r/t anxiety, excessive sympathetic discharge

Risk for **Injury**: eye damage: Risk factor: exophthalmos

Hyperventilation

Ineffective **Breathing** pattern r/t anxiety, acid-base imbalance

Hypocalcemia

Activity intolerance r/t neuromuscular irritability

Imbalanced **Nutrition**: less than body requirements r/t effects of vitamin D deficiency, renal failure, malabsorption, laxative use

Ineffective **Breathing** pattern r/t laryngospasm

Hypoglycemia

Disturbed **Thought** processes r/t insufficient blood glucose to brain

Imbalanced **Nutrition**: less than body requirements r/t imbalance of glucose and insulin level

Ineffective **Health** maintenance r/t deficient knowledge regarding disease process, self-care

Risk for unstable blood **Glucose** (See **Glucose**, unstable blood, risk for, Section III)

See Diabetes Mellitus; Diabetes Mellitus, Juvenile

Hypokalemia

Activity intolerance r/t muscle weakness

Decreased **Cardiac** output r/t possible dysrhythmia from electrolyte imbalance

Hypomagnesemia

Imbalanced **Nutrition**: less than body requirements r/t deficient knowledge of nutrition, alcoholism

See Alcoholism

Hypomania

Insomnia r/t psychological stimulus

See Manic Disorder, Bipolar I

Hyponatremia

Disturbed **Thought** processes r/t electrolyte imbalance

Excess **Fluid** volume r/t excessive intake of hypotonic fluids

Risk for **Injury**: Risk factors: seizures, new onset of confusion

Hypoplastic Left Lung

See Congenital Heart Disease/Cardiac Anomalies

Hypotension

Decreased **Cardiac** output r/t decreased preload, decreased contractility

Ineffective **Tissue** perfusion: cerebral/cardiopulmonary or peripheral r/t hypovolemia, decreased contractility, decreased afterload

Risk for deficient **Fluid** volume: Risk factor: excessive fluid loss

See cause of Hypotension

Hypothermia

Hypothermia (See **Hypothermia**, Section III)

Hypothyroidism

Activity intolerance r/t muscular stiffness, shortness of breath on exertion

Constipation r/t decreased gastric motility

Disturbed **Thought** processes r/t altered metabolic process

Imbalanced **Nutrition**: more than body requirements r/t decreased metabolic process

Impaired **Gas** exchange r/t possible respiratory depression

Impaired **Skin** integrity r/t edema, dry or scaly skin

Ineffective **Health** maintenance r/t deficient knowledge regarding disease process and self-care

Hypovolemic Shock

Deficient **Fluid** volume r/t trauma, third spacing, loss of fluid from body

See Shock

Hypoxia

Acute **Confusion** r/t decreased oxygen supply to brain

Disturbed **Thought** processes r/t decreased oxygen supply to brain

Fear r/t breathlessness

Impaired **Gas** exchange r/t altered oxygen supply, inability to transport oxygen

Hysterectomy

Acute **Pain** r/t surgical injury

Constipation r/t opioids, anesthesia, bowel manipulation during surgery

Ineffective **Coping** r/t situational crisis of surgery

Grieving r/t change in body image, loss of reproductive status

Ineffective **Health** maintenance r/t deficient knowledge regarding precautions and self-care after surgery

Risk for **Constipation**: Risk factors: narcotics, anesthesia, bowel manipulation during surgery

Risk for deficient **Fluid** volume: Risk factors: abnormal blood loss, hemorrhage

Risk for ineffective **Tissue** perfusion: Risk factor: thromboembolism

Risk for urge urinary **Incontinence**: Risk factors: edema in area, anesthesia, narcotics, pain

Sexual dysfunction r/t disturbance in self-concept

Urinary retention r/t edema in area, anesthesia, opioids, pain

See Surgery, Perioperative; Surgery, Preoperative; Surgery, Postoperative

I

IBS (Irritable Bowel Syndrome)

Chronic **Pain** r/t spasms, increased motility of bowel

Constipation r/t low-residue diet, stress

Diarrhea r/t increased motility of intestines associated with stress

Ineffective **Health** maintenance r/t deficient knowledge regarding self-care with IBS

Ineffective **Therapeutic** regimen management r/t deficient knowledge, powerlessness

Readiness for enhanced **Therapeutic** regimen management: r/t expressed desire to manage illness and prevent onset of symptoms

ICD (Implantable Cardioverter/ Defibrillator)

Ineffective **Health** maintenance r/t deficient knowledge regarding self-care, action of internal cardiac defibrillator

Decreased **Cardiac** output r/t possible dysrhythmia

IDDM (Insulin-Dependent Diabetes)

See Diabetes Mellitus

Identity Disturbance

Disturbed personal **Identity** r/t situational crisis, psychological impairment, chronic illness, pain

Readiness for enhanced **Coping** r/t seeking social support

Spiritual distress r/t expression of alienation from others

Idiopathic Thrombocytopenic Purpura

See ITP (Idiopathic Thrombocytopenic Purpura)

Ileal Conduit

Deficient **Knowledge** r/t care of stoma

Disturbed **Body** image r/t presence of stoma

Ineffective **Sexuality** pattern r/t altered body function and structure

Ineffective **Therapeutic** regimen management r/t new skills required to care for appliance and self

Readiness for enhanced **Therapeutic** regimen management: r/t expressed desire to care for stoma

Risk for impaired **Skin** integrity: Risk factor: difficulty obtaining tight seal of appliance

Risk for latex **Allergy** response: Risk factor: repeated exposures to latex associated with treatment and management of disease

Social isolation r/t alteration in physical appearance, fear of accidental spill of ostomy contents

Ileostomy

Constipation r/t dietary changes, change in intestinal motility

Deficient **Knowledge** r/t limited practice of stoma care, dietary modifications

Diarrhea r/t dietary changes, alteration in intestinal motility

Disturbed **Body** image r/t presence of stoma

Ineffective **Sexuality** pattern r/t altered body function and structure

Ineffective **Therapeutic** regimen management r/t new skills required to care for appliance and self

Risk for impaired **Skin** integrity: Risk factors: difficulty obtaining tight seal of appliance, caustic drainage

Social isolation r/t alteration in physical appearance, fear of accidental spill of ostomy contents

Ileus

Acute **Pain** r/t pressure, abdominal distention

Constipation r/t decreased gastric motility

Deficient **Fluid** volume r/t loss of fluids from vomiting, fluids trapped in bowel

Nausea r/t gastrointestinal irritation

Immobility

Adult **Failure** to thrive r/t limited physical mobility

Constipation r/t immobility

Disturbed **Thought** processes r/t sensory deprivation from immobility

Impaired physical **Mobility** r/t medically imposed bedrest

Impaired **Transfer** ability r/t limited physical mobility

Impaired **Walking** r/t limited physical mobility

Ineffective **Breathing** pattern r/t inability to deep breathe in supine position

Ineffective **Tissue** perfusion: peripheral r/t interruption of venous flow

Powerlessness r/t forced immobility from health care environment

Risk for **Disuse** syndrome: Risk factor: immobilization

Risk for impaired **Skin** integrity: Risk factors: pressure on immobile parts, shearing forces when moved

Immunization

Readiness for enhanced **Immunization** status (See **Immunization** status, readiness for enhanced, Section III)

Immunosuppression

Ineffective **Protection** r/t medications, treatments, or pathology suppressing immune system function

Risk for **Infection**: Risk factor: immunosuppression

Impaction of Stool

Constipation r/t decreased fluid intake, less than adequate amounts of fiber and bulk-forming foods in diet, medication effect, or immobility

Imperforate Anus

Anxiety r/t ability to care for newborn

Deficient **Knowledge** r/t home care for newborn

Impaired **Skin** integrity r/t pruritus

Risk for impaired **Skin** integrity: Risk factor: presence of stool at surgical repair site

Impetigo

Ineffective **Health** maintenance r/t parental deficient knowledge regarding care of impetigo

See Communicable Diseases, Childhood

Implantable Cardioverter/Defibrillator

See ICD (Implantable Cardioverter/Defibrillator)

I

I

Impotence

Readiness for enhanced **Knowledge**: treatment information for erectile dysfunction

Self-esteem disturbance r/t physiological crisis, inability to practice usual sexual activity

Sexual dysfunction r/t altered body function

See Erectile Dysfunction

Inactivity

Activity intolerance r/t imbalance between oxygen supply and demand, sedentary lifestyle, weakness, immobility

Impaired physical **Mobility** r/t intolerance to activity, decreased strength and endurance, depression, severe anxiety, musculoskeletal impairment, perceptual or cognitive impairment, neuromuscular impairment, pain, discomfort

Risk for **Constipation**: Risk factor: insufficient physical activity

Incompetent Cervix

See Premature Dilation of the Cervix (Incompetent Cervix)

Incontinence of Stool

Bowel incontinence r/t decreased awareness of need to defecate, loss of sphincter control

Deficient **Knowledge** r/t lack of information on normal bowel elimination

Disturbed **Body** image r/t inability to control elimination of stool

Risk for impaired **Skin** integrity: Risk factor: presence of stool

Situational low **Self-esteem** r/t inability to control elimination of stool

Toileting **Self-care** deficit r/t toileting needs

Incontinence of Urine

Functional urinary **Incontinence** r/t altered environment; sensory, cognitive, or mobility deficits

Overflow urinary **Incontinence** r/t relaxation of pelvic muscles and changes in urinary structures

Reflex urinary **Incontinence** r/t neurological impairment

Risk for impaired **Skin** integrity: Risk factor: presence of urine

Toileting **Self-care** deficit r/t neuromuscular dysfunction

Situational low **Self-esteem** r/t inability to control passage of urine

Stress urinary **Incontinence** (See **Incontinence**, stress urinary, Section III)

Total urinary **Incontinence** (See **Incontinence**, total urinary, Section III)

Urge urinary **Incontinence** (See **Incontinence**, urge urinary, Section III)

Indigestion

Imbalanced **Nutrition**: less than body requirements r/t discomfort when eating

Nausea r/t gastrointestinal irritation

Induction of Labor

Anxiety r/t medical interventions

Decisional **Conflict** r/t perceived threat to idealized birth

Ineffective **Coping** r/t situational crisis of medical intervention in birthing process

Readiness for enhanced **Family** processes: family support during induction of labor

Risk for **Injury**: maternal and fetal: Risk factors: hypertonic uterus, potential prematurity of newborn

Self-esteem disturbance r/t inability to carry out normal labor

Infant Apnea

See Premature Infant (Child); Respiratory Conditions of the Neonate; SIDS (Sudden Infant Death Syndrome)

Infant Behavior

Disorganized **Infant** behavior r/t pain, oral/motor problems, feeding intolerance, environmental overstimulation, lack of containment or boundaries, prematurity, invasive or painful procedures

Readiness for enhanced organized **Infant** behavior r/t prematurity, pain

Risk for disorganized **Infant** behavior: Risk factors: pain, oral/motor problems, environmental overstimulation, lack of containment or boundaries

Infant Feeding Pattern, Ineffective

Ineffective **Infant** feeding pattern r/t prematurity, neurological impairment or delay, oral hypersensitivity, prolonged nothing-by-mouth order

Infant of Diabetic Mother

Deficient **Fluid** volume r/t increased urinary excretion and osmotic diuresis

Delayed **Growth** and development r/t prolonged and severe postnatal hypoglycemia

Imbalanced **Nutrition**: less than body requirements r/t hypotonia, lethargy, poor sucking, postnatal metabolic changes from hyperglycemia to hypoglycemia and hyperinsulinism

Risk for decreased **Cardiac** output: Risk factor: increased incidence of cardiomegaly

Risk for delayed **Development**: Risk factors: prolonged and severe postnatal hypoglycemia

Risk for disproportionate **Growth**: Risk factors: prolonged and severe postnatal hypoglycemia

Risk for impaired **Gas** exchange: Risk factors: increased incidence of cardiomegaly, prematurity

See Premature Infant (Child); Respiratory Conditions of the Neonate

Infant of Substance-Abusing Mother (Fetal Alcohol Syndrome, Crack Baby, Other Drug Withdrawal Infants)

Delayed **Growth** and development r/t effects of maternal use of drugs, effects of neurological impairment, decreased attentiveness to environmental stimuli or inadequate stimuli

Diarrhea r/t effects of withdrawal, increased peristalsis from hyperirritability

Disturbed **Sensory** perception r/t hypersensitivity to environmental stimuli

Imbalanced **Nutrition**: less than body requirements r/t feeding problems; uncoordinated or ineffective suck and swallow; effects of diarrhea, vomiting, or colic associated with maternal substance abuse

Impaired **Parenting** r/t impaired or absent attachment behaviors, inadequate support systems

Ineffective **Airway** clearance r/t pooling of secretions from the lack of adequate cough reflex, effects of viral or bacterial lower airway infection as a result of altered protective state

Ineffective **Infant** feeding pattern r/t uncoordinated or ineffective sucking reflex

Ineffective **Protection** r/t effects of maternal substance abuse

Insomnia r/t hyperirritability or hypersensitivity to environmental stimuli

Interrupted **Breastfeeding** r/t use of drugs or alcohol by mother

Risk for delayed **Development**: Risk factor: substance abuse

Risk for disproportionate **Growth**: Risk factor: substance abuse

Risk for **Infection**: skin, meningeal, respiratory: Risk factor: effects of withdrawal

See Cerebral Palsy; Child with Chronic Condition; Crack Baby; Failure to Thrive, Nonorganic; Hospitalized Child; Hyperactive Syndrome; Premature Infant (Child); SIDS (Sudden Infant Death Syndrome)

Infantile Polyarteritis
See Kawasaki Disease

Infantile Spasms
See Seizure Disorders, Childhood

Infection
Hyperthermia r/t increased metabolic rate

Ineffective **Protection** r/t inadequate nutrition, abnormal blood profiles, drug therapies, treatments

Infection, Potential for
Risk for **Infection** (See **Infection**, risk for, Section III)

Infertility
Chronic **Sorrow** r/t inability to conceive a child

Ineffective **Therapeutic** regimen management r/t deficient knowledge about infertility

Powerlessness r/t infertility

Spiritual distress r/t inability to conceive a child

Inflammatory Bowel Disease (Child and Adult)
Acute **Pain** r/t abdominal cramping and anal irritation

Deficient **Fluid** volume r/t frequent and loose stools

Diarrhea r/t effects of inflammatory changes of the bowel

Imbalanced **Nutrition**: less than body requirements r/t anorexia, decreased absorption of nutrients from gastrointestinal tract

Impaired **Skin** integrity r/t frequent stools, development of anal fissures

Ineffective **Coping** r/t repeated episodes of diarrhea

Social isolation r/t diarrhea

See Child with Chronic Condition; Crohn's Disease; Hospitalized Child; Maturational Issues, Adolescent

Influenza
Acute **Pain** r/t inflammatory changes in joints

Deficient **Fluid** volume r/t inadequate fluid intake

Hyperthermia r/t infectious process

Ineffective **Health** maintenance r/t deficient knowledge regarding self-care

Ineffective **Therapeutic** regimen management r/t lack of knowledge regarding preventive immunizations

Readiness for enhanced **Knowledge**: about information to prevent or treat influenza

Inguinal Hernia Repair
Acute **Pain** r/t surgical procedure

Impaired physical **Mobility** r/t pain at surgical site and fear of causing hernia to rupture

Risk for **Infection**: Risk factor: surgical procedure

Urinary retention r/t possible edema at surgical site

Injury
Risk for **Falls**: Risk factors: orthostatic hypertension, impaired physical mobility, diminished mental status

Risk for **Injury**: Risk factor: environmental conditions interacting with client's adaptive and defensive resources

Insomnia
Insomnia (See **Insomnia**, Section III)

Insulin Shock
See Hypoglycemia

Intermittent Claudication
Acute **Pain** r/t decreased circulation to extremities with activity

Deficient **Knowledge** r/t lack of knowledge of cause and treatment of peripheral vascular diseases

Ineffective **Tissue** perfusion: peripheral r/t interruption of arterial flow

Readiness for enhanced **Knowledge**: prevention of pain and impaired circulation

Risk for **Injury**: Risk factor: tissue hypoxia

Risk for **Peripheral** neurovascular dysfunction: Risk factor: disruption in arterial flow

See Peripheral Vascular Disease

Internal Cardioverter/Defibrillator
See ICD (Implantable Cardioverter/Defibrillator)

I

Internal Fixation

Impaired **Walking** r/t repair of fracture

Risk for **Infection**: Risk factors: traumatized tissue, broken skin

See Fracture

Interstitial Cystitis

Acute **Pain** r/t inflammatory process

Impaired **Urinary** elimination r/t inflammation of bladder

Risk for **Infection**: Risk factor: suppressed inflammatory response

Intervertebral Disk Excision

See Laminectomy

Intestinal Obstruction

See Ileus

Intoxication

Acute **Confusion** r/t alcohol abuse

Anxiety r/t loss of control of actions

Disturbed **Sensory** perception r/t neurochemical imbalance in brain

Disturbed **Thought** processes r/t effect of substance on central nervous system

Impaired **Memory** r/t effects of alcohol on mind

Ineffective **Coping** r/t use of mind-altering substances as a means of coping

Risk for **Falls**: Risk factor: diminished mental status

Risk for other-directed **Violence**: Risk factor: inability to control thoughts and actions

Intraaortic Balloon Counterpulsation

Anxiety r/t device providing cardiovascular assistance

Compromised family **Coping** r/t seriousness of significant other's medical condition

Decreased **Cardiac** output r/t failing heart needing counterpulsation

Impaired physical **Mobility** r/t restriction of movement because of mechanical device

Risk for **Peripheral** neurovascular dysfunction: Risk factors: vascular obstruction of balloon catheter, thrombus formation, emboli, edema

Intracranial Pressure, Increased

Acute **Confusion** r/t increased intracranial pressure

Adult **Failure** to thrive r/t undetected changes from increased intracranial pressure

Decreased **Intracranial** adaptive capacity r/t sustained increase in intracranial pressure

Disturbed **Sensory** perception r/t pressure damage to sensory centers in brain

Disturbed **Thought** processes r/t pressure damage to brain

Impaired **Memory** r/t neurological disturbance

Ineffective **Breathing** pattern r/t pressure damage to breathing center in brainstem

Ineffective **Tissue** perfusion: cerebral r/t effects of increased intracranial pressure

See cause of Increased Intracranial Pressure

Intrauterine Growth Retardation

Anxiety: maternal r/t threat to fetus

Delayed **Growth** and development r/t insufficient supply of oxygen and nutrients

Imbalanced **Nutrition**: less than body requirements r/t insufficient placenta

Impaired **Gas** exchange r/t insufficient placental perfusion

Ineffective **Coping**: maternal r/t situational crisis, threat to fetus

Risk for delayed **Development**: Risk factor: insufficient supply of oxygen and nutrients

Risk for disproportionate **Growth**: Risk factor: insufficient supply of oxygen and nutrients

Risk for **Injury**: Risk factor: insufficient supply of oxygen and nutrients

Risk for **Powerlessness**: Risk factor: unknown outcome of fetus

Situational low **Self-esteem**: maternal r/t guilt about threat to fetus

Spiritual distress r/t unknown outcome of fetus

Intubation, Endotracheal or Nasogastric

Acute **Pain** r/t presence of tube

Disturbed **Body** image r/t altered appearance with mechanical devices

Imbalanced **Nutrition**: less than body requirements r/t inability to ingest food because of the presence of tubes

Impaired **Oral** mucous membrane r/t presence of tubes

Impaired verbal **Communication** r/t endotracheal tube

Irregular Pulse

See Dysrhythmia

Irritable Bowel Syndrome

See IBS (Irritable Bowel Syndrome)

Isolation

Social isolation (See **Social** isolation, Section III)

Itching

Risk for **Infection**: Risk factor: potential break in skin

Pruritus r/t inflammation of the skin

ITP (Idiopathic Thrombocytopenic Purpura)

Deficient **Diversional** activity r/t activity restrictions, safety precautions

Ineffective **Protection** r/t decreased platelet count

Risk for **Injury**: Risk factors: decreased platelet count, developmental level, age-appropriate play

See Hospitalized Child

J

Jaundice

Disturbed **Thought** processes r/t toxic blood metabolites

Pruritus r/t toxic metabolites excreted in the skin

Risk for impaired **Liver** function: Risk factor: possible viral infection

Risk for impaired **Skin** integrity: Risk factors: pruritus, itching

See Cirrhosis; Hepatitis

Jaundice, Neonatal

Readiness for enhanced **Therapeutic** regimen management: r/t expresses desire to manage treatment: assessment of jaundice when infant is discharged from the hospital, when to call the physician, and possible preventive measures such as frequent breastfeeding

See Hyperbilirubinemia

Jaw Pain and Heart Attacks

See Angina Pectoris; Chest Pain; MI (Myocardial Infarction)

Jaw Surgery

Acute **Pain** r/t surgical procedure

Deficient **Knowledge** r/t emergency care for wired jaws (e.g., cutting bands and wires), oral care

Imbalanced **Nutrition**: less than body requirements r/t jaws wired closed

Impaired **Swallowing** r/t edema from surgery

Risk for **Aspiration**: Risk factor: wired jaws

Jet Lag Prevention

Readiness for enhanced **Knowledge** r/t getting adequate sleep before travel, drinking extra water, avoiding caffeine and alcohol, engaging in regular exercise (but not at bedtime)

Jittery

Anxiety r/t unconscious conflict about essential values and goals, threat to or change in health status

Death Anxiety r/t unresolved issues relating to end of life

Risk for **Post-trauma** syndrome: Risk factors: occupation, survivor's role in event, inadequate social support

Jock Itch

Impaired **Skin** integrity r/t moisture and irritating or tight-fitting clothing

Ineffective **Therapeutic** regimen management r/t prevention and treatment

See Itching

Joint Dislocation

See Dislocation

Joint Inflammation

See Arthritis; JRA (Juvenile Rheumatoid Arthritis)

Joint Pain

See Arthritis; Bursitis; JRA (Juvenile Rheumatoid Arthritis); Osteoarthritis; Rheumatoid Arthritis

Joint Replacement

Risk for **Peripheral** neurovascular dysfunction: Risk factor: orthopedic surgery

See Total Joint Replacement

JRA (Juvenile Rheumatoid Arthritis)

Acute **Pain** r/t swollen or inflamed joints, restricted movement, physical therapy

Delayed **Growth** and development r/t effects of physical disability, chronic illness

Fatigue r/t chronic inflammatory disease

Impaired physical **Mobility** r/t pain, restricted joint movement

Risk for compromised human **Dignity**: Risk factors: perceived intrusion by clinicians, invasion of privacy

Risk for impaired **Skin** integrity: Risk factors: splints, adaptive devices

Risk for **Injury**: Risk factors: impaired physical mobility, splints, adaptive devices, increased bleeding potential from antiinflammatory medications

Risk for situational low **Self-esteem**: Risk factor: disturbed body image

Self-care deficits: feeding, bathing/hygiene, dressing, grooming, toileting r/t restricted joint movement, pain

See Child with Chronic Condition; Hospitalized Child

Juvenile Onset Diabetes

See Diabetes Mellitus, Juvenile

K

Kaposi's Sarcoma

Risk for Complicated **Grieving**: Risk factor: loss of social support

Risk for compromised human **Dignity**: Risk factor: use of undefined medical terms

Risk for impaired **Religiosity**: Risk factors: illness/hospitalization, ineffective coping

See AIDS (Acquired Immune Deficiency Syndrome)

Kawasaki Disease (Formerly Mucocutaneous Lymph Node Syndrome)

Acute **Pain** r/t enlarged lymph nodes; erythematous skin rash that progresses to desquamation, peeling, denuding of skin

Anxiety: parental r/t progression of disease, complications of arthritis, and cardiac involvement

Hyperthermia r/t inflammatory disease process

Imbalanced **Nutrition**: less than body requirements r/t impaired oral mucous membranes

Impaired **Oral** mucous membranes r/t inflamed mouth and pharynx; swollen lips that become dry, cracked, fissured

Impaired **Skin** integrity r/t inflammatory skin changes

See Hospitalized Child

Kegel Exercise

Health-seeking behavior r/t desire for information to relieve incontinence

Risk for urge urinary Incontinence: Risk factors: effects of alcohol, caffeine, decreased bladder capacity, irritation of bladder stretch receptors causing spasm, increased urine concentration, overdistention of bladder

Stress urinary Incontinence r/t degenerative change in pelvic muscles

Urge urinary Incontinence r/t decreased bladder capacity

Keloids

Disturbed Body image r/t presence of scar tissue at site of a healed skin injury

Readiness for enhanced Therapeutic regimen management: desire to have information to decrease discoloration of skin from sun exposure

Keratoconjunctivitis Sicca

Risk for Infection r/t dry eyes

See Conjunctivitis

Keratoplasty

See Corneal Transplant

Ketoacidosis, Diabetic

Deficient Fluid volume r/t excess excretion of urine, nausea, vomiting, increased respiration

Imbalanced Nutrition: less than body requirements r/t body's inability to use nutrients

Impaired Memory r/t fluid and electrolyte imbalance

Ineffective Therapeutic regimen management r/t denial of illness, lack of understanding of preventive measures, and adequate blood sugar control

Noncompliance: diabetic regimen r/t ineffective coping with chronic disease

Risk for Powerlessness: Risk factor: illness-related regimen

Risk for unstable Glucose Level: Risk factor: deficient knowledge of diabetes management (e.g., action plan)

See Diabetes Mellitus

Ketoacidosis: Alcoholic

See Alcohol Withdrawal; Alcoholism

Keyhole Heart Surgery

See MIDCAB (Minimally Invasive Direct Coronary Artery Bypass)

Kidney Failure

See Renal Failure

Kidney Stone

Acute Pain r/t obstruction from renal calculi

Deficient Knowledge r/t fluid requirements and dietary restrictions

Impaired Urinary elimination: urgency and frequency r/t anatomical obstruction, irritation caused by stone

Overflow urinary Incontinence r/t bladder outlet obstruction

Risk for deficient Fluid volume: Risk factors: nausea, vomiting

Risk for Infection: Risk factor: obstruction of urinary tract with stasis of urine

Kidney Transplant

Decisional Conflict r/t acceptance of donor kidney

Ineffective Protection r/t immunosuppressive therapy

Readiness for enhanced Decision making: expresses desire to enhance understanding of choices

Readiness for enhanced Family processes: adapting to life without dialysis

Readiness for enhanced Spiritual well-being: heightened coping, living without dialysis

Readiness for enhanced Therapeutic regimen management: desire to manage the treatment and prevention of complications post transplant

See Nephrectomy; Renal Failure; Renal Transplantation, Donor; Renal Transplantation, Recipient; Surgery, Perioperative Care; Surgery, Postoperative Care; Surgery, Preoperative Care

Kidney Tumor

See Wilms' Tumor

Kissing Disease

See Mononucleosis

Knee Replacement

See Total Joint Replacement

Knowledge

Readiness for enhanced Knowledge (See **Knowledge**, readiness for enhanced, Section III)

Knowledge, Deficient

Deficient Knowledge (See **Knowledge**, deficient, Section III)

Ineffective Health maintenance r/t lack of or significant alteration in communication skills (written, verbal, and/or gestural)

Ineffective Therapeutic regimen management r/t complexity of therapeutic regimen

Kock Pouch

See Continent Ileostomy (Kock Pouch)

Korsakoff's Syndrome

Acute Confusion r/t alcohol abuse

Dysfunctional Family processes: alcoholism r/t possible cause of syndrome

Impaired Memory r/t neurological changes

Risk for Falls: Risk factor: cognitive impairment

Risk for imbalanced Nutrition: less than body requirements: Risk factor: lack of adequate balanced intake

Risk for impaired Liver function: Risk factor: substance abuse (alcohol)

Risk for Injury: Risk factors: sensory dysfunction, lack of coordination when ambulating

L

Labor, Induction of

See Induction of Labor

Labor, Normal

Acute **Pain** r/t uterine contractions, stretching of cervix and birth canal

Anxiety r/t fear of the unknown, situational crisis

Deficient **Knowledge** r/t lack of preparation for labor

Fatigue r/t childbirth

Health-seeking behaviors healthy outcome of pregnancy, prenatal care, and childbirth education

Impaired **Tissue** integrity r/t passage of infant through birth canal, episiotomy

Readiness for enhanced family **Coping** r/t significant other providing support during labor

Readiness for enhanced **Power**: expresses readiness to enhance participation in choices regarding treatment during labor

Risk for deficient **Fluid** volume: Risk factor: excessive loss of blood

Risk for **Infection**: Risk factors: multiple vaginal examinations, tissue trauma, prolonged rupture of membranes

Risk for **Injury**: Risk factor: fetal, r/t hypoxia

Risk for **Post-trauma** syndrome: Risk factors: trauma or violence associated with labor pains, birth process, medical or surgical interventions, history of sexual abuse

Risk for **Powerlessness**: Risk factor: labor process

Labyrinthitis

Risk for **Injury** r/t dizziness

Ineffective **Therapeutic** regimen management r/t delay in seeking treatment for respiratory and ear infections

Readiness for enhanced **Therapeutic** regimen management: management of episodes

Lactation

See Breastfeeding, Effective; Breastfeeding, Ineffective; Breastfeeding, Interrupted

Lactic acidosis

Decreased **Cardiac** output r/t altered heart rate/rhythm, preload, and contractility

See Ketoacidosis, Diabetic

Lactose Intolerance

Readiness for enhanced **Knowledge** r/t interest in identifying lactose intolerance, treatment, and substitutes for milk products

See Abdominal Distention; Diarrhea

Laminectomy

Acute **Pain** r/t localized inflammation and edema

Anxiety r/t change in health status, surgical procedure

Deficient **Knowledge** r/t appropriate postoperative and post-discharge activities

Disturbed **Sensory** perception: tactile r/t possible edema or nerve injury

Impaired physical **Mobility** r/t neuromuscular impairment

Risk for impaired **Tissue** perfusion: Risk factors: edema, hemorrhage, embolism

Risk for perioperative positioning **Injury**: Risk factor: prone position

Urinary retention r/t competing sensory impulses, effects of narcotics or anesthesia

See Scoliosis; Surgery, Perioperative; Surgery, Postoperative; Surgery, Preoperative

Laparoscopic Laser Cholecystectomy

See Cholecystectomy; Laser Surgery

Laparoscopy

Acute **Pain**: shoulder r/t gas irritating the diaphragm

Urge urinary **Incontinence** r/t pressure on the bladder from gas

Laparotomy

See Abdominal Surgery

Laryngectomy

Grieving r/t loss of voice, fear of death

Chronic **Sorrow** r/t change in body image

Death **Anxiety** r/t unknown results of surgery

Disturbed **Body** image r/t change in body structure and function

Imbalanced **Nutrition**: less than body requirements r/t absence of oral feeding, difficulty swallowing, increased need for fluids

Impaired **Oral** mucous membranes r/t absence of oral feeding

Impaired **Swallowing** r/t edema, laryngectomy tube

Impaired verbal **Communication** r/t removal of larynx

Ineffective **Airway** clearance r/t surgical removal of glottis, decreased humidification of air

Ineffective **Health** maintenance r/t deficient knowledge regarding self-care with laryngectomy

Interrupted **Family** processes r/t surgery, serious condition of family member, difficulty communicating

Risk for complicated **Grieving**: Risk factors: loss, major life event

Risk for compromised human **Dignity**: Risk factor: loss of control of body function

Risk for **Infection**: Risk factors: invasive procedure, surgery

Risk for **Powerlessness**: Risk factors: chronic illness, change in communication

Risk for situational low **Self-esteem**: Risk factor: disturbed body image

Laser Surgery

Acute **Pain** r/t heat from laser

Constipation r/t laser intervention in vulval and perianal areas

Deficient **Knowledge** r/t preoperative and postoperative care associated with laser procedure

L

Risk for **Infection**: Risk factor: delayed heating reaction of tissue exposed to laser

Risk for **Injury**: Risk factor: accidental exposure to laser beam

LASIK Eye Surgery (Laser-Assisted in Situ Keratomileusis)

Decisional **Conflict** r/t decision to have the surgery

Readiness for enhanced **Therapeutic** regimen management: surgical procedure pre- and postoperative teaching and expectations

Latex Allergy

Latex **Allergy** response (See **Allergy** response, latex, Section III)

Readiness for enhanced **Knowledge** of prevention and treatment of exposure to latex products

Risk for latex **Allergy** response (See **Allergy** response, latex, risk for, Section III)

Laxative Abuse

Perceived **Constipation** r/t health belief, faulty appraisal, impaired thought processes

Lead Poisoning

Contamination r/t flaking, peeling paint in presence of young children

Impaired **Home** maintenance r/t presence of lead paint

Risk for delayed **Development**: Risk factor: lead poisoning

Legionnaires' Disease

Contamination r/t contaminated water in air-conditioning systems

Ineffective community **Therapeutic** regimen management r/t contaminated air systems in large buildings

See Pneumonia

Lens Implant

See Cataract Extraction; Vision Impairment

Lethargy/Listlessness

Adult **Failure** to thrive r/t apathy

Insomnia r/t internal or external stressors

Fatigue r/t decreased metabolic energy production

Ineffective **Tissue** perfusion: cerebral r/t lack of oxygen supply to brain

See cause of Lethargy/Listlessness

Leukemia

Ineffective **Protection** r/t abnormal blood profile

Risk for deficient **Fluid** volume: Risk factors: nausea, vomiting, bleeding, side effects of treatment

Risk for **Infection**: Risk factor: ineffective immune system

See Cancer; Chemotherapy

Leukopenia

Ineffective **Protection** r/t leukopenia

Risk for **Infection** r/t low white blood cell count

Level of Consciousness, Decreased

See Confusion, Acute; Confusion, Chronic

Lice

Pruritus r/t inflammation

Impaired **Home** maintenance r/t close unsanitary, overcrowded conditions

Readiness for enhanced **Therapeutic** regimen management: r/t preventing and treating infestation

See Communicable Diseases, Childhood

Lifestyle, sedentary

Sedentary **Lifestyle** (See **Lifestyle**, sedentary, Section III)

Lightheadedness

See Dizziness; Vertigo

Limb Reattachment Procedures

Anxiety r/t unknown outcome of reattachment procedure, use and appearance of limb

Disturbed **Body** image r/t unpredictability of function and appearance of reattached body part

Grieving r/t unknown outcome of reattachment procedure

Risk for deficient **Fluid** volume: hemorrhage: Risk factor: severed vessels

Risk for impaired **Religiosity**: Risk factors: suffering, hospitalization

Risk for perioperative positioning **Injury**: Risk factor: immobilization

Risk for **Peripheral** neurovascular dysfunction: Risk factors: trauma, orthopedic and neurovascular surgery, compression of nerves and blood vessels

Risk for **Powerlessness**: Risk factor: unknown outcome of procedure

Spiritual distress r/t anxiety about condition

Stress overload r/t multiple coexisting stressors, physical demands

See Surgery, Postoperative Care

Liposuction

Disturbed **Body** image r/t dissatisfaction with unwanted fat deposits in body

Readiness for enhanced **Decision** making r/t expressed desire to make decision regarding liposuction

Readiness for enhanced **Self-concept** r/t satisfaction with new body image

See Surgery, Perioperative Care; Surgery, Postoperative Care; Surgery, Preoperative Care

Lithotripsy

Readiness for enhanced **Therapeutic** regimen management: expresses desire for information related to procedure and after care and prevention of stones

See Kidney Stone

Liver Biopsy

Anxiety r/t procedure and results

Risk for deficient **Fluid** volume r/t hemorrhage from biopsy site

Risk for **Powerlessness** r/t inability to control outcome of procedure

Liver Disease

See Cirrhosis; Hepatitis

Liver Function

Risk for impaired **Liver** function: Risk factors (See **Liver** function, risk for impaired, Section III)

Liver Transplant

Decisional **Conflict** r/t acceptance of donor liver

Ineffective **Protection** r/t immunosuppressive therapy

Readiness for enhanced **Family** processes: change in physical needs of family member

Readiness for enhanced **Spiritual** well-being: heightened coping

Readiness for enhanced **Therapeutic** regimen management: desire to manage the treatment and prevention of complications posttransplant

Risk for impaired **Liver** function: Risk factors: possible rejection, infection

See Surgery, Perioperative Care; Surgery, Postoperative Care; Surgery, Preoperative Care

Living Will

Moral distress r/t end-of-life decisions

Readiness for enhanced **Decision Making**: expresses desire to enhance understanding of choices for decision making

Readiness for enhanced **Religiosity** r/t request to meet with religious leaders or facilitators

Readiness for enhanced **Spiritual** well-being r/t acceptance of and preparation for end of life

See Advance Directives

Lobectomy

See Thoracotomy

Loneliness

Readiness for enhanced **Hope** r/t expresses desire to enhance interconnectedness with others

Risk for impaired **Religiosity**: Risk factor: lack of social interaction

Risk for **Loneliness**: Risk factors (See **Loneliness**, risk for, Section III)

Risk for situational low **Self-esteem**: Risk factors: failure, rejection

Spiritual distress r/t loneliness, social alienation

Loose Stools

Diarrhea r/t increased gastric motility

See cause of Loose Stools

Loss of Bladder Control

See Incontinence of Urine

Loss of Bowel Control

See Incontinence of Stool

Lou Gehrig's Disease

See ALS (Amyotrophic Lateral Sclerosis)

Low Back Pain

Chronic **Pain** r/t degenerative processes, musculotendinous strain, injury, inflammation, congenital deformities

Impaired physical **Mobility** r/t back pain

Ineffective **Health** maintenance r/t deficient knowledge regarding self-care with back pain

Readiness for enhanced **Therapeutic** regimen management: expressed desire for information to manage pain

Risk for **Powerlessness**: Risk factor: living with chronic pain

Urinary retention r/t possible spinal cord compression

Lumbar Puncture

Acute **Pain**: headache r/t possible loss of cerebrospinal fluid

Anxiety r/t invasive procedure and unknown results

Deficient **Knowledge** r/t information about procedure

Risk for **Infection**: Risk factor: invasive procedure

Lumpectomy

Decisional **Conflict** r/t treatment choices

Readiness for enhanced **Knowledge** r/t preoperative and postoperative care

Readiness for enhanced **Spiritual** well-being r/t hope of benign diagnosis

See Cancer

Lung Cancer

See Cancer; Chemotherapy; Radiation Therapy; Thoracotomy

Lupus Erythematosus

Acute **Pain** r/t inflammatory process

Chronic **Sorrow** r/t presence of chronic illness

Disturbed **Body** image r/t change in skin, rash, lesions, ulcers, mottled erythema

Fatigue r/t increased metabolic requirements

Impaired **Religiosity** r/t ineffective coping with disease

Ineffective **Health** maintenance r/t deficient knowledge regarding medication, diet, activity

Powerlessness r/t unpredictability of course of disease

Risk for impaired **Skin** integrity: Risk factors: chronic inflammation, edema, altered circulation

Spiritual distress r/t chronicity of disease, unknown etiology

Lyme Disease

Acute **Pain** r/t inflammation of joints, urticaria, rash

Deficient **Knowledge** r/t lack of information concerning disease, prevention, treatment

Fatigue r/t increased energy requirements

Risk for decreased **Cardiac** output: Risk factor: dysrhythmia

Risk for **Powerlessness**: Risk factor: possible chronic condition

L

Lymphedema

Deficient **Knowledge** r/t management of condition

Disturbed **Body** image r/t change in appearance of body part with edema

Excess **Fluid** volume r/t compromised regulatory system; inflammation, obstruction, or removal of lymph glands

Risk for situational low **Self-esteem** r/t disturbed body image

Lymphoma

See Cancer

Macular Degeneration

Compromised **Family** coping r/t deteriorating vision of family member

Disturbed **Sensory** perception: visual r/t blurred, distorted, dim, or absent central vision

Effective management of **Therapeutic** regimen: appropriate choices of daily activities for meeting the goals of a treatment program

Hopelessness r/t deteriorating vision

Ineffective **Coping** r/t visual loss

Risk for **Falls**: Risk factor: visual difficulties

Risk for impaired **Religiosity**: Risk factor: possible lack of transportation

Risk for **Injury**: Risk factor: inability to distinguish traffic lights

Risk for **Powerlessness**: Risk factor: deteriorating vision

Risk prone health **Behavior** r/t deteriorating vision

Sedentary **Lifestyle** r/t visual loss

Social isolation r/t inability to drive because of visual changes

Magnetic Resonance Imaging

See MRI (Magnetic Resonance Imaging)

Major Depressive Disorder

Interrupted **Family** processes r/t change in health status of family member

Risk for **Loneliness**: Risk factors: social isolation associated with feelings of sadness, hopelessness

See Depression (Major Depressive Disorder)

Malabsorption Syndrome

Deficient **Knowledge** r/t lack of information about diet and nutrition

Diarrhea r/t lactose intolerance, gluten sensitivity, resection of small bowel

Imbalanced **Nutrition**: less than body requirements r/t inability of body to absorb nutrients because of biological factors

Risk for deficient **Fluid** volume: Risk factor: diarrhea

Risk for disproportionate **Growth**: Risk factor: malnutrition from malabsorption

See Abdominal Distention

Maladaptive Behavior

See Crisis; Post-trauma Syndrome; Suicide Attempt

Malaise

See Fatigue

Malaria

Contamination r/t geographic area

Readiness for enhanced community **Coping**: Uses resources available for problem solving

Readiness for enhanced **Immunization** status: expresses desire to enhance immunization status and knowledge of immunization standards

Risk for **Contamination**: Risk factors: increased environmental exposure (not wearing protective clothing, not using insecticide or repellant on skin and in room in areas where infected mosquitoes are present); inadequate defense mechanisms (inappropriate use of prophylactic regimen)

See Anemia

Malignancy

See Cancer

Malignant Hypertension (Arteriolar Nephrosclerosis)

Decreased **Cardiac** output r/t altered afterload, altered contractility

Disturbed **Sensory** perception: visual r/t altered sensory reception from papilledema

Excess **Fluid** volume r/t decreased renal function

Fatigue r/t disease state, increased blood pressure

Readiness for enhanced **Therapeutic** regimen: management expresses desire to manage the illness, high blood pressure

Risk for acute **Confusion**: Risk factors: increased blood urea nitrogen or creatine levels

Risk for imbalanced **Fluid** volume: Risk factors: hypertension, altered renal function

Malignant Hyperthermia

Effective **Therapeutic** regimen management: verbalizes desire to manage the treatment of illness; informs health care providers of anesthesia problems

Hyperthermia r/t anesthesia reaction associated with inherited condition

Malnutrition

Adult **Failure** to thrive r/t undetected malnutrition

Deficient **Knowledge** r/t misinformation about normal nutrition, social isolation, lack of food preparation facilities

Imbalanced **Nutrition**: less than body requirements r/t inability to ingest food, digest food, or absorb nutrients because of biological, psychological, or economic factors; institutionalization (i.e., lack of menu choices)

Ineffective **Protection** r/t inadequate nutrition

Ineffective **Therapeutic** regimen management r/t economic difficulties

Risk for disproportionate **Growth**: Risk factor: malnutrition

Risk for **Powerlessness**: Risk factor: possible inability to provide adequate nutrition

Mammography

Effective **Therapeutic** regimen management: verbalizes desire to manage prevention of sequelae; follows guidelines for mammograms

Health-seeking behaviors: information regarding mammograms

Manic Disorder, Bipolar I

Anxiety r/t change in role function

Deficient **Fluid** volume r/t decreased intake

Disturbed **Thought** processes r/t mania

Imbalanced **Nutrition**: less than body requirements r/t lack of time and motivation to eat, constant movement

Impaired **Home** maintenance r/t altered psychological state, inability to concentrate

Ineffective **Coping** r/t situational crisis

Ineffective **Denial** r/t fear of inability to control behavior

Ineffective **Role** performance r/t impaired social interactions

Interrupted **Family** processes r/t family member's illness

Ineffective **Therapeutic** regimen management r/t lack of social supports

Ineffective **Therapeutic** regimen management: families r/t unpredictability of client, excessive demands on family, chronicity of condition

Insomnia r/t constant anxious thoughts

Noncompliance r/t denial of illness

Readiness for enhanced **Hope** r/t expresses desire to enhance problem-solving goals

Risk for **Caregiver** role strain r/t unpredictability of condition

Risk for impaired **Religiosity**: Risk factor: depression

Risk for **Powerlessness**: Risk factor: inability to control changes in mood

Risk for self- or other-directed **Violence**: Risk factors: hallucinations, delusions

Risk for **Spiritual** distress: Risk factor: depression

Risk for **Suicide**: Risk factor: bipolar disorder

Sleep deprivation r/t hyperagitated state

Manipulation of Organs, Surgical Incision

Deficient **Knowledge** r/t lack of exposure to information regarding care after surgery and at home

Risk for **Infection**: Risk factor: presence of urinary catheter

Urinary retention r/t swelling of urinary meatus

Manipulative Behavior

Defensive **Coping** r/t superior attitude toward others

Impaired **Social** interaction r/t self-concept disturbance

Ineffective **Coping** r/t inappropriate use of defense mechanisms

Risk for **Loneliness**: Risk factor: inability to interact appropriately with others

Risk for **Self-mutilation**: Risk factor: inability to cope with increased psychological or physiological tension in healthy manner

Risk for situational low **Self-esteem** Risk factor: history of learned helplessness

Self-mutilation r/t use of manipulation to obtain nurturing relationship with others

Marasmus

See Failure to Thrive, Nonorganic

Marfan Syndrome

Decreased **Cardiac** output r/t dilation of the aortic root, dissection or rupture of the aorta

Disturbed **Sensory** perception; visual r/t myopia associated with Marfan syndrome

Effective **Therapeutic** regimen management: Verbalizes desire to manage the treatment of illness and intent to reduce risk factors for progression of illness

Readiness for enhanced **Therapeutic** regimen management: Describes reduction of risk factors

See Mitral Valve Prolapse; Scoliosis

Marshall-Marchetti-Krantz Operation

PREOPERATIVE

Stress urinary **Incontinence** r/t weak pelvic muscles and pelvic supports

POSTOPERATIVE

Acute **Pain** r/t manipulation of organs, surgical incision

Deficient **Knowledge** r/t lack of exposure to information regarding care after surgery and at home

Risk for **Infection** r/t presence of urinary catheter

Urinary retention r/t swelling of urinary meatus

Mastectomy

Acute **Pain** r/t surgical procedure

Chronic **Sorrow** r/t disturbed body image, unknown long-term health status

Death **Anxiety** r/t threat of mortality associated with breast cancer

Deficient **Knowledge** r/t self-care activities

Disturbed **Body** image r/t loss of sexually significant body part

Fear r/t change in body image, prognosis

Nausea r/t chemotherapy

Risk for impaired physical **Mobility**: Risk factors: nerve or muscle damage, pain

Risk for **Post-trauma** syndrome: Risk factors: loss of body part, surgical wounds

Risk for **Powerlessness**: Risk factor: fear of unknown outcome of procedure

Sexual dysfunction r/t change in body image, fear of loss of femininity

Spiritual distress r/t change in body image

See Cancer; Modified Radical Mastectomy; Surgery, Perioperative; Surgery, Postoperative; Surgery, Preoperative

Mastitis

Acute **Pain** r/t infectious disease process, swelling of breast tissue

Anxiety r/t threat to self, concern over safety of milk for infant

Deficient **Knowledge** r/t antibiotic regimen, comfort measures

Ineffective **Breastfeeding** r/t breast pain, conflicting advice from health care providers

Ineffective **Role** performance r/t change in capacity to function in expected role

Maternal Infection

Ineffective **Protection** r/t invasive procedures, traumatized tissue

See Postpartum, Normal Care

Maturational Issues, Adolescent

Deficient **Knowledge**: potential for enhanced health maintenance r/t information misinterpretation, lack of education regarding age-related factors

Impaired **Social** interaction r/t ineffective, unsuccessful, or dysfunctional interaction with peers

Ineffective **Coping** r/t maturational crises

Interrupted **Family** processes r/t developmental crises of adolescence resulting from challenge of parental authority and values, situational crises from change in parental marital status

Readiness for enhanced **Communication**: expressing willingness to communicate with parental figures

Risk for **Injury/Trauma**: Risk factor: thrill-seeking behaviors

Risk for situational low **Self-esteem**: Risk factor: developmental changes

Risk-prone health **Behavior** r/t inadequate comprehension, negative attitude toward health care

Social isolation r/t perceived alteration in physical appearance, social values not accepted by dominant peer group

See Sexuality, Adolescent; Substance Abuse (if relevant)

Maze III Procedure

See Open Heart Surgery; Dysrhythmia

Measles (Rubeola)

See Communicable Diseases, Childhood

Meconium Aspiration

See Respiratory Conditions of the Neonate

Melanoma

Acute **Pain** r/t surgical incision

Disturbed **Body** image r/t altered pigmentation, surgical incision

Fear r/t threat to well-being

Ineffective **Health** maintenance r/t deficient knowledge regarding self-care and treatment of melanoma

See Cancer

Melena

Fear r/t presence of blood in feces

Risk for deficient **Fluid** volume: Risk factor: hemorrhage

See GI Bleed (Gastrointestinal Bleeding)

Memory Deficit

Impaired **Memory** (See **Memory**, impaired, Section III)

Ménière's Disease

Effective management of **Therapeutic** regimen; prompt treatment of ear infection

Readiness for enhanced **Therapeutic** regimen management: expresses desire to manage illness

Risk for **Injury**: r/t symptoms from disease

See Dizziness; Nausea; Vertigo

Meningitis/Encephalitis

Acute **Pain** r/t biological injury

Decreased **Intracranial** adaptive capacity r/t sustained increase in intracranial pressure of 10 to 15 mm Hg

Delayed **Growth** and development r/t effects of physical disability

Disturbed **Sensory** perception: hearing r/t central nervous system infection, ear infection

Disturbed **Sensory** perception: kinesthetic r/t central nervous system infection

Disturbed **Sensory** perception: visual r/t photophobia attributable to central nervous system infection

Disturbed **Thought** processes r/t inflammation of brain, fever

Excess **Fluid** volume r/t increased intracranial pressure, syndrome of inappropriate secretion of antidiuretic hormone

Impaired **Mobility** r/t neuromuscular or central nervous system insult

Ineffective **Airway** clearance r/t seizure activity

Ineffective **Tissue** perfusion: cerebral r/t inflamed cerebral tissues and meninges, increased intracranial pressure

Readiness for enhanced **Immunization** status r/t expresses desire to enhance immunization status and knowledge of immunization standards

Risk for acute **Confusion** r/t infection of brain

Risk for **Aspiration**: Risk factor: seizure activity

Risk for **Falls**: Risk factor: neuromuscular dysfunction

Risk for **Injury**: Risk factor: seizure activity

See Hospitalized Child

M

Meningocele

See Neural Tube Defects

Menopause

Health-seeking behavior: expresses desire for increased control of health practice

Impaired **Memory** r/t change in hormonal levels

Ineffective **Sexuality** pattern r/t altered body structure, lack of physiological lubrication, lack of knowledge of artificial lubrication

Ineffective **Thermoregulation** r/t changes in hormonal levels

Readiness for enhanced **Spiritual** well-being r/t desire for harmony of mind, body, and spirit

Readiness for enhanced **Therapeutic** regimen management: verbalized desire to manage menopause

Readiness for enhanced **Self-care**: expresses satisfaction with body image

Risk for imbalanced **Nutrition**: more than body requirements: Risk factor: change in metabolic rate caused by fluctuating hormone levels

Risk for **Powerlessness**: Risk factor: changes associated with menopause

Risk for situational low **Self-esteem**: Risk factors: developmental changes: menopause

Risk for urge urinary **Incontinence**: Risk factor: changes in hormonal levels affecting bladder function

Menorrhagia

Fear r/t loss of large amounts of blood

Risk for deficient **Fluid** volume r/t excessive loss of menstrual blood

Mental Illness

Chronic **Sorrow** r/t presence of mental illness

Compromised family **Coping** r/t lack of available support from client

Defensive **Coping** r/t psychological impairment, substance abuse

Disabled family **Coping** r/t chronically unexpressed feelings of guilt, anxiety, hostility, or despair

Disturbed **Thought** processes: inaccurate interpretation of environment, inappropriate thinking

Ineffective community **Therapeutic** regimen management: insufficient health care resources/programs

Ineffective **Coping** r/t situational crisis, coping with mental illness

Ineffective **Denial** r/t refusal to acknowledge abuse problem, fear of the social stigma of disease

Ineffective family **Therapeutic** regimen management r/t chronicity of condition, unpredictability of client, unknown prognosis

Risk for **Loneliness**: Risk factor: social isolation

Risk for **Powerlessness**: Risk factor: lifestyle of helplessness

Stress overload r/t multiple coexisting stressors

Mental Retardation

Delayed **Growth** and development r/t cognitive or perceptual impairment, developmental delay

Grieving r/t loss of perfect child, birth of child with congenital defect or subsequent head injury

Impaired **Home** maintenance r/t insufficient support systems

Impaired **Swallowing** r/t neuromuscular impairment

Impaired verbal **Communication** r/t developmental delay

Interrupted **Family** processes r/t crisis of diagnosis and situational transition

Readiness for enhanced family **Coping**: adaptation and acceptance of child's condition and needs

Risk for delayed **Development**: Risk factor: cognitive or perceptual impairment

Risk for disproportionate **Growth**: Risk factor: mental retardation

Risk for impaired **Religiosity**: Risk factor: social isolation

Risk for **Self-mutilation**: Risk factors: separation anxiety, depersonalization

Self-care deficit: bathing, hygiene, dressing, grooming, feeding, toileting r/t perceptual or cognitive impairment

Self-mutilation r/t inability to express tension verbally

Spiritual distress r/t chronic condition of child with special needs

Stress overload r/t intense, repeated stressor (chronic condition)

See Child with Chronic Condition; Safety, Childhood

Metabolic Acidosis

See Ketoacidosis, Diabetic; Ketoacidosis, Alcoholic

Metabolic Alkalosis

Deficient **Fluid** volume r/t fluid volume loss, vomiting, gastric suctioning, failure of regulatory mechanisms

Metastasis

See Cancer

MI (Myocardial Infarction)

Acute **Pain** r/t myocardial tissue damage from inadequate blood supply

Anxiety r/t threat of death, possible change in role status

Constipation r/t decreased peristalsis from decreased physical activity, medication effect, change in diet

Death **Anxiety** r/t seriousness of medical condition

Decreased **Cardiac** output r/t ventricular damage, ischemia, dysrhythmias

Fear r/t threat to well-being

Ineffective **Denial** r/t fear, deficient knowledge about heart disease

Ineffective family **Coping** r/t spouse or significant other's fear of partner loss

Ineffective **Health** maintenance r/t deficient knowledge regarding self-care and treatment

M

Ineffective **Sexuality** pattern r/t fear of chest pain, possibility of heart damage

Ineffective **Therapeutic** regimen management r/t knowledge deficit

Interrupted **Family** processes r/t crisis, role change

Readiness for enhanced **Knowledge**: expresses an interest in learning about condition

Risk for **Powerlessness**: Risk factor: acute illness

Risk for **Spiritual** distress: Risk factors: physical illness: MI

Situational low **Self-esteem** r/t crisis of MI

MIDCAB (Minimally Invasive Direct Coronary Artery Bypass)

Readiness for enhanced **Therapeutic** regimen management: pre- and postoperative care associated with the surgery

Risk for **Infection**: Risk factor: large breasts on incision line

See Angioplasty, Coronary; Coronary Artery Bypass Grafting

Midlife Crisis

Ineffective **Coping** r/t inability to deal with changes associated with aging

Powerlessness r/t lack of control over life situation

Readiness for enhanced **Spiritual** well-being: desire to find purpose and meaning to life

Spiritual distress r/t questioning beliefs or value system

Migraine Headache

Acute **Pain**: headache r/t vasodilation of cerebral and extracerebral vessels

Disturbed **Energy** field r/t pain, disruption of normal flow of energy

Ineffective **Health** maintenance r/t deficient knowledge regarding prevention and treatment of headaches

Readiness for enhanced **Therapeutic** regimen management: expressed desire to manage the illness

Milk Intolerance

See Lactose Intolerance

Minimally Invasive Heart Surgery

See MIDCAB (Minimally Invasive Direct Coronary Artery Bypass); OPCAB (Off-Pump Coronary Artery Bypass)

Miscarriage

See Pregnancy Loss

Mitral Stenosis

Activity intolerance r/t imbalance between oxygen supply and demand

Anxiety r/t possible worsening of symptoms, activity intolerance, fatigue

Decreased **Cardiac** output r/t incompetent heart valves, abnormal forward or backward blood flow, flow into a dilated chamber, flow through an abnormal passage between chambers

Fatigue r/t reduced cardiac output

Ineffective **Health** maintenance r/t deficient knowledge regarding self-care with disorder

Mitral Valve Prolapse

Acute **Pain** r/t mitral valve regurgitation

Anxiety r/t symptoms of condition: palpitations, chest pain

Effective management of **Therapeutic** regimen: verbalizes desire to manage prevention of sequelae

Fatigue r/t abnormal catecholamine regulation, decreased intravascular volume

Fear r/t lack of knowledge about mitral valve prolapse, feelings of having a heart attack

Ineffective **Health** maintenance r/t deficient knowledge regarding methods to relieve pain and treat dysrhythmia and shortness of breath, need for prophylactic antibiotics before invasive procedures

Ineffective **Tissue** perfusion: cerebral r/t postural hypotension

Readiness for enhanced **Knowledge**: expresses an interest in learning about condition

Risk for **Infection**: Risk factor: invasive procedures

Risk for **Powerlessness**: Risk factor: unpredictability of onset of symptoms

Mobility, Impaired Bed

Impaired bed **Mobility** (See **Mobility**, impaired bed, Section III)

Mobility, Impaired Physical

Impaired physical **Mobility** (See **Mobility**, impaired physical, Section III)

Risk for **Falls** r/t impaired physical mobility

Mobility, Impaired Wheelchair

Impaired wheelchair **Mobility** (See **Mobility**, impaired wheelchair, Section III)

Modified Radical Mastectomy

Decisional **Conflict** r/t treatment of choice

Readiness for enhanced **Communication**: willingness to enhance communication

See Mastectomy

Mononucleosis

Activity intolerance r/t generalized weakness

Acute **Pain** r/t enlargement of lymph nodes, oropharyngeal edema

Fatigue r/t disease state, stress

Hyperthermia r/t infectious process

Impaired **Swallowing** r/t enlargement of lymph nodes, oropharyngeal edema

Ineffective **Health** maintenance r/t deficient knowledge concerning transmission and treatment of disease

Risk for **Injury**: Risk factor: possible rupture of spleen

Risk for **Loneliness**: Risk factor: social isolation

Mood Disorders

Caregiver role strain r/t symptoms associated with disorder of care receiver

Readiness for enhanced **Communication**: expresses feelings

Risk for situational low **Self-esteem**: Risk factor: unpredictable changes in mood

Risk-prone health **Behavior** r/t hopelessness, altered locus of control

Social isolation r/t alterations in mental status

See Specific Disorder: Depression; Dysthymic Disorder; Hypomania; Manic Disorder, Bipolar I

Moon Face

Disturbed **Body** image r/t change in appearance from disease and medication

Risk for situational low **Self-esteem**: Risk factor: change in body image

See Cushing's Syndrome

Moral/Ethical Dilemmas

Decisional **Conflict** r/t questioning personal values and belief, which alter decision

Moral Distress r/t conflicting information guiding moral or ethical decision making

Readiness for enhanced **Decision** making: expresses desire to enhance congruency of decisions with personal values and goals

Readiness for enhanced **Religiosity**: requests assistance in expanding religious options

Readiness for enhanced **Spiritual** well-being: request for interaction with others regarding difficult decisions

Risk for **Powerlessness**: Risk factor: lack of knowledge to make a decision

Risk for **Spiritual** distress: Risk factor: moral or ethical crisis

Morning Sickness

See Hyperemesis Gravidarum; Pregnancy, Normal

Mottling of Peripheral Skin

Ineffective **Tissue** perfusion: peripheral r/t interruption of arterial flow, decreased circulating blood volume

Mourning

See Grieving

Mouth Lesions

See Mucous Membranes, Impaired Oral

MRI (Magnetic Resonance Imaging)

Anxiety r/t fear of being in closed spaces

Deficient **Knowledge** r/t unfamiliarity with information resources; exam information

Readiness for enhanced **Knowledge**: expresses interest in learning about exam

Readiness for enhanced **Therapeutic** regimen management: describes reduction of risk factors associated with exam

Mucocutaneous Lymph Node Syndrome

See Kawasaki Syndrome

Mucous Membranes, Impaired Oral

Impaired **Oral** mucous membranes (See **Oral** mucous membranes, impaired, Section III)

Multiinfarct Dementia

See Dementia

Multiple Gestation

Anxiety r/t uncertain outcome of pregnancy

Death **Anxiety** r/t maternal complications associated with multiple gestation

Deficient **Knowledge** r/t caring for more than one infant

Fatigue r/t physiological demands of a multifetal pregnancy and/or care of more than one infant

Imbalanced **Nutrition**: less than body requirements r/t physiological demands of a multifetal pregnancy

Impaired **Home** maintenance r/t fatigue

Impaired physical **Mobility** r/t increased uterine size

Impaired **Transfer** ability r/t enlarged uterus

Insomnia r/t impairment of normal sleep pattern; parental responsibilities

Readiness for enhanced **Family** processes: family adapting to change with more than one infant

Risk for **Constipation**: Risk factor: enlarged uterus

Risk for delayed **Development**: fetus: Risk factor: multiple gestation

Risk for disproportionate **Growth**: fetus: Risk factor: multiple gestation

Risk for ineffective **Breastfeeding**: Risk factors: lack of support, physical demands of feeding more than one infant

Stress overload r/t multiple coexisting stressors, family demands

Stress urinary **Incontinence** r/t increased pelvic pressure

Multiple Personality Disorder (Dissociative Identity Disorder)

Anxiety r/t loss of control of behavior and feelings

Chronic low **Self-esteem** r/t rejection, failure

Defensive **Coping** r/t unresolved past traumatic events, severe anxiety

Disturbed **Body** image r/t psychosocial changes

Disturbed personal **Identity** r/t severe child abuse

Hopelessness r/t long-term stress

Ineffective **Coping** r/t history of abuse

Readiness for enhanced **Communication**: willingness to discuss problems associated with condition

Risk for **Self-mutilation**: Risk factor: need to act out to relieve stress

See Dissociative Identity Disorder (Not Otherwise Specified)

Multiple Sclerosis (MS)

Chronic **Sorrow** r/t loss of physical ability

Disturbed **Energy** field r/t disruption in energy flow resulting from disharmony between mind and body

Disturbed **Sensory** perception: specify r/t pathology in sensory tracts

M

Impaired physical **Mobility** r/t neuromuscular impairment

Ineffective **Airway** clearance r/t decreased energy or fatigue

Powerlessness r/t progressive nature of disease

Readiness for enhanced **Self-care**: expresses desire to enhance knowledge of strategies and responsibility for self-care

Readiness for enhanced **Spiritual** well-being: struggling with chronic debilitating condition

Readiness for enhanced **Therapeutic** regimen management: expresses a desire to manage condition

Risk for **Disuse** syndrome: Risk factor: physical immobility

Risk for imbalanced **Nutrition**: less than body requirements: Risk factors: impaired swallowing, depression

Risk for impaired **Religiosity**: Risk factor: illness

Risk for **Injury**: Risk factors: altered mobility, sensory dysfunction

Risk for latex **Allergy** response: Risk factor: possible repeated exposures to latex associated with intermittent catheterizations

Risk for **Powerlessness**: Risk factor: chronic illness

Self-care deficit: specify r/t neuromuscular impairment

Sexual dysfunction r/t biopsychosocial alteration of sexuality

Spiritual distress r/t perceived hopelessness of diagnosis

Urinary retention r/t inhibition of the reflex arc

See Neurological Disorders

Mumps

See Communicable Diseases, Childhood

Murmurs

Decreased **Cardiac** output r/t altered preload/afterload

Muscular Atrophy/Weakness

Risk for **Disuse** syndrome: Risk factor: impaired physical mobility

Risk for **Falls**: Risk factor: impaired physical mobility

Muscular Dystrophy (MD)

Activity intolerance r/t fatigue

Constipation r/t immobility

Decreased **Cardiac** output r/t effects of congestive heart failure

Disturbed **Energy** field r/t illness

Fatigue r/t increased energy requirements to perform activities of daily living

Imbalanced **Nutrition**: less than body requirements r/t impaired swallowing or chewing

Imbalanced **Nutrition**: more than body requirements r/t inactivity

Impaired **Mobility** r/t muscle weakness and development of contractures

Impaired **Transfer** ability r/t muscle weakness

Impaired **Walking** r/t muscle weakness

Ineffective **Airway** clearance r/t muscle weakness and decreased ability to cough

Readiness for enhanced **Self-concept**: acceptance of strength and abilities

Risk for **Aspiration**: Risk factor: impaired swallowing

Risk for **Disuse** syndrome: Risk factor: complications of immobility

Risk for **Falls**: Risk factor: muscle weakness

Risk for impaired **Gas** exchange: Risk factor: ineffective airway clearance and ineffective breathing pattern caused by muscle weakness

Risk for impaired **Religiosity**: Risk factor: illness

Risk for impaired **Skin** integrity: Risk factors: immobility, braces, or adaptive devices

Risk for ineffective **Breathing** pattern: Risk factor: muscle weakness

Risk for **Infection**: Risk factor: pooling of pulmonary secretions as a result of immobility and muscle weakness

Risk for **Injury**: Risk factor: muscle weakness and unsteady gait

Risk for **Powerlessness**: Risk factor: chronic condition

Risk for situational low **Self-esteem**: Risk factor: presence of chronic condition

Self-care deficits: feeding, bathing, dressing, toileting r/t muscle weakness and fatigue

See Child with Chronic Condition; Hospitalized Child

MVA (Motor Vehicle Accident)

See Fracture; Head Injury; Injury; Pneumothorax

Myasthenia Gravis

Fatigue r/t paresthesia, aching muscles

Imbalanced **Nutrition**: less than body requirements r/t difficulty eating and swallowing

Impaired physical **Mobility** r/t defective transmission of nerve impulses at the neuromuscular junction

Impaired **Swallowing** r/t neuromuscular impairment

Ineffective **Airway** clearance r/t decreased ability to cough and swallow

Ineffective **Therapeutic** regimen management r/t lack of knowledge of treatment, uncertainty of outcome

Interrupted **Family** processes r/t crisis of dealing with diagnosis

Readiness for enhanced **Spiritual** well-being: heightened coping with serious illness

Risk for **Caregiver** role strain: Risk factor: severity of illness of client

Risk for impaired **Religiosity**: Risk factor: illness

See Neurological Disorders

Mycoplasma Pneumonia

See Pneumonia

Myelocele

See Neural Tube Defects

Myelogram, Contrast

Acute **Pain** r/t irritation of nerve roots

Risk for deficient **Fluid** volume: Risk factor: possible dehydration

Risk for ineffective **Tissue** perfusion: cerebral: Risk factors: hypotension, loss of cerebrospinal fluid

Urinary retention r/t pressure on spinal nerve roots

Myelomeningocele

See Neural Tube Defects

Myocardial Infarction

See MI (Myocardial Infarction)

Myocarditis

Activity intolerance r/t reduced cardiac reserve and prescribed bed rest

Decreased **Cardiac** output r/t altered preload/afterload

Deficient **Knowledge** r/t treatment of disease

Readiness for enhanced **Knowledge** of treatment of disease

See CHF (Congestive Heart Failure), if appropriate

Myringotomy

Acute **Pain** r/t surgical procedure

Disturbed **Sensory** perception r/t possible hearing impairment

Fear r/t hospitalization, surgical procedure

Ineffective **Health** maintenance r/t deficient knowledge regarding care after surgery

Risk for **Infection**: Risk factor: invasive procedure

Myxedema

See Hypothyroidism

N

Narcissistic Personality Disorder

Decisional **Conflict** r/t lack of realistic problem-solving skills

Defensive **Coping** r/t grandiose sense of self

Disturbed **Personal** identity r/t psychological impairment

Impaired **Social** interaction r/t self-concept disturbance

Interrupted **Family** processes r/t taking advantage of others to achieve own goals

Risk for **Loneliness** r/t inability to interact appropriately with others

Risk-prone health **Behavior**: Risk factor: low self-efficacy

Risk for **Self-mutilation**: Risk factor: inadequate coping

Narcolepsy

Anxiety r/t fear of lack of control over falling asleep

Insomnia r/t uncontrollable desire to sleep

Readiness for enhanced **Sleep**: expression of willingness to enhance sleep

Risk for **Trauma**: Risk factor: falling asleep during potentially dangerous activity

Narcotic Use

Risk for **Constipation**: Risk factor: effects of opioids on peristalsis

See Substance Abuse (if relevant)

Nasogastric Suction

Impaired **Oral** mucous membrane r/t presence of nasogastric tube

Risk for deficient **Fluid** volume: Risk factor: loss of gastrointestinal fluids without adequate replacement

Nausea

Nausea: biophysical, situational, treatment related (See **Nausea**, Section III)

Near-Drowning

Aspiration r/t aspiration of fluid into the lungs

Fear: parental r/t possible death of child, possible permanent and debilitating sequelae

Grieving/Risk for Complicated **Grieving** r/t potential death of child, unknown sequelae, guilt about accident

Hypothermia r/t central nervous system injury, prolonged submersion in cold water

Impaired **Gas** exchange r/t laryngospasm, holding breath, aspiration

Ineffective **Airway** clearance r/t aspiration, impaired gas exchange

Ineffective **Health** maintenance r/t parental deficient knowledge regarding safety measures appropriate for age

Readiness for enhanced **Spiritual** well-being: struggle with survival of life-threatening situation

Risk for delayed **Development** and disproportionate growth: Risk factors: hypoxemia, cerebral anoxia

Risk for **Infection**: Risk factors: aspiration, invasive monitoring

See Child with Chronic Condition; Hospitalized Child; Safety, Childhood; Terminally Ill Child/Death of Child, Parent

Nearsightedness

Effective **Therapeutic** regimen management: early diagnosis and appropriate referral for eyeglasses or contact lenses when nearsightedness is suspected; signs that may indicate a vision problem, including sitting close to television, holding books very close when reading, or having difficulty reading the blackboard in school or signs on a wall

Nearsightedness; Corneal Surgery

See LASIK Eye Surgery (Laser-Assisted in Situ Keratomileusis)

Neck Vein Distention

Decreased **Cardiac** output r/t decreased contractility of heart resulting increased preload

Excess **Fluid** volume r/t excess fluid intake, compromised regulatory mechanisms

See CHF (Congestive Heart Failure)

Necrosis, Renal Tubular; ATN (Acute Tubular Necrosis); Necrosis, Acute Tubular

See Renal Failure

Necrotizing Enterocolitis (NEC)

Deficient **Fluid** volume r/t vomiting, gastrointestinal bleeding

Disturbed **Energy** field r/t illness

Imbalanced **Nutrition**: less than body requirements r/t decreased ability to absorb nutrients, decreased perfusion to gastrointestinal tract

Ineffective **Breathing** pattern r/t abdominal distention, hypoxia

Ineffective **Tissue** perfusion: gastrointestinal r/t shunting of blood away from mesenteric circulation and toward vital organs as a result of perinatal stress, hypoxia

Risk for **Infection**: Risk factors: bacterial invasion of gastrointestinal tract, invasive procedures

See Hospitalized Child; Premature Infant (Child)

Necrotizing Fasciitis (Flesh-Eating Bacteria)

Acute **Pain** r/t toxins interfering with blood flow

Decreased **Cardiac** output r/t tachycardia and hypotension

Fear r/t possible fatal outcome of disease

Grieving r/t poor prognosis associated with disease

Hyperthermia r/t presence of infection

Ineffective **Protection** r/t cellulites resistant to treatment

Ineffective **Tissue** perfusion: peripheral r/t thrombosis of the subcutaneous blood vessels, leading to necrosis of nerve fibers

See Renal Failure; Septicemia; Shock

Negative Feelings About Self

Chronic low **Self-esteem** r/t longstanding negative self-evaluation

Readiness for enhanced **Self-concept** r/t expresses willingness to enhance self-concept

Self-esteem disturbance r/t inappropriate learned negative feelings about self

Neglect, Unilateral

See Neglect, Unilateral Section III

Neglectful Care of Family Member

Caregiver role strain r/t care demands of family member, lack of social or financial support

Deficient **Knowledge** r/t care needs

Disabled family **Coping** r/t highly ambivalent family relationships, lack of respite care

Ineffective community **Therapeutic** regimen management r/t deficits in community for support of caregivers, detection of client neglect

Interrupted **Family** processes r/t situational transition or crisis

Risk for compromised human **Dignity**: Risk factor: inadequate participation in decision making

Neonate

See Newborn, Normal; Newborn, Postmature; Newborn, Small for Gestational Age (SGA)

Neoplasm

Fear r/t possible malignancy

See Cancer

Nephrectomy

Acute **Pain** r/t incisional discomfort

Anxiety r/t surgical recovery, prognosis

Constipation r/t lack of return of peristalsis

Impaired **Urinary** elimination r/t loss of kidney

Ineffective **Breathing** pattern r/t location of surgical incision

Risk for deficient **Fluid** volume: Risk factors: vascular losses, decreased intake

Risk for **Infection** Risk factors: invasive procedure, lack of deep breathing because of location of surgical incision

Spiritual distress r/t chronic illness

Nephrostomy, Percutaneous

Acute **Pain** r/t invasive procedure

Impaired **Urinary** elimination r/t nephrostomy tube

Risk for **Infection**: Risk factor: invasive procedure

Nephrotic Syndrome

Activity intolerance r/t generalized edema

Disturbed **Body** image r/t edematous appearance and side effects of steroid therapy

Excess **Fluid** volume r/t edema resulting from oncotic fluid shift caused by serum protein loss and renal retention of salt and water

Imbalanced **Nutrition**: less than body requirements r/t anorexia, protein loss

Imbalanced **Nutrition**: more than body requirements r/t increased appetite attributable to steroid therapy

Risk for impaired **Skin** integrity: Risk factor: edema

Risk for **Infection**: Risk factor: altered immune mechanisms caused by disease and effects of steroids

Risk for **Noncompliance**: Risk factor: side effects of home steroid therapy

Social isolation r/t edematous appearance

See Child with Chronic Condition; Hospitalized Child

Nerve Entrapment

See Carpal Tunnel Syndrome

Neural Tube Defects (Meningocele, Myelomeningocele, Spina Bifida, Anencephaly)

Chronic low **Self-esteem** r/t perceived differences, decreased ability to participate in physical and social activities at school

Constipation r/t immobility or less than adequate mobility

Delayed **Growth** and development r/t physical impairments, possible cognitive impairment

Disturbed **Sensory** perception: visual r/t altered reception caused by strabismus

Grieving r/t loss of perfect child, birth of child with congenital defect

Impaired **Mobility** r/t neuromuscular impairment

Impaired **Skin** integrity r/t incontinence

Readiness for enhanced family **Coping**: effective adaptive response by family members

Readiness for enhanced **Family** processes: family supports each other

Reflex **Incontinence** r/t neurogenic impairment

Risk for imbalanced **Nutrition**: more than body requirements: Risk factors: diminished, limited, or impaired physical activity

Risk for impaired **Skin** integrity: lower extremities: Risk factor: decreased sensory perception

Risk for latex **Allergy** response: Risk factor: multiple exposures to latex products

Risk for **Powerlessness**: Risk factor: debilitating disease

Total urinary **Incontinence** r/t neurogenic impairment

Urge urinary **Incontinence** r/t neurogenic impairment

See Child with Chronic Condition; Premature Infant (Child)

Neuritis

Activity intolerance r/t pain with movement

Acute **Pain** r/t stimulation of affected nerve endings, inflammation of sensory nerves

Ineffective **Health** maintenance r/t deficient knowledge regarding self-care with neuritis

Neurofibromatosis

Compromised **Family** coping r/t cost and emotional needs of disease

Disturbed **Energy** field r/t disease

Disturbed **Sensory** perception r/t optic nerve gliomas associated with disease

Effective **Therapeutic** regimen management: evaluate visual disturbances associated with NF1 optic pathway tumors: dimness of vision, headache, visual field defects, nystagmus and distortion of binocular fixation, decreased visual acuity, proptosis or a droopy eyelid

Impaired **Skin** integrity r/t café-au-lait spots

Readiness for enhanced **Decision** making: expresses desire to enhance understanding of choices and meaning of choices, genetic counseling

Readiness for enhanced **Therapeutic** regimen management: seeks cancer screening, education and genetic counseling

Risk for delayed **Development**: learning disorders including attention deficit–hyperactivity disorder, low intelligent quotient scores, and developmental delay: Risk factor: genetic disorder

Risk for decreased **Cardiac** output: Risk factor: hypertension associated with condition

Risk for **Constipation**: Risk factor: intestinal neurofibromas

Risk for disproportionate **Growth**: short stature, precocious puberty, delayed maturation, thyroid disorders: Risk factor: genetic disorder

Risk for **Injury**: Risk factor: possible problems with balance

Risk for **Spiritual** distress: Risk factor: possible severity of disease

See Abdominal Distension; Surgery, Perioperative; Surgery, Postoperative; Surgery, Preoperative

Neurogenic Bladder

Overflow urinary **Incontinence** r/t detrusor external sphincter dyssynergia

Reflex **Incontinence** r/t neurological impairment

Risk for latex **Allergy** response: Risk factors: repeated exposures to latex associated with possible repeated catheterizations

Urinary retention r/t interruption in the lateral spinal tracts

Neurological Disorders

Acute **Confusion** r/t dementia, alcohol abuse, drug abuse, delirium

Disturbed **Energy** field r/t illness

Grieving r/t loss of usual body functioning

Imbalanced **Nutrition**: less than body requirements r/t impaired swallowing, depression, difficulty feeding self

Impaired **Home** maintenance r/t client's or family member's disease

Impaired **Memory** r/t neurological disturbance

Impaired physical **Mobility** r/t neuromuscular impairment

Impaired **Swallowing** r/t neuromuscular dysfunction

Ineffective **Airway** clearance r/t perceptual or cognitive impairment, decreased energy, fatigue

Ineffective **Coping** r/t disability requiring change in lifestyle

Interrupted **Family** processes r/t situational crisis, illness, or disability of family member

Powerlessness r/t progressive nature of disease

Risk for **Disuse** syndrome: Risk factors: physical immobility, neuromuscular dysfunction

Risk for impaired **Religiosity**: Risk factor: life transition

Risk for impaired **Skin** integrity: Risk factors: altered sensation, altered mental status, paralysis

Risk for **Injury**: Risk factors: altered mobility, sensory dysfunction, cognitive impairment

Self-care deficit: specify r/t neuromuscular dysfunction

Sexual dysfunction r/t biopsychosocial alteration of sexuality

Social isolation r/t altered state of wellness

Wandering r/t cognitive impairment

Neuropathy, Peripheral

Chronic **Pain** r/t damage to nerves in the peripheral nervous system as a result of medication side effects, vitamin deficiency, or diabetes

Ineffective **Thermoregulation** r/t decreased ability to regulate body temperature

Risk for **Injury**: Risk factors: lack of muscle control, decreased sensation

Risk for **Peripheral** neurovascular dysfunction: Risk factors: compression, entrapment

See Peripheral Vascular Disease

Neurosurgery

See Craniectomy/Craniotomy

Newborn, Normal

Effective **Breastfeeding** r/t normal oral structure and gestational age greater than 34 weeks

Ineffective **Protection** r/t immature immune system

Ineffective **Thermoregulation** r/t immaturity of neuroendocrine system

Readiness for enhanced organized **Infant** behavior r/t pain

Readiness for enhanced **Parenting**: providing emotional and physical needs of infant

Risk for **Infection**: Risk factor: open umbilical stump

Risk for **Injury**: Risk factors: immaturity, need for caretaking

Risk for sudden infant **Death** syndrome: Risk factors: lack of knowledge regarding infant sleeping in prone or side-lying position, prenatal or postnatal infant smoke exposure, infant overheating or overwrapping, loose articles in the sleep environment

Newborn, Postmature

Hypothermia r/t depleted stores of subcutaneous fat

Impaired **Skin** integrity r/t cracked and peeling skin as a result of decreased vernix

Risk for ineffective **Airway** clearance: Risk factor: meconium aspiration

Risk for unstable **Glucose** level: Risk factor: depleted glycogen stores

Risk for **Injury**: Risk factor: hypoglycemia caused by depleted glycogen stores

Newborn, Small for Gestational Age (SGA)

Imbalanced **Nutrition**: less than body requirements r/t history of placental insufficiency

Ineffective **Thermoregulation** r/t decreased brown fat, subcutaneous fat

Risk for delayed **Development**: Risk factor: history of placental insufficiency

Risk for disproportionate **Growth**: Risk factor: history of placental insufficiency

Risk for **Injury**: Risk factors: hypoglycemia, perinatal asphyxia, meconium aspiration

Risk for sudden infant **Death** syndrome: Risk factor: low birth weight

Nicotine Addiction

Ineffective **Health** maintenance r/t lack of ability to make a judgment about smoking cessation

Powerlessness r/t perceived lack of control over ability to give up nicotine

Readiness for enhanced **Decision** making: expresses desire to enhance understanding and meaning of choices

Readiness for enhanced **Therapeutic** regimen management: expresses desire to learn measures to stop smoking

NIDDM (Non-Insulin-Dependent Diabetes Mellitus)

Health-seeking behaviors r/t desiring information on exercise and diet to manage diabetes

See Diabetes Mellitus

Nightmares

Disturbed **Energy** field r/t disharmony of body and mind

Post-trauma syndrome r/t disaster, war, epidemic, rape, assault, torture, catastrophic illness, or accident

Rape-trauma syndrome: compound reaction or silent reaction r/t forced violent sexual penetration against the victim's will and consent

Nipple Soreness

Acute **Pain** r/t injury to nipples

See Painful Breasts, Sore Nipples

Nocturia

Impaired **Urinary** elimination r/t sensory motor impairment, urinary tract infection

Risk for **Powerlessness**: Risk factor: inability to control nighttime voiding

Total **Urinary** incontinence r/t neuropathy preventing transmission of reflex indicating bladder fullness; neurological dysfunction causing triggering of micturition at unpredictable times; independent contraction of detrusor reflex as result of surgery, trauma, or disease affecting spinal cord nerves; anatomical fistula

Urge urinary **Incontinence** r/t decreased bladder capacity, irritation of bladder stretch receptors causing spasm, alcohol, caffeine, increased fluids, increased urine concentration, overdistention of bladder

Nocturnal Myoclonus

See Restless Leg Syndrome; Stress

Nocturnal Paroxysmal Dyspnea

See PND (Paroxysmal Nocturnal Dyspnea)

Noncompliance

Noncompliance (See **Noncompliance**, Section III)

Non-Insulin-Dependent Diabetes Mellitus (NIDDM)

See Diabetes Mellitus

Normal Pressure Hydrocephalus (NPH)

Acute **Confusion** r/t dementia caused by obstruction to flow of cerebrospinal fluid

Impaired **Memory** r/t neurological disturbance

Impaired verbal **Communication** r/t obstruction of flow of cerebrospinal fluid

Ineffective **Tissue** perfusion: cerebral r/t obstruction to flow of cerebrospinal fluid as a result of closed-head injury, craniotomy, meningitis, or subarachnoid hemorrhage

Risk for **Falls**: Risk factor: unsteady gait as a result of obstruction of cerebrospinal fluid

Norwalk Virus

See Viral Gastroenteritis

NSTEMI (non-ST-elevation myocardial infarction)

See MI (Myocardial Infarction)

Nursing

See Breastfeeding, Effective; Breastfeeding, Ineffective; Breastfeeding, Interrupted

Nutrition

Readiness for enhanced **Nutrition** (See **Nutrition**, readiness for enhanced, Section III)

Nutrition, Imbalanced

Imbalanced **Nutrition**: less than body requirements (See **Nutrition**, imbalanced: less than body requirements, Section III)

Imbalanced **Nutrition**: more than body requirements (See **Nutrition**, imbalanced: more than body requirements, Section III)

Risk for imbalanced **Nutrition**: more than body requirements (See **Nutrition**, risk for imbalanced: more than body requirements, Section III)

Obesity

Chronic low **Self-esteem** r/t ineffective coping, overeating

Disturbed **Body** image r/t eating disorder, excess weight

Imbalanced **Nutrition**: more than body requirements r/t caloric intake exceeding energy expenditure

Readiness for enhanced **Nutrition**: expresses willingness to enhance nutrition

OBS (Organic Brain Syndrome)

See Organic Mental Disorders

Obsessive-Compulsive Disorder

Anxiety r/t threat to self-concept, unmet needs

Decisional **Conflict** r/t inability to make a decision for fear of reprisal

Disabled family **Coping** r/t family process being disrupted by client's ritualistic activities

Disturbed **Thought** processes r/t persistent thoughts, ideas, impulses that seem irrelevant and will not relent

Ineffective **Coping** r/t expression of feelings in an unacceptable way, ritualistic behavior

Powerlessness r/t unrelenting repetitive thoughts to perform irrational activities

Risk for situational low **Self-esteem**: Risk factor: inability to control repetitive thoughts and actions

Risk-prone health **Behavior** r/t inadequate comprehension associated with repetitive thoughts

Obstruction, Bowel

See Bowel Obstruction

Obstructive Sleep Apnea

Health-seeking behaviors r/t seeking nutritional information to control weight that may be contributing to sleep apnea

Imbalanced **Nutrition**: more than body requirements r/t excessive intake related to metabolic need

Insomnia r/t blocked airway

See PND (Paroxysmal Nocturnal Dyspnea)

ODD

See Oppositional Defiant Disorder (ODD)

Older Adult

See Aging

Oligohydramnios

Anxiety: maternal r/t fear of unknown, threat to fetus

Risk for **Injury**: fetal: Risk factor: decreased umbilical cord blood flow as a result of compression

Oliguria

Deficient **Fluid** volume r/t active fluid loss, failure of regulatory mechanism

See Cardiac Output Decrease; Renal Failure; Shock

Omphalocele

See Gastroschisis/Omphalocele

Onychomycosis

See Ringworm of Nails

Oophorectomy

Risk for ineffective **Sexuality** pattern: Risk factor: altered body function

See Surgery, Perioperative; Surgery, Postoperative; Surgery, Preoperative

OPCAB (Off-Pump Coronary Artery Bypass)

Acute **Confusion** r/t possible decreased cerebral tissue perfusion

Acute **Pain** r/t possible gastrointestinal dysfunction

Decreased **Cardiac** output r/t increased vasodilation

Impaired **Gas** exchange r/t alveolar-capillary membrane changes

Impaired **Memory** r/t possible decreased cerebral tissue perfusion

Readiness for enhanced **Therapeutic** regimen management r/t preoperative and postoperative care associated with surgery

Risk for deficient **Fluid** volume: Risk factor: bleeding associated with anticoagulant therapy

See Angioplasty, Coronary; Coronary Artery Bypass Grafting

O

Open Heart Surgery

Decreased **Cardiac** output r/t altered preload or afterload

Impaired **Gas** exchange r/t cardiac surgery

See Coronary Artery Bypass Grafting; Dysrhythmia

Open Reduction of Fracture with Internal Fixation (Femur)

Anxiety r/t outcome of corrective procedure

Impaired physical **Mobility** r/t postoperative position, abduction of leg, avoidance of acute flexion

Powerlessness r/t loss of control, unanticipated change in lifestyle

Risk for perioperative positioning **Injury**: Risk factor: immobilization

Risk for **Peripheral** neurovascular dysfunction: Risk factors: mechanical compression, orthopedic surgery, immobilization

See Surgery, Postoperative Care

Opiate Use

Risk for **Constipation**: Risk factor: effects of opiates on peristalsis

See Drug Abuse; Drug Withdrawal

Opportunistic Infection

Delayed **Surgical** recovery r/t abnormal blood profiles, impaired healing

Risk for **Infection**: Risk factor: abnormal blood profiles

See AIDS (Acquired Immune Deficiency Syndrome); HIV (Human Immunodeficiency Virus)

Oppositional Defiant Disorder (ODD)

Anxiety r/t feelings of anger and hostility toward authority figures

Chronic or situational low **Self-esteem** r/t poor self-control and disruptive behaviors

Disabled **Family** coping r/t feelings of anger, hostility; defiant behavior toward authority figures

Disturbed **Thought** processes r/t difficulty thinking, making appropriate decisions

Impaired **Social** interaction r/t being touchy or easily annoyed, blaming others for own mistakes, constant trouble in school

Ineffective **Coping** r/t lack of self-control or perceived lack of self-control

Ineffective family **Therapeutic** regimen management r/t difficulty in limit setting and managing oppositional behaviors

Risk for impaired **Parenting**: Risk factors: children's difficult behaviors and inability to set limits

Risk for other-directed **Violence**: Risk factors: history of violence, threats of violence against others; history of antisocial behavior; history of indirect violence

Risk for **Powerlessness**: Risk factor: inability to deal with difficulty behaviors

Risk for **Spiritual** distress: Risk factors: anxiety and stress in dealing with difficulty behaviors

Risk prone Health **Behavior** r/t multiple stressors associated with condition

Social isolation r/t unaccepted social behavior

Oral Mucous Membrane, Impaired

Impaired **Oral** mucous membrane (See **Oral**, mucous membrane, impaired, Section III)

Oral Thrush

See Candidiasis, Oral

Orchitis

Readiness for enhanced **Therapeutic** regimen management r/t follows recommendations for mumps vaccination

See Epididymitis

Organic Mental Disorders

Adult **Failure** to thrive r/t undetected organic mental disorder

Impaired **Social** interaction r/t disturbed thought processes

Risk for **Injury**: Risk factors: disorientation to time, place, person

See Dementia

Orthopedic Traction

Impaired **Social** interaction r/t limited physical mobility

Impaired **Transfer** ability r/t limited physical mobility

Ineffective **Role** performance r/t limited physical mobility

Risk for impaired **Religiosity**: Risk factor: immobility

See Traction and Casts

Orthopnea

Decreased **Cardiac** output r/t inability of heart to meet demands of body

Ineffective **Breathing** pattern r/t inability to breathe with head of bed flat

Orthostatic Hypotension

See Dizziness

Osteoarthritis

Activity intolerance r/t pain after exercise or use of joint

Acute **Pain** r/t movement

Impaired **Transfer** ability r/t pain

See Arthritis

Osteomyelitis

Acute **Pain** r/t inflammation in affected extremity

Deficient **Diversional** activity r/t prolonged immobilization, hospitalization

Fear: parental r/t concern regarding possible growth plate damage caused by infection, concern that infection may become chronic

Hyperthermia r/t infectious process

Impaired physical **Mobility** r/t imposed immobility as a result of infected area

Ineffective **Health** maintenance r/t continued immobility at home, possible extensive casts, continued antibiotics

Risk for **Constipation**: Risk factor: immobility

Risk for impaired **Skin** integrity: Risk factor: irritation from splint or cast

Risk for **Infection**: Risk factor: inadequate primary and secondary defenses

See Hospitalized Child

Osteoporosis

Acute **Pain** r/t fracture, muscle spasms

Deficient **Knowledge** r/t diet, exercise, need to abstain from alcohol and nicotine

Effective **Therapeutic** regimen management: individual: appropriate choices for diet and exercise to prevent and manage condition

Imbalanced **Nutrition**: less than body requirements r/t inadequate intake of calcium and vitamin D

Impaired physical **Mobility** r/t pain, skeletal changes

Readiness for enhanced **Therapeutic** regimen management: expresses desire to manage the treatment of illness and prevent complications

Risk for **Injury**: fracture: Risk factors: lack of activity, risk of falling resulting from environmental hazards, neuromuscular disorders, diminished senses, cardiovascular responses, responses to drugs

Risk for **Powerlessness**: Risk factor: debilitating disease

Ostomy

See Child with Chronic Condition; Colostomy; Ileal Conduit; Ileostomy

Otitis Media

Acute **Pain** r/t inflammation, infectious process

Disturbed **Sensory** perception: auditory r/t incomplete resolution of otitis media, presence of excess drainage in middle ear

Readiness for enhanced **Knowledge** of information: information on treatment and prevention of disease

Risk for delayed speech and language **Development**: Risk factor: frequent otitis media

Risk for **Infection**: Risk factors: eustachian tube obstruction, traumatic eardrum perforation, infectious disease process

Ovarian Carcinoma

Death **Anxiety** r/t unknown outcome, possible poor prognosis

Fear r/t unknown outcome, possible poor prognosis

Ineffective **Health** maintenance r/t deficient knowledge regarding self-care, treatment of condition

See Chemotherapy; Hysterectomy; Radiation Therapy

Oxyuriasis

See Pinworms

P

Pacemaker

Acute **Pain** r/t surgical procedure

Anxiety r/t change in health status, presence of pacemaker

Death **Anxiety** r/t worry over possible malfunction of pacemaker

Deficient **Knowledge** r/t self-care program, when to seek medical attention

Readiness for enhanced **Therapeutic** regimen management appropriate health care management of pacemaker

Risk for decreased **Cardiac** output: Risk factor: malfunction of pacemaker

Risk for **Infection**: Risk factors: invasive procedure, presence of foreign body (catheter and generator)

Risk for **Powerlessness**: Risk factor: presence of electronic device to stimulate heart

Paget's Disease

Chronic **Sorrow** r/t chronic condition with altered body image

Deficient **Knowledge** r/t appropriate diet high in protein and calcium, mild exercise

Disturbed **Body** image r/t possible enlarged head, bowed tibias, kyphosis

Risk for **Trauma**: fracture r/t excessive bone destruction

Pain, Acute

Acute **Pain** (See **Pain**, acute, Section III)

Disturbed **Energy** field r/t unbalanced energy field

Pain, Chronic

Chronic **Pain** (See **Pain**, chronic, Section III)

Disturbed **Energy** field r/t unbalanced energy field

Painful Breasts, Engorgement

Acute **Pain** r/t distention of breast tissue

Impaired **Tissue** integrity r/t excessive fluid in breast tissues

Ineffective **Role** performance r/t change in physical capacity to assume role of breastfeeding mother

Risk for ineffective **Breastfeeding**: Risk factors: pain, infant's inability to latch on to engorged breast

Risk for **Infection**: Risk factor: milk stasis

Painful Breasts, Sore Nipples

Acute **Pain** r/t cracked nipples

Impaired **Skin** integrity r/t mechanical factors involved in suckling, breastfeeding management

Ineffective **Breastfeeding** r/t pain

Ineffective **Role** performance r/t change in physical capacity to assume role of breastfeeding mother

Risk for **Infection**: Risk factor: break in skin

P

P

Pallor of Extremities

Ineffective **Tissue** perfusion: peripheral r/t interruption of vascular flow

Palpitations (Heart Palpitations)

See Dysrhythmia

Pancreatic Cancer

Death **Anxiety** r/t possible poor prognosis of disease process

Deficient **Knowledge** r/t disease-induced diabetes, home management

Fear r/t poor prognosis of the disease

Grieving r/t shortened life span

Ineffective family **Coping** r/t poor prognosis

Spiritual distress r/t poor prognosis

See Cancer; Chemotherapy; Radiation Therapy; Surgery, Perioperative; Surgery, Postoperative; Surgery, Preoperative

Pancreatitis

Acute **Pain** r/t irritation and edema of the inflamed pancreas

Adult **Failure** to thrive r/t pain

Chronic **Sorrow** r/t chronic illness

Diarrhea r/t decrease in pancreatic secretions resulting in steatorrhea

Deficient **Fluid** volume r/t vomiting, decreased fluid intake, fever, diaphoresis, fluid shifts

Imbalanced **Nutrition**: less than body requirements r/t inadequate dietary intake, increased nutritional needs as a result of acute illness, increased metabolic needs caused by increased body temperature

Ineffective **Breathing** pattern r/t splinting from severe pain

Ineffective **Denial** r/t ineffective coping, alcohol use

Ineffective **Health** maintenance r/t deficient knowledge concerning diet, alcohol use, medication

Nausea r/t irritation of gastrointestinal system

Readiness for enhanced **Comfort** r/t expresses desire to enhance comfort

Panic Disorder

Anxiety r/t situational crisis

Ineffective **Coping** r/t personal vulnerability

Post-trauma syndrome r/t previous catastrophic event

Readiness for enhanced **Coping**: seeks problem-oriented and emotion-oriented strategies to manage condition

Risk for **Loneliness**: Risk factor: inability to socially interact because of fear of losing control

Risk for **Post-trauma** syndrome: Risk factors: perception of the event, diminished ego strength

Risk for **Powerlessness**: Risk factor: ineffective coping skills

Social isolation r/t fear of lack of control

See Anxiety; Anxiety Disorder

Paralysis

Acute **Pain** r/t prolonged immobility

Chronic **Sorrow** r/t loss of physical mobility

Constipation r/t effects of spinal cord disruption, inadequate fiber in diet

Disturbed **Body** image r/t biophysical changes, loss of movement, immobility

Impaired **Home** maintenance r/t physical disability

Impaired physical **Mobility** r/t neuromuscular impairment

Impaired **Transfer** ability r/t paralysis

Impaired wheelchair **Mobility** r/t neuromuscular impairment

Ineffective **Health** maintenance r/t deficient knowledge regarding self-care with paralysis

Powerlessness r/t illness-related regimen

Readiness for enhanced **Self-care**: expresses desire to enhance knowledge and responsibility for strategies for self-care

Reflex **Incontinence** r/t neurological impairment

Risk for **Disuse** syndrome: Risk factor: paralysis

Risk for **Falls**: Risk factor: paralysis

Risk for impaired **Religiosity**: Risk factors: immobility, possible lack of transportation

Risk for impaired **Skin** integrity: Risk factors: altered circulation, altered sensation, immobility

Risk for **Injury**: Risk factors: altered mobility, sensory dysfunction

Risk for latex **Allergy** response: Risk factor: possible repeated urinary catheterizations

Risk for **Post-trauma** syndrome: Risk factor: event causing paralysis

Risk for situational low **Self-esteem**: Risk factor: change in body image and function

Self-care deficit: specify r/t neuromuscular impairment

Sexual dysfunction r/t loss of sensation, biopsychosocial alteration

See Child with Chronic Condition; Hemiplegia; Hospitalized Child; Neural Tube Defects; Spinal Cord Injury

Paralytic Ileus

Acute **Pain** r/t pressure, abdominal distention

Constipation r/t decreased gastric motility

Deficient **Fluid** volume r/t loss of fluids from vomiting, retention of fluid in bowel

Impaired **Oral** mucous membrane r/t presence of nasogastric tube

Nausea r/t gastrointestinal irritation

Paranoid Personality Disorder

Anxiety r/t uncontrollable intrusive, suspicious thoughts

Chronic low **Self-esteem** r/t inability to trust others

Disturbed personal **Identity** r/t difficulty with reality testing

Disturbed **Sensory** perception: specify r/t psychological dysfunction, suspicious thoughts

Disturbed **Thought** processes r/t psychological conflicts

Risk-prone health **Behavior** r/t intense emotional state

Risk for **Loneliness**: Risk factor: social isolation

Risk for other-directed **Violence**: Risk factor: being suspicious of others and others' actions

Risk for **Post-trauma** syndrome: Risk factor: exaggerated sense of responsibility

Risk for **Suicide**: Risk factor: psychiatric illness

Social isolation r/t inappropriate social skills

Paraplegia

See Spinal Cord Injury

Parathyroidectomy

Anxiety r/t surgery

Risk for impaired verbal **Communication**: Risk factors: possible laryngeal damage, edema

Risk for ineffective **Airway** clearance: Risk factors: edema or hematoma formation, airway obstruction

Risk for **Infection**: Risk factor: surgical procedure

See Hypocalcemia

Parent Attachment

Chronic **Sorrow** r/t difficult parent-child relationship

Risk for impaired parent/child **Attachment** (See **Attachment**, impaired parent/child, risk for, Section III)

Risk for **Spiritual** distress: Risk factor: altered relationships

Parental Role Conflict

Chronic **Sorrow** r/t difficult parent-child relationship

Parental role **Conflict** r/t (See **Conflict**, parental role, Section III)

Readiness for enhanced **Parenting**: willingness to enhance parenting

Risk for **Spiritual** distress: Risk factor: altered relationships

Parenting

Readiness for enhanced **Parenting** (See **Parenting**, readiness for enhanced, Section III)

Parenting, Impaired

Chronic **Sorrow** r/t difficult parent-child relationship

Impaired **Parenting** (See **Parenting**, impaired, Section III)

Risk for **Spiritual** distress: Risk factor: altered relationships

Parenting, Risk for Impaired

Chronic **Sorrow** r/t difficult parent-child relationship

Risk for impaired **Parenting** (See **Parenting**, impaired, risk for, Section III)

Risk for **Spiritual** distress: Risk factors: altered relationships

Paresthesia

Disturbed **Sensory** perception: tactile r/t altered sensory reception, transmission, integration

Risk for **Injury** r/t inability to feel temperature changes, pain

Parkinson's Disease

Chronic **Sorrow** r/t loss of physical capacity

Constipation r/t weakness of defecation muscles, lack of exercise, inadequate fluid intake, decreased autonomic nervous system activity

Imbalanced **Nutrition**: less than body requirements r/t tremor, slowness in eating, difficulty in chewing and swallowing

Impaired verbal **Communication** r/t decreased speech volume, slowness of speech, impaired facial muscles

Risk for **Injury**: Risk factors: tremors, slow reactions, altered gait

See Neurological Disorders

Paroxysmal Nocturnal Dyspnea

See PND (Paroxysmal Nocturnal Dyspnea)

Patent Ductus Arteriosus (PDA)

See Congenital Heart Disease/Cardiac Anomalies

Patient-Controlled Analgesia

See PCA (Patient-Controlled Analgesia)

Patient Education

Deficient **Knowledge** r/t lack of exposure to information, information misinterpretation, unfamiliarity with information resources

Effective **Therapeutic** regimen management: verbalizes desire to manage illness

Health-seeking behaviors: expresses desire to seek control of health practices

Readiness for enhanced **Decision** making: expresses desire to enhance understanding of choices for decision making

Readiness for enhanced **Knowledge** (specify): interest in learning

Readiness for enhanced **Spiritual** well-being: desires to reach harmony with self, others, higher power/God

Readiness for enhanced **Therapeutic** regimen management: expresses desire for information to manage the illness

PCA (Patient-Controlled Analgesia)

Deficient **Knowledge** r/t self-care of pain control

Effective **Therapeutic** regimen management: ability to manage pain with appropriate use of PCA

Pruritus r/t side effects of medication

Nausea r/t side effects of medication

Readiness for enhanced **Knowledge**: appropriate management of PCA

Risk for **Injury**: Risk factors: possible complications associated with PCA

Pediculosis

See Lice

Pelvic Inflammatory Disease

See PID (Pelvic Inflammatory Disease)

Penile Prosthesis

Health-seeking behaviors r/t information regarding use and care of prosthesis

Ineffective **Sexuality** pattern r/t use of penile prosthesis

Risk for **Infection**: Risk factor: invasive surgical procedure

Risk for situational low **Self-esteem**: Risk factors: ineffective sexuality pattern

See Impotence; Erectile Dysfunction (ED)

P

Peptic Ulcer

See Ulcer, Peptic (Duodenal or Gastric)

Percutaneous Transluminal Coronary Angioplasty (PTCA)

See Angioplasty, Coronary

Pericardial Friction Rub

Acute **Pain** r/t inflammation, effusion

Decreased **Cardiac** output r/t inflammation in pericardial sac, fluid accumulation compressing heart

Delayed **Surgical** recovery r/t complications associated with cardiac problems

Pericarditis

Activity intolerance r/t reduced cardiac reserve, prescribed bed rest

Acute **Pain** r/t biological injury, inflammation

Decreased **Cardiac** output r/t inflammation in pericardial sac, fluid accumulation compressing heart function

Delayed **Surgical** recovery r/t complications associated with cardiac problems

Deficient **Knowledge** r/t unfamiliarity with information sources

Ineffective **Tissue** perfusion: cardiopulmonary/peripheral r/t risk for development of emboli

Risk for imbalanced **Nutrition**: less than body requirements r/t fever, hypermetabolic state associated with fever

Perioperative Positioning

Risk for perioperative positioning **Injury**: Risk factors: (See **Injury**, perioperative, risk for, Section III)

Peripheral Neuropathy

See Neuropathy, Peripheral

Peripheral Neurovascular Dysfunction

Risk for **Peripheral** neurovascular dysfunction: Risk factors: (See **Peripheral** neurovascular dysfunction, risk for, Section III)

See Neuropathy, Peripheral; Peripheral Vascular Disease

Peripheral Vascular Disease

Activity intolerance r/t imbalance between peripheral oxygen supply and demand

Chronic **Pain**: intermittent claudication r/t ischemia

Ineffective **Health** maintenance r/t deficient knowledge regarding self-care and treatment of disease

Ineffective **Tissue** perfusion: peripheral r/t interruption of vascular flow

Readiness for enhanced **Therapeutic** regimen management; self-care and treatment of disease

Risk for **Falls**: Risk factor: altered mobility

Risk for impaired **Skin** integrity: Risk factor: altered circulation or sensation

Risk for **Injury**: Risk factors: tissue hypoxia, altered mobility, altered sensation

Risk for **Peripheral** neurovascular dysfunction: Risk factor: possible vascular obstruction

See Neuropathy, Peripheral; Peripheral Neurovascular Dysfunction

Peritoneal Dialysis

Acute **Pain** r/t instillation of dialysate, temperature of dialysate

Chronic **Sorrow** r/t chronic disability

Deficient **Knowledge** r/t treatment procedure, self-care with peritoneal dialysis

Impaired **Home** maintenance r/t complex home treatment of client

Risk for **Fluid** volume excess: Risk factor: retention of dialysate

Risk for ineffective **Breathing** pattern: Risk factor: pressure from dialysate

Risk for ineffective **Coping**: Risk factor: disability requiring change in lifestyle

Risk for **Infection**: peritoneal: Risk factor: invasive procedure, presence of catheter, dialysate

Risk for **Powerlessness**: Risk factor: chronic condition and care involved

See Child with Chronic Condition; Hospitalized Child; Renal Failure; Renal Failure, Acute/Chronic, Child

Peritonitis

Acute **Pain** r/t inflammation, stimulation of somatic nerves

Constipation r/t decreased oral intake, decrease of peristalsis

Deficient **Fluid** volume r/t retention of fluid in bowel with loss of circulating blood volume

Imbalanced **Nutrition**: less than body requirements r/t nausea, vomiting

Ineffective **Breathing** pattern r/t pain, increased abdominal pressure

Nausea r/t gastrointestinal irritation

Pernicious Anemia

Diarrhea r/t malabsorption of nutrients

Effective **Therapeutic** regimen management r/t follows treatment plan; lifelong replacement of vitamin B_{12}

Fatigue r/t imbalanced nutrition: less than body requirements

Imbalanced **Nutrition**: less than body requirements r/t lack of appetite associated with nausea and altered oral mucous membrane

Impaired **Memory** r/t anemia; lack of adequate red blood cells

Impaired **Oral** mucous membranes r/t vitamin deficiency; inability to absorb vitamin B_{12} associated with lack of intrinsic factor

Nausea r/t altered oral mucous membrane; sore tongue, bleeding gums

Risk for **Peripheral** neurovascular dysfunction: Risk factor: anemia

Risk for **Falls**: Risk factor: dizziness, lightheadedness

Persistent Fetal Circulation

See Congenital Heart Disease/Cardiac Anomalies

Personal Identity Problems

Disturbed personal **Identity** r/t situational crisis, psychological impairment, chronic illness, pain

Personality Disorder

Chronic low **Self-esteem** r/t inability to set and achieve goals

Compromised family **Coping** r/t inability of client to provide positive feedback to family, chronicity exhausting family

Decisional **Conflict** r/t low self-esteem, feelings that choices will always be wrong

Disturbed personal **Identity** r/t lack of consistent positive self-image

Impaired **Social** interaction r/t knowledge or skill deficit regarding ways to interact effectively with others, self-concept disturbances

Readiness for enhanced **Self-concept**: expresses willingness to enhance self-concept

Risk for **Loneliness**: Risk factor: inability to interact appropriately with others

Risk for **Self-mutilation**: Risk factors: disturbed interpersonal relationships, borderline personality disorders

Risk for situational low **Self-esteem**: Risk factor: history of learned helplessness

Risk-prone health **Behavior** r/t ambivalent behavior toward others, testing of others' loyalty

Spiritual distress r/t lack of identifiable values, lack of meaning to life

See Antisocial Personality Disorder; Borderline Personality Disorder; Obsessive-Compulsive Disorder; Paranoid Personality Disorder

Pertussis (Whooping Cough)

See Respiratory Infections, Acute Childhood

Pesticide Contamination

Contamination r/t use of environmental contaminants; pesticides

Effective **Therapeutic** regimen management: verbalizes intent to reduce risk factors associated with environmental toxins; meticulous hand hygiene

Health-seeking behaviors r/t expression of concern about environmental conditions

Risk for disproportionate **Growth**: Risk factor: environmental contamination

Petechiae

See Clotting Disorder; Anticoagulant Therapy; DIC (Disseminated Intravascular Coagulation); Hemophilia

Petit Mal Seizure

Effective **Therapeutic** regimen management r/t follows prescribed medication regimen

Readiness for enhanced **Therapeutic** regimen management: wears medical alert bracelet; limits hazardous activities such as driving, swimming, working at heights, operating equipment

See Epilepsy

Pharyngitis

See Sore Throat

Phenylketonuria

See PKU (Phenylketonuria)

Pheochromocytoma

Anxiety r/t symptoms from increased catecholamines—headache, palpitations, sweating, nervousness, nausea, vomiting, syncope

Ineffective **Health** maintenance r/t deficient knowledge regarding treatment and self-care

Insomnia r/t high levels of catecholamines

Nausea r/t increased catecholamines

Risk for ineffective **Tissue** perfusion: cardiopulmonary and renal: Risk factor: episodes of hypertension

See Surgery, Perioperative; Surgery, Postoperative; Surgery, Preoperative

Phlebitis

See Thrombophlebitis

Phobia (Specific)

Anxiety r/t inability to control emotions when dreaded object or situation is encountered

Fear r/t presence or anticipation of specific object or situation

Ineffective **Coping** r/t transfer of fears from self to dreaded object situation

Powerlessness r/t anxiety about encountering unknown or known entity

Readiness for enhanced **Communication**: willingness to discuss situation

Readiness for enhanced **Power**: expresses readiness to enhance identification of choices that can be made for change

Risk for **Post-trauma** syndrome: Risk factor: exposure to dreaded object or situation

Risk for **Powerlessness**: Risk factor: inadequate coping patterns

Risk for situational low **Self-esteem**: Risk factor: decreased power/control over fears

See Anxiety; Anxiety Disorder; Panic Disorder

Photosensitivity

Ineffective **Health** maintenance r/t deficient knowledge regarding medications inducing photosensitivity

Risk for impaired **Skin** integrity: Risk factor: exposure to sun

Physical Abuse

See Abuse, Child; Abuse, Spouse, Parent, or Significant Other

Pica

Anxiety r/t stress from urge to eat nonnutritive substances

Imbalanced **Nutrition**: less than body requirements r/t eating nonnutritive substances

Impaired **Parenting** r/t lack of supervision, food deprivation

Risk for **Constipation**: Risk factor: presence of undigestible materials in gastrointestinal tract

Risk for **Infection**: Risk factor: ingestion of infectious agents via contaminated substances

Risk for **Poisoning**: Risk factor: ingestion of substances containing lead

PID (Pelvic Inflammatory Disease)

Acute **Pain** r/t biological injury; inflammation, edema, congestion of pelvic tissues

Ineffective **Health** maintenance r/t deficient knowledge regarding self-care, treatment of disease

Ineffective **Sexuality** pattern r/t medically imposed abstinence from sexual activities until acute infection subsides, change in reproductive potential

Risk for **Infection**: Risk factors: insufficient knowledge to avoid exposure to pathogens; proper hygiene, nutrition, other health habits

Risk for urge urinary **Incontinence**: Risk factors: inflammation, edema, congestion of pelvic tissues

See Maturational Issues, Adolescent

PIH (Pregnancy-Induced Hypertension/Preeclampsia)

Anxiety r/t fear of the unknown, threat to self and infant, change in role functioning

Death **Anxiety** r/t threat of preeclampsia

Deficient **Diversional** activity r/t bed rest

Deficient **Knowledge** r/t lack of experience with situation

Excess **Fluid** volume r/t decreased renal function

Impaired **Home** maintenance r/t bed rest

Impaired **Parenting** r/t bed rest

Impaired physical **Mobility** r/t medically prescribed limitations

Impaired **Social** interaction r/t imposed bed rest

Ineffective **Role** performance r/t change in physical capacity to assume role of pregnant woman or resume other roles

Interrupted **Family** processes r/t situational crisis

Powerlessness r/t complication threatening pregnancy, medically prescribed limitations

Readiness for enhanced **Knowledge**: desire for information on managing condition

Risk for imbalanced **Fluid** volume: Risk factors: hypertension, altered renal function

Risk for **Injury**: fetal: Risk factors: decreased uteroplacental perfusion, seizures

Risk for **Injury**: maternal: Risk factors: vasospasm, high blood pressure

Situational low **Self-esteem** r/t loss of idealized pregnancy

See Malignant Hypertension

Piloerection

Hypothermia r/t exposure to cold environment

Pimples

See Acne

Pinworms

Effective **Therapeutic** regimen management: adheres to guidelines for infected person and appropriate care

Impaired **Home** maintenance r/t inadequate cleaning of bed linen and toilet seats

Insomnia r/t discomfort

Pruritus r/t inflammation of skin

Readiness for enhanced **Therapeutic** regimen: proper hand washing; short clean fingernails; avoiding hand, mouth, nose contact with unwashed hands; appropriate cleaning of bed linen and toilet seats

Pituitary Cushing's

See Cushing's Syndrome

PKU (Phenylketonuria)

Effective management of **Therapeutic** regimen: testing of newborn for PKU and following prescribed dietary regimen if test is positive

Risk for delayed **Development**: Risk factors: not following strict dietary program; eating foods extremely low in phenylalanine; avoiding eggs, milk, any foods containing aspartame (Nutrasweet)

Placenta Abruptio

Acute **Pain**: abdominal/back r/t premature separation of placenta before delivery

Death **Anxiety** r/t threat of mortality associated with bleeding

Fear r/t threat to self and fetus

Ineffective **Health** maintenance r/t deficient knowledge regarding treatment and control of hypertension associated with placenta abruptio

Risk for deficient **Fluid** volume r/t maternal blood loss

Risk for **Powerlessness**: Risk factors: complications of pregnancy and unknown outcome

Risk for **Spiritual** distress: Risk factor: fear from unknown outcome of pregnancy

Placenta Previa

Death **Anxiety** r/t threat of mortality associated with bleeding

Deficient **Diversional** activity r/t long-term hospitalization

Disturbed **Body** image r/t negative feelings about body and reproductive ability, feelings of helplessness

Fear r/t threat to self and fetus, unknown future

Impaired **Home** maintenance r/t maternal bed rest, hospitalization

Impaired physical **Mobility** r/t medical protocol, maternal bed rest

Ineffective **Coping** r/t threat to self and fetus

Ineffective **Role** performance r/t maternal bed rest, hospitalization

Ineffective **Tissue** perfusion: placental r/t dilation of cervix, loss of placental implantation site

Interrupted **Family** processes r/t maternal bed rest, hospitalization

Risk for **Constipation**: Risk factor: bed rest, pregnancy

Risk for deficient **Fluid** volume: Risk factor: maternal blood loss

Risk for imbalanced **Fluid** volume: Risk factor: maternal blood loss

Risk for impaired **Parenting**: Risk factors: maternal bed rest, hospitalization

Risk for **Injury**: fetal and maternal: Risk factors: threat to uteroplacental perfusion, hemorrhage

Risk for **Powerlessness**: Risk factors: complications of pregnancy and unknown outcome

Situational low **Self-esteem** r/t situational crisis

Spiritual distress r/t inability to participate in usual religious rituals, situational crisis

Pleural Effusion

Acute **Pain** r/t inflammation, fluid accumulation

Excess **Fluid** volume r/t compromised regulatory mechanisms; heart, liver, or kidney failure

Hyperthermia r/t increased metabolic rate secondary to infection

Ineffective **Breathing** pattern r/t pain

Pleural Friction Rub

Acute **Pain** r/t inflammation, fluid accumulation

Ineffective **Breathing** pattern r/t pain

See cause of Pleural Friction Rub

Pleural Tap

See Pleural Effusion

Pleurisy

Acute **Pain** r/t pressure on pleural nerve endings associated with fluid accumulation or inflammation

Impaired **Gas** exchange r/t ventilation perfusion imbalance

Ineffective **Breathing** pattern r/t pain

Risk for impaired physical **Mobility**: Risk factors: activity intolerance, inability to "catch breath"

Risk for ineffective **Airway** clearance: Risk factors: increased secretions, ineffective cough because of pain

PMS (Premenstrual Tension Syndrome)

Acute **Pain** r/t hormonal stimulation of gastrointestinal structures

Deficient **Knowledge** r/t methods to deal with and prevent syndrome

Excess **Fluid** volume r/t alterations of hormonal levels inducing fluid retention

Fatigue r/t hormonal changes

Readiness for enhanced **Communication**: willingness to express thoughts and feelings about PMS

Readiness for enhanced **Therapeutic** regimen management: desire for information to manage and prevent symptoms

Risk for **Powerlessness**: Risk factors: lack of knowledge and ability to deal with symptoms

PND (Paroxysmal Nocturnal Dyspnea)

Anxiety r/t inability to breathe during sleep

Decreased **Cardiac** output r/t failure of the left ventricle

Ineffective **Breathing** pattern r/t increase in carbon dioxide levels, decrease in oxygen levels

Insomnia r/t suffocating feeling from fluid in lungs on awakening from sleep

Readiness for enhanced **Sleep**: expresses willingness to learn measures to enhance sleep

Risk for **Powerlessness**: Risk factor: inability to control nocturnal dyspnea

Sleep deprivation r/t inability to breathe during sleep

Pneumonia

Activity intolerance r/t imbalance between oxygen supply and demand

Deficient **Knowledge** r/t Risk factors predisposing person to pneumonia, treatment

Hyperthermia r/t dehydration, increased metabolic rate, illness

Imbalanced **Nutrition**: less than body requirements r/t loss of appetite

Impaired **Gas** exchange r/t decreased functional lung tissue

Impaired **Oral** mucous membrane r/t dry mouth from mouth breathing, decreased fluid intake

Ineffective **Airway** clearance r/t inflammation and presence of secretions

Ineffective **Health** maintenance r/t deficient knowledge regarding self-care and treatment of disease

Risk for deficient **Fluid** volume: Risk factor: inadequate intake of fluids

See Respiratory Infections, Acute Childhood

Pneumothorax

Acute **Pain** r/t recent injury, coughing, deep breathing

Fear r/t threat to own well-being, difficulty breathing

Impaired **Gas** exchange r/t ventilation-perfusion imbalance

Risk for **Injury**: Risk factor: possible complications associated with closed chest drainage system

Poisoning, Risk for

External/Internal

Risk for **Poisoning**: Risk factors: (See **Poisoning**, risk for, Section III)

Polydipsia

Readiness for enhanced **Fluid** balance: no excessive thirst when diabetes is controlled

See Diabetes Mellitus

Polyphagia

Readiness for enhanced **Nutrition**: knowledge of appropriate diet for diabetes

See Diabetes Mellitus

P

Polyuria

Readiness for enhanced **Urinary** elimination: willingness to learn measures to enhance urinary elimination

See Diabetes Mellitus

Postoperative Care

See Surgery, Postoperative

Postpartum Blues

Anxiety r/t new responsibilities of parenting

Chronic **Sorrow** r/t loss of ideal postpartum experience or ideal parent-infant relationship

Deficient **Knowledge** r/t lifestyle changes

Disturbed **Body** image r/t normal postpartum recovery

Fatigue r/t childbirth, postpartum state

Impaired **Home** maintenance r/t fatigue, care of newborn

Impaired **Parenting** r/t hormone-induced depression

Impaired **Social** interaction r/t change in role functioning

Ineffective **Coping** r/t hormonal changes, maturational crisis

Ineffective **Role** performance r/t new responsibilities of parenting

Readiness for enhanced **Hope**: Expresses desire to enhance hope and interconnectedness with others

Risk for **Post-trauma** syndrome: Risk factors: trauma or violence associated with labor and birth process, medical/surgical interventions, history of sexual abuse

Risk for situational low **Self-esteem**: Risk factor: decreased power over feelings of sadness

Risk for **Spiritual** distress: Risk factors: altered relationships, social isolation

Risk-prone health **Behavior** r/t lack of support systems

Sexual dysfunction r/t fear of another pregnancy, postpartum pain, lochia flow

Sleep deprivation r/t environmental stimulation of newborn

Postpartum Hemorrhage

Activity intolerance r/t anemia from loss of blood

Acute **Pain** r/t nursing and medical interventions to control bleeding

Death **Anxiety** r/t threat of mortality associated with bleeding

Decreased **Cardiac** output r/t hypovolemia

Deficient **Fluid** volume r/t uterine atony, loss of blood

Deficient **Knowledge** r/t lack of exposure to situation

Disturbed **Body** image r/t loss of ideal childbirth

Fear r/t threat to self, unknown future

Impaired **Home** maintenance r/t lack of stamina

Ineffective **Tissue** perfusion r/t hypovolemia

Interrupted **Breastfeeding** r/t separation from infant for medical treatment

Risk for imbalanced **Fluid** volume: Risk factor: maternal blood loss

Risk for **Infection**: Risk factors: loss of blood, depressed immunity

Risk for impaired **Parenting**: Risk factor: weakened maternal condition

Risk for **Powerlessness**: Risk factor: acute illness

Postpartum, Normal Care

Acute **Pain** r/t episiotomy, lacerations, bruising, breast engorgement, headache, sore nipples, epidural or intravenous (IV) site, hemorrhoids

Anxiety r/t change in role functioning, parenting

Constipation r/t hormonal effects on smooth muscles, fear of straining with defecation, effects of anesthesia

Deficient **Knowledge**: infant care r/t lack of preparation for parenting

Effective **Breastfeeding** r/t basic breastfeeding knowledge, support of partner and health care provider

Fatigue r/t childbirth, new responsibilities of parenting, body changes

Health-seeking behaviors r/t postpartum recovery and adaptation

Impaired **Skin** integrity r/t episiotomy, lacerations

Impaired **Urinary** elimination r/t effects of anesthesia, tissue trauma

Ineffective **Breastfeeding** r/t lack of knowledge, lack of support, lack of motivation

Ineffective **Role** performance r/t new responsibilities of parenting

Readiness for enhanced family **Coping**: adaptation to new family member

Readiness for enhanced **Parenting**: expressing willingness to enhance parenting skills

Risk for **Constipation**: Risk factors: hormonal effects on smooth muscles, fear of straining with defecation, effects of anesthesia

Risk for imbalanced **Fluid** volume: Risk factors: shift in blood volume, edema

Risk for impaired **Parenting**: Risk factors: lack of role models, deficient knowledge

Risk for **Infection**: Risk factors: tissue trauma, blood loss

Risk for **Post-trauma** syndrome: Risk factors: trauma or violence associated with labor and birth process, medical/surgical interventions, history of sexual abuse

Risk for urge urinary **Incontinence**: Risk factors: effects of anesthesia or tissue trauma

Sexual dysfunction r/t fear of pain or pregnancy

Sleep deprivation r/t care of infant

Post-Trauma Syndrome

Post-trauma syndrome r/t (See **Post-trauma** syndrome, Section III)

Post-Trauma Syndrome, Risk for

Risk for **Post-trauma** syndrome: Risk factors: (See **Post-trauma** syndrome, risk for, Section III)

Post-Traumatic Stress Disorder

Anxiety r/t exposure to internal or external cues that symbolize or resemble an aspect of the traumatic event

Death **Anxiety** r/t psychological stress associated with traumatic event

Disturbed **Energy** field r/t disharmony of mind, body, spirit

Disturbed **Sensory** perception r/t psychological stress

Disturbed **Thought** processes r/t sense of reliving the experience (flashbacks)

Ineffective **Breathing** pattern r/t hyperventilation associated with anxiety

Ineffective **Coping** r/t extreme anxiety

Insomnia r/t recurring nightmares

Post-trauma syndrome r/t exposure to a traumatic event

Readiness for enhanced **Comfort**: expresses desire to enhance relaxation

Readiness for enhanced **Communication**: willingness to express feelings and thoughts

Readiness for enhanced **Spiritual** well-being: desire for harmony after stressful event

Risk for **Powerlessness**: Risk factors: flashbacks, reliving event

Risk for self- or other-directed **Violence**: Risk factors: fear of self or others

Sleep deprivation r/t nightmares associated with traumatic event

Spiritual distress r/t feelings of detachment or estrangement from others

Potassium, Increase/Decrease

See Hyperkalemia; Hypokalemia

Power/Powerlessness

Powerlessness r/t (See **Powerlessness**, Section III)

Readiness for enhanced **Power** (See **Power**, readiness for enhanced, Section III)

Risk for **Powerlessness** Risk factors: (See **Powerlessness**, risk for, Section III)

Preeclampsia

See PIH (Pregnancy-Induced Hypertension/Preeclampsia)

Pregnancy, Cardiac Disorders

See Cardiac Disorders in Pregnancy

Pregnancy-Induced Hypertension/Preeclampsia

See PIH (Pregnancy-Induced Hypertension/Preeclampsia)

Pregnancy Loss

Acute **Pain** r/t surgical intervention

Anxiety r/t threat to role functioning, health status, situational crisis

Chronic **Sorrow** r/t loss of a fetus or child

Complicated **Grieving** r/t sudden loss of pregnancy, fetus, or child

Compromised family **Coping** r/t lack of support by significant other because of personal suffering

Ineffective **Coping** r/t situational crisis

Grieving r/t loss of pregnancy, fetus, or child

Complicated **Grieving** r/t sudden loss of pregnancy, fetus, or child

Ineffective **Role** performance r/t inability to assume parenting role

Ineffective **Sexuality** pattern r/t self-esteem disturbance resulting from pregnancy loss and anxiety about future pregnancies

Readiness for enhanced **Communication**: willingness to express feelings and thoughts about loss

Readiness for enhanced **Hope**: expresses desire to enhance hope

Readiness for enhanced **Spiritual** well-being: desire for acceptance of loss

Risk for deficient **Fluid** volume: blood loss

Risk for complicated **Grieving**: Risk factor: loss of pregnancy

Risk for **Infection**: Risk factor: retained products of conception

Risk for **Powerlessness**: Risk factor: situational crisis

Risk for **Spiritual** distress: Risk factor: intense suffering

Spiritual distress r/t intense suffering

Pregnancy, Normal

Deficient **Knowledge** r/t primiparity

Disturbed **Body** image r/t altered body function and appearance

Fear r/t labor and delivery

Health-seeking behaviors r/t desire to promote optimal fetal and maternal health

Imbalanced **Nutrition**: less than body requirements r/t growing fetus, nausea

Imbalanced **Nutrition**: more than body requirements r/t deficient knowledge regarding nutritional needs of pregnancy

Ineffective **Coping** r/t personal vulnerability, situational crisis

Interrupted **Family** processes r/t developmental transition of pregnancy

Nausea r/t hormonal changes of pregnancy

Readiness for enhanced family **Coping**: satisfying partner relationship, attention to gratification of needs, effective adaptation to developmental tasks of pregnancy

Readiness for enhanced **Parenting**: expresses willingness to enhance parenting skills

Sexual dysfunction r/t altered body function, self-concept, body image with pregnancy

Sleep deprivation r/t sleep deprivation secondary to uncomfortable pregnancy state

See Discomforts of Pregnancy

P

Premature Dilation of the Cervix (Incompetent Cervix)

Deficient **Diversional** activity r/t bed rest

Deficient **Knowledge** r/t treatment regimen, prognosis for pregnancy

Fear r/t potential loss of infant

Grieving r/t potential loss of infant

Ineffective **Coping** r/t bed rest, threat to fetus

Ineffective **Role** performance r/t inability to continue usual patterns of responsibility

Impaired physical **Mobility** r/t imposed bed rest to prevent preterm birth

Impaired **Social** interaction r/t bed rest

Powerlessness r/t inability to control outcome of pregnancy

Risk for **Infection**: Risk factors: invasive procedures to prevent preterm birth

Risk for **Injury**: fetal: Risk factors: preterm birth, use of anesthetics

Risk for **Injury**: maternal: Risk factors: surgical procedures to prevent preterm birth (e.g., cerclage)

Risk for **Spiritual** distress: Risk factors; physical/psychological stress

Sexual dysfunction r/t fear of harm to fetus

Situational low **Self-esteem** r/t inability to complete normal pregnancy

Premature Infant (Child)

Delayed **Growth** and development: developmental lag r/t prematurity, environmental and stimulation deficiencies, multiple caretakers

Disorganized **Infant** behavior r/t prematurity

Disturbed **Sensory** perception r/t noxious stimuli, noisy environment

Insomnia r/t noisy and noxious intensive care environment

Imbalanced **Nutrition**: less than body requirements r/t delayed or understimulated rooting reflex, easy fatigue during feeding, diminished endurance

Impaired **Gas** exchange r/t effects of cardiopulmonary insufficiency

Impaired **Swallowing** r/t decreased or absent gag reflex, fatigue

Ineffective **Thermoregulation** r/t large body surface/weight ratio, immaturity of thermal regulation, state of prematurity

Readiness for enhanced organized **Infant** behavior: prematurity

Risk for delayed **Development**: Risk factor: prematurity

Risk for disproportionate **Growth**: Risk factor: prematurity

Risk for **Infection**: Risk factors: inadequate, immature, or undeveloped acquired immune response

Risk for **Injury**: Risk factor: prolonged mechanical ventilation, retinopathy of prematurely (ROP) secondary to 100% oxygen environment

Premature Infant (Parent)

Chronic **Sorrow** r/t threat of loss of a child, prolonged hospitalization

Complicated **Grieving** (prolonged) r/t unresolved conflicts

Compromised family **Coping** r/t disrupted family roles and disorganization, prolonged condition exhausting supportive capacity of significant persons

Decisional **Conflict** r/t support system deficit, multiple sources of information

Grieving r/t loss of perfect child possibly leading to complicated grieving

Ineffective **Breastfeeding** r/t disrupted establishment of effective pattern secondary to prematurity or insufficient opportunities

Parental role **Conflict** r/t expressed concerns, expressed inability to care for child's physical, emotional, or developmental needs

Readiness for enhanced **Family** process: adaptation to change associated with premature infant

Risk for impaired parent/child **Attachment**: Risk factors: separation, physical barriers, lack of privacy

Risk for **Powerlessness**: Risk factor: inability to control situation

Risk for **Spiritual** distress: Risk factors: challenged belief or value systems regarding moral or ethical implications of treatment plans

Spiritual distress r/t challenged belief or value systems regarding moral or ethical implications of treatment plans

See Child with Chronic Condition; Hospitalized Child

Premature Rupture of Membranes

Anxiety r/t threat to infant's health status

Disturbed **Body** image r/t inability to carry pregnancy to term

Grieving r/t potential loss of infant

Ineffective **Coping** r/t situational crisis

Risk for **Infection**: Risk factor: rupture of membranes

Risk for **Injury**: fetal r/t risk of premature birth

Situational low **Self-esteem** r/t inability to carry pregnancy to term

Premenstrual Tension Syndrome

See PMS (Premenstrual Tension Syndrome)

Prenatal Care, Normal

Anxiety r/t unknown future, threat to self secondary to pain of labor

Constipation r/t decreased gastrointestinal motility secondary to hormonal stimulation

Deficient **Knowledge** r/t lack of experience with pregnancy and care

Fatigue r/t increased energy demands

Health-seeking behaviors r/t consistent prenatal care and education

Imbalanced **Nutrition**: less than body requirements r/t nausea from normal hormonal changes

Impaired **Urinary** elimination r/t frequency caused by increased pelvic pressure and hormonal stimulation

Ineffective **Breathing** pattern r/t increased intrathoracic pressure and decreased energy secondary to enlarged uterus

Insomnia r/t discomforts of pregnancy and fetal activity

Interrupted **Family** processes r/t developmental transition

Readiness for enhanced **Knowledge**: appropriate prenatal care

Readiness for enhanced **Nutrition**: desire for knowledge of appropriate nutrition during pregnancy

Readiness for enhanced **Parenting**: realistic expectations of new role as parent

Readiness for enhanced **Spiritual** well-being: new role as parent

Risk for **Activity** intolerance: Risk factors: enlarged abdomen, increased cardiac workload

Risk for **Constipation**: Risk factors: decreased gastrointestinal motility secondary to hormonal stimulation

Risk for **Injury**: maternal: Risk factors: change in balance and center of gravity secondary to enlarged abdomen

Risk for **Sexual** dysfunction: Risk factors: enlarged abdomen, fear of harm to infant

Prenatal Testing

Acute **Pain** r/t invasive procedures

Anxiety r/t unknown outcome, delayed test results

Health-seeking behaviors r/t desire to have information regarding prenatal testing

Risk for **Infection** r/t invasive procedures during amniocentesis or chorionic villi sampling

Risk for **Injury**: fetal r/t invasive procedures

Preoperative Teaching

Health-seeking behaviors: preoperative regimens, postoperative precautions, expectations of role of client during preoperative or postoperative time

See Surgery, Preoperative Care

Pressure Ulcer

Acute **Pain** r/t tissue destruction, exposure of nerves

Imbalanced **Nutrition**: less than body requirements r/t limited access to food, inability to absorb nutrients because of biological factors, anorexia

Impaired bed **Mobility** r/t intolerance to activity, pain, cognitive impairment, depression, severe anxiety

Impaired **Skin** integrity: stage I or II pressure ulcer r/t physical immobility, mechanical factors, altered circulation, skin irritants

Impaired **Tissue** integrity: stage III or IV pressure ulcer r/t altered circulation, impaired physical mobility

Risk for **Infection**: Risk factors: physical immobility, mechanical factors (shearing forces, pressure, restraint, altered circulation, skin irritants)

Total urinary **Incontinence** r/t neurological dysfunction

Preterm Labor

Anxiety r/t threat to fetus, change in role functioning, change in environment and interaction patterns, use of tocolytic drugs

Deficient **Diversional** activity r/t long-term hospitalization

Grieving r/t loss of idealized pregnancy, potential loss of fetus

Impaired **Home** maintenance r/t medical restrictions

Impaired physical **Mobility** r/t medically imposed restrictions

Impaired **Social** interaction r/t prolonged bed rest or hospitalization

Ineffective **Coping** r/t situational crisis, preterm labor

Ineffective **Role** performance r/t inability to carry out normal roles secondary to bed rest or hospitalization, change in expected course of pregnancy

Readiness for enhanced **Comfort**: expresses desire to enhance relation

Readiness for enhanced **Communication**: willingness to discuss thoughts and feelings about situation

Risk for **Injury**: Risk factors: fetal: premature birth, immature body systems

Risk for **Injury**: Risk factor: maternal: use of tocolytic drugs

Risk for **Powerlessness**: Risk factor: lack of control over preterm labor

Sexual dysfunction r/t actual or perceived limitation imposed by preterm labor and/or prescribed treatment, separation from partner because of hospitalization

Situational low **Self-esteem** r/t threatened ability to carry pregnancy to term

Sleep deprivation r/t change in usual pattern secondary to contractions, hospitalization, treatment regimen

Problem-Solving Ability

Defensive **Coping** r/t situational crisis

Ineffective **Coping** r/t situational crisis

Readiness for enhanced **Communication** r/t willingness to share ideas with others

Readiness for enhanced **Spiritual** well-being: desires to draw on inner strength and find meaning and purpose to life

Risk-prone health **Behavior** r/t altered locus of control

Projection

Anxiety r/t threat to self-concept

Chronic low **Self-esteem** r/t failure

Defensive **Coping** r/t inability to acknowledge that own behavior may be a problem, blaming others

Impaired **Social** interaction r/t self-concept disturbance, confrontational communication style

Risk for **Loneliness**: Risk factor: blaming others for problems

Risk for **Post-trauma** syndrome: Risk factor: diminished ego strength

Prolapsed Umbilical Cord

Fear r/t threat to fetus, impending surgery

Ineffective **Tissue** perfusion: fetal r/t interruption in umbilical blood flow

Risk for **Injury**: fetal: Risk factors: cord compression, ineffective tissue perfusion

Risk for **Injury**: maternal: Risk factor: emergency surgery

P

Prolonged Gestation

Anxiety r/t potential change in birthing plans, need for increased medical intervention, unknown outcome for fetus

Defensive **Coping** r/t underlying feeling of inadequacy regarding ability to give birth normally

Imbalanced **Nutrition**: less than body requirements (fetal) r/t aging of placenta

Powerlessness r/t perceived lack of control over outcome of pregnancy

Situational low **Self-esteem** r/t perceived inadequacy of body functioning

Prostatectomy

See TURP (Transurethral Resection of the Prostate)

Prostatic Hypertrophy

Ineffective **Health** maintenance r/t deficient knowledge regarding self-care and prevention of complications

Insomnia r/t nocturia

Risk for **Infection**: Risk factors: urinary residual after voiding, bacterial invasion of bladder

Risk for urge urinary **Incontinence**: Risk factor: small bladder capacity

Urinary retention r/t obstruction

See BPH (Benign Prostatic Hypertrophy)

Prostatitis

Ineffective **Health** maintenance r/t deficient knowledge regarding treatment

Ineffective **Protection** r/t depressed immune system

Risk for urge **Incontinence** r/t irritation of bladder

Protection, Altered

Ineffective **Protection** r/t (See **Protection**, ineffective, Section III)

Pruritus

Deficient **Knowledge** r/t methods to treat and prevent itching

Pruritus r/t (See **Pruritus**, Section III)

Risk for impaired **Skin** integrity: Risk factor: scratching from pruritus

Psoriasis

Disturbed **Body** image r/t lesions on body

Impaired **Skin** integrity r/t lesions on body

Ineffective **Health** maintenance r/t deficient knowledge regarding treatment modalities

Powerlessness r/t lack of control over condition with frequent exacerbations and remissions

Psychosis

Anxiety r/t unconscious conflict with reality

Chronic **Sorrow** r/t chronic mental illness

Disturbed **Thought** processes r/t inaccurate interpretations of environment

Fear r/t altered contact with reality

Imbalanced **Nutrition**: less than body requirements r/t lack of awareness of hunger, disinterest toward food

Impaired **Home** maintenance r/t impaired cognitive or emotional functioning, inadequate support systems

Impaired **Social** interaction r/t impaired communication patterns, self-concept disturbance, disturbed thought processes

Impaired verbal **Communication** r/t psychosis, inaccurate perceptions, hallucinations, delusions

Ineffective **Coping** r/t inadequate support systems, unrealistic perceptions, disturbed thought processes, impaired communication

Ineffective **Health** maintenance r/t cognitive impairment, ineffective individual and family coping

Insomnia r/t sensory alterations contributing to fear and anxiety

Interrupted **Family** processes r/t inability to express feelings, impaired communication

Readiness for enhanced **Hope**: expresses desire to enhance problem-solving to meet goals

Risk for **Post-trauma** syndrome: Risk factor: diminished ego strength

Risk for self- or other-directed **Violence**: Risk factors: lack of trust, panic, hallucinations, delusional thinking

Risk for **Suicide**: Risk factors: psychiatric illness/disorder

Self-care deficit r/t loss of contact with reality, impairment of perception

Self-esteem disturbance r/t excessive use of defense mechanisms (e.g., projection, denial, rationalization)

Social isolation r/t lack of trust, regression, delusional thinking, repressed fears

See Schizophrenia

PTCA (Percutaneous Transluminal Coronary Angioplasty)

See Angioplasty, Coronary

Pulmonary Edema

Anxiety r/t fear of suffocation

Impaired **Gas** exchange r/t extravasation of extravascular fluid in lung tissues and alveoli

Ineffective **Breathing** pattern r/t presence of tracheobronchial secretions

Ineffective **Health** maintenance r/t deficient knowledge regarding treatment regimen

Sleep deprivation r/t inability to breathe

See CHF (Congestive Heart Failure)

Pulmonary Embolism

Acute **Pain** r/t biological injury, lack of oxygen to cells

Decreased **Cardiac** output r/t right ventricular failure secondary to obstructed pulmonary artery

Deficient **Knowledge** r/t activities to prevent embolism, self-care after diagnosis of embolism

Delayed **Surgical** recovery r/t complications associated with respiratory difficulty

P

Fear r/t severe pain, possible death

Impaired **Gas** exchange r/t altered blood flow to alveoli secondary to lodged embolus

Ineffective **Tissue** perfusion: pulmonary r/t interruption of pulmonary blood flow secondary to lodged embolus

See Anticoagulant Therapy

Pulmonary Stenosis

See Congenital Heart Disease/Cardiac Anomalies

Pulse Deficit

Decreased **Cardiac** output r/t dysrhythmia

See Dysrhythmia

Pulse Oximetry

Readiness for enhanced **Knowledge**: information associated with treatment regimen

See Hypoxia

Pulse Pressure, Increased

See Intracranial Pressure, Increased

Pulse Pressure, Narrowed

See Shock

Pulses, Absent or Diminished Peripheral

Ineffective **Tissue** perfusion: peripheral r/t interruption of arterial flow

Risk for **Peripheral** neurovascular dysfunction: Risk factors: fractures, mechanical compression, orthopedic surgery trauma, immobilization, burns, vascular obstruction

See cause of Absent or Diminished Peripheral Pulses

Purpura

See Clotting Disorder

Pyelonephritis

Acute **Pain** r/t inflammation and irritation of urinary tract

Impaired **Urinary** elimination r/t irritation of urinary tract

Ineffective **Health** maintenance r/t deficient knowledge regarding self-care, treatment of disease, prevention of further urinary tract infections

Insomnia r/t urinary frequency

Risk for urge urinary **Incontinence**: Risk factor: irritation of urinary tract

Pyloric Stenosis

Acute **Pain** r/t surgical incision

Deficient **Fluid** volume r/t vomiting, dehydration

Imbalanced **Nutrition**: less than body requirements r/t vomiting secondary to pyloric sphincter obstruction

Ineffective **Health** maintenance r/t parental deficient knowledge regarding home care feeding regimen, wound care

See Hospitalized Child

Q

Quadriplegia

Disturbed **Energy** field r/t illness, grieving for loss of normal function

Grieving r/t loss of normal lifestyle, severity of disability

Impaired **Transfer** ability r/t quadriplegia

Impaired wheelchair **Mobility** r/t quadriplegia

Ineffective **Breathing** pattern r/t inability to use intercostal muscles

Readiness for enhanced **Spiritual** well being: r/t heightened coping associated with disability

Risk for **Autonomic** dysreflexia: Risk factors: bladder distention, bowel distention, skin irritation, lack of client and caregiver knowledge

Risk for impaired **Religiosity**: Risk factors: immobility, possible lack of transportation

See Spinal Cord Injury

R

RA (Rheumatoid Arthritis)

See Rheumatoid Arthritis

Rabies

Acute **Pain** r/t multiple immunization injections

Health-seeking behaviors r/t prophylactic immunization of domestic animals, avoidance of contact with wild animals

Hopelessness r/t poor prognosis

Ineffective **Health** maintenance r/t deficient knowledge regarding care of wound, isolation, and observation of infected animal

Radial Nerve Dysfunction

Acute **Pain** r/t trauma to hand or arm

See Neuropathy, Peripheral

Radiation Therapy

Activity intolerance r/t fatigue from possible anemia

Deficient **Knowledge** r/t what to expect with radiation therapy

Diarrhea r/t irradiation effects

Disturbed **Body** image r/t change in appearance, hair loss

Imbalanced **Nutrition**: less than body requirements r/t anorexia, nausea, vomiting, irradiation of areas of pharynx and esophagus

Impaired **Oral** mucous membrane r/t irradiation effects

Ineffective **Protection** r/t suppression of bone marrow

Nausea r/t side effects of radiation

Risk for impaired **Skin** integrity: Risk factor: irradiation effects

R

Risk for **Powerlessness**: Risk factors: medical treatment and possible side effects

Risk for **Spiritual** distress: Risk factors: radiation treatment, prognosis

Radical Neck Dissection

See Laryngectomy

Rage

Risk for other-directed **Violence**: Risk factors: panic state, manic excitement, organic brain syndrome

Risk for **Self-mutilation**: Risk factor: command hallucinations

Risk for **Suicide**: Risk factor: desire to kill oneself

Risk-prone health **Behavior** r/t multiple stressors

Stress overload r/t multiple coexisting stressors

Rape-Trauma Syndrome

Chronic **Sorrow** r/t forced loss of virginity

Rape-trauma syndrome (See **Rape-trauma** syndrome, Section III)

Rape-trauma syndrome: compound reaction (See **Rape-trauma** syndrome, compound reaction, Section III)

Rape-trauma syndrome: silent reaction (See **Rape-trauma** syndrome, silent reaction, Section III)

Risk for **Post-trauma** syndrome: Risk factors: trauma or violence associated with rape

Risk for **Powerlessness**: Risk factor: inability to control thoughts about incident

Risk for **Spiritual** distress: Risk factor: forced loss of virginity

Rash

Impaired **Skin** integrity r/t mechanical trauma

Pruritus r/t inflammation of skin

Risk for **Infection**: Risk factors: traumatized tissue, broken skin

Risk for latex **Allergy**: Risk factor: allergy to products associated with latex

Rationalization

Defensive **Coping** r/t situational crisis, inability to accept blame for consequences of own behavior

Ineffective **Denial** r/t fear of consequences, actual or perceived loss

Readiness for enhanced **Communication**: expressing desire to share thoughts and feelings

Readiness for enhanced **Spiritual** well-being: possibility of seeking harmony with self, others, higher power, God

Risk for **Post-trauma** syndrome: Risk factor: survivor's role in event

Rats, Rodents in the Home

Impaired **Home** maintenance r/t lack of knowledge, insufficient finances

See Filthy Home Environment

Raynaud's Disease

Deficient **Knowledge** r/t lack of information about disease process, possible complications, self-care needs regarding disease process and medication

Ineffective **Tissue** perfusion: peripheral r/t transient reduction of blood flow

RDS (Respiratory Distress Syndrome)

See Respiratory Conditions of the Neonate

Rectal Fullness

Constipation r/t decreased activity level, decreased fluid intake, inadequate fiber in diet, decreased peristalsis, side effects from antidepressant or antipsychotic therapy

Risk for **Constipation**: Risk factor: habitual denial or ignoring of urge to defecate

Rectal Lump

See Hemorrhoids

Rectal Pain/Bleeding

Acute **Pain** r/t pressure of defecation

Constipation r/t pain on defecation

Deficient **Knowledge** r/t possible causes of rectal bleeding, pain, treatment modalities

Risk for deficient **Fluid** volume: bleeding: Risk factor: untreated rectal bleeding

Rectal Surgery

See Hemorrhoidectomy

Rectocele Repair

Acute **Pain** r/t surgical procedure

Constipation r/t painful defecation

Ineffective **Health** maintenance r/t deficient knowledge of postoperative care of surgical site, dietary measures, exercise to prevent constipation

Risk for **Infection**: Risk factors: surgical procedure, possible contamination of site with feces

Risk for urge urinary **Incontinence**: Risk factor: edema from surgery

Urinary retention r/t edema from surgery

Reflex Incontinence

Reflex **Incontinence** r/t neurological impairment

Regression

Anxiety r/t threat to or change in health status

Defensive **Coping** r/t denial of obvious problems, weaknesses

Ineffective **Role** performance r/t powerlessness over health status

Powerlessness r/t health care environment

See Hospitalized Child; Separation Anxiety

Regretful

Anxiety r/t situational or maturational crises

Death **Anxiety** r/t feelings of not having accomplished goals in life

Risk for **Spiritual** distress: Risk factor: inability to forgive

R

Rehabilitation

Impaired physical **Mobility** r/t injury, surgery, psychosocial condition warranting rehabilitation

Ineffective **Coping** r/t loss of normal function

Readiness for enhanced **Comfort**: expresses desire to enhance feeling of comfort

Readiness for enhanced **Self-concept**: accepts strengths and limitations

Readiness for enhanced **Therapeutic** regimen management: expression of desire to manage rehabilitation

Self-care deficit r/t impaired physical mobility

Relaxation Techniques

Anxiety r/t disturbed energy field

Health-seeking behaviors r/t requesting information about ways to relieve stress

Readiness for enhanced **Comfort**: expresses desire to enhance relaxation

Readiness for enhanced **Religiosity**: requests religious materials or experiences

Readiness for enhanced **Self-concept**: willingness to enhance self-concept

Readiness for enhanced **Spiritual** well-being: seeking comfort from higher power

Religiosity

Impaired **Religiosity** (See **Religiosity**, impaired, Section III)

Readiness for enhanced **Religiosity** (See **Religiosity**, readiness for enhanced, Section III)

Risk for impaired **Religiosity** (See **Religiosity**, risk for impaired, Section III)

Religious Concerns

Readiness for enhanced **Spiritual** well-being: desire for increased spirituality

Risk for impaired **Religiosity**: Risk factors: ineffective support, coping, caregiving

Risk for **Spiritual** distress: Risk factors: physical or psychological stress

Spiritual distress r/t separation from religious or cultural ties

Relocation Stress Syndrome

Relocation stress syndrome (See **Relocation** stress syndrome, Section III)

Risk for **Relocation** stress syndrome (See **Relocation** stress syndrome, risk for, Section III)

Renal Failure

Activity intolerance r/t effects of anemia, congestive heart failure

Chronic **Sorrow** r/t chronic illness

Death **Anxiety** r/t unknown outcome of disease

Decreased **Cardiac** output r/t effects of congestive heart failure, elevated potassium levels interfering with conduction system

Excess **Fluid** volume r/t decreased urine output, sodium retention, inappropriate fluid intake

Fatigue r/t effects of chronic uremia and anemia

Imbalanced **Nutrition**: less than body requirements r/t anorexia, nausea, vomiting, altered taste sensation, dietary restrictions

Impaired **Oral** mucous membranes r/t irritation from nitrogenous waste products

Impaired **Urinary** elimination r/t effects of disease, need for dialysis

Ineffective **Coping** r/t depression resulting from chronic disease

Pruritus r/t effects of uremia

Risk for impaired **Oral** mucous membranes: Risk factors: dehydration, effects of uremia

Risk for **Infection**: Risk factor: altered immune functioning

Risk for **Injury**: Risk factors: bone changes, neuropathy, muscle weakness

Risk for **Noncompliance**: Risk factor: complex medical therapy

Risk for **Powerlessness**: Risk factor: chronic illness

Spiritual distress r/t dealing with chronic illness

Renal Failure, Acute/Chronic, Child

Deficient **Diversional** activity r/t immobility during dialysis

Disturbed **Body** image r/t growth retardation, bone changes, visibility of dialysis access devices (shunt, fistula), edema

See Child with Chronic Condition; Hospitalized Child; Renal Failure

Renal Failure, Nonoliguric

Anxiety r/t change in health status

Risk for deficient **Fluid** volume: Risk factor: loss of large volumes of urine

See Renal Failure

Renal Transplantation, Donor

Decisional **Conflict** r/t harvesting of kidney from traumatized donor

Moral Distress r/t conflict among decision makers, end-of-life decisions, time constraints for decision making

Readiness for enhanced **Communication**: r/t expressing thoughts and feelings about situation

Readiness for enhanced family **Coping**: decision to allow organ donation

Readiness for enhanced **Decision making**: expresses desire to enhance understanding and meaning of choices

Readiness for enhanced **Spirituality**: inner peace resulting from allowance of organ donation

Spiritual distress r/t grieving from loss of significant person

See Nephrectomy

Renal Transplantation, Recipient

Anxiety r/t possible rejection, procedure

Deficient **Knowledge** r/t specific nutritional needs, possible paralytic ileus, fluid or sodium restrictions

R

Impaired **Health** maintenance r/t long-term home treatment after transplantation, diet, signs of rejection, use of medications

Impaired **Urinary** elimination r/t possible impaired renal function

Ineffective **Protection** r/t immunosuppression therapy

Readiness for enhanced **Spiritual** well-being: acceptance of situation

Risk for **Infection**: Risk factor: use of immunosuppressive therapy to control rejection

Risk for **Spiritual** distress: Risk factor: obtaining transplanted kidney from someone's traumatic loss

See Kidney Transplant

Respiratory Acidosis

See Acidosis, Respiratory

Respiratory Conditions of the Neonate (Respiratory Distress Syndrome [RDS], Meconium Aspiration, Diaphragmatic Hernia)

Fatigue r/t increased energy requirements and metabolic demands

Impaired **Gas** exchange r/t decreased surfactant, immature lung tissue

Ineffective **Airway** clearance r/t sequelae of attempts to breathe in utero resulting in meconium aspiration

Ineffective **Breathing** pattern r/t prolonged ventilator dependence

Risk for **Infection**: Risk factors: tissue destruction or irritation as a result of aspiration of meconium fluid

See Bronchopulmonary Dysplasia; Hospitalized Child; Premature Infant, Child

Respiratory Distress

See Dyspnea

Respiratory Distress Syndrome (RDS)

See Respiratory Conditions of the Neonate

Respiratory Infections, Acute Childhood (Croup, Epiglottitis, Pertussis, Pneumonia, Respiratory Syncytial Virus)

Activity intolerance r/t generalized weakness, dyspnea, fatigue, poor oxygenation

Anxiety/Fear r/t oxygen deprivation, difficulty breathing

Deficient **Fluid** volume r/t insensible losses (fever, diaphoresis), inadequate oral fluid intake

Hyperthermia r/t infectious process

Imbalanced **Nutrition**: less than body requirements r/t anorexia, fatigue, generalized weakness, poor sucking and breathing coordination, dyspnea

Impaired **Gas** exchange r/t insufficient oxygenation as a result of inflammation or edema of epiglottis, larynx, bronchial passages

Ineffective **Airway** clearance r/t excess tracheobronchial secretions

Ineffective **Breathing** pattern r/t inflamed bronchial passages, coughing

Risk for **Aspiration**: Risk factors: inability to coordinate breathing, coughing, sucking

Risk for **Infection**: transmission to others: Risk factor: virulent infectious organisms

Risk for **Injury** (to pregnant others): Risk factors: exposure to aerosolized medications (e.g., ribavirin, pentamidine), resultant potential fetal toxicity

Risk for **Suffocation**: Risk factors: inflammation of larynx, epiglottis

See Hospitalized Child

Respiratory Syncytial Virus

See Respiratory Infections, Acute Childhood

Restless Leg Syndrome

Insomnia r/t leg discomfort during sleep relieved by frequent leg movement

Sleep deprivation r/t frequent leg movements

See Stress

Retarded Growth and Development

See Growth and Development Lag

Retching

Imbalanced **Nutrition**: less than body requirements r/t inability to ingest food

Nausea r/t chemotherapy, postsurgical anesthesia, irritation to gastrointestinal system, stimulation of neuropharmacological mechanisms

Retinal Detachment

Anxiety r/t change in vision, threat of loss of vision

Deficient **Knowledge** r/t symptoms, need for early intervention to prevent permanent damage

Disturbed **Sensory** perception: visual r/t changes in vision, sudden flashes of light, floating spots, blurring of vision

Risk for impaired **Home** maintenance: Risk factors: postoperative care, activity limitations, care of affected eye

See Vision Impairment

Retinopathy, Diabetic

See Diabetic Retinopathy

Retinopathy of Prematurity (ROP)

Effective **Therapeutic** regimen management: r/t eye examinations by a qualified ophthalmologist

Risk for **Injury**: Risk factors: prolonged mechanical ventilation, ROP secondary to 100% oxygen environment

See Retinal Detachment

Reye's Syndrome

Compromised family **Coping** r/t acute situational crisis

Deficient **Fluid** volume r/t vomiting, hyperventilation

Disturbed **Sensory** perception r/t cerebral edema

Disturbed **Thought** processes r/t degenerative changes in fatty brain tissue, encephalopathy

R

Excess **Fluid** volume: cerebral r/t cerebral edema

Grieving r/t uncertain prognosis and sequelae

Imbalanced **Nutrition**: less than body requirements r/t effects of liver dysfunction, vomiting

Impaired **Gas** exchange r/t hyperventilation, sequelae of increased intracranial pressure

Impaired **Skin** integrity r/t effects of decorticate or decerebrate posturing, seizure activity

Ineffective **Breathing** pattern r/t neuromuscular impairment

Ineffective **Health** maintenance r/t deficient knowledge regarding use of salicylates during viral illness of child

Risk for **Injury**: Risk factors: combative behavior, seizure activity

Situational low **Self-esteem**: family r/t negative perceptions of self, perceived inability to manage family situation, expressions of guilt

See Hospitalized Child

Rh Factor Incompatibility

Anxiety r/t unknown outcome of pregnancy

Deficient **Knowledge** r/t treatment regimen from lack of experience with situation

Effective **Therapeutic** regimen management: r/t following recommended protocol

Health-seeking behaviors: r/t prenatal care, compliance with diagnostic and treatment regimen

Powerlessness r/t perceived lack of control over outcome of pregnancy

Risk for fetal **Injury**: Risk factors: intrauterine destruction of red blood cells, transfusions

Rhabdomyolysis

Impaired physical **Mobility** r/t myalgia and muscle weakness

Impaired **Urinary** elimination r/t presence of myoglobin in the kidneys

Ineffective **Coping** r/t seriousness of condition

Readiness for enhanced **Therapeutic** regimen management: r/t seeks information to avoid condition

Risk for deficient **Fluid** volume: Risk factor: reduced blood flow to kidneys

See Renal Failure

Rheumatic Fever

See Endocarditis

Rheumatoid Arthritis

Chronic **Pain** r/t swollen or inflamed joints, restricted movement, physical therapy

Effective **Therapeutic** regimen management: following prescribed medication and adhering to exercise program; physical therapy

Fatigue r/t chronic inflammatory disease

Impaired physical **Mobility** r/t pain, limited range of motion

Imbalanced **Nutrition**: less than body requirements r/t loss of appetite

Risk for impaired **Skin** integrity: Risk factors: splints, adaptive devices

Risk for **Injury**: Risk factors: impaired physical mobility, splints, adaptive devices, increased bleeding potential as a result of antiinflammatory medications

Risk for situational low **Self-esteem**: Risk factor: disturbed body image

Self-care deficits: feeding, bathing, hygiene, dressing, grooming, toileting r/t restricted joint movement, pain

See Arthritis; JRA (Juvenile Rheumatoid Arthritis)

Rib Fracture

Acute **Pain** r/t movement, deep breathing

Ineffective **Breathing** pattern r/t fractured ribs

See Ventilator Client (if relevant)

Ridicule of Others

Defensive **Coping** r/t situational crisis, psychological impairment, substance abuse

Risk for **Post-trauma** syndrome: Risk factor: perception of the event

Ringworm of Body

Impaired **Skin** integrity r/t presence of macules associated with fungus

Ineffective **Therapeutic** regimen management r/t deficient knowledge of prevention, treatment

See Itching; Pruritus

Ringworm of Nails

Disturbed **Body** image r/t appearance of nails, removed nails

Ineffective **Therapeutic** regimen management r/t deficient knowledge of prevention, treatment

Ringworm of Scalp

Disturbed **Body** image r/t possible hair loss (alopecia)

Ineffective **Therapeutic** regimen management r/t deficient knowledge of prevention, treatment

See Itching; Pruritus

Risk for Relocation Stress Syndrome

See Relocation Stress Syndrome, Section II

Roaches, Invasion of Home with

Impaired **Home** maintenance r/t lack of knowledge, insufficient finances

See Filthy Home Environment

Role Performance, Altered

Ineffective **Role** performance (See **Role** performance, ineffective, Section III)

ROP

See Retinopathy of Prematurity (ROP)

RSV (Respiratory Syncytial Virus)

See Respiratory Infection, Acute Childhood

R

Rubella

See Communicable Diseases, Childhood

Rubor of Extremities

Ineffective **Tissue** perfusion: peripheral r/t interruption of arterial flow

See Peripheral Vascular Disease

Ruptured Disk

See Low Back Pain

S

SAD (Seasonal Affective Disorder)

Effective **Therapeutic** regimen management: uses SAD lights during winter months

See Depression (Major Depressive Disorder)

Sadness

Adult **Failure** to thrive r/t depression, apathy

Complicated **Grieving** r/t actual or perceived loss

Readiness for enhanced **Communication**: willingness to share feelings and thoughts

Readiness for enhanced **Spiritual** well-being: desire for harmony after actual or perceived loss

Risk for **Powerlessness**: Risk factor: actual or perceived loss

Risk for **Spiritual** distress: Risk factor: loss of loved one

Spiritual distress r/t intense suffering

See Depression (Major Depressive Disorder); Major Depressive Disorder

Safe Sex

Effective **Therapeutic** regimen management: taking appropriate precautions during sexual activity to keep from contacting a sexually transmitted disease

See Sexuality, Adolescent; STD (Sexually Transmitted Disease)

Safety, Childhood

Deficient **Knowledge**: potential for enhanced health maintenance r/t parental knowledge and skill acquisition regarding appropriate safety measures

Health-seeking behaviors r/t enhanced parenting r/t adequate support systems, appropriate requests for help, desire and request for safety information

Readiness for enhanced **Immunization** status: expresses desire to enhance immunization status

Risk for altered **Health** maintenance: Risk factors: parental deficient knowledge regarding appropriate safety needs per developmental stage, child-proofing house

Risk for **Aspiration** (See **Aspiration**, risk for, Section III)

Risk for impaired **Parenting**: Risk factors: lack of available and effective role model, lack of knowledge, misinformation from other family members (old wives' tales)

Risk for **Injury/Trauma**: Risk factors: developmental age, altered home maintenance

Risk for **Poisoning**: Risk factors: use of lead-based paint; presence of asbestos or radon gas; drugs not locked in cabinet; household products left in accessible area (bleach, detergent, drain cleaners, household cleaners); alcohol and perfume within reach of child; presence of poisonous plants; atmospheric pollutants

Salmonella

Readiness for enhanced **Therapeutic** regimen management: avoiding improperly prepared or stored food, wearing gloves when handling pet reptiles or their feces

Impaired **Home** maintenance r/t improper preparation or storage of food, lack of safety measures when caring for pet reptile

See Gastroenteritis; Gastroenteritis, Child

Salpingectomy

Decisional **Conflict** r/t sterilization procedure

Grieving r/t possible loss from tubal pregnancy

Risk for impaired **Urinary** elimination: Risk factor: trauma to ureter during surgery

See Hysterectomy; Surgery, Perioperative Care; Surgery, Postoperative Care; Surgery, Preoperative Care

Sarcoidosis

Acute **Pain** r/t possible disease affecting joints

Anxiety r/t change in health status

Decreased **Cardiac** output r/t dysrhythmias

Impaired **Gas** exchange r/t ventilation-perfusion imbalance

Ineffective **Health** maintenance r/t deficient knowledge regarding home care and medication regimen

SARS (Severe Acute Respiratory Syndrome)

Risk for **Infection**: Risk factor: increased environmental exposure (travelers in close proximity to infected persons, traveling when a fever is present)

Readiness for enhanced **Knowledge** r/t information regarding travel and precautions to avoid exposure to SARS

Effective **Therapeutic** regimen management r/t uses appropriate hand hygiene

See Pneumonia

SBE (Self Breast Examination)

Effective **Therapeutic** regimen management r/t practices SBE per recommended protocol

Health-seeking behaviors r/t desires to have information about SBE

Readiness for enhanced **Knowledge**: self-breast examination

Scabies

See Communicable Diseases, Childhood

Scared

Anxiety r/t threat of death, threat to or change in health status

Death **Anxiety** r/t unresolved issues surrounding end-of-life decisions

Fear r/t hospitalization, real or imagined threat to own well-being

Readiness for enhanced **Communication**: willingness to share thoughts and feelings

Schizophrenia

Anxiety r/t unconscious conflict with reality

Chronic **Sorrow** r/t chronic mental illness

Deficient **Diversional** activity r/t social isolation, possible regression

Disturbed **Sensory** perception r/t biochemical imbalances for sensory distortion (illusions, hallucinations)

Disturbed **Thought** processes r/t inaccurate interpretations of environment

Fear r/t altered contact with reality

Imbalanced **Nutrition**: less than body requirements r/t fear of eating, lack of awareness of hunger, disinterest toward food

Impaired **Home** maintenance r/t impaired cognitive or emotional functioning, insufficient finances, inadequate support systems

Impaired **Social** interaction r/t impaired communication patterns, self-concept disturbance, disturbed thought processes

Impaired verbal **Communication** r/t psychosis, disorientation, inaccurate perception, hallucinations, delusions

Ineffective **Coping** r/t inadequate support systems, unrealistic perceptions, inadequate coping skills, disturbed thought processes, impaired communication

Ineffective **Health** maintenance r/t cognitive impairment, ineffective individual and family coping, lack of material resources

Ineffective family **Therapeutic** regimen management r/t chronicity and unpredictability of condition

Insomnia r/t sensory alterations contributing to fear and anxiety

Interrupted **Family** processes r/t inability to express feelings, impaired communication

Readiness for enhanced **Hope**: expresses desire to enhance interconnectedness with others and problem-solve to meet goals

Readiness for enhanced **Power**: expresses willingness to enhance participation in choices for daily living and health and enhance knowledge for participation in change

Risk for **Caregiver** role strain: Risk factors: bizarre behavior of client, chronicity of condition

Risk for compromised human **Dignity**: Risk factor: stigmatizing label

Risk for impaired **Religiosity**: Risk factors: ineffective coping, lack of security

Risk for **Loneliness**: Risk factor: inability to interact socially

Risk for **Post-trauma** syndrome: Risk factor: diminished ego strength

Risk for **Powerlessness**: Risk factor: intrusive, distorted thinking

Risk for self- and other-directed **Violence**: Risk factors: lack of trust, panic, hallucinations, delusional thinking

Risk for **Suicide**: Risk factor: psychiatric illness

Self-care deficit r/t loss of contact with reality, impairment of perception

Sleep deprivation r/t intrusive thoughts, nightmares

Social isolation r/t lack of trust, regression, delusional thinking, repressed fears

Spiritual distress r/t loneliness, social alienation

Sciatica

See Neuropathy, Peripheral

Scoliosis

Acute **Pain** r/t musculoskeletal restrictions, surgery, reambulation with cast or spinal rod

Chronic **Sorrow** r/t chronic disability

Disturbed **Body** image r/t use of therapeutic braces, postsurgery scars, restricted physical activity

Impaired **Gas** exchange r/t restricted lung expansion as a result of severe presurgery curvature of spine, immobilization

Impaired physical **Mobility** r/t restricted movement, dyspnea caused by severe curvature of spine

Impaired **Skin** integrity r/t braces, casts, surgical correction

Ineffective **Breathing** pattern r/t restricted lung expansion caused by severe curvature of spine

Ineffective **Health** maintenance r/t deficient knowledge regarding treatment modalities, restrictions, home care, postoperative activities

Readiness for enhanced **Therapeutic** regimen management r/t desire for knowledge regarding treatment for condition

Risk for **Infection**: Risk factor: surgical incision

Risk for perioperative positioning **Injury**: Risk factor: prone position

Risk-prone health **Behavior** r/t lack of developmental maturity to comprehend long-term consequences of noncompliance with treatment procedures

See Hospitalized Child; Maturational Issues, Adolescent

Sedentary Lifestyle

Activity intolerance r/t sedentary lifestyle

Readiness for enhanced **Coping** r/t seeking knowledge of new strategies to adjust to sedentary lifestyle

Sedentary **Lifestyle** (See **Lifestyle**, sedentary, Section III)

Seizure Disorders, Adult

Acute **Confusion** r/t postseizure state

Impaired **Memory** r/t seizure activity

Ineffective **Health** maintenance r/t lack of knowledge regarding anticonvulsive therapy

Readiness for enhanced **Knowledge** r/t anticonvulsive therapy

Readiness for enhanced **Self-care**: expresses desire to enhance knowledge and responsibility for self-care

Risk for disturbed **Thought** processes: Risk factor: effects of anticonvulsant medications

Risk for **Falls**: Risk factor: uncontrolled seizure activity

Risk for ineffective **Airway** clearance: Risk factor: accumulation of secretions during seizure

S

Risk for **Injury**: Risk factors: uncontrolled movements during seizure, falls, drowsiness caused by anticonvulsants

Risk for **Powerlessness**: Risk factor: possible seizure

Social isolation r/t unpredictability of seizures, community-imposed stigma

See Epilepsy

Seizure Disorders, Childhood (Epilepsy, Febrile Seizures, Infantile Spasms)

Ineffective **Health** maintenance r/t lack of knowledge regarding anticonvulsive therapy, fever reduction (febrile seizures)

Risk for delayed **Development** and disproportionate growth: Risk factors: effects of seizure disorder, parental overprotection

Risk for disturbed **Thought** processes: Risk factor: effects of anticonvulsant medications

Risk for **Falls**: Risk factor: possible seizure

Risk for ineffective **Airway** clearance: Risk factor: accumulation of secretions during seizure

Risk for **Injury**: Risk factors: uncontrolled movements during seizure, falls, drowsiness caused by anticonvulsants

Social isolation r/t unpredictability of seizures, community-imposed stigma

See Epilepsy

Self Breast Examination

See SBE (Self Breast Examination)

Self-Care

Readiness for enhanced **Self-Care** (See **Self-care**, readiness for enhanced, Section III)

Self-Care Deficit, Bathing/Hygiene

Bathing/hygiene **Self-care** deficit (See **Self-care** deficit, bathing, hygiene, Section III)

Self-Care Deficit, Dressing/Grooming

Dressing/grooming **Self-care** deficit (See **Self-care** deficit, dressing/grooming, Section III)

Self-Care Deficit, Feeding

Feeding **Self-care** deficit (See **Self-care** deficit, feeding, Section III)

Self-Care Deficit, Toileting

Toileting **Self-care** deficit (See **Self-care** deficit, toileting, Section III)

Self-Concept

Readiness for enhanced **Self-concept** (See **Self-concept**, readiness for, Section III)

Self-Destructive Behavior

Post-trauma response r/t unresolved feelings from traumatic event

Risk for self-directed **Violence**: Risk factors: panic state, history of child abuse, toxic reaction to medication

Risk for **Self-mutilation**: Risk factors: feelings of depression, rejection, self-hatred, depersonalization; command hallucinations

Risk for **Suicide**: Risk factor: history of self-destructive behavior

Self-Esteem, Chronic Low

Chronic low **Self-esteem** (See **Self-esteem**, chronic low, Section III)

Self-Esteem, Situational Low

Risk for situational low **Self-esteem** (See **Self-esteem**, situational low, risk for, Section III)

Self-esteem disturbance r/t inappropriate and learned negative feelings about self

Situational low **Self-esteem** (See **Self-esteem**, situational low, Section III)

Self-Mutilation, Risk for

Risk for **Self-mutilation** (See **Self-mutilation**, risk for, Section III)

Self-mutilation (See **Self-mutilation**, Section III)

Senile Dementia

Sedentary **lifestyle** r/t lack of interest

See Dementia

Sensory/Perceptual Alterations

Disturbed **Sensory** perception: visual, auditory, kinesthetic, gustatory, tactile, olfactory (See **Sensory** perception, disturbed, Section III)

Separation Anxiety

Ineffective **Coping** r/t maturational and situational crises, vulnerability related to developmental age, hospitalization, separation from family and familiar surroundings, multiple caregivers

Insomnia r/t separation for significant others

Risk for impaired parent/child **Attachment**: Risk factor: separation

See Hospitalized Child

Sepsis, Child

Delayed **Surgical** recovery r/t presence of infection

Imbalanced **Nutrition**: less than body requirements r/t anorexia, generalized weakness, poor sucking reflex

Ineffective **Thermoregulation** r/t infectious process, septic shock

Ineffective **Tissue** perfusion: cardiopulmonary, peripheral r/t arterial or venous blood flow exchange problems, septic shock

Risk for impaired **Skin** integrity: Risk factors: desquamation caused by disseminated intravascular coagulation

See Hospitalized Child; Premature Infant, Child

Septicemia

Deficient **Fluid** volume r/t vasodilation of peripheral vessels, leaking of capillaries

Imbalanced **Nutrition**: less than body requirements r/t anorexia, generalized weakness

Ineffective **Tissue** perfusion r/t decreased systemic vascular resistance

See Sepsis, Child; Shock; Shock, Septic

S

Severe Acute Respiratory Syndrome

See SARS (Severe Acute Respiratory Syndrome); Pneumonia

Sexual Dysfunction

Chronic **Sorrow** r/t loss of ideal sexual experience, altered relationships

Sexual dysfunction (See **Sexual** dysfunction, Section III)

See Erectile Dysfunction

Sexuality, Adolescent

Decisional **Conflict**: sexual activity r/t undefined personal values or beliefs, multiple or divergent sources of information, lack of relevant information

Deficient **Knowledge**: potential for enhanced health maintenance r/t multiple or divergent sources of information or lack of relevant information regarding sexual transmission of disease, contraception, prevention of toxic shock syndrome

Disturbed **Body** image r/t anxiety caused by unachieved developmental milestone (puberty) or deficient knowledge regarding reproductive maturation as manifested by amenorrhea or expressed concerns regarding lack of growth of secondary sex characteristics

Risk for **Rape-trauma** syndrome: Risk factors: date rape, campus rape, insufficient knowledge regarding self-protection mechanisms

See Maturational Issues, Adolescent

Sexuality Pattern, Ineffective

Ineffective **Sexuality** pattern (See **Sexuality**, ineffective pattern, Section III)

Sexually Transmitted Disease

See STD (Sexually Transmitted Disease)

Shaken Baby Syndrome

Decreased **Intracranial** adaptive capacity r/t brain injury

Impaired **Parenting** r/t stress, history of being abusive

Risk for other-directed **Violence**: Risk factors: history of violence against others, perinatal complications

Stress overload r/t intense repeated family stressors, family violence

See Child Abuse; Suspected Child Abuse and Neglect (SCAN), Child; Suspected Child Abuse and Neglect (SCAN), Parent

Shakiness

Anxiety r/t situational or maturational crisis, threat of death

Shame

Self-esteem disturbance r/t inability to deal with past traumatic events, blaming of self for events not under one's control

Shingles

Acute **Pain** r/t vesicular eruption along the nerves

Ineffective **Protection** r/t abnormal blood profiles

Pruritus r/t inflammation

Risk for **Infection**: Risk factor: tissue destruction

Social isolation r/t altered state of wellness, contagiousness of disease

See Itching

Shivering

Hypothermia r/t exposure to cool environment

Shock

Fear r/t serious threat to health status

Ineffective **Tissue** perfusion: cardiopulmonary; peripheral r/t arterial/venous blood flow exchange problems

Risk for **Injury**: Risk factor: prolonged shock resulting in multiple organ failure or death

See Shock, Cardiogenic; Shock, Hypovolemic; Shock, Septic

Shock, Cardiogenic

Decreased **Cardiac** output r/t decreased myocardial contractility, dysrhythmia

See Shock

Shock, Hypovolemic

Deficient **Fluid** volume r/t abnormal loss of fluid

See Shock

Shock, Septic

Deficient **Fluid** volume r/t abnormal loss of fluid through capillaries, pooling of blood in peripheral circulation

Ineffective **Protection** r/t inadequately functioning immune system

See Sepsis, Child; Septicemia; Shock

Shoulder Repair

Risk for perioperative positioning **Injury**: Risk factor: immobility

Self-care deficit: bathing, hygiene, dressing, grooming, feeding r/t immobilization of affected shoulder

See Surgery, Preoperative; Surgery, Perioperative; Surgery, Postoperative; Total Joint Replacement

Sickle Cell Anemia/Crisis

Activity intolerance r/t fatigue, effects of chronic anemia

Acute **Pain** r/t viscous blood, tissue hypoxia

Deficient **Fluid** volume r/t decreased intake, increased fluid requirements during sickle cell crisis, decreased ability of kidneys to concentrate urine

Impaired physical **Mobility** r/t pain, fatigue

Risk for ineffective **Tissue** perfusion: renal, cerebral, cardiac, gastrointestinal, peripheral: Risk factors: effects of red cell sickling, infarction of tissues

Risk for **Infection**: Risk factor: alterations in splenic function

See Child with Chronic Condition; Hospitalized Child

SIDS (Sudden Infant Death Syndrome)

Anxiety/Fear: parental r/t life-threatening event

Deficient **Knowledge**: potential for enhanced health maintenance r/t knowledge or skill acquisition of cardiopulmonary resuscitation and home apnea monitoring

S

Grieving r/t potential loss of infant

Insomnia: parental/infant r/t home apnea monitoring

Interrupted **Family** processes r/t stress as a result of special care needs of infant with apnea

Risk for **Powerlessness**: Risk factor: unanticipated life-threatening event

Risk for sudden infant **Death** syndrome (See **Death** syndrome, sudden infant, risk for, Section III)

See Terminally Ill Child/Death of Child, Parent

Situational Crisis

Ineffective **Coping** r/t situational crisis

Interrupted **Family** processes r/t situational crisis

Readiness for enhanced **Communication**: willingness to share feelings and thoughts

Readiness for enhanced **Religiosity**: requests religious material and/or experiences

Readiness for enhanced **Spiritual** well-being: desire for harmony following crisis

SJS (Stevens-Johnson Syndrome)

See Stevens-Johnson Syndrome

Skin Cancer

Impaired **Skin** integrity r/t abnormal cell growth in skin, treatment of skin cancer

Ineffective **Health** maintenance r/t deficient knowledge regarding self-care with skin cancer

Readiness for enhanced **Knowledge** r/t self-care to prevent and treat skin cancer

Skin Disorders

Internal/External

Impaired **Skin** integrity (See **Skin** integrity, impaired, Section III)

Skin Integrity, Risk for Impaired

Internal/External

Risk for impaired **Skin** integrity (See **Skin** integrity, impaired, risk for, Section III)

Skin Turgor, Change in Elasticity

Deficient **Fluid** volume r/t active fluid loss (decreased skin turgor can be a normal finding in the elderly)

Sleep

Readiness for enhanced **Sleep** (See **Sleep**, readiness for enhanced, Section III)

Sleep Apnea

See PND (Paroxysmal Nocturnal Dyspnea)

Sleep Deprivation

Disturbed **Sensory** perception r/t lack of sleep

Fatigue r/t lack of sleep

Sleep deprivation (See **Sleep** deprivation, Section III)

Sleep Pattern Disorders

Insomnia (See **Insomnia**, Section III)

Sleep Pattern, Disturbed, Parent/Child

Insomnia: child r/t anxiety or fear

Insomnia: parent r/t parental responsibilities, stress

See Suspected Child Abuse and Neglect

Slurring of Speech

Impaired verbal **Communication** r/t decrease in circulation to brain, brain tumor, anatomical defect, cleft palate

Situational low **Self-esteem** r/t speech impairment

See Communication Problems

Small Bowel Resection

See Abdominal Surgery

Smell, Loss of Ability to

Risk for **Injury**: Risk factors: inability to detect gas fumes, smoke smells

See Anosmia

Smoke Inhalation

Impaired **Gas** exchange r/t ventilation perfusion imbalance

Ineffective **Airway** clearance r/t smoke inhalation

Readiness for effective **Therapeutic** regimen management: functioning smoke detectors and carbon monoxide detectors in home and work, plan for escape route worked out and reviewed

Risk for acute **Confusion**: Risk factor: decreased oxygen supply

Risk for **Poisoning**: Risk factor: exposure to carbon monoxide

See Atelectasis; Burns; Pneumonia

Smoking Behavior

Altered **Health** maintenance r/t denial of effects of smoking, lack of effective support for smoking withdrawal

Readiness for enhanced **Knowledge** r/t smoking cessation

Social Interaction, Impaired

Impaired **Social** interaction (See **Social** interaction, impaired, Section III)

Social Isolation

Social isolation (See **Social** isolation, Section III)

Sociopathic Personality

See Antisocial Personality Disorder

Sodium, Decrease/Increase

See Hyponatremia/Hypernatremia

Somatization Disorder

Anxiety r/t unresolved conflicts channeled into physical complaints or conditions

Chronic **Pain** r/t unexpressed anger, multiple physical disorders, depression

Ineffective **Coping** r/t lack of insight into underlying conflicts

Ineffective **Denial** r/t displaces psychological stress to physical symptoms

S

Sore Nipples, Breastfeeding

Ineffective **Breastfeeding** r/t deficient knowledge regarding correct feeding procedure

See Painful Breasts, Sore Nipples

Sore Throat

Acute **Pain** r/t inflammation, irritation, dryness

Deficient **Knowledge** r/t treatment, relief of discomfort

Impaired **Oral** mucous membrane r/t inflammation or infection of oral cavity

Impaired **Swallowing** r/t irritation of oropharyngeal cavity

Sorrow

Chronic **Sorrow** (See **Sorrow**, chronic, Section III)

Grieving r/t loss of significant person, object, or role

Readiness for enhanced **Communication**: expresses thoughts and feelings

Readiness for enhanced **Spiritual** well-being: desire to find purpose and meaning of loss

Spastic Colon

See IBS (Irritable Bowel Syndrome)

Speech Disorders

Anxiety r/t difficulty with communication

Delayed **Growth** and development r/t effects of physical or mental disability

Disturbed **Sensory** perception (auditory) r/t altered sensory reception, transmission, and/or integration

Impaired verbal **Communication** r/t anatomical defect, cleft palate, psychological barriers, decrease in circulation to brain

Spina Bifida

See Neural Tube Defects

Spinal Cord Injury

Chronic **Sorrow** r/t immobility, change in body function

Complicated **Grieving** r/t loss of usual body function

Constipation r/t immobility, loss of sensation

Deficient **Diversional** activity r/t long-term hospitalization, frequent lengthy treatments

Disturbed **Body** image r/t change in body function

Fear r/t powerlessness over loss of body function

Impaired **Home** maintenance r/t change in health status, insufficient family planning or finances, deficient knowledge, inadequate support systems

Impaired physical **Mobility** r/t neuromuscular impairment

Impaired wheelchair **Mobility** r/t neuromuscular impairment

Ineffective **Health** maintenance r/t deficient knowledge regarding self-care with spinal cord injury

Readiness for enhanced **Self-care**: expresses desire to enhance independence in maintaining well-being

Reflex **Incontinence** r/t spinal cord lesion interfering with conduction of cerebral messages

Risk for **Autonomic** dysreflexia: Risk factors: bladder or bowel distention, skin irritation, deficient knowledge of patient and caregiver

Risk for **Disuse** syndrome: Risk factor: paralysis

Risk for impaired **Religiosity**: Risk factor: lack of transportation

Risk for impaired **Skin** integrity: Risk factors: immobility, paralysis

Risk for ineffective **Breathing** pattern: Risk factor: neuromuscular impairment

Risk for **Infection**: Risk factors: chronic disease, stasis of body fluids

Risk for latex **Allergy** response: Risk factor: continuous or intermittent catheterization

Risk for **Loneliness**: Risk factor: physical immobility

Risk for **Powerlessness**: Risk factor: loss of function

Self-care deficit r/t neuromuscular impairment

Sedentary **lifestyle** r/t lack of resources or interest

Sexual dysfunction r/t altered body function

Urinary retention r/t inhibition of reflex arc

See Child with Chronic Condition; Hospitalized Child; Neural Tube Defects

Spinal Fusion

Impaired bed **Mobility** r/t impaired ability to turn side to side while keeping spine in proper alignment

Impaired physical **Mobility** r/t musculoskeletal impairment associated with surgery, possible back brace

Readiness for enhanced **Knowledge** r/t expresses interest in information associated with surgery

See Acute Back; Back Pain; Scoliosis; Surgery, Preoperative Care; Surgery, Perioperative Care; Surgery, Postoperative Care

Spiritual Distress

Risk for **Spiritual** distress (See **Spiritual** distress, risk for, Section III)

Spiritual distress (See **Spiritual** distress, Section III)

Spiritual Well-Being

Readiness for enhanced **Spiritual** well-being (See **Spiritual** well-being, readiness for enhanced, Section III)

Splenectomy

See Abdominal Surgery

Sprains

Acute **Pain** r/t physical injury

Effective **Therapeutic** regimen management: not exercising when tired or in pain; maintaining healthy weight; wearing properly fitting shoes; using appropriate warm-up, stretching, and cool down exercises; wearing protective equipment; running on even surfaces; staying physically fit

Impaired physical **Mobility** r/t injury

Stapedectomy

Acute **Pain** r/t headache

Disturbed **Sensory** perception: auditory r/t hearing loss caused by edema from surgery

S

Risk for **Falls**: Risk factor: dizziness

Risk for **Infection**: Risk factor: invasive procedure

Stasis Ulcer

Impaired **Tissue** integrity r/t chronic venous congestion

See CHF (Congestive Heart Failure); Varicose Veins

STD (Sexually Transmitted Disease)

Acute **Pain** r/t biological or psychological injury

Fear r/t altered body function, risk for social isolation, fear of incurable illness

Ineffective **Health** maintenance r/t deficient knowledge regarding transmission, symptoms, treatment of STD

Ineffective **Sexuality** pattern r/t illness, altered body function

Readiness for enhanced **Knowledge** r/t prevention and treatment of STDs

Risk for **Infection**/spread of infection: Risk factor: lack of knowledge concerning transmission of disease

Social isolation r/t fear of contracting or spreading disease

See Maturational Issues, Adolescent

STEMI (ST-Elevation Myocardial Infarction)

See MI (Myocardial Infarction)

Stent (Coronary Artery Stent)

Decrease **Cardiac** output r/t possible restenosis

Readiness for enhanced **Decision** making: expresses desire to enhance risk benefit analysis, understanding and meaning of choices, and decisions regarding treatment

Risk for **Injury**: Risk factor: complications associated with stent placement

See Angioplasty Coronary, Cardiac Catheterization

Sterilization Surgery

Decisional **Conflict** r/t multiple or divergent sources of information, unclear personal values or beliefs

See Surgery, Preoperative Care; Surgery, Perioperative Care; Surgery, Postoperative Care; Tubal Ligation; Vasectomy

Stertorous Respirations

Ineffective **Airway** clearance r/t pharyngeal obstruction

Stevens-Johnson Syndrome (SJS)

Acute **Pain** r/t painful skin lesions and painful oral mucosa lesions

Impaired **Oral** mucous membrane r/t immunocompromised condition associated with allergic medication reaction

Impaired **Skin** integrity r/t allergic medication reaction

Risk for acute **Confusion**: Risk factors: dehydration, electrolyte disturbances

Risk for deficient **Fluid** volume: Risk factors: factors affecting fluid needs (hypermetabolic state, hyperthermia), excessive losses through normal routes (vomiting and diarrhea)

Stillbirth

See Pregnancy Loss

Stoma

See Colostomy; Ileostomy

Stomatitis

Impaired **Oral** mucous membrane r/t pathological conditions of oral cavity

Stone, Kidney

See Kidney Stone

Stool, Hard/Dry

Constipation r/t inadequate fluid intake, inadequate fiber intake, decreased activity level, decreased gastric motility

Straining with Defecation

Constipation r/t less than adequate fluid intake, less than adequate dietary intake

Risk for decreased **Cardiac** output r/t vagal stimulation with dysrhythmia resulting from Valsalva maneuver

Stress

Anxiety r/t feelings of helplessness, feelings of being threatened

Disturbed **Energy** field r/t low energy level, feelings of hopelessness

Fear r/t powerlessness over feelings

Ineffective **Coping** r/t ineffective use of problem-solving process, feelings of apprehension or helplessness

Readiness for enhanced **Communication** r/t willingness to share thoughts and feelings

Readiness for enhanced **Spiritual** well-being r/t desire for harmony and peace in stressful situation

Risk for **Post-trauma** syndrome: Risk factors: perception of event, survivor's role in event

Self-esteem disturbance r/t inability to deal with life events

Stress overload r/t intense or multiple stressors

Stress Overload

Stress overload (See **Stress** overload, Section III)

Stress Urinary Incontinence

Risk for urge urinary **Incontinence** r/t involuntary sphincter relaxation

Stress urinary **Incontinence** r/t degenerative change in pelvic muscles

See Incontinence of Urine

Stridor

Ineffective **Airway** clearance r/t obstruction, tracheobronchial infection, trauma

Stroke

See CVA (Cerebrovascular Accident)

Stuttering

Anxiety r/t impaired verbal communication

Impaired verbal **Communication** r/t anxiety, psychological problems

Subarachnoid Hemorrhage

Acute **Pain**: headache r/t irritation of meninges from blood, increased intracranial pressure

Ineffective **Tissue** perfusion: cerebral r/t bleeding from cerebral vessel

See Intracranial Pressure, Increased

Substance Abuse

Anxiety r/t loss of control

Compromised/disabled family **Coping** r/t codependency issues

Defensive **Coping** r/t substance abuse

Dysfunctional **Family** processes: alcohol r/t inadequate coping skills

Imbalanced **Nutrition**: less than body requirements r/t anorexia

Ineffective **Coping** r/t use of substances to cope with life events

Ineffective **Denial** r/t refusal to acknowledge substance abuse problem

Ineffective **Protection** r/t malnutrition, sleep deprivation

Insomnia r/t irritability, nightmares, tremors

Powerlessness r/t substance addiction

Readiness for enhanced **Coping**: seeking social support and knowledge of new strategies

Readiness for enhanced **Self-concept**: accepting strengths and limitations

Risk for impaired parent/child **Attachment**: Risk factor: substance abuse

Risk for **Injury**: Risk factor: alteration in sensory perception

Risk for self- or other-directed **Violence**: Risk factors: reactions to substances used, impulsive behavior, disorientation, impaired judgment

Risk for **Suicide**: Risk factor: substance abuse

Self-esteem disturbance r/t failure at life events

Social isolation r/t unacceptable social behavior or values

See Maturational Issues, Adolescent

Substance Abuse, Adolescent

See Alcohol Withdrawal; Maturational Issues, Adolescent; Substance Abuse

Substance Abuse in Pregnancy

Defensive **Coping** r/t denial of situation, differing value system

Deficient **Knowledge** r/t lack of exposure to information regarding effects of substance abuse in pregnancy

Health-seeking behaviors (substance abuse counseling) r/t desire to provide child with substance-free perinatal period

Ineffective **Health** maintenance r/t addiction

Noncompliance r/t differing value system, cultural influences, addiction

Risk for fetal **Injury** r/t effects of drugs on fetal growth and development

Risk for impaired parent/child **Attachment**: Risk factors: substance abuse, inability of parent to meet infant's or own personal needs

Risk for impaired **Parenting**: Risk factor: lack of ability to meet infant's needs

Risk for **Infection**: Risk factors: intravenous drug use, lifestyle

Risk for maternal **Injury**: Risk factor: drug use

See Substance Abuse

Sucking Reflex

Effective **Breastfeeding** r/t regular and sustained sucking and swallowing at breast

Sudden Infant Death Syndrome (SIDS)

See SIDS (Sudden Infant Death Syndrome)

Suffocation, Risk for

Internal/External

Risk for **Suffocation** (See **Suffocation**, risk for, Section III)

Suicide Attempt

Hopelessness r/t perceived or actual loss, substance abuse, low self-concept, inadequate support systems

Ineffective **Coping** r/t anger, complicated grieving

Post-trauma response r/t history of traumatic events, abuse, rape, incest, war, torture

Readiness for enhanced **Communication**: willingness to share thoughts and feelings

Readiness for enhanced **Spiritual** well-being: desire for harmony and inner strength to help redefine purpose for life

Risk for **Post-trauma** syndrome: Risk factor: survivor's role in suicide attempt

Risk for **Suicide** (See **Suicide**, risk for, Section III)

Self-esteem disturbance r/t guilt, inability to trust, feelings of worthlessness or rejection

Social isolation r/t inability to engage in satisfying personal relationships

Spiritual distress r/t hopelessness, despair

See Violent Behavior

Support System

Readiness for enhanced family **Coping**: ability to adapt to tasks associated with care, support of significant other during health crisis

Readiness for enhanced **Family** processes: activities support the growth of family members

Readiness for enhanced **Parenting**: children or other dependent person(s) expressing satisfaction with home environment

Suppression of Labor

See Preterm Labor; Tocolytic Therapy

Surgery, Perioperative Care

Risk for imbalanced **Fluid** volume: Risk factor: surgery

Risk for perioperative positioning **Injury**: Risk factors: predisposing condition, prolonged surgery

S

Surgery, Postoperative Care

Activity intolerance r/t pain, surgical procedure

Acute **Pain** r/t inflammation or injury in surgical area

Anxiety r/t change in health status, hospital environment

Deficient **Knowledge** r/t postoperative expectations, lifestyle changes

Delayed **Surgical** recovery r/t extensive surgical procedure, postoperative surgical infection

Imbalanced **Nutrition**: less than body requirements r/t anorexia, nausea, vomiting, decreased peristalsis

Nausea r/t manipulation of gastrointestinal tract, postsurgical anesthesia

Risk for **Constipation**: Risk factors: decreased activity, decreased food or fluid intake, anesthesia, pain medication

Risk for deficient **Fluid** volume: Risk factors: hypermetabolic state, fluid loss during surgery, presence of indwelling tubes

Risk for ineffective **Breathing** pattern: Risk factors: pain, location of incision, effects of anesthesia or narcotics

Risk for ineffective **Tissue** perfusion: peripheral: Risk factors: hypovolemia, circulatory stasis, obesity, prolonged immobility, decreased coughing, decreased deep breathing

Risk for **Infection**: Risk factors: invasive procedure, pain, anesthesia, location of incision, weakened cough as a result of aging

Urinary retention r/t anesthesia, pain, fear, unfamiliar surroundings, client's position

Surgery, Preoperative Care

Anxiety r/t threat to or change in health status, situational crisis, fear of the unknown

Deficient **Knowledge** r/t preoperative procedures, postoperative expectations

Insomnia r/t anxiety about upcoming surgery

Readiness for enhanced **Knowledge** of r/t preoperative and postoperative expectations for self-care

Surgical Recovery, Delayed

Delayed **Surgical** recovery (See **Surgical** recovery, delayed, Section III)

Suspected Child Abuse and Neglect (SCAN), Child

Acute **Pain** r/t physical injuries

Anxiety/Fear: child r/t threat of punishment for perceived wrongdoing

Chronic low **Self-esteem** r/t lack of positive feedback, excessive negative feedback

Deficient **Diversional** activity r/t diminished or absent environmental or personal stimuli

Delayed **Growth** and development: regression versus delayed r/t diminished or absent environmental stimuli, inadequate caretaking, inconsistent responsiveness by caretaker

Imbalanced **Nutrition**: less than body requirements r/t inadequate caretaking

Impaired **Skin** integrity r/t altered nutritional state, physical abuse

Insomnia r/t hypervigilance, anxiety

Post-trauma response r/t physical abuse, incest, rape, molestation

Rape-trauma syndrome: compound/silent reaction r/t altered lifestyle because of abuse, changes in residence

Readiness for enhanced community **Coping**: obtaining resources to prevent child abuse, neglect

Risk for **Poisoning**: Risk factors: inadequate safeguards, lack of proper safety precautions

Risk for **Suffocation**: secondary to aspiration: Risk factors: propped bottle, unattended child

Risk for **Trauma**: Risk factors: inadequate precautions, cognitive or emotional difficulties

Social isolation: family-imposed r/t fear of disclosure of family dysfunction and abuse

See Hospitalized Child; Maturational Issues, Adolescent

Suspected Child Abuse and Neglect (SCAN), Parent

Chronic low **Self-esteem** r/t lack of successful parenting experiences

Disabled family **Coping** r/t dysfunctional family, underdeveloped nurturing parental role, lack of parental support systems or role models

Dysfunctional **Family** processes: alcoholism r/t inadequate coping skills

Impaired **Home** maintenance r/t disorganization, parental dysfunction, neglect of safe and nurturing environment

Impaired **Parenting** r/t unrealistic expectations of child; lack of effective role model; unmet social, emotional, or maturational needs of parents; interruption in bonding process

Ineffective **Health** maintenance r/t deficient knowledge of parenting skills as a result of unachieved developmental tasks

Powerlessness r/t inability to perform parental role responsibilities

Risk for **Violence** toward child r/t inadequate coping mechanisms, unresolved stressors, unachieved maturational level by parent

Suspicion

Impaired **Social** interaction r/t disturbed thought processes, paranoid delusions, hallucinations

Powerlessness r/t repetitive paranoid thinking

Risk for self- or other-directed **Violence**: Risk factor: inability to trust

Swallowing Difficulties

Impaired **Swallowing** (See **Swallowing**, impaired, Section III)

Syncope

Anxiety r/t fear of falling

Decreased **Cardiac** output r/t dysrhythmia

Impaired physical **Mobility** r/t fear of falling

Ineffective **Tissue** perfusion: cerebral r/t interruption of blood flow

Risk for **Falls**: Risk factor: syncope

Risk for **Injury**: Risk factors: altered sensory perception, transient loss of consciousness, risk for falls

Social isolation r/t fear of falling

Syphilis

See STD (Sexually Transmitted Disease)

Systemic Lupus Erythematosus

See Lupus Erythematosus

T

T & A (Tonsillectomy and Adenoidectomy)

Acute **Pain** r/t surgical incision

Deficient **Knowledge**: potential for enhanced health maintenance r/t insufficient knowledge regarding postoperative nutritional and rest requirements, signs and symptoms of complications, positioning

Ineffective **Airway** clearance r/t hesitation or reluctance to cough because of pain

Nausea r/t gastric irritation, pharmaceuticals, anesthesia

Risk for **Aspiration/Suffocation**: Risk factors: postoperative drainage and impaired swallowing

Risk for deficient **Fluid** volume: Risk factors: decreased intake because of painful swallowing, effects of anesthesia (nausea, vomiting), hemorrhage

Risk for imbalanced **Nutrition**: less than body requirements: Risk factors: hesitation or reluctance to swallow

Tachycardia

See Dysrhythmia

Tachypnea

Ineffective **Breathing** pattern r/t pain, anxiety

See cause of Tachypnea

Tardive Dyskinesia

Deficient **Knowledge** r/t cognitive limitation in assimilating information relating to side effects associated with neuroleptic medications

Disturbed sensory **Perception** r/t tardive dyskinesia

Ineffective management of **Therapeutic** regimen r/t complexity of therapeutic regimen or medications

Risk for **Injury** r/t drug-induced abnormal body movements

Taste Abnormality

Adult **Failure** to thrive r/t imbalanced nutrition: less than body requirements associated with taste abnormality

Disturbed **Sensory** perception: gustatory r/t medication side effects; altered sensory reception, transmission, integration; aging changes

TB (Pulmonary Tuberculosis)

Fatigue r/t disease state

Hyperthermia r/t infection

Impaired **Gas** exchange r/t disease process

Impaired **Home** maintenance management r/t client or family member with disease

Ineffective **Airway** clearance r/t increased secretions, excessive mucus

Ineffective **Breathing** pattern r/t decreased energy, fatigue

Ineffective **Therapeutic** regimen management r/t deficient knowledge of prevention and treatment regimen

Readiness for enhanced **Therapeutic** regimen management r/t taking medications according to prescribed protocol for prevention and treatment

Risk for **Infection**: Risk factors: insufficient knowledge regarding avoidance of exposure to pathogens

TBI (Traumatic Brain Injury)

Acute **Confusion** r/t brain injury

Chronic **Sorrow** r/t change in health status and functional ability

Decreased **Intracranial** adaptive capacity r/t brain injury

Disturbed **Sensory** perception: specify r/t pressure damage to sensory centers in brain

Disturbed **Thought** processes r/t pressure damage to brain

Impaired **Memory** r/t neurological disturbances

Ineffective **Tissue** perfusion: cerebral r/t effects of increased intracranial pressure

Ineffective **Breathing** pattern r/t pressure damage to breathing center in brainstem

Interrupted **Family** processes r/t traumatic injury to family member

Risk for impaired **Religiosity**: Risk factor: impaired physical mobility

Risk for **Post-trauma** syndrome: Risk factor: perception of event causing TBI

TD (Traveler's Diarrhea)

Risk for deficient **Fluid** volume r/t excessive loss of fluids, diarrhea

Risk for **Infection**: Risk factors: insufficient knowledge regarding avoidance of exposure to pathogens (water supply, iced drinks, local cheeses, ice cream, undercooked meat, fish and shellfish, uncooked vegetables, unclean eating utensils, improper handwashing)

Temperature, Decreased

Hypothermia r/t exposure to cold environment

Temperature, Increased

Hyperthermia r/t dehydration, illness, trauma

Temperature Regulation, Impaired

Ineffective **Thermoregulation** r/t trauma, illness

TEN (Toxic Epidermal Necrolysis)

See Toxic Epidermal Necrolysis

Tension

Anxiety r/t threat to or change in health status, situational crisis

T

Disturbed **Energy** field r/t change in health status, discouragement, pain

Readiness for enhanced **Communication**: r/t willingness to share feelings and thoughts

See Stress

Terminally Ill Adult

Compromised family **Coping** r/t inability to discuss impending death

Death **Anxiety** r/t unresolved issues relating to death and dying

Decisional **Conflict** r/t planning for advance directives

Disturbed **Energy** field r/t impending disharmony of mind, body, spirit

Grieving r/t loss of self or significant other

Readiness for enhanced **Religiosity**: requests religious material and/or experiences

Readiness for enhanced **Spiritual** well-being: desire to achieve harmony of mind, body, spirit

Risk for **Spiritual** distress: Risk factor: impending death

Spiritual distress r/t suffering before death

Terminally Ill Child, Adolescent

Disturbed **Body** image r/t effects of terminal disease, already critical feelings of group identity and self-image

Impaired **Social** interaction/social isolation r/t forced separation from peers

Ineffective **Coping** r/t inability to establish personal and peer identity because of the threat of being different or not being healthy, inability to achieve maturational tasks

See Child with Chronic Condition; Hospitalized Child

Terminally Ill Child, Infant/Toddler

Ineffective **Coping** r/t separation from parents and familiar environment attributable to inability to understand dying process

See Child with Chronic Condition

Terminally Ill Child, Preschool Child

Fear r/t perceived punishment, bodily harm, feelings of guilt caused by magical thinking (i.e., believing that thoughts cause events)

See Child with Chronic Condition

Terminally Ill Child, School-Age Child/Preadolescent

Fear r/t perceived punishment, body mutilation, feelings of guilt

See Child with Chronic Condition

Terminally Ill Child/Death of Child, Parent

Compromised family **Coping** r/t inability or unwillingness to discuss impending death and feelings with child or support child through terminal stages of illness

Decisional **Conflict** r/t continuation or discontinuation of treatment, do-not-resuscitate decision, ethical issues regarding organ donation

Grieving r/t death of child

Hopelessness r/t overwhelming stresses caused by terminal illness

Impaired **Parenting** r/t risk for overprotection of surviving siblings

Impaired **Social** interaction r/t complicated grieving

Ineffective **Denial** r/t complicated grieving

Insomnia r/t grieving process

Interrupted **Family** processes r/t situational crisis

Powerlessness r/t inability to alter course of events

Readiness for enhanced family **Coping**: r/t impact of crisis on family values, priorities, goals, or relationships; expressed interest or desire to attach meaning to child's life and death

Risk for complicated **Grieving**: Risk factors: prolonged, unresolved, obstructed progression through stages of grief and mourning

Social isolation: imposed by others r/t feelings of inadequacy in providing support to grieving parents

Social isolation: self-imposed r/t unresolved grief, perceived inadequate parenting skills

Spiritual distress r/t sudden and unexpected death, prolonged suffering before death, questioning the death of youth, questioning the meaning of one's own existence

Tetralogy of Fallot

See Congenital Heart Disease/Cardiac Anomalies

Therapeutic Regimen Management, Effective

Effective **Therapeutic** regimen management (See **Therapeutic** regimen management, effective, Section III)

Therapeutic Regimen Management, Ineffective

Ineffective **Therapeutic** regimen management (See **Therapeutic** regimen management, ineffective, Section III)

Therapeutic Regimen Management, Ineffective: Community

Ineffective community **Therapeutic** regimen management (See **Therapeutic** regimen management, ineffective community, Section III)

Therapeutic Regimen Management, Ineffective: Family

Ineffective family **Therapeutic** regimen management (See **Therapeutic** regimen management, ineffective family, Section III)

Therapeutic Regimen Management, Readiness for Enhanced

Readiness for enhanced **Therapeutic** regimen management (See **Therapeutic** regimen management, readiness for enhanced, Section III)

Therapeutic Touch

Disturbed **Energy** field r/t low energy levels, disturbance in energy fields, pain, depression, fatigue

Thermoregulation, Ineffective

Ineffective **Thermoregulation** (See **Thermoregulation**, ineffective, Section III)

Thoracentesis

See Pleural Effusion

Thoracotomy

Activity intolerance r/t pain, imbalance between oxygen supply and demand, presence of chest tubes

Acute **Pain** r/t surgical procedure, coughing, deep breathing

Deficient **Knowledge** r/t self-care, effective breathing exercises, pain relief

Ineffective **Airway** clearance r/t drowsiness, pain with breathing and coughing

Ineffective **Breathing** pattern r/t decreased energy, fatigue, pain

Risk for **Infection**: Risk factor: invasive procedure

Risk for **Injury**: Risk factor: disruption of closed-chest drainage system

Risk for perioperative positioning **Injury**: Risk factor: lateral positioning, immobility

Thought Disorders

Disturbed **Thought** processes r/t disruption in cognitive thinking, processing

See Schizophrenia

Thought Processes, Disturbed

Disturbed **Thought** processes (See **Thought** processes, disturbed, Section III)

Thrombocytopenic Purpura

See ITP (Idiopathic Thrombocytopenic Purpura)

Thrombophlebitis

Acute **Pain** r/t vascular inflammation, edema

Constipation r/t inactivity, bed rest

Deficient **Diversional** activity r/t bed rest

Deficient **Knowledge** r/t pathophysiology of condition, self-care needs, treatment regimen and outcome

Delayed **Surgical** recovery r/t complication associated with inactivity

Impaired physical **Mobility** r/t pain in extremity, forced bed rest

Ineffective **Tissue** perfusion: peripheral r/t interruption of venous blood flow

Risk for **Injury**: Risk factor: possible embolus

Sedentary **Lifestyle** r/t deficient knowledge of benefits of physical exercise

See Anticoagulant Therapy

Thyroidectomy

Risk for altered verbal **Communication**: Risk factors: edema, pain, vocal cord of laryngeal nerve damage

Risk for ineffective **Airway** clearance: Risk factors: edema or hematoma formation, airway obstruction

Risk for **Injury**: Risk factor: possible parathyroid damage or removal

See Surgery, Preoperative Care; Surgery, Perioperative Care; Surgery, Postoperative Care

TIA (Transient Ischemic Attack)

Acute **Confusion** r/t hypoxia

Decreased **Cardiac** output r/t dysrhythmia contributing to inadequate oxygen supply to brain

Health-seeking behaviors r/t obtaining knowledge regarding treatment, prevention of inadequate oxygenation

Ineffective **Tissue** perfusion: cerebral r/t lack of adequate oxygen supply to brain

Risk for **Falls**: Risk factor: hypoxia

Risk for **Injury**: Risk factor: possible syncope

See Syncope

Tic Disorder

See Tourette Syndrome (TS)

Tinea Capitis

Pruritus r/t inflammation

See Ringworm of Scalp

Tinea Corporis

See Ringworm of Body

Tinea Cruris

See Jock Itch; Itching; Pruritus

Tinea Pedis

See Athlete's Foot; Itching; Pruritus

Tinea Unguium (Onychomycosis)

See Ringworm of Nails

Tinnitus

Disturbed **Sensory** perception: auditory r/t altered sensory reception, transmission, integration

Ineffective **Health** maintenance r/t deficient knowledge regarding self-care with tinnitus

Tissue Damage, Corneal, Integumentary, or Subcutaneous

Impaired **Tissue** integrity (See **Tissue** integrity, impaired, Section III)

Tissue Perfusion, Decreased

Ineffective **Tissue** perfusion (See **Tissue** perfusion, ineffective, Section III)

Tocolytic Therapy

Ineffective **Health** maintenance r/t deficient knowledge regarding management of preterm labor, treatment regimen

Risk for **Fluid** volume excess: Risk factor: effects of tocolytic drugs

See Preterm Labor

T

Toilet Training

Health-seeking behaviors: bladder/bowel training r/t achievement of developmental milestone as a result of enhanced parenting skills

Deficient **Knowledge**: parent r/t signs of readiness for training

Risk for **Constipation**: Risk factor: withholding stool

Risk for **Incontinence**: Risk factor: difficulty in maintaining bladder/bowel control

Risk for **Infection**: Risk factor: withholding urination

Toileting Problems

Impaired **Transfer** ability r/t neuromuscular deficits

Self-care deficit: toileting r/t impaired transfer ability, impaired mobility status, intolerance of activity, neuromuscular impairment, cognitive impairment

Tonsillectomy and Adenoidectomy

See T & A (Tonsillectomy and Adenoidectomy)

Toothache

Acute **Pain** r/t inflammation, infection

Impaired **Dentition** r/t ineffective oral hygiene, barriers to self-care, economic barriers to professional care, nutritional deficits, lack of knowledge regarding dental health

Total Anomalous Pulmonary Venous Return

See Congenital Heart Disease/Cardiac Anomalies

Total Joint Replacement (Total Hip/Total Knee/Shoulder)

Acute **Pain** r/t possible edema, physical injury, surgery

Deficient **Knowledge** r/t self-care, treatment regimen, outcomes

Disturbed **Body** image r/t large scar, presence of prosthesis

Impaired physical **Mobility** r/t musculoskeletal impairment, surgery, prosthesis

Risk for **Infection**: Risk factors: invasive procedure, anesthesia, immobility

Risk for **Injury**: neurovascular: Risk factors: altered peripheral tissue perfusion, altered mobility, prosthesis

See Surgery, Preoperative Care; Surgery, Perioperative Care; Surgery, Postoperative Care

Total Parenteral Nutrition

See TPN (Total Parenteral Nutrition)

Total Urinary Incontinence

Total urinary **Incontinence** (See **Incontinence**, total urinary, Section III)

Tourette Syndrome (TS)

Hopelessness r/t inability to control behavior

Risk for situational low **Self-esteem** r/t uncontrollable behavior, motor and phonic tics

See Attention Deficit Disorder

Toxemia

See PIH (Pregnancy-Induced Hypertension/Preeclampsia)

Toxic Epidermal Necrolysis

Death **Anxiety** r/t uncertainty of prognosis

Disturbed **Sensory** perception (visual) r/t altered sensory reception associated with visual changes from conjunctival inflammation and scarring

See Stevens-Johnson syndrome

TPN (Total Parenteral Nutrition)

Imbalanced **Nutrition**: less than body requirements r/t inability to ingest or digest food or absorb nutrients as a result of biological or psychological factors

Risk for **Fluid** volume excess: Risk factor; rapid administration of TPN

Risk for **Infection**: Risk factors: concentrated glucose solution, invasive administration of fluids

Tracheoesophageal Fistula

Imbalanced **Nutrition**: less than body requirements r/t difficulties in swallowing

Ineffective **Airway** clearance r/t aspiration of feeding because of inability to swallow

Risk for **Aspiration**: Risk factors: common passage of air and food

See Respiratory Conditions of the Neonate; Hospitalized Child

Tracheostomy

Acute **Pain** r/t edema, surgical procedure

Anxiety r/t impaired verbal communication, ineffective airway clearance

Deficient **Knowledge** r/t self-care, home maintenance management

Disturbed **Body** image r/t abnormal opening in neck

Impaired verbal **Communication** r/t presence of mechanical airway

Risk for **Aspiration** r/t presence of tracheostomy

Risk for ineffective **Airway** clearance: Risk factors: increased secretions, mucous plugs

Risk for **Infection**: Risk factors: invasive procedure, pooling of secretions

Traction and Casts

Acute **Pain** r/t immobility, injury, or disease

Constipation r/t immobility

Deficient **Diversional** activity r/t immobility

Impaired physical **Mobility** r/t imposed restrictions on activity because of bone or joint disease injury

Impaired **Transfer** ability r/t presence of traction, casts

Risk for **Disuse** syndrome: Risk factor: mechanical immobilization

Risk for impaired **Skin** integrity: Risk factor: contact of traction or cast with skin

Risk for **Peripheral** neurovascular dysfunction: Risk factor: mechanical compression

Self-care deficit: feeding, dressing, grooming, bathing, hygiene, toileting r/t degree of impaired physical mobility, body area affected by traction or cast

Transfer Ability

Impaired **Transfer** ability (See **Transfer** ability, impaired, Section III)

Transient Ischemic Attack

See TIA (Transient Ischemic Attack)

Transposition of Great Vessels

See Congenital Heart Disease/Cardiac Anomalies

Transurethral Resection of the Prostate

See TURP (Transurethral Resection of the Prostate)

Trauma in Pregnancy

Acute **Pain** r/t trauma

Anxiety r/t threat to self or fetus, unknown outcome

Deficient **Knowledge** r/t lack of exposure to situation

Impaired **Skin** integrity r/t trauma

Risk for deficient **Fluid** volume: Risk factor: blood loss

Risk for fetal **Injury**: Risk factor: premature separation of placenta

Risk for **Infection**: Risk factor: traumatized tissue

Trauma, Risk for

Internal/External

Risk for **Trauma** (See **Trauma**, risk for, Section III)

Traumatic Brain Injury (TBI)

See TBI (Traumatic Brain Injury); Intracranial Pressure, Increased

Traumatic Event

Post-trauma syndrome r/t previously experienced trauma

Traveler's Diarrhea (TD)

See TD (Traveler's Diarrhea)

Trembling of Hands

Anxiety/Fear r/t threat to or change in health status, threat of death, situational crisis

Tricuspid Atresia

See Congenital Heart Disease/Cardiac Anomalies

Trigeminal Neuralgia

Acute **Pain** r/t irritation of trigeminal nerve

Imbalanced **Nutrition**: less than body requirements r/t pain when chewing

Ineffective **Therapeutic** regimen management r/t deficient knowledge regarding prevention of stimuli that trigger pain

Risk for **Injury** (eye): Risk factor: possible decreased corneal sensation

Truncus Arteriosus

See Congenital Heart Disease/Cardiac Anomalies

TS (Tourette's Syndrome)

See Tourette's Syndrome (TS)

TSE (Testicular Self-Examination)

Health-seeking behaviors: testicular self-examinations

Tubal Ligation

Decisional **Conflict** r/t tubal sterilization

See Laparoscopy

Tube Feeding

Risk for **Aspiration**: Risk factors: improperly administered feeding, improper placement of tube, improper positioning of client during and after feeding, excessive residual feeding or lack of digestion, altered gag reflex

Risk for deficient **Fluid** volume: Risk factor: inadequate water administration with concentrated feeding

Risk for imbalanced **Nutrition**: less than body requirements: Risk factors: intolerance to tube feeding, inadequate calorie replacement to meet metabolic needs

Tuberculosis

See TB (Pulmonary Tuberculosis)

TURP (Transurethral Resection of the Prostate)

Acute **Pain** r/t incision, irritation from catheter, bladder spasms, kidney infection

Deficient **Knowledge** r/t postoperative self-care, home maintenance management

Risk for deficient **Fluid** volume: Risk factors: fluid loss, possible bleeding

Risk for **Infection**: Risk factors: invasive procedure, route for bacteria entry

Risk for urge urinary **Incontinence**: Risk factor: edema from surgical procedure

Risk for **Urinary** retention: Risk factor: obstruction of urethra or catheter with clots

U

Ulcer, Peptic (Duodenal or Gastric)

Acute **Pain** r/t irritated mucosa from acid secretion

Fatigue r/t loss of blood, chronic illness

Ineffective **Health** maintenance r/t lack of knowledge regarding health practices to prevent ulcer formation

Nausea r/t gastrointestinal irritation

See GI Bleed (Gastrointestinal Bleeding)

Ulcerative Colitis

See Inflammatory Bowel Disease (Child and Adult)

Ulcers, Stasis

See Stasis Ulcer

Unilateral Neglect of One Side of Body

Unilateral **Neglect** (See **Neglect**, unilateral, Section III)

Unsanitary Living Conditions

Impaired **Home** maintenance r/t impaired cognitive or emotional functioning, lack of knowledge, insufficient finances

Urgency to Urinate

Risk for urge urinary **Incontinence** (See **Incontinence**, urge urinary, risk for, Section III)

Urge urinary **Incontinence** (See **Incontinence**, urge urinary, Section III)

Urinary Diversion

See Ileal Conduit

Urinary Elimination, Impaired

Impaired **Urinary** elimination (See **Urinary** elimination, impaired, Section III)

Urinary Incontinence

See Incontinence of Urine

Urinary Readiness

Readiness for enhanced **Urinary** elimination (See **Urinary** elimination, readiness for enhanced, Section III)

Urinary Retention

Urinary retention (See **Urinary** retention, Section III)

Urinary Tract Infection (UTI)

See UTI (Urinary Tract Infection)

Urolithiasis

See Kidney Stone

Uterine Atony in Labor

See Dystocia

Uterine Atony in Postpartum

See Postpartum Hemorrhage

Uterine Bleeding

See Hemorrhage; Postpartum Hemorrhage; Shock

UTI (Urinary Tract Infection)

Acute **Pain**: dysuria r/t inflammatory process in bladder

Impaired **Urinary** elimination: frequency r/t urinary tract infection

Ineffective **Health** maintenance r/t deficient knowledge regarding methods to treat and prevent UTIs

Risk for urge urinary **Incontinence**: Risk factor: hyperreflexia from cystitis

V

VAD

See Ventricular Assist Device (VAD)

Vaginal Hysterectomy

Risk for **Infection** r/t surgical site

Risk for **Perioperative** positioning injury: Risk factor: lithotomy position

Risk for urge urinary **Incontinence**: Risk factors: edema, congestion of pelvic tissues

Urinary retention r/t edema at surgical site

See Postpartum Hemorrhage

Vaginitis

Acute **Pain**: pruritus r/t inflamed tissues, edema

Ineffective **Health** maintenance r/t deficient knowledge regarding self-care with vaginitis

Ineffective **Sexuality** pattern r/t abstinence during acute stage, pain

Pruritus r/t inflammation

Vagotomy

See Abdominal Surgery

Value System Conflict

Decisional **Conflict** r/t unclear personal values or beliefs

Readiness for enhanced **Spiritual** well-being: desire for harmony with self, others, higher power, God

Spiritual distress r/t challenged value system

Varicose Veins

Chronic **Pain** r/t impaired circulation

Ineffective **Health** maintenance r/t deficient knowledge regarding health care practices, prevention, treatment regimen

Ineffective **Tissue** perfusion: peripheral r/t venous stasis

Risk for impaired **Skin** integrity: Risk factor: altered peripheral tissue perfusion

Vascular Dementia (Formerly Called Multiinfarct Dementia)

See Dementia

Vascular Obstruction, Peripheral

Acute **Pain** r/t vascular obstruction

Anxiety r/t lack of circulation to body part

Ineffective **Tissue** perfusion: peripheral r/t interruption of circulatory flow

Risk for **Peripheral** neurovascular dysfunction: Risk factor: vascular obstruction

Vasectomy

Decisional **Conflict** r/t surgery as method of permanent sterilization

Effective **Therapeutic** regimen management: r/t verbalizes desire to manage prevention of sequelae

Vasocognopathy

See Alzheimer's Type Dementia

Venereal Disease

See STD (Sexually Transmitted Disease)

Ventilation, Impaired Spontaneous

Impaired spontaneous **Ventilation** (See **Ventilation**, impaired spontaneous, Section III)

Ventilator Client

Dysfunctional **Ventilatory** weaning response r/t psychological, situational, physiological factors

Fear r/t inability to breathe on own, difficulty communicating

Impaired **Gas** exchange r/t ventilation-perfusion imbalance

Impaired spontaneous **Ventilation** r/t metabolic factors, respiratory muscle fatigue

Impaired verbal **Communication** r/t presence of endotracheal tube, decreased mentation

Ineffective **Airway** clearance r/t increased secretions, decreased cough and gag reflex

Ineffective **Breathing** pattern r/t decreased energy and fatigue as a result of possible altered nutrition: less than body requirements

Powerlessness r/t health treatment regimen

Risk for **Infection**: Risk factors: presence of endotracheal tube, pooled secretions

Risk for latex **Allergy** response: Risk factors: repeated exposure to latex products

Social isolation r/t impaired mobility, ventilator dependence

See Child with Chronic Condition; Hospitalized Child; Respiratory Conditions of the Neonate

Ventilatory, Dysfunctional Weaning Response (DVWR)

Dysfunctional **Ventilatory** weaning response (See **Ventilatory** weaning response, dysfunctional, Section III)

Ventricular Assist Device (VAD)

Readiness for enhanced **Decision** making: r/t Expresses desire to enhance the understanding of the meaning of choices regarding implanting a ventricular assist device

See Open Heart Surgery

Ventricular Fibrillation

See Dysrhythmia

Vertigo

Disturbed **Sensory** perception: kinesthetic r/t altered sensory reception, transmission, integration; medications

Ineffective **Tissue** perfusion: cerebral r/t decreased blood supply to brain

Risk for **Falls**: Risk factor: vertigo

Risk for **Injury**: Risk factor: disturbed sensory perception

Violent Behavior

Risk for other-directed **Violence** (See **Violence**, other directed, risk for, Section III)

Risk for self-directed **Violence**: Risk factors: (See **Violence**, self-directed, risk for, Section III)

Viral Gastroenteritis

Diarrhea r/t infectious process, rotavirus, Norwalk virus

Ineffective **Therapeutic** regimen management r/t inadequate handwashing

Ineffective community **Therapeutic** regimen management r/t contaminated food and/or water

See Gastroenteritis, Child

Vision Impairment

Disturbed **Sensory** perception r/t altered sensory reception associated with impaired vision

Fear r/t loss of sight

Risk for **Injury**: Risk factor: disturbed sensory perception

Self-care deficit: specify r/t perceptual impairment

Social isolation r/t altered state of wellness, inability to see

See Blindness

Vomiting

Nausea r/t chemotherapy, postsurgical anesthesia, irritation to the gastrointestinal system, stimulation of neuropharmacological mechanisms

Risk for deficient **Fluid** volume: Risk factor: decreased intake, loss of fluids with vomiting

Risk for imbalanced **Nutrition**: less than body requirements: Risk factor: inability to ingest food

von Recklinghausen's Disease

See Neurofibromatosis

W

Walking Impairment

Impaired **Walking** (See **Walking**, impaired, Section III)

Wandering

Wandering (See **Wandering**, Section III)

Weakness

Fatigue r/t decreased or increased metabolic energy production

Risk for **Falls**: Risk factor: weakness

Weight Gain

Imbalanced **Nutrition**: more than body requirements r/t excessive intake in relation to metabolic need

Weight Loss

Imbalanced **Nutrition**: less than body requirements r/t inability to ingest food because of biological, psychological, economic factors

Wellness-Seeking Behavior

Health-seeking behaviors r/t expressed desire for increased control of health practice

Wernicke Korsakoff Syndrome

See Korsakoff's Syndrome

West Nile Virus

Effective **Therapeutic** regimen management: avoid mosquito bites, use mosquito-repellant products containing DEET, wear long sleeves and pants, mosquito-proof the home, community spray for mosquitos

See Meningitis/Encephalitis

Wheelchair Use Problems

Impaired wheelchair **Mobility** (See **Mobility**, impaired wheelchair, Section III)

Wheezing

Ineffective **Airway** clearance r/t tracheobronchial obstructions, secretions

Wilms' Tumor

Acute **Pain** r/t pressure from tumor

Constipation r/t obstruction associated with presence of tumor

See Chemotherapy; Hospitalized Child; Radiation Therapy; Surgery, Preoperative Care; Surgery, Perioperative Care; Surgery, Postoperative Care

Withdrawal from Alcohol

See Alcohol Withdrawal

Withdrawal from Drugs

See Drug Withdrawal

Wound Debridement

Acute **Pain** r/t debridement of wound

Impaired **Tissue** integrity r/t debridement, open wound

Risk for **Infection**: Risk factors: open wound, presence of bacteria

Wound Dehiscence, Evisceration

Fear r/t client fear of body parts "falling out," surgical procedure not going as planned

Imbalanced **Nutrition**: less than body requirements r/t inability to digest nutrients, need for increased protein for healing

Risk for deficient **Fluid** volume: Risk factors: inability to ingest nutrients, obstruction, fluid loss

Risk for delayed **Surgical** recovery: Risk factors: separation of wound, exposure of abdominal contents

Risk for **Injury**: Risk factor: exposed abdominal contents

Wound Infection

Disturbed **Body** image r/t dysfunctional open wound

Hyperthermia r/t increased metabolic rate, illness, infection

Imbalanced **Nutrition**: less than body requirements r/t biological factors, infection, hyperthermia

Impaired **Tissue** integrity r/t wound, presence of infection

Risk for deficient **Fluid** volume: Risk factor: increased metabolic rate

Risk for delayed **Surgical** recovery: Risk factor: presence of infection

Risk for **Infection**: spread of: Risk factor: imbalanced nutrition: less than body requirements

W

Guide to Planning Care

Section III is a listing of nursing diagnosis care plans according to NANDA-I. The care plans are arranged alphabetically by diagnostic concept.

MAKING AN ACCURATE NURSING DIAGNOSIS

Verify the accuracy of the previously suggested nursing diagnoses (from Section II) for the client. To do this:

- Read the definition for the suggested nursing diagnosis and determine if it sounds appropriate
- Compare the Defining Characteristics with the symptoms that were identified from the client data collected or
- Compare the Risk Factors with the symptoms that were identified from the client data collected (if it is a "Risk for" Nursing Diagnosis, they do not have defining characteristics)

WRITING OUTCOMES, STATEMENTS, AND NURSING INTERVENTIONS

After selecting the appropriate nursing diagnosis, use this section to write outcomes and interventions:

- Use the NOC/NIC outcomes and interventions with the associated rating scales or
- Use the Client Outcomes/Nursing Interventions as written by the authors and contributors
- Read the rationales; the majority of rationales are based on nursing or clinical research that validates the efficacy of the interventions.

Following these steps, you will be able to write a nursing care plan:

- Follow this care plan to administer nursing care to the client.
- Document all steps and evaluate and update the care plan as needed.

A

Activity intolerance *Betty Ackley, MSN, EdS, RN*

NANDA **Definition**

Insufficient physiological or psychological energy to endure or complete required or desired daily activities

Defining Characteristics

Abnormal blood pressure response to activity; abnormal heart rate response to activity; electrocardiographic changes reflecting arrhythmias; electrocardiographic changes reflecting ischemia; exertional discomfort; exertional dyspnea; verbal report of fatigue; verbal report of weakness

Related Factors (r/t)

Bed rest; generalized weakness; imbalance between oxygen supply/demand; immobility, sedentary lifestyle

NOC **Outcomes (Nursing Outcomes Classification)**

Suggested NOC Outcomes

Activity Tolerance, Endurance, Energy Conservation, Self-Care: Instrumental Activities of Daily Living (IADLs)

> ### Example NOC Outcome with Indicators
>
> **Endurance** as evidenced by the following indicators: Performance of usual routine/Activity/Rested appearance/ Concentration/Interest in surroundings/Muscle endurance/Eating pattern/Libido/Energy restored after rest/Blood oxygen level/Hemoglobin/Hematocrit/Blood glucose/Serum electrolytes (Rate the outcome and indicators of **Endurance:** 1 = severely compromised, 2 = substantially compromised, 3 = moderately compromised, 4 = mildly compromised, 5 = not compromised [see Section I].)

Client Outcomes

Client Will (Specify Time Frame):

- Participate in prescribed physical activity with appropriate changes in heart rate, blood pressure, and breathing rate; maintains monitor patterns (rhythm and ST segment) within normal limits
- State symptoms of adverse effects of exercise and report onset of symptoms immediately
- Maintain normal skin color and skin is warm and dry with activity
- Verbalize an understanding of the need to gradually increase activity based on testing, tolerance, and symptoms
- Demonstrate increased tolerance to activity

NIC **Interventions (Nursing Interventions Classification)**

Suggested NIC Interventions

Activity Therapy, Energy Management

> ### Example NIC Activities—Energy Management
>
> Monitor cardiorespiratory response to activity (e.g., tachycardia, other dysrhythmias, dyspnea, diaphoresis, pallor, hemodynamic pressures, respiratory rate); Monitor location and nature of discomfort or pain during movement/activity

Nursing Interventions and *Rationales*

- Determine cause of activity intolerance (see Related Factors) and determine whether cause is physical, psychological, or motivational. *Determining the cause of a disease can help direct appropriate interventions.*

• = Independent; ▲ = Collaborative; EBN = Evidence-Based Nursing; EB = Evidence-Based

A

- If mainly on bed rest, minimize cardiovascular deconditioning by positioning the client in an upright position several times daily. *Deconditioning of the cardiovascular system occurs within days and involves fluid shifts, fluid loss, decreased cardiac output, decreased peak oxygen uptake, and increased resting heart rate (Fletcher, 2005; Kasper et al, 2005).*
- Assess the client daily for appropriateness of activity and bed rest orders. **EB:** *A study utilizing tomography demonstrated significant decreased strength in the hip, thigh, and calf muscles in elderly orthopedic clients, as well as bone mineral loss (Berg et al, 2007). Bed rest for treatment of medical conditions is associated with worse outcomes than early mobilization (Allen, Glasziou & Del Mar, 1999).*
- If client is mostly immobile, consider use of a transfer chair, a chair that becomes a stretcher. *Using a transfer chair where the client is pulled onto a flat surface and then seated upright in the chair can help previously immobile clients get out of bed (Nelson et al, 2003).*
- When appropriate, gradually increase activity, allowing the client to assist with positioning, transferring, and self-care as possible. Progress from sitting in bed to dangling, to standing, to ambulation. *Always have the client dangle at the bedside before trying standing to evaluate for postural hypotension. Postural hypotension can be detected in up to 30% of elderly clients. These methods can help prevent falls (Tinetti, 2003).*
- When getting a client up, observe for symptoms of intolerance such as nausea, pallor, dizziness, visual dimming, and impaired consciousness, as well as changes in vital signs. *When an adult rises to the standing position, 300 to 800 mL of blood pools in the lower extremities. As a result, symptoms of central nervous system hypoperfusion may occur, including feelings of weakness, nausea, headache, neck ache, lightheadedness, dizziness, blurred vision, fatigue, tremulousness, palpitations, and impaired cognition (Bradley & Davis, 2003).*
- ▲ If a client experiences syncope with activity, refer for evaluation by a physician. *Syncope has many causes, including benign vasovagal, but can also be due to serious cardiac disease, resulting in death (Hauer, 2003).*
- Perform range-of-motion (ROM) exercises if the client is unable to tolerate activity or is mostly immobile. See care plan for **risk for Disuse syndrome.**
- Monitor and record the client's ability to tolerate activity: note pulse rate, blood pressure, monitor pattern, dyspnea, use of accessory muscles, and skin color before and after activity. If the following signs and symptoms of cardiac decompensation develop, activity should be stopped immediately (Wenger, 2001):
  - Onset of chest discomfort
  - Dyspnea
  - Palpitations
  - Excessive fatigue
  - Lightheadedness, confusion, ataxia, pallor, cyanosis, nausea, or any peripheral circulatory insufficiency
  - Dysrhythmia (symptomatic supraventricular tachycardia, ventricular tachycardia, exercise-induced intraventricular conduction defect, second- or third-degree atrioventricular block, frequent premature ventricular contractions)
  - Exercise hypotension (drop in systolic blood pressure of 10 mm Hg from baseline blood pressure despite an increase in workload)
  - Excessive rise in blood pressure (systolic >180 mm Hg or diastolic >110 mm Hg) NOTE: These are upper limits; activity may be stopped before reaching these values
  - Inappropriate bradycardia (drop in heart rate >10 beats/min or <50 beats/min)
  - Increased heart rate above 100 beats/min
- ▲ Instruct the client to stop the activity immediately and report to the physician if the client is experiencing the following symptoms: new or worsened intensity or increased frequency of discomfort; tightness or pressure in chest, back, neck, jaw, shoulders, and/or arms; palpitations; dizziness; weakness; unusual and extreme fatigue; excessive air hunger. *These are common symptoms of angina and are caused by a temporary insufficiency of coronary blood supply. Symptoms typically last for minutes as opposed to momentary twinges. If symptoms last longer than 5 to 10 minutes, the client should be evaluated by a physician.*
- Observe and document skin integrity several times a day. *Activity intolerance may lead to pressure*

ulcers. Mechanical pressure, moisture, friction, and shearing forces all predispose to their development (Kasper et al, 2005).

- Assess for constipation. If present, refer to care plan for **Constipation. Activity intolerance** *is associated with increased risk of constipation.*
- ▲ Refer the client to physical therapy to help increase activity levels and strength.
- ▲ Consider dietitian referral to assess nutritional needs related to activity intolerance. Recognize that undernutrition causes significant morbidity due to the loss of lean body mass. *The decline in body mass, with physical weakness, inhibits mobility, increasing liability to deep vein thrombosis and pressure ulcers. Respiratory muscle weakness causes difficulty in expectorating, increasing susceptibility to chest infection. Immunocompetence declines, increasing the risk of infection, which in turn reduces nutritional status (Holmes, 2003).*
- Identify the factors that contribute to malnutrition in hospital clients, especially in older clients. **EB:** *Underweight elderly clients who had difficulty feeding themselves or bathing were at greatest risk to die in the hospital (Thomas, Kamel & Azharrudin, 2005).*
- Provide emotional support and encouragement to the client to gradually increase activity. *Fear of breathlessness, pain, or falling may decrease willingness to increase activity.*
- Observe for pain before activity. If possible, treat pain before activity and ensure that the client is not heavily sedated. *Pain restricts the client from achieving a maximal activity level and is often exacerbated by movement.*
- ▲ Obtain any necessary assistive devices or equipment needed before ambulating the client (e.g., walkers, canes, crutches, portable oxygen). *Assistive devices can increase mobility by helping the client overcome limitations.*
- Use a gait walking belt when ambulating the client. *Gait belts improve the caregiver's grasp, reducing the incidence of injuries (Nelson, 2003).*
- ▲ Work with the client to set mutual goals that increase activity levels.
- ▲ If the client is scheduled for a surgical intervention that will result in bed rest in intensive care, consider referring to physical therapy for a program including warm-up, aerobic conditioning, strength building, and flexibility enhancement to increase strength and endurance before surgery. **EBN:** *Increasing a client's functional capacity before hospitalization can be a helpful means of modifying the predictable deconditioning that happens with intensive care unit (ICU) admission (Topp et al, 2002).*

Activity Intolerance Due to Respiratory Disease

- If the client is able to walk and has chronic obstructive pulmonary disease (COPD), consider the use of an accelerometer to assess walking ability or use the traditional 6-minute walk distance. **EBN and EB:** *Use of the accelerometer was very predictive of maximum distance walked during a 6-minute walk test (Belza et al, 2001). The 6-minute walk test predicted mortality in COPD clients (Pinto-Plata et al, 2004).*
- ▲ Ensure that the chronic pulmonary client has oxygen saturation testing with exercise. Use supplemental oxygen to keep oxygen saturation 90% or above or as prescribed with activity. *Clients with COPD may suffer from inadequate gas exchange, cor pulmonale, and other factors limiting oxygen transport. The use of oxygen increases survival, lowers pressure and pulmonary vascular resistance, and improves cardiac function, exercise capacity, and tolerance of ADLs (Garvey, 2001).*
- Monitor a COPD client's response to activity by observing for symptoms of respiratory intolerance such as increased dyspnea, loss of ability to control breathing rhythmically, use of accessory muscles, and skin tone changes such as pallor and cyanosis.
- Instruct and assist a COPD client in using conscious, controlled breathing techniques, including pursed-lip breathing, and inspiratory muscle training. **EB:** *Pursed-lip breathing reduces end expiratory volume and breathlessness (Bianchi et al, 2004). A systematic review found that inspiratory muscle training was effective in increasing endurance of the client and decreasing dyspnea (Crowe et al, 2005).*
- ▲ Refer the COPD client to a pulmonary rehabilitation program. **EB:** *Pulmonary rehabilitation has been shown to relieve dyspnea and fatigue, help the clients deal with emotions, and enhance the clients' sense of control over the disease (Lacasse et al, 2006).*

• = Independent;   ▲ = Collaborative;   EBN = Evidence-Based Nursing;   EB = Evidence-Based

Activity Intolerance Due to Cardiovascular Disease

- If the client is able to walk and has heart failure, consider use of the 6-minute walk test to determine physical ability. **EBN and EB:** *The distance walked in 6 minutes was useful in clients with left ventricular dysfunction, as well as those with preserved function, and that distance walked was directly related to rates of rehospitalization and death for 100 clients with dilated cardiomyopathy (Ford et al, 2004). The 6-minute walk test was shown to be highly reproducible in determining ability to ambulate in a client in heart failure (Demers et al, 2001).*
- Allow for periods of rest before and after planned exertion periods such as meals, baths, treatments, and physical activity. *Both physical and emotional rest helps lower arterial pressure and reduce the workload of the myocardium (Kasper et al, 2005).*
- ▲ Refer to heart failure program or cardiac rehabilitation program for education, evaluation, and guided support to increase activity and rebuild life. **EB:** *Exercise can help many clients with heart failure. A carefully monitored exercise program can improve both exercise capacity and quality of life in mild to moderate heart failure clients (Rees et al, 2004). Exercise-based cardiac rehabilitation is effective in reducing the number of cardiac deaths, also decreasing cholesterol levels, systolic blood pressure, and self-reported smoking (Taylor et al, 2004).*
- See care plan for **Decreased Cardiac output** for further interventions.

Geriatric

- Slow the pace of care. Allow the client extra time to carry out activities.
- Encourage families to help/allow an elderly client to be independent in whatever activities possible. *Sometimes families believe they are assisting by allowing clients to be sedentary. Encouraging activity not only enhances good functioning of the body's systems but also promotes a sense of worth (Kasper et al, 2005).*
- ▲ Evaluate medications the client is taking to see if they could be causing activity intolerance. Medications such as beta-blockers, lipid-lowering agents, which can damage muscle, and some antihypertensives such as Clonidine and lowering the blood pressure to normal in the elderly can result in decreased functioning. *Elderly clients may need a blood pressure of 140/80 or higher in order to walk without dizziness. It is important that medications be reviewed to ensure not resulting in less function of the elderly client (Haque, 2007). Many of the medications found on the Beers List of medications, which are inappropriate to prescribe for elderly clients, can result in decreased function (Fick et al, 2003).*
- ▲ If the client has heart disease causing activity intolerance, refer for cardiac rehabilitation. **EB:** *Studies indicate that elderly clients with coronary heart disease who participate in prevention clinics have significant improvement in function, pain, and general health (Murchie et al, 2004).*
- ▲ Refer the client to physical therapy for resistance exercise training as able, including abdominal crunch, leg press, leg extension, leg curl, calf press, and more. **EB:** *Six months of resistance exercise for the elderly greatly increased their aerobic capacity, possibly from increased skeletal muscle strength (Vincent et al, 2002).*
- When mobilizing the elderly client, watch for orthostatic hypotension accompanied by dizziness and fainting. *Postural hypotension can be detected in up to 30% of elderly clients. These methods can help prevent falls (Tinetti, 2003).*
- Once the client is able to walk independently and needs an exercise program, suggest the client enter an exercise program with a friend. **EBN:** *Findings from a study of exercise behavior found that friends have the strongest influence to keep on an exercise program, more than family members or experts (Resnick et al, 2002).*

Home Care

- ▲ Begin discharge planning as soon as possible with case manager or social worker to assess need for home support systems and the need for community or home health services.
- ▲ Assess the home environment for factors that contribute to decreased activity tolerance such as stairs or distance to the bathroom. Refer to occupational therapy if needed to assist the client in restructuring the home and ADL patterns. *During hospitalization, clients and families often estimate energy requirements at home inaccurately because the hospital's availability of staff support distorts the level of care that will be needed.*

A

▲ Refer to physical therapy for strength training and possible weight training, to regain strength, increase endurance, and improve balance. If the client is homebound, the physical therapist can also initiate cardiac rehabilitation.

▲ Support strength training program prescribed by physical therapist.

• Normalize the client's activity intolerance; encourage progress with positive feedback. *The client's experience should be validated as within expected norms. Recognition of progress enhances motivation.* **EBN:** *In qualitative studies, fatigued women reported that they felt distressed when healthcare providers invalidated their experiences of fatigue (Asbring & Narvanen, 2004; Patusky, 2002).*

• Teach the client/family the importance of and methods for setting priorities for activities, especially those having a high energy demand (e.g., home/family events). Instruct in realistic expectations. **EBN:** *Unrealistic expectations provoke guilt feelings in the client, leading to efforts that can exceed the client's energy capacity (Patusky, 2002).*

• Provide the client/family with resources such as senior centers, exercise classes, educational and recreational programs, and volunteer opportunities that can aid in promoting socialization and appropriate activity. *Social isolation can be an outcome of and contribute to activity intolerance.*

• Discuss the importance of sexual activity as part of daily living. Instruct the client in adaptive techniques to conserve energy during sexual interactions.

• Instruct the client and family in the importance of maintaining proper nutrition. Instruct in use of dietary supplements as indicated. *Illness may suppress appetite, leading to inadequate nutrition.*

▲ Refer to medical social services as necessary to assist the family in adjusting to major changes in patterns of living.

▲ Assess the need for long-term supports for optimal activity tolerance of priority activities (e.g., assistive devices, oxygen, medication, catheters, massage), especially for a hospice client. Evaluate intermittently.

▲ Refer to home health aide services to support the client and family through changing levels of activity tolerance. Introduce aide support early. Instruct the aide to promote independence in activity as tolerated.

• Allow terminally ill clients and their families to guide care. *Many African American families are composed of large networks, and often it is thought that such large networks tend to be very supportive during times of crises such as during death and the dying process (Dowd et al, 1998). However, large-network groups can have both positive and negative effects on wellness, illness, and recovery behaviors. Two researchers found that network size was positively related to distress; the more informal helpers there were, the higher the distress score was on the instrument used in the survey. One conclusion of the study is that network size is not a good measure of perceived social support. Control by the client or family respects their autonomy and promotes effective coping.*

• Provide increased attention to comfort and dignity of the terminally ill client in care planning. *Interventions should be provided as much for psychological effect as for physiological support. For example, oxygen may be more valuable as a support to the client's psychological comfort than as a booster of oxygen saturation.*

▲ Institute case management of frail elderly to support continued independent living.

Client/Family Teaching

• Instruct the client on rationale and techniques for avoiding activity intolerance.

• Teach the client to use controlled breathing techniques with activity.

• Teach the client the importance and method of coughing, clearing secretions.

• Instruct the client in the use of relaxation techniques during activity.

• Help the client with energy conservation and work simplification techniques in ADLs.

▲ Describe to the client the symptoms of activity intolerance, including which symptoms to report to the physician.

▲ Explain to the client how to use assistive devices, oxygen, or medications before or during activity.

• Help client set up an activity log to record exercise and exercise tolerance.

evolve See the EVOLVE website for World Wide Web resources for client education.

• = Independent; ▲ = Collaborative; EBN = Evidence-Based Nursing; EB = Evidence-Based

REFERENCES

Allen C, Glasziou P, Del Mar C: Bed rest: a potentially harmful treatment needing more careful evaluation, *Lancet* 354(9186):1229, 1999.

Asbring P, Narvanen A: Patient power and control: a study of women with uncertain illness trajectories, *Qual Health Res* 14(2):226, 2004.

Belza B, Steele BG, Hunziker J et al: Correlates of physical activity in chronic obstructive pulmonary disease, *Nurs Res* 50(4):195, 2001.

Berg HE, Eiken O, Miklavcic L et al: Hip, thigh and calf muscle atrophy and bone loss after 5-week bed rest inactivity, *Eur J Appl Physiol* 99(3):283-289, 2007.

Bianchi R, Gigliotti F, Romagnoli I et al: Chest wall kinematics and breathlessness during pursed-lip breathing in patients with COPD, *Chest* 125(2):459, 2004.

Bradley JG, Davis KA: Orthostatic hypotension, *Am Fam Physician* 68(12):2393, 2003.

Crowe J, Reid WD, Geddes EL et al: Inspiratory muscle training compared with other rehabilitation interventions in adults with chronic obstructive pulmonary disease: a systematic literature review and meta-analysis, *COPD* 2(3):319-329, 2005.

Demers C, McKelvie RS, Negassa A et al: Reliability, validity, and responsiveness of the six-minute walk test in patients with heart failure, *Am Heart J* 142(4):698, 2001.

Dowd S, Poole V, Davidhizar R et al: Death, dying and grieving in a transcultural context: application of the Giger and Davidhizar model, *Hosp J* 13(4):33-56, 1998.

Fick DM, Cooper JW, Wade WE et al. Updating the Beers criteria for potentially inappropriate medication use in older adults: results of a US consensus panel of experts, *Arch Intern Med* 163(22):2716-2724, 2003.

Fletcher K: Immobility: geriatric self-learning module, *Medsurg Nurs* 14(1):35, 2005.

Ford CM, Pruitt R, Parker V et al: CHF: effects of cardiac rehabilitation and brain natriuretic peptide, *Nurse Pract* 29(3):36, 2004.

Garvey C: Pulmonary rehabilitation for the elderly client, *Topics Adv Prac Nurse J* 1(2):2001. Available at www.medscape.com/viewarticle/408409, accessed on April 5, 2005.

Haque R: *Polypharmacy in the elderly—cardiovascular component,* Presentation at conference: New Directions in Cardiovascular Disease, March 10, 2007. Jackson, Michigan.

Hauer KE: Discovering the cause of syncope, *Postgrad Med* 113(1):31, 2003.

Holmes S: Undernutrition in hospital patients, *Nurs Stand* 17(19):45, 2003.

Jackson J, Neighbors H, Gurin G: Findings from a national survey on Black mental health: implications for practice and training, 1986, National Institute of Mental Health.

Kasper DL, Braunwald E, Fauci AS et al: *Harrison's principles of internal medicine*, ed 16, New York, 2005, McGraw-Hill.

Lacasse Y, Goldstein R, Lasserson T et al: Pulmonary rehabilitation for chronic obstructive pulmonary disease, *Cochrane Database Syst Rev* (3):CD003793, 2006.

Murchie P, Campbell NC, Ritchie LD et al: Effects of secondary prevention clinics on health status in patients with coronary heart disease: 4 year follow-up of a randomized trial in primary care, *Fam Pract* 21(5):567-574, 2004.

Nelson A, Owen B, Lloyd JD et al: Safe patient handling and movement, *Am J Nurs* 103(3):32, 2003.

Patusky KL: Relatedness theory as a framework for the treatment of fatigued women, *Arch Psychiatr Nurs* 5:224, 2002.

Pinto-Plata VM, Cote C, Cabral H et al: The 6-min walk distance: change over time and value as a predictor of survival in severe COPD, *Eur Respir J* 23(1):23, 2004.

Rees K, Taylor RS, Singh S et al: Exercise based rehabilitation for heart failure, *Cochrane Database Syst Rev* (3):CD003331, 2004.

Resnick B, Orwig D, Magaziner J: The effect of social support on exercise behavior in older adults, *Clin Nurs Res* 11(1):52, 2002.

Taylor RS, Brown A, Ebrahim S et al: Exercise-based rehabilitation for patients with coronary heart disease: systematic review and meta-analysis of randomized controlled trials, *Am J Med* 116(10):682, 2004.

Thomas DR, Kamel H, Azharrudin M et al: The relationship of functional status, nutritional assessment, and severity of illness to in-hospital mortality, *J Nutr Health Aging* 9(3):169-175, 2005.

Tinetti ME: Preventing falls in elderly persons, *N Engl J Med* 348(1):421, 2003.

Topp R, Ditmyer M, King K et al: The effect of bed rest and potential of prehabilitation on patients in the intensive care unit, *AACN Clin Issues* 13(2):263, 2002.

Vincent KR, Braith RW, Feldman RA et al: Improved cardiorespiratory endurance following 6 months of resistance exercise in elderly men and women, *Arch Intern Med* 162(6):673, 2002.

Wenger NK: Rehabilitation of the patient with coronary heart disease. In Fuster V et al, editors: *Hurst's the heart,* ed 10, New York, 2001, McGraw-Hill.

Risk for Activity intolerance   *Betty J. Ackley, MSN, EdS, RN*

NANDA   Definition

At risk for experiencing insufficient physiological or psychological energy to endure or complete required or desired daily activities

Risk Factors

Deconditioned status; history of previous intolerance; inexperience with activity; presence of circulatory problems; presence of respiratory problems

NOC   Outcomes (Nursing Outcomes Classification)

Suggested NOC Outcomes

Activity Tolerance, Endurance, Energy Conservation

• = Independent;   ▲ = Collaborative;   EBN = Evidence-Based Nursing;   EB = Evidence-Based

A

Endurance as evidenced by the following indicators: Performance of usual routine/Activity/Rested appearance/Blood oxygen level within normal limits/Concentration/Interest in surroundings/Muscle endurance/Eating pattern/Libido/Energy restored after rest/Blood oxygen level/Hemoglobin/Hematocrit/Blood glucose/Serum electrolytes (Rate the outcome and indicators of **Endurance**: 1 = severely compromised, 2 = substantially compromised, 3 = moderately compromised, 4 = mildly compromised, 5 = not compromised [see Section I].)

NIC   Interventions (Nursing Interventions Classification)

Suggested NIC Interventions

Energy Management, Exercise Promotion: Strength Training, Activity Therapy

Example NIC Activities—Energy Management

Monitor cardiorespiratory response to activity (e.g., tachycardia, other dysrhythmias, dyspnea, diaphoresis, pallor, hemodynamic pressures, respiratory rate); Monitor location and nature of discomfort or pain during movement/activity

Client Outcomes, Nursing Interventions and *Rationales,* and Client/Family Teaching

See care plan for **Activity intolerance.**

Ineffective Airway clearance   *Julie T. Sanford, MSN, RN, and Mike Jacobs, DNS, RN*   evolve

NANDA   Definition

Inability to clear secretions or obstructions from the respiratory tract to maintain a clear airway

Defining Characteristics

Absent or ineffective cough; adventitious breath sounds; changes in respiratory rate; changes in respiratory rhythm; cyanosis; difficulty vocalizing diminished breath sounds; dyspnea; excessive sputum; orthopnea; restlessness; wide-eyed

Related Factors (r/t)

Environmental

Second-hand smoke; smoking; smoke inhalation

Obstructed Airway

Airway spasm; excessive mucus; exudates in the alveoli; foreign body in airway; presence of artificial airway; retained secretions; secretions in the bronchi

Physiological

Allergic airways; asthma; chronic obstructive pulmonary disease; hyperplasia of the bronchial walls; infection; neuromuscular dysfunction

NOC   Outcomes (Nursing Outcomes Classification)

Suggested NOC Outcomes

Aspiration Prevention, Respiratory Status: Airway Patency, Gas Exchange, Ventilation

• = Independent;   ▲ = Collaborative;   EBN = Evidence-Based Nursing;   EB = Evidence-Based

---

Example NOC Outcome with Indicators

Respiratory Status: Ventilation as evidenced by the following indicators: Respiratory rate/Moves sputum out of airway/Adventitious breath sounds not present/SOB not present/Auscultated breath sounds/Auscultated vocalization/Chest x-ray findings (Rate the outcome and indicators of **Respiratory Status: Ventilation:** 1 = severely compromised, 2 = substantially compromised, 3 = moderately compromised, 4 = mildly compromised, 5 = not compromised [see Section I].)

SOB, Shortness of breath.

Client Outcomes

Client Will (Specify Time Frame):

- Demonstrate effective coughing and clear breath sounds
- Cyanotic free skin
- Maintain a patent airway at all times
- Relate methods to enhance secretion removal
- Relate the significance of changes in sputum to include color, character, amount, and odor
- Identify and avoid specific factors that inhibit effective airway clearance

NIC   Interventions (Nursing Interventions Classification)

Suggested NIC Interventions

Airway Management, Airway Suctioning, Cough Enhancement

Example NIC Activities—Airway Management

Instruct how to cough effectively; Auscultate breath sounds, noting areas of decreased or absent ventilation and presence of adventitious sounds

Nursing Interventions and *Rationales*

- Auscultate breath sounds q1 to 4 hours. Breath sounds are normally clear or scattered fine crackles at bases, which clear with deep breathing. *The presence of coarse crackles during late inspiration indicates fluid in the airway; wheezing indicates a narrowed airway (Simpson, 2006).*
- Monitor respiratory patterns, including rate, depth, and effort. *A normal respiratory rate for an adult without dyspnea is 12 to 16. With secretions in the airway, the respiratory rate will increase (Simpson, 2006).*
- Monitor blood gas values and pulse oxygen saturation levels as available. *An oxygen saturation of less than 90% (normal: 95% to 100%) or a partial pressure of oxygen of less than 80 (normal: 80 to 100) indicates significant oxygenation problems (Clark, Giuliano & Chen, 2006).*
- Position the client to optimize respiration (e.g., head of bed elevated 45 degrees and repositioned at least every 2 hours). *An upright position allows for maximal lung expansion; lying flat causes abdominal organs to shift toward the chest, which crowds the lungs and makes it more difficult to breathe.* **EB:** *In a mechanically ventilated client, there is a decreased incidence of pneumonia if the client is positioned at a 45-degree semirecumbent position as opposed to a supine position (Seckel, 2007).*
- If the client has unilateral lung disease, alternate a semi-Fowler's position with a lateral position (with a 10- to 15-degree elevation and "good lung down") for 60 to 90 minutes. This method is contraindicated for a client with a pulmonary abscess or hemorrhage or with interstitial emphysema. *Gravity and hydrostatic pressure allow the dependent lung to become better ventilated and perfused, which increases oxygenation (Marklew, 2006).*
- Help the client deep breathe and perform controlled coughing. Have the client inhale deeply, hold breath for several seconds, and cough two or three times with mouth open while tightening the upper abdominal muscles. *This technique can help increase sputum clearance and decrease cough*

• = Independent;   ▲ = Collaborative;   EBN = Evidence-Based Nursing;   EB = Evidence-Based

spasms (Donahue, 2002; Nursing2004). Controlled coughing uses the diaphragmatic muscles, making the cough more forceful and effective.

- If the client has COPD, cystic fibrosis, or bronchiectasis, consider helping the client use the forced expiratory technique, the "huff cough." The client does a series of coughs while saying the word "huff." *This technique prevents the glottis from closing during the cough and is effective in clearing secretions in the central airways (Goodfellow & Jones, 2002; Pruitt & Jacobs, 2005).*

- Encourage the client to use an incentive spirometer. *The incentive spirometer is an effective tool that can help prevent atelectasis and retention of bronchial secretions (Guimarães & Atallah, 2007).* **EB:** *A study of postoperative abdominal surgery clients demonstrated that coughing and deep breathing clients vs. use of an incentive spirometer resulted in no significant difference in oxygenation (Genc et al, 2004).*

- Assist with clearing secretions from pharynx by offering tissues and gentle suction of the oral pharynx if necessary. *In the debilitated client, gentle suctioning of the posterior pharynx may stimulate coughing and remove secretions.*

- Observe sputum, noting color, odor, and volume. *Normal sputum is clear or gray and minimal; abnormal sputum is green, yellow, or bloody; malodorous; and often copious.*

- When suctioning an endotracheal tube or tracheostomy tube for a client on a ventilator, do the following:
  - Explain the process of suctioning before and ensure the client is not in pain or overly anxious. *Suctioning can be a frightening experience; an explanation along with adequate pain relief or needed sedation can reduce stress, anxiety, and pain (Smith-Temple & Johnson, 2005).*
  - Hyperoxygenate before and between endotracheal suction sessions. **EBN:** *Hyperoxygenation helps prevent oxygen desaturation in a suctioned client (Choi & Jones, 2005).*
  - Use a closed, in-line suction system. **EB:** *Endotracheal suctioning using a closed system resulted in less deoxygenation of the client than when disconnecting the tubing for suctioning (Maggiore et al, 2003). A study demonstrated that using a closed system for suctioning, using pressure support as a recruitment measure, and avoiding disconnecting the tubing resulted in decreased collapse of alveoli with suctioning and increased oxygenation (Maggiore et al, 2003).*
  - Avoid saline instillation during suctioning. **EBN:** *Saline instillation before suctioning has an adverse effect on oxygen saturation in both adults and children (Celik & Kanan, 2006; Ridling, Martin & Bratton, 2003). Instillation of saline into the endotracheal tube increased the number of colonies of bacteria dislodged from the tube to enter the lower airways, which can result in pneumonia (Freytag et al, 2003; Hagler & Traver, 1994).*
  - Document results of coughing and suctioning, particularly client tolerance and secretion characteristics such as color, odor, and volume.

- Encourage activity and ambulation as tolerated. If unable to ambulate the client, turn the client from side to side at least every 2 hours. *Body movement helps mobilize secretions and can be a powerful means to maintain lung health (Pruitt, 2006).* **EB:** *Changes of postoperative position from sitting to standing are very important to improve outcomes, and the supine position should be avoided (Nielsen, Holte & Kehlet, 2003).* See interventions for **Impaired Gas exchange** for further information on positioning a respiratory client.

- ▲ If client is intubated, consider use of kinetic therapy, using a kinetic bed that slowly moves the client with 40-degree turns. **EBN:** *Use of the kinetic bed versus turning clients every 2 hours resulted in decreased ventilator-associated pneumonia and atelectasis (Ahrens et al, 2004). Rotational therapy decreases the incidence of pneumonia, but had little effect on mortality rates, number of days on ventilator, or number of days in ICU (Goldhill et al, 2007).*

- Encourage fluid intake of up to 2500 mL/day within cardiac or renal reserve. *Fluids help minimize mucosal drying and maximize ciliary action to move secretions (Smith-Sims, 2001). Some clients cannot tolerate increased fluids because of underlying disease.*

- ▲ Administer oxygen as ordered. *Oxygen has been shown to correct hypoxemia, which can be caused by retained respiratory secretions.*

- ▲ Administer medications such as bronchodilators or inhaled steroids as ordered. Watch for side effects such as tachycardia or anxiety with bronchodilators, or inflamed pharynx with inhaled steroids. *Bronchodilators decrease airway resistance secondary to bronchoconstriction.*

▲ Provide postural drainage, percussion, and vibration only as ordered. **EB:** *There is no advantage of chest physiotherapy over other airway clearance techniques for cystic fibrosis clients (Main, Prasad & van der Schans, 2005). There is not enough evidence to support or refute the use of bronchial hygiene physical therapy in COPD or bronchiectasis clients (Jones & Rowe, 2000).*

▲ Refer for physical therapy or respiratory therapy for further treatment.

Geriatric

- Encourage ambulation as tolerated without causing exhaustion. *Immobility is often harmful to the elderly because it decreases ventilation and increases stasis of secretions, leading to atelectasis or pneumonia (Fletcher, 2005).*

- Actively encourage the elderly to deep breathe and cough. *Cough reflexes are blunted, and coughing is decreased in the elderly (Miller, 2004).*

- Ensure adequate hydration within cardiac and renal reserves. *The elderly are prone to dehydration and therefore more viscous secretions because they frequently use diuretics or laxatives and forget to drink adequate amounts of water (Miller, 2004).*

Home Care

- Some of the above interventions may be adapted for home care use.

▲ Begin discharge planning as soon as possible with case manager or social worker to assess need for home support systems, assistive devices, and community or home health services.

- Assess home environment for factors that exacerbate airway clearance problems (e.g., presence of allergens, lack of adequate humidity in air, poor air flow, stressful family relationships). **EBN:** *Home environmental triggers of asthma have been found to include dust/dust mites, animal dander, mold, perfumes/detergents, and cigarette smoke. Psychosocial triggers included family tensions, physical activity, anxiety/stress, and friends/peer pressure (Navaie-Waliser et al, 2004).*

- Assess affective climate within family and family support system. *Problems with respiratory function and resulting anxiety can provoke anger and frustration in the client. Feelings may be displaced onto caregiver and require intervention to ensure continued caregiver support.* Refer to care plan for **Caregiver role strain.**

▲ Refer to GOLD and ACP-ASIM/ACCP guidelines for management of home care and indications of hospital admission criteria (Chojnowski, 2003).

- Provide the client with emotional support in dealing with symptoms of respiratory distress. **EBN:** *Social support was identified as a reason for non-adherence in asthmatics (Elliott, 2006).*

- When respiratory procedures are being implemented, explain equipment and procedures to family members, and provide needed emotional support. *Family members assuming responsibility for respiratory monitoring often find this stressful. They may not have been able to assimilate fully any instructions provided by hospital staff (McNeal, 2000).*

- When electrically based equipment for respiratory support is being implemented, evaluate home environment for electrical safety, proper grounding, and so on. Ensure that notification is sent to the local utility company, the emergency medical team, and police and fire departments. *Notification is important to provide for priority service (NHLB, 2006).*

- Support clients' efforts at self-care. Ensure they have all the information they need to participate in care. **EBN:** *Self-care study participants showed competence at managing care of their own asthma (Makinen et al, 2000).*

- Provide family with support for care of a client with chronic or terminal illness. *Breathing difficulty can provoke extreme anxiety, which can interfere with the client's ability or willingness to adhere to the treatment plan.* Refer to care plan for **Anxiety.** *Witnessing breathing difficulties and facing concerns of dealing with chronic or terminal illness can create fear in caregiver. Fear inhibits effective coping.* **EBN:** *Parents of a child with cystic fibrosis particularly benefit from nursing support. Parents deal with devastation upon receiving the diagnosis, a sense of fear and isolation, an overwhelming sense of guilt and powerlessness, vigilance, and returning to normalcy (Carpenter & Narsavage, 2004).* Refer to care plan for **Powerlessness.**

A

▲ Instruct the client to avoid exposure to persons with upper respiratory infections.

▲ Provide/teach percussion and postural drainage per physician orders. Teach adaptive breathing techniques.

• Determine client adherence to medical regimen. Instruct the client and family in importance of reporting effectiveness of current medications to physician.

• Teach the client when and how to use inhalant or nebulizer treatments at home.

▲ Teach the client/family importance of maintaining regimen and having PRN drugs easily accessible at all times. *Success in avoiding emergency or institutional care may rest solely on medication compliance or availability.* **EBN:** *Parents/family have been found to have inadequate knowledge about recognition of asthma attacks, triggers, and management (Navaie-Waliser et al, 2004).*

• Teach the client/family the importance of and methods for setting priorities for activities, especially those having a high energy demand (e.g., home/family events). Instruct in realistic expectations. **EBN:** *Client and/or family may assume a higher degree of energy than is actually present. Assistance may be needed to ensure accuracy of expectations for the client. Unrealistic expectations provoke guilt feelings in the client, leading to efforts that can exceed the client's energy capacity (Patusky, 2002).*

• Instruct the client and family in the importance of maintaining proper nutrition, adequate fluids, rest, and behavioral pacing for energy conservation and rehabilitation.

• Instruct in use of dietary supplements as indicated. *Illness may suppress appetite, leading to inadequate nutrition. Pacing activities to energy capacity and rest are important to ensure the client does not overdo his or her capability. Low fluid intake can increase the thickness of respiratory secretions.*

• Identify an emergency plan, including criteria for use. *Ineffective airway clearance can be life-threatening.*

▲ Refer for home health aide services for assistance with ADLs. *Clients with decreased oxygenation and copious respiratory secretions are often unable to maintain energy for ADLs.*

▲ Assess family for role changes and coping skills. Refer to medical social services as necessary. *Clients with decreased oxygenation are unable to maintain role activities and therefore experience frustration and anger, which may pose a threat to family integrity. Family counseling to adapt to role changes may be needed.*

Client/Family Teaching

▲ Teach importance of not smoking. Be aggressive in approach, ask to set a date for smoking cessation, and recommend nicotine replacement therapy (nicotine patch or gum). Refer to smoking cessation programs, and encourage clients who relapse to keep trying to quit. *All healthcare clinicians should be aggressive in helping smokers quit (CDC, 2007).* **EB:** *The combination of nicotine therapy and an intensive, prolonged relapse prevention program are effective in promoting long-term abstinence from smoking (Wagena et al, 2004).*

▲ Teach the client how to use a flutter clearance device if ordered, which vibrates to loosen mucus and gives positive pressure to keep airways open. **EB:** *This device has been shown to effectively decrease mucous viscosity and elasticity (App et al, 1998), increase amount of sputum expectorated (Bellone et al, 2000), and increase peak expiratory flow rate (Burioka et al, 1998). Daily use of the flutter device was shown to be as effective as the active cycle of breathing technique and was a preferred technique by clients (Thompson et al, 2002). Use of the mucus clearance device had improved exercise performance compared with COPD clients who use a sham device (Wolkove et al, 2004).*

▲ Teach the client how to use peak expiratory flow rate (PEFR) meter if ordered and when to seek medical attention if PEFR reading drops. Also teach how to use metered dose inhalers and self-administer inhaled corticosteroids as ordered following precautions to decrease side effects.

• Teach the client how to deep breathe and cough effectively. **EB:** *Controlled coughing uses the diaphragmatic muscles, making the cough more forceful and effective (Donahue, 2002; Nursing 2004).*

- Teach the client/family to identify and avoid specific factors that exacerbate ineffective airway clearance, including known allergens and especially smoking (if relevant) or exposure to second-hand smoke.
- Educate the client and family about the significance of changes in sputum characteristics, including color, character, amount, and odor. *With this knowledge, the client and family can identify early the signs of infection and seek treatment before acute illness occurs.*
- Teach the client/family the need to take ordered antibiotics until the prescription has run out. *Taking the entire course of antibiotics helps to eradicate bacterial infection, which decreases lingering, chronic infection.*

evolve   See the EVOLVE website for World Wide Web resources for client education.

REFERENCES

Ahrens T, Kollef M, Stewart J et al: Effect of kinetic therapy on pulmonary complications, *Am J Crit Care* 13(5):376, 2004.

App EM, Kieselmann R, Reinhardt D et al: Sputum rheology changes in cystic fibrosis lung disease following two different types of physiotherapy: flutter vs. autogenic drainage, *Chest* 114(1):171, 1998.

Bellone A, Lascioli R, Raschi S et al: Chest physical therapy in patients with acute exacerbation of chronic bronchitis: effectiveness of three modes, *Arch Phys Med Rehabil* 81(5):558, 2000.

Burioka N, Sugimoto Y, Suyama H et al: Clinical efficacy of the FLUTTER device for airway mucus clearance in patients with diffuse panbronchiolitis, *Respirology* 3(3):183, 1998.

Carpenter DR, Narsavage GL: One breath at a time: living with cystic fibrosis, *J Pediatr Nurs* 19(1):25, 2004.

Celik SA, Kanan N: A current conflict: use of isotonic sodium chloride solution on endotracheal suctioning in critically ill patients, *Dimens Crit Care Nurs* 25(1):11, 2006.

Centers for Disease Control (CDC): *Smoking and tobacco use*, Retrieved from http://www.cdc.gov/doc.do/id/0900f3ec802346d8, 2007.

Choi JS, Jones AY: Effects of manual hyperinflation and suctioning on respiratory mechanics in mechanically ventilated patients with ventilator-associated pneumonia, *Aust J Physio* 51:25, 2005.

Chojnowski D: "GOLD" standards for acute exacerbation in COPD, *Nurs Pract* 28(5):26, 2003.

Clark AP, Giuliano K, Chen, HM: Pulse oximetry revisited: "but his O(2) sat was normal!", *Clin Nurs Spec* 20(6):268-272, 2006.

Donahue M: "Spare the cough, spoil the airway": back to the basics in airway clearance, *Pediatr Nurs* 28(2):119, 2002.

Elliott RA: Poor adherence to anti-inflammatory medication in asthma: reasons, challenges, and strategies for improved disease management, *Dis Manage Health Outcomes* 14(4):223-233, 2006.

Fletcher K: Immobility: geriatric self-learning module, *Medsurg Nurs* 14(1):35, 2005.

Freytag CC, Thies FL, Konig W et al: Prolonged application of closed in-line suction catheters increases microbial colonization of the lower respiratory tract and bacterial growth on catheter surface, *Infection* 31(1):31-37, 2003.

Genc A, Yildirim Y, Gnerli A: Researching of the effectiveness of deep breathing and incentive spirometry in postoperative early stage, *Fizyoterapi Rehabil* 15(1), 2004.

Goldhill DR, Imhoff M, McLean B et al: Rotational bed therapy to prevent and treat respiratory complications: a review and meta-analysis, *Am J Crit Care* 16(1):50-61, 2007.

Goodfellow LT, Jones M: Bronchial hygiene therapy, *Am J Nurs* 102(1):37-43, 2002.

Guimarães MF, Atallah AN, El Dib RP: Incentive spirometer for prevention of postoperative pulmonary complications in upper abdominal surgery. (Protocol) *Cochrane Database Syst Rev* (2):CD006058, 2007.

Hagler DA, Traver GA: Endotracheal saline and suction catheters: sources of lower airway contamination, *Am J Crit Care* 3(6):444, 1994.

Jones AP, Rowe BH: Bronchopulmonary hygiene physical therapy for chronic obstructive pulmonary disease and bronchiectasis, *Cochrane Database Syst Rev* (2):CD000045, 2000.

Maggiore SM, Lellouche F, Pigeot J et al: Prevention of endotracheal suctioning-induced alveolar decruitement in acute lung injury, *Am J Respir Crit Care Med* 167(9):1215, 2003.

Main E, Prasad A, van der Schans C: Conventional chest physiotherapy compared to other airway clearance techniques for cystic fibrosis, *Cochrane Database Syst Rev*, (1):CD002011, 2005.

Makinen S, Suominen T, Lauri S: Self-care in adults with asthma: how they cope, *J Clin Nurs* 9:557, 2000.

Marklew A: Body positioning and its effect on oxygenation—a literature review, *Br Assoc Crit Care Nurs* 11(1):16, 2006.

McNeal GJ: *AACN guide to acute care procedures in the home*, Philadelphia, 2000, Lippincott.

Miller CA: *Nursing for wellness in older adults*, ed 4, Philadelphia, 2004, Lippincott.

National Heart, Lung, and Blood Institute (NHLB): *Living with COPD*. Retrieved from http://www.nhlbi.nih.gov/health/dci/Diseases/Copd/Copd_WhatIs.html, 2006.

Navaie-Waliser M, Misener M, Mersman C et al: Evaluating the needs of children with asthma in home care: the vital role of nurses as caregivers and educators, *Public Health Nurs* 21(4):306, 2004.

Nielsen KG, Holte K, Kehlet H: Effects of posture on postoperative pulmonary function, *Acta Anaesthesiol Scand* 47(10):1270, 2003.

Nursing2004: Respiratory challenge, *Nursing* 34(11):70, 2004.

Patusky KL: Relatedness theory as a framework for the treatment of fatigued women, *Arch Psychiatr Nurs* 5:224, 2002.

Pruitt B: Help your patient combat postoperative atelectasis, *Nursing* 36(5):64, 2006.

Pruitt B, Jacobs M: Clearing away pulmonary secretions, *Nursing* 35(7):36, 2005.

Ridling DA, Martin LD, Bratton SL: Endotracheal suctioning with or without instillation of isotonic sodium chloride solution in critically ill children, *Am J Crit Care* 12(3):212, 2003.

Seckel M: Implementing evidence-based practice guidelines to minimize ventilator-associated pneumonia, *AACN News* 24(1):8-10, 2007.

Simpson H: Respiratory assessment, *Br J Nurs* 15(9):484-488, 2006.

Smith-Sims K: Hospital-acquired pneumonia, *Am J Nurs* 101(1):24AA, 2001.

Smith-Temple AJ, Johnson JY: *Nurses' guide to clinical procedures*, ed 5 Philadelphia, 2005, Lippincott Williams & Wilkins.

Thompson CS, Harrison S, Ashley J: Randomised crossover study of the flutter device and the active cycle of breathing technique in noncystic fibrosis bronchiectasis, *Thorax* 57:446, 2002.

Wagena EJ, van der Meer RM, Ostelo RJ et al: The efficacy of smoking cessation strategies in people with chronic obstructive pulmo-

nary disease: results from a systematic review, *Respir Med* 98(9):805, 2004.

Wolkove N, Baltzan MA Jr, Kamel H et al: A randomized trial to evaluate the sustained efficacy of a mucus clearance device in ambulatory patients with chronic obstructive pulmonary disease, *Can Respir J* 11(8):567, 2004.

Latex Allergy response   *Leslie H. Nicoll, PhD, MBA, RN, B, and DeLancey Nicoll, SN*

NANDA   Definition

A hypersensitive reaction to natural latex rubber products

Defining Characteristics

Life-threatening reactions occurring <1 hour after exposure to latex protein: Bronchospasm; cardiac arrest; contact urticaria progressing to generalized symptoms; dyspnea; edema of the lips; edema of the throat; edema of the tongue; edema of the uvula; hypotension; respiratory arrest; syncope; tightness in chest; wheezing

Orofacial characteristics: Edema of eyelids; edema of sclera; erythema of the eyes; facial erythema; facial itching; itching of the eyes; oral itching; nasal congestion; nasal erythema; nasal itching; rhinorrhea; tearing of the eyes

Gastrointestinal characteristics: Flushing; generalized discomfort; generalized edema; increasing complaint of total body warmth; restlessness

Generalized characteristics: Flushing; generalized discomfort; generalized edema; increasing complaint of total body warmth; restlessness

Type 1V reactions occurring >1 hour after exposure to latex protein: Discomfort reaction to additives such as thiurams and carbamates; eczema; irritation; redness

Related Factors (r/t)

Hypersensitivity to natural latex rubber protein

NOC   Outcomes (Nursing Outcomes Classification)

Suggested NOC Outcomes

Allergic Response: Localized, Systemic; Immune Hypersensitivity Response

Example NOC Outcome with Indicators
Allergic Response: Systemic as evidenced by the following indicators: Laryngeal edema/dyspnea at rest/wheezing/tachycardia/decreased blood pressure/hives/petechiae/erythema (Rate the outcome and indicators of **Allergic Response: Systemic:** 1 = severe, 2 = substantial, 3 = moderate, 4 = mild, 5 = none [see Section I].)

Client Outcomes

Client Will (Specify Time Frame):

• Identify presence of NRL allergy
• List history of risk factors
• Identify type of reaction
• State reasons not to use or to have anyone use latex products
• Experience a latex-safe environment for all healthcare procedures
• Avoid areas where there is powder from NRL gloves
• State the importance of wearing a Medic-Alert bracelet and wear one
• State the importance of carrying an emergency kit with a supply of nonlatex gloves, antihistamines, and an autoinjectable epinephrine syringe (Epi-pen), and carry one

NIC   Interventions (Nursing Interventions Classification)   A

Suggested NIC Interventions
Allergy Management, Latex Precautions

Example NIC Activities—Latex Precautions
Question patient or appropriate other about history of systemic reaction or sensitization to NRL (e.g., facial or scleral edema, tearing eyes, urticaria, rhinitis, and wheezing); Place allergy band on patient

Nursing Interventions and *Rationales*

- Identify clients at risk: those persons who are most likely to exhibit a sensitivity to NRL that may result in varying degrees of reactivity. Consider the following client groups:
  - Persons with neural tube defects including spina bifida, myelomeningocele/meningocele. **EB:** *Clients with spina bifida represent the highest-risk group for developing NRL hypersensitivity.* **EB:** *Recognized risk factors for these clients are repeated surgeries and an atopic disposition (Buck et al, 2000).* **EB:** *Incidence of latex allergy in clients with spina bifida varies between 28% and 67% (Gulbahar et al, 2004).* **EB:** *Spina bifida, even in the absence of multiple surgeries, seems to be an independent risk factor for latex sensitization (Hochleitner et al, 2001).*
  - Children who have experienced three or more surgeries, particularly as a neonate. **EB:** *A significant correlation between the total number of surgeries, particularly during the first year of life, and degree of sensitization has been established (Degenhardt et al, 2001; Sparta et al, 2004).*
  - Children with chronic renal failure. **EB:** *Children with chronic renal failure are at risk because of their intense exposure to latex through catheters, gloves, and anesthetic equipment during frequent hospitalizations from early life on (Dehlink et al, 2004).*
  - Atopic individuals (persons with a tendency to have multiple allergic conditions) including allergies to food products. Particular allergies to fruits and vegetables including bananas, avocado, celery, fig, chestnut, papaya, potato, tomato, melon, and passion fruit are significant. **EB:** *Atopy is an important risk for the development of latex allergy (Proietti et al, 2005).* **EB:** *Class I chitinases, related to plant defense, are the panallergens in these foods and are associated with latex-fruit syndrome (Perkin, 2000; Salcedo et al, 2001).*
  - Persons who possess a known or suspected NRL allergy by having exhibited an allergic or anaphylactic reaction, positive skin testing, or positive IgE antibodies against latex. **EB:** *Persons who are sensitized or have demonstrated an NRL allergy are at risk, even when a latex-free environment is adopted (Mazon et al, 2000; Taylor & Erkek, 2004).*
  - Persons who have had an ongoing occupational exposure to NRL, including healthcare workers, rubber industry workers, bakers, laboratory personnel, food handlers, hairdressers, janitors, policemen, and firefighters. **EB:** *The predominant pattern of allergen reactivity in healthcare workers and others with occupational exposure is different from that among children with spina bifida; it has been suggested that occupational exposure is from NRL glove proteins inhaled through powders as opposed to particle bound latex proteins in urinary catheters (Sutherland et al, 2002; Barbara et al, 2004).* **EB:** *HCWs have an increased risk of sensitization and allergic symptoms to latex (Bousquet et al, 2006).* **EB:** *Estimates of prevalence in healthcare workers range from 2% to 17% (Ahmed et al, 2004).* **EB:** *Allergic reactions to NRL have increased during the past 10 years, especially in healthcare workers who have high exposure to latex allergens both by direct skin contact and by inhalation of latex particles from powdered gloves (Jones et al, 2004).* **EB:** *The prevalence of a type I allergy to NRL in dental hygienists appears similar to that reported for other oral healthcare professionals and is greater than the general population (Hamann et al, 2005).* **EB:** *While many argue that the implementation of universal precautions is a driving factor behind the increase of latex allergy in healthcare workers, researchers at the University of Minnesota dispute that claim (McCall et al, 2003).*
- Take a thorough history of the client at risk. **EB:** *A complete and thorough history remains as the most reliable screening test to predict the likelihood of an anaphylactic reaction (Hepner & Castells,*

A

2003). **EB:** *Those at risk may be identified through a thorough medical history and allergy testing (Binkley et al J 2003).* **EB:** *Skin prick tests and serum IgE are of limited value in epidemiological studies of NRL allergy; questionnaires about local symptoms are more relevant (Galobardes et al, 2001).* **EB:** *It is possible to make a diagnosis of type I NRL allergy by taking an accurate history, including questions on atopic status, food allergy, and possible reactions to latex devices (Toraason et al, 2000).*

- Question the client about associated symptoms of itching, swelling, and redness after contact with rubber products such as rubber gloves, balloons, and barrier contraceptives, or swelling of the tongue and lips after dental examinations. **EB:** *Dermatitis, itching, erythema, contact urticaria, asthma and/or rhinitis were significantly related to skin prick tests that were positive for latex (Larese Filon et al, 2001; Ylitalo et al, 2000).*

- Consider a skin prick test with NRL extracts to identify IgE-mediated immunity. **EB:** *Skin prick tests with well-characterized latex extracts are highly sensitive and specific predictors of latex-specific IgE antibodies (Ownby, 2003).*

- All latex-sensitive clients are treated as if they have NRL allergy. **EB:** *Even if a person has not experienced an NRL reaction, if it can be documented that he or she has been sensitized, then he or she should be treated as if he or she has an NRL allergy. Every hospital and scientific research facility should institute a comprehensive emergency treatment program for NRL allergic clients and workers, latex-safe areas in their facilities, and a prevention program that includes the wide use of latex-free gloves and absence of powdered gloves throughout these facilities (Edlich et al, 2003).* **EB:** *Reducing exposure to latex is a safe and more economical alternative to complete removal of the individual from the place of employment (Ranta & Ownby, 2004).*

- Clients with spina bifida and others with a positive history of NRL sensitivity or NRL allergy should have all medical/surgical/dental procedures performed in a latex-controlled environment. **EB:** *Allergen avoidance and substitution and the use of latex-safe devices including synthetic gloves are essential for the affected client (Lukesova, 2005).* **EB:** *A latex-controlled environment is defined as one in which no latex gloves are used in the room or surgical suite and no latex accessories (catheters, adhesives, tourniquet, and anesthesia equipment) come in contact with the client (Joint Task Force on Practice Parameters, 1998).* **EB:** *The American Society of Anesthesiologists Task Force of Latex Sensitivity recommends that clients who are latex allergic have a surgical procedure performed as the first case in the morning, when the levels of latex aeroallergens are the smallest (Berry et al, 1999).*

- The most effective approach to preventing NRL anaphylaxis is complete latex avoidance. Medications may reduce certain symptoms. **EB:** *Safe and readily available immunotherapy for NRL allergy is currently lacking (Brehler & Kutting, 2001; Sutherland et al, 2002).* **EB:** *Prevention is the cornerstone in the management of latex sensitization (Hepner & Castells, 2003).*

- Materials and items that contain NRL must be identified, and latex-free alternatives must be found. **EB:** *The development of a guide listing latex-containing drugs is essential for the primary prevention of allergic reactions to this substance in hospital (Navarrete et al, 2006).* **EB:** *Effective September 1998, all medical devices must be labeled regarding their latex content (Hubbard, 1997).* **EB:** *Substitution of powdered latex gloves with low-protein powder-free NRL gloves or latex-free gloves promises benefits to both workers' health and cost and human resource savings for employers (LaMontagne, 2006).*

- In healthcare settings, general use of latex gloves having negligible allergen content, powder-free latex gloves, and nonlatex gloves and medical articles should be considered in an effort to minimize exposure to latex allergen. **EB:** *Simple measures such as the avoidance of unnecessary glove use, the use of non-powdered latex gloves by all workers, and use of non-latex gloves by sensitized subjects can stop the progression of latex symptoms and can avoid new cases of sensitization (Filon & Radman 2006).* **EB:** *Surgical powdered latex gloves were the major predisposing factor for latex sensitization measured by latex-specific IgE among anesthesiologists (Tatsumi et al, 2005).*

▲ If latex gloves are chosen for protection from blood or body fluids, a reduced-protein, powder-free glove should be selected. **EB:** *Until well-accepted standardized tests are available, total protein serves as a useful indicator of the exposure of concern. Protein levels below 50 mg/g are considered the least allergenic (Muller, 2003).*

• = Independent;   ▲ = Collaborative;   EBN = Evidence-Based Nursing;   EB = Evidence-Based

A

- See Box III-1 for examples of products that may contain NRL and safe alternatives that are available. **EB:** *Anaphlaxis from NRL allergy is a medical emergency and must be treated as such. Latex is a potent allergen, and a type I anaphylactic reaction may be immediate in sensitized individuals. Acute treatment must be carried out in a latex-free environment (Hepner & Castells, 2003).*

 ### Home Care

- Assess the home environment for presence of NRL products (e.g., balloons, condoms, gloves, and products of related allergies, such as bananas, avocados, and poinsettia plants). **EB:** *Strict compliance with latex avoidance instructions is essential both inside and outside the hospital. Greater emphasis should be placed on reducing latex exposure in the home and school environments, as such contact could maintain positive IgE-antibody levels (Dieguez et al, 2006).*
- At onset of care, assess client history and current status of NRL allergy response. **EBN:** *A complete and thorough history remains as the most reliable screening test to predict the likelihood of an anaphylactic reaction (American Association of Nurse Anesthetists, 1998).*
- ▲ Seek medical care as necessary.

BOX III-1 PRODUCTS THAT MAY CONTAIN LATEX AND LATEX-FREE ALTERNATIVES USED IN HEALTHCARE SETTINGS

Frequently Contain Latex	Latex-Free Alternative
Ace wraps	Teds, pneumatic boots
Airways	Hudson airways, oxygen masks
Ambu (bag-valve) masks (black or blue reusable)	Clear, disposable ambu-bags
Bandaids	Sterile dressing with plastic tape or tegaderm
Blood pressure cuffs	Dura-Cuf Critikon Vital Answers or use over gown or stockinetter
Catheter, indwelling	Silocone foley (Kendall, Argyle, Baxter)
Catheter, straight	Plastic (Mentor, Bard)
Chux	Double, triple lumen (Bard, Rusch)
Disposable gloves, latex, non-sterile	Disposable underpads
Dressings—Moleskin, Micropore, Coban (3M)	Sensicare gloves
Dressings—Moleskin, Micropore, Coban (3M)	Tegaderm (3M), Steri-strips
Endotracheal tubes	3M, Baxter electrocardiogram pads
Gloves, sterile and exam, surgical and medical	Dantec surface electrocardiogram pads
Heplock-PRN adapter	Mallinckrodt, Sheridan, Portex tube styletes
IV solutions and tubing systems	Laryngeal mask airway
Medication syringes	Vinyl, neoprene gloves (Neolon, Tachylon, Tru-touch, Elastryn)
Medication vial	Use stopcock to inject medications
Oral and nasal airways	Baxter, Abbott, Walrus tubing
OR caps with elastic (bouffant)	Walrus anesthesia sets are latex-free
Oxygen tubing	Abbott IV fluid
Stethoscope tubing	Becton Dickinson angiocaths and syringes
Suction tubing	Concord Portex, Bard syringes
Tape—cloth, adhesive, paper	Remove latex stopper
Tourniquets	Hudson airways, oxygen masks
	Caps with ties
	Nasal, face mask
	Do not let tubing touch client, cover with web roll
	Mallinckrodt, Yankauer, Davol suction catheters
	Plastic, silk, 3M Microfoam Blenderm, Durapore
	Latex-free tourniquet (blue)

A

- Do not use NRL products in caregiving.
- Assist the client in identifying and obtaining alternatives to NRL products. **EB:** *Preventing exposure to latex is the key to managing and preventing this allergy. Providing a safe environment for clients with NRL allergy is the responsibility of all healthcare professionals (American Association of Nurse Anesthetists, 1998).* **EB:** *Avoidance management should be individualized, taking into consideration factors such as age, activity, occupation, hobbies, residential conditions, and the client's level of personal anxiety (Joint Task Force on Practice Parameters, 1998).*

Client/Family Teaching

- Provide written information about NRL allergy and sensitivity. **EB:** *Client education is the most important preventive strategy. Clients should be carefully instructed about "hidden" latex, cross-reactions, particularly foods, and unforeseen risks during medical procedures (Joint Task Force on Practice Parameters, 1998).*
- ▲ Instruct the client to inform healthcare professionals if he or she has an NRL allergy, particularly if he or she is scheduled for surgery. **EB:** *It is essential to recognize which clients and colleagues are sensitized to latex to provide appropriate treatment and to establish adequate prevention (Hepner & Castells, 2003).*
- Teach the client what products contain NRL and to avoid direct contact with all latex products and foods that trigger allergic reactions. **EBN:** *Once an individual becomes allergic to latex, special precautions are needed to prevent exposures. Teaching is an effective strategy (Society of Gastroenterology Nurses and Associates, Inc., 2004).*
- See Box III-2 for examples of products found in the community that may contain NRL and safe alternatives that are available.
- Teach the client to avoid areas where powdered latex gloves are used, as well as where latex bal-

---

BOX III-2 LATEX PRODUCTS AND SAFE ALTERNATIVES OUTSIDE OF THE HEALTHCARE SETTING

Containing Latex Latex	Free Alternative
Balloons	Mylar balloons
Balls, koosh ball	Vinyl, thornton sport ball
Belt for clothing	Leather or cloth belts
Beach shoes	Cotton socks
Bungee cords	Rope or twine
Cleaning/kitchen gloves	Vinyl gloves
Condoms	Polyurethane avanti for males
Crib mattress pads	Polyurethane reality for females
Elastic bands	Heavy cotton pads
Elastic on legs, waist of clothing, disposable diapers, rubber pants	Paper clips, staples, twine
Halloween rubber masks	Velcro closures
Pacifiers	Cloth diapers
Racquet handles	Plastic mask or water based paints
Raincoats/slickers	Plastic pacifier "The First Years"
Swim fins	Silicone—Pur, Gerber, Soft-Flex
Telephone cords	Leather handles
	Nylon or synthetic waterproof coats
	Clear plastic fins
	Clear cords

Data on boxes 1 and 2 from: American Association of Nurse Anesthetists: *AANA latex protocol,* Park Ridge, Ill, 1998, The Association, pp 1-9; National Institute for Occupational Safety and Health: *Preventing allergic reactions to natural rubber latex in the workplace,* Cincinnati, July 1998, The Institute; Hepner DL, Castells MC: Latex allergy: an update, *Anesth Analg* 96(4):1219-1229, 2003.

• = Independent;   ▲ = Collaborative;   EBN = Evidence-Based Nursing;   EB = Evidence-Based

loons are inflated or deflated. **EB:** *Powder from gloves acts as a carrier for latex protein (Hepner &*
Castells, 2003).

- Instruct the client with NRL allergy to wear a medical identification bracelet and/or carry a
  medical identification card. **EB:** *Identification of the client with NRL allergy is critical for prevent-*
  ing problems and for early intervention with appropriate treatment if an exposure occurs (Joint Task
  Force on Practice Parameters, 1998; Hepner & Castells, 2003).
- Instruct the client to carry an emergency kit with a supply of nonlatex gloves, antihistamines,
  and an autoinjectable epinephrine syringe (Epi-Pen). **EB:** *An autoinjectable epinephrine syringe*
  should be prescribed to sensitized clients who are at risk for an anaphylactic episode with accidental latex
  exposure (Joint Task Force on Practice Parameters, 1998; National Institute for Occupational Safety
  and Health, 1998; Tarlo, 1998).

evolve   See the EVOLVE website for World Wide Web resources for client education.

REFERENCES

Ahmed SM, Aw TC, Adisesh A: Toxicological and immunological aspects of occupational latex allergy, *Toxicol Rev* 23(2):123-134, 2004.

American Association of Nurse Anesthetists: *AANA latex protocol,* Park Ridge, Ill, 1998, The Association.

Barbara J, Santais MC, Levy DA et al: Inhaled cornstarch glove powder increases latex-induced airway hyper-sensitivity in guinea pigs, *Clin Exp Allergy* 34(6):978-983, 2004.

Berry AJ, Katz JD, Brown RH et al: *Natural rubber latex allergy: considerations for anesthesiologists,* Park Ridge, Ill, 1999, American Society of Anesthesiologists.

Binkley HM, Schroyer T, Catalfano J: Latex allergies: a review of recognition, evaluation, management, prevention, education, and alternative product use, *J Athl Train* 38(2):133-140, 2003.

Bousquet J, Flahault A, Vandenplas O et al: Natural rubber latex allergy among health care workers: a systematic review of the evidence, *J Allergy Clin Immunol* 118(2):447-454, 2006.

Brehler R, Kutting B: Natural rubber latex allergy: a problem of interdisciplinary concern in medicine, *Arch Intern Med* 161(8):1057-1064, 2001.

Buck D, Michael T, Wahn U et al: Ventricular shunts and the prevalence of sensitization and clinically relevant allergy to latex in patients with spina bifida, *Pediatr Allergy Immunol* 11(2):111-115, 2000.

Degenhardt P, Golla S, Wahn F et al: Latex allergy in pediatric surgery is dependent on repeated operations in the first year of life, *J Pediatr Surg* 36(10):1535-1539, 2001.

Dehlink E, Prandstetter C, Eiwegger T et al: Increased prevalence of latex-sensitization among children with chronic renal failure, *Allergy* 59(7):734-738, 2004.

Dieguez Pastor MC, Anton Girones M et al: Latex allergy in children: a follow-up study, *Allergol Immunopathol (Madr)* 34(1):17-22, 2006.

Edlich RF, Woodard CR, Hill LG et al: Latex allergy: a life-threatening epidemic for scientists, healthcare personnel, and their patients, *J Long Term Eff Med Implants* 13(1):11-19, 2003.

Filon FL, Radman G: Latex allergy: a follow-up study of 1040 healthcare workers, *Occup Environ Med* 63(2):121-125, 2006.

Galobardes B, Quiliquini AM, Roux N et al: Influence of occupational exposure to latex on the prevalence of sensitization and allergy to latex in a Swiss hospital, *Dermatology* 203(3):226-232, 2001.

Gulbahar O, Demir F, Mete N et al: Latex allergy and associated risk factors in a group of Turkish patients with spina bifida, *Turk J Pediatr* 46(3):226-231, 2004.

Hamann CP, Rodgers PA, Sullivan KM: Prevalence of type I natural rubber latex allergy among dental hygienists, *J Dent Hyg* 79(2):7, 2005.

Hepner DL, Castells MC: Latex allergy: an update, *Anesth Analg* 96(4):1219-1229, 2003.

Hochleitner BW, Menardi G, Haussler B et al: Spina bifida as an independent risk factor for sensitization to latex, *J Urol* 166(6):2370-2373, 2001.

Hubbard WK: Department of Health and Human Services. Food and Drug Administration: natural rubber-containing medical devices—user labeling, *Federal Register* 62:189, 1997.

Joint Task Force on Practice Parameters; American Academy of Allergy, Asthma and Immunology; American College of Allergy, Asthma and Immunology; and the Joint Council of Allergy, Asthma and Immunology: The diagnosis and management of anaphylaxis, *J Allergy Clin Immunol* 101(6 Pt 2):S465, 1998.

Jones KP, Rolf S, Stingl C et al: Longitudinal study of sensitization to natural rubber latex among dental school students using powder-free gloves, *Ann Occup Hyg* 48(5):455-457, 2004.

LaMontagne AD, Radi S, Elder DS et al: Primary prevention of latex related sensitization and occupational asthma: a systematic review, *Occup Environ Med* 63(5):359-364, 2006.

Larese Filon F, Bosco A, Fiorito A et al: Latex symptoms and sensitization in healthcare workers, *Int Arch Occup Environ Health* 74(3):219-223, 2001.

Lukesova S, Krcmova I, Kopecky O: Latex allergy—report on two cases, *Cas Lek Cesk* 144(9):641-643, 2005.

Mazon A, Nieto A, Linana JJ et al: Latex sensitization in children with spina bifida: follow-up comparative study after two years, *Ann Allergy Asthma Immunol* 84(2):207, 2000.

McCall BP, Horwitz IB, Kammeyer-Mueller JD: Have health conditions associated with latex increased since the issuance of universal precautions? *Am J Public Health* 93(4):599-604, 2003.

Muller BA: Minimizing latex exposure and allergy: how to avoid or reduce sensitization in the healthcare setting, *Postgrad Med* 113(4):91-96, 2003.

National Institute for Occupational Safety and Health: *Preventing allergic reactions to natural rubber latex in the workplace,* Cincinnati, The Institute, 1998.

Navarrete MA, Salas A, Palacios L et al: Latex allergy, *Farm Hosp* 30(3):177-186, 2006.

Ownby DR: Strategies for distinguishing asymptomatic latex sensitization from true occupational allergy or asthma, *Ann Allergy Asthma Immunol* 90(5 Suppl 2):42-46, 2003.

Perkin JE: The latex and food allergy connection, *J Am Diet Assoc* 100(11):1381-1384, 2000.

Proietti L, Gueli G, La Rocca G et al: Latex allergy prevalence and atopy in 1300 health care workers, *Recenti Prog Med* 96(10):478-482, 2005.

Ranta PM, Ownby DR: A review of natural-rubber latex allergy in healthcare workers, *Clin Infect Dis* 38(2):252-256, 2004.

Salcedo G, Diaz-Perales A, Sanchez-Monge R: The role of plant pan-allergens in sensitization to natural rubber latex, *Curr Opin Allergy Clin Immunol* 1(2):177-183, 2001.

Society for Gastroenterology Nurses and Associates, Inc: SGNA Guidelines for preventing sensitivity and allergic reactions to natural rubber latex in the workplace, *Gastroenterol Nurs* 27(4):191-197, 2004.

Sparta G, Kemper MJ, Gerber AC et al: Latex allergy in children with urological malformation and chronic renal failure, *J Urol* 171(4):1647-1649, 2004.

Sutherland MF, Suphioglu C, Rolland JM et al: Latex allergy: towards immunotherapy for healthcare workers, *Clin Exp Allergy* 32(5):667-673, 2002.

Tarlo SM: Latex allergy: a problem for both healthcare professionals and patients, *Ostomy Wound Manage* 44(8):80-88, 1998.

Tatsumi K, Ide T, Kitaguchi K et al: Prevalence and risk factors for latex sensitization among anesthesiologists, *Masui* 54(2):195-201, 2005.

Taylor JS, Erkek E: Latex allergy: diagnosis and management, *Dermatol Ther* 17(4):289-301, 2004.

Toraason M, Sussman G, Biagini R et al: Latex allergy in the workplace, *Toxicol Sci* 58(1):5-14, 2000.

Ylitalo L, Alenius H, Turjanmaa K et al: Natural rubber latex allergy in children: a follow-up study, *Clin Exp Allergy* 30(11):1611-1617, 2000.

Risk for latex Allergy response

Leslie H. Nicoll, PhD, MBA, RN, B, and DeLancey Nicoll, SN

NANDA Definition

At risk for allergic response to natural rubber latex (NRL) products

Risk Factors

Children with three or more surgeries, especially as a neonate; neural tube defects (e.g., spina bifida); children with chronic renal failure; allergies to bananas, avocados, tropical fruits, kiwis, chestnuts, apples, carrots, celery, potatoes, tomatoes; professions with daily exposure to latex (e.g., healthcare workers, rubber industry workers, food handlers, hairdressers, janitors, police, firefighters); conditions needing continuous or intermittent catheterization; history of reactions to latex (e.g., balloons, condoms, gloves); atopic individuals (persons with a tendency to have multiple allergic conditions)

NOC Outcomes (Nursing Outcomes Classification)

Suggested NOC Outcomes

Allergic Response: Systemic, Immune Hypersensitivity Response, Knowledge: Health Behavior

Example NOC Outcome with Indicators
Immune Hypersensitivity Response as evidenced by the following indicators: Respiratory function/Cardiac function/Gastrointestinal function/Renal function/Neurological function/Allergic reactions (Rate the outcome and indicators of **Immune Hypersensitivity Response:** 1 = severely compromised, 2 = substantially compromised, 3 = moderately compromised, 4 = mildly compromised, 5 = not compromised [see Section I].)

IER, In expected range.

Client Outcomes

Client Will (Specify Time Frame):

* State risk factors for NRL allergy
* Request latex-free environment
* Demonstrate knowledge of plan to treat NRL allergic reaction

NIC Interventions (Nursing Interventions Classification)

Suggested NIC Interventions

Allergy Management, Latex Precautions

• = Independent;   ▲ = Collaborative;   EBN = Evidence-Based Nursing;   EB = Evidence-Based

A

Example NIC Activities—Latex Precautions

Question patient or appropriate other about history of systemic reaction to NRL (e.g., facial or scleral edema, tearing eyes, urticaria, rhinitis, and wheezing); Place allergy band on patient

---

Nursing Interventions and *Rationales*

- Clients at high risk need to be identified, such as those with frequent bladder catheterizations, occupational exposure to latex, past history of atopy (hay fever, asthma, dermatitis, or food allergy to fruits such as bananas, avocados, papaya, chestnut, or kiwi); those with a history of anaphylaxis of uncertain etiology, especially if associated with surgery; healthcare workers; and females exposed to barrier contraceptives and routine examinations during gynecological and obstetric procedures. **EB:** *Latex allergy is an increasingly common condition because the use of latex products is widespread (Eustachio et al, 2003).* **EB:** *Healthcare professionals, hospital clients, and rubber industry workers have noted a marked increase in allergic reactions to NRL in the past 10 years (Ranta & Ownby, 2004).* **EB:** *Allergy to NRL is significantly associated with hypersensitivity to certain foods, including avocados, chestnuts, papayas, kiwis, potatoes, tomatoes, and bananas (Isola et al, 2003).* **EB:** *A latex-directed history is the primary method of identifying latex sensitivity, although both skin and serum testing are available and are increasingly accurate (American Association of Nurse Anesthetists, 1998; Hepner & Castells, 2003; Society of Gastroenterology Nurses and Associates, Inc., 2004).*
- Clients with spina bifida are a high-risk group for NRL allergy and should remain latex free from the first day of life. **EB:** *The SB population bears a disease-associated propensity for latex sensitization. This effect cannot be explained exclusively by a higher number of operations and differences related to atopy, age, or gender (Eiwegger et al, 2006).* **EB:** *Clients with spina bifida represent the highest risk group for developing NRL hypersensitivity. Recognized risk factors for these clients are repeated surgeries and an atopic disposition (Buck et al, 2000).* **EB:** *Latex-free precautions from birth in children with spina bifida are more effective in preventing latex sensitization than the same precautions instituted in later life (Nieto et al, 2002).*
- Children who are on home ventilation should be assessed for NRL allergy. **EB:** *There is a high incidence of NRL allergy in children on home ventilation. All children on home ventilation should be screened for NRL allergy to prevent untoward reactions from exposure to latex (Nakamura et al, 2000).*
- Children with chronic renal failure should be assessed for NRL allergy. **EB:** *This study demonstrated a high incidence of NRL in children with chronic renal failure. Children with chronic renal failure are at risk because of their intense exposure to latex through catheters, gloves, and anesthetic equipment during frequent hospitalizations from early life on (Dehlink et al, 2004).*
- Assess for NRL allergy in clients who are exposed to "hidden" latex. **EB:** *Case studies have reported on serious complications in clients exposed to latex through hair glue (Cogen & Beezhold, 2002) and microdermabrasion (Farris & Rietschel, 2002).*
- See care plan for **Latex Allergy response.**

Home Care

- ▲ Ensure that the client has a medical plan if a response develops. *Prompt treatment decreases potential severity of response.*
- See care plan for **Latex Allergy response.** Note client history and environmental assessment.

Client/Family Teaching

- ▲ A client who has had symptoms of NRL allergy or who suspects he or she is allergic to latex should tell his or her employer and contact his or her institution's occupational health services. **EB:** *Occupational health services can arrange testing by an allergist. If an allergy is present, measures to protect the client's well-being in the workplace should be instituted (National Institute for Occupational Safety and Health, 1998).*
- Provide written information about latex allergy and sensitivity. **EB:** *Client education is the most important preventive strategy. Clients should be carefully instructed about "hidden" latex; cross-reactions,*

particularly foods; and unforeseen risks during medical procedures (Joint Task Force on Practice Parameters, 1998).

- Healthcare workers should avoid the use of latex gloves and seek alternatives such as gloves made from nitrile. **EB:** *The risk of NRL allergy appears to be largely linked to occupational exposure, and NRL-associated occupational asthma is due almost solely to powdered glove use. Airborne NRL is dependent on the use of powdered NRL gloves; conversion to non-NRL or nonpowdered NRL substitutes result in predictable rapid disappearance of detectable levels of aeroallergen (Brown et al, 2004; Charous et al, 2002).* **EB:** *Preliminary reports of primary preventive strategies suggest that avoidance of high-protein, powdered gloves in healthcare facilities can be cost-effective and is associated with a decline in sensitized workers (Tarlo et al, 2001).* **EB:** *A case study report of two nurses indicated worsening symptoms when they worked in an environment with powdered gloves, even though they avoided direct skin contact with latex (Amr & Suk, 2004).* **EBN:** *Nitrile examination gloves offer better protection than latex types when handling lipid-soluble substances and chemicals (Russell-Fell, 2000).* **EB:** *The level of dexterity provided by latex and nitrile SafeSkin gloves for tasks on a gross dexterity level are comparable and health workers will benefit from the non-allergenic properties of nitrile (Sawyer & Bennett 2006).*
- Healthcare institutions should develop prevention programs for the use of latex-free gloves and the absence of powdered gloves; they should also establish latex-safe areas in their facilities. **EB:** *Latex allergy has become a global epidemic, affecting clients, healthcare workers, and scientific personnel (Edlich, Woodard, Hill et al, 2003).*

REFERENCES

American Association of Nurse Anesthetists: *AANA latex protocol,* Park Ridge, Ill, 1998, The Association.

Amr S, Suk WA: Latex allergy and occupational asthma in healthcare workers: adverse outcomes, *Environ Health Perspect* 112(3):378-381, 2004.

Brown RH, Taenkhum K, Buckley TJ et al: Different latex aeroallergen size distributions between powdered surgical and examination gloves: significance for environmental avoidance, *J Allergy Clin Immunol* 114(2):358-363, 2004.

Buck D, Michael T, Wahn U et al: Ventricular shunts and the prevalence of sensitization and clinically relevant allergy to latex in patients with spina bifida, *Pediatr Allergy Immunol* 11(2):111-115, 2000.

Charous BL, Blanco C, Tarlo S et al: Natural rubber latex allergy after 12 years: recommendations and perspectives, *J Allergy Clin Immunol* 109(1):31-34, 2002.

Cogen FC, Beezhold DH: Hair glue anaphylaxis: a hidden latex allergy, *Ann Allergy Asthma Immunol* 88(1):61-63, 2002.

Dehlink E, Prandstetter C, Eiwegger T et al: Increased prevalence of latex-sensitization among children with chronic renal failure, *Allergy* 59(7):734-738, 2004.

Edlich RF, Woodard CR, Hill LG et al: Latex allergy: a life-threatening epidemic for scientists, healthcare personnel, and their patients, *J Long Term Eff Med Implants* 13(1):11-19, 2003.

Eiwegger T, Dehlink E, Schwindt J et al: Early exposure to latex products mediates latex sensitization in spina bifida but not in other diseases with comparable latex exposure rates, *Clin Exp Allergy* 36(10):1242-1246, 2006.

Eustachio N, Cristina CM, Antonio F et al: A discussion of natural rubber latex allergy with special reference to children: clinical considerations, *Curr Drug Targets Immune Endocr Metabol Disord* 3(3):171-180, 2003.

Farris PK, Rietschel RL: An unusual acute urticarial response following microdermabrasion, *Dermatol Surg* 28(7):606-608, 2002.

Hepner DL, Castells MC: Latex allergy: an update, *Anesth Analg* 96(4):1219-1229, 2003.

Isola S, Ricciardi L, Saitta S et al: Latex allergy and fruit cross-reaction in subjects who are nonatopic, *Allergy Asthma Proc* 24(3):193-197, 2003.

Joint Task Force on Practice Parameters; American Academy of Allergy, Asthma and Immunology; American College of Allergy, Asthma and Immunology; and the Joint Council of Allergy, Asthma and Immunology: The diagnosis and management of anaphylaxis, *J Allergy Clin Immunol* 101(6 Pt 2):S465, 1998.

Nakamura CT, Ferdman RM, Keens TG et al: Latex allergy in children on home mechanical ventilation, *Chest* 118(4):1000-1003, 2000.

National Institute for Occupational Safety and Health: *Preventing allergic reactions to natural rubber latex in the workplace,* Cincinnati, 1998, The Institute.

Nieto A, Mazon A, Pamies R et al: Efficacy of latex avoidance for primary prevention of latex sensitization in children with spina bifida, *J Pediatr* 140(3):370-372, 2002.

Perkin JE: The latex and food allergy connection, *J Am Diet Assoc* 100(11):1381-1384, 2000.

Ranta PM, Ownby DR: A review of natural-rubber latex allergy in healthcare workers, *Clin Infect Dis* 38(2):252-256, 2004.

Russell-Fell R: Avoiding problems: evidence-based selection of medical gloves, *Br J Nurs* 9(3):139-142, 144-146, 2000.

Sawyer J, Bennett A: Comparing the level of dexterity offered by latex and nitrile SafeSkin gloves, *Ann Occup Hyg* 50(3):289-296, 2006.

Society for Gastroenterology Nurses and Associates, Inc: SGNA Guidelines for preventing sensitivity and allergic reactions to natural rubber latex in the workplace, *Gastroenterol Nurs* 27(4):191-197, 2004.

Tarlo SM, Easty A, Eubanks K et al: Outcomes of a natural rubber latex control program in an Ontario teaching hospital, *J Allergy Clin Immunol* 108(4):628-633, 2001.

Anxiety   *Ruth McCaffrey, DNP, ARNP, BC*   **evolve**   A

NANDA   Definition

A vague uneasy feeling of discomfort or dread accompanied by an autonomic response (the source often nonspecific or unknown to the individual); a feeling of apprehension caused by anticipation of danger. It is an alerting signal that warns of impending danger and enables the individual to take measures to deal with threat

Defining Characteristics

Behavioral

Diminished productivity; expressed concerns due to change in life events; extraneous movement; fidgeting; glancing about; insomnia; poor eye contact; restlessness; scanning; vigilance

Affective

Apprehensive; anguish; distressed; fearful; feelings of inadequacy; focus on self; increased wariness; irritability; jittery; overexcited; painful increased helplessness; persistent increased helplessness; rattled; regretful; scared; uncertainty; worried

Physiological

Facial tension; hand tremors; increased perspiration; increased tension; shakiness; trembling; voice quivering

Sympathetic

Anorexia; cardiovascular excitation; diarrhea; dry mouth; facial flushing; heart pounding; increased blood pressure; increased pulse; increased reflexes; increased respiration; pupil dilation; respiratory difficulties; superficial vasoconstriction; twitching; weakness

Parasympathetic

Abdominal pain; decreased blood pressure; decreased pulse; diarrhea; faintness; fatigue; nausea; sleep disturbance; tingling in extremities; urinary frequency; urinary hesitancy; urinary urgency

Cognitive

Awareness of physiologic symptoms; blocking of thought; confusion; decreased perceptual field; difficulty concentrating; diminished ability to learn; diminished ability to problem solve; fear of unspecified consequences; forgetfulness; impaired attention; preoccupation; rumination; tendency to blame others

Related Factors (r/t)

Change in: economic status, environment, health status, interaction patterns, role function, role status; exposure to toxins; familial association; heredity; interpersonal contagion; interpersonal transmission; maturational crises; situational crises; stress; substance abuse; threat of death; threat to: economic status, environment, health status, interaction patterns, role function, role status; threat to self-concept; unconscious conflict about essential goals of life; unconscious conflict about essential values; unmet needs

NOC   Outcomes (Nursing Outcomes Classification)

Suggested NOC Outcomes

Aggression Self-Control, Anxiety Level, Anxiety Self-Control, Coping, Impulse Self-Control

Example NOC Outcome with Indicators
Anxiety Self-Control as evidenced by the following indicators: Eliminates precursors of anxiety/Monitors physical manifestations of anxiety/Controls anxiety response (Rate the outcome and indicators of **Anxiety Self-Control**: 1 = never demonstrated, 2 = rarely demonstrated, 3 = sometimes demonstrated, 4 = often demonstrated, 5 = consistently demonstrated [see Section I].)

• = Independent;   ▲ = Collaborative;   EBN = Evidence-Based Nursing;   EB = Evidence-Based

A **Client Outcomes**

Client Will (Specify Time Frame):

- Identify and verbalize symptoms of anxiety
- Identify, verbalize, and demonstrate techniques to control anxiety
- Verbalize absence of or decrease in subjective distress
- Have vital signs that reflect baseline or decreased sympathetic stimulation
- Have posture, facial expressions, gestures, and activity levels that reflect decreased distress
- Demonstrate improved concentration and accuracy of thoughts
- Identify and verbalize anxiety precipitants, conflicts, and threats
- Demonstrate return of basic problem-solving skills
- Demonstrate increased external focus
- Demonstrate some ability to reassure self

NIC **Interventions (Nursing Interventions Classification)**

Suggested NIC Intervention

Anxiety Reduction

Example NIC Activities—Anxiety Reduction
Use a calm, reassuring approach; Explain all procedures, including sensations likely to be experienced during the procedure

Nursing Interventions and *Rationales*

- Assess the client's level of anxiety and physical reactions to anxiety (e.g., tachycardia, tachypnea, nonverbal expressions of anxiety). Consider using The Face Anxiety Scale. *It is an easy to use and accurate way to measure anxiety in critically ill clients (Gustad, Chaboyer & Wallis, 2005).* **EBN:** *Anxiety is known to intensify physical symptoms (DeVane, 2005). In adolescents, anxiety symptoms were correlated with physical complaints and depression (DeVane, 2005).*
- Rule out withdrawal from alcohol, sedatives, or smoking as the cause of anxiety. **EB:** *One third of respondents in this study with an alcohol use disorder (abuse or dependence) were three times more likely to have an anxiety disorder (Hasin, 2006).*
- Identify and limit, discontinue, or be aware of the use of any stimulants such as caffeine, nicotine, theophylline, terbutaline sulfate, amphetamines, and cocaine. *Many substances cause or potentially cause anxiety symptoms (Lawton-Craddock, Nixon & Tivis, 2003).*
- If the situational response is rational, use empathy to encourage the client to interpret the anxiety symptoms as normal. **EBN:** *The way a nurse interacts with a client influences his/her quality of life. Enhancing self-esteem and providing information and psychological support promotes the client's well-being and his or her quality of life (Alasad & Ahmad, 2005).*
- If irrational thoughts or fears are present, offer the client accurate information and encourage him or her to talk about the meaning of the events contributing to the anxiety. **EBN:** *During the diagnosis and management of cancer, highlighting the importance of the meaning of events to an individual is an important factor in helping clients to identify what makes them anxious. Acknowledgment of this meaning may help to reduce anxiety (Antoni, 2006).*
- Encourage the client to use positive self-talk such as, "Anxiety won't kill me," "I can do this one step at a time," "Right now I need to breathe and stretch," "I don't have to be perfect." **EBN:** *Cognitive therapies focus on changing behaviors and feelings by changing thoughts. Replacing negative self-statements with positive self-statements helps to decrease anxiety (Roemer & Orsillo, 2007).*
- Intervene when possible to remove sources of anxiety. **EBN:** *Anxiety has a negative effect on quality of life that persists over time (Sareen et al, 2006).*
- Explain all activities, procedures, and issues that involve the client; use nonmedical terms and calm, slow speech. Do this in advance of procedures when possible, and validate the client's understanding. *Triad communication or talking to another staff or family member in front of the client is a way to provide additional information to assist in understanding (Davidhizar & Dowd, 2003).*

- Ascertain client preferences about the desire to be distracted before and during noxious medical procedures. **EBN:** *Clients have individual preferences for the use of distraction during anxiety-provoking procedures (Kwekkeboom, 2003).*
- Provide backrubs/massage for the client to decrease anxiety. **EBN:** *Massage and aromatherapy significantly decreased anxiety or perception of tension (Mansky & Wallerstedt, 2006).*
- Use therapeutic touch and healing touch techniques. **EBN:** *Various techniques that involve intention to heal, laying on of hands, clearing the energy field surrounding the body, and transfer of healing energy from the environment through the healer to the subject can reduce anxiety (Mansky & Wallerstedt, 2006).* **EBN:** *Anxiety was significantly reduced in a therapeutic touch placebo condition. Healing touch may be one of the most useful nursing interventions available to reduce anxiety (Krucoff et al, 2005).*
- Guided imagery can be used to decrease anxiety. **EBN:** *Anxiety was decreased with the use of guided imagery using audiotape intervention for postoperative pain (Antall & Kresevic, 2004).*
- Provide clients with a means to listen to music of their choice or audiotapes. Provide a quiet place and encourage clients to listen for 20 minutes. **EBN:** *Music listening reduces anxiety and pain (McCaffrey & Locsin, 2006).* **EBN:** *Chemotherapy clients who used audiotapes had lower anxiety than a control group (Williams & Schreier, 2004).*

Geriatric

▲ Monitor the client for depression. Use appropriate interventions and referrals. **EB:** *Anxiety often accompanies or masks depression in elderly adults. Clients who have depression and anxiety, are socially isolated, or are severely ill should be asked whether they've been thinking about ending their life or wanting to die (Conner et al, 2006).* **EB:** *Anxiety and depression are associated with overall health status, emotional and cognitive functioning, and fatigue (Smith, Gomm & Dickens, 2003).*

- Older adults report less worry than younger adults. **EB:** *There were no age differences in the report of somatic and affective symptoms. Thus, worry appears to play a less prominent role in the presentation of anxiety in older adults. These findings suggest that older adults do experience anxiety differently than younger adults (Brenes, 2006).*
- Observe for adverse changes if anti-anxiety drugs are taken. *Age renders clients more sensitive to both the clinical and toxic effects of many agents (Le Couteur, 2004).*
- Provide a quiet environment with diversion. *Excessive noise increases anxiety; involvement in a quiet activity can be soothing to the elderly (Chaudhury, 2006).*
- Provide alternative interventions such as massage therapy, guided imagery, aroma therapy to complement traditional medical regimens. *Effective nursing practice for reducing anxiety in elderly clients provides a challenge and an opportunity for nurses and family caregivers to blend alternative therapies with technology to provide more individualized and holistic client care.* **EBN:** *Massage intervention significantly reduced pain and anxiety in elderly clients (Mok & Woo, 2004).*

Multicultural

- Assess for the presence of culture-bound anxiety states. **EBN:** *The context in which anxiety is experienced and the response to anxiety are culturally mediated (Emery, 2006; Kuipers, 2004). African-American women have historically been through heartbreaking experiences as they have fought to maintain their family and survive the subjugation and horror of the slavery experience. Even for those African-American women who were not personally involved, the anxiety lives on in family stories and by association with the culture (Cherry & Giger, 2008, in press).*
- Identify how anxiety is manifested in the culturally diverse client. **EBN:** *Anxiety is manifested differently from culture to culture through cognitive to somatic symptoms (Kisely & Simon, 2006).*
- Acknowledge that value conflicts from acculturation stresses may contribute to increased anxiety. **EBN:** *Challenges to traditional beliefs and values are anxiety provoking (Halbreich et al, 2006).*
- For the diverse client experiencing preoperative anxiety, provide music of their choice. **EBN:** *Music intervention was found to have cross-cultural validity in the reduction of preoperative anxiety in Chinese male clients (Twiss, Seaver & McCaffrey, 2006).*

A

Home Care

- Above interventions may be adapted for home care use.
- ▲ Assess for suicidal ideation. Implement emergency plan as indicated. *Suicidal ideation may occur in response to co-occurring depression or a sense of hopelessness over severe anxiety symptoms or once antidepressant medications have been started (Yigletu, 2004).* Refer to care plan for **Risk for Suicide.**
- Assess for influence of anxiety on medical regimen. **EBN:** *The ability to direct attention is necessary for self-care and independence and was reduced for several months after surgery in older women newly diagnosed with breast cancer (Stark & Cimprich, 2003).*
- Assess for presence of depression. *Depression and anxiety co-occur frequently (Covera-Tindel, 2004).*
- Assist family to be supportive of the client in the face of anxiety symptoms. **EBN:** *Social support, self-esteem, and optimism were all positively related to positive health practices, and social support was positively related to self-esteem and optimism (Cooper et al, 2006).*
- ▲ Consider referral for the prescription of anti-anxiety or antidepressant medications for clients who have panic disorder (PD) or other anxiety-related psychiatric disorders. **EBN:** *The use of antidepressants, especially SSRI medications, is effective in many cases of anxiety (Jackson & Lipman, 2004).*
- ▲ Assist the client/family to institute medication regimen appropriately. Instruct in side effects, importance of taking medications as ordered, and effects to report immediately to nurse or physician. *Anti-anxiety and antidepressant medications have side effects that may prompt the client to discontinue use, sometimes with additional uncomfortable effects. Some medications may be used to overdose. Antidepressant medications can take up to several weeks for full effect, and the client may discontinue use prematurely if there is little effect or if the medication is effective and the client considers it no longer necessary (Antai-Otong, 2006).*
- ▲ Refer for psychiatric home healthcare services for client reassurance and implementation of a therapeutic regimen. **EBN:** *Psychiatric home care nurses can address issues relating to the client's anxiety, including agoraphobia, with or without coexisting depression. Behavioral interventions in the home can assist the client to participate more effectively in the treatment plan (Brown et al, 2006).*

Client/Family Teaching

- ▲ Teach use of appropriate community resources in emergency situations (e.g., suicidal thoughts), such as hotlines, emergency departments, law enforcement, and judicial systems. **EB:** *The method of suicide prevention found to be most effective is a systematic, direct-screening procedure that has a high potential for institutionalization (Simon et al, 2007).*
- Teach the client/family the symptoms of anxiety. **EBN:** *Information is empowering and reduces anxiety (Godfrey, Parten & Buchner, 2006).*
- Help client to define anxiety levels (from "easily tolerated" to "intolerable") and select appropriate interventions. **EBN:** *Mild anxiety enhances learning and adaptation, but moderate to severe anxiety may impede or immobilize progress (Kolcaba, Tilton & Drouin, 2006).*
- Teach the client techniques to self-manage anxiety. **EBN:** *Teaching clients anxiety reduction techniques can help them manage side effects with self-care behaviors (Blanchard, Courneya & Laing, 2001).*
- Teach progressive muscle relaxation techniques. **EBN:** *A significant reduction in anxiety level was obtained by using progressive muscle relaxation interventions (Schaffer & Yucha, 2004).*
- Teach relaxation breathing for occasional use: client should breathe in through nose, fill slowly from abdomen upward while thinking "re," and then breathe out through mouth, from chest downward, and think "lax." **EBN:** *Anxiety management training effectively treats both specific and generalized anxiety (Schaffer & Yucha, 2004).*
- Teach the client to visualize or fantasize about the absence of anxiety or pain, successful experience of the situation, resolution of conflict, or outcome of procedure. **EBN:** *Use of guided imagery has been useful for reducing anxiety (Krucoff et al, 2005).*

- Teach relationship between a healthy physical and emotional lifestyle and a realistic mental attitude. **EBN:** *Exercise is an excellent means of decreasing anxiety (DeMoor et al, 2006).*
- ▲ Provide family members with information to help them to distinguish between a panic attack and serious physical illness symptoms. Instruct family members to consult a healthcare professional if they have questions. **EBN:** *Education on managing anxiety disorders must include family members because they are the ones usually called on to take the client for emergency care. Family members can be expert informants because of their familiarity with the client's history and symptoms (Schaffer & Yucha, 2004).*

evolve See the EVOLVE website for World Wide Web resources for client education.

REFERENCES

Alasad J, Ahmad M: Communication with critically ill patients, *J Adv Nurs* 50(3):256-262, 2005.

Antai-Otong D: The art of prescribing antidepressants in late-life depression: prescribing principals, *Perspect Psychiatr Care* 42(2):149-153, 2006.

Antall GF, Kresevic D: The use of guided imagery to manage pain in an elderly orthopaedic population, *Orthop Nurs* 23(5):335-340, 2004.

Antoni M: Reduction of cancer-specific thought intrusions and anxiety symptoms with a stress management intervention among women undergoing treatment for breast cancer, *Am J Psychiatr* 163(10):1791-1797, 2006.

Blanchard CM, Courneya KS, Laing D: Effects of acute exercise on state anxiety in breast cancer survivors, *Oncol Nurs Forum* 28(10):1617-1621, 2001.

Brenes G: Age differences in the presentation of anxiety, *Aging Men Health* 19(3):298-302, 2006.

Brown E, Raue P, Schulberg H et al: Clinical competencies: caring for late-life depression in home care patients, *J Gerontol Nurs* 32(9):10-14, 2006.

Chaudhury H: Nurses' perception of single-occupancy versus multioccupancy rooms in acute care environments: an exploratory comparative assessment, *Appl Nurs Res* 19(3):118-125, 2006.

Cherry B, Giger J: African-Americans. In Giger J, Davidhizar R, editors: *Transcultural nursing: assessment and intervention.* St Louis, (in press), Mosby.

Conner K, Duberstein P, Beckman A et al: Planning of suicide attempts among depressed inpatients ages 50 and over, *J Affect Disord* 96(1-2):212-220, 2006.

Cooper C, Katona C, Orrell M et al: Coping strategies and anxiety in caregivers of people with Alzheimer's disease: the LASER-AD study, *J Affect Disord* 90(1):15-20, 2006.

Covera-Tindel T: Predictors of noncompliance to exercise training in heart failure, *J Cardiovasc Nurs* 19(4):269-279, 2004.

Davidhizar R, Dowd S: Using a triad to facilitate communication in radiology *RT* 16(48):1, 2003.

DeMoor MHM, Beem AL, Stubbe D et al: Regular exercise, anxiety, depression and personality: a population-based study, *Prev Med* 42(4):273-279, 2006.

DeVane C: Anxiety disorders in the 21st century: status, challenges, opportunities, and comorbidity with depression, *Am J Manag Care* 11(12 Suppl):S344-S353, 2005.

Emery P: Building a new culture of aging: revolutionizing long-term care, *J Christ Nurs* 23(1):16-24, 2006.

Godfrey B, Parten C, Buckner E: Identification of special care needs: the comparison of the cardiothoracic intensive care unit patient and nurse, *Dimens Crit Care Nurs* 25(6):275-282, 2006.

Gustad L, Chaboyer W, Wallis M: Performance of the Faces Anxiety

Scale in patients transferred from the ICU, *Intensive Crit Care Nurs* 21(6):355-360, 2005.

Halbreich Y, Alarcon RD, Calil H et al: Culturally-sensitive complaints of depressions and anxieties in women, *J Affect Disord* Nov 6 [Epub ahead of print], 2006.

Hasin D: Diagnosis of comorbid psychiatric disorders in substance users assessed with the psychiatric research interview for substance and mental disorders for DSM-IV, *Am J Psychiatry* 163(4):689-696, 2006.

Jackson K, Lipman AC: Drug therapy for anxiety in palliative care, *Cochrane Database Syst Rev* (1):CD004596, 2004.

Kisely S, Simon G: An international study comparing the effect of medically explained and unexplained somatic symptoms on psychosocial outcome, *J Psychosom Res* 60(2):125-130, 2006.

Kolcaba K, Tilton C, Drouin C: Comfort theory: a unifying framework to enhance the practice environment, *J Nurs Admin* 36(11):538-544, 2006.

Krucoff MW, Crater SW, Gallup D et al: Music, imagery, touch, and prayer as adjuncts to interventional cardiac care: the Monitoring and Actualization of Noetic Trainings (MANTRA) II randomized study, *Lancet* 366(9481):211-217, 2005.

Kuipers J: Mexican Americans. In Giger J, Davidhizar R: *Transcultural nursing: assessment and intervention*, St Louis, 2004, Mosby.

Kwekkeboom KL: Music versus distraction for procedural pain and anxiety in patients with cancer, *Oncol Nurs Forum* 30(3):433-440, 2003.

Lawton-Craddock A, Nixon SJ, Tivis R: Cognitive efficiency in stimulant abusers with and without alcohol dependence, *Alcohol Clin Exp Res* 27(3):457-464, 2003.

Le Couteur D: Prescribing in older people, *Aust Fam Physician* 33(10):777-781, 2004.

Mansky PJ, Wallerstedt DB: Complementary medicine in palliative care and cancer symptom management, *Cancer J* 12(5):425-431, 2006.

McCaffrey R, Locsin R: The effect of music on pain and acute confusion in older adults undergoing hip and knee surgery, *Holist Nurs Pract*, 20(5):218-224, 2006.

Mok E, Woo CP: The effects of slow-stroke back massage on anxiety and pain in elderly stroke patients, *Complemen Ther Nurs Midwifery*, 10(4):209-216, 2004.

Roemer L, Orsillo SM: An open trial of acceptance-based behavior therapy for generalized anxiety disorder, *Behav Ther* 38(1):72-85, 2006.

Sareen J, Jacobi F, Cox BJ et al: Disability and poor quality of life associated with comorbid anxiety disorders and physical conditions, *Arch Intern Med* 166(19):2109-2116, 2006.

Schaffer S, Yucha C: Relaxation & pain management: the relaxation

A

response can play a role in managing chronic and acute pain, *Am J Nurs* 104(8):75-82, 2004.

Simon N, Zalta A, Otto, M et al: The association of comorbid anxiety disorders with suicide attempts and suicidal ideation in outpatients with bipolar disorder, *J Psychiatr Res* 41(3-4):255-264, 2007.

Smith EM, Gomm SA, Dickens CM: Assessing the independent contribution to quality of life from anxiety and depression in patients with advanced cancer, *Palliat Med* 17(6):509-513, 2003.

Stark MA, Cimprich B: Promoting attentional health: importance to women's lives, *Health Care Women Int* 24(2):93-102, 2003.

Twiss E, Seaver J, McCaffrey R: The effect of music listening on anxiety and postoperative ventilation in older adults undergoing cardiovascular surgery, *Nurs Crit Care* 23(5):245-251, 2006.

Williams SA, Schreier AM: The effects of education in managing side effects in women receiving chemotherapy for management of breast cancer, *Oncol Nurs Forum* 31(1):E16-E23, 2004.

Yigletu H: Assessing suicide ideation: comparing self-report versus clinician report, *J Am Psychiatr Nurses Assoc* 10(1):9-15, 2004.

Death Anxiety   *Ruth McCaffrey, DNP, ARNP, BC*

NANDA   Definition

Vague uneasy feeling of discomfort or dread generated by perceptions of a real or imagined threat to one's existence

Defining Characteristics

Reports concerns of overworking the caregiver; reports deep sadness; reports fear of developing terminal illness; reports fear of loss of mental abilities when dying; reports fear of pain related to dying; reports fear of premature death; reports fear of the process of dying; reports fear of prolonged dying; reports fear of suffering related to dying; reports feeling powerless over dying; reports negative thoughts related to death and dying; reports worry about the impact on one's own death on significant others

Related Factors (r/t)

Anticipating adverse consequences of general anesthesia; anticipating impact of death on others; anticipating pain; anticipating suffering; confronting reality of terminal disease; discussions on topic of death; experiencing dying process; near death experience; nonacceptance of own mortality; observations related to death; perceived proximity of death; uncertainty about an encounter with a higher power; uncertainty about the existence of a higher power; uncertainty about life after death; uncertainty of prognosis

NOC   Outcomes (Nursing Outcomes Classification)

Suggested NOC Outcomes

Dignified Life Closure, Fear, Self-Control, Health Beliefs: Perceived Threat

Example NOC Outcome with Indicators
Dignified Life Closure as evidenced by the following indicators: Expresses readiness for death/Resolves important issues and concerns/Shares feelings about dying/Discusses spiritual concerns (Rate the outcome and indicators of **Dignified Life Closure:** 1 = never demonstrated, 2 = rarely demonstrated, 3 = sometimes demonstrated, 4 = often demonstrated, 5 = consistently demonstrated [see Section I].)

Client Outcomes

Client Will (Specify Time Frame):

- State concerns about impact of death on others
- Express feelings associated with dying
- Seek help in dealing with feelings
- Discuss concerns about God or higher being
- Discuss realistic goals
- Use prayer or other religious practice for comfort

• = Independent;   ▲ = Collaborative;   EBN = Evidence-Based Nursing;   EB = Evidence-Based

NIC   Interventions (Nursing Interventions Classification)   A

Suggested NIC Interventions

Dying Care, Grief Work Facilitation, Spiritual Support

Example NIC Activities—Dying Care
Communicate willingness to discuss death; Support patient and family through stages of grief

Nursing Interventions and *Rationales*

- Assess the psychosocial maturity of the individual. **EB:** *As psychosocial maturity and age increase, death anxiety decreases. Findings have shown that psychosocial maturity is a better predictor of death anxiety than is age (Chochinov, 2004).*
- Assess clients for pain and provide pain relief measures. **EBN:** *Barriers to optimal care of the dying, according to family members contacted by phone interview, include level of pain and management of pain (Deffner & Bell, 2005).*
- Assess client for fears related to death. **EBN:** *Acknowledging and responding to these fears is the core of end-of-life palliative care (Dunne, 2005).*
- Assist clients with life planning: consider and redefine main life goals, focus on areas of strength and/or goals that will provide satisfaction, adopt realistic goals and recognize those that are impossible to achieve. **EB:** *Life planning processes affect self-esteem and self-concept by changing unrealistic goals (Skilbeck & Payne, 2003).* **EB:** *Increased levels of death anxiety may block future thoughts (Martz & Livneh, 2003).*
- Assist clients with life review and reminiscence. **EB:** *Life reviewing can foster the integration of past conflicts. It can improve ego integrity and life satisfaction, lower depression, and reduce stress (Heyland et al, 2006).*
- Provide music of a client's choosing. **EBN:** *Music therapy is a nonpharmacological nursing intervention that may be used to promote relaxation (McCaffrey & Locsin, 2004).* **EB:** *Music may be beneficial in easing emotional, physical, and spiritual distress as death approaches (Hogan, 2003).*
- Provide social support for families, understanding what is most important to families who are caring for clients at the end of life. **EBN:** *The elements rated as extremely important at the end of life of a family member were (1) to have trust and confidence in the doctors, (2) to be honestly told about the prognosis of the family member, and (3) resolving conflicts with the dying family member and saying goodbye (Heyland et al, 2006).*
- Encourage clients to pray. **EBN:** *Prayer, scripture reading, and clergy visits were found to comfort some hospice clients, but sometimes specific religious tenets may be troubling and need to be resolved before the client can find peace (Forbes & Rosdahl, 2003).*

Geriatric

- Carefully assess older adults for issues regarding death anxiety. **EBN:** *Elders differ in their readiness for death. Some still have goals that they want to reach. These goals may not always be realistic (Bente et al, 2006). As client advocate, nurses can be confident the decisions made by older adults are accurate and reflect a lifelong set of values that were important to the decision making process (Martin & Roberto, 2006).* **EB:** *Old age raises questions for many adults, such as whether we face a painful death, what happens after death, and if our lives had meaning (Goldsteen et al, 2006).*
- Provide back massage for clients who have anxiety regarding issues such as death. **EBN:** *Massage significantly decreased anxiety or perception of tension (Smith et al, 2002).*
- Refer to care plan for **Anticipatory Grieving.**

Multicultural

- Assist clients to identify with their culture and its values. **EB:** *The process of identification with one's culture is identified as a coping mechanism that may protect the individual from increased death*

A

anxiety (Lobar, Youngblut & Brooten, 2006). **EBN:** *Practices related to life support, DNR, advanced directives, and routines and rituals at the end of life are related to cultural orientation. Depending on the cultural orientation, specific members are responsible for communication related to death and dying (Fordham, Giger & Davidhizar, 2006).*

- Refer to care plans for **Anxiety** and **Anticipatory Grieving.**

Home Care

- Above interventions may be adapted for home care.
- Identify times and places when anxiety is greatest. Provide for psychological support at those times, using such strategies as personal contact, telephone contact, diversionary activities, or therapeutic self. *Anxiety may be related to earlier events associated with home setting or daily patterns that created pain and now serve as triggers (Jakobsson et al, 2006).*
- Support religious beliefs; encourage client to participate in services and activities of choice. *Belief in a supreme being/higher power provides a feeling of ever-present help (Puchalski, Dorff & Hendi, 2004).*
- ▲ Refer to medical social services or mental health services, including support groups as appropriate (e.g., anticipatory grieving groups from hospice, visiting volunteers of hospice). *Referral to specialty groups may be a key part of the nursing plan (Jakobsson et al, 2006).*
- Encourage the client to verbalize feelings to family/caregivers, counselors, and self. *Expression of feelings relieves fear burden and allows examination and validation of feelings (Fry, 2003).*
- Identify client's preferences for end-of-life care; provide assistance in honoring preferences as much as practicable. **EB:** *A review of issues with malignant mesothelioma found that many such clients expressed the preference of dying at home, but were often hospitalized in the days prior to death without returning home (Hawley & Monk, 2004).*
- ▲ Assist the client in making contact with death-related planning organizations, if appropriate, such as the Cremation Society and funeral homes. *Planning and direct action (contracting for after-death care) often relieve anxiety and provide the client with a measure of control (Bente et al, 2006).*
- With client, create a memento book reflecting life achievements. Leave in the home for regular review by client. If family will be the recipient, a memento book serves as both an opportunity for life review and a means of proactively leaving something behind for survivors. *Memento books and written life goals are tangible milestones related to life and death. They provide comfort, reassurance, hope, and direction for the client and more definition for client/caregiver expectations. It gives client a sense of focus, decreasing feelings of powerlessness over death (Eliott & Olver, 2007).*
- ▲ Refer for psychiatric home healthcare services for client reassurance and implementation of a therapeutic regimen. Psychiatric home care nurses can address issues relating to client's death anxiety, including family relationships. *Behavioral interventions in the home can assist client to participate more effectively in the treatment plan (Jakobsson et al, 2006).*
- Refer to care plan for **Powerlessness.**

Client/Family Teaching

- Promote more effective communication to family members engaged in the care giving role. Encourage them to talk to their loved one about areas of concern. *Both caregivers and care receivers avoid discussing.* **EBN:** *Increasing the knowledge of and access to palliative care decreases suffering before death (Jakobsson et al, 2006).*
- Allow family members to be physically close to their dying loved one, giving them permission, instruction, and opportunities to touch. Keep family members informed. **EBN:** *Tertiary care centers are criticized for not providing a peaceful death experience (Nelson et al, 2006).*
- To increase clients' knowledge about end-of-life issues, teach them and their family members about options for care, such as advance directives. **EBN:** *Educating clients and families about end-of-life options will provide security and reduce anxiety (Sinclair, 2005).*

evolve See the EVOLVE website for World Wide Web resources for client education.

REFERENCES

Bente A, Swane C, Halberg I et al: Being given a cancer diagnosis in old age: a phenomenological study, *Int J Nurs Stud* 43(8):1101-1109, 2006.

Chochinov H: Dignity and the eye of the beholder, *J Clin Oncol* 22(7):1336-1340, 2004.

Deffner J, Bell S: Nurses' death anxiety, comfort level during communication with patients and families regarding death, and exposure to communication education: a quantitative study, *J Nurses Staff Dev* 21(1):19-23, 2005.

Dunne K: Effective communication in palliative care, *Nurs Stand* 20(13):57-64, 2005.

Eliott J, Olver I: Hope and hoping in the talk of dying cancer patients, *Soc Sci Med* 64(1):138-149, 2007.

Forbes MA, Rosdahl DR: The final journey of life, *J Hospice Palliative Nurs* 5(4):213-220, 2003.

Fordham P, Giger J, Davidhizar R: Multi-cultural and multi-ethnic considerations and advanced directives: developing cultural competency, *J Cult Divers* 13(1):3-9, 2006.

Fry PS: Perceived self-efficacy domains as predictors of fear of the unknown and fear of dying among older adults, *Psychol Aging* 18(3):474-486, 2003.

Goldsteen M, Houtepen R, Proot I et al: What is a good death? Terminally ill patients dealing with normative expectations around death and dying, *Patient Educ Couns* 64(1-3):378-386, 2006.

Hawley R, Monk A: Malignant mesothelioma: current practice and research directions, *Collegian* 11(2):22, 2004.

Heyland D, Dodek P, Groll D et al: What matters most in end-of-life care: perceptions of seriously ill patients and their family members *CMAJ* 174(5):627-633, 2006.

Hogan BE: Soul music in the twilight years: music therapy and the dying process, *Top Geriatr Rehabil* 19(4):275-281, 2003.

Jakobsson E, Bergh I, Ohlen J et al: Utilization of health-care services at the end-of-life, *Health Policy* 80(2):245-250, 2006.

Lobar S, Youngblut J, Brooten D: Cross-cultural beliefs, ceremonies, and rituals surrounding death of a loved one, *Pediatr Nurs* 32(1):44-50, 2006.

Martin V, Roberto K: Assessing the stability of values and health care preferences of older adults: a long term comparison study, *J Gerontol Nurs* 32(11):23-31, 2006.

Martz E, Livneh H: Death anxiety as a predictor of future time orientation among individuals with spinal cord injuries, *Disabil Rehabil* 25(18):1024-1032, 2003.

McCaffrey R, Locsin R: The effects of music on older adults after hip and knee surgery, *J Clin Nurs* 13(96b):91-96, 2004.

Nelson J, Angus D, Weissfeld L et al: End-of-life care for the critically ill: a national intensive care unit survey, *Crit Care Med* 34(10):2547-2553, 2006.

Puchalski C, Dorff E, Hendi I: (2004) Spirituality, religion, and healing in palliative care, *Clin Geriatr Med* 20(4):689-714, 2004.

Sinclair C: End-of-life decision making: a cross-national study, *JAMA* 294(10):1278-1279, 2005.

Skilbeck J, Payne S: Emotional support and the role of Clinical Nurse Specialists in palliative care. *J Adv Nurs* 43(5):521-530, 2003.

Smith M, Kemp J, Hemphill L et al. Outcomes of therapeutic massage for hospitalized cancer patients, *J Nurs Schol* 34(3):257-262, 2002.

Risk for Aspiration   Betty J. Ackley, MSN, EdS, RN

NANDA   Definition

At risk for entry of gastrointestinal secretions, oropharyngeal secretions, solids, or fluids into the tracheobronchial passages

Risk Factors

Decreased gastrointestinal motility; delayed gastric emptying; depressed cough; depressed gag reflex; facial surgery; facial trauma; gastrointestinal tubes; incompetent lower esophageal sphincter; increased gastric residual; increased intragastric pressure; impaired swallowing; medication administration; neck trauma; neck surgery; oral surgery; oral trauma; presence of endotracheal tube; presence of tracheostomy tube; reduced level of consciousness; situations hindering elevation of upper boy; tube feedings; wired jaws

NOC   Outcomes (Nursing Outcomes Classification)

Suggested NOC Outcomes

Aspiration Prevention, Respiratory Status: Ventilation, Swallowing Status

• = Independent;   ▲ = Collaborative;   EBN = Evidence-Based Nursing;   EB = Evidence-Based

A

Example NOC Outcome with Indicators
Respiratory Status: Ventilation as evidenced by the following indicators: Respiratory rate/Moves sputum out of airway/Adventitious breath sounds not present/SOB not present/Auscultated breath sounds/Auscultated vocalization/Chest x-ray findings (Rate the outcome and indicators of **Respiratory Status: Ventilation**: 1 = severely compromised, 2 = substantially compromised, 3 = moderately compromised, 4 = mildly compromised, 5 = not compromised [see Section I].)

SOB, Shortness of breath.

Client Outcomes

Client Will (Specify Time Frame):
- Swallow and digest oral, nasogastric, or gastric feeding without aspiration
- Maintain patent airway and clear lung sounds

NIC   Interventions (Nursing Interventions Classification)

Suggested NIC Intervention
Aspiration Precautions

Example NIC Activities—Aspiration Precautions
Monitor level of consciousness, cough reflex, gag reflex, and swallowing ability; Check nasogastric or gastrostomy residual before feeding

Nursing Interventions and *Rationales*

- Monitor respiratory rate, depth, and effort. Note any signs of aspiration such as dyspnea, cough, cyanosis, wheezing, or fever. *Signs of aspiration should be detected as soon as possible to prevent further aspiration and to initiate treatment that can be lifesaving. Because of laryngeal pooling and residue in clients with dysphagia, silent aspiration (i.e., not manifested by choking or coughing) may occur (Smith & Connolly, 2003; Ramsey, Smithard & Kalra, 2005).*
- Auscultate lung sounds frequently and before and after feedings; note any new onset of crackles or wheezing. **EB:** *Bronchial auscultation of lung sounds was shown to be specific in identifying clients at risk for aspirating (Shaw et al, 2004).*
- Take vital signs frequently, noting onset of a temperature.
- Before initiating oral feeding, check client's gag reflex and ability to swallow by feeling the laryngeal prominence as the client attempts to swallow. *It is important to check client's ability to swallow before feeding. A client can aspirate even with an intact gag reflex (Smith & Connolly, 2003).*
- When feeding client, watch for signs of impaired swallowing or aspiration, including coughing, choking, spitting food, or excessive drooling. If client is having problems swallowing, see Nursing Interventions for **Impaired Swallowing.**
- Have suction machine available when feeding high-risk clients. If aspiration does occur, suction immediately. *A client with aspiration needs immediate suctioning and may need further lifesaving interventions such as intubation.*
- Keep head of bed elevated when feeding and for at least an hour afterward. *Maintaining a sitting position after meals can help decrease aspiration pneumonia in the elderly.* **EB:** *The number of clients developing a fever was significantly reduced when kept sitting upright after eating (Matsui et al, 2002).*
- ▲ Note presence of any nausea, vomiting, or diarrhea. Treat nausea promptly with antiemetics.
- Listen to bowel sounds frequently, noting if they are decreased, absent, or hyperactive. *Decreased or absent bowel sounds can indicate an ileus with possible vomiting and aspiration; increased high-pitched bowel sounds can indicate mechanical bowel obstruction with possible vomiting and aspiration (Kasper et al, 2005).*

• = Independent;   ▲ = Collaborative;   EBN = Evidence-Based Nursing;   EB = Evidence-Based

- Note new onset of abdominal distention or increased rigidity of abdomen. *Abdominal distention or rigidity can be associated with paralytic or mechanical obstruction and an increased likelihood of vomiting and aspiration (Kasper et al, 2005).*
▲ If client has a tracheostomy, ask for referral to speech pathologist for swallowing studies before attempting to feed. After evaluation, decision should be made to have cuff either inflated or deflated when client eats. **EBN and EB:** *Clients who had aspiration following a tracheostomy had aspiration before the tracheostomy, and if the client did not aspirate before the tracheostomy, they also did not aspirate after the tracheostomy procedure was done (Leder & Ross, 2000). For some clients, inflating the cuff may help decrease aspiration; for others, the inflated cuff will interfere with swallowing. This decision should be made following swallowing studies for the safety of the client's airway (Murray & Brzozowski, 1998).*
- If client shows symptoms of nausea and vomiting, position on side.
- If client needs to be fed, feed slowly and allow adequate time for chewing and swallowing. Position upright during and after feedings.

Enteral Feedings

- Insert nasogastric feeding tube using the internal nares to distallower esophageal-sphincter distance, an updated version of the Hanson method. *The ear to nose to xiphoid process is often inaccurate.* **EBN:** *The revised Hanson's method was more accurate in predicting the correct distance than the traditional method (Ellet et al, 2005).*
▲ Check to make sure initial nasogastric feeding tube placement was confirmed by x-ray, with the openings of the tube in the stomach, not the esophagus. This is especially important if a small-bore feeding tube is used, although larger tubes used for feedings or medication administration should be verified by x-ray also. If unable to use x-ray for verification, check the pH of the aspirate. If pH reading is 4 or less, the tube is probably in the stomach. *X-ray verification of placement remains the gold standard for determining safe placement of feeding tubes (Metheny, 2006).* **EBN:** *Use of pH has generally been found to be predictive of correct placement of feeding tubes (Metheny, Smith & Stewart, 2000).*
- Keep nasogastric tube securely taped.
- Measure and record the length of the tube that is outside of the body at defined intervals to help ensure correct placement. *As part of maintaining correct placement, it is helpful to note the length of the tube outside of the body; it is possible for a tube to slide out and be in the esophagus, without obvious disruption of the tape (Metheny, 2006).*
- Note the placement of the tube on any x-rays that are done on the client. *This is needed to verify that the tube is in the correct place (Metheny, 2006).*
- Determine placement of feeding tube before each feeding or every 4 hours if client is on continuous feeding. Note length of tube outside of body, any recent x-ray results, and characteristic appearance of aspirate; do not rely on air insufflation method. **EBN:** *The auscultatory air insufflation method is not reliable for differentiating between gastric or respiratory placement (Metheny et al, 1990; Metheny, 2006). Testing the pH may not be helpful with ongoing tube feeding, since the feeding can change the pH of gastric secretions (Metheny, 2006).*
▲ Check for gastric residual volume during continuous feedings or before feedings; if residual is greater than 200 mL, hold feedings following institutional protocol. **EBN:** *Monitoring gastric residual as evidence of risk for aspiration may or may not be effective (Metheny et al, 2006; McClave et al, 2005), but still should be done at intervals (ASPEN, 2002), especially if there is a question of tube feeding intolerance. The practice of holding tube feedings if increased residual reduces the amount of calories given to the client. If the client has a small-bore feeding tube, it is difficult to check gastric residual volume and may be inaccurate (Metheny et al, 2005).* **EBN:** *A study of the effectiveness of either returning gastric residual volumes to the client or discarding it resulted in inconclusive findings with complications when either action was taken; more research is needed in the area (Booker, Niedringhaus & Eden, 2000).*
▲ Test for the presence of glucose in tracheobronchial secretions or the presence of pepsin to detect aspiration of enteral feedings. *Recognize that the glucose test may not be accurate if there is blood in the aspirate or if a low glucose feeding is being used (St. John, 2000).* **EBN:** *Tracheobronchial secretions*

A

that test positive for glucose can indicate aspiration of enteral feedings (Metheny, St. John & Clouse, 1998). The detection of pepsin in tracheal secretions is considered an indicator of aspiration of gastric contents; a flat position is strongly associated with the presence of pepsin in secretions (Metheny et al, 2002).

▲ Do not use blue dye to tint enteral feedings. *The presence of blue and green skin and urine and serum discoloration from use of blue dye has been associated with the death of two clients (Maloney et al, 2002; Lucarelli et al, 2004). The FDA has reported at least 12 deaths from the use of blue dye in enteral feedings (USFDA, 2003). The use of a multiple-use bottle may result in contamination of feedings and spread bacteria (Fellows et al, 2000). Use of the blue dye is not consistently effective in identifying tracheal aspiration (Metheny et al, 2002).*

• During enteral feedings, position client with head of bed elevated 30 to 45 degrees; maintain for 30 to 45 minutes after feeding. **EBN and EB:** *A study of mechanically ventilated clients receiving tube feedings demonstrated there was an increase of the presence of pepsin (from gastric contents) in pulmonary secretions if the client was in a flat position versus being positioned with head elevated (Metheny et al, 2000; Metheny et al, 2006). A review of aspiration in ventilator clients who were being tube fed found support for elevating the head of the bed at least 30 degrees (Bowman et al, 2005). A similar study of clients receiving enteral feedings demonstrated a decreased incidence of nosocomial pneumonia if the client was positioned at a 45-degree semirecumbent position as opposed to a supine position (Drakulovic et al, 1999).*

• Use a closed versus an open enteral delivery system of tube feeding if possible. **EB:** *The closed delivery system did not result in contamination of the feeding; use of the open bags resulted in several tube feeding formulas becoming contaminated (Vanek, 2000).*

• Stop continual feeding temporarily when turning or moving client. *When turning or moving a client, it is difficult to keep the head elevated to prevent regurgitation and possible aspiration.*

Geriatric

• Carefully check elderly client's gag reflex and ability to swallow before feeding. *Laryngeal nerve endings are reduced in the elderly, which diminishes the gag reflex (Miller, 2004).*

• Watch for signs of aspiration pneumonia in the elderly with cerebrovascular accidents, even if there are no apparent signs of difficulty swallowing or of aspiration. *Bedside evaluation for swallowing and aspiration can be inaccurate; silent aspiration can occur in this population (Smith & Connolly, 2003).*

▲ Use central nervous system depressants cautiously; elderly clients may have an increased incidence of aspiration with altered levels of consciousness. *Elderly clients have altered metabolism, distribution, and excretion of drugs. Some medications can interfere with the swallowing reflex (Miller, 2004).*

• Keep the elderly, mostly bedridden client sitting upright for 2 hours following meals. **EB:** *The number of clients developing a fever was significantly reduced when kept sitting upright after eating (Matsui et al, 2002).*

▲ Recommend to families that tube feedings not be used for clients with dementia; instead use increased feeding assistance, modified food consistency as needed, or environmental alterations. **EBN:** *Tube feedings in this population do not prevent malnutrition or aspiration, improve survival, or reduce infections, instead there is an increased risk for aspiration pneumonia (Keithley & Swanson, 2004).*

Home Care

• Above interventions may be adapted for home care use.

▲ For clients at high risk for aspiration, obtain complete information from the discharging institution regarding institutional management.

• Assess the client and family for willingness and cognitive ability to learn and cope with swallowing, feeding, and related disorders.

• Assess caregiver understanding and reinforce teaching regarding positioning and assessment of the client for possible aspiration.

• Provide the client with emotional support in dealing with fears of aspiration. *Fear of choking can provoke extreme anxiety, which can interfere with the client's ability or willingness to adhere to the treatment plan.* Refer to care plan for **Anxiety.**

- Establish emergency and contingency plans for care of client. *Clinical safety of client between visits is a primary goal of home care nursing.*
- ▲ Have a speech and occupational therapist assess client's swallowing ability and other physiological factors and recommend strategies for working with client in the home (e.g., pureeing foods served to client; providing adaptive equipment for independence in eating). *Successful strategies allow the client to remain part of the family.*
- Obtain suction equipment for the home as necessary.
- Teach caregivers safe, effective use of suctioning devices. Inform client and family that only individuals instructed in suctioning should perform the procedure.
- ▲ Institute case management of frail elderly to support continued independent living.

Client/Family Teaching

- Teach the client and family signs of aspiration and precautions to prevent aspiration.
- Teach the client and family how to safely administer tube feeding.

evolve   See the EVOLVE website for World Wide Web resources for client education.

REFERENCES

ASPEN Board of Directors, Section VIII: Access for administration of nutritional support. *J Parenter Enteral Nutr,* 26(1 Suppl):33SA-35SA, 2002.

Booker KJ, Niedringhaus L, Eden B: Comparison of 2 methods of managing gastric residual volumes from feeding tubes, *Am J Crit Care* 9(5):318, 2000.

Bowman A, Greiner JE, Doerschug KC et al: Implementation of an evidenced-based feeding protocol and aspiration risk reduction algorithm, *Crit Care Nurs Q,* 28(4):324-333, 2005.

Drakulovic MB, Torres A, Bauer TT et al: Supine body position as a risk factor for nosocomial pneumonia in mechanically ventilated patients: a randomised trial, *Lancet* 354(9193):1851, 1999.

Ellett ML, Beckstrand J, Flueckiger J et al: Predicting the insertion distance for placing gastric tubes, *Clin Nurs Res* 14(1):11, 2005.

Fellows LS, Miller EH, Frederickson M et al: Evidence-based practice for enteral feedings: aspiration prevention strategies, bedside detection, and practice change, *Medsurg Nurs* 9(1):27, 2000.

Kasper DL, Braunwald E, Fauci AS et al: *Harrison's principles of internal medicine,* ed 16, New York, McGraw-Hill, 2005.

Keithley JK, Swanson B: Enteral nutrition: an update on practice recommendations, *Medsurg Nurs* 13(2):131, 2004.

Leder SB, Ross DA: Investigation of the causal relationship between tracheostomy and aspiration in the acute care setting, *Laryngoscope* 100(4):641, 2000.

Lucarelli MR, Shirk MB, Julian MW et al: Toxicity of Food Drug and Cosmetic Blue No. 1 dye in critically ill patients, *Chest* 125(2):793, 2004.

Maloney JP, Ryan TA, Brasel KJ et al: Food dye use in enteral feedings: a review and a call for a moratorium, *Nutr Clin Pract* 17(3):169, 2002.

Matsui T, Yamaya M, Ohrui T et al: Sitting position to prevent aspiration in bed-bound patients, *Gerontology* 48(3):194, 2002.

McClave SA, Lukan JK, Stefater JA et al: Poor validity of residual volumes as a marker for risk of aspiration in critically ill patients, *Crit Care Med,* 33(2):324-330, 2005.

Metheny N, McSweeney M, Wehrle MA et al: Effectiveness of the auscultatory method in predicting feeding tube location, *Nurs Res* 39(5):262, 1990.

Metheny NA: Preventing respiratory complications of tube feedings: evidence-based practice, *Am J Crit Care* 15(4):360-369, 2006.

Metheny NA, Chang YH, Ye JS et al: Pepsin as a marker for pulmonary aspiration, *Am J Crit Care* 11(2):150, 2002.

Metheny NA, Clouse RE, Chang YH et al. Tracheobronchial aspiration of gastric contents in critically ill tube-fed patients: frequency, outcomes, and risk factors, *Crit Care Med* 34(4):1007-1015, 2006.

Metheny NA, Dahms TE, Stewart BJ et al: Efficacy of dye-stained enteral formula in detecting pulmonary aspiration, *Chest* 122(1):276-281, 2002.

Metheny NA, Smith L, Stewart BJ: Development of a reliable and valid bedside test for bilirubin and its utility for improving prediction of feeding tube location, *Nurs Res* 49(6):302, 2000.

Metheny NA, Stewart J, Nuetzel G et al: Effect of feeding-tube properties on residual volume measurements in tube-fed patients, *J Parenter Enteral Nutr* 29(3):192-197, 2005.

Metheny NA, St John RE, Clouse RE: Measurement of glucose in tracheobronchial secretions to detect aspiration of enteral feedings, *Heart Lung* 27(5):285, 1998.

Miller CA: *Nursing for wellness in older adults,* ed 4, Philadelphia, 2004, Lippincott.

Murray KA, Brzozowski LA: Swallowing in patients with tracheotomies, *AACN Clin Issues* 9(3):416, 1998.

Ramsey D, Smithard D, Kalra L: Silent aspiration: what do we know? *Dysphagia* 20(3):218-225, 2005.

Shaw JL, Sharpe S, Dyson SE et al: Bronchial auscultation: an effective adjunct to speech and language therapy bedside assessment when detecting dysphagia and aspiration? *Dysphagia* 19(4):211-218, 2004.

Smith HA, Connolly MJ: Evaluation and treatment of dysphagia following stroke, *Topics Geriatr Rehab* 19(1):43, 2003.

St John RE: Ask the experts, *Crit Care Nurse* 20(4):100, 2000.

US Food and Drug Administration (USFDA): Reports of blue discoloration and death in patients receiving enteral feedings tinted with the dye, FD&C Blue no. 1. *FDA Public Health Advisory,* 2003, Accessed March 11, 2007. Available online: http://www.cfsan.fda.gov/.

Vanek VW: Closed versus open enteral delivery systems: a quality improvement study, *Nutr Clin Pract* 15(5):234, 2000.

Risk for impaired parent/child Attachment

Mary DeWys, BS, RN, and Peg Padnos, AB, BSN, RN

NANDA   Definition

Disruption of the interactive process between parent/significant other and infant/child that fosters the development of a protective and nurturing reciprocal relationship

Risk Factors

Anxiety associated with the parent role; ill infant/child who is unable to effectively initiate parental contact due to altered behavioral organization; inability of parents to meet personal needs; lack of privacy; parental conflict due to altered behavioral organization; physical barriers; premature infant who is unable to effectively initiate parental contact due to altered behavioral organization; separation; substance abuse

NOC   Outcomes (Nursing Outcomes Classification)

Suggested NOC Outcomes

Caregiver Adaptation to Patient Institutionalization, Child Development, Coping, Parent-Infant Attachment, Parenting Performance

Example NOC Outcomes with Indicators
Demonstrates appropriate **Child Development: 2 Months** as evidenced by the following indicators: Coos and vocalizes/Shows interest in visual stimuli/Shows interest in auditory stimuli/Smiles/Shows pleasure in interactions, especially with primary caregivers. **4 Months:** Looks at and becomes excited by mobile/Recognizes parents' voices/Smiles, laughs, and coos. **6 months:** Smiles, laughs, squeals, imitates noise/Shows beginning of stranger anxiety. **12 Months:** Plays social games/Imitates vocalizations/Pulls to stand (Rate the outcome and indicators of appropriate **Child Development:** 1 = never demonstrated, 2 = rarely demonstrated, 3 = sometimes demonstrated, 4 = often demonstrated, 5 = consistently demonstrated [see Section I].)

Client Outcomes

Parent(s)/Caregiver(s) Will (Specify Time Frame):

- Be willing to consider pumping breast milk (and storing appropriately) or breastfeeding, if feasible
- Demonstrate behaviors that indicate secure attachment to infant/child
- Provide a safe environment, free of physical hazards
- Provide nurturing environment sensitive to infant/child's need for nutrition/feeding, sleeping, comfort, and social play
- Read and respond contingently to infant/child's behavior cues that signal approach/engagement or avoidance/disengagement
- Be able to calm and relieve infant/child's distress
- Support infant's self-regulation capabilities, intervening when needed
- Engage in mutually satisfying interactions that provide opportunities for attachment
- Give infant nurturing sensory experiences (e.g., holding, cuddling, stroking, rocking)
- Demonstrate an awareness of developmentally appropriate activities that are pleasurable, emotionally supportive, and growth fostering
- Avoid physical and emotional abuse and/or neglect as retribution for parent's perception of infant/child's misbehavior
- Be knowledgeable of appropriate community resources and support services

NIC   Interventions (Nursing Interventions Classification)

Suggested NIC Interventions

Anticipatory Guidance, Attachment Process, Attachment Promotion, Coping Enhancement, Developmental Care, Attachment Process, Parent Education: Infant

---

• = Independent;   ▲ = Collaborative;   EBN = Evidence-Based Nursing;   EB = Evidence-Based

Example NIC Activities—Anticipatory Guidance
Instruct about normal development and behavior, as appropriate; Provide information on realistic expectations related to the patient's behavior; Use case examples to enhance the patient's problem-solving skills, as appropriate

Nursing Interventions and *Rationales*

- Establish a trusting relationship with parent/caregiver. *The quality of the nurse-client relationship was found to be a key to success or failure (Barnard, 1998). Interventions must address both the infant's needs for a stimulating, responsive, and secure environment and meet the parent's developmental and emotional challenges (Barnard, 1998).*
- Encourage mothers to breastfeed their infants, and provide support. *Mothers who choose to breastfeed display enhanced sensitivity during early infancy that, in turn, may foster secure attachment (Britton et al, 2006). Successful breastfeeding has been significantly associated with help from hospital staff (Rajan, 1993).*
- ▲ Identify factors related to postpartum depression (PPD) and major depression and offer appropriate interventions and referrals. **EB:** *The "Postpartum Bonding Questionnaire" (PBQ) is an effective instrument for identifying mothers with PPD (Brockington et al, 2006).* **EBN:** *Depressive symptoms in low-income mothers have been shown to affect infant development negatively. Treatment in the home by masters-prepared psychiatric nurses was helpful in reducing depressive symptoms (Beeber et al, 2004).*
- Nurture parents so that they in turn can nurture their infant/child. **EBN:** *Provide relationship-based caregiving; when working with parents the nurse is nurturing the developing mother-infant relationship (Lawhon, 2002). "Minding the Baby" is an interdisciplinary, relationship-based home visiting program that addresses the relationship disruptions stemming from mothers' early trauma and history of derailed attachment (Slade et al, 2005).*
- Offer a safe, nonjudgmental environment in which parents can express their feelings. **EB:** *Acknowledge and support the strengths of the infant/child, parent, and family members (Goodfriend, 1993).*
- Offer parents opportunities to verbalize their childhood fears. *"Ghosts in the nursery" are parents' early memories of fearful experiences from childhood that may surface when they themselves become parents. "Hearing a mother's cries" is necessary to help her "hear her child's cries" and is an important aspect of therapeutic healing (Fraiberg, Adelson & Shapiro, 1975).*
- Suggest journaling as a way for parents of hospitalized infants to cope with their stress and emotional reactions. **EBN:** *A study of parents of preterm infants, who kept journals as a means to cope with the most stressful aspects of the NICU experience, reported that the practice promoted their willingness to involve themselves in their infants' care (Macnab et al, 1998).*
- Offer parent-to-parent support to parents of NICU hospitalized infants. **EBN:** *One-to-one support, by veteran parents "who have been there," in a nurse-managed program, may influence maternal and maternal-infant interaction outcomes (Roman et al, 1995).*
- Support parents' behaviors that will result in "secure" rather than "avoidant" or "ambivalent" attachment. *A mother's warmth, sensitivity, and consistency in responding to the infant's stress/cries will facilitate secure attachment (Karen, 1998).*
- Encourage parents of hospitalized infants to "personalize the baby" by bringing in clothing, pictures of themselves, toys, and tapes of their voices. **EBN:** *These actions help parents claim the infant as their own. Neonatal nurses are in a unique position to support families' competence and confidence in caring for their infants at their own pace and to encourage the developing mother-infant relationship (Lawhon, 2002).*
- Encourage physical closeness using skin-to-skin experiences for parents and infants as appropriate. **EBN:** *"Kangaroo care" is one of several effective bonding and attachment strategies; others include swaddling, offering pacifier, listening to heartbeat sounds and sounds of mother's voice, rhythmic movement, and decreasing external stimuli (Ludington-Hoe et al, 2002). Placing the newborn skin-to-skin on the mother's chest immediately after delivery until the infant latches on for the first feeding, encouraging continued breastfeeding, and keeping the mother and infant always together in the first hours and days after delivery helps to establish a bond between mother and infant (Kennell & McGrath, 2005).*

• = Independent;   ▲ = Collaborative;   EBN = Evidence-Based Nursing;   EB = Evidence-Based

A

- Assist parents in developing new caregiving competencies and/or revising and extending old ones. **EBN:** *Five caregiving domains have been identified: (1) being with the infant, (2) knowing the infant as a person, (3) giving care to the infant, (4) communicating and engaging with others about needs (both infant and parental), and (5) problem-solving/decision-making/learning (Pridham et al, 1998).*
- Plan ways for parents to interact/assist with caregiving for their hospitalized/institutionalized infant/child. **EBN:** *Seeing the infant in the delivery room prior to admission to the NICU may decrease parental stress, which can be a significant barrier to attachment (Shields-Poe & Pinelli, 1997). The most stressful aspect of parental role alteration is the feeling of helplessness in not being able to protect or help the infant/child, but by allowing parents to touch and/or hold as soon as possible, the attachment process will be strengthened (Miles et al, 1999).*
- Educate parents about reading and responding sensitively to their infant's unique "body language" (behavior cues) that communicate approach ("I'm ready to play"), avoidance/stress ("I'm unhappy. I need a change."), and self-calming ("I'm helping myself"). *Providing knowledge of how infants communicate their feelings and needs offers parents guidelines for choosing their own behavioral responses (Boris, Aoki & Zeanah, 1999). Infants may be more difficult to console if they are not responded to within 90 seconds (Johnson & Johnson Pediatric Institute, Ltd, 1998).*
- Educate and support parent's ability to relieve infant/child's stress/distress. **EB:** *The more that the infant of a nonresponsive mother cries at two months of age, the more likely is the establishment of a negative feedback cycle that can impair attachment and feelings of security at 18 months of age (Gunnar et al, 1996).*
- Guide parents in adapting their behaviors and activities with infant/child cues and changing needs. **EBN:** *Assisting parents to be responsive to infant/child cues and helping parents to be sensitive to their responsiveness to those cues are growth-fostering activities that nurses can encourage (Barnard, 1994). Model calming interventions to provide parents with tools for positive interactions with their infant/child (Karl, 1999).*
- Attend to both the parent and infant/child in an effort to strengthen high-quality parent-infant interactions. **EB:** *Enabling and facilitating attunement and synchrony between infant and mother in the earliest years of life will enhance secure attachment, resulting in a substantial buffer against life's "slings and arrows" (Svanberg, 1998).* **EBN:** *Identifying the infant/child's strengths and limitations can provide parents with information regarding ways to encourage optimal growth and development (Barnard, Morisset & Spieker, 1993).*
- Assist parents with providing pleasurable sensory learning experiences (i.e. sight, sound, movement, touch, and body awareness). **EBN:** *Various studies of hospitalized preterm infants who received gentle human touch (GHT) and massage showed similar positive findings: lower morbidity, shorter length of stay, fewer days on supplemental oxygen, lower neurobiologic risk scores, and higher average daily weight gain than control counterparts (Harrison, 2001).*
- Encourage parents and caregivers to massage their infants and children. *Infant massage enhances attachment through stimulation of mature sensory systems (tactile/kinesthetic) and has been shown to be an effective "low-tech" means of providing developmentally appropriate care for premature infants (Beachy, 2003; Field, 2002).* **EB:** *Having grandparents and parents provide the therapy was shown to enhance their own wellness and provided a cost-effective treatment for stress relief for infants/children (Field, 1995).*

Infant

- Recognize and support infant/child's capacity for self-regulation and intervene when appropriate. *Infants must learn to take in sensory information while simultaneously managing not to become overaroused and overwhelmed by stimuli (Greenspan, 1992; DeGangi & Breinbauer, 1997).*
- Provide lyrical, soothing music in the nursery and home that is appropriate for age (i.e., corrected, in the case of premature infants) and contingent with state and behavioral cues. **EBN:** *Overall beneficial effects of music therapy have been observed in preterm infants (Standley, 2002).*
- Recognize and support infant/child's attention capabilities. *"The ability to take an interest in the*

• = Independent;   ▲ = Collaborative;   EBN = Evidence-Based Nursing;   EB = Evidence-Based

*sights, sounds, and sensations of the world" is a significant developmental milestone (Greenspan &
Weider, 1998).*

- Encourage opportunities for mutually satisfying interactions between infant and parent. *The
process of attachment involves communication and patterns of interactions between parent and infant
that are synchronous and rhythmic (Rosetti, 1990). Opportunities should be provided for infants to be
with their parents and hear their voices naturally (Graven, 2000).*
- Encourage opportunities for physical closeness. **EB:** *The neurodevelopmental profile was more
mature for infants receiving Kangaroo Care. Results underscore the role of early skin-to-skin contact in
the maturation of the autonomic and circadian systems in preterm infants (Feldman & Eidelman,
2003).*

 ## Multicultural

- Discuss cultural norms with families to provide care that is appropriate for enhancing attachment
with the infant/child. **EBN:** *Misinterpretation of parenting behaviors can occur when the nurse and
parent are from different cultures. It is inappropriate to pressure parents to relate to the infant/child in a
way that is culturally unacceptable/abnormal for the family (Guarnaccia, 1998).*
- Promote the attachment process in women who have abused substances by providing a treatment
environment that is culturally based and women-centered. **EBN:** *Pregnant and postpartum Asian/
Pacific Islander women in substance abuse treatment identified provisions for the newborn, infant
health care, parent education, and infant mother bonding as conducive to their treatment (Morelli, Fong
& Oliveria, 2001).*
- Empower family members to draw on personal strengths in which multiple worldviews and
values of individual members are recognized, incorporated, and negotiated. **EB:** *A respectful intervention process can reiterate a parallel process in the family in which multiple worldviews among different members are explored, accepted, appreciated, and negotiated for the benefit of the family (Lee &
Mjelde-Mossey, 2004).*
- Encourage positive involvement and relationship development between children and noncusto-
dial fathers to enhance health and development. **EB:** *Research with low-income African American
fathers has shown that these fathers are strongly committed to their children, but there is a need for
outside facilitation to overcome barriers that interfere with their positive involvement (Dubowitz et al,
2004).*

 ## Home Care

- Above interventions may be adapted for home care use.
- Assess quality of interaction between parent and infant/child. *The infant/child needs to be lovingly
attached to a reliable parental figure and this need is a primary motivation force in human life.
"Attachment evolves from the need for proximity, for felt security, for love: the need to be held, to be understood, to work through our losses; these basic themes of attachment are to some degree built into us bi-
ologically" (Karen, 1998).*
- Use "interaction coaching" (i.e., teaching mother to let the infant lead) so that the mother will
match her style of interaction to the baby's cues. **EBN:** *Mothers with postpartum depressive symptoms who received interaction coaching demonstrated significantly greater responsiveness to their infants
(Horowitz et al, 2001).*
- ▲ Provide home visitation for infants with depressed mothers and for highly stressed parents of
preterm infants. **EB:** *Several studies identified home visitation as an effective intervention for depressed and stressed parents/caregivers. Such programs offered support, counseling, and developmental
guidance to facilitate early attachment and bonding (Barnard, 1997; NCAST, 1994). NSTEP-P was
developed to assist parents in understanding preterm infant behavior and caregiving practices for families (Barnard, 1994).*
- ▲ Identify community resources and supportive network systems for mothers showing depressive
symptoms. **EBN:** *Identifying maternal depressive symptoms leading to early intervention and treatment of women at risk for depression can decrease the negative effects on infant development (Mew
et al, 2003).*

evolve See the EVOLVE website for World Wide Web resources for client education.

• = Independent;   ▲ = Collaborative;   EBN = Evidence-Based Nursing;   EB = Evidence-Based

A

REFERENCES

Barnard KE: *Caregiver/parent-child interaction feeding and teaching manual,* Seattle, 1994, NCAST Publications.

Barnard KE, editor: Developing, implementing, and documenting interventions with parents and young children, *Zero to Three,* February and March, 1998, 23-29.

Barnard KE: Influencing parent-child interactions. In Guralnick MJ, editor: *The effectiveness of early intervention,* Baltimore, 1997, Brooks Publishing, pp 249-268.

Barnard KE, Morisset CE, Spieker SJL: Preventive interventions: enhancing parent-infant relationship. In Zeanah C, editor: *Handbook on infant mental health,* New York, 1993, The Guilford Press, pp 386-401.

Beachy JM: Premature infant massage in the NICU, *Neonatal Netw* 22(3):39-45, 2003.

Beeber LS, Holditch-Davis D, Belyea MJ et al: In-home intervention for depressive symptoms with low-income mothers of infants and toddlers in the United States, *Health Care Women Int* 25(6):561-580, 2004.

Boris NW, Aoki Y, Zeanah CH: The development of infant-parent attachment: considerations for assessment, *Infants Young Child* 11(4):1, 1999.

Britton JR, Britton HL, Gronwaldt V: Breastfeeding, sensitivity, and attachment. *Pediatrics* 118(5):e1436-1443, 2006.

Brockington IF, Fraser C, Wilson D: The postpartum bonding questionnaire: a validation, *Arch Womens Ment Health* 9:233-242, 2006.

DeGangi GA, Breinbauer C: The symptomatology of infants and toddlers with regulatory disorders, *J Development Learning Dis* 1(1):183-215, 1997.

Dubowitz H, Lane W, Ross K et al: The involvement of low-income African American fathers in their children's lives, and the barriers they face, *Ambul Pediatr* 4(6):505-508, 2004.

Feldman R, Eidelman A: Skin-to-skin contact (kangaroo care) accelerates autonomic and neurobehavioural maturation in preterm infants, *Dev Med Child Neurol* 45(4):274, 2003.

Field T: Massage, *Med Clin North Am* 86(1):163-167, 2002.

Field T: Massage therapy for infants and children, *J Dev Behav Pediatr* 16(2):105-111, 1995.

Fraiberg S, Adelson E, Shapiro V: Ghosts in the nursery: a psychoanalytic approach to the problems of impaired infant-mother relationships, *J Am Acad Child Psychiatry* 14:387-421, 1975.

Goodfriend MS: Treatment of attachment disorder of infancy in a neonatal intensive care unit, *Pediatrics,* 9(1):139-142, 1993.

Graven S: Sound and the developing infant in the NICU: conclusions and recommendations for care, *J Perinatol* 20(8)(Pt2):S88-S93, 2000.

Greenspan SI: *Infancy and early childhood: the practice of clinical assessment and intervention with emotional and developmental challenges.* Madison, Conn, 1992, International Universities Press.

Greenspan SI, Wieder S: *The child with special needs: encouraging intellectual and emotional growth,* Reading, Mass, 1998, Perseus Books.

Guarnaccia P: Multicultural experiences of family caregiving: a study of African American, European American, and Hispanic American families, *New Dir Ment Health Serv* 77:45-61, 1998.

Gunnar MR, Brodersen L, Nachmias M et al: Stress reactivity and attachment security, *Dev Psychobiol* 29(3):191-204, 1996.

Harrison LL: The use of comforting touch and massage to reduce stress for preterm infants in the neonatal intensive care unit, *Newborn Infant Nurs Rev* 1:235-241, 2001.

Horowitz JA, Bell M, Trybulski J et al: Promoting responsiveness between mothers with depressive symptoms and their infants, *J Nurs Schol* 33(4):323-329, 2001.

Johnson & Johnson Pediatric Institute, Ltd: *Amazing talents of the newborn. Emerging perspectives in perinatal care: a reference guide for the healthcare professional.* Skillman, NJ, 1998, Author.

Karen R: *Becoming attached, first relationships and how they shape our capacity to love,* New York and Oxford, 1998, Oxford University Press, pp 444-445.

Karl D: The interactive newborn bath, *MCN Am J Matern Child Nurs* 24(6):280-286, 1999.

Kennell J, McGrath S: Starting the process of mother-infant bonding, *Acta Paediatr* 94(6):775-777, 2005.

Lawhon G: Integrated nursing care: vital issues important in the humane care of the newborn, *Semin Neonatol* 7:441-446, 2002.

Lee MY, Mjelde-Mossey L: Cultural dissonance among generations: a solution-focused approach with East Asian elders and their families, *J Marital Fam Ther* 30(4):497-513, 2004.

Ludington-Hoe SM, Cong X, Hashemi F: Infant crying: nature, physiologic consequences, and select interventions, *Neonatal Netw* 21(2):29-36, 2002.

Macnab AJ, Beckett LY, Park CC et al: Journal writing as a social support strategy for parents of premature infants: a pilot study, *Patient Educ Couns* 33:149-159, 1998.

Mew AM, Holditch-Davis D, Belyea M et al: Correlates of depressive symptoms in mothers of preterm infants, *Neonatal Netw* 22(5):51-60, 2003.

Miles MS, Holditch-Davis D, Burchinal P et al: Distress and growth outcomes in mothers of medically fragile infants, *Nurs Res* 48(3):129-140, 1999.

Morelli PT, Fong R, Oliveria J: Culturally competent substance abuse treatment for Asian/Pacific Islander women, *J Hum Behav Soc Environ* 3(3/4):263, 2001.

NCAST: *Keys to caregiving: a video program,* Seattle, 1994, NCAST Publications.

Pridham KF: Guided participation and development of care-giving competencies for families of low birth-weight infants, *J Adv Nurs* 28(5):948-958, 1998.

Rajan L: The contribution of professional support, information and consistent correct advice to successful breast feeding, *Midwifery* 9:197-209, 1993.

Roman LA, Lindsay JD, Boger RP et al: Parent-to-parent support initiated in the neonatal intensive care unit, *Res Nurs Health* 18: 385-394, 1995.

Rossetti LM: *Infant-toddler assessment,* Boston, 1999, Little-Brown and Company.

Shields-Poe D, Pinelli J: Variables associated with parental stress in neonatal intensive care units, *Neonat Netw* 16(1):29, 1997.

Slade A, Sadler L, De Dios-Kenn C et al: Minding the baby: a reflective parenting program, *Psychoanal Study Child,* 60:74-100, 2005.

Standley JM: A meta-analysis of the efficacy of music for premature infants, *Pediatr Nurs* 17(2):107-113, 2002.

Svanberg PG: Attachment, resilience and prevention, *J Ment Health.* 7(6):543-578, 1998.

• = Independent;   ▲ = Collaborative;   EBN = Evidence-Based Nursing;   EB = Evidence-Based

Autonomic dysreflexia   *Paula Sherwood, PhD, RN, CNRN, and Elizabeth A. Crago, MSN, CEN, CCRN, RN*

A

NANDA   Definition

Life-threatening, uninhibited sympathetic response of the nervous system to a noxious stimulus after a spinal cord injury at T7 or above

Defining Characteristics

Blurred vision; bradycardia; chest pain, chilling; conjunctival congestion; diaphoresis (above the injury); headache (a diffuse pain in different portions of the head and not confined to any nerve distribution area); Horner's syndrome; metallic taste in mouth; nasal congestion; pallor (below the injury); paroxysmal hypertension; pilomotor reflex; red splotches on skin (above the injury); tachycardia

Related Factors (r/t)

Bladder distention; bowel distention; deficient caregiver knowledge; deficient patient knowledge; skin irritation

NOC   Outcomes (Nursing Outcomes Classification)

Suggested NOC Outcomes

Neurological Status, Neurological Status: Autonomic

Example NOC Outcome with Indicators
Neurological Status: Autonomic as evidenced by the following indicators: Systolic blood pressure/Diastolic blood pressure/Apical heart rate/Perspiration response pattern/Goose bump response pattern/Pupil reactivity/Peripheral tissue perfusion (Rate the outcome and indicators of **Neurological Status: Autonomic:** 1 = severely compromised, 2 = substantially compromised, 3 = moderately compromised, 4 = mildly compromised, 5 = not compromised [see Section I].)

Client Outcomes/Goals

Client Will (Specify Time Frame):

- Maintain normal vital signs
- Remain free of dysreflexia symptoms
- Explain symptoms, prevention, and treatment of dysreflexia

NIC   Interventions (Nursing Interventions Classification)

Suggested NIC Intervention

Dysreflexia Management

Example NIC Activities—Dysreflexia Management
Identify and minimize stimuli that may precipitate dysreflexia; Monitor for signs and symptoms of autonomic dysreflexia

Nursing Interventions and *Rationales*

- Monitor the client for symptoms of dysreflexia, particularly those with high-level and more extensive spinal cord injuries. See Defining Characteristics. **EB:** *Some clients are mostly asymptomatic (Dunn, 2004), although AD is more common in those with higher and more complete injuries (Frisbie, 2006; Rabchevsky, 2006).*

• = Independent;   ▲ = Collaborative;   EBN = Evidence-Based Nursing;   EB = Evidence-Based

A

▲ Collaborate with healthcare practitioners to identify the cause of dysreflexia (e.g., distended bladder, impaction, pressure ulcer, urinary calculi, bladder infection, acute condition in the abdomen, penile pressure, ingrown toenail, or other source of noxious stimuli). *Noxious stimuli cause an uncontrolled sympathetic nervous system response (Widerstrom-Noga, Cruz-Almeida & Krassioukov, 2004).*

▲ If symptoms of dysreflexia are present, place client in high Fowler's position, remove all support hoses or binders, and immediately determine the noxious stimuli causing the response. If blood pressure cannot be decreased within 1 minute, notify the physician STAT (Walker, 2002; Dunn, 2004). *These steps promote venous pooling, decrease venous return, and decrease blood pressure. The client should be rapidly evaluated by both the physician and nurse to find the possible cause (Kavchak-Keyes, 2000).*

▲ To determine the stimulus for dysreflexia:
  ■ First, assess bladder function. Check for distention, and if present, catheterize using an anesthetic jelly as a lubricant. Do not use Valsalva maneuver or Crede's method to empty the bladder. Ensure existing catheter patency. Also note signs of urinary tract infection. **EB:** *AD may be associated with bladder care for 30% of persons with a spinal cord injury (Anderson et al, 2006).*
  ■ Second, assess bowel function. Numb the bowel area with a topical anesthetic as ordered, and once agent is effective (5 minutes), check for impaction. **EB:** *AD may be associated with bowel care for 23% of persons with a spinal cord injury (Anderson et al, 2006).*
  ■ Third, assess the skin, looking for any points of pressure. **EB:** *Stimuli for dysreflexia are commonly bladder distention, bowel impaction, pressure on the skin, and pain (Essat, 2003; Krassioukov, Furlan & Fehlings, 2003; Widerstrom-Noga, Cruz-Almeida & Krassioukov, 2004).*

▲ Initiate antihypertensive therapy as soon as ordered. *A severely elevated blood pressure must be decreased for client safety, particularly given the client with AD's increased susceptibility to ventricular arrhythmias (Collins, Rodenbaugh & DiCarlo, 2006).*

▲ Be careful not to increase noxious sensory stimuli. If numbing agent is ordered, use it on anus and 1 inch of rectum before attempting to remove a fecal impaction. Also spray pressure ulcer with it. If necessary to replace an obstructed catheter, use an anesthetic jelly as ordered. *Increased noxious sensory stimuli can exacerbate the abnormal response and worsen the client's prognosis (Walker, 2002; Dunn, 2004).* **EB:** *The use of topical lidocaine did not limit the development of autonomic dysreflexia during anorectal procedures in spinal cord injury clients (Cosman, Vu & Plowman, 2002). AD may be associated with bladder and bowel care for persons with a spinal cord injury (Anderson et al, 2006).*

• Monitor vital signs every 3 to 5 minutes during acute event; continue to monitor vital signs after event is resolved. *It is possible for the client to develop rebound hypotension after the acute event because of the use of antihypertensive medications, or symptoms of dysreflexia may reoccur (Kasper, Braunwald & Fauci, 2005).*

▲ Watch for complications of dysreflexia, including signs of cerebral hemorrhage, seizures, MI, or intraocular hemorrhage. *Extremely high blood pressure can cause intracranial hemorrhage and death (Kasper, Braunwald & Fauci, 2005).*

• Accurately and completely record any incidences of dysreflexia; especially note the precipitating stimuli. *It is imperative to determine both the causes of the condition and whether the condition is persistent, requiring the client to take medications routinely to prevent repeat incidences (Kavchak-Keyes, 2000).*

• Use the following interventions to prevent dysreflexia:
  ■ Ensure that drainage from Foley catheter is good and that bladder is not distended.
  ■ Ensure a regular pattern of defecation to prevent fecal impaction. **EB:** *Bladder distention and bowel impaction are most common causes of dysreflexia (Krassioukov, Furlan & Fehlings, 2003; Widerstrom-Noga, Cruz-Almeida & Krassioukov et al, 2004).*
  ■ Frequently change position of client to relieve pressure and prevent the formation of pressure ulcers.

▲ If ordered, apply an anesthetic agent to any wound below level of injury before performing

---

• = Independent;   ▲ = Collaborative;   EBN = Evidence-Based Nursing;   EB = Evidence-Based

wound care. **EB:** *Pain is a common cause of dysreflexia (Widerstrom-Noga, Cruz-Almeida & Krassioukov, 2004).*

▲ Because episodes can reoccur, notify all healthcare team members of the possibility of a dysreflexia episode. **EB:** *All healthcare personnel working with the client should be aware of the condition because symptoms could begin while the client is away from the nursing unit (Karlsson, 2006).*

▲ For female clients with spinal cord injury who become pregnant, collaborate with obstetrical healthcare practitioners to monitor for signs and symptoms of dysreflexia. **EB:** *Autonomic dysreflexia may signal the onset of labor or be a sign of preterm labor, and obstetrical healthcare personnel should monitor potential cardiovascular complications (Osgood & Kuczkowski, 2006).*

 ### Home Care

• Above interventions may be adapted for home care use.

• Instruct the client with any known proclivity toward dysreflexia to wear a medical alert bracelet and carry a medical alert wallet card when not in a safe environment (i.e., not with someone who knows client has the condition and can respond appropriately). *Autonomic dysreflexia is life-threatening response (Karlsson, 2006).*

▲ Establish an emergency plan: obtain physician orders for medications to be used in situations in which first aid does not work and plans to identify potential stimuli (Assadi, Czech & Palmisano, 2004). *Medication administered immediately can reverse early stage dysreflexia. Dysreflexia that is not recognized and treated can result in death (Kasper, Braunwald & Fauci, 2005).*

▲ If orders have not been obtained or client does not have medications, use emergency medical services.

• When episode of dysreflexia is resolved, monitor blood pressure every 30 to 60 minutes for next 5 hours or admit to institution for observation. *After an episode of autonomic dysreflexia, it is not uncommon for a second episode or rebound to occur (Kasper, Braunwald & Fauci, 2005).*

 ### Client/Family Teaching

• Teach recognition of the earliest symptoms of dysreflexia, the actions that should be taken when they occur, and the need to summon help immediately. Give client a written card that contains this information. *The client must know the symptoms and treatment well enough to instruct people in his or her environment how to relieve the symptoms (Kavchak-Keyes, 2000).*

• Teach steps to prevent dysreflexia episodes: care of bladder, bowel, and skin and prevention of other forms of noxious stimuli (i.e., not wearing clothing that is too tight). *Dysreflexia can occur anytime after discharge. Of clients with spinal cord lesions above C6, 85% experience dysreflexia (Kasper, Braunwald, & Fauci, 2005).*

• Discuss the potential impact of sexual intercourse and pregnancy on autonomic dysreflexia. **EB:** *Autonomic dysreflexia has been shown to be triggered by preterm and full-term labor for women (Osgood & Kuczkowski, 2006) and by ejaculation for men (Elliott & Krassioukov, 2006). Clients who develop AD during bowel and bladder care may be at higher risk for developing AD during sexual activity (Anderson et al, 2006).*

 See the EVOLVE website for World Wide Web resources for client education.

REFERENCES

Anderson KD, Borisoff JF, Johnson RD et al: The impact of spinal cord injury on sexual function: concerns of the general population, *Spinal Cord* 10:1-10, 2006.

Assadi F, Czech K, Palmisano J: Autonomi dysreflexia manifested by severe hypertension, *Med Sci Monit* 10(12):CS77-CS79, 2004.

Collins HL, Rodenbaugh DW, DiCarlo SE: Spinal cord injury alters cardiac electrophysiology and increases the susceptibility to ventricular arrhythmias, *Prog Brain Res* 152:275-288, 2006.

Cosman BC, Vu TT, Plowman BK: Topical lidocaine does not limit autonomic dysreflexia during anorectal procedures in spinal cord injury: a prospective, double-blind study, *Int J Colorectal Dis* 17(2):104, 2002.

Dunn KL: Identification and management of autonomic dysreflexia in the emergency department, *Top Emerg Med* 26(3):254, 2004.

Elliot S, Krassioukov A: Malignant autonomic dysreflexia in spinal cord injured men, *Spinal Cord* 44:386-392, 2006.

Essat Z: Management of autonomic dysreflexia, *Nurs Stand* 17(32):42, 2003.

Frisbie JH: Unstable baseline blood pressure in chronic tetraplegia, *Spinal Cord* Mar 28:1-4, 2006.

Kasper DL, Braunwald E, Fauci AS: *Harrison's principles of internal medicine,* ed 16, New York, 2005, McGraw-Hill.

Karlsson AK: Autonomic dysfunction in spinal cord injury: clinical presentation of symptoms and signs, *Prog Brain Res* 152:1-8, 2006.

Kavchak-Keyes MA: Autonomic hyperreflexia, *Rehabil Nurs* 25(1):31, 2000.

Krassioukov A, Furlan J, Fehlings M: Autonomic dysreflexia in acute spinal cord injury: an under-recognized clinical entity, *J Neurotrauma* 20(8):707-713, 2003.

Osgood SL, Kuczkowski KM: Autonomic dysreflexia in a patient with spinal cord injury, *Acta Anaesthesiol Belg* 57(2):161-162, 2006.

Rabchevsky AG: Segmental organization of spinal reflexes mediating autonomic dysreflexia after spinal cord injury, *Prog Brain Res* 152:265-274, 2006.

Walker JA: Autonomic dysreflexia, *Prof Nurse* 17(9):519-520, 2002.

Widerstrom-Noga, E, Cruz-Almeida Y, Krassioukov A: Is there a relationship between chronic pain and autonomic dysreflexia in persons with cervical spinal cord injury? *J Neurotrauma* 21(2):195-204, 2004.

Risk for Autonomic dysreflexia *Betty J. Ackley, MSN, EdS, RN*

NANDA Definition

At risk for life-threatening, uninhibited response of the sympathetic nervous system; post-spinal shock; in an individual with spinal cord injury or lesion at T6 or above (has been demonstrated in clients with injuries at T7 and T8)

Defining Characteristics (Risk Factors)

An injury/lesion at T6 or above and at least one of the following noxious stimuli:

- **Cardiac/pulmonary problems:** pulmonary emboli; deep vein thrombosis
- **Gastrointestinal stimuli:** bowel distention; constipation; difficult passage of stool; digital stimuli; enemas; esophageal reflux; fecal impaction; gallstones; gastric ulcers; GI system pathology; hemorrhoids; suppositories
- **Musculoskeletal**-integumentary stimuli: cutaneous stimulations (e.g., pressure ulcer, ingrown toenail, dressings, burns, rash); fractures, heterotrophic bone; pressure over bony prominences or genitalia; range-of-motion exercises; spasm; sunburns; wounds
- **Neurological stimuli:** painful/irritating stimuli below the level of injury
- **Regulatory stimuli:** extreme environmental temperatures; temperature fluctuations
- **Reproductive stimuli:** ejaculation; labor and delivery; menstruation; ovarian cyst; pregnancy; sexual intercourse
- **Situational stimuli:** constrictive clothing (e.g., straps, stockings, shoes); drug reactions (e.g., decongestants, sympathomimetics, vasoconstrictors); positioning; surgical procedures
- **Urological stimuli:** bladder distention; bladder spasms; calculi; catheterization; cystitis; detrusor sphincter dyssynergia; epididymitis; instrumentation; surgery; urethritis; urinary tract infection

NOC Outcomes (Nursing Outcomes Classification)

Suggested NOC Outcomes

Neurological Status, Neurological Status: Autonomic

Example NOC Outcome with Indicators
Neurological Status: Autonomic as evidenced by the following indicators: Systolic blood pressure/Diastolic blood pressure/Apical heart rate/Perspiration response pattern/Goose bumps response pattern/Pupil reactivity size/Peripheral tissue perfusion (Rate the outcome and indicators with regard to **Neurological Status: Autonomic:** 1 = severely compromised, 2 = substantially compromised, 3 = moderately compromised, 4 = mildly compromised, 5 = not compromised [see Section I].)

NIC Interventions (Nursing Interventions Classification)

Suggested NIC Intervention

Dysreflexia Management

• = Independent;   ▲ = Collaborative;   EBN = Evidence-Based Nursing;   EB = Evidence-Based

Example NIC Activities—Dysreflexia Management
Identify and minimize stimuli that may precipitate dysreflexia; monitor for signs and symptoms of autonomic dysreflexia

B

Client Outcomes, Nursing Interventions and *Rationales*

Refer to care plan for **Autonomic dysreflexia**

Risk-prone health Behavior   *Gail Ladwig, MSN, CHTP, RN*

NANDA   Definition

Inability to modify lifestyle/behavior in a manner consistent with a change in health status

Defining Characteristics

Demonstrates nonacceptance of health status change; failure to achieve optimal sense of control; failure to take action that prevents health problems; minimizes health status change

Related Factors (r/t)

Inadequate comprehension; inadequate social support; low self-efficacy; low socioeconomic status; multiple stressors; negative attitude toward health status change

NOC   Outcomes (Nursing Outcomes Classification)

Suggested NOC Outcomes

Acceptance: Health Status, Health-Seeking Behavior, Participation in Health Care Decisions, Psychosocial Adjustment: Life Change

Example NOC Outcome with Indicators
Acceptance: Health Status as evidenced by the following indicators: Appears peaceful/Relinquishes previous concept of personal health/Reports decreased need to verbalize about feelings about health/Recognizes reality of health situation/Copes with health situation (Rate the outcome and indicators of **Acceptance: Health Status:** 1 = never demonstrated, 2 = rarely demonstrated, 3 = sometimes demonstrated, 4 = often demonstrated, 5 = consistently demonstrated [see Section I].)

Client Outcomes

Client Will (Specify Time Frame):

- State acceptance of change in health status
- Request assistance in altering behaviors to adapt to change
- State personal goals for dealing with change in health status and means to prevent further health problems
- State experience of a period of grief that is proportional to the actual or perceived effect of the loss
- Report and/or demonstrate behavior changes mutually agreed upon with nurse as evidence of positive adaptation

NIC   Interventions (Nursing Interventions Classification)

Suggested NIC Intervention

Coping Enhancement

• = Independent;   ▲ = Collaborative;   EBN = Evidence-Based Nursing;   EB = Evidence-Based

B

Example NIC Activities—Coping Enhancement
Assist the patient with developing an objective appraisal of the event; Explore with the patient previous methods of dealing with life problems

Nursing Interventions and *Rationales*

- Assess the client's perception about the illness/event. Ask the client to state feelings related to the change in health status. **EBN:** *Negative responses to a need for change in behavior related to an alteration in health status can be understood only following a thorough assessment of the client's appraisal framework (Dudley-Brown, 2002).*

- Assess for negative affect and internalization of problems. **EBN:** *Exploring the meaning of health status change and the adjustments required for a successful adaptation within the client's life experience fosters positive growth (Norris & Spelic, 2002; Richer & Ezer, 2002).*

- Allow the client adequate time to express feelings about the change in health status. **EBN:** *Nurses need to provide an opportunity for clients to address all aspects of the impact of a health status change on their lives (Richer & Ezer, 2002).*

- Use open-ended questions to allow the client free expression (e.g., "Tell me about your last hospitalization" or "How does this time compare?"). **EBN:** *Active listening aimed at clarifying family concerns regarding the change in health status will facilitate nursing interventions that promote positive coping behaviors (Weiss & Chen, 2002).*

- Help the client work through the stages of grief. Denial is usually the initial response and may be an adaptive coping mechanism. Acknowledge that grief takes time, and give the client permission to grieve; accept crying. *The process of grieving is integral to adaptation to a disruption of health status. Denial is the initial phase of the grieving response and would be expected when a client is told of a significant change in health status (Norris & Spelic, 2002).*

- Discuss resources (e.g., the client's support system) that have worked previously when dealing with changes in lifestyle or health status. **EBN:** *Integration of a client's repertoire of coping strategies into an intervention program to facilitate adaptation to a change in health status will facilitate positive coping (Wassem, Beckham & Dudley, 2001).*

- Discuss the client's current goals. If appropriate, have the client list goals so that they can be referred to and steps can be taken to accomplish them. Support hope that the goals will be accomplished. **EBN:** *Clarification of the client/family goals and expectations will allow the nurse to clarify what is possible and to identify measures that can facilitate achievement of the goals (Northouse et al, 2002). "Hope theory" may facilitate recovery and clearer and more sustainable goals (Snyder et al, 2006).*

- Allow the client choices in daily care, particularly choices that result from the change in health status. **EBN:** *A client will demonstrate a more positive adaptation if the resources, and interventions offered by the nurse are adapted to the client's perceived circumstances and needs (LeClere et al, 2002).*

- List the client activities that may require assistance and those that can be performed independently. **EBN:** *Clarification of behaviors conducive to a positive adjustment to a change in health status and the resources available to the client facilitates positive coping behaviors toward adaptation (Northouse et al, 2002).*

- Give the client positive feedback for accomplishments, no matter how small. **EBN:** *The nurse's provision of a climate of acceptance and encouragement facilitates a positive adaptation (Richer & Ezer, 2002).*

- Manipulate the environment to decrease stress; allow the client to display personal items that have meaning. **EBN:** *Appraisal uncertainty is a risk factor for a negative adaptation to health change (Dudley-Brown, 2002).*

- Maintain consistency and continuity in daily schedule. When possible, provide the same caregiver. **EBN:** *The predictability of interaction with the same nurses as a part of treatment facilitates trust, confidence, and positive adaptation (Richer & Ezer, 2002).*

- Foster communication between the client/family and medical staff. **EBN:** *Family members of in-*

• = Independent;   ▲ = Collaborative;   EBN = Evidence-Based Nursing;   EB = Evidence-Based

dividuals undergoing cardiopulmonary resuscitation expressed a need to be involved and present or informed at all times during the process (Wagner, 2004). **EB:** *Psychotherapeutic interventions should not only address the clients' problems but also the support-givers' questions, needs, and psychosocial burdens (Frick et al, 2005).*

- Promote use of positive spiritual influences. *Spiritual coping strategies may facilitate a positive adaptation to a change in health status (Baldacchino & Draper, 2001).*
- ▲ Refer to community resources. Provide general and contact information for ease of use. **EBN:** *Social support is necessary to coordinate all possible resources that may assist the client and/or family in their adjustment to a change in health status (Wassem, Beckham & Dudley, 2001).*

Geriatric

- ▲ Assess for signs of depression resulting from illness-associated changes and make appropriate referral. **EBN:** *Signs and symptoms of depression when evident would assist the nurse in the individualization of interventions to a particular client (Reynaud & Meeker, 2002).*
- Monitor the client for agitation associated with health problems. Support family caring for elders with agitation. **EB:** *The findings in this study suggest that some symptoms, such as agitation/ aggression and irritability/lability, may affect the caregivers significantly, although their frequency and severity are low (Matsumoto et al, 2007).*

Multicultural

- Assess for the influence of cultural beliefs, norms, and values on the client's ability to modify health behavior. **EBN:** *What the client considers normal and abnormal health behavior may be based on cultural perceptions (Leininger & McFarland, 2002).*
- Assess the role of fatalism on the client's ability to modify health behavior. **EB:** *Fatalistic perspectives, which involve the belief that you cannot control your own fate, may influence health behaviors in some African-American, Asian, and Latino populations (Phillips, Cohen & Moses, 1999; Powe & Finnie, 2003).*
- ▲ Assess for signs of depression and level of social support and make appropriate referrals. **EB:** *Increased depressed feelings and lower levels of available social support were reported by minorities in this study who had mild to moderate traumatic brain injury (Brown et al, 2004).*
- Identify which family members the client can rely on for support. **EBN:** *A variety of different cultures rely on family members to cope with stress (White et al, 2002).*
- Encourage spirituality as a source of support for coping. **EBN:** *Many African-Americans and Latinos identify spirituality, religiousness, prayer, and church-based approaches as coping resources (Samuel-Hodge et al, 2000).*
- Negotiate with the client regarding the aspects of health behavior that will need to be modified. **EBN:** *Give-and-take with the client will lead to culturally congruent care (Leininger & McFarland, 2002).*

Home Care

- Above interventions may be adapted for home care use.
- Take the client's perspective into consideration, and use a holistic approach in assessing and responding to client planning for the future. **EBN:** *Caring for women post-myocardial infarction (MI), researchers concluded, must approach health as being more than the absence of illness (Johansson, Dahlberg & Ekebergh, 2003).*
- Assist client to recognize and exercise power in using self-care management to adjust to health change. **EBN:** *Women post-myocardial infarction reported that not participating in their health process increased their suffering and left them feeling powerless (Johansson, Dahlberg & Ekebergh, 2003).*
- ▲ Refer the client to counselor or therapist for follow-up care. Initiate community referrals as needed (e.g., grief counseling, self-help groups). **EBN:** *Families need assistance in coping with health changes. The nurse is often perceived as the individual who can help them obtain necessary social support (Northouse et al, 2002).*
- Refer to care plan for **Powerlessness.**

B

 Client/Family Teaching

- Assess family/caregivers for coping and teaching/learning styles. **EBN:** *The degree of optimism and pessimism influences the coping and health outcomes of caregivers of clients with Parkinson's disease (Lyons et al, 2004).*
- Educate and prepare families regarding the appearance of the client and the environment before initial exposure. *Successful adaptation requires a coordination of efforts to fit the nursing interventions to the client's perception of the threat, personal values and beliefs, and recognition of personal strengths (Norris & Spelic, 2002).*
- Teach the client to maintain a positive outlook by listing current strengths. **EBN:** *Successful adaptation requires a coordination of efforts to fit the nursing interventions to the client's perception of the threat, personal values and beliefs, and recognition of personal strengths (Norris & Spelic, 2002). Parents of critically ill children demonstrated fewer complications following their participation in a structured hospital-based intervention (Melnyk et al, 2004).*
- Teach a client and his or her family relaxation techniques (controlled breathing, guided imagery) and help them practice. **EBN:** *Relaxation training has been demonstrated to improve self-efficacy in Alzheimer family caregivers (Fisher & Laschinger, 2001).*
- Allow the client to proceed at own pace in learning; provide time for return demonstrations (e.g., self-injection of insulin). **EBN:** *Use clear and distinct language free of medical jargon and meaningless values (Wagner, 2004). Successful adaptation requires a coordination of efforts to fit the nursing interventions to the client's perception of the threat, personal values and beliefs, and recognition of personal strengths (Norris & Spelic, 2002).*
- Involve significant others in planning and teaching. **EBN:** *Parents of critically ill children demonstrated fewer complications following their participation in a structured hospital-based intervention (Melnyk et al, 2004). Successful adaptation requires a coordination of efforts to fit the nursing interventions to the client's perception of the threat, personal values and beliefs, and recognition of personal strengths (Norris & Spelic, 2002).*
- If long-term deficits are expected, inform the family as soon as possible. **EBN:** *An honest assessment shared by the nurse of a particular situation is important to the family's sense of what is expected of them in adapting to a healthcare change (Weiss & Chen, 2002).*
- Teach families intervention techniques for family members such as setting limits, communicating acceptable behavior, and having time-outs. *Psychological, social, and behavioral interventions are effective in mediating aggressive behavior (Harper-Jaques & Reimer, 2002). Parents of critically ill children demonstrated fewer complications following their participation in a structured hospital-based intervention (Melnyk et al, 2004).*
- Provide clients with information on how to access and evaluate available health information via the internet. *Client access to health information and personal health records is becoming increasingly important in today's healthcare society. MedlinePlus, NIH Senior Health, and ClinicalTrials.gov are designed to get medical information directly into the hands of clients (Koonce et al, 2007).*

evolve See the EVOLVE website for World Wide Web resources for client education.

REFERENCES

Baldacchino D, Draper P: Spiritual coping strategies: a review of the EBN literature, *J Adv Nurs* 34(6):833, 2001.

Brown SA, McCauley SR, Levin HS et al: Perception of health and quality of life in minorities after mild-to-moderate traumatic brain injury, *Appl Neuropsychol* 11(1):54-64, 2004.

Dudley-Brown S: Prevention of psychological distress in persons with inflammatory bowel disease, *Issues Ment Health Nurs* 23:403, 2002.

Fisher PA, Laschinger HS: A relaxation training program to increase self-efficacy for anxiety control in Alzheimer family caregivers, *Holist Nurs Pract* 15(2):47-58, 2001.

Frick E, Rieg-Appleson C, Tyroller M et al: Social support, affectivity, and the quality of life of patients and their support-givers

prior to stem cell transplantation, *J Psychosoc Oncol* 23(4):15-34, 2005.

Harper-Jaques S, Reimer M: Management of aggression. In Boyd MA, editor: *Psychiatric nursing in contemporary practice*, ed 2, Philadelphia, 2002, Lippincott.

Johansson A, Dahlberg K, Ekebergh M: Living with experiences following a myocardial infarction, *Euro J Cardiovasc Nurs* 2:229, 2003.

Koonce T, Giuse D, Beauregard J et al: Toward a more informed patient: bridging health care information through an interactive communication portal, *J Med Libr Assoc* 95(1):77, 2007.

LeClere CM, Wells DL, Craig D et al: Falling short of the mark, *Clin Nurs Res* 11(3):242-263, 2002.

• = Independent;   ▲ = Collaborative;   EBN = Evidence-Based Nursing;   EB = Evidence-Based

Leininger MM, McFarland MR: *Transcultural nursing: concepts, theories, research and practices,* ed 3, New York, 2002, McGraw-Hill.

Lyons KS, Stewart BJ, Archbold PG et al: Pessimism and optimism as early warning signs for compromised health for caregivers of patients with Parkinson's disease, *Nurs Res* 53(6):354-362, 2004.

Matsumoto N, Ikeda M, Fukuhara R et al: Caregiver burden associated with behavioral and psychological symptoms of dementia in elderly people in the local community, *Dement Geriatr Cogn Disord,* 23(4): e219-224, 2007.

Melnyk BM, Alpert-Gillis L, Feinstein NF et al: Creating opportunities for parent empowerment: program effects on the mental health/coping outcomes of critically ill young children and their mothers, *Pediatrics* 113(6):e597-607, 2004.

Norris J, Spelic SS: Supporting adaption to body image disruption, *Rehabil Nurs* 27(1):8-12, 2002.

Northouse L, Walker J, Schafenacker A et al: A family-based program of care for women with recurrent breast cancer and their family members, *Oncol Nurs Forum* 29(10):1411-1419, 2002.

Phillips JM, Cohen MZ, Moses G: Breast cancer screening and African American women: fear, fatalism, and silence, *Oncol Nurs Forum* 26(3):561, 1999.

Powe BD, Finnie R: Cancer fatalism: the state of the science, *Cancer Nurs* 26(6):454-465, 2003.

Reynaud SN, Meeker BJ: Coping styles of older adults with ostomies, *J Gerontol Nurs* 28(5):30-6, May 2002.

Richer MC, Ezer H: Living in it, living with it, and moving on: dimensions of meaning during chemotherapy, *Oncol Nurs Forum* 29(1):113-119, 2002.

Samuel-Hodge CD, Headen SW, Skelly AH et al: Influences on day-to-day self-management of type 2 diabetes among African-American women: spirituality, the multi-caregiver role, and other social context factors, *Diabetes Care* 23(7):928-933, 2000.

Snyder CR, Lehman KA, Kluck B et al: Hope for rehabilitation and vice versa, *Rehab Psychol* 51(2):89-112, 2006.

Wagner JM: Lived experience of critically ill patients' family members during cardiopulmonary resuscitation: *Am J Crit Care* 13(5): 416-420, 2004.

Wassem R, Beckham N, Dudley W: Test of a nursing intervention to promote adjustment to fibromyalgia, *Orthop Nurs* 20(3):33-45, 2001.

Weiss SJ, Chen JL: Factors influencing maternal mental health and family functioning during the low birthweight infant's first year of life, *J Pediatr Nurs* 17(2):114-125, 2002.

White N, Bichter J, Koeckeritz J et al: A cross-cultural comparison of family resiliency in hemodialysis patients, *J Transcult Nurs* 13(3):218-227, 2002.

Disturbed Body image   *Dale Nasby, RNCNS, and Gail B. Ladwig, MSN, CHTP, RN*

NANDA   Definition

Confusion in mental picture of one's physical self

Defining Characteristics

Behaviors of acknowledgment of one's body; behaviors of avoidance on one's body; behaviors of monitoring one's body; nonverbal response to actual change in body (e.g., appearance, structure, or function); nonverbal response to perceived change in body (e.g., appearance, structure, or function); verbalization of feelings that reflect an altered view of one's body (e.g. appearance, structure, function); verbalization of perceptions that reflect an altered view of one's body appearance

Objective

Actual change in function; actual change in structure; behaviors of acknowledging one's body; behaviors of monitoring one's body; change in ability to estimate spatial relationship of body to environment; change in social involvement; extension of body boundary to incorporate environmental objects; intentional hiding of body part; intentional overexposure of body part; missing body part; not looking at body part; not touching body part; trauma to nonfunctioning part; unintentional hiding of body part; unintentional overexposing of body part

Subjective

Depersonalization of loss by impersonal pronouns; depersonalization of part by impersonal pronouns; emphasis of remaining strengths; fear of reaction by others; fear of rejection by others; focus on past appearance; focus on past function; focus on past strength; heightened achievement; negative feelings about body (e.g., feeling of helplessness, hopelessness, or powerlessness); personalization of loss; personalization of part by name; preoccupation with change; preoccupation with loss; refusal to verify actual change; verbalization of change in lifestyle

Related Factors (r/t)

Biophysical; cognitive; cultural; developmental changes; illness; illness treatment; injury; perceptual; psychosocial; spiritual; surgery; trauma

• = Independent;   ▲ = Collaborative;   EBN = Evidence-Based Nursing;   EB = Evidence-Based

B

Suggested NOC Outcomes

Body Image, Self-Control, Psychosocial Adjustment: Life Change, Self-Esteem

NOC Outcome with Indicators
Body Image as evidenced by the following indicators: Congruence between body reality, body ideal, and body presentation/Satisfaction with body appearance/Adjustment to changes in physical appearance (Rate the outcome and indicators of **Body Image:** 1 = never positive, 2 = rarely positive, 3 = sometimes positive, 4 = often positive, 5 = consistently positive [see Section I].)

Client Outcomes

Client Will (Specify Time Frame):

- Demonstrate adaptation to changes in physical appearance or body function as evidenced by adjustment to lifestyle change
- Identify and change irrational beliefs and expectations regarding body size or function
- Verbalize congruence between body reality and body perception
- Describe, touch, or observe affected body part
- Demonstrate social involvement rather than avoidance and utilize adaptive coping and/or social skills
- Utilize cognitive strategies or other coping skills to improve perception of body image and enhance functioning
- Utilize strategies to enhance appearance (e.g., wig, clothing)

NIC   Interventions (Nursing Interventions Classification)

Suggested NIC Intervention

Body Image Enhancement

Example NIC Activities—Body Image Enhancement
Determine patient's body image expectations based on developmental stage; Assist patient to identify actions that will enhance appearance

Nursing Interventions and *Rationales*

- Incorporate psychosocial questions related to body image as part of nursing assessment to identify clients at risk for body image disturbance (e.g., body builders, cancer survivors, clients with eating disorders, burns, skin disorders, polycystic ovary disease, or those with stomas/ostomies/colostomies or other disfiguring conditions). **EB:** *Assessment of psychosocial issues can help to identify clients at risk for body image concerns as a result of a disfiguring condition (Rumsey, et al, 2004).*
- If client is at risk for body image disturbance, consider using a tool such as the Body Image Quality of Life Inventory (BIQLI), which quantifies both the positive and negative effects of body image on one's psychosocial quality of life. **EB:** *A favorable body image quality of life was related to higher self-esteem, optimism, and social support in both sexes and less eating disturbance among women (Cash, Jakatdar & Williams, 2003).* **EBN:** *Using a body image scale can help nurses to identify possible body image disturbances and to plan individual nursing interventions (Souto & Garcia, 2002).*
- ▲ Assess for body dysmorphic disorder (BDD) and refer to psychiatry or other appropriate provider. *BDD is characterized by a preoccupation with an imagined defect in appearance that causes significant distress or impairment in social, occupational, or other areas of functioning.* **EB:** *Clients with BDD often seek medical treatment in dermatology or other areas to correct the imagined defect and thus*

• = Independent;   ▲ = Collaborative;   EBN = Evidence-Based Nursing;   EB = Evidence-Based

may be seen by many healthcare providers. Phillips & Diaz (1997) found that approximately 20% of clients receiving psychiatric treatment for BDD had cosmetic surgery.

▲ Assess for the possibility of muscle dysmorphia (pathological preoccupation with muscularity and leanness; occurs more often in males than in females) and make appropriate referrals. **EB:** *This condition is often seen among body builders or those in sports that emphasize size and bulk (e.g., wrestling) and will likely continue to increase with the societal focus on body image. Fluoxetine alone or in combination with CBT may be an effective treatment (Leone, Sedory & Grayl, 2005).*

• Assess client and family response to surgery that results in a change in body and offer support. **EBN:** *A qualitative study by Notter and Burnard (2006) revealed that although many clients and family members received education before surgery, most felt the reality of it differed significantly from their expectations.*

• If nursing assessment reveals body image concerns related to a disfiguring condition, assist client in voicing his/her concerns and if appropriate, coaching the client in how to respond to questions from others in social situations. If within the nurse's level of expertise, may assist client in graded practice in social situations (e.g., going to hairdresser, swimming pool). **EB:** *Many clients with disfiguring conditions are concerned about and may avoid exposing the disfigurement to others' gaze and displays of ignorance and negative comments by others (Rumsey et al, 2004; Newell, 1999).*

▲ Refer clients with body image disturbance for CBT and/or social skills training if indicated. **EB:** *CBT and social skills training help clients learn new mental scripts for interacting with others, challenge negative thoughts and replacing these with new thoughts, and applying new behaviors and thoughts in social situations (Jarry & Ip, 2005; Newell & Clarke, 2000).*

• Acknowledge denial, anger, or depression as normal feelings when adjusting to changes in body and lifestyle. However, allow client to share emotions when they are ready, rather than rushing them. **EB:** *The influence of emotion-focused coping (venting emotions and mental disengagement) on distress following disfiguring injury was associated with less body image disturbance (Fauerbach et al, 2002).*

• Encourage the client to discuss interpersonal and social conflicts that may arise. **EB:** *Changes in physical appearance and function associated with disease processes (and sometimes treatment) need to be integrated into the interaction that occurs between clients and lay caregivers (Price, 2000).*

• Explore opportunities to assist the client to develop a realistic perception of his or her body image. **EB:** *Actual body size may not be consistent with the client's perceived body size. Inaccurate perception by the client can be unhealthy (Townsend, 2003).*

• Help client describe self-ideal, and identify self-criticisms, to foster acceptance of self. **EB:** *The perception of self-image involves knowing the self and what is important and valued. Disability causes individuals to live as changed human beings regardless of whether they are willing to do so (Pohl & Winland-Brown, 1992).*

• Encourage clients to verbalize treatment preferences and play a role in treatment decisions. **EB:** *Women who received the treatment they preferred for stage 1 or 2 breast cancer had better body image (and mental health) than women who did not. Good communication between physicians and women improved outcomes (Figueiredo et al, 2004).*

• Encourage the clients to write a narrative description of their changes. **EB:** *One's experience of coping or adjustment to a disability is represented as narratives about himself or herself. Each person with traumatic brain injury (TBI) reconstructed certain self-narratives when coping with their changed self-images and daily lives (Nochi, 2000).*

• Take cues from clients regarding readiness to look at wound (may ask if client has seen wound yet) and utilize client's questions or comments as way to teach about wound care and healing. **EB:** *Clients with disfiguring conditions, in this case burns, respond in a variety of ways, and the severity of the disfigurement does not always predict impact on body image. Tailoring interventions to individual clients and reading their nonverbal cues likely contributes to clients' ability to heal emotionally from impact of wound on body image (Birdsall & Weinberg, 2001).*

• Encourage the client to continue same personal care routine that was followed before the change in body image. It is preferable that this care be completed in the bathroom and not in bed. **EBN:** *This routine gives the client privacy and also prevents the client from settling into an "invalid" role. Women who resume familiar routines and habits heal better and suffer less depression than those who settle into the role of client (Johnson, 1994).*

• = Independent; ▲ = Collaborative; EBN = Evidence-Based Nursing; EB = Evidence-Based

B

- Encourage the client to purchase clothes that are attractive and that deemphasize their disability. **EB:** *Individuals with osteoporosis are not usually disabled but may perceive themselves as unattractive and experience social isolation as a result of ill-fitting clothes that accentuate the physical changes (Sedlak & Doheny, 2000).*
- Encourage client to participate in regular aerobic exercise when feasible. **EB:** *A systematic review of exercise during and after cancer treatment found that exercise may be an effective intervention to improve body image but depends on many factors (e.g., stage of treatment, client lifestyle) (Knols, Aaronson & Uebelhart, 2005).* **EB:** *A meta-analysis examined research regarding the impact of exercise on body image and concluded that exercise was associated with improved body image (Hausenblas & Fallon, 2006).*
- ▲ Provide client with a list of appropriate community resources (e.g., Reach to Recovery, Ostomy Association). **EB:** *Motivation, sharing of experiences, camaraderie with and support from peers, and knowledge of not being alone have been identified as advantages of group learning (Payne, 1993).*

Geriatric

- Focus on remaining abilities. Have client make a list of strengths. **EB:** *Results from unstructured interviews with women aged 61 to 92 years regarding their perceptions and feelings about their aging bodies suggest that women exhibit the internalization of ageist beauty norms, even as they assert that health is more important to them than physical attractiveness and comment on the "naturalness" of the aging process (Hurd, 2000).*
- Encourage regular exercise for the elderly. **EB:** *Researchers in this study conclude that regular exercise had positive effects on the self-esteem and body image of elderly women (Anonymous, 2001).*

Multicultural

- Assess for the influence of cultural beliefs, norms, and values on the client's body image. **EBN:** *The client's body image may be based on cultural perceptions, as well as influences from the larger social context. Use of pan-ethnic status such as Asian or Hispanic may obscure important ethnic group differences (Yates, Edman & Aruguete, 2004).* **EBN:** *Body image is affected by relationships between tactile space and visual space, special behavior, and proximity to others (Giger & Davidhizar, 2004). Each client should be assessed for body image based on the phenomenon of communication, time, space, social organization, environmental control, and biological variations (Giger & Davidhizar, 2004).*
- Assess for the presence of conflicting cultural demands. **EBN:** *Poor peer socialization and family rigidity were found to be related to the preoccupation with body size and slimness in a young female Mexican-American population (Kuba & Harris, 2001).*
- Assess for the presence of depressive symptoms. **EBN:** *Body image attitudes were significantly related to depressive symptoms in a study of diverse postpartum women (Walker et al, 2002).*
- Acknowledge that body image disturbances can affect all individuals regardless of culture, race, or ethnicity. **EBN:** *Body image disturbances are pervasive across western cultures and appear to increase in other cultures with acculturation to western ideals (Hebl, King & Lin, 2004).* **EB:** *Non-Caucasian girls were found to report higher internalization of the thin ideal than their Caucasian peers (Hermes & Keele, 2003).*

Home Care

- Above interventions may be adapted for home care use.
- Assess client's level of social support as it is one of the determinants of client's recovery and emotional health. **EBN:** *Females who perceived they have good social support were found to adapt better to changes in body image after stoma surgery (Brown & Randle, 2005).*
- Assess family/caregiver level of acceptance of client's body changes. **EB:** *Family members' expressions and reactions were found to impact women's coping, and negative reactions in particular increased the women's level of anxiety. Negative feedback from family/caregiver can influence client's reactions and ability to adjust to body changes negatively (Brown & Randle, 2005).*

• = Independent;   ▲ = Collaborative;   EBN = Evidence-Based Nursing;   EB = Evidence-Based

- Recognize that older women may continue their younger preoccupation with weight and recurrent dieting, despite being at normal weight. Assess source of low weight or weight loss with this in mind. **EB:** *Reports suggest that elderly women continue to be preoccupied with being thin. Increased awareness of eating habits and weight preoccupation in elderly women has been recommended (Fallaz et al, 1999).*
- Encourage client to discuss concerns related to sexuality and provide support or information as indicated. Many conditions that affect body image also affect sexuality. **EB:** *Brown & Randall (2005) found that clients (particularly females) with stomas often believe they are less sexually attractive after surgery, though their sexual partner may not share that view. However, clients who underwent urostomy surgery often experienced a decrease in sexual functioning.*
- Teach all aspects of care. Involve client and caregivers in self-care as soon as possible. Do this in stages if client still has difficulty looking at or touching changed body part. *Involvement in self-care improves likelihood of acceptance of body change, and improved body image and self-esteem.*
- ▲ Refer for prosthetic device if appropriate. **EB:** *Swanson, Stube, and Edman (2005) found that use of the C-Leg for lower limb amputees improved body image due to feeling more secure in public (stability of device) and ability to walk with a more natural gait.*

Client/Family Teaching

- Teach appropriate care of surgical site (e.g., mastectomy site, amputation site, ostomy site). *Client teaching by enterostomal therapist (ET) nurses may alleviate problems associated with altered body image in relation to the presence of an ostomy (Tomaselli, Jenks & Morin, 1991).*
- Inform client of available community support groups; offer to make initial phone call. *Motivation, sharing of experiences, camaraderie with and support from peers, and knowledge of not being alone have been identified as advantages of group learning (Payne, 1993).*
- ▲ Refer the client to counseling for help adjusting to body change. *Counseling is important for a client who is trying to create a new body ideal or work through a grief process (Price, 1990).*
- Provide printed material and didactic information for significant others. *Some significant others prefer to receive didactic material rather than vent their feelings as a way of showing support (Northouse & Peters-Golden, 1993).*
- Encourage significant others to offer support. *Social support from significant others enhances both emotional and physical health (Badger, 1990).*
- Direct social support as follows: instruct regarding practical care (bandaging); encourage appraisal support (listening); encourage self-esteem support (favorable comparisons between client's and others' appearance); and encourage sense of belonging (assist with socializing). *The preceding are four categories of support recognized in the body-image care model. Clients with an active social support network are likely to make better progress than those without support (Price, 1990).*
- ▲ Refer clients who are having difficulty with personal acceptance, personal and social body image disruption, sexual concerns, reduced self-care skills, and the management of surgical complications to an interdisciplinary team or specialist (e.g. ostomy nurse) if available. **EB:** *A multidisciplinary team approach that includes an ET nurse, psychologist, and surgeon work together to assist clients deal with body image concerns. The multidisciplinary approach has been demonstrated to be successful in facilitating adaptation to an altered body image (Walsh et al, 1995).* **EB:** *Clients who had a stoma had problems with body image (Ross et al, 2006).*

evolve   See the EVOLVE website for World Wide Web resources for client education.

REFERENCES

Anonymous: Active seniors less susceptible to depression, *J Phys Educ Recreat Dance* 72(1):9-11, 2001.

Badger V: Men with cardiovascular disease and their spouses: coping, health and marital adjustment, *Arch Psychiatr Nurs* 4:319, 1990.

Birdsall C, Weinberg K: Adult clients looking at their burn injuries for the first time, *J Burn Care Rehabal* 22(5):360-364, 2001.

Brown H, Randle J: Living with a stoma: a review of the literature, *J Clin Nurs* 14(1):74-81, 2005.

Cash TF, Jakatdar TA, Williams, EF: The body image quality of life inventory: further validation with college men and women, *Body Image* 11(4):279-287, 2003.

Fallaz AF, Bernstein M, Van Nes MC et al: Weight loss preoccupation in aging women: a review, *J Nutr Health Aging* 3:177-181, 1999.

Fauerbach JA, Heinberg LJ, Lawrence JW et al: Coping with body image changes following a disfiguring burn injury, *Health Psychol* 21(2):115-121, 2002.

Figueiredo MI, Cullen J, Yi-Ting H et al: Breast cancer treatment in older women: does getting what you want improve your long-term body image and mental health? *J Clin Oncol* 22(19):4002-4009, 2004.

Giger J, Davidhizar R: *Transcultural nursing: assessment and intervention*, ed 4, St. Louis, 2004, Mosby.

Hausenblas HA, Fallon E: Exercise and body image: a meta-analysis, *Psychol Health* 21(1):33-47, 2006.

Hebl MR, King EB, Lin J: The swimsuit becomes us all: ethnicity, gender, and vulnerability to self-objectification, *Pers Soc Psychol Bull* 30(10):1322-1331, 2004.

Hermes SF, Keel PK: The influence of puberty and ethnicity on awareness and internalization of the thin ideal, *Int J Eat Disord* 33(4):465-467, 2003.

Hurd LC: Older women's body image and embodied experience: an exploration, *J Women Aging* 12(3-4):77-97, 2000.

Jarry JL, Ip K: The effectiveness of stand-alone cognitive-behavioural therapy for body image: a meta-analysis, *Body Image* 2(4):317-331, 2005.

Johnson J: Caring for the woman who's had a mastectomy, *Am J Nurs* 94:24-31, 1994.

Knols R, Aaronson NK, Uebelhart D: Physical exercise in cancer clients during and after medical treatment: a systematic review of randomized and controlled clinical trials, *J Clin Oncol* 23(19):3830-3842, 2005.

Kuba SA, Harris DJ: Eating disturbances in women of color: an exploratory study of contextual factors in the development of disordered eating in Mexican American women, *Health Care Women Int* 22(3):281-298, 2001.

Leone JE, Sedory EJ, Gray, KA: Recognition and treatment of muscle dysmorphia and related body image disorders, *J Athl Train* 40(4):352-359, 2005.

Newell R, Clarke M: Evaluation of a self help leaflet in treatment of social difficulties following facial disfigurement, *Int J Nurs Studies* 37(5):381-388, 2000.

Newell RJ: Altered body image: a fear-avoidance model of psychosocial difficulties following disfigurement, *J Adv Nurs* 30(5):1230-1238, 1999.

Nochi M: Reconstructing self-narratives in coping with traumatic brain injury, *Soc Sci Med* 51(12):1795-1804, 2000.

Northouse L, Peters-Golden H: Cancer and the family: strategies to assist spouses, *Semin Oncol Nurs* 9:74-82, 1993.

Notter J, Burnard P: Preparing for loop ileostomy surgery: women's accounts from a qualitative study, *Int J Nurs Studies* 43(2):147-159, 2006.

Payne J: The contribution of group learning to the rehabilitation of spinal cord injured adults, *Rehabil Nurs* 18:375-379, 1993.

Phillips KA, Diaz S: Gender differences in body dysmorphic disorder, *J Nerv Ment Dis* 185(9):570–577, 1997.

Pohl C, Winland-Brown J: The meaning of disability in a caring environment, *J Nurs Adm* 22(6):29-35, 1992.

Price B: A model for body-image care, *J Adv Nurs* 15(5):585-593, 1990.

Price B: Altered body image: managing social encounters, *Int J Palliat Nurs* 6(4):179-185, 2000.

Ross L, Abild-Nielsen AG, Thomsen BL et al: Quality of life of Danish colorectal cancer patients with and without a stoma, *Support Care Cancer*, Nov. 14, 2006 (Epub ahead of print).

Rumsey N, Clarke A, White P et al: Altered body image: appearance related concerns of people with visible disfigurement, *J Adv Nursing* 48(5):443-453, 2004.

Sedlak CA, Doheny MO: Fashion tips for women with osteoporosis, *Orthop Nurs* 19(5):31-35, 2000.

Souto CMR, Garcia TR: Construction and validation of a body image rating scale: a preliminary study, *Int J Nurs Terminol Classif* 13(4):117-126, 2002.

Swanson E, Stube J, Edman, P: Function and body image levels in individuals with transfemoral amputation using the C-Leg, *JPO* 17(3):80-84, 2005.

Tomaselli N, Jenks J, Morin K: Body image in clients with stomas: a critical review of the literature, *J ET Nurs* 18(3):95-99, 1991.

Townsend MC: *Psychiatric mental health nursing: concepts of care*, Saddle River, NJ, 2003, FA Davis.

Walker L, Timmerman GM, Kim M et al: Relationships between body image and depressive symptoms during postpartum in ethnically diverse, low income women, *Women Health* 36(3):101-121, 2002.

Walsh BA, Grunert BK, Telford GL et al: Multidisciplinary management of altered body image in the client with an ostomy, *J Wound Ostomy Continence Nurs* 22(5):227-236, 1995.

Yates A, Edman J, Aruguete M: Ethnic differences in BMI and body/self-dissatisfaction among Whites, Asian subgroups, Pacific Islanders, and African-Americans, *J Adolesc Health* 34(4):300-307, 2004.

Risk for imbalanced Body temperature   *Betty J. Ackley, MSN, EdS, RN*

NANDA   Definition

At risk for failure to maintain body temperature within a normal range

Risk Factors

Altered metabolic rate; dehydration; exposure to cold/cool environments; exposure to warm/hot environments; extremes of age or weight; illness affecting temperature regulation; inactivity; inappropriate clothing for environmental temperature; medications causing vasoconstriction; medications causing vasodilation; sedation; trauma affecting temperature regulation; vigorous activity

NOC   Outcomes (Nursing Outcomes Classification)

Suggested NOC Outcomes

Thermoregulation, Thermoregulation: Newborn

• = Independent;   ▲ = Collaborative;   EBN = Evidence-Based Nursing;   EB = Evidence-Based

B

Example NOC Outcome with Indicators
Thermoregulation as evidenced by the following indicators: Increased or decreased skin temperature/ Hyperthermia/Hypothermia/Skin color changes/Dehydration (Rate the outcome and indicators of **Thermoregulation:** 1 = severe, 2 = substantial, 3 = moderate, 4 = mild, 5 = none [see Section I].)

Client Outcomes

Client Will (Specify Time Frame):

- Maintain temperature within normal range
- Explain measures needed to maintain normal temperature
- Identify symptoms of hypothermia or hyperthermia

NIC   Interventions (Nursing Interventions Classification)

Suggested NIC Interventions

Temperature Regulation, Temperature Regulation: Intraoperative, Vital Signs Monitoring

Example NIC Activities—Temperature Regulation
Institute a continuous core temperature monitoring device as appropriate; Promote adequate fluid and nutritional intake

Nursing Interventions and *Rationales*

Refer to the interventions and rationales for **Ineffective Thermoregulation**

Bowel incontinence   *Mikel Gray, PhD, CUNP, CCCN, FAAN*

NANDA   Definition

Change in normal bowel elimination habits characterized by involuntary passage of stool

Defining Characteristics

Constant dribbling of soft stool, fecal odor; inability to delay defecation; rectal urgency; self-report of inability to feel rectal fullness or presence of stool in bowel; fecal staining of underclothing; recognition of rectal fullness but reported inability to expel formed stool; inattention to urge to defecate; inability to recognize urge to defecate; irritation of perianal skin

Related Factors (r/t)

Change in stool consistency (diarrhea, constipation, fecal impaction); abnormal motility (metabolic disorders, inflammatory bowel disease, infectious disease, drug-induced motility disorders, food intolerance); defects in rectal vault function (low rectal compliance from ischemia, fibrosis, radiation, infectious proctitis, Hirschprung's disease, local or infiltrating neoplasm, severe rectocele); sphincter dysfunction (obstetric- or traumatic-induced incompetence, fistula or abscess, prolapse, third-degree hemorrhoids, high-tone pelvic floor muscle dysfunction); neurological disorders impacting gastrointestinal motility, rectal vault function, and sphincter function (cerebrovascular accident, spinal injury, traumatic brain injury, central nervous system tumor, advanced stage dementia, encephalopathy, profound mental retardation, multiple sclerosis, myelodysplasia and related neural tube defects, gastroparesis of diabetes mellitus, heavy metal poisoning, chronic alcoholism, infectious or autoimmune neurological disorders, myasthenia gravis)

• = Independent;   ▲ = Collaborative;   EBN = Evidence-Based Nursing;   EB = Evidence-Based

B

NOC   Outcomes (Nursing Outcomes Classification)

Suggested NOC Outcomes

Bowel Continence, Bowel Elimination

Example NOC Outcome with Indicators
Bowel Continence as evidenced by the following indicators: Maintains predictable pattern of stool evacuation/ Maintains control of stool passage/Evacuates stool at least every 3 days (Rate the outcome and indicators of **Bowel Continence:** 1 = never demonstrated, 2 = rarely demonstrated, 3 = sometimes demonstrated, 4 = often demonstrated, 5 = consistently demonstrated [see Section I].)

Client Outcomes

Client Will (Specify Time Frame):

- Have regular, complete evacuation of fecal contents from the rectal vault (pattern may vary from every day to every 3 to 5 days) (Roig et al, 1993)
- Have regulation of stool consistency (soft, formed stools)
- Reduce or eliminate frequency of incontinent episodes
- Demonstrate intact skin in the perianal/perineal area
- Demonstrate the ability to isolate, contract, and relax pelvic muscles (when incontinence related to sphincter incompetence or high-tone pelvic floor dysfunction)
- Increase pelvic muscle strength (when incontinence related to sphincter incompetence)

NIC   Interventions (Nursing Interventions Classification)

Suggested NIC Interventions

Bowel Incontinence Care, Bowel Incontinence Care: Encopresis, Bowel Training

Example NIC Interventions—Bowel Incontinence Care
Determine physical or psychological cause of fecal incontinence; Instruct patient/family to record fecal output, as appropriate

Nursing Interventions and *Rationales*

- In a private setting, directly question any client at risk about the presence of fecal incontinence. If the client reports altered bowel elimination patterns, problems with bowel control, or "uncontrollable diarrhea," complete a focused nursing history including previous and present bowel elimination routines, dietary history, frequency and volume of uncontrolled stool loss, and aggravating and alleviating factors. *Unless questioned directly, clients are unlikely to report the presence of fecal incontinence (Schultz, Dickey & Skoner, 1997). The nursing history determines the patterns of stool elimination, to characterize involuntary stool loss, and the likely etiology of the incontinence (Norton & Chelvanayagam, 2000).*
- Women who have been pregnant and have delivered one or more children vaginally should be routinely screened for fecal incontinence. **EB:** *A study of women during a routine gynecologic exam revealed a 26.8% prevalence of anal and urinary incontinence symptoms, and the majority stated a desire to receive professional advice and assistance with these symptoms. However, 67% were not asked about their condition (Griffiths, Makam & Edwards, 2006).*
- ▲ In close consultation with a physician or advanced practice nurse, consider routine use of a validated tool that focuses on bowel elimination patterns. *More than 23 validated symptom questionnaires have been developed and validated for the evaluation of urinary and fecal incontinence (Avery et al, 2007).*
- Complete a focused physical assessment including inspection of perineal skin, pelvic muscle

---

• = Independent;   ▲ = Collaborative;   EBN = Evidence-Based Nursing;   EB = Evidence-Based

strength assessment, digital examination of the rectum for presence of impaction and anal sphincter strength, and evaluation of functional status (mobility, dexterity, visual acuity). *A focused physical examination (including a vaginal examination to determine coexisting pelvic organ prolapse) assists in determining the severity of fecal leakage and its likely etiology; it should be completed prior to functional testing such as anorectal manometry or anal sphincter electromyography (Rao, 2006). A functional assessment provides important information concerning the impact of functional status on stool elimination patterns and incontinence (Gray & Burns, 1996).*

- Complete an assessment of cognitive function. *Dementia, acute confusion, and mental retardation are risk factors for fecal incontinence (O'Donnell et al, 1992; Norton & Chelvanaygam, 2000).*
- Document patterns of stool elimination and incontinent episodes through a bowel record, including frequency of bowel movements, stool consistency, frequency and severity of incontinent episodes, precipitating factors, and dietary and fluid intake. *This document, used to confirm the verbal history, assists in determining the likely etiology of stool incontinence and serves as a baseline to evaluate treatment efficacy (Norton & Chelvanayagam, 2000).*
- Assess stool consistency and its influence on risk for stool loss. *Several classification systems for stool have been promulgated (Bliss et al, 2001b). They assist the nurse and client to differentiate between normal soft, formed stool, hardened stools associated with constipation, and liquid stools associated with diarrhea.* **EBN:** *A study of stool consistency found good reliability when evaluated by professional nurses, student nurses, and clients. Word-only descriptors yielded equivocal consistency when assessed by subjects as did tools that combined words with illustrations of various stool consistencies (Bliss et al, 2001B).*
- Identify conditions contributing to or causing fecal incontinence. *Fecal incontinence is frequently multifactorial. Accurate assessment of the probable etiology of fecal incontinence is necessary to select a treatment plan likely to control or eliminate the condition (Norton & Chelvanayagam, 2000).*
- Improve access to toileting:
  - Identify usual toileting patterns among persons in the acute care or long-term care facility and plan opportunities for toileting accordingly.
  - Provide assistance with toileting for clients with limited access or impaired functional status (mobility, dexterity, access).
  - Institute a prompted toileting program for persons with impaired cognitive status (retardation, dementia).
  - Provide adequate privacy for toileting.
  - Respond promptly to requests for assistance with toileting.
  Acute or transient fecal incontinence frequently occurs in the acute care or long-term care facility because of inadequate access to toileting facilities, insufficient assistance with toileting, or inadequate privacy when attempting to toilet (Bliss et al, 2000; Gray and Burns, 1996).
- Counsel clients with fecal incontinence associated with liquid stools (diarrhea) about methods to normalize stool consistency via dietary fiber or fiber supplements. *A liquid stool is associated with an increased likelihood of fecal incontinence (Bliss et al, 2000).* **EBN:** *Daily supplementation of dietary fiber using a product containing psyllium improved stool consistency and reduced frequency of incontinent stools (Bliss et al, 2001a).*
- For the client with intermittent episodes of fecal incontinence related to acute changes in stool consistency, begin a bowel reeducation program consisting of:
  - Cleansing the bowel of impacted stool if indicated
  - Normalizing stool consistency by adequate intake of fluids (30 mL/kg of body weight/day) and dietary or supplemental fiber
  - Establishing a regular routine of fecal elimination based on established patterns of bowel elimination (patterns established prior to onset of incontinence)
  Bowel reeducation is designed to reestablish normal defecation patterns and to normalize stool consistency in order to reduce or eliminate the risk of recurring fecal incontinence associated with changes in stool consistency (Doughty & Jensen, 2006).
- Begin a prompted defecation program for the adult with dementia, mental retardation, or related learning disabilities. *Prompted urine and fecal elimination programs have been shown to reduce or eliminate incontinence in the long-term care facility and in community settings (Doughty & Jensen, 2006; Smith et al, 1994).*

• = Independent;   ▲ = Collaborative;   EBN = Evidence-Based Nursing;   EB = Evidence-Based

B

- Begin a scheduled stimulation defecation program for persons with neurological conditions causing fecal incontinence including the following steps:
  - Cleanse the bowel of impacted fecal material before beginning the program.
  - Implement strategies to normalize stool consistency including adequate intake of fluid and fiber and avoidance of foods associated with diarrhea.
  - Determine a regular schedule for bowel elimination (typically every day or every other day) based on prior patterns of bowel elimination whenever feasible.
  - Provide a stimulus before assisting the client to a position on the toilet; digital stimulation, a stimulating suppository, "mini-enema," or pulsed evacuation enema may be used for stimulation.

  The scheduled, stimulated program relies on consistency of stool, and a mechanical or chemical stimulus to produce a bolus contraction of the rectum with evacuation of fecal material (Doughty & Jensen, 2006; Dunn & Galka; 1994; King, Currie & Wright, 1994, Munchiando & Kendall, 1993).

▲ Begin a reeducation or pelvic floor muscle exercise program for the person with sphincter incompetence or high-tone pelvic floor muscle dysfunction of the pelvic muscles, or refer persons with fecal incontinence related to sphincter dysfunction to a nurse specialist or other therapist with clinical expertise in these techniques of care. **EB:** *There is insufficient evidence to conclude that bowel reeducation or pelvic floor muscle exercise programs are effective for the management of fecal incontinence in adults, but the existing evidence does provide adequate support to consider implementing this intervention in selected clients, particularly given the potential for benefit in the absence of harmful side effects (Norton, Hosker & Brazzelli, 2006). A nonrandomized cohort study of 281 clients with fecal incontinence revealed modest improvement in most clients undergoing pelvic floor muscle rehabilitation and profound improvement in a minority of subjects (Terra et al, 2006).*

- Begin a pelvic muscle biofeedback program among clients with urgency to defecate and fecal incontinence related to recurrent diarrhea. *Pelvic muscle reeducation, including biofeedback, can reduce uncontrolled loss of stool among persons who experience urgency and diarrhea as provocative factors for fecal incontinence (Chiarioni et al, 1993).*

- Institute a structured skin care regimen that incorporates three essential steps: cleanse, moisturize, and protect. Select a cleanser with a pH range comparable to that of normal skin (usually labeled "pH balanced"), moisturize with an emollient to replace lipids removed with cleansing, and protect with a skin protectant containing a petrolatum, dimethicone, or zinc oxide base, or a no-sting skin barrier. Skin that is exposed to urine and/or stool should be cleansed daily and following major incontinence episodes. When feasible, select a product that combined two or all three of these processes into a single step. Ensure that products are available at the bedside when caring for a client with total incontinence in an inpatient facility. *Urinary incontinence, particularly when combined with fecal incontinence or use of absorptive pads or adult containment briefs, increases the risk of incontinence-associated dermatitis.* **EBN:** *A structured skin care regimen based on a three-step process (cleanse, moisturize, and protect) is effective for the prevention of incontinence-associated dermatitis (Gray et al, 2007).*

- Cleanse the perineal and perianal skin following each episode of fecal incontinence. *Frequent cleaning with soap and water may compromise perianal skin integrity and enhance the irritation produced by fecal leakage (Gray et al, 2007).*

- Apply a moisture barrier containing dimethicone or zinc oxide to clients with severe urinary incontinence or those with double urinary and fecal incontinence. *Clients with very severe incontinence and those with double fecal and urinary incontinence (particularly when the stool is liquefied) typically require a product with vigorous moisture barrier qualities. Petrolatum-based products containing dimethicone or zinc oxide are preferred (Gray et al, 2007).*

▲ Consult the physician or advanced practice nurse concerning use of a moisture barrier with active healing ingredients when perineal dermatitis exists. Apply and teach care providers to use the product sparingly when applying to affected areas. **EBN:** *Xenaderm contains active ingredients (Balsam Peru, trypsin, and castor oil) that have been shown more effective than placebo for the management of partial thickness wounds in clients with urinary or fecal incontinence (Gray & Jones, 2004). A thin layer of an antifungal powder may be layered beneath the ointment, but excessive application may paradoxically retain moisture and diminish its effectiveness (Evans & Gray, 2003; Gray, Ratliff & Donovan, 2002).*

B

- Assist the client to select and apply a containment device for occasional episodes of fecal incontinence. *A fecal containment device will prevent soiling of clothing and reduce odors in the client with uncontrolled stool loss (Brazzelli, Shirran & Vale, 2003).*
- Teach the caregiver of the client with frequent episodes of fecal incontinence and limited mobility to regularly monitor the sacrum and perineal area for pressure ulcerations. *Limited mobility, particularly when combined with fecal incontinence, increases the risk of pressure ulceration. Routine cleansing, pressure reduction techniques, and management of fecal and urinary incontinence reduce this risk (Johanson, Irizarry & Doughty, 1997; Schnelle et al, 1997).*
- ▲ Teach the client with more frequent stool loss to apply an anal continence plug in consultation with the physician. *The anal continence plug is a device that can reduce or eliminate persistent liquid or solid stool incontinence in selected clients (Doherty, 2004).*
- Apply a fecal pouch to the critically ill client with frequent stool loss, particularly when fecal incontinence produces altered perianal skin integrity. *Fecal pouches contain stool loss, reduce odor, and protect the perianal skin from chemical irritation related to contact with stool (Fiers & Thayer, 2000; Waldrop & Doughty, 2000).*
- ▲ Consult a physician or advanced practice nurse about insertion of a bowel management system in the critically ill client with frequent stool loss, particularly when fecal incontinence produces altered perianal skin integrity. *Introduction of the Zassi Bowel Management system coincided with a clinically relevant decline in perineal and perianal skin damage among critical care clients managed in a university-based hospital system (Benoit & Watts, 2007).*

Geriatric

- Evaluate all elderly clients for established or acute fecal incontinence when the elderly client enters the acute or long-term care facility and intervene as indicated. *The prevalence of fecal incontinence, which often coexists with urinary incontinence, is approximately 50% in long-term care and 20% in acute care facilities (Hunskaar et al, 2005; Junkin & Selekof, 2007).*
- Evaluate cognitive status in the elderly person with a NEECHAM confusion scale (Neelan et al, 1992) for acute cognitive changes, a Folstein Mini-Mental Status Examination (Folstein, Folstein & McHugh, 1975), or other tool as indicated. *Acute or established dementias increase the risk of fecal incontinence among the elderly.*

Home Care

- Above interventions may be adapted for home care use.
- Assess and teach a bowel management program to support continence. Address timing, diet, fluids, and actions taken independently to deal with bowel incontinence. *Identifying factors that change level of incontinence may guide interventions. If client has been taking over-the-counter medications or home remedies, it is important to consider their influence.*
- Instruct caregiver to provide clothing that is nonrestrictive, can be manipulated easily for toileting, and can be changed with ease. *Avoidance of complicated maneuvers increases the chance of success in toileting programs and decreases the client's risk for embarrassing incontinent episodes.*
- Evaluate self-care strategies of community-dwelling elders; strengthen adaptive behaviors and counsel elders about altering strategies that compromise general health. **EBN:** *A survey of 242 community-dwelling elders reveals multiple self-care strategies designed to alleviate or prevent intermittent episodes of fecal incontinence. The most common included use of containment or protective devices and dietary alterations designed to normalize stool consistency. However, elders also reported reductions in physical activity and exercise, potentially compromising overall mobility and health (Bliss, Fischer & Savik, 2005).*
- Assist the family in arranging care in a way that allows the client to participate in family or favorite activities without embarrassment. *Careful planning can both help client retain dignity and maintain integrity of family patterns.*
- ▲ If the client is limited to bed (or bed and chair), provide a commode or bedpan that can be easily accessed. If necessary, refer the client to physical therapy services to learn side transfers and to build strength for transfers.
- ▲ If the client is frequently incontinent, refer for home health aide services to assist with hygiene and skin care.

B

- Teach the client and family to perform a bowel reeducation program; scheduled, stimulated program; or other strategies to manage fecal incontinence.
- Teach the client and family about common dietary sources for fiber, as well as supplemental fiber or bulking agents as indicated.
▲ Refer the family to support services to assist with in-home management of fecal incontinence as indicated.
- Teach nursing colleagues and nonprofessional care providers the importance of providing toileting opportunities and adequate privacy for the client in an acute or long-term care facility.

NOTE: Refer to nursing diagnoses **Diarrhea** and **Constipation** for detailed management of these related conditions.

evolve   See the EVOLVE website for World Wide Web resources for client education.

REFERENCES

Avery KN, Bosch JL, Gotoh M et al: Questionnaires to assess urinary and anal incontinence: review and recommendations, *J Urol* 177(1):39-49, 2007.

Benoit RA, Watts CY: The effect of a pressure ulcer prevention program and a bowel management program (BMS) in reducing pressure ulcer prevalence in an ICU setting, *J Wound Ostomy* 34(2):163-175, 2007.

Bliss DZ, Fischer LR, Savik K: Managing fecal incontinence: self-care practices of older adults. *J Gerontol Nurs* 31(7):35-44, 2005.

Bliss DZ, Johnson S, Savik K et al: Fecal incontinence in hospitalized patients who are acutely ill, *Nurs Res* 49(2):101-108, 2000a.

Bliss DZ, Jung HJ, Savik K et al: Supplementation with dietary fiber improves fecal incontinence, *Nurs Res* 50(4):203-213, 2001b.

Bliss DZ, Larson SJ, Burr JK et al: Reliability of a stool consistency classification system, *J Wound Ostomy Cont Nurs* 28(6):305-313, 2001.

Brazzelli M, Shirran E, Vale L: Absorbent products for containing urinary and/or fecal incontinence in adults, *Cochrane Database Syst Rev* 3:CD001406, 2003.

Chiarioni G, Scattolini C, Bonfante F et al: Liquid stool incontinence with severe urgency: anorectal function and effective biofeedback treatment, *Gut* 34(11):1576-1580, 1993.

Doherty W: Managing fecal incontinence or leakage: the Peristeen Anal Plug, *Br J Nurs* 13(21):1293-1297, 2004.

Doughty DB, Jensen LL: Assessment and management of the patient with fecal incontinence and related bowel dysfunction. In Doughty DB, editor: *Urinary and fecal incontinence: current management concepts*, ed 2, St Louis, 2006, Elsevier.

Dunn KL, Galka ML: A comparison of the effectiveness of Therevac SB and bisacodyl suppositories in SCI patients' bowel programs, *Rehabil Nurs* 19:334-338, 1994.

Evans EC, Gray M: What interventions are effective for the prevention and treatment of cutaneous candidiasis? *J Wound Ostomy Continence Nurs* 30(1):11-16, 2003.

Fiers S, Thayer D: Management of intractable incontinence. In: Doughty DB, editor: *Urinary and fecal incontinence: nursing management*, ed 2, St Louis, 2000, Mosby.

Folstein MF, Folstein EF, McHugh P: Mini Mental State: a practical method of grading the cognitive status of the patient for the clinician, *J Psychiatric Rev* 12:189, 1975.

Gray M, Bliss DZ, Doughty DB et al: Incontinence-associated dermatitis: a consensus, *J Wound Ostomy Continence Nurs* 34(1):45-54, 2007.

Gray M, Jones DP: The effect of different formulations of equivalent active ingredients on the performance of two topical wound treatment products, *Ostomy Wound Manage* 50(3):34-44, 2004.

Gray M, Ratliff C, Donovan A: Perineal skin care for the incontinent patient, *Adv Skin Wound Care* 15(4):170-175, 2002.

Gray ML, Burns SM: Continence management, *Crit Care Nurs Clin North Am* 8:29, 1996.

Griffiths AN, Makam A, Edwards GJ: Should we actively screen for urinary and anal incontinence in the general gynecology outpatients setting? A prospective observational study, *J Obstet Gynecol* 26(5):442-444, 2006.

Hunskaar S et al: Epidemiology of urinary (UI) and fecal (FI) incontinence and pelvic organ prolapse (POP) *3rd International Consultation on Incontinence*, ed 3, Plymouth, England, 2005, Health Publication, Plymbridge Distributors.

Johanson JF, Irizarry F, Doughty A: Risk factors for fecal incontinence in a nursing home population, *J Clin Gastroenterol* 24:156, 1997.

Junkin J, Selekof J: Prevalence of incontinence and associated skin injury in an acute care population, *J Wound Ostomy Continence Nurs* 24(3), 2007 (in press).

King JC, Currie DM, Wright E: Bowel training in spina bifida: importance of education, patient compliance, age, and anal reflexes, *Arch Phys Med Rehabil* 75:243, 1994.

Munchiando JF, Kendall K: Comparison of the effectiveness of two bowel programs for CVA patients, *Rehabil Nurs* 18:168, 1993.

Neelan VJ et al: Use of the NEECHAM confusion scale to assess acute confusional states of hospitalized older patients. In Funk SG et al, editors: *Key aspects of elder care: managing falls, incontinence and cognitive impairment*, New York, 1992, Springer.

Norton C, Chelvanayagam S: A nursing assessment tool for adult with fecal incontinence, *J Wound Ostomy Cont Nurs* 27:279, 2000.

Norton C, Hosker G, Brazzelli M: Biofeedback and/or sphincter exercises for the treatment of faecal incontinence in adults, *Cochrane Database Syst Rev* 2:CD002111, 2006.

O'Donnell BF, Drachman DA, Barnes HJ et al: Incontinence and troublesome behaviors predict institutionalization in dementia, *J Geriatr Psychiatry Neurol* 5(1):45-52, 1992.

Rao SS: A balancing view: fecal incontinence: test or treat empirically: which strategy is best? *Am J Gastroenterol* 101(12):2683-2684, 2006.

Roig Vila JV, Garcia Garcia A, Flors Alandi C et al: The defecation habits in a normal working population, *Rev Esp Enferm Dig* 84(4):224-230, 1993.

Schnelle JF, Adamson GM, Cruise PA et al: Skin disorders and moisture in incontinent nursing home residents: intervention implications, *J Am Geriatr Soc* 45(10):1182-1188, 1997.

Schultz A, Dickey G, Skoner M: Self-report of incontinence in acute care, *Urol Nurs* 17(1):23-28, 1997.

• = Independent;   ▲ = Collaborative;   EBN = Evidence-Based Nursing;   EB = Evidence-Based

Smith LJ, Franchetti B, McCoull K et al: A behavioural approach to retraining bowel function after long-standing constipation and faecal impaction in people with learning disabilities, *Dev Med Child Neurol* 36(1):41-49, 1994.

Terra MP, Dobben AC, Berghmans B et al: Electrical stimulation and pelvic floor muscle training with biofeedback in patients with fecal incontinence: a cohort study of 281 patients, *Dis Colon Rectum* 49(8):1149-1159, 2006.

Waldrop J, Doughty DB: Pathophysiology of bowel dysfunction and fecal incontinence. In Doughty DB, editor: *Urinary and fecal incontinence: nursing management*, ed 2, St Louis, 2000, Mosby.

Effective Breastfeeding   Arlene Farren, RN, MA, AOCN, and Teresa Howell, MSN, ARHP

NANDA   Definition

Mother-infant dyad/family exhibits adequate proficiency and satisfaction with the breastfeeding process

Defining Characteristics

Adequate infant elimination patterns for age; appropriate infant weight pattern for age; eagerness of infant to nurse; effective mother/infant communication patterns; infant content after feeding; maternal verbalization of satisfaction with the breastfeeding process; mother able to position infant at breast to promote a successful latching-on response; regular and sustained suckling at the breast; regular and sustained swallowing at the breast; signs of oxytocin release; symptoms of oxytocin release

Related Factors (r/t)

Basic breastfeeding knowledge; infant gestational age >34 weeks; maternal confidence; normal breast structure; normal infant oral structure; support

NOC   Outcomes (Nursing Outcomes Classification)

Suggested NOC Outcomes

Breastfeeding Establishment: Infant, Maternal, Breastfeeding Maintenance

Example NOC Outcome with Indicators
Breastfeeding Establishment: Infant as evidenced by the following indicators: Proper alignment and latch-on/Proper areolar grasp/Proper areolar compression/Correct suck and tongue placement/Swallowing a minimum of 5 to 10 minutes per breast/Minimum eight feedings per day/Urinations per day appropriate for age/Weight gain appropriate for age (Rate the outcome and indicators of **Breastfeeding Establishment: Infant:** 1 = not adequate, 2 = slightly adequate, 3 = moderately adequate, 4 = substantially adequate, 5 = totally adequate [see Section I].)

Client Outcomes

Client Will (Specify Time Frame):

- Maintain effective breastfeeding
- Maintain normal growth patterns (infant)
- Verbalize satisfaction with breastfeeding process (mother)

NIC   Interventions (Nursing Interventions Classification)

Suggested NIC Interventions

Breastfeeding Assistance, Lactation Counseling

Example NIC Activities—Breastfeeding Assistance
Discuss with parents an estimate of effort and length of time they would like to put toward breastfeeding; Provide early mother/infant contact opportunity to breastfeed within 2 hours after birth

---

• = Independent;   ▲ = Collaborative;   EBN = Evidence-Based Nursing;   EB = Evidence-Based

B

Nursing Interventions and *Rationales*

- Encourage and facilitate early skin-to-skin contact (SSC) (position includes contact of the naked baby with the mother's bare chest within 2 hours after birth). *Early SSC is thought to assist with maternal milk production, aid in establishing breastfeeding, and have a positive effect on duration of breastfeeding (Anderson et al, 2003; Spatz, 2004).* **EBN:** *Benefits of SSC have been supported in the literature (Anderson et al, 2003).*
- Encourage rooming-in and breastfeeding on demand. **EBN:** *Demand feedings have been associated with continuation of breastfeeding 4 to 6 weeks postpartum in comparison to restricted feeding intervals (Renfew et al, 2001).* **EB:** *A U.S. national survey and a Canadian team reporting a systematic review conclude that there is good evidence to recommend rooming-in as an effective intervention to promote breastfeeding (Levitt et al, 2004).*
- Monitor the breastfeeding process. **EBN:** *Breastfeeding should be observed by nurses and lactation consultants while the woman is hospitalized to identify ineffective breastfeeding patterns prior to discharge (Lewallen et al, 2006).* **EB:** *Breastfeeding support is recommended and findings indicate there is a beneficial effect on any breastfeeding and exclusive breastfeeding when extra professional support is provided (Maternity Center Association, 2004).*
- Identify opportunities to enhance knowledge and experience regarding breastfeeding. Support and teaching must be individualized to the client's level of understanding. *Exposure to a variety of sources of information is an important predictor of breastfeeding duration (Palda et al, 2004).* **EB:** *Findings from a systematic review indicate there is a beneficial effect on any breastfeeding and exclusive breastfeeding when extra professional support is provided (Sikorski et al, 2002).*
- Give encouragement/positive feedback related to breastfeeding mother-infant interactions. *Effective breastfeeding is influenced by maternal state and the mother's knowledge of breastfeeding (Mulder, 2006).* **EBN:** *A precursor to effective breastfeeding is a comfortable and relaxed maternal state (Mulder, 2006).*
- Monitor for signs and symptoms of nipple pain and/or trauma. *These factors have been identified as impacting the continuation of breastfeeding in the first weeks of motherhood (Lewallen et al, 2006).* **EBN:** *Ensuring proper latch-on is a key intervention to decrease sore nipples (Lewallen et al, 2006).*
- Discuss prevention and treatment of common breastfeeding problems. **EBN:** *Evidence-based practice guidelines support the need to evaluate breastfeeding women's knowledge regarding the prevention and management of common problems (e.g., sore nipples, breast engorgement) associated with breastfeeding (Registered Nurses Association of Ontario, 2003).*
- Monitor infant responses to breastfeeding. *Ongoing evaluation of the adequacy of infant intake such as weight, number of excretions (urine and stool) per 24 hours, and assessment of the presence of jaundice is important to support ongoing effective breastfeeding and for early detection of problems (Registered Nurses Association of Ontario, 2003).* **EBN:** *Evidence-based practice guidelines include monitoring infant responses as described above (Registered Nurses Association of Ontario, 2003).*
- Identify current support person network and opportunities for continued breastfeeding support. **EBN:** *Mothers receiving support through a peer support program were continuing to breastfeed longer and reported greater satisfaction with their breastfeeding experience than their counterparts receiving conventional care (Dennis et al, 2002).*
- Avoid supplemental bottle feedings and do not provide samples of formula on discharge. **EBN:** *Supplemental feedings can contribute to decreased milk supply (Lewallen et al, 2006).* **EB:** *Use of commercial discharge packages have been shown to decrease breastfeeding rates (Palda et al, 2004).*
- ▲ Provide follow-up contact; as available provide home visits and/or peer counseling. **EB:** *Evidence suggests that practitioners providing extra support and attention to mothers is the key to breastfeeding success (Winterburn, 2005).*

Multicultural

- Assess for the influence of cultural beliefs, norms, and values on current breastfeeding practices. *The client's knowledge of breastfeeding may be based on cultural perceptions, as well as influences from the larger social context (Cricco-Lizza, 2004; Gill et al, 2004; Kong & Lee, 2004).* **EBN:** *A study of African-American women revealed formula-feeding experiences were the norm and infant-feeding beliefs reflected responses to life experiences (Cricco-Lizza, 2004).* **EBN:** *The Hispanic mother may believe stress and anger makes bad milk, which makes a breastfeeding infant ill. Some Hispanic women neutralize the bowel when weaning from breast to bottle by feeding only anise tea for 24 hours (Gonzalez, Owens & Esperat, 2008, in press.)* **EBN:** *Each client should be assessed for ability to*

• = Independent;   ▲ = Collaborative;   EBN = Evidence-Based Nursing;   EB = Evidence-Based

breastfeed based on a culturally competent assessment of the phenomenon of communication, time, space, social organization, environmental control, and biological variations (Giger & Davidhizar, 2004).

- Assess mothers' timing preference to begin breastfeeding. *Women from different cultures may have different beliefs about the best time to begin breastfeeding (Purnell & Paulanka, 2003).* **EBN:** *Although usual hospital practice is to begin breastfeeding immediately, some cultures (e.g., Arab heritage) do not regard colostrum as appropriate for newborns and may prefer to wait until milk is present at about 3 days of age (Purnell & Paulanka, 2003).*
- Validate the client's concerns about the amount of milk taken. **EBN:** *Provide information about physical signs that baby is getting enough milk (Lewallen et al, 2006).*

Home Care

- Above interventions may be adapted for home care use.

Client/Family Teaching

- Include the father and other family members in education about breastfeeding. *Allaying the misconceptions and the social embarrassment associated with breastfeeding can encourage fathers to be more supportive (Shepherd et al, 2000; Wolfberg et al, 2004).* **EB:** *Researchers conducting a randomized controlled trial with a 2-hour intervention class on infant care and breastfeeding promotion found that the fathers in the intervention group were influential advocates for breastfeeding (Wolfberg et al, 2004).*
- Teach the client the importance of maternal nutrition. **EB:** *Generally, no special diet is required; however, 500 calories above the nonpregnant recommendations (or adjusting caloric intake to need) is thought to assist in sustaining breastfeeding, and consuming a healthy diet using foods from a variety of sources is recommended (Breslin & Lucas, 2003; US Department of Health and Human Services & US Department of Agriculture, 2005).*
- Reinforce the infant's subtle hunger cues (e.g., quiet-alert state, rooting, sucking, hand-to-mouth activity) and encourage the client to nurse whenever signs are apparent. *Parents need to know infant characteristics and the early feeding readiness cues of infants so that they can respond appropriately (Karl, 2004).* **EBN:** *Evidence-based practice guidelines support the teaching/reinforcement of these skills as important to effective breastfeeding (Association of Women's Health Obstetric and Neonatal Nurses, 2000).*
- Review guidelines for frequency (every 2 to 3 hours, or 8 to 12 feedings per 24 hours) and duration (until suckling and swallowing slow down and satiety is reached) of feeding times. *In the first few days, frequent and regular stimulation of the breasts is important to establish an adequate milk supply; after breastfeeding is established, feeding lasts until the breasts are drained (Association of Women's Health Obstetric and Neonatal Nurses, 2000; Neifert, 2004).* **EBN:** *Evidence-based guidelines recommend assessment of infant satisfaction/satiety including infant cues and patterns of weight (Association of Women's Health Obstetric and Neonatal Nurses, 2000).*
- Provide anticipatory guidance about common infant behaviors. *Being able to anticipate and manage behaviors and problems promotes parental confidence (Association of Women's Health Obstetric and Neonatal Nurses, 2000; Milligan et al, 2000).* **EBN:** *Lack of knowledge about infant growth spurts, temperament, sleep/wake cycles, and introduction of other foods can create parental anxiety and lead to premature termination of breastfeeding (Milligan et al, 2000).*
- Provide information about additional breastfeeding resources. **EBN:** *Evidence-based clinical practice guidelines suggest that breastfeeding books, materials, websites, and breastfeeding support groups, which provide current and accurate information, can enhance maternal success and satisfaction with the breastfeeding process (Association of Women's Health Obstetric and Neonatal Nurses, 2000).*

evolve See the EVOLVE website for World Wide Web resources for client education.

REFERENCES

Anderson GC, Moore E, Hepworth J et al: Early skin-to-skin contact for mothers and their healthy newborn infants, *Cochrane Database Syst Rev* (2):CD003519, 2003.

Association of Women's Health Obstetric and Neonatal Nurses: *Evidence-based clinical practice guideline: breastfeeding support: prenatal care through the first year (practice guideline),* Washington, DC, 2000, The Association.

Breslin ET, Lucas VA: *Women's health nursing: toward evidence-based practice,* St Louis, 2003, WB Saunders.

Cricco-Lizza R: Infant-feeding beliefs and experiences of black women enrolled in WIC in the New York metropolitan area, *Qual Health Res* 14(9):1197-1210, 2004.

Dennis CL, Hodnett E, Gallop R: The effect of peer support on

• = Independent; ▲ = Collaborative; EBN = Evidence-Based Nursing; EB = Evidence-Based

breast-feeding duration among primiparous women: a randomized controlled trial, *CMAJ* 166(1):21-28, 2002.

Giger J, Davidhizar R: *Transcultural nursing: assessment and intervention*, St Louis, 2004, Mosby.

Gill SL, Reifsnider E, Mann AR et al: Assessing infant breastfeeding belief among low-income Mexican Americans, *J Perinat Educ* 13:29, 2004.

Gonzalez E, Owens D, Esperat C: Mexican Americans. In Giger J, Davidhizar R, editors: *Transcultural nursing: assessment and intervention*. St Louis, 2008, Mosby, in press.

Karl DJ: Using principles of newborn behavioral state organization to facilitate breastfeeding, *MCN Am J Matern Child Nurs* 29(5): 292-298, 2004.

Kong SK, Lee DT: Factors influencing decision to breastfeed, *J Adv Nurs* 46(4):369-379, 2004.

Levitt C et al: Systematic review of the literature on postpartum care: methodology and literature search results, *Birth* 31(3):196-202, 2004.

Lewallen LP, Dick MJ, Flowers J et al: Breastfeeding support and early cessation, *J Obstet Gynecol Neonatal Nurs* 35(2):166-172, 2006.

Milligan RA et al: Breastfeeding duration among low income women, *J Midwif Womens Health* 45(3):246-252, 2000.

Mulder PJ: A concept analysis of effective breastfeeding, *J Obstet Gynecol Neonatal Nurs* 35(3):332-339, 2006.

Neifert MR: Breastmilk transfer: positioning, latch-on, and screening for problems in milk transfer, *Clin Obstet Gynecol* 47(3):656-675, 2004.

Palda VA, Guise JM, Wathen CN et al: Interventions to promote breast-feeding: applying the evidence in clinical practice, *CMAJ* 170(6):976-978, 2004.

Purnell LD, Paulanka BJ: *Transcultural health care: a culturally competent approach*, ed 2, Philadelphia, 2003, FA Davis.

Registered Nurses Association of Ontario (RNAO): *Breastfeeding best practice guidelines for nurses*, Toronto, 2003, The Association.

Renfrew M et al: Feeding schedules in hospitals for newborn infants. In Neilson J et al, editors: *Pregnancy and childbirth module of the Cochrane Database of Systematic Reviews*. Available in The Cochrane Library (data-base on disk and CD ROM). The Cochrane Collaboration, Issue 1. Oxford, UK: Updata Software (updated quarterly), 2001.

Shepherd CK, Power KG, Carter H: Examining the correspondence of breastfeeding and bottle-feeding couples' infant feeding attitudes, *J Adv Nurs* 31(3):651-660, 2000.

Sikorski J, Renfrew MJ, Pindoria S et al: Support for breastfeeding mothers, *Cochrane Database Syst Rev* (1):CD001141, 2002.

Spatz DL: Ten steps for promoting and protecting breastfeeding for vulnerable infants, *J Perinat Neonatal Nurs* 18(4):385-396, 2004.

US Department of Health and Human Services and US Department of Agriculture: *Dietary guidelines for Americans 2005*, Washington, DC, 2005, The Departments.

Winterburn SA: Breastfeeding support plans: an evidenced-based approach, *Prim Health Care* 15(4):36-39, 2005.

Wolfberg AJ, Michels KB, Shields W et al: Dads as breastfeeding advocates: results from a randomized controlled trial of an educational intervention, *Am J Obstet Gynecol* 191(3):708-712, 2004.

Ineffective Breastfeeding   Arlene Farren, RN, MA, AOCN, and Teresa Howell, MSN, ARHP

NANDA   Definition

Dissatisfaction or difficulty a mother, infant, or child experiences with the breastfeeding process

Defining Characteristics

Inadequate milk supply; infant arching at the breast; infant crying at the breast; infant inability to latch on to maternal breast correctly; infant exhibiting crying within the first hour after breastfeeding; infant exhibiting fussiness within the first hour after breastfeeding; insufficient emptying of each breast per feeding; insufficient opportunity for suckling at the breast; no observable signs of oxytocin release; nonsustained suckling at the breast; observable signs of inadequate infant intake; perceived inadequate milk supply, persistence of sore nipples beyond first week of breastfeeding; resisting latching on; unresponsive to other comfort measures; unsatisfactory breastfeeding process

Related Factors (r/t)

Infant anomaly; infant receiving supplemental feedings with artificial nipple; interruption in breastfeeding; knowledge deficit; maternal ambivalence; maternal anxiety; maternal breast anomaly; nonsupportive family; nonsupportive partner; poor infant reflex; prematurity; previous breast surgery; previous history of breastfeeding failure

NOC   Outcomes (Nursing Outcomes Classification)

Suggested NOC Outcomes

Breastfeeding Establishment: Infant, Maternal, Breastfeeding Maintenance, Breastfeeding Weaning, Knowledge: Breastfeeding

• = Independent;   ▲ = Collaborative;   EBN = Evidence-Based Nursing;   EB = Evidence-Based

---

Example NOC Outcome with Indicators

Breastfeeding Establishment: Infant as evidenced by the following indicators: Proper alignment and latch-on/Proper areolar grasp/Proper areolar compression/Correct suck and tongue placement/Swallowing a minimum of 5 to 10 minutes per breast/Minimum eight feedings per day/Urinations per day appropriate for age/Weight gain appropriate for age (Rate the outcome and indicators of **Breastfeeding Establishment: Infant**: 1 = not adequate, 2 = slightly adequate, 3 = moderately adequate, 4 = substantially adequate, 5 = totally adequate [see Section I].)

Client Outcomes

Client Will (Specify Time Frame):

- Achieve effective breastfeeding (dyad)
- Verbalize/demonstrate techniques to manage breastfeeding problems (mother)
- Manifest signs of adequate intake at the breast (infant)
- Manifest positive self-esteem in relation to the infant feeding process (mother)
- Explain alternative method of infant feeding if unable to continue exclusive breastfeeding (mother)

NIC   Interventions (Nursing Interventions Classification)

Suggested NIC Interventions

Breastfeeding Assistance, Lactation Counseling

Example NIC Activities—Breastfeeding Assistance

Discuss with parents an estimate of effort and length of time they would like to put toward breastfeeding; Provide early mother/infant contact opportunity to breastfeed within 2 hours after birth

---

Nursing Interventions and *Rationales*

- Identify women with risk factors for lower breastfeeding initiation and continuation rates (age <20 years, low socioeconomic status) as well as factors contributing to ineffective breastfeeding as early as possible in the perinatal experience. **EB:** *The prenatal period is a favorable time for interventions to encourage breastfeeding (Lee et al, 2005).*
- Provide time for clients to express expectations and concerns and give emotional support. **EBN:** *Nurses provide psychosocial support and three consecutive skin-to-skin breastfeedings with positive outcomes (Burkhammer, Anderson & Chiu, 2004).*
- Use valid and reliable tools to measure breastfeeding performance and to predict early discontinuance of breastfeeding whenever possible/feasible. **EB:** *Breastfeeding Assessment Score (BAS) has been used to identify infants at risk for early cessation of breastfeeding and may predict exclusive breastfeeding failure (Gianni et al, 2004).*
- Observe a full breastfeeding session (every 8 hours in the early postpartum and once per visit on follow-up). **EBN:** *Women identified nurses' activities such as assessment, teaching, and assistance as being sources of emotional, informational, and tangible support (Hong et al, 2003).*
- Provide evidence-based teaching and breastfeeding assistance appropriate to the client's individualized needs (see Client/Family Teaching). **EBN:** *In an expert review of one teaching video, the content and medium were evaluated as meeting the needs of breastfeeding mothers of babies being cared for in the NICU (Hayes, 2003).*
- Promote comfort and relaxation to reduce pain and anxiety. *Discomfort and increased tension are factors associated with reduced let-down reflex and premature discontinuance of breastfeeding. Anxiety and fear are associated with decreased milk production (Mezzacappa & Katkin, 2002).*
- Avoid supplemental feedings. **EBN:** *Supplementation with formula feedings has been associated with early weaning of the infant (Araujo et al, 2007).*

• = Independent;   ▲ = Collaborative;   EBN = Evidence-Based Nursing;   EB = Evidence-Based

B

- Monitor infant behavioral cues and responses to breastfeeding. **EBN:** *Infant behaviors contribute to oxytocin release and let-down, contribute to effective feeding, indicate effective breastfeeding, manifest satiety, and indicate adequacy of the feeding while contributing to positive maternal–infant attachment (White, Simon & Bryan, 2002).*
- Provide necessary equipment/instruction/assistance for milk expression as needed. **EBN:** *Breast massage using the Oketani method (first reported in Japan) was associated with improved quality of milk and growth and development patterns (Foda et al, 2004).*
- ▲ Provide referrals and resources: lactation consultants, nurse and peer support programs, community organizations, and written and electronic sources of information. **EBN:** *Evidenced-based guidelines and systematic reviews support the use of professionals with special skills in breastfeeding and other support programs to promote continued breastfeeding (Association of Women's Health Obstetric and Neonatal Nurses, 2000b).*
- If unsuccessful in achieving effective breastfeeding, help client accept and learn an alternate method of infant feeding. **EBN:** *Once the decision has been made to provide an alternate method of infant feeding, the mother needs support and education (Mozingo et al, 2000).*
- See care plan for **Effective Breastfeeding.**

Multicultural

- Assess whether the client's concerns about the amount of milk taken during breastfeeding is contributing to dissatisfaction with the breastfeeding process. **EBN:** *Some cultures may add semi-solid food within the first month of life as a result of concerns that the infant is not getting enough to eat and the perception that "big is healthy" (Higgins, 2000).*
- Assess the influence of family support on the decision to continue or discontinue breastfeeding. **EBN:** *Women are the keepers and transmitters of culture in families. Female family members can play a dominant role in how infants are fed (Cesario, 2001).* **EB:** *In one Italian study, a description of mother's characteristics that may indicate the need for more support included mothers that smoke and have had their first newborn (Bertini et al, 2003). Recent research has found that the mother's partner and family are most influential in the choice of infant feeding method and, thus, should be included in breastfeeding promotion programs for ethnically diverse women (Rose et al, 2004).*
- Assess for the influence of mother's weight on attempts to initiate and sustain breastfeeding. **EB:** *Prepregnant overweight and obesity have been associated with failure to initiate and to sustain breastfeeding among Caucasian and Hispanic women (Kugyelka, Rasmussen & Frongillo, 2004).*
- See care plan for **Effective Breastfeeding.**

Home Care

- Above interventions may be adapted for home care use.
- Provide anticipatory guidance in relation to home management of breastfeeding. *Mothers who are prepared for the needs of home management and possible problems (such as fatigue) can institute self-care measures, will feel more confident, and will be less likely to discontinue breastfeeding (Ertem, Votto & Leventhal, 2001).*
- Investigate availability/refer to public health department, hospital home follow-up breastfeeding program, or other postdischarge support. **EBN:** *Some hospitals and public health departments have follow-up breastfeeding programs, particularly for high-risk mothers (e.g., older mothers, past history substance use, risk of physical abuse) (McNaughton, 2004).*
- Monitor for specific difficulties contributing to bonding difficulties between mother and infant. Refer to care plan for **Risk for impaired parent/child Attachment.**

Client/Family Teaching

- Review maternal and infant benefits of breastfeeding. **EBN:** *Information about benefits of breastfeeding can assist women/families to make informed decisions about breastfeeding (Association of Women's Health Obstetric and Neonatal Nurses, 2000ab; U.S. Department of Health and Human Services, 2000).*
- Instruct the client on maternal breastfeeding behaviors/techniques (preparation for, positioning, initiation of/promoting latch-on, burping, completion of session, and frequency of feeding).

• = Independent;   ▲ = Collaborative;   EBN = Evidence-Based Nursing;   EB = Evidence-Based

Consider use of a video. **EBN:** *Difficulties in these practices contribute to ineffective breastfeeding (Foda et al, 2004). Researchers found preliminary support for a teaching intervention in the form of a breastfeeding promotion video addressing barriers to breastfeeding for low-income women (Khoury et al, 2002).*

- Teach the client self-care measures for the breastfeeding woman (e.g., breast care, management of breast/nipple discomfort, nutrition/fluid, rest/activity). **EBN:** *Nipple trauma, pain, mastitis, and fatigue are some of the problems a breastfeeding woman may experience (Foda et al, 2004).*
- Provide information regarding infant cues and behaviors related to breastfeeding and appropriate maternal responses (e.g., cues that infant is ready to feed, behaviors during feeding that contribute to effective breastfeeding, measures of infant feeding adequacy). **EBN:** *Nurses are vital to helping parents understand infant states, cues, and behaviors and by providing that information postnatally, will foster a mutually satisfying interaction between parent and infant (White, Simon & Bryan, 2002).*
- Provide education to father/family/significant others as needed. *Informed support people may be needed to assist mothers with breastfeeding management issues (e.g., fatigue and sleep pattern disturbances) (Quillin & Glenn, 2004; Wolfberg et al, 2004).* **EB:** *An educational intervention demonstrated the critical role of dads in encouraging women to breastfeed her newborn (Wolfberg et al, 2004).*

evolve See the EVOLVE website for World Wide Web resources for client education.

REFERENCES

See **Effective Breastfeeding** for additional references.

Araujo EC, Lopes ND, Vasconcelos MGL et al: Risk for ineffective breastfeeding: an ethnographic report, *Int J Adv Nurs Pract* 7(2). Available at http://www.ispub.com/ostia/index. php?xmlFilePath5journals/ijanp/vol7n2/breast.xml, accessed on March 5, 2007.

Association of Women's Health Obstetric and Neonatal Nurses: *Evidence-based clinical practice guideline: breastfeeding support: pre-natal care through the first year (practice guideline)*, Washington, DC, 2000a, The Association.

Association of Women's Health Obstetric and Neonatal Nurses: Evidence-based clinical practice guideline: breastfeeding support: prenatal care through the first year (monograph), Washington, DC, 2000b, The Association.

Bertini G, Perugi S, Dani C et al: Maternal education and the incidence and duration of breast feeding: a prospective study, *J Pediatr Gastroenterol Nutr* 37(4):447-452, 2003.

Burkhammer MD, Anderson GC, Chiu SH: Grief, anxiety, stillbirth, and perinatal problems: healing with kangaroo care, *J Obstet Gynecol Neonat Nurs* 33(6):774-782, 2004.

Cesario S: Care of the Native American woman: strategies for practice, education, and research, *J Obstet Gynecol Neonatal Nurs* 30(1):13-19, 2001.

Ertem IO, Votto N, Leventhal JM: The timing and predictors of the early termination of breastfeeding, *Pediatrics* 107(3):543-548, 2001.

Foda MI, Kawashima T, Nakamura S et al: Composition of milk obtained from unmassaged versus massaged breasts of lactating mothers, *J Pediatr Gastroentrol Nutr* 38(5):484-487, 2004.

Gianni ML, Vegni C, Ferraris G et al: 96 usefulness of an early breastfeeding assessment score to predict exclusive breastfeeding failure, *Pediatr Res* 56:480, 2004.

Hayes B: A premie needs his mother: first steps to breastfeeding your premature baby, *Birth* 30(1):69, 2003.

Higgins B: Puerto Rican cultural beliefs: influence on infant feeding practices in western New York, *J Transcult Nurs* 11(1):19-30, 2000.

Hong TM, Callister LC, Schwartz R: First-time mothers' views of breastfeeding support from nurses, *MCN Am J Matern Child Nurs* 28:10, 2003.

Khoury AJ, Mitra AK, Hinton A et al: An innovative video succeeds in addressing barriers to breastfeeding among low-income women, *J Hum Lact* 18(2):125-131, 2002.

Kugyelka JG, Rasmussen KM, Frongillo EA: Maternal obesity is negatively associated with breastfeeding success among Hispanic but not Black women, *J Nutr* 134(7):1746-1753, 2004.

Lee HG, Rubio MR, Elo IT et al: Factors associated with intention to breastfeed among low-income, inner-city pregnant women, *Matern Child Health J* 9(3):253-261, 2005.

McNaughton DB. Nurse home visits to maternal-child clients: a review of intervention research. *Public Health Nurs* 21(3):207-219, 2004.

Mezzacappa ES, Katkin ES: Breast-feeding is associated with reduced perceived stress and negative mood in mothers, *Health Psychol* 21(2):187-193, 2002.

Mozingo JN, Davis MW, Droppleman PG et al: "It wasn't working." Women's experiences with short-term breastfeeding, *MCN Am J Matern Child Nurs* 25(3):120-126, 2000.

Rose VA, Warrington VO, Linder R et al: Factors influencing infant feeding method in an urban community, *J Natl Med Assoc* 96(3):325-331, 2004.

US Department of Health and Human Services: *HHS blueprint for action on breastfeeding*, Washington, DC, 2000, US Department of Health and Human Services, Office on Women's Health.

White C, Simon M, Bryan A: Using evidence to educate birthing center nursing staff: about infant states, cues, and behaviors, *MCN Am J Matern Child Nurs* 27(5):294-298, 2002.

Wolfberg AJ, Michels KB, Shields W et al: Dads as breastfeeding advocates: results from a randomized controlled trial of an educational intervention, *Am J Obstet Gynecol* 191(3):708-712, 2004.

B

Interrupted Breastfeeding   *Arlene Farren, RN, MA, AOCN, and Teresa Howell, MSN, ARHP*

NANDA   Definition

Break in the continuity of the breastfeeding process as a result of inability or inadvisability to put baby to breast for feeding

Defining Characteristics

Infant receives no nourishment at the breast for some or all feedings; lack of knowledge regarding expression of breast milk; lack of knowledge regarding storage of breast milk; maternal desire to eventually provide breast milk for infant/child's nutritional needs; maternal desire to maintain breastfeeding for infant/child's nutritional needs; maternal desire to provide breast milk for infant/child's nutritional needs; separation of mother and infant

Related Factors (r/t)

Contraindications to breastfeeding; infant illness; maternal employment; maternal illness; need to abruptly wean infant; prematurity

NOC   Outcomes (Nursing Outcomes Classification)

Suggested NOC Outcomes

Breastfeeding Establishment: Infant, Maternal, Breastfeeding Maintenance, Knowledge: Breastfeeding, Parent-Infant Attachment

Example NOC Outcome with Indicators
Breastfeeding Establishment: Infant as evidenced by the following indicators: Proper alignment and latch on/Proper areolar grasp/Proper areolar compression/Correct suck and tongue placement/Swallowing a minimum of 5 to 10 minutes per breast/Minimum eight feedings per day/Urinations per day appropriate for age/Weight gain appropriate for age (Rate the outcome and indicators of **Breastfeeding Establishment: Infant:** 1 = not adequate, 2 = slightly adequate, 3 = moderately adequate, 4 = substantially adequate, 5 = totally adequate [see Section I].)

Client Outcomes

Client Will (Specify Time Frame):

Infant

• Receive mother's breast milk if not contraindicated by maternal conditions (e.g., certain drugs, infections) or infant conditions (e.g., true breast milk jaundice)

Maternal

• Maintain lactation
• Achieve effective breastfeeding or satisfaction with the breastfeeding experience
• Demonstrate effective methods of breast milk collection and storage

NIC   Interventions (Nursing Interventions Classification)

Suggested NIC Interventions

Bottle Feeding, Breastfeeding Assistance, Emotional Support, Kangaroo Care, Lactation Counseling

Example NIC Activities—Lactation Counseling
Instruct parents on how to differentiate between perceived and actual insufficient milk supply; Encourage employers to provide opportunities for and private facilities for lactating mothers to pump and store breast milk during the workday

• = Independent;   ▲ = Collaborative;   EBN = Evidence-Based Nursing;   EB = Evidence-Based

Nursing Interventions and *Rationales*

- Discuss mother's desire/intention to begin or resume breastfeeding. **EBN:** *It is very important that key personnel in the hospital (lactation consultants and nurses) assist mothers with getting breastfeeding off to a good start, especially with first-time breastfeeders who have no experience to rely on (Lewallen et al, 2006). Interventions to enhance a mother's confidence in breastfeeding should be initiated by healthcare providers (Dunn et al, 2006).*

- Provide anticipatory guidance to the mother/family regarding potential duration of the interruption when possible/feasible. *When conditions require a temporary interruption of breastfeeding, every opportunity should be taken to address the primary reason and provide nursing intervention (Lewallen et al, 2006).* **EBN:** *The likelihood of continuing/resuming breastfeeding decreases the longer feeding is delayed and formula supplements are used (Lewallen et al, 2006). Women with a history of breast augmentation should be monitored for the possible complication of lactation insufficiency (Hill et al, 2004).*

- Reassure mother/family that early measures to sustain lactation and promote parent-infant attachment can make it possible to resume breastfeeding when the condition/situation requiring interruption is resolved. **EBN:** *Dunn et al 2006 suggest that a predictor of early cessation of breastfeeding is a low level of confidence by the mother.*

- Reassure the mother/family that the infant will benefit from any amount of breast milk provided. **EBN:** *The perception of insufficient milk supply is a common reason women discontinue breastfeeding (Lewallen et al, 2006).* **EB:** *Exclusive breastfeeding is recommended because of beneficial effects in relation to growth and development, protection from asthma, allergies (Fulhan, Collier & Duggan, 2003; O'Connor, Merko & Brennan, 2004).*

- ▲ Collaborate with the mother/family/healthcare providers/employers (as needed) to develop a plan for expression of breast milk/infant feeding/kangaroo care/SSC. **EBN:** *Nurses should collaborate with women to develop a plan for pumping and maintaining lactation, and providing support (Rojjanasrirat, 2004).*

- Monitor for signs indicating infants' ability to and interest in breastfeeding. **EBN:** *An infant's contentedness and ability to be soothed (aspects of responsiveness) contribute to mothers' evaluation of self in relation to confidence and competence (Pridham, Lin & Brown, 2001).*

- Observe mother performing psychomotor skill (expression, storage, alternative feeding, kangaroo care, and/or breastfeeding) and assist as needed. *The nurse's presence and involvement allow for identification of those areas for which assistance, clarification, and/or support are needed and promote maternal confidence (Hong et al, 2003).*

- ▲ Provide and/or assist with arrangements and/or necessary equipment. **EBN:** *Working women and those with chronic illness have specific needs including assistance with arrangement of space and time for milk expression (hand or pump) and anticipatory guidance for planning for pumping schedules, using alternative feeding positions/approaches to promote successful breastfeeding (Ortiz, McGilligan & Kelly, 2004; Rojjanasrirat, 2004; Schaefer, 2004).*

- ▲ Use supplementation only as medically indicated. **EB:** *If human milk can be provided and fed to the infant, it is preferable (Fulhan, Collier & Duggan, 2003; O'Connor, Merko & Brennan, 2004).*

- Provide anticipatory guidance for common problems associated with interrupted breastfeeding (e.g., incomplete emptying of milk glands, diminishing milk supply, infant difficulty with resuming breastfeeding, or infant refusal of alternative feeding method). **EBN:** *The most common reason for discontinuation of breastfeeding was the perception of insufficient milk supply (Lewallen et al, 2006).*

- ▲ Initiate follow-up and make appropriate referrals. **EBN:** *Breastfeeding women receiving nurse and peer counselor support had longer duration of breastfeeding, and infants had fewer sick visits and reported use of fewer medications than those receiving usual care (Pugh et al, 2002).*

- Assist the client to accept and learn an alternative method of infant feeding if effective breastfeeding is not achieved. **EBN:** *If it is clear that breastfeeding cannot be achieved after the interruption and an alternative feeding method must be instituted, the mother needs support and education (Mozingo et al, 2000).*

- See care plans for **Effective Breastfeeding** and **Ineffective Breastfeeding**.

• = Independent;   ▲ = Collaborative;   EBN = Evidence-Based Nursing;   EB = Evidence-Based

Multicultural

- Assess for the influence of cultural beliefs, norms, and values on current decision to stop breast-feeding. **EBN:** *The client's decision to halt breastfeeding may be based on cultural perceptions, as well as influences from the larger social context (Cricco-Lizza, 2004; Newton, 2004). A study of Thai nurses suggests that beliefs about breastfeeding and postpartum practices of the nurse care provider may also have implications for clients' breastfeeding experiences (Kaewsarn, Moyle & Creedy, 2003). The Hispanic mother may believe stress and anger makes bad milk, which makes a breastfeeding infant ill (Gonzalez, Owens & Esperat, 2008). Some Hispanics neutralize the bowel when weaning from breast to bottle by feeding only anise tea for 24 hours (White, Linhart & Medley, 1996).*
- Teach culturally appropriate techniques for maintaining lactation. **EBN:** *The Oketani method of breast massage is used by Japanese and other Asian women. Oketani breast massage improved quality of human milk by increasing total solids, lipids, casein concentration, and gross energy (Foda et al, 2004).*
- Validate the client's feelings with regard to the difficulty of or her dissatisfaction with breastfeeding. **EBN:** *In a Scandinavian study the first 5 weeks was a vulnerable period and found factors associated with continuing to breastfeed. They concluded that interventions should be aimed at improving self-efficacy and resources available to those at risk (Kronborg & Vaeth, 2004).*
- See care plans for **Effective Breastfeeding** and **Ineffective Breastfeeding**.

Home Care

- Above interventions may be adapted for home care use.

Client/Family Teaching

- Teach mother effective methods to express breast milk. *There are a variety of methods of expression, and these involve psychomotor skills requiring instruction; breast stimulation is essential to continuing lactation (Foda et al, 2004).* **EBN:** *Those using the electric pump had shorter expression times but produced no more milk than those using the manual pump (Fewtrell et al, 2001).*
- Teach mother/parents about kangaroo care. **EBN:** *Indirect stimulation of lactation through close contact with the infant can occur, and kangaroo care has been associated with positive neonatal outcomes (Mellien, 2001).*
- Instruct mother on safe breast milk handling techniques. **EBN:** *Storage and handling practices can optimize the nutritional value and provide protection against contaminants (Phillipp, 2003).*
- See care plans for **Effective Breastfeeding** and **Ineffective Breastfeeding.**

 See the EVOLVE website for World Wide Web resources for client education.

REFERENCES

See **Effective Breastfeeding** for additional references.

Cricco-Lizza R: Infant-feeding beliefs and experiences of black women enrolled in WIC in the New York metropolitan area, *Qual Health Res* 14(9):1197-1210, 2004.

Dunn S, Davies B, McCleary L et al: The relationship between vulnerability factors and breastfeeding outcomes, *J Obstet Gynecol Neonat Nurs* 35(1):87-97, 2006.

Fewtrell MS, Lucas P, Collier S et al: Randomized trial comparing the efficacy of a novel manual breast pump with a standard electric breast pump in mothers who delivered preterm infants, *Pediatrics* 107(6):1291-1297, 2001.

Foda MI, Kawashima T, Nakamura S et al: Composition of milk obtained from unmassaged versus massaged breasts of lactating mothers, *J Pediatr Gastroenterol Nutr* 38(5):484-487, 2004.

Fulhan J, Collier S, Duggan C: Update on pediatric nutrition: breastfeeding, infant nutrition, and growth, *Curr Opin Pediatr* 15(3): 323-332, 2003.

Gonzalez E, Owens D, Esperat C: Mexican Americans. In Giger J, Davidhizar R, editors: Transcultural nursing: assessment and intervention. St. Louis, 2008, Mosby.

Hill PD, Wilhelm PA, Aldag JC et al: Breast augmentation and lactation outcomes: a case report, *MCN Am J Matern Child Nurs* 29:238, 2004.

Hong TM, Callister LC, Schwartz R: First-time mothers' views of breastfeeding support from nurses, *MCN Am J Matern Child Nurs* 28:10, 2003.

Kaewsarn P, Moyle W, Creedy D: Thai nurses' beliefs about breastfeeding and postpartum practices, *J Clin Nurs* 12:467, 2003.

Kronborg H, Vaeth M: The influence of psychosocial factors on the duration of breastfeeding, *Scand J Public Health* 32:210, 2004.

Lewallen LP, Dick MJ, Flowers J et al: Breastfeeding support and early cessation, *J Obstet Gynecol Neonatal Nurs* 35(2):166-172, 2006.

Mellien AC: Incubators versus mothers' arms: body temperature conservation in very-low-birth-weight premature infants, *J Obstet Gynecol Neonatal Nurs* 30(2):157-164, 2001.

Mozingo JN, Davis MW, Droppleman PG et al: "It wasn't working." Women's experiences with short-term breastfeeding, *MCN Am J Matern Child Nurs* 25(3):120-126, 2000.

Newton ER: The epidemiology of breastfeeding, *Clin Obstet Gynecol* 47:613, 2004.

O'Connor DL, Merko S, Brennan J: Human milk feeding of very low birth weight infants during initial hospitalization and after discharge, *Nutr Today* 39:102, 2004.

Ortiz J, McGilligan K, Kelly P: Duration of breast milk expression among working mothers enrolled in an employer-sponsored lactation program, *Pediatric Nurs* 30:111, 2004.

Philipp B: Encouraging patients to use a breast pump, *Contemp Ob Gyn* 1:88-100, 2003.

Pridham K, Lin CY, Brown R: Mothers' evaluation of their caregiving for premature and full-term infants through the first year: contributing factors, *Res Nurs Health* 24(3):157-169, 2001.

Pugh LC, Milligan RA, Frick KD et al: Breastfeeding duration, costs,

and benefits of a support program for low-income breast-feeding women, *Birth* 29(2):95-100, 2002.

Rojjanasrirat W: Working women's breastfeeding experiences, *MCN Am J Matern Child Nurs* 29:222, 2004.

Schaefer KM: Breastfeeding in chronic illness: the voices of women with fibromyalgia, *MCN Am J Matern Child Nurs* 29:248, 2004.

White J, Linhart J, Medley L: Culture, diet and the maternity, *Adv Nurse Pract* 4:26-28, 1996.

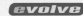

Ineffective Breathing pattern   *Julie T. Sanford, MSN, RN, and Mike Jacobs, DNS, RN*   evolve

NANDA   Definition

Inspiration and/or expiration that does not provide adequate ventilation

Defining Characteristics

Alterations in depth of breathing; altered chest excursion; assumption of a 3-point position; bradypnea; decreased expiratory pressure; decreased inspiratory pressure; decreased minute ventilation; decreased vital capacity; dyspnea; increased anterior-posterior diameter; nasal flaring; orthopnea; prolonged expiration phase; pursed-lip breathing; tachypnea; timing ratio; use of accessory muscles to breathe

Related Factors (r/t)

Anxiety; body position; bony deformity; chest wall deformity; cognitive impairment; fatigue hyperventilation; hypoventilation syndrome; musculoskeletal impairment; neurological immaturity; neuromuscular dysfunction; obesity; pain; perception impairment; respiratory muscle fatigue; spinal cord injury

NOC   Outcomes (Nursing Outcomes Classification)

Suggested NOC Outcomes

Respiratory Status: Airway Patency, Ventilation, Vital Signs

Example NOC Outcome with Indicators
Respiratory Status: Ventilation as evidenced by the following indicators: Respiratory rate/Respiratory rhythm/Depth of inspiration/Symmetrical chest expansion/Ease of breathing/Auscultated breath sounds/Tidal volume/Vital capacity (Rate the outcome and indicators of **Respiratory Status: Ventilation:** 1 = severely compromised, 2 = substantially compromised, 3 = moderately compromised, 4 = mildly compromised, 5 = not compromised [see Section I].)

Client Outcomes

Client Will (Specify Time Frame):

• Demonstrate a breathing pattern that supports blood gas results within the client's normal parameters
• Report ability to breathe comfortably
• Demonstrate ability to perform pursed-lip breathing and controlled breathing and use relaxation techniques effectively
• Identify and avoid specific factors that exacerbate episodes of ineffective breathing patterns

NIC   Interventions (Nursing Interventions Classification)

Suggested NIC Interventions

Airway Management, Respiratory Monitoring

• = Independent;   ▲ = Collaborative;   EBN = Evidence-Based Nursing;   EB = Evidence-Based

B

| **Example NIC Activities—Airway Management** |
| Encourage slow, deep breathing; turning; and coughing; Monitor respiratory and oxygenation status as appropriate |

Nursing Interventions and *Rationales*

- Monitor respiratory rate, depth, and ease of respiration. Normal respiratory rate is 12 to 16 breaths/min in the adult. *When the respiratory rate exceeds 24 breaths/min, significant respiratory or cardiovascular disease is generally evident.* See Defining Characteristics for guidelines for children.
- Note pattern of respiration. If client is dyspneic, note what seems to cause the dyspnea, the way in which the client deals with the condition, and how the dyspnea resolves or gets worse. Note amount of anxiety associated with the dyspnea. *A normal respiratory pattern is regular in a healthy adult. To assess dyspnea, it is important to consider all of its dimensions, including antecedents, mediators, reactions, and outcomes (Holt, 2005).* **EBN:** *A qualitative study demonstrated that experienced nurses working with COPD clients frequently used the degree of anxiety as an indicator of an acute exacerbation of COPD (Bailey, Colella & Mossey, 2004).*
- Attempt to determine if client's dyspnea is physiological or psychological in cause. *Psychological dyspnea includes dyspnea caused by anxiety or fear and can be associated with a panic attack (Meuret, Wilhelm & Roth, 2004).*

Psychological Dyspnea—Hyperventilation

- Assess cause of hyperventilation by asking client about current emotions and psychological state. **EB:** *Clients with idiopathic hyperventilation were more anxious and had a higher depression score than control subjects (Jack et al, 2004).*
- Ask the client to breathe with you to slow down respiratory rate. Maintain eye contact and give reassurance. *By making the client aware of respirations and giving support, the client may gain control of the breathing rate.*
- ▲ If pain is the cause of hyperventilation, provide medication routinely as ordered to prevent severe pain. Use distraction techniques to help client deal with pain. See interventions for **Acute Pain.** *An increased respiratory rate is one sign of pain. Providing pain relief will cause the respiratory rate to return to normal.*
- ▲ If client has chronic problems with hyperventilation, numbness and tingling in extremities, dizziness, and other signs of panic attacks, refer for counseling. *Cognitive behavioral therapy can be helpful for panic attacks, as can respiratory feedback utilizing measurement of CO_2 levels using a capnometry device to give the client feedback on rate and depth of breathing (Meuret, Wilhelm & Roth, 2004).* **EB:** *Findings from a study of advanced-stage cancer clients showed that when clients complaining of dyspnea were administered air and oxygen via nasal cannula, both groups reported decreased feelings of breathlessness with no significant differences (Philip et al, 2006).*

Physiological Dyspnea

- Ensure that client in acute dyspneic state has received medications, oxygen, and any other treatment needed. *Pharmacological treatment of dyspnea exists but may not suffice to relieve dyspnea (Holt, 2005).*
- Determine severity of dyspnea using a rating scale such as the modified Borg scale, rating dyspnea 0 (best) to 10 (worst) in severity. Alternative scales are the Visual Analogue Scale (VAS) with dyspnea rated as 0 (best) to 100 (worst), or the Medical Research Council Dyspnea Scale. **EB:** *In a study in an emergency room, the modified Borg scale correlated well with clinical measurements of respiratory function and was found helpful by both clients and nurses (Kendrick, Baxi & Smith, 2000). Another study comparing dyspnea scales in clients with COPD found that the Medical Research Council Dyspnea Scale most effectively measured breathlessness in this client group (Ozalevli, 2006).*
- Note abdominal breathing, use of accessory muscles, nasal flaring, retractions, irritability, confusion, or lethargy. *These symptoms signal increasing respiratory difficulty and increasing hypoxia.*

• = Independent;   ▲ = Collaborative;   EBN = Evidence-Based Nursing;   EB = Evidence-Based

- Observe color of tongue, oral mucosa, and skin. *Cyanosis of the tongue and oral mucosa is central cyanosis and generally represents a medical emergency. Peripheral cyanosis of nail beds or lips may or may not be serious (Kasper et al, 2005).*
- Auscultate breath sounds, noting decreased or absent sounds, crackles, or wheezes. *These abnormal lung sounds can indicate a respiratory pathology associated with an altered breathing pattern.*
- ▲ Monitor client's oxygen saturation and blood gases. *An oxygen saturation of less than 90% (normal: 95% to 100%) or a partial pressure of oxygen of less than 80 (normal: 80 to 100) indicates significant oxygenation problems (Clark, Giuliano & Chen, 2006).*
- ▲ Monitor for presence of pain and provide pain medication for comfort as needed. *Pain causes the client to hypoventilate and take shallow breaths that predispose the client to atelectasis.*
- Using touch on the shoulder, coach the client to slow respiratory rate, demonstrating slower respirations; making eye contact with the client; and communicating in a calm, supportive fashion. *The nurse's presence, reassurance, and help in controlling the client's breathing can be very beneficial in decreasing anxiety (Syrett & Taylor, 2003).* **EBN:** *Anxiety can exacerbate dyspnea, causing the client to enter into a dyspneic panic state (Holt, 2005). A study demonstrated that anxiety is an important indicator of severity of client's disease with COPD (Bailey, 2004).*
- Support the client in using pursed-lip and controlled breathing techniques. *Pursed-lip breathing results in increased use of intercostal muscles, decreased respiratory rate, increased tidal volume, and improved oxygen saturation levels (Dechman & Wilson, 2004).* **EB:** *Pursed-lip breathing is effective in decreasing breathlessness (Bianchi et al, 2004).*
- Position the client in an upright or semi-Fowler's position. *An upright position facilitates lung expansion.* See Nursing Interventions and Rationales for **Impaired Gas exchange** for further information on positioning.
- ▲ Administer oxygen as ordered. *Oxygen therapy helps decrease dyspnea through reduction in the central drive mediated via peripheral chemoreceptors in the carotid body (Dahlin, 2006).*
- Increase client's activity to walking three times per day as tolerated. Assist the client to use oxygen during activity as needed. See Nursing Interventions and Rationales for **Activity intolerance.** *Supervised exercise has been shown to decrease dyspnea and increase tolerance to activity (Kasper et al, 2005).* **EB:** *Clients with COPD who experienced desaturation with exercise may or may not also experience dysrthymias (Jones et al, 2006).*
- Schedule rest periods before and after activity. *Respiratory clients with dyspnea are easily exhausted and need additional rest.*
- ▲ Evaluate the client's nutritional status. Refer to a dietitian if needed. Use nutritional supplements to increase nutritional level if need indicated. *Improved nutrition may help increase inspiratory muscle function and decrease dyspnea (Bauldoff & Diaz, 2006).*
- Provide small, frequent feedings. *Small feedings are given to avoid compromising ventilatory effort and to conserve energy. Clients with dyspnea often do not eat sufficient amounts of food because their priority is breathing.*
- Offer a fan to move the air in the environment. *The movement of cool air on the face may help relieve dyspnea in pulmonary clients.* **EB:** *COPD clients who participated in a qualitative study reported that they found the use of fans to be very helpful (Booth, 2006).*
- Encourage the client to take deep breaths at prescribed intervals and do controlled coughing.
- Help the client with chronic respiratory disease to evaluate dyspnea experience to determine if similar to previous incidences of dyspnea and to recognize that he or she made it through those incidences. Encourage the client to be self-reliant if possible, use problem-solving skills, and maximize use of social support. *The focus of attention on sensations of breathlessness has an impact on judgment used to determine the intensity of the sensation (Meek, 2000).* **EBN:** *The most frequently used coping styles for clients with COPD are being optimistic and self-reliant, using problem-solving skills, and receiving social support (Baker & Scholz, 2002).*
- See **Ineffective Airway clearance** if client has a problem with increased respiratory secretions.
- ▲ Refer COPD client for pulmonary rehabilitation. **EB:** *Pulmonary rehabilitation has been shown to improve dyspnea and result in increased quality of life for clients diagnosed with COPD (Verrill et al, 2005) and reduce the use of healthcare resources (California Pulmonary Rehabilitation Collaborative Group, 2004).*

• = Independent;   ▲ = Collaborative;   EBN = Evidence-Based Nursing;   EB = Evidence-Based

B

 Geriatric

- Encourage ambulation as tolerated. *Immobility is harmful to the elderly because it decreases ventilation and increases stasis of secretions (Fletcher, 2005).*
- Encourage elderly clients to sit upright or stand and to avoid lying down for prolonged periods during the day. *Thoracic aging results in decreased lung expansion; an erect position fosters maximal lung expansion (Fletcher, 2005).*

Home Care

- Above interventions may be adapted for home care use.
- Assist the client and family with identifying other factors that precipitate or exacerbate episodes of ineffective breathing patterns (i.e., stress, allergens, stairs, activities that have high energy requirements). *Awareness of precipitating factors helps clients avoid them and decreases risk of ineffective breathing episodes.*
- Assess client knowledge of and compliance with medication regimen. *Client/family may need repetition of instructions received at hospital discharge and may require reiteration as fear of a recent crisis decreases. Fear interferes with the ability to assimilate new information.*
- Teach the client and family the importance of maintaining regimen and having PRN drugs easily accessible at all times. *Appropriate and timely use of medications can decrease the risk of exacerbating ineffective breathing.* **EBN:** *Parents/family have been found to have inadequate knowledge about recognition of asthma attacks, triggers, and management (Navaie-Waliser et al, 2004).*
- Provide the client with emotional support in dealing with symptoms of respiratory difficulty. Provide family with support for care of a client with chronic or terminal illness. Refer to care plan for **Anxiety.** *Witnessing breathing difficulties and facing concerns of dealing with chronic or terminal illness can create fear in caregiver. Fear inhibits effective coping.* **EBN:** *Social support was identified as a reason for nonadherence in asthmatics (Elliott, 2006).*
- When respiratory procedures (e.g., apneic monitoring for an infant) are being implemented, explain equipment and procedures to family members, and provide needed emotional support. *Family members assuming responsibility for respiratory monitoring often find this stressful. They may not have been able to assimilate fully any instructions provided by hospital staff (McNeal, 2000).*
- ▲ When electrically based equipment for respiratory support is being implemented, evaluate home environment for electrical safety, proper grounding, etc. Ensure that notification is sent to the local utility company, the emergency medical team, and police and fire departments. *Notification is important to provide for priority service (McNeal, 2000).*
- Refer to GOLD and ACP-ASIM/ACCP guidelines for management of home care and indications of hospital admission criteria (Chojnowski, 2003).
- Support clients' efforts at self-care. Ensure they have all the information they need to participate in care. **EBN:** *Self-care study participants showed competence at managing care of their own asthma (Makinen, Suominen & Lauri, 2000).* **EB:** *In another study of asthma clients, less self-efficacy, more depressive symptoms, expectation to be cured of asthma, having difficult access to care, and being Hispanic or African-American predicted lower scores on quality-of-life questionnaires (Mancuso et al, 2001).*
- Identify an emergency plan including when to call the physician or 911.
- ▲ Refer the client to an outpatient pulmonary rehabilitation program or a home-based training program for COPD. **EB:** *Outpatient rehabilitation programs can achieve worthwhile benefits including decreased perception of dyspnea, increased physical performance, and improved quality of life (Verrill et al, 2005). Pulmonary rehabilitation programs resulted in an improvement in depression, a decrease in symptoms, increase in ADLs, and an improvement in complaints of dyspnea (Pan-Diaz et al, 2007).*
- ▲ Refer to occupational therapy for evaluation and teaching of energy conservation techniques.
- ▲ Refer to home health aide services as needed to support energy conservation.
- ▲ Institute case management of frail elderly to support continued independent living.

 Client/Family Teaching

- Teach pursed-lip and controlled breathing techniques. *Pursed-lip breathing results in increased use of intercostal muscles, decreased respiratory rate, increased tidal volume, and improved oxygen saturation*

levels (Dechman & Wilson, 2004). **EB:** *Pursed-lip breathing was effective in decreasing breathlessness (Bianchi et al, 2004).*

- Using a prerecorded tape, teach client progressive muscle relaxation techniques. **EB:** *Relaxation therapy can help reduce dyspnea and anxiety (National Lung Health Education Program, 2007).*
- Teach about dosage, actions, and side effects of medications. *Inhaled steroids and bronchodilators can have undesirable side effects, especially when taken in inappropriate doses.*
- Teach the client to identify and avoid specific factors that exacerbate ineffective breathing patterns, such as exposure to other sources of air pollution, especially smoking.

evolve   See the EVOLVE website for World Wide Web resources for client education.

REFERENCES

Bailey PH: The dyspnea-anxiety-dyspnea cycle—COPD patients stories of breathlessness: "It's scary when you can't breathe," *Qual Health Res* 14(6):760, 2004.

Bailey PH, Colella T, Mossey S: COPD-intuition or template: nurses' stories of acute exacerbations of chronic obstructive pulmonary disease, *J Clin Nurs* 13(6):756, 2004.

Baker CF, Scholz JA: Coping with symptoms of dyspnea in chronic obstructive pulmonary disease, *Rehabil Nurs* 27(2):67, 2002.

Bauldoff GS, Diaz PT: Improving outcomes for COPD patients, *Nurs Prac* 31(8):26, 2006.

Bianchi R, Gigliotti F, Romagnoli I et al: Chest wall kinematics and breathlessness during pursed-lip breathing in patients with COPD, *Chest* 125(2):459, 2004.

Booth S: The impact of a breathlessness intervention service (BIS) on the lives of patients with intractable dyspnea: a qualitative phase 1 study, *Palliative Sup Care* 4(3):287, 2006.

California Pulmonary Rehabilitation Collaborative Group: Effects of pulmonary rehabilitation on dyspnea, quality of life and healthcare costs in California, *J Cardiopulm Rehabil* 24(1):52, 2004.

Chojnowski D: "GOLD" standards for acute exacerbation in COPD, *Nurse Pract* 28(5):26, 2003.

Clark AP, Giuliano K, Chen HM: Pulse oximetry revisited, *Clin Nurse Spec* 20(6):268-272, 2006.

Dahlin C: End-stage COPD: it takes my breath away. Part 2: Pharmacologic and nonpharmacologic management of dyspnea and other symptoms, *Home Health Nurs* 24(4):218, 2006.

Dechman G, Wilson CR: Evidence underlying breathing retraining in people with stable chronic obstructive pulmonary disease, *Phys Ther* 84(12):1189, 2004.

Elliott RA: Poor adherence to anti-inflammatory medication in asthma: reasons, challenges, and strategies for improved disease management, *Dis Manage Health Outcomes* 14(4):223, 2006.

Fletcher K: Immobility: geriatric self-learning module, *Medsurg Nurs* 14(1):35, 2005.

Holt K: Managing breathlessness, *Prim Health Care* 15(7):33, 2005.

Jack S, Rossiter HB, Pearson MG et al: Ventilatory responses to inhaled carbon dioxide, hypoxia, and exercise in idiopathic hyperventilation, *Am J Respir Crit Care Med* 170(2):118, 2004.

Jones AY, Yu WC, Mok NS et al: Exercise-induced desaturation and electrocardiogram changes in people with severe lung disease: an exploratory investigation of 25 serial cases, *Heart Lung* 35(6):397-404, 2006.

Kasper DL et al: *Harrison's principles of internal medicine,* ed 16, New York, 2005, McGraw-Hill.

Kendrick KR, Baxi SC, Smith RM: Usefulness of the modified 1-10 Borg scale in assessing the degree of dyspnea in patients with COPD and asthma, *J Emerg Nurs* 26(3):216, 2000.

Makinen S, Suominen T, Lauri S: Self-care in adults with asthma: how they cope, *J Clin Nurs* 9:557, 2000.

Mancuso CA, Rincon M, McCulloch CE et al: Self-efficacy, depressive symptoms, and patients' expectations predict outcomes in asthma, *Med Care* 39(12):1326, 2001.

McNeal GJ: *AACN guide to acute care procedures in the home,* Philadelphia, 2000, Lippincott.

Meek PM: Influence of attention and judgment on perception of breathlessness in healthy individuals and patients with chronic obstructive pulmonary disease, *Nurs Res* 49(1):11, 2000.

Meuret AE, Wilhelm FH, Roth WT: Respiratory feedback for treating panic disorder, *J Clin Psychol* 60(2):197, 2004.

National Lung Health Education Program: A breath of fresh air, *Consum Rep Hlth* 19(2):3-6, 2007.

Navaie-Waliser M, Misener M, Mersman C et al: Evaluating the needs of children with asthma in home care: the vital role of nurses as caregivers and educators, *Public Health Nurs* 21(4):306, 2004.

Ozalevli S: The comparison of different dyspnea scales in patients with COPD, *J Eval Clin Pract* 12(5):532-538, 2006.

Pan-Diaz H, Montes di Oca MM, Lopez JM et al: Pulmonary rehabilitation improves depression, anxiety, dyspnea and health status in patients with COPD, *Am J Phys Med Rehabil* 86(1):30-36, 2007.

Philip J, Pall D, Gold M et al: A randomized, double-blind, crossover trial of the effect of oxygen on dyspnea in patients with advanced cancer, *J Pain Symptom Manage* 32(6):541-550, 2006.

Syrett E, Taylor J: Non-pharmacological management of breathlessness: a collaborative nurse-physiotherapist approach, *Int J Palliat Nurs* 9(4):150-156, 2003.

Verrill D, Barton C, Beasley W et al: The effects of short-term and long-term pulmonary rehabilitation on functional capacity, perceived dyspnea, and quality of life, *Chest* 128(2):673-683, 2005.

C

Decreased Cardiac output

evolve

Marian Crowther, MSN, RN, APNC, CCRN, and Betty Ackley, MSN, EdS, RN

NANDA   Definition

Inadequate volume of blood pumped by the heart per minute to meet metabolic demands of the body

Defining Characteristics

Altered heart rate/rhythm: Arrhythmias; bradycardia; electrocardiographic changes; palpitations; tachycardia

Altered preload: Edema; decreased central venous pressure (CVP); decreased pulmonary artery wedge pressure (PAWP); fatigue; increased central venous pressure (CVP); increased pulmonary artery wedge pressure (PAWP); jugular vein distention; murmurs; weight gain

Altered afterload: Clammy skin; dyspnea; decreased peripheral pulses; decreased pulmonary vascular resistance (PVR); decreased systemic vascular resistance (SVR); increased pulmonary vascular resistance (PVR); increased systemic vascular resistance (SVR); oliguria, prolonged capillary refill; skin color changes; variations in blood pressure readings

Altered contractility: Crackles; cough; decreased ejection fraction; decreased left ventricular stroke work index (LVSWI); decreased stroke volume index (SVI); decreased cardiac index; decreased cardiac output; orthopnea; paroxysmal nocturnal dyspnea; S3 sounds; S4 sounds

Behavioral/emotional: Anxiety; restlessness

Related Factors (r/t)

Altered heart rate; altered heart rhythm; altered stroke volume: altered preload, altered afterload, altered contractility

NOC   Outcomes (Nursing Outcomes Classification)

Suggested NOC Outcomes

Cardiac Pump Effectiveness, Circulation Status, Tissue Perfusion: Abdominal Organs, Peripheral, Vital Signs

Example NOC Outcome with Indicators
Cardiac Pump Effectiveness as evidenced by the following indicators: Blood pressure/Heart rate/Cardiac index/Ejection fraction/Activity tolerance/Peripheral pulses strong/NVD not present/Dysrhythmias not present/Abnormal heart sounds not present/Angina not present/Peripheral edema not present/Pulmonary edema not present (Rate the outcome and indicators of **Cardiac Pump Effectiveness:** 1 = severely compromised, 2 = substantially compromised, 3 = moderately compromised, 4 = mildly compromised, 5 = not compromised [see Section I].)

Client Outcomes

Client Will (Specify Time Frame):

- Demonstrate adequate cardiac output as evidenced by blood pressure and pulse rate and rhythm within normal parameters for client; strong peripheral pulses; and an ability to tolerate activity without symptoms of dyspnea, syncope, or chest pain
- Remain free of side effects from the medications used to achieve adequate cardiac output
- Explain actions and precautions to take for primary or secondary prevention of cardiac disease

NIC   Interventions (Nursing Interventions Classification)

Suggested NIC Interventions

Cardiac Care, Cardiac Care: Acute

> **Example NIC Activities—Cardiac Care**
>
> Evaluate chest pain (e.g., intensity, location, radiation, duration, and precipitating and alleviating factors); Document cardiac dysrhythmias

Nursing Interventions and *Rationales*

- Monitor for symptoms of heart failure and decreased cardiac output; listen to heart sounds, lung sounds; note symptoms, including dyspnea, orthopnea, paroxysmal nocturnal dyspnea, Cheyne-Stokes respirations, fatigue, weakness, third and fourth heart sounds, crackles in lungs, increased venous pressure greater than 16 cm H_2O, and positive hepatojugular reflex. *These are major criteria for diagnosis of heart failure—the Framingham Criteria (Kasper et al, 2005).*

▲ Recognize the importance of cardiac index estimated by thermodilution in the intensive care unit (ICU) client. **EBN:** *The cardiac index reflects with good precision the cardiac output of ICU clients and provides immediate results; in addition, the measurements are easy to repeat (Oliva & Monteiro da Cruz, 2003).* **EB:** *Cardiac index is preferred to cardiac output to attenuate the effects of body mass index (BMI) (Stelfox et al, 2006).*

▲ When using pulmonary arterial catheter technology, be sure to appropriately level and zero the equipment, use minimal tubing, maintain system patency, perform square wave testing, position the client appropriately, and consider correlation to respiratory and cardiac cycles when assessing waveforms and integrating data into client assessment. **EB:** *Hemodynamic parameters are analyzed to assess cellular oxygen delivery, and cardiac output is a major determinant of oxygen delivery. Proper technique is imperative to accurate data collection (Adams, 2004).* **EBN:** *A study that assessed three different bed rest positions when measuring cardiac output by continuous method (using a heated filament in the PA catheter) at 0, 5, and 10 minutes after position changes demonstrated no differences in cardiac index across measurement conditions (Giuliano et al, 2003).*

▲ Hemodynamic pressure and parameters can be obtained either before or after cardiac output measurement. **EBN:** *A study assessing hemodynamic parameter differences between precardiac and postcardiac output measurement found minimal differences between groups and concluded that hemodynamic parameters may be accurately obtained at either time (Urquhart & Jensen, 2003).* **EBN:** *A study assessing normal variations in hemodynamic parameters demonstrated normal fluctuations with values that vary under 8% for pulmonary artery systolic pressure, under 11% for pulmonary artery diastolic pressure, and under 12% for pulmonary artery wedge pressure in clients with left ventricular systolic dysfunction (Moser et al, 2002).*

▲ Be aware of the utilization of impedance cardiography in noninvasive hemodynamic monitoring of heart failure. **EB:** *Impedance cardiography has demonstrated diagnostic and prognostic value in emergent and chronic heart failure. It has been shown to aid in the diagnosis of cardiac versus noncardiac heart failure clients (Yancy & Abraham, 2003).* **EBN:** *Impedance cardiography has been well correlated with thermodilution in clients with decompensated complex heart failure (Albert, Hail & Li, 2004).*

▲ Be aware of the utilization of other cardiac output techniques including the Fick Method and esophageal Doppler imaging. **EBN:** *A study assessing various methods for measuring cardiac output including bioimpedance, Fick, and thermodilution methods seem not to be interchangeable, although each can be trended separately, with the least accurate being the bioimpedance cardiography (Engoren & Barbee, 2005).* **EBN:** *There is good correlation between thermodilution and esophageal Doppler imaging methods (Iregui et al, 2003) and between thermodilution and bioimpedance methods for obtaining cardiac output (Albert, Hail & Li, 2004).*

- Recognize the effect of sleep disordered breathing in heart failure. **EBN:** *Sleep disordered breathing, including obstructive sleep apnea and Cheyne-Stokes with central sleep apnea, are common organic sleep disorders in clients with chronic heart failure and are a poor prognostic sign associated with higher mortality (Brostrom et al, 2004).*

- Observe for chest pain or discomfort; note location, radiation, severity, quality, duration, associated manifestations such as nausea, indigestion, and diaphoresis; also note precipitating and re-

C

lieving factors. *Chest pain/discomfort is generally indicative of an inadequate blood supply to the heart, which can compromise cardiac output. Clients with heart failure can continue to have chest pain with angina or can reinfarct.*

▲ If chest pain is present, have client lie down, monitor cardiac rhythm, give oxygen, check vital signs, run a monitor strip, medicate for pain, and notify the physician. *Prompt assessment of the client with acute coronary symptoms is critical because the incidence of ventricular fibrillation is 15 times greater during the first hour after symptoms of an acute myocardial infarction (Newberry, 2003).*

• Monitor intake and output. If client is acutely ill, measure hourly urine output and note decreases in output. *Decreased cardiac output results in decreased perfusion of the kidneys, with a resulting decrease in urine output.*

▲ Note results of electrocardiography and chest radiography. *Heart failure is strongly suggested by the presence of cardiomegaly or pulmonary vascular congestion on the chest radiograph. The probability of heart failure is increased by anterior Q waves or left bundle branch block on the electrocardiogram (Dosh, 2004).*

▲ Note results of diagnostic imaging studies such as echocardiogram, radionuclide imaging, or dobutamine stress echocardiography. *The echocardiogram is of critical importance in determining the cause and severity of heart failure (Kasper et al, 2005). The ejection fraction (EF) is often quoted as a measure of left ventricular function, with an EF <40% indicating clinical heart failure (Williams & Kearney, 2002).*

▲ Watch laboratory data closely, especially arterial blood gases, electrolytes including potassium, and B-type natriuretic peptide (BNP assay). *Client may be receiving cardiac glycosides and the potential for toxicity is greater with hypokalemia; hypokalemia is common in heart clients because of diuretic use (Kasper et al, 2005).* **EB:** *Rapid measurement of BNP is useful in establishing or eliminating the diagnosis of heart failure in the client with dyspnea (Kasper et al, 2005; Maisel et al, 2002).*

▲ Monitor laboratory work such as complete blood count (CBC), sodium level, and serum creatinine. *Routine blood work can provide insight into the etiology of heart failure and extent of decompensation. A low serum sodium level often is observed with advanced heart failure and can be a poor prognostic sign (Kasper et al, 2005). Serum creatinine levels will elevate in clients with severe heart failure because of decreased perfusion to the kidneys.*

▲ Administer oxygen as needed per physician's order. *Supplemental oxygen increases oxygen availability to the myocardium.*

• Place client in semi-Fowler's or high Fowler's position with legs down or position of comfort. *Elevating the head of the bed and legs down position may decrease the work of breathing and may also decrease venous return and preload.*

▲ Check blood pressure, pulse, and condition before administering cardiac medications such as angiotensin-converting enzyme (ACE) inhibitors, digoxin, calcium channel blockers, and beta-blockers such as Carvedilol. Notify physician if heart rate or blood pressure is low before holding medications. *It is important that the nurse evaluate how well the client is tolerating current medications before administering cardiac medications; do not hold medications without physician input. The physician may decide to have medications administered even though the blood pressure or pulse rate has lowered.*

• During acute events, ensure client remains on short-term bed rest or maintains activity level that does not compromise cardiac output. *In severe heart failure, restriction of activity reduces the workload of the heart (Kasper et al, 2005).*

• Gradually increase activity when client's condition is stabilized by encouraging slower paced activities or shorter periods of activity with frequent rest periods following exercise prescription; observe for symptoms of intolerance. Take blood pressure and pulse before and after activity and note changes. *Activity of the cardiac client should be closely monitored.* See **Activity intolerance.**

▲ Serve small sodium-restricted, low-cholesterol meals. *Sodium-restricted diets help decrease fluid volume excess. Low-cholesterol diets help decrease atherosclerosis, which causes coronary artery disease. Clients with cardiac disease tolerate smaller meals better because they require less cardiac output to digest.*

• Serve only small amounts of coffee or caffeine-containing beverages if requested (no more than four cups per 24 hours) if no resulting dysrhythmia. **EBN and EB:** *A review of studies on caffeine* *and cardiac arrhythmias concluded that moderate caffeine consumption does not increase the frequency or severity of cardiac arrhythmias (Hogan, Hornick & Bouchoux, 2002; Myers & Harris, 1990; Schneider, 1987).*

▲ Monitor bowel function. Provide stool softeners as ordered. Caution client not to strain when defecating. *Decreased activity can cause constipation, as well as pain medication. Straining when defecating that results in the Valsalva maneuver can lead to dysrhythmia, decreased cardiac function, and sometimes death.*

• Have clients use a commode or urinal for toileting and avoid use of a bedpan. *Getting out of bed to use a commode or urinal does not stress the heart any more than staying in bed to toilet. In addition, getting the client out of bed minimizes complications of immobility and is often preferred by the client (Winslow, 1992).*

• Provide a restful environment by minimizing controllable stressors and unnecessary disturbances. Schedule rest periods after meals and activities. *Rest helps lower arterial pressure and reduce the workload of the myocardium by diminishing the requirements for cardiac output (Kasper et al, 2005).*

• Weigh client at same time daily (after voiding). *An accurate daily weight is needed to guide the administration of diuretics (Kasper et al, 2005). Daily weight is also a good indicator of fluid balance. Increased weight and severity of symptoms can signal decreased cardiac function with retention of fluids.*

▲ Apply graduated compression stockings as ordered. Ensure proper fit by measuring accurately. Remove the stocking at least once a day, then reapply. Assess the condition of the extremity frequently. **EB:** *Graduated compression stockings, alone or used in conjunction with other prevention modalities, help promote venous return and prevent deep vein thrombosis in hospitalized clients (Amarigiri & Lees, 2005).*

• Assess for presence of anxiety. Consider using music to decrease anxiety and improve cardiac function. See Nursing Interventions and Rationales for **Anxiety** to facilitate reduction of anxiety in clients and family. **EBN:** *Music has been shown to reduce heart rate, blood pressure, anxiety, and cardiac complications (Guzzetta, 1994). Watch for signs of depression: flat affect, poor sleeping, loss of appetite, listlessness.*

▲ Refer for treatment if anxiety is present. *Depression is very common in heart failure clients and can result in increased mortality (Thomas et al, 2003).*

▲ Closely monitor fluid intake, including intravenous lines. Maintain fluid restriction if ordered. *In clients with decreased cardiac output, poorly functioning ventricles may not tolerate increased fluid volumes.*

▲ If intravenous fluid is ordered for circulatory failure, administer cautiously and observe for signs of fluid overload. Administering excessive volume is detrimental to cardiac output. **EB:** *The response to rapid fluid loading can be predicted noninvasively by changes in pulse pressure during passive leg raising in clients with acute circulatory failure who were receiving mechanical ventilation (Boulain et al, 2002).*

▲ Observe for symptoms of cardiogenic shock, including impaired mentation, hypotension with blood pressure lower than 90 mm Hg, decreased peripheral pulses, cold clammy skin, signs of pulmonary congestion, and decreased organ function. If present, notify physician immediately. *Cardiogenic shock is a state of circulatory failure from loss from cardiac function associated with inadequate organ perfusion with a high mortality rate (Fuster et al, 2005).* **EBN:** *In a study the defining characteristics of decreased cardiac output were best indicated by decreased peripheral pulses and decreased peripheral perfusion (Oliva & Monteiro da Cruz, 2003).*

▲ If shock is present, monitor hemodynamic parameters for an increase in pulmonary wedge pressure, an increase in systemic vascular resistance, or a decrease in cardiac output and index. *Hemodynamic parameters give a good indication of cardiac function (Sole, Lamborn & Hartshorn, 2001).*

▲ Titrate inotropic and vasoactive medications within defined parameters to maintain contractility, preload, and afterload per physician's order. *By following parameters, the nurse ensures maintenance of a delicate balance of medications that stimulate the heart to increase contractility, while maintaining adequate perfusion of the body.*

▲ Be aware that intraaortic balloon counterpulsation is implemented to treat cardiogenic shock by decreasing the workload of the left ventricle and improving myocardial perfusion (Reid & Cottrell, 2005).

C

▲ Be aware that mechanical ventilation can decrease cardiac output. **EB:** *High-frequency oscillation ventilation in adults leads to significantly decreased cardiac output (Mehta et al, 2004).*

▲ Refer to heart failure program or cardiac rehabilitation program for education, evaluation, and guided support to increase activity and rebuild life. **EB:** *Exercise can help many clients with heart failure. Inactivity can worsen the skeletal muscle myopathy in these clients. A carefully monitored exercise program can improve both exercise capacity and quality of life in mild to moderate heart failure clients (Rees et al, 2004). Exercise-based cardiac rehabilitation is effective in reducing the number of cardiac deaths, decreasing cholesterol levels and systolic blood pressure, and reduced self-reported smoking (Taylor et al, 2004; Jolliffe et al, 2001).*

▲ Be aware that cardiac resynchronization therapy improves cardiac output and may be ordered for appropriate clients. **EB:** *A study of both ischemic and nonischemic clients had increases in cardiac output after cardiac resynchronization therapy (Woo et al, 2005).*

▲ Be aware that pregnancy increases cardiac output and take into consideration when assessing nutritional needs. **EB:** *A study that assessed changes in basal metabolic rate during pregnancy found that by gestational week 32, weight gain and the percentage of total body fat must be considered when calculating energy requirements in pregnancy (Lof et al, 2005).*

Geriatric

• Observe for atypical pain; the elderly often have jaw pain instead of chest pain or may have silent myocardial infarctions (MIs) with symptoms of dyspnea or fatigue. *Symptoms, when present in older clients with an acute MI, may be extremely vague, and, as with myocardial ischemia, the diagnosis may be easily missed. Atypical symptoms of MI include dyspnea, neurologic symptoms, or gastrointestinal (GI) symptoms (Aronow, 2003).*

▲ If client has heart disease causing activity intolerance, refer for cardiac rehabilitation. **EB:** *The anxiety experienced after hospitalization is higher in elderly clients with heart disease compared to that of younger clients participating in exercise programs. (Twiss, Seaver & McCaffrey, 2006).*

• Consider the use of graphic feedback with the elderly in exercise adherence. **EBN:** *The graphic format may be especially helpful because graphs provide a clear picture of the client's exercise goals and recent progress (Duncan & Pozehl, 2003).*

• Observe for syncope, dizziness, palpitations, or feelings of weakness associated with an irregular heart rhythm. *Dysrhythmias are common in the elderly.*

▲ Observe for side effects from cardiac medications. *The elderly have difficulty with metabolism and excretion of medications due to decreased function of the liver and kidneys; therefore toxic side effects are more common.*

Pediatrics/Newborn

• Monitor heart rate continuously in the newborn and report abnormalities immediately. **EBN:** *Cardiac output in the newborn is dependent on heart rate, but has a decreased ability to maximize and vary heart rate (Sherman et al, 2002).*

Home Care

• Some of the above interventions may be adapted for home care use.

▲ Begin discharge planning as soon as possible with case manager or social worker to assess home support systems and the need for community or home health services. Consider referral for advanced practice nurse (APN) follow-up. Support services may be needed to assist with home care, meal preparations, housekeeping, personal care, transportation to doctor visits, or emotional support. *Clients often need help on discharge.* **EBN:** *In a randomized control trial, the assignment of an APN to assist with transition to the home for elders with heart failure resulted in greater length of time between hospitalizations, fewer total hospitalizations, and decreased healthcare costs. A study of transitional care using nonspecialist nurses found an improvement in the quality of life and a reduction in the number of emergency department visits with congestive heart failure (CHF) clients (Clark & Nadash, 2004).*

▲ Adopt a clinical pathway to address focused interventions with CHF, coronary artery bypass graft (CABG). National Practice Guidelines for Cardiac Home Care are available to direct intervention for the client post-CABG who is recovering at home (Frantz & Walters, 2001).

• = Independent;   ▲ = Collaborative;   EBN = Evidence-Based Nursing;   EB = Evidence-Based

EBN: *Study of the outcome of a CHF clinical pathway revealed a 45% reduction in rehospitalization (Hoskins et al, 2001; Young et al, 2004).*

▲ Assess or refer to case manager or social worker to evaluate client ability to pay for prescriptions. *The cost of drugs may be a factor in filling prescriptions and adhering to a treatment plan.*

• Continue to monitor client closely for exacerbation of heart failure when discharged home. *Transition to home can create increased stress and physiological instability related to diagnosis.* **EBN:** *Home visits and phone contacts that emphasize client education and recognition of early symptoms of exacerbation can decrease rehospitalization (Gorski & Johnson, 2003).*

• Monitor women for differential symptoms of MI and institute emergency treatment measures as indicated. **EBN:** *Continuing research is exploring differences in MI symptoms between men and women. A qualitative study of 40 women following MI noted prodromal symptoms. Most frequent were unusual fatigue, discomfort in the shoulder blade area, and chest sensations. Most common acute symptoms were chest sensations, shortness of breath, feeling hot and flushed, and unusual fatigue. Severe pain during the acute phase was experienced by only 11 women (McSweeney & Crane, 2000). African-American and Caucasian women have different physical recovery trajectories from acute MI (prolonged) but similar psychosocial recovery trajectories (Rankin, 2002).*

• Instruct women in the differential symptoms of MI in women, and the need to take symptoms seriously and seek help as indicated. **EBN:** *Women delay seeking help a median of 6.25 hours. Help-seeking behavior was influenced by beliefs about women's susceptibility to MI and differential symptom awareness. Symptoms presenting in this study were rarely consistent with those described in the health promotion literature (Holliday, Lowe & Outram, 2000).*

▲ Assess client for understanding of and compliance with medical regimen, including medications, activity level, and diet. Client/family may need repetition of instructions received at hospital discharge, and may require reiteration as fear of a recent crisis decreases. *Fear interferes with the ability to assimilate new information.*

▲ Assess and monitor for signs of depression (particularly in adults age 65 years or older) or social isolation. Refer for mental health treatment as indicated. **EBN:** *Mood disturbance, social isolation, low socioeconomic status, and nonwhite ethnicity predicted lower functional status of clients with left ventricular dysfunction after 1 year (Clarke et al, 2000).* **EB:** *Depression has been noted as prevalent after acute MI in clients over age 65. Depression has been shown to be an independent risk factor for heart failure in elderly women but not in elderly men (Williams et al, 2002).*

• Assess for signs/symptoms of cognitive impairment. **EBN:** *Cognitive function may decline in late-stage CHF (Quaglietti et al, 2004).*

• Assess for fatigue and weakness frequently. Assess home environment for safety, as well as resources/obstacles to energy conservation. Instruct client and family members on need for behavioral pacing and energy conservation. **EBN:** *Fatigue and weakness limit activity level and quality of life. Assistive devices and other techniques of work simplification can help the client participate in and respond to the healthcare regimen more effectively (Quaglietti et al, 2004).*

• Instruct family and client about the disease process, complications of disease process, information on medications, need for weighing daily, and when it is appropriate to call doctor. *Early recognition of symptoms facilitates early problem solving and prompt treatment. Decreased cardiac output can be life threatening.* **EBN:** *Clients with heart failure need intensive education about these topics to help prevent readmission to the hospital (Moser, 2000).*

• Help family adapt daily living patterns to establish life changes that will maintain improved cardiac functioning in the client. Take the client's perspective into consideration, and use a holistic approach in assessing and responding to client planning for the future. *Transition to the home setting can cause risk factors such as inappropriate diet to reemerge.* **EBN:** *A study of women recovering from MI revealed that these women lived with a feeling of insecurity, based on a new inability to trust their bodies. Caring for women post-MI, researchers concluded, must approach health as being more than the absence of illness (Johansson, Dahlberg & Ekebergh, 2003).*

• Assist client to recognize and exercise power in using self-care management to adjust to health change. **EBN:** *Women post-MI reported that not participating in their health process increased their suffering and left them feeling powerless (Johansson, Dahlberg & Ekebergh, 2003).* Refer to care plan for **Powerlessness.**

• = Independent;   ▲ = Collaborative;   EBN = Evidence-Based Nursing;   EB = Evidence-Based

- Support client self-efficacy to increase physical activity by creating a supportive environment, offering encouragement, providing anticipatory guidance, and supplying a realistic assessment of the client's abilities. *Increasing self-efficacy takes time, but can lead to increased physical activity, decreased symptomology, and improved quality of life for the client (Borsody et al, 1999).*
▲ Explore barriers to medical regimen adherence. Review medications and treatment regularly for needed modifications. Take complaints of side effects seriously and serve as client advocate to address changes as indicated. *The presence of uncomfortable side effects frequently motivates clients to deviate from the medication regimen (Erhardt, 1999).*
▲ Refer for cardiac rehabilitation, strengthening exercises if client is not involved in outpatient cardiac rehabilitation. **EB:** *Exercise improves hemodynamic responsiveness in clients after uncomplicated acute myocardial infarction (Motohiro et al, 2005).*
▲ Refer to medical social services as necessary for counseling about the impact of severe or chronic cardiac disease. *Social workers can assist the client and family with acceptance of life changes.*
▲ Institute case management of frail elderly to support continued independent living.
▲ As client condition warrants, refer to hospice. *The multidisciplinary hospice team can reduce hospital readmission, increase functional capacity, and improve quality of life in end-stage heart failure (Coviello, Hricz & Masulli, 2002).*
- Identify emergency plan, including use of cardiopulmonary resuscitation (CPR). Encourage family members to become certified in cardiopulmonary resuscitation. **EBN:** *CPR training significantly increased perceived control in spouses of recovering cardiac clients (Moser & Dracup, 2000).*

Client/Family Teaching

- Teach symptoms of heart failure and appropriate actions to take if client becomes symptomatic.
- Teach importance of smoking cessation and avoidance of alcohol intake. *Smoking is a well-established risk factor for coronary artery disease. Help clients who smoke stop by informing them of potential consequences and by helping them find an effective cessation method. Excessive intake of alcohol can produce alcoholic cardiomyopathy or worsen heart failure (Caboral & Mitchell, 2003).* **EB:** *Smoking cessation advice and counsel given by nurses can be effective, and should be available to clients to help stop smoking (Rice & Stead, 2000).* **EBN:** *Newborns of mothers who smoked during gestation had limited ability to maximize and vary their heart rates, and as cardiac output in the newborn is primarily dependent on heart rate, may be potentially at risk for morbidity and mortality (Sherman et al, 2002).* **EB:** *A study assessing right heart hemodynamic values and respiratory function among chronic smokers found that cardiac output and respiratory function worsened significantly in this sample (Gulbaran et al, 2004).*
- Teach stress reduction (e.g., imagery, controlled breathing, muscle relaxation techniques).
- Explain necessary restrictions, including consumption of a sodium-restricted diet, guidelines on fluid intake, and the avoidance of Valsalva maneuver. Teach the importance of pacing activities, work simplification techniques, and the need to rest between activities to prevent becoming overly fatigued. *Sodium retention leading to fluid overload is a common cause of hospital readmission (Bennett et al, 2000).*
▲ Teach the client actions, side effects, and importance of consistently taking cardiovascular medications. **EBN:** *A research study demonstrated that heart failure clients were not knowledgeable of the medications or for the need for weight monitoring and recognizing the definition for heart failure (Artinian et al, 2002).*
- Provide client/family with advance directive information to consider. Allow client to give advance directions about medical care or designate who should make medical decisions if he or she should lose decision-making capacity.
▲ Instruct the client on importance of getting a pneumonia shot (usually one per lifetime) and yearly influenza shots as prescribed by physician. *Clients with decreased cardiac output are considered higher risk for complications or death if they do not get immunization injections.*
- Instruct client/family on the need to weigh daily and keep a weight log. Ask if client has a scale at home; if not, assist in getting one. Instruct on establishing baseline weight on own scale when gets home. *Daily weighing is an essential aspect of self-management. A scale is necessary. Scales vary; the client needs to establish a baseline weight on his or her home scale.*
- Provide specific written materials and self-care plan for client/caregivers to use for reference.

- ▲ Consult dietitian or assist client in understanding the need for a sodium-restricted diet. Provide alternatives for salt such as spices, herbs, lemon juice, or vinegar. *Although the initial elimination of salt from the diet is very difficult, the taste of salt can be unlearned. The spices and seasonings above can enhance the taste appeal of food while the preference for salt is changing (Cataldo, DeBruyne & Whitney, 2003). Taste sensation is often diminished as a function of age, producing a greater desire for salty foods (Forman & Rich, 2003).*
- • Instruct family regarding cardiopulmonary resuscitation.

evolve   See the EVOLVE website for World Wide Web resources for client education.

REFERENCES

Adams KL: Hemodynamic assessment: the physiologic basis for turning data into clinical information, *AACN Clinical Issues*, 15(4):534-546, 2004.

Albert NM, Hail MD, Li J: Equivalence of the bioimpedance and thermodilution methods in measuring cardiac output in hospitalized patients with advanced, decompensated chronic heart failure, *Am J Crit Care* 13(6):469, 2004.

Amarigiri SV, Lees TA: Elastic compression stockings for prevention of deep vein thrombosis, *Cochrane Database Syst Rev* (3): CD001484, 2005.

Aronow W, Silent MI: Prevalence and prognosis in older patients diagnosed by routine electrocardiograms, *Geriatrics* 58(1):24-26, 36-38, 40, 2003.

Artinian NT, Magnan M, Christian W et al: What do patients know about their heart failure? *Appl Nurs Res* 15(4):200, 2002.

Bennett SJ, Cordes DK, Westmoreland G et al: Self-care strategies for symptom management in patients with chronic heart failure, *Nurs Res* 49(3):139, 2000.

Borsody JM, Courtney M, Taylor K et al: Using self-efficacy to increase physical activity in patients with heart failure, *Home Healthc Nurse* 17:113, 1999.

Boulain T, Achard J, Teboul J et al: Changes in blood pressure induced by passive leg raising predict response to fluid loading in critically ill patients, *Chest* 121(4):1245-1253, 2002.

Brostrom A, Stromberg A, Dahlstrom U et al: Sleep difficulties, daytime sleepiness, and health-related quality of life in patients with chronic heart failure, *J Cardiovasc Nurs* 19(4):234, 2004.

Caboral M, Mitchell J: New guidelines for heart failure focus on prevention, *Nurse Pract* 28(1):13, 16, 22-23, 2003.

Cataldo CB, DeBruyne LK, Whitney EN: *Nutrition and diet therapy*, ed 6, Belmont, 2003, Thomson Wadsworth.

Clark A, Nadash P: The effectiveness of a nurse-led transitional care model for patients with congestive heart failure, *Home Healthc Nurs* 22(3):160, 2004.

Clarke SP, Frasure-Smith N, Lesperance F et al: Psychosocial factors as predictors of functional status at 1 year in patients with left ventricular dysfunction, *Res Nurs Health* 23:290-300, 2000.

Coviello JS, Hricz L, Masulli PS: Client challenge: accomplishing quality of life in end-stage heart failure: a hospice multidisciplinary approach, *Home Healthc Nurs* 20:195, 2002.

Dosh S: Diagnosis of heart failure in adults, *Am Fam Physician* 70(11):2145, 2004.

Duncan K, Pozehl B: Effects of an exercise adherence intervention on outcomes in patients with heart failure, *Cardiac Rehab* 28(4):117, 2003.

Engoren M, Barbee D: Comparison of cardiac output determined by bioimpedance, thermodilution, and the Fick method, *Am J Crit Care* 14(1):40, 2005.

Erhardt ER: The essence of effective treatment and compliance is simplicity, *Am J Hypertens* 12(10 Pt 2):105SS, 1999.

Forman D, Rich M: Heart failure in the elderly, *Congest Heart Fail* 9(6):311, 2003.

Frantz AK, Walters JI: Recovery from coronary artery bypass grafting at home: is your practice current? *Home Healthc Nurs* 19:417, 2001.

Fuster V et al: *Hurst's the heart*, ed 11, vol 2, New York, 2005, McGraw Hill.

Giuliano KK, Scott SS, Brown V et al: Backrest angle and cardiac output measurement in critically ill patients, *Nurs Res* 52(4):242-248, 2003.

Gorski LA, Johnson K: A disease management program for heart failure: collaboration between a home care agency and a care management organization, *Home Healthc Nurs* 21(11):734, 2003.

Gulbaran M, Cagatay T, Gurman T et al: Right heart haemodynamic values and respiratory function test parameters in chronic smokers, *Eastern Mediterr Health J* 10(1/2):90-95, 2004.

Guzzetta CE: Soothing the ischemic heart, *Am J Nurs* 94:24, 1994.

Hogan E, Hornick B, Bouchoux A: Communicating the message: clarifying the controversies about caffeine, *Nutr Today* 37(1):28, 2002.

Holliday JE, Lowe JM, Outram S: Women's experience of myocardial infarction, *Intl J Nurs Pract* 6:307, 2000.

Hoskins LM, Clark HM, Schroeder MA et al: A clinical pathway for congestive heart failure, *Home Healthc Nurs* 19:207, 2001.

Iregui MG, Prentice D, Sherman G et al: Physicians' estimates of cardiac index and intravascular volume based on clinical assessment versus transesophageal Doppler measurements obtained by critical care nurses, *Am J Crit Care* 12(4):336-343, 2003.

Johansson A, Dahlberg K, Ekebergh M: Living with experiences following a myocardial infarction, *Euro J Cardiovasc Nurs* 2:229, 2003.

Jolliffe, Rees K, Taylor RS et al: Exercise-based rehabilitation for coronary heart disease, *Cochrane Database Syst Rev* (1):CD001800, 2001.

Kasper DL et al: *Harrison's principles of internal medicine*, ed 16, New York, 2005, McGraw-Hill.

Lof M, Olausson H, Bostrom K et al: Changes in basal metabolic rate during pregnancy in relation to changes in body weight and composition, cardiac output, insulin growth factor-I and thyroid hormones and in relation to fetal growth, *Am J Clin Nutr* 81(3):678-685, 2005.

Maisel AS, Krishnaswamy P, Nowak RM et al: Rapid measurement of B-type natriuretic peptide in the emergency diagnosis of heart failure, *N Engl J Med* 347(3):11, 2002.

McSweeney JC, Crane PB: Challenging the rules: women's prodromal and acute symptoms of myocardial infarction, *Res Nurs Health* 23:135, 2000.

Mehta S, Granton J, Macdonald RJ et al: High frequency oscillaroty ventilation in adults: the Toronto experience, *Chest* 126(2):518-527, 2004.

Moser DK: Heart failure management: optimal health care delivery programs, *Annu Rev Nurs Res* 18:91, 2000.

Moser DK, Dracup K: Impact of cardiopulmonary resuscitation training on perceived control in spouses of recovering cardiac patients, *Res Nurs Health* 23:270, 2000.

Moser DK, Frazier SK, Woo MA et al: Normal fluctuations in pulmonary artery pressures and cardiac output in patients with severe left ventricular dysfunction, *Eur J Cardiovasc Nurs* 1(2):131-137, 2002.

Motohiro M, Yuasa F, Hattori T et al: Cardiovascular adaptations to exercise training after uncomplicated acute myocardial infarction, *Am J Phys Med Rehabil* 84(9):684-691, 2005.

Myers MG, Harris L: High dose caffeine and ventricular arrhythmias, *Can J Cardiol* 6(3):95, 1990.

Newberry L: *Sheehy's emergency nursing,* ed 5, St Louis, 2003, Mosby.

Oliva AP, Cruz DAL: Decreased cardiac output: validation with postoperative heart surgery patients, *Dimens Crit Care Nurs* 22(1):39-44, 2003.

Quaglietti S, Lovett S, Hawthorne C et al: Management of the patient with congestive heart failure in the home care and palliative care setting, *Ann Long Term Care* 12(1):33, 2004.

Rankin SH: Women recovering from acute myocardial infarction: psychosocial and physical functioning outcomes for 12 months after acute myocardial infarction, *Heart Lung* 31(6):399, 2002.

Reid MB, Cottrell D: Nursing care of patients receiving intraaortic balloon counterpulsation, *Crit Care Nurse* 25(5):40-49, 2005.

Rees K, Taylor RS, Singh S et al: Exercise based rehabilitation for heart failure, *Cochrane Database Syst Rev* (3):CD003331, 2004.

Rice VH, Stead LF: Nursing interventions for smoking cessation, *Cochrane Database Syst Rev* (2):CD001188, 2000.

Schneider JR: Effects of caffeine ingestion on heart rate, blood pressure, myocardial oxygen consumption, and cardiac rhythm in acute myocardial infarction patients, *Heart Lung* 16:167, 1987.

Sherman J, Young A, Sherman MP et al: Prenatal smoking and alterations in newborn heart rate during transition, *J Obstet Gynecol Neonatal Nurs* 31(6):680-687, 2002.

Sole ML, Lamborn ML, Hartshorn JC: *Introduction to critical care nursing,* ed 3, Philadelphia, 2001, WB Saunders.

Stelfox H, Ahmed S, Ribeiro RA et al: Hemodynamic monitoring in obese patients: the impact of body mass index on cardiac output and stroke volume, *Crit Care Med* 34(4):1243-1246, 2006.

Taylor RS, Brown A, Ebrahim S et al: Exercise-based rehabilitation for patients with coronary heart disease: systematic review and meta-analysis of randomized controlled trials, *Am J Med* 116(10):682, 2004.

Thomas SA, Friedmann E, Khatta M et al: Depression in patients with heart failure: physiologic effects, incidence, and relation to mortality, *AACN Clin Issues* 14(1):3, 2003.

Twiss E, Seaver J, McCaffrey R: The effects of music listening on older adults undergoing cardiovascular surgery, *Nurs Crit Care* 11(5):224-231, 2006.

Urquhart G, Jensen L: Timing of hemodynamic pressure measurements on derived hemodynamic parameters, *Dynamics* 14(3):13-20, 2003.

Williams H, Kearney M: Chronic heart failure, *Pharma J* 269:325, 2002

Williams SA, Kasl SV, Heiat A et al: Depression and risk of heart failure among the elderly: a prospective community-based study, *Psychosom Med* 64(1):6, 2002.

Winslow EH: Panning bedpans, *Am J Nurs* 92:16G, 1992.

Woo GW, Petersen-Stejskal S, Johnson JW et al: Ventricular reverse remodeling and 6-month outcomes in patients receiving cardiac re-synchronization therapy: analysis of the MIRACLE study, *J Interv Card Electrophysiol* 12(2):107-13, 2005.

Yancy C, Abraham W: Noninvasive hemodynamic monitoring in heart failure: utilization of impedance cardiography, *Congest Heart Fail* 9(5):241, 2003.

Young W, McShane J, O'Connor T et al: Registered nurses' experiences with an evidence-based home care pathway for myocardial infarction clients, *Can J Cardiovasc Nurs* 14(3):24, 2004.

Caregiver role strain   *evolve*

Barbara Given, PhD, RN, FAAN, and Paula Sherwood, PhD, RN, CNRN

NANDA   Definition

Difficulty in performing family caregiver role

Defining Characteristics

Caregiving Activities

Apprehension about care receiver's care if caregiver unable to provide care; apprehension about the future regarding care receiver's health; apprehension about the future regarding caregiver's ability to provide care; apprehension about possible institutionalization of care receiver; difficulty completing required tasks; difficulty performing required tasks; dysfunctional change in caregiving activities; preoccupation with care routine

Caregiver Health Status—Physical

Cardiovascular disease; diabetes; fatigue; GI upset; headaches; hypertension; rash; weight change

Caregiver Health Status—Emotional

Anger; disturbed sleep; feeling depressed; frustration; impaired individual coping; impatience; increased emotional lability; increased nervousness; lack of time to meet personal needs; somatization; stress

---

• = Independent;   ▲ = Collaborative;   EBN = Evidence-Based Nursing;   EB = Evidence-Based

Socioeconomic

Changes in leisure activities; low work productivity; refuses career advancement; withdraws from social life

Caregiver–Care Receiver Relationship

Difficulty watching care receiver go through the illness; grief regarding changed relationship with care receiver; uncertainty regarding changed relationship with care receiver

Family Processes

Concerns about family members; family conflict

Related Factors (r/t)

Care Receiver Health Status

Addiction; codependence; cognitive problems; dependency; illness chronicity; illness severity; increasing care needs; instability of care receiver's health; problem behaviors; psychological problems; unpredictability of illness course

Socioeconomic Factors

Isolation from others; competing role commitments; alienation from family, friends, and coworkers; insufficient recreation

Caregiver Health Status

Addiction; codependency; cognitive problems; inability to fulfill one's own expectations; inability to fulfill other's expectations; marginal coping patterns; physical problems; psychological problems; unrealistic expectations of self

Caregiver–Care Receiver Relationship

History of poor relationship; mental status of elder inhibiting conversation presence of abuse or violence; unrealistic expectations of caregiver by care receiver

Caregiving Activities

24-hour care responsibilities; amount of activities; complexity of activities; discharge of family members to home with significant care needs; ongoing changes in activities; unpredictability of care situation; years of caregiving

Family Processes

History of family dysfunction; history of marginal family coping

Resources

Caregiver is not developmentally ready for caregiver role; deficient knowledge about community resources; difficulty accessing community resources; emotional strength; formal assistance; formal support; inadequate community resources (e.g., respite services, recreational resources); inadequate equipment for providing care; inadequate physical environment for providing care (e.g., housing, temperature, safety); inadequate transportation; inexperience with caregiving; informal assistance; informal support; insufficient finances; insufficient time; lack of caregiver privacy; lack of support; physical energy

Socioeconomic

Alienation from others; competing role commitments; insufficient recreation; isolation from others

NOC   Outcomes (Nursing Outcomes Classification)

Suggested NOC Outcomes

Caregiver Emotional Health, Caregiver Lifestyle Disruption, Caregiver Performance: Direct Care, Indirect Care, Caregiver Physical Health, Caregiver Stressors, Caregiver Well-Being, Role

---

• = Independent;   ▲ = Collaborative;   EBN = Evidence-Based Nursing;   EB = Evidence-Based

Performance, Caregiver Self-Esteem, Caregiver Mastery, Caregiver Competence, Caregiver Role Adjustment

Example NOC Outcome with Indicators

Caregiver Emotional Health with plans for a positive future as evidenced by the following indicators: Satisfaction with life/Sense of control/Self-esteem/Free of anger/Free of guilt/Free of depression/Perceived social connectedness/Perceived spiritual well-being (Rate the outcome and indicators of **Caregiver Emotional Health:** 1 = severely compromised, 2 = substantially compromised, 3 = moderately compromised, 4 = mildly compromised, 5 = not compromised [see Section I].)

Client Outcomes

- Caregiver will feel supported
- Caregiver will report low or no feelings of burden or distress
- Caregiver will maintain own physical and psychological/emotional health
- Caregiver will identify resources available to help in giving care
- Caregiver will verbalize mastery of the care situation, feeling confident and competent to provide care
- Care receiver will obtain quality and safe care

NIC   Interventions (Nursing Interventions Classification)

Suggested NIC Intervention

Caregiver Support

Example NIC Activities—Caregiver Support

Determine caregiver's acceptance of role; Accept expressions of negative emotion

Nursing Interventions and *Rationales*

- Watch for signs of depression and deteriorating physical health in the caregiver, especially if the marital relationship is poor, the care recipient has cognitive or neuropsychiatric symptoms, there is little social support available, the caregiver becomes enmeshed in the care situation, the caregiver is elderly, female, or has poor preexisting physical or emotional health. Refer to the care plan for **Hopelessness** when appropriate. **EB:** *Caregiving may weaken the immune system and predispose the caregiver to illness in some situations (Mills et al, 2004; Redwine et al, 2004). The incidence of depression in family caregivers is estimated to be 40% to 50% (Schulz & Martire, 2004; Knop, Bergman-Evans & McCabe, 1998).* **EBN:** *Intervening early to help the caregiver can result in improved care for the stroke client and, it is hoped, improved health for the caregiver (Bakas & Burgener, 2002; Teel, Duncan & Lai, 2001).*
- The impact of providing care on the caregiver's emotional health should be assessed at regular intervals using a reliable and valid instrument such as the Caregiver Strain Index, Caregiver Burden Inventory, Caregiver Reaction Assessment, Screen for Caregiver Burden, and the Subjective and Objective Burden Scale (Deeken et al, 2003; Given et al, 1992; Vitaliano et al, 1991). **EBN and EB:** *Research has validated the effectiveness of a number of evaluation tools for caregiver stress, including the Caregiver Reaction Assessment (Given et al, 1992), Burden Interview (Zarit et al, 1980), the Caregiver Strain Index (Robinson, 1983), and the Caregiver Burden Inventory (Novak & Guest, 1989). Caregiver assessment tools should be multidimensional and evaluate the impact of providing care on multiple aspects of the caregiver's life (Hudson & Hayman-White, 2006).*
- Identify potential caregiver resources such as mastery, social support, optimism, and positive aspects of care. **EB:** *Research has shown that caregivers can have simultaneous positive and negative responses to providing care. Positive responses may help to buffer the negative effects of providing care on caregivers' emotional health (Pinquart & Sorenson, 2003).*
- Screen for caregiver role strain at the onset of the care situation, at regular intervals throughout

• = Independent;   ▲ = Collaborative;   EBN = Evidence-Based Nursing;   EB = Evidence-Based

the care situation, and with changes in care recipient status and care transitions. **EB:** *Care situations that last for several months or years can cause wear and tear that exhaust caregivers' coping mechanisms and available resources. In addition, changes in the care recipient's health status necessitate new skills and monitoring from the caregiver and affect the caregiver's ability to continue to provide care (Burton et al, 2003). Providing caregiver support throughout the care situation may decrease care recipient institutionalization (Mittelman et al, 2006).*

- Watch for caregivers who become enmeshed in the care situation (e.g., becoming overinvolved or unable to disentangle themselves from the caregiver role). **EB:** *Role training (assisting caregivers to understand and define their role) may prevent caregivers from becoming enmeshed, which can in turn prevent burden and depression (Hepburn et al, 2001).*
- Arrange for intervals of respite care for the caregiver; encourage use if available. **EB:** *Respite care provides time away from the care situation and can help alleviate distress (Sorensen, Pinquart & Duberstein, 2002).*
- Help the caregiver to identify and utilize support systems. **EBN:** *Caregivers sometimes feel abandoned and need assistance to activate their support systems (Borg & Hallberg, 2006).*
- Encourage the caregiver to grieve over changes in the care receiver's condition and give the caregiver permission to share angry feelings in a safe environment. Refer to nursing interventions for **Grieving. EBN:** *Caregivers grieve the loss of function of their loved one, especially when dementia is involved (Narayan et al, 2001; Schulz et al, 2006).*
- Help the caregiver find personal time to meet his or her needs, learn stress management techniques, schedule regular health screenings, and schedule regular respite time. **EB:** *Self-care is important for the caregiver (Belle et al, 2006). Maintaining personal wellness can increase stamina, energy, and self-esteem and enhance the quality of care given.*
- Encourage the caregiver to schedule and keep routine healthcare appointments (i.e., annual physicals and screening tests). **EB:** *Caregivers who report being strained are at risk for lower perceptions of their own health status, increased risky behaviors such as smoking, and higher use of prescription drugs (Beach et al, 2000).*
- Encourage the caregiver to talk about feelings, concerns, uncertainties, and fears. Acknowledge the frustration associated with caregiver responsibilities. **EBN:** *Caregivers need a safe outlet for their feelings regarding the care situation (Narayan et al, 2001).*
- Observe for any evidence of caregiver or care receiver violence or abuse; if evidence is present, speak with the caregiver and care receiver separately. **EB:** *Caregiver violence is possible, particularly when high levels of care demands or caregiver distress are present (Hansberry, Chen & Gorbien, 2005).*
- ▲ Involve the family in care transitions; use a multidisciplinary team to provide medical and social services for instruction and planning. **EBN:** *Caregivers who reported involvement in discharge planning, particularly when discharge planning was done by an interdisciplinary team, report better acceptance of the caregiving role and better health (Bull, Hansen & Gross, 2000; Bull & Roberts, 2001).*
- ▲ Encourage regular communication with the care recipient and with the healthcare team. **EB:** *Caregivers' preferential communication method and communication needs should be addressed at regular intervals to improve their sense of mastery over the care situation (Iconomou, Vagenakis & Kalofonos, 2001).*
- Help caregiver assess his/or her socioeconomic status (services reimbursed by insurance, available support through community and religious organizations). **EB and EBN:** *Low incomes and limited financial resources can cause strain for the caregiver, particularly if there are substantial out-of-pocket costs involved in providing care (Nijboer et al, 2001; Hayman et al, 2001).*
- Help the caregiver identify competing occupational demands and potential ways to modify the work role in order to provide care (enact the Family Leave Act, change from full to part time, work from home, take a leave of absence or early retirement). **EB:** *Employed caregivers report missed days, interruptions at work, leaves of absence, and reduced productivity due to providing care (Cameron et al, 2002).*
- When necessary, help the caregiver transition the care recipient to a long-term care facility. **EB:** *Placing a loved one in an extended care facility can relieve the burden of care but does not relieve the stress resulting from financial concerns, guilt, loss of control, or lack of support (Schulz et al, 2004).*

• = Independent; ▲ = Collaborative; EBN = Evidence-Based Nursing; EB = Evidence-Based

- Help the caregiver problem solve to meet the care recipient's needs. **EBN:** *Using a problem solving intervention—helping the caregiver identify the problem, its sources, and generating potential solutions—has been shown to lower distress in caregivers of persons with cancer (Given et al, 2006).*

Geriatric

- Monitor the caregiver for psychological distress and signs of depression, especially if caring for a mentally impaired elder or if there was an unsatisfactory marital relationship before caregiving. **EBN:** *A difficult marriage before caregiving predisposes the caregiver to depression (Hansberry, Chen & Gorbien, 2005).* **EBN:** *Older adults in long-term marriages need to be considered as individuals as well as members of a couple in both assessment and planning interventions (Padula & Sullivan, 2006).*
- Assess the health of caregivers at intervals, especially if they have their own chronic illness in addition to caregiving role. **EB:** *Caregivers who report feeling burdened have an increased risk of mortality, risk that may be particularly high in elderly caregivers with comorbid conditions (Beach et al, 2000; Schulz & Beach, 1999).*
- Assess social support and encourage the use of secondary caregivers with elderly caregivers. **EBN:** *Older caregivers often become enmeshed in the care situation (often because they provide care by themselves) and isolate themselves from social and family support to become completely focused on providing care for their spouse (Borg & Hallberg, 2006).*
- Provide skills training related to direct care, performing complex monitoring tasks, supervision interpreting client symptoms, assisting with decision making, providing emotional support and comfort, and coordinating care. **EBN:** *Each task demands different skills and knowledge, organizational capacities, role demands, and social and psychological strengths from family members (Schumacher et al, 2000).*
- Teach symptom management techniques (assessment, potential causes, aggravating factors, potential alleviating factors, reassessment), particularly for fatigue, constipation, anorexia, and pain. **EB and EBN:** *Certain client symptoms such as fatigue, constipation, anorexia, pain, and depression have been associated with caregiver strain (Kurtz et al, 2004; Newton et al, 2002; Yurk et al, 2002).*

Multicultural

- Assess for the influence of cultural beliefs, norms, and values on the client's ability to modify health behavior. **EBN:** *What the client considers normal and abnormal health behavior may be based on cultural perceptions (Doswell & Erlen, 1998; Leininger & McFarland, 2002; Giger & Davidhizar, 2004).* **EBN:** *Each client should be assessed for ability to modify health behavior based on the phenomenon of communication, time, space, social organization, environmental control, and biological variations (Giger & Davidhizar, 2004).*
- Encourage spirituality as a source of support for coping. **EBN:** *Many African-Americans and Latinos identify spirituality, religiousness, prayer, and church-based approaches as coping resources (Samuel-Hodge et al, 2000).* **EBN:** *Socioeconomic status, geographical location, and risks associated with health-seeking behavior all influence the likelihood that clients will seek health care and modify health behavior (Appel, Giger & Davidhizar, 2005).*
- Negotiate with the client regarding the aspects of health behavior that will need to be modified. **EBN:** *Give-and-take with the client will lead to culturally congruent care (Leininger & McFarland, 2002).*
- Assess the role of fatalism on the client's ability to modify health behavior. **EB:** *Fatalistic perspectives, which involve the belief that you cannot control your own fate, influenced health behaviors in some African-American, Asian, and Latino populations (Joiner et al, 2001; Powe & Finnie, 2003; Giger & Davidhizar, 2004).*
- Identify which family members the client can rely on for support. **EBN:** *A variety of different cultures rely on family members to cope with stress (Aziz & Rowland, 2002; Donnelly, 2002; Gleeson-Kreig, Bernal & Woolley, 2002; White et al, 2002).* **EBN:** *For clients from Afghanistan adjustment to the United States has been particularly difficult, and family members have needed to lean on the immediate family who are available for support (Giger & Davidhizar, 2002).*
- ▲ Assess for signs of depression and level of social support and make appropriate referrals. **EB:** *Increased depressed feelings and lower levels of available social support were reported by minorities following injury (Brown et al, 2004).*
- Assess for the presence of conflicting values within the culture. **EBN:** *Whereas sharing and caring is*

part of the Amish community, females with breast cancer were found to value privacy issues related to their body image and health status and to prefer this was shared in the closed community (Schwartz, 2002).

 Home Care

- Identify client and caregiver factors that necessitate the use of formal home care services, that may affect provision of care, or that need to be addressed before the client can be safely discharged from home care. **EBN:** *Although home care resources can be useful in decreasing caregiver distress, they are not used with regularity across client populations. Healthcare practitioners should assess for the need for support resources prior to discharge and at routine intervals throughout the care situation, particularly in the first 2 years following diagnosis and with changes in the care recipient's condition (King & Semik, 2006).*

- Collaborate with the caregiver and discuss the care needs of the client, disease processes, medications, and what to expect; use a variety of instructional techniques (e.g., explanations, demonstrations, visual aids) until the caregiver is able to express a degree of comfort with care delivery. **EB:** *Knowledge and confidence are separate concepts. Self-assurance in caregiving will improve performance of the role in client maintenance that caregivers assume (Scott, 2000).*

- Assist the caregiver and client in arranging care so that it is compatible with other household patterns. **EBN:** *Caregivers of elders have been identified as using home environmental modification strategies for specific purposes: organizing the home, supplementing the elder's function, structuring the elder's day, protecting the elder, working around limitations or deficits in the home environment, enriching the home environment, and transitioning to a new home setting (Messecar et al, 2002).*

- Assess family caregiving skill. The identification of caregiver difficulty with any of a core set of processes highlights areas for intervention. **EBN:** *The ability to engage effectively and smoothly in nine processes has been identified as constituting family caregiving skill: monitoring client behavior, interpreting changes accurately, making decisions, taking action, making adjustment to care, accessing resources, providing hands-on care, working together with the ill person, and negotiating the healthcare system (Schumacher et al, 2000).* **EBN:** *Caregiver skills training has been shown to reduce burden in caregivers of persons with dementia (Davis et al, 2004).*

- Assess the client and caregiver at every visit for quality of care provided, functional disability of care recipient, caregiver coping, and signs of caregiver stress. **EB:** *A study of caregiver burden found that caregivers are most burdened by client behavior, with client physical and cognitive impairments and amount of care provision contributing. Coping processes and caregiver receipt of social support may moderate the relationship between caregiving demands and caregiving outcomes. The researchers concluded that caregivers need interventions that will reduce client behavior problems and increase caregivers' skills in handling behavioral difficulties (Pinquart & Sorensen, 2003).*

- Assess the client and caregiver at every visit for quality of relationship, and for the quality of caring that exists. **EBN:** *Quality of the caregiver/care recipient relationship and the impact of the care situation on that relationship can be an important source of distress or support for the caregiver (Cheung & Hocking, 2004; Clark et al, 2004; Krause & Rook, 2003; Martire et al, 2002). Chronic illness, especially dementia, can represent a gradual and devastating loss of the marital relationship as it existed formerly. An understanding of the prior relationship is needed before the couple can be helped to anticipate continuing care needs or deterioration (Zarit, 2001).*

- Assess preexisting strengths and weaknesses the caregiver brings to the situation, as well as current responses, depression, and fatigue levels. **EBN:** *Low individual and family hardiness was found to foster depression and fatigue in caregivers; coping strategies did not mediate the relationship (Clark, 2002). The type of empathy shown by caregivers can influence outcomes. Caregivers with high cognitive empathy (i.e., ability to understand another's feelings while maintaining emotional distance) viewed caregiving as less stressful, were less depressed, and reported higher life satisfaction than those with low cognitive empathy. Emotional empathy (i.e., vicarious emotional response to the perceived feelings of others) was associated with lower life satisfaction, presumably because caregivers were unable to detach themselves from the clients' feelings (Lee, Brennan & Daly, 2001).*

- Identify and support strengths and weaknesses of the caregiver and efforts to gain control of unpredictable situations. **EB:** *The use of external services may be helpful to gain control of the situation, and should be implemented when caregivers show signs of depressive symptomatology (Bookwala et al, 2004).* **EB:** *Caregivers with high levels of neuroticism may be less likely to benefit from interventions to alleviate caregiver burden (Jang et al, 2004).*

• = Independent;   ▲ = Collaborative;   EBN = Evidence-Based Nursing;   EB = Evidence-Based

C

- Form a trusting and supportive relationship with the caregiver. Allow the caregiver to verbalize frustrations. **EB:** *Building a supportive relationship between the healthcare provider and family caregiver is vital to meeting caregivers' needs (Kimberlin et al, 2004).*
- Explore with the spouse the process of understanding the client's behavior that the spouse has been undergoing; assist with reframing that understanding to be as realistic and positive as possible. Consider use of the Progressively Lowered Stress Threshold psychoeducational nursing intervention to help the spouse understand and handle the behavior changes associated with Alzheimer's disease. **EBN:** *In a qualitative study, wives of clients with Alzheimer's disease described a process of recognizing changes, drawing inferences about their observations, rewriting identities for themselves and their husbands as they took on the husbands' roles and responsibilities, and constructing a new daily life. Reframing interventions can help caregivers consider positive aspects of caring along with grief and frustration (Perry, 2002). Nurses can help caregivers normalize events, making these events more manageable and less threatening (Ayres, 2000a, 2000b). The Progressively Lowered Stress Threshold psychoeducational nursing intervention has been shown to have a positive effect in decreasing the frequency of disruptive behavior and improving the response of the caregiver to the behaviors of the Alzheimer's client (Gerdner, Buckwalter & Reed, 2002).*
- ▲ Refer the client to home health aide services for assistance with ADLs and light housekeeping. Allow the caregiver to gain confidence in the respite provider. *Home health aide services can provide physical relief and respite for the caregiver.* **EB:** *The greatest caregiver burden was reported to occur as physical demands increased, especially during the last 3 months of the client's life (Brazil et al, 2003).*
- ▲ Identify appropriate individual and group interventions for the caregiver; assess for appropriateness of referrals given the caregiver's needs and mobility. **EBN:** *Individual interventions (family-focused individual therapy, cognitive behavioral therapy, cognitive stimulation training, professional and peer counseling, stress management and problem solving) and group interventions (professional versus self-help support groups, stress management, respite care, multimedia training groups, caregiver training in behavior management and social skills) have been identified as effective in reducing caregiver stress (Yin, Zhou & Bashford, 2002).*
- ▲ Refer to a caregivers' support group if available or recommend an online support group—see suggested websites listed on the Evolve website. **EBN:** *Sharing concerns with others can mitigate loneliness. When nurses assist with online support groups, the groups can help caregivers learn, give them a sense of community, and encourage a sense of empowerment (White & Dorman, 2000).*
- Assess the caregiver for over-involvement with the client and client's illness. Encourage the caregiver to address an enmeshed relationship with the client prompted by concerns over the client's illness and altered quality of life by discussing the issue, seeking respite, and attending support groups. **EBN:** *In one study of women caring for husbands with chronic obstructive pulmonary disease, women had difficulty separating themselves from their husbands (Bergs, 2002).*
- ▲ Refer for homemaker or psychiatric home healthcare services for respite, client reassurance, and implementation of a therapeutic regimen. **EB:** *Homecare services have been shown to decrease caregiver stress and improve the mental health of caregivers (Shu, Lung & Huang, 2002; Tribaldi et al, 2004).*
- As indicated by client status, assist the caregiver in examining the option of adult day care and maintaining realistic expectations of adult day care. **EB:** *Studies have not shown a major impact of day care on the anxiety or depression of older adults, or on caregiver burden. However, a study did find subjective reports of reduced loneliness, anxiety, and depression among clients, and decreased perceived burden on caregivers (Baumgarten et al, 2002).*
- ▲ As indicated by deterioration of the client's condition, assist the caregiver in examining options for institutional placement. **EB:** *Caregiver overload can lead to decreased physical health and increased anxiety over time (Schulz et al, 1999). The caregiver may require instruction in the client's need for formal supports as condition deteriorates.*
- Assess the caregiver's emotional response to placement of the client and provide support, cognitive interventions, and problem solving as needed. *A variety of difficulties may impede the caregiver's acceptance of the need for the client's placement, including financial concerns, inability to accept the client's level of need for increased supervision, guilt, or unresolved relationship issues. It is important to identify the relevant concerns and options, as well to address psychological issues.* **EBN:** *Placement of a family member involves a struggle to make a decision, find reassurance, and remain connected to the client (Butcher et al, 2001).*
- Be aware that physical and emotional demands on the caregiver tend to increase during the last

---

• = Independent;   ▲ = Collaborative;   EBN = Evidence-Based Nursing;   EB = Evidence-Based

C

3 months of a care recipient's life, which may require more frequent or intense intervention. **EB:** *Families of terminally ill clients are especially vulnerable to caregiver role strain because the timing of the impending death is unpredictable, caregiver effort and resources are disproportionately spent early in the caregiving process, and increased physical care demands are associated with caregiver burden (Brazil et al, 2003).*

Caregiver/Family Teaching

- Assess the caregiver's need for information such as information on symptom management, disease progression, specific skills, and available support. **EBN:** *Using problem solving to help the caregiver manage clients' symptoms has been shown to significantly lower caregiver distress (Given et al, 2006).*
- Teach the caregiver warning signs for burnout, depression, and anxiety. Help them identify a resource in case they begin to feel overwhelmed.
- Teach the caregiver methods for managing disruptive behavioral symptoms if present. Refer to the care plan for **Chronic Confusion.** *Multicomponent interventions can be particularly effective in caregivers of persons with neurologic sequelae (Gitlin et al, 2003).*
- Teach the caregiver how to provide the care needed and put a plan in place for monitoring the care provided.
- Provide ongoing support and evaluation of care skills as the care situation and care demands change.
- Provide information regarding the care recipient's diagnosis, treatment regimen, and expected course of illness. **EB:** *An internet- and telephone-based education and support network for caregivers of individuals with progressive dementia has been developed (AlzOnline), and preliminary results demonstrate reductions in caregiver burden and improvements in caregiver mastery (Glueckauf et al, 2004).*
- ▲ Refer to counseling or support groups to assist in adjusting to the caregiver role and periodically evaluate not only the caregiver's emotional response to care but the safety of the care delivered to the care recipient.

evolve See the EVOLVE website for World Wide Web resources for caregiver education.

REFERENCES

Appel SJ, Giger JN, Davidhizar RE: Opportunity cost: the impact of contextual risk factors on the cardiovascular health of low-income rural southern African American women, *J Cardiovasc Nurs* 20:315-324, 2005.

Ayres L: Narratives of family caregiving: four story types, *Res Nurs Health* 23(5):359-371, 2000a.

Ayres L: Narratives of family caregiving: the process of making meaning, *Res Nurs Health* 23(6):424-434, 2000b.

Aziz NM, Rowland JH: Cancer survivorship research among ethnic minority and medically underserved groups, *Oncol Nurs Forum* 29(5):789-801, 2002.

Bakas T, Burgener S: Predictors of emotional distress, general health, and caregiving outcomes in family caregivers of stroke survivors, *Top Stroke Rehabil* 9(1):34-45, 2002.

Baumgarten M, Lebel P, Laprise H et al: Adult day care for the frail elderly: outcomes, satisfaction, and cost, *J Aging Health* 14(2): 237-259, 2002.

Beach S, Schulz R, Yee J et al: Negative and positive health effects of caring for a disabled spouse: longitudinal findings from the caregiver health effects study, *Psychol Aging* 15(2):259-271, 2000.

Belle SH, Burgio L, Burns R et al: Enhancing the quality of life of dementia caregivers from different ethnic or racial groups: a randomized, controlled trial, *Ann Intern Med* 145(10):727-738, 2006.

Bergs D: "The hidden client"—women caring for husbands with COPD: their experience of quality of life, *J Clin Nurs* 11(5):613-621, 2002.

Bookwala J, Zdaniuk B, Burton L et al: Concurrent and long-term predictors of older adults' use of community-based long-term care services: the Caregiver Health Effects Study, *J Aging Health* 16(1):88-115, 2004.

Borg C, Hallberg I: Life satisfaction among informal caregivers in comparison with non-caregivers, *Scand J Caring Sci* 20(4):427-438, 2006.

Brazil K, Bedard M, Willison K et al: Caregiving and its impact on families of the terminally ill, *Aging Ment Health* 7(5):376-382, 2003.

Brown SA et al: Perception of health and quality of life in minorities after mild-to-moderate traumatic brain injury, *Appl Neuropsychol* 11(1):54-64, 2004.

Bull MJ, Hansen HE, Gross CR: Differences in family caregiver outcomes by their level of involvement in discharge planning, *Appl Nurs Res* 13(2):76-82, 2000.

Bull MJ, Roberts J: Components of a proper hospital discharge for elders, *J Adv Nurs* 35(4):571-581, 2001.

Burton LC et al: Transitions in spousal caregiving, *Gerontologist* 43(2):230-241, 2003.

Butcher HK, Holkup PA, Park M et al: Thematic analysis of the experience of making a decision to place a family member with Alzheimer's disease in a special care unit, *Res Nurs Health* 24(6):470-480, 2001.

Cameron J, Franche RL, Cheung AM et al: Lifestyle interference and emotional distress in family caregivers of advanced cancer patients, *Cancer* 94(2):521-527, 2002.

Cheung J, Hocking P: Caring as worrying: the experience of spousal carers, *J Adv Nurs* 47(5):475-482, 2004.

Clark MC: A causal functional explanation of maintaining a dependent elder in the community, *Res Nurs Health* 20(6):515-526, 1997.

Clark PC: Effects of individual and family hardiness on caregiver depression and fatigue, *Res Nurs Health* 25(1):37-48, 2002.

Clark PC, Dunbar SB, Shields CG et al: Influence of stroke survivor characteristics and family conflict surrounding recovery on caregivers' mental and physical health, *Nurs Res* 53(6):406-413, 2004.

• = Independent;   ▲ = Collaborative;   EBN = Evidence-Based Nursing;   EB = Evidence-Based

Davis LL, Burgio LD, Buckwalter KC et al: A comparison of in-home and telephone-based skill training interventions with caregivers of persons with dementia, *J Men Health Aging* 10(1):31-44, 2004.

Deeken J, Taylor K, Mangan P et al: Care for the caregivers: a review of self-report instruments developed to measure the burden, needs, and quality of life of informal caregivers, *J Pain Symptom Manage* 26(4):922-953, 2003.

Donnelly TT: Contextual analysis of coping: implications for immigrants' mental health care, *Issues Ment Health Nurs* 23(7):715-732, 2002.

Doswell W, Erlen J: Multicultural issues and ethical concerns in the delivery of nursing care interventions, *Nurs Clin North Am* 33(2):353-361, 1998.

Giger J, Davidhizar R: Culturally competent care: emphasis on understanding the people of Afghanistan, Afghanistan Americans, and Islamic culture and religion, *Int Nurs Rev* 49(2):79-86, 2002.

Giger J, Davidhizar R: *Transcultural nursing: assessment and intervention,* St Louis, 2004, Mosby.

Gerdner LA, Buckwalter KC, Reed D: Impact of a psychoeducational intervention on caregiver response to behavior problems, *Nurs Res* 51(6):363-374, 2002.

Gitlin L, Belle SH, Burgio LD et al: Effect of multicomponent interventions on caregiver burden and depression: the REACH multisite initiative at 6-month follow-up, *Psychol Aging* 18(3):361-374, 2003.

Given B, Given CW, Sikorskii A et al: The impact of providing symptom management assistance on caregiver reaction: results of a randomized trial, *J Pain Symptom Manage* 32(5):433-443, 2006.

Given CW, Given B, Stommel M et al: The caregiver reaction assessment (CRA) for caregivers to persons with chronic physical and mental impairments, *Res Nurs Health* 15(4):271-383, 1992.

Gleeson-Kreig J et al: The role of social support in the self-management of diabetes mellitus among a Hispanic population, *Public Health Nurs* 19(3):215-222, 2002.

Glueckauf R, Ketterson T, Loomis J et al: Online support and education for dementia caregivers: overview, utilization, and initial program evaluation, *Telemed J E Health* 10(2):223-232, 2004.

Hansberry MR, Chen E, Gorbien MJ: Dementia and elder abuse, *Clin Geriatr Med* 21(2):315-332, 2005.

Hayman J, Langa KM, Kabeto MU et al: Estimating the cost of informal caregiving for elderly patients with cancer, *J Clin Oncol* 19(13):3219-3225, 2001.

Hepburn K, Tornatore J, Center B et al: Dementia family caregiver training: affecting beliefs about caregiving and caregiver outcomes, *J Am Geriatr Soc* 49(4):450-457, 2001.

Hudson PL, Hayman-White K: Measuring the psychosocial characteristics of family caregivers of palliative care patients: psychometric properties of nine self-report instruments, *J Pain Symptom Manage* 31(3):215-228, 2006.

Iconomou G, Vagenakis AG, Kalofonos HP: The informational needs, satisfaction with communication, and psychological status of primary caregivers of cancer patients receiving chemotherapy, *Support Care Cancer* 9(8):591-596, 2001.

Jang Y, Clay O, Roth D et al: Neurotocism and longitudinal change in caregiver depression: impact of a spouse-caregiver intervention, *Gerontologist* 44(3):311-317, 2004.

Joiner T, Perez M, Wagner K et al: On fatalism, pessimism, and depressive symptoms among Mexican-American and other adolescents attending an obstetrics-gynecology clinic. *Behav Res Ther* 39(8):887-896, 2001.

Kimberlin C, Brushwood D, Allen W et al: Cancer patient and caregiver experiences: communication and pain management issues, *J Pain Symptom Manage* 28(6):566-578, 2004.

King RB, Semik PE: Stroke caregiving: difficult times, resource use, and needs during the first 2 years, *J Gerontol Nurs* 32(4):37-44, 2006.

Knop DS, Bergman-Evans B, McCabe BW: In sickness and in health: an exploration of the perceived quality of the marital relationship, coping, and depression in caregivers of spouses with Alzheimer's disease, *J Psychosoc Nurs Ment Health Serv* 36(1):16-21, 1998.

Krause N, Rook K: Negative interaction in late life: issues in the stability and generalizability of conflict across relationships, *J Ge-ontol B Psychol Sci Soc Sci* 58(2):P88-99, 2003.

Kurtz M, Kurtz JC, Given CW et al: Depression and physical health among family caregivers of geriatric patients with cancer—a longitudinal view, *Med Sci Monit* 10(8):CR447-456, 2004.

Lee HS et al: Relationship of empathy to appraisal, depression, life satisfaction, and physical health in informal caregivers of older adults, *Res Nurs Health* 24(1):44-56, 2001.

Leininger MM, McFarland MR: *Transcultural nursing: concepts, theories, research and practices,* ed 3, New York, 2002, McGraw-Hill.

Martire LM, Stephens MA, Druley JA et al: Negative reactions to received spousal care: predictors and consequences of miscarried support, *Health Psychol* 21(2):167-276, 2002.

Messecar DC, Archbold PG, Stewart BJ et al: Home environmental modification strategies used by caregivers of elders, *Res Nurs Health* 25(5):357-370, 2002.

Mills P, Adler KA, Dimsdale JE et al: Vulnerable caregivers of Alzheimer disease patients have a deficit in beta 2-adrenergic receptor sensitivity and density, *Am J Geriatr Psychiatry* 12(3):281-286, 2004.

Mittelman, MS et al: Improving caregiver well-being delays nursing home placement of patients with Alzheimer disease, *Neurology* 67(9):1592-1595, 2006.

Narayan S, Lewis M, Tornatore J et al: Subjective responses to caregiving for a spouse with dementia, *J Gerontol Nurs* 27(3):19-28, 2001.

Newton M, Bell D, Lambert S et al: Concerns of hospice patient caregivers. *ABNF J,* 13(6):140-144, 2002.

Nijboer C, Tempelaar R, Triemstra M et al: The role of social and psychologic resources in caregiving of cancer patients, *Cancer* 91(5):1029-1039, 2001.

Novak M, Guest C: Application of a multidimensional caregiver burden inventory, *Gerontologist* 29(6):798-803, 1989.

Padula C, Sullivan M: Long term married couples health promotion behaviors. *J Gerontol Nurs* 32(10):37-47, 2006.

Perry J: Wives giving care to husbands with Alzheimer's disease: a process of interpretive caring, *Res Nurs Health* 25(4):307-316, 2002.

Pinquart M, Sorensen S: Associations of stressors and uplifts of caregiving with caregiver burden and depressed mood: a meta-analysis, *J Gerontol B Psychol Sci Soc Sci* 58(2):P112-P128, 2003.

Powe, BD, Finnie R: Cancer fatalism: the state of the science, *Cancer Nurs* 26(6):454-465, 2003.

Redwine L, Mills P, Sada M et al: Differential immune cell chemotaxis responses to acute psychological stress in Alzheimer care-givers compared to non-caregiver controls, *Psychosom Med* 66(5):770-775, 2004.

Robinson B: Validation of a Caregiver Strain Index, *J Gerontol* 38(3):344-348, 1983.

Samuel-Hodge CD et al: Influences on day-to-day self-management of type 2 diabetes among African-American women: spirituality, the multi-caregiver role, and other social context factors, *Diabetes Care,* 23(7):928-933, 2000.

Schulz R, Beach SR: Caregiving as a risk factor for mortality: the Caregiver Health Effects Study, *JAMA* 282(23):2215-2219, 1999.

Schulz R, Belle S, Czaja S et al: Long-term care placement of dementia patients and caregiver health and well-being, *JAMA* 292(8):961-967, 2004.

Schulz R, Boerner K, Shear K et al: Predictors of complicated grief among dementia caregivers: A prospective study of bereavement, *Am J Geriatr Psychiatr* 14(8):650-658, 2006.

Schulz R, Martire L: Family caregiving of persons with dementia: prevalence, health effects, and support strategies, *Am J Geriatr Psychiatry* 12(3):240-249, 2004.

Schumacher KL, Stewart BJ, Archbold PG et al: Family caregiving skill: development of the concept, *Res Nurs Health* 23(3):191-203, 2000.

Schwartz K: Breast cancer and health care beliefs, values, and practices of Amish women, *Diss Abstr* 29(1):587, 2002.

Scott LD: Caregiving and care receiving among a technologically dependent heart failure population, *Adv Nurs Sci* 23(2):82-97, 2000.

Shu BC, Lung FW, Huang C: Mental health of primary caregivers with children with intellectual disability who receive a home care programme, *J Intellec Disabil Res* 46(Pt 3):257-263, 2002.

Sorensen S, Pinquart M, Duberstein P: How effective are interventions with caregivers? An updated meta-analysis, *Gerontologist* 42(3):356-372, 2002.

Teel CS, Duncan P, Lai SM: Caregiving experiences after stroke, *Nurs Res* 50(1):53, 2001.

Thornton M, Travis SS: Analysis of the reliability of the Modified Caregiver Strain Index, *Gerontol B Psychol Sci Soc Sci* 58(2):S127-S132, 2003.

Tribaldi V, Aimonino N, Ponzetto M et al: A randomized controlled trial of a home hospital intervention for frail elderly demented patients: behavioral disturbances and caregiver's stress, *Arch Gerontol Geriatr* (Suppl 9):431-436, 2004.

Vitaliano P, Russo J, Young H et al: The screen for caregiver burden, *Gerontologist* 31(1):76-83, 1991.

White MH, Dorman SM: Online support for caregivers: analysis of an internet Alzheimer mailgroup, *Comput Nurs* 18(4):168-176, 2000.

Yin T, Zhou Q, Bashford C: Burden on family members: caring for frail elderly: a meta-analysis of interventions, *Nurs Res* 51(3):199-208, 2002.

Yurk R, Morgan D, Franey S et al: Understanding the continuum of palliative care for patients and their caregivers, *J Pain Symptom Manage* 24(5):459-470, 2002.

Zarit SH, Leitsch SA: Developing and evaluating community based intervention programs for Alzheimer's patients and their caregivers, *Aging Ment Health* Suppl 1:S84-S98, 2001.

Zarit SH, Reever KE, Bach-Peterson J et al: Relatives of the impaired elderly: correlates of feelings of burden, *Gerontologist* 20(6):649-655, 1980.

Risk for Caregiver role strain   Betty J. Ackley, MSN, EdS, RN

NANDA   Definition

Caregiver is vulnerable for felt difficulty in performing the family caregiver role

Risk Factors

Addiction; amount of caregiving tasks; care receiver exhibits bizarre behavior; care receiver exhibits deviant behavior; caregiver's competing role commitments; caregiver health impairment; caregiver is female; caregiver is spouse; caregiver isolation; caregiver not developmentally ready for caregiver role; codependency; cognitive problems in care receiver; complexity of caregiving tasks; congenital defect; developmental delay of the care receiver; developmental delay of the caregiver; discharge of family member with significant home care needs; duration of caregiving required; family dysfunction prior to the caregiving situation; family isolation; illness severity of the care receiver; inadequate physical environment for providing care (e.g., housing, transportation, community services, equipment); inexperience with caregiving; instability in the care receiver's health; lack of recreation for caregiver; lack of respite for caregiver; marginal caregiver's coping patterns; marginal family adaptation; past history of poor relationship between caregiver and care receiver; premature birth; presence of abuse; presence of situational stressors that normally affect families (e.g., significant loss, disaster or crisis, economic vulnerability, major life events); presence of violence; psychological problems in care receiver; retardation of the care receiver; retardation of the caregiver; unpredictable illness course

NOC   Outcomes (Nursing Outcomes Classification)

Suggested NOC Outcomes

Caregiver Emotional Health, Caregiver Lifestyle Disruption, Caregiver Performance: Direct Care, Caregiver Performance: Indirect Care, Caregiver Physical Health, Caregiver Stressors, Caregiver Well-Being, Role Performance

Example NOC Outcome with Indicators

Caregiver Emotional Health with plans for a positive future as evidenced by the following indicators: Satisfaction with life/Sense of control/Self-esteem/Free of anger/Free of guilt/Free of depression/Perceived social connectedness/Perceived spiritual well-being (Rate the outcome and indicators of **Caregiver Emotional Health:** 1 = severely compromised, 2 = substantially compromised, 3 = moderately compromised, 4 = mildly compromised, 5 = not compromised [see Section I].)

C

Client Outcomes

Client/Caretaker Will (Specify Time Frame):
- Maintain physical and psychological health
- Identify resources available to help in giving care
- Obtain appropriate care

NIC   Interventions (Nursing Interventions Classification)

Suggested NIC Interventions

Caregiver Support, Family Support, Home Maintenance Assistance, Normalization Promotion, Respite Care, Support Group

Example NIC Activities—Caregiver Support
Determine caregiver's acceptance of role; Accept expressions of negative emotion

Nursing Interventions and *Rationales* and Client/Family Teaching

Refer to the care plan for **Caregiver role strain**

Readiness for enhanced Comfort

Barbara Kraynyak Luise, EdD, RN, and Scott C. Lamont, BSN, RN, PhD(c)

NANDA   Definition

A pattern of ease, relief and transcendence in physical, psycho spiritual, environmental, and social dimensions that can be strengthened

Defining Characteristics

Expresses desire to enhance comfort; expresses desire to enhance feelings of contentment; expresses desire to enhance relaxation; expresses desire to enhance resolution of complaints

NOC   Outcomes (Nursing Outcomes Classification)

Suggested NOC Outcomes

Client Satisfaction: Caring, Symptom Control, Comfort Level, Coping, Decision Making, Health Beliefs, Hope, Motivation, Pain Control, Participation in Healthcare Decisions, Personal Well-Being, Sensory Function Status, Social Support, Spiritual Health

Example NOC Outcomes with Indicators
Comfort Level as evidenced by the following indicators: Physical well-being/Symptom control/Psychological well-being/Pain control (Rate the outcome and indicators of **Comfort Level:** 1 = not at all satisfied, 2 = somewhat satisfied, 3 = moderately satisfied, 4 = very satisfied, 5 = completely satisfied.)

Client Outcomes

Client Will (Specify Time Frame):
- Assess current level of comfort as acceptable
- Express the need to achieve an enhanced level of comfort
- Identify strategies to enhance comfort

• = Independent; ▲ = Collaborative; EBN = Evidence-Based Nursing; EB = Evidence-Based

- Perform appropriate interventions as needed for increased comfort
- Evaluate the effectiveness of interventions at regular intervals
- Maintain an enhanced level of comfort when possible

NIC   Interventions (Nursing Interventions Classification)

Suggested NIC Interventions

Acupressure, Animal Assisted Therapy, Aroma Therapy, Art Therapy, Biblio Therapy, Biofeedback, Calming Technique, Cutaneous Stimulation, Environmental Management, Comfort, Financial Resources Assistance, Heat/Cold Application, Hope Inspiration, Humor, Meditation Facilitation, Music Therapy, Pain Management, Presence, Religious Ritual Enhancement, Simple Guided Imagery, Simple Massage, Simple Relaxation Therapy, Spiritual Growth Facilitation, Spiritual Support, Therapeutic Play, Therapeutic Touch, Touch, TENS, Distraction, Hypnosis, Activity Therapy

Example NIC Activities—Hope Inspiration

Assist the patient/family to identify areas of hope in life; Help the patient expand spiritual self; involve the patient actively in own care

Nursing Interventions and *Rationales*

- Assess client's current level of comfort. *This is the first step in helping clients to achieve enhanced comfort. Sources of assessment data to determine level of comfort can be subjective, objective, primary, secondary, focused, or even special needs (Wilkinson & VanLeuven, 2007). While clinicians are assessing pain more frequently, this has not resulted in widespread pain reduction. A solution may be to establish comfort-function goals for clients, reminding clients to tell their nurse when pain interferes with function (Pasero & McCaffrey, 2004).*
- Help clients understand that enhanced comfort is a desirable, positive, and achievable goal. *Human beings strive to have their basic comfort needs met, but comfort is more than just the absence of pain (Kolcaba, 2003). Comfort is best recognized when a person leaves the state of discomfort and nurses can enhance their client's comfort in everyday practice (Malinowski & Stamler, 2002).*
- ▲ Enhance feelings of trust between the client and the healthcare provider. *To attain the highest comfort level a client must be able to trust their nurse (Morse, 2000).* **EBN:** *This study demonstrates the importance of promoting open relationships with clients, which helps to acknowledge their individuality. Knowing the client and family proved to be pivotal in the provision of optimum palliative and terminal care (Luker et al, 2000).* **EB:** *Delivering care that reflects a person's wants and needs becomes critical at the end of life (Cavinsky et al, 2000).*
- Manipulate the environment as necessary to enhance comfort. *Comforting strategies are measures taken that help to alleviate distress. Examples might be making the environment warmer, quieter, or darker. Dimming the lights, warm blankets, and pillows can help to enhance comfort levels (Morse, 2000).*
- Use therapeutic massage for enhancement of comfort. **EBN:** *This study determined the effects of hand massage on clients near the end of life, with clients reporting feeling special and that the massage felt good. Also, meaningful connectedness was achieved (Kolcaba et al, 2004). Massage is helpful for low back pain and other orthopaedic problems (Dryden, Baskwill & Preyde, 2004).* **EB:** *This study described a program for sleep enhancement, at bedtime nonpharmacologic techniques such as back massage and relaxation tapes were used. The interventions substantially reduced the use of sedative drugs for sleep enhancement and proved to be an effective and nontoxic alternative to the use of sedative drugs in elder hospitalized clients (Inouye et al, 2000).*
- Teach and encourage use of guided imagery. **EBN:** *Guided imagery is an effective intervention that resulted in increased comfort (Kolcaba & Steiner, 2000). Guided imagery can be helpful on pain level, physical functional status, and self-efficacy on persons with fibromyalgia (Menzies, Taylor & Bourguignon, 2006).*

• = Independent;   ▲ = Collaborative;   EBN = Evidence-Based Nursing;   EB = Evidence-Based

C

- Foster and instill hope in clients whenever possible.
- See the care plan for **Hopelessness.**
- Provide opportunities for and enhance spiritual care activities. **EBN:** *Clients may find a life event such as illness and suffering becomes a meaningful trigger of a spiritual life event. These moments can provide nurses with the opportunity to enhance spirituality and promote coping and support for their clients (Cavendish et al, 2000). The need for comfort and reassurance may be perceived as spiritual needs. To meet these needs, nurses engaged in interaction when they comforted assured clients. Participants also identified absolution as a spiritual need, and there is evidence that forgiveness may bring one feelings of joy, peace, elation, and a sense of renewed self-worth (Narayanasomy et al, 2004). In this study, although clients did not perceive nurses as providers of spiritual care, spirituality was an innate need in their lives that helped them to connect with others; guide decisions; and to accept, reorder, and transcend life events (Cavendish et al, 2000).*
- ▲ Enhance social support and family involvement. **EBN:** *Increased social support was found to lead to positive health practices in middle-aged adults (McNicholas, 2002).* **EBN:** *Methods to help terminally ill clients and their families transition from cure to comfort care included spending an increased amount of time with one's family, appointing one close friend to act as a contact person for other friends, and establishing an e-mail list serve for updates of a client's status and care (Duggleby & Berry, 2005).* **EBN:** *Clients who are ill need to preserve their personal integrity, including "being able" and connectedness or "being with." Clients first wanted to connect with family members and then friends, neighbors, or other individuals. Ongoing contact was best achieved through personal visits, telephone calls, or establishing new connections (Leidy & Haase, 1999).*
- Encourage mind-body therapies such as meditation as an enhanced comfort activity. **EB:** *The most common therapies used were meditation, imagery, and yoga. Research demonstrating the connection between the mind and body has therefore increased interest in the potential use of these therapies (Wolsko et al, 2004).* **EBN:** *Meditation has been shown to reduce anxiety, relieve pain, decrease depression, enhance mood and self-esteem, decrease stress, and generally improve clinical symptoms (Bonadonna, 2003).*
- ▲ Promote participation in creative arts and activity programs. **EBN:** *A creative arts program for caregivers of cancer clients was shown to lower anxiety, and positive emotions were expressed (Walsh, Martin & Schmidt, 2004). The use of an individualized music protocol program by elderly women was shown to promote and maintain sleep (Johnson, 2003).*
- ▲ Encourage clients to use Health Information Technology (HIT) as needed. Client services can now include management of medications, symptoms, emotional support, health education, and health information (Moody, 2005). **EBN:** *Computer-mediated support groups as a means of self-help were found to help in getting information, sharing experiences, receiving general support, venting feelings, gaining accessibility, and using writing in the comfort of their own home (Han & Belcher, 2001).*
- Evaluate the effectiveness of all interventions at regular intervals and adjust therapies as necessary. *It is important for nurses to determine comfort and pain management goals because comfort goals will change with circumstances. Ask questions and ask them frequently, such as "How is your comfort?" Establish guidelines for frequency of assessment and document responses noting if goals are being met (Kolcaba, 2003).* **EB:** *A comprehensive palliative care project was conducted at 11 sites. The interdisciplinary review process built trust, endorsed creativity, and ultimately resulted in better meeting the needs of clients, families, and the community (London et al, 2005). Evaluation must be planned for, ongoing, and systematic. Evaluation demonstrates caring and responsibility on the part of the nurse (Wilkinson & VanLeuven, 2007).*

Pediatric

- Assess and evaluate child's level of comfort at frequent intervals. *Comfort needs should be individually assessed and planned for. With assessment of pain in children, it is best to use input from the parents or a primary care provider. Use only accepted scales for standardized pain assessment (Remke & Chrastek, 2007).*
- Provide gentle, soothing touch, which may be well-suited for clients who cannot tolerate more stimulating interventions such as simple massage. **EBN:** *A study of 1- to 3-week-old neonates in a level III neonatal intensive care unit (NICU) found that infants receiving gentle human touch showed evidence of being soothed compared with a control group but that the intervention must be carefully*

monitored in this client group because episodes of physiological instability were experienced by some subjects (Harrison et al, 2000).

- Skin-to-skin contact (SSC) and selection of most effective method improves the comfort of newborns during routine blood draws. **EB:** *A small, randomized clinical trial of healthy, full-term infants showed a decrease in pain reactions in the group receiving SSC with their mothers during heel lancing (Gray, Watt & Blass, 2000).*

- Lower fevers with medication rather than sponging alone or in combination with medication unless there is a clear need to rapidly lower the client's temperature. **EBN:** *Medications such as acetaminophen reduce fever more quickly than sponging alone, and some studies found that children perceived sponging as discomforting (Joanna Briggs Institute, 2001).*

- Adjust the environment as needed to enhance comfort. *Environmental comfort measures include maintaining orderliness; quiet; minimizing furniture; special attention to temperature, light and sound, color, and landscape (Kolcaba & DeMarco, 2005).*

- Encourage parental presence whenever possible. The same basic principles for managing pain in adults and children apply to neonates. *In addition to other comfort measures, parental presence should be encouraged whenever possible (Pasero, 2004).* **EBN:** *This study reported the effects of co-residence and caregiving on the parents of children dying with AIDS. Although parents who did more caregiving did experience anxiety, insomnia, and fatigue, the caregiving experiences for many parents gave them an opportunity to fulfill their perceived duty as parents before their child died. This in turn resulted in better physical and emotional health outcomes (Kespichayawattana & VanLandingham, 2003).*

- Promote use of alternative comforting strategies such as positioning, presence, massage, spiritual care, music therapy, art therapy, and story-telling to enhance comfort when needed. *In addition to oral sucrose, other comfort measures should be used to alleviate pain such as swaddling, skin-to-skin contact with mother, nursing, rocking, and holding (Pasero, 2004).* **EBN:** *Building on the belief that parents are the primary care providers and healthcare resource for families, the blended infant massage parenting program is effective for both mother and infant (Porter & Porter, 2004). Children are born with an intrinsic spiritual essence that can be enhanced. Spirituality promotes a sense of hope, comfort, and strength and creates a sense of being loved and nurtured by a higher power (Elkins & Cavendish, 2004).* **EBN:** *In this study, focus groups were conducted with Moroccan pediatric oncology nurses and physicians to better understand how pain management was achieved in children with cancer. When no medication was available to relieve pain, other techniques were used to comfort clients. These included use of cold therapy, presence, holding a child's hand, utilizing distraction techniques, playing with them, story-telling, and encouraging parental engagement activities (McCarthy et al, 2004).*

Multicultural

- Identify cultural beliefs, values, lifestyles, practices, and problem-solving strategies when assessing clients. *Cultural sensitivity must always be a component of pain assessment. The nurse must remember that pain expression will vary among clients and that variation must also be acknowledged within cultures (Andrews & Boyle, 2003).* **EBN:** *In a qualitative study that identified issues in pain management, cultural beliefs were cited as impediments or barriers to pain management, for example, some Moroccan physicians felt illness-related pain was inevitable, that suffering was normal, and that it had to be endured, especially by boys (McCarthy et al, 2004).*

- Enhance cultural knowledge by actively seeking out information regarding different cultural and ethnic groups. *Cultural knowledge is the process of actively seeking information about different cultural and ethnic groups such as their world views, health conditions, health practices, use of home remedies or self-medication, barriers to healthcare, and risk taking or health-seeking behaviors (Institute of Medicine, 2002).*

- Recognize the impact of culture on communication styles and techniques. *Communication and culture are closely intertwined and communication is the way culture is transmitted and preserved. It influences how feelings are expressed, decisions are made, and what verbal and nonverbal expressions are acceptable. By the age of 5, cultural patterns of communication can be identified in children (Giger & Davidhizar, 2004).*

- Provide culturally competent care to clients from different cultural groups. *Cultural competency re-*

quires healthcare providers to act appropriately in the context of daily interactions with people who are different from themselves. Providers need to honor and respect the beliefs, interpersonal styles, attitudes and behaviors of others. This level of cultural awareness requires providers to refrain from forming stereotypes and judgments based on one's own cultural framework (Institute of Medicine, 2002). **EBN:** *The findings from a review of two studies of Japanese and American women suggest that although there were common ethical concerns between the two cultures, the cultural context of the underlying values may create very different meanings and result in different nursing practices (Wros, Doutrich & Izumi, 2004).*

Home Care

- The nursing interventions described previously in **Readiness for enhanced Comfort** may be used with clients in the home care setting. When needed, adaptations can be made to meet the needs of specific clients, families, and communities.
- ▲ Make appropriate referrals to other organizations or providers as needed to enhance comfort. *Referrals should have merit, be practical, timely, individualized, coordinated, and mutually agreed upon by all involved (Hunt, 2005).*
- ▲ Promote an interdisciplinary approach to home care. *Members of the interdisciplinary team who provide specialized care to enhance comfort can include the physician, physical therapist, occupational therapist, nutritionist, music therapist, social worker, etc. (Stanhope & Lancaster, 2006).*
- Evaluate regularly if enhanced comfort is attainable in the home care setting. *Home health agencies monitor client outcomes closely. Evaluation is an ongoing process and is essential for the provision of quality care (Stanhope & Lancaster, 2006).*

Client/Family Teaching

- Teach client how to regularly assess levels of comfort.
- Instruct client that a variety of interventions may be needed at any given time to enhance comfort.
- Help clients to understand that enhanced comfort is an achievable goal.
- Teach techniques to enhance comfort as needed.
- ▲ When needed, empower clients to seek out other health professionals as members of the interdisciplinary team to assist with comforting measures and techniques.
- Encourage self-care activities and continued self-evaluation of achieved comfort levels to ensure enhanced comfort will be maintained.

REFERENCES

Andrews M, Boyle J: *Transcultural concepts in nursing*, ed 4, Philadelphia, 2003, Lippincott, Williams and Wilkins.

Bonadonna R: Meditation's impact on chronic illness, *Holist Nurs Pract* 17(6):309-319, 2003.

Cavendish R, Luise B, Home K et al: Opportunities for enhanced spirituality relevant to well adults, *Int J Nurs Lang Classification* 11(4):151-162, 2000.

Cavinsky K, Fuller J, Yaffe K et al: Communication and decision-making in seriously ill patients: findings of the support project, *J Am Geriatr Soc* 48:187-193, 2000.

Dryden T, Baskwill A, Preyde M: Massage therapy for the orthopoedic patient: a review, *Orthop Nurs* 23:327-332, 2004.

Duggleby W, Berry P: Transitions and shifting goals of care for palliative patients and their families, *Clin J Oncol Nurs* 9(4):425-428, 2005.

Elkins M, Cavendish R: Developing a plan for pediatric spiritual care, *Holist Nurs Pract* 18(4):179-184, 2004.

Giger J, Davidhizar R: *Transcultural nursing: assessment and intervention*, ed 4, St. Louis, 2004, Mosby.

Gray L et al: Skin-to-skin contact is analgesic in healthy newborns, *Pediatrics* 105(1):e14, 2000.

Han H, Belcher A: Computer mediated support group use among parents of children with cancer: an exploratory study, *Comput Nurs* 19:27-33, 2001.

Harrison LL et al: Physiologic and behavioral effects of gentle human touch on preterm infants, *Res Nurs Health* 23(6):435-446, 2000.

Hunt R: *Introduction to community-based nursing*, ed. 3, Philadelphia, 2005, Lippincott.

Inouye S, Bogardus S, Baker D et al: The hospital elder life program: a model of care to prevent cognitive and functional decline in older hospitalized patients, *J Am Geriatr Soc* 48(12):1697-1706, 2000.

Institute of Medicine: *Speaking of health*, Washington, 2002, The National Academies Press.

The Joanna Briggs Institute for Evidence Based Nursing and Midwifery: *Management of the child with fever, best practice* 5(5), Australia, 2001, Blackwell Science.

Johnson J: The use of music to promote sleep in older women, *J Community Health Nurs* 20:27-35, 2003.

Kespichayawattana J, VanLandingham M: Effects of coresidence and caregiving on health of Thai parents of adult children with AIDS, *J Nurs Schol* 35(3):217-224, 2003.

Kolcaba K: *Comfort theory and practice*, New York, 2003, Springer.

Kolcaba K, DeMarco M: Comfort theory and application to pediatric nursing, *Pediatr Nurs* 31(3):187-194: 2005.

Kolcaba K, Dowd T, Steiner R et al: Efficacy of hand massage for enhancing the comfort of hospice patients, *Int J Palliat Nurs* 6(2):91-102, 2004.

• = Independent;   ▲ = Collaborative;   EBN = Evidence-Based Nursing;   EB = Evidence-Based

Kolcaba K, Steiner R: Empirical evidence for the nature of holistic comfort, *J Holist Nurs* 18(1):46-62, 2000.

Leidy N, Haase J: Functional status from the patient's perspective: the challenge of preserving personal integrity, *Res Nurs Health* 22:67-77, 1999.

London M, McSkimming S, Drew N et al: Evaluation of a comprehensive, adaptable, life-affirming, longitudinal palliative care project, *J Palliat Med* 8(6):1214-1225, 2005.

Luker K, Austin L, Caress A et al: The importance of "knowing the patient": community nurses constructions of quality in providing palliative care, *J Adv Nurs* 31(4):775-782, 2000.

Malinowski A, Stamler L: Comfort: exploration of the concept in nursing, *J Adv Nurs* 39(6):599-606, 2002.

McCarthy P, Chammas G, Wilimas J et al: Managing children's cancer pain in Morocco, *J Nurs Scholarsh* 36(1):11-15, 2004.

McNicholas S: Social support and positive health practices, *West J Nurs Res* 24(7):772-787, 2002.

Menzies V, Taylor A, Bourguignon C: Effects of guided imagery on outcomes of pain, functional status, and self-efficacy in persons diagnosed with fibromyalgia, *J Altern Complement Med* 12(1):23-30, 2006.

Moody L: E-health web portals: delivering holistic healthcare and making home the point of care, *Holist Nurs Pract* 19(4):156-160, 2005.

Morse J: On comfort and comforting, *Am J Nurs* 100(9):34-37, 2000.

Narayanasomy A, Clissett P, Parumal L et al: Responses to the spiritual needs of older people, *J Adv Nurs* 48(1):6-16, 2004.

Pasero C: Pain relief for neonates, *Am J Nurs* 104(5):44-47, 2004.

Pasero C, McCaffrey M: Comfort—function goals, *Am J Nurs* 104(9):77-81, 2004.

Porter L, Porter B: A blended infant massage-parenting enhancement program for recovering substance abusing mothers, *Pediatr Nurs* 30(5):363-401, 2004.

Remke S, Chrastek J: Improving care in the home for children with palliative care needs, *Home Healthc Nurse* 25(1):45-51, 2007.

Stanhope M, Lancaster J: *Foundation of nursing in the community*, ed. 2, St. Louis, 2006, Mosby.

Walsh S, Martin S, Schmidt L: Testing the efficacy of a creative-arts intervention with family caregivers of patients with cancer, *J Nurs Scholarsh* 36(3):214-219, 2004.

Wilkinson J, VanLeuven K: *Fundamentals of nursing*, Philadelphia, 2007, FA Davis.

Wolsko P, Eisenberg D, Davis R et al: Use of mind-body medical therapies, *J Gen Intern Med* 19:43-50, 2004.

Wros P, Doutrich D, Izumi S: Ethical concerns: comparison of values from two cultures, *Nurs Health Sci* 6(2):131-140, 2004.

Impaired verbal Communication   *Gail B. Ladwig, MSN, CHTP, RN, and Stacey Carroll, PHD, RN*

NANDA   Definition

Decreased, delayed, or absent ability to receive, process, transmit, and use a system of symbols

Defining Characteristics

Absence of eye contact; cannot speak; difficulty in comprehending usual communication pattern; difficulty expressing thoughts verbally (e.g., aphasia, dysphasia, apraxia, dyslexia); difficulty forming sentences; difficulty forming words (e.g., aphonia, dyslalia, dysarthria); difficulty in maintaining usual communication pattern; difficulty in selective attending; difficulty in use of body expressions; difficulty in use of facial expressions; disorientation to person; disorientation to space; disorientation to time; does not speak; dyspnea; inability to speak language of caregiver; inability to use body expressions; inability to use facial expressions; inappropriate verbalization; partial visual deficit; slurring; speaks with difficulty; stuttering; total visual deficit; verbalizes with difficulty; willful refusal to speak

Related Factors (r/t)

Absence of significant others; altered perceptions; alteration in self-concept; alteration in self-esteem; alteration of central nervous system; anatomical defect (e.g., cleft palate, alteration of the neuromuscular visual system, auditory system, phonatory apparatus); brain tumor; cultural differences; decrease in circulation to brain; differences related to development age; emotional conditions; environmental barriers; lack of information; physical barrier (e.g., tracheostomy, intubation); physiological conditions; psychological barriers (e.g., psychosis, lack of stimuli); side effects of medication; stress; weakening of the musculoskeletal system

NOC   Outcomes (Nursing Outcomes Classification)

Suggested NOC Outcomes

Communication, Communication: Expressive, Receptive

• = Independent;   ▲ = Collaborative;   EBN = Evidence-Based Nursing;   EB = Evidence-Based

C

Example NOC Outcome with Indicators

Communication as evidenced by the following indicators: Use of spoken language/Use of written language/Acknowledgment of messages received/Exchanges messages accurately with others (Rate the outcome and indicators of **Communication:** 1 = Severely compromised, 2 = substantially compromised, 3 = moderately compromised, 4 = mildly compromised, 5 = not compromised [see Section I].)

Client Outcomes

Client Will (Specify Time Frame):

- Use effective communication techniques
- Use alternative methods of communication effectively
- Demonstrate congruency of verbal and nonverbal behavior
- Demonstrate understanding even if not able to speak
- Express desire for social interactions

NIC   Interventions (Nursing Interventions Classification)

Suggested NIC Interventions

Active Listening; Communication Enhancement: Hearing Deficit; Communication Enhancement: Speech Deficit

Example NIC Activities—Communication Enhancement: Hearing Deficit

Listen attentively; Validate understanding of messages by asking client to repeat what was said

Nursing Interventions and *Rationales*

▲ When the client is having difficulty communicating, assess and refer for consultation for hearing loss. Suspect hearing loss when:
  - Client frequently complains that people mumble, speech is not clear, or client hears only parts of conversations when people are talking.
  - Client often asks people to repeat what they said.
  - Client's friends or relatives tell them that client doesn't seem to hear very well.
  - Client does not laugh at jokes because client misses too much of the story.
  - Client needs to ask others about the details of a meeting that the client just attended.
  - Others say that the client plays the television or radio too loudly.
  - Client cannot hear the doorbell or the telephone.
  - Client finds that looking at people when they talk to them makes it somewhat easier to understand, especially when clients are in a noisy place or where there are competing conversations.

  People with hearing disorders do not hear sounds clearly. Such disorders may range from hearing speech sounds faintly or in a distorted way to profound deafness (American Speech-Language-Hearing Association, 2007).
- Involve a familiar person when attempting to communicate with a client who has difficulty with communication, if accepted by the client. **EB:** *Conversation partners of individuals with aphasia, including healthcare professionals, families, and others, play a role that is important for communication for individuals with aphasia (Roth, 2004).*
- Avoid making assumptions about the communication choice of those with hearing loss. **EB:** *Clients with hearing loss and their physicians had different perceptions about what constituted effective communication, and clients recommended that physicians ask them about their preferred communication approach (Iezonni et al, 2004).*
▲ Identify the language spoken; obtain a language dictionary or interpreter if possible and accepted by the client. **EB:** *Professional interpreters are able to communicate medical terms while reducing the*

• = Independent;   ▲ = Collaborative;   EBN = Evidence-Based Nursing;   EB = Evidence-Based

ever-present risk of breaching client privacy and confidentiality (Greenbaum & Flores, 2004). Bilingual hospital staff members have as high as 50% inaccuracy when interpreting (Elderkin-Thompson, Silver & Waitzkin, 2001). The CLAS Standards recommend asking individuals to rate their primary language and capacity in English, and to use qualified institutional interpreters (Pope, 2005).

- Listen carefully. Validate verbal and nonverbal expressions particularly when dealing with pain. **EBN:** *Listening to a client was identified as a caring behavior of nurses (Gregg, 2004).* **EBN:** *Nonverbal indicators of pain observed by nurses of clients with intellectual disabilities: moaning, crying, painful facial expression, swelling and screaming during manipulation, not using (affected) body part, and moving the body in a specific way of behaving (Zwakhalen et al, 2004).*

- When communicating with a client with a hearing loss, face toward his or her unaffected side or better ear while allowing client to see speaker's face at a reasonably close distance. *Correct positioning increases the client's awareness of the interaction and enhances the client's ability to communicate (Alexander Graham Bell Association for the Deaf and Hard of Hearing, 2007).*

- Provide sufficient light and do not stand in front of window when communicating with a person with a hearing loss. *Light illuminates the speaker's face, making expressions and lip movements clearer. Standing in front of a window causes glare, which impedes the client's ability to clearly see the speaker (Alexander Graham Bell Association for the Deaf and Hard of Hearing, 2006).*

- Use simple communication; speak in a well-modulated voice, smile, and show concern for the client. **EBN:** *Affective questions and tentative speech, together with continuers, facilitated active participation by clients receiving health counseling (Kettunen, Poskiparta & Karhila, 2003).*

- Maintain eye contact at the client's level. **EBN:** *Good communication involves many familiar concepts, including good eye contact (Summers, 2002).*

- When working with clients who have hearing impairments, remove masks or use see-through masks and reduce background noise whenever possible. *Information on see-through masks: www.amphl.org.* **EB:** *Background noise had a negative effect on the ability to process speech and on perceived effort, especially for those with hearing loss (Larsby et al, 2005).*

- Use touch as appropriate. **EBN:** *The use of touch by the nurse conveys caring to the client (Gregg, 2004).*

- Use presence. Spend time with the client, allow time for responses, and make the call light readily available. **EBN:** *Attentive presence makes explicit that the other is cherished; it is a universal lived experience that is important to health and quality of life (Carroll, 2002).* **EBN:** *Time with the nurse had a positive effect on the healing process and recovery (Rudolfsson et al, 2003).*

- Explain all healthcare procedures. **EBN:** *Clients who were nonvocal and ventilated were attuned to everything occurring around them, and they appreciated explanations from the nurse (Carroll, 2004).*

- Be persistent in deciphering what the client is saying, and do not pretend to understand when the message is unclear. *When clients are truly understood, they experience greater satisfaction with nursing care (Shattell & Hogan, 2005).* **EBN:** *Persons who were nonvocal and ventilated stated that they appreciated persistence on the nurses' part with respect to being understood, and that it was bothersome to them when others pretended to understand them (Carroll, 2004).*

- ▲ Obtain communication equipment such as electronic devices, letter boards, picture boards, and magic slates. **EBN:** *Communication technology enables humanness (Dickerson et al, 2002).* **EBN:** *Use of voice output communication aids is possible with selected critically ill adults and may contribute to greater ease of communication during respiratory tract intubation, particularly with family members (Happ, Roesch & Garrett, 2004).*

- ▲ Consider the use of a lipreader translator (LRT) for those who are intubated via a tracheostomy. *LRTs are proficient lipreaders who determine what a nonvocal client is mouthing and then verbalize the client's words verbatim to others, in order to facilitate communication (Carroll, 2003).*

- Using an individualized approach, establish an alternative method of communication such as writing or pointing to letters, word phrases, picture cards, or simple drawings of basic needs. **EB:** *Alternative methods of communication are necessary when the client is unable to speak verbally (Happ, Roesch & Kagan, 2005).*

- ▲ Consider use of an intelligent keyboard to facilitate communication for clients unable to express themselves verbally. **EBN:** *Clients and nurses considered the "intelligent keyboard" to be significantly better than the traditional letter board (van den Boogaard & van Grunsven, 2004).*

• = Independent;   ▲ = Collaborative;   EBN = Evidence-Based Nursing;   EB = Evidence-Based

C

▲ Consultation with a speech pathologist may be helpful. Supplement the work of the speech pathologist with appropriate exercises. *Speech pathologists consider interventions optimizing communication in people with hearing loss (Hickson, Worrall & Donaldson-Scarinci, 2005).* **EB:** *Consultation and collaboration with a speech pathologist may provide the best approach to improving communication in clients with aphasia (Greener, Enderby & Whurr, 2006).*

• Establish an understanding of the client's symbolic speech, especially with clients who have schizophrenia. Ask the client to clarify particular statements. *Good communication with healthcare professionals was identified by people with schizophrenia as helping them learn to live with their illness (Schneider et al, 2004).*

• If a comprehension deficit is present, keep the environment quiet when communicating and get the client's attention before attempting to communicate (e.g., touch the client's shoulder, call the client's name). **EB:** *Conditions that are tolerable for hearing adults in casual conversation can be intolerable for persons with deficits of hearing, language, attention, or processing. Sound-field amplification can improve the speech audibility index for all listeners in a noisy room (Boothroyd, 2004).*

• Do not raise your voice or shout at the client. *A loud voice can distort the voice, be frightening, and decrease communication.*

Pediatric

• Observe behavioral communication cues in infants. **EBN:** *Infant pain is encoded into observable manifestations through which an infant communicates behavioral and physiological changes such as altered vital signs, characteristic cries, and facial expressions (Byers & Thornley, 2004).*

• Identify and define variations of communication that may be used by children with significant disabilities. Teach at least two new forms of socially acceptable communication alternatives to teach as repairs when communication breaks down. Example: Teach use of one-word requests or teach the child to point, reinforce appropriate responses. **EB:** *Young children with significant disability often have limited communicative repertoires. The means they have available to communicate with others might include natural gesturing, vocalizing, and occasionally challenging behavior (Halle, Brady & Drasgow, 2004).*

• Teach children with severe disabilities functional communication skills. **EB:** *Children with severe disabilities can be taught new forms of communication to replace prelinguistic behaviors associated with escape or avoidance (Sigafoos et al, 2004).*

▲ Refer children with primary speech and language delay/disorder for speech and language therapy interventions. **EBN:** *Speech and language therapy interventions showed a positive effect on children with expressive phonological and expressive vocabulary difficulties (Law, Garrett & Nye, 2003).*

Geriatric

• Carefully assess all clients for hearing difficulty using an audiometer. **EB:** *Healthy People 2010 encourages early identification of people with hearing loss. Despite a high prevalence of hearing loss in the elderly, there is a low incidence of audiological evaluation (Milstein & Weinstein, 2002).*

• Avoid use of "elderspeak." **EBN:** *Care providers unknowingly may communicate messages of dependence, incompetence, and control to older adults by using elderspeak, a speech style similar to baby talk that fails to communicate appropriate respect (Williams, Kemper & Hummert, 2004).*

• Initiate communication with the client with dementia. *The responsibility to initiate communication with clients who have dementia lies with the clinician. Identifying the client's communication pattern and deficits is helpful in understanding the client (Frazier-Rios & Zembrzuski, 2005).*

• Encourage the client to wear hearing aids, if appropriate. **EB:** *Identifying individuals with hearing loss and supplying appropriate hearing aids or other listening devices and teaching coping strategies may have a positive effect on quality of life for older people (Dalton et al, 2003).* **EB:** *Disability from hearing impairment was reduced when clients with dementia were screened for hearing impairment and fitted with hearing aids (Allen et al, 2003).*

• Facilitate communication and reminiscing with remembering boxes that contain objects, photographs, and writings that have meaning for the client. **EB:** *These communication tools helped staff* *learn more about clients and enhanced interactions with staff and client's families (Hagens, Beaman & Ryan, 2003). Reminiscence therapy is an appropriate intervention for communication and to relieve stress in elders (Stokes & Gordon, 2003).*

 Multicultural

- Nurses should become more sensitive to the meaning of a culture's nonverbal communication modes, such as eye contact, facial expression, touching, and body language. *Nurses should realize that their good intentions and their usual nonverbal communication style may sometimes be interpreted as offensive and insulting by a specific cultural group.* **EBN:** *To give a client a positive signal during a therapy session, a nurse may display the American sign of thumbs up. In Iran, however, thumbs extended upward is considered a vulgar gesture (Campinha-Bacote, 1998).* **EBN:** *Years of watching animal behavior for survival needs have made the Eskimo people experts in the interpretation of nonverbal language. For the traditional Eskimo, a raised eyebrow may mean "yes" and a wrinkled nose "no." Disagreeing in public is seldom done. Nodding may not indicate agreement (Sanders & Davidhizar, 2004).*
- Assess for the influence of cultural beliefs, norms, and values on the client's communication process. **EBN:** *What the client considers normal and abnormal communication may be based on cultural perceptions (Leininger & McFarland, 2002; Giger & Davidhizar, 2004). The nurse must be aware of personal beliefs about communication and control personal reactions by a broadened understanding of the beliefs and behaviors of others (Giger & Davidhizar, 2004). An affirmative answer does not necessarily mean "yes"; a client may be showing respect to the caregiver or avoiding the embarrassment of saying "no" (Galanti, 1997).*
- Assess personal space needs, acceptable communication styles, acceptable body language, interpretation of eye contact, perception of touch, and use of paraverbal modes when communicating with the client. **EBN:** *Nurses need to consider multiple factors when interpreting verbal and nonverbal messages (Giger & Davidhizar, 2004). Native Americans may consider avoiding direct eye contact to be a sign of respect and asking questions to be rude and intrusive (Seiderman et al, 1996). Empirical findings suggest that Chinese Americans and European Americans differ in the ways that they describe emotional experience, with Chinese Americans using more somatic and social words than Americans (Tsai, Simeonova & Watanabe, 2004).*
- Assess for how language barriers contribute to health disparities among ethnic and racial minorities. **EBN:** *Language barriers are associated with longer visit time per clinic visit, fewer frequent clinic visits, less understanding of physician's explanation, more laboratory tests, more emergency department visits, less follow-up, and less satisfaction with health services (Yeo, 2004).*
- Although touch is generally beneficial, there may be certain instances where it may not be advisable due to cultural considerations. **EBN:** *Touch is largely culturally defined (Leininger & McFarland, 2002). Touch is believed by some cultures to be a source of illness. Touching a baby's head requires parental permission in some Southeast Asian cultures. Many Latinos believe that excessive admiration of a child without touching will result in physical illness of the child (mal de ojo—"evil eye"). In some Islamic and Latino cultures, physical touch between a nurse and client is acceptable only if the individuals are of the same sex (Kelley, 1998). Some Asian cultures believe that touching the head is a sign of disrespect (Galanti, 1997).*
- Modify and tailor the communication approach in keeping with the client's particular culture. **EBN:** *Modification of communication will convey respect to the client and may increase client's satisfaction with care (Taylor & Lurie, 2004). Culturally tailored communication interventions were positively viewed by African-American women (Kreuter et al, 2004).*
- Use reminiscence therapy as a language intervention. **EBN:** *Reminiscence therapy is well-suited as a language intervention for older adults from culturally and linguistically diverse backgrounds (Harris, 1997).*
- Use of the Office of Minority Health (OMH) of the U.S. Department of Health and Human Services (DHHS) standards on culturally and linguistically appropriate services (CLAS) in healthcare should be used as needed. **EB:** *The recommended standards cover three broad areas of competence requirements for health care for racial or ethnic minorities: (1) culturally competent care, (2) language access services, and (3) organizational support for cultural competence (CLAS, 2007).*

• = Independent;   ▲ = Collaborative;   EBN = Evidence-Based Nursing;   EB = Evidence-Based

C

Home Care

- The interventions described previously may be adapted for home care use.

Client/Family Teaching

- Teach the client and family techniques to increase communication, including the use of communication devices. *Alternative methods of communication are necessary when the client is unable to use verbal communication.*
- Encourage significant others to use touch, such as holding the client's hand or stroking the arm. **EBN:** *Touch can be useful for improving comfort and communication among terminally ill older adults and their loved ones (Bush, 2001).*
- ▲ Refer the client to a speech-language pathologist (SLP) or audiologist. Audiological assessment quantifies and qualifies hearing in terms of the degree of hearing loss, the type of hearing loss, and the configuration of the hearing loss. Once a particular hearing loss has been identified, a treatment and management plan can be put into place by an SLP (American Speech-Language-Hearing Association, 2004).
- ▲ Refer to a specialist for possible surgical intervention when clients have surgical defects caused by cancer of the maxillary sinus and alveolar ridge. **EB:** *Obturators have been developed for surgical defects caused by cancer of the maxillary sinus and alveolar ridge. Clients' mean self-perceived communication effectiveness with the obturator in place was 75% of what it was before the diagnosis of cancer (Sullivan et al, 2002).*

    See the EVOLVE Website for World Wide Web resources for client education.

REFERENCES

Alexander Graham Bell Association for the Deaf and Hard of Hearing: *Communicating with people who have a hearing loss.* Available at www.agbell.org/docs/CWPWHHL.pdf, accessed on March 9, 2007.

Allen NH, Burns A, Newton V et al: The effects of improving hearing in dementia, *Age Ageing,* 32(2):189-193, 2003.

American Speech-Language-Hearing Association: *Hearing assessment.* Available at www.asha.org/public/hearing/testing/assess.htm, accessed on March 9, 2007.

American Speech-Language-Hearing Association: *How do I know if I have a hearing loss?* Available at www.asha.org/public/hearing/disorders/how_know.htm, accessed on March 9, 2007.

Boothroyd A: Room acoustics and speech perception, *Semin Hear* 25(2):55-166, 2004.

Bush E: The use of human touch to improve the well-being of older adults: a holistic nursing intervention, *J Holist Nurs* 19(3):256-270, 2001.

Byers JF, Thornley K: Cueing into infant pain, *MCN Am J Matern Child Nurs* 29(2):84-91, 2004.

Campinha-Bacote J: *A model of practice to address cultural competence in rehabilitation nursing,* Continuing Education, Association of Rehabilitation Nurses, 1998. Available at www.rehabnurse.org/ce/010201/010201_a.htm, accessed on March 9, 2007.

Carroll KA: Attentive presence: a lived experience of human becoming. Loyola University of Chicago doctoral dissertation (136 p). UMI Order #AAI3056410, 2002.

Carroll, SM: Lip-reading translating for non-vocal ventilated patients. *JAMPHL Online* 1(2): 2003. Available at www.amphl.org, accessed on November 26, 2006.

Carroll SM: Silent, slow lifeworld: a phenomenological study of the communication experience of nonvocal ventilated patients. Boston College doctoral dissertation (173p). CINAHL AN: 2009027345, 2004.

CLAS (Culturally and appropriate Linguistic Services): available at http://www.omhrc.gov/templates/browse.aspx?lvl52&lvlID515 accessed on February 24, 2007.

Dalton DS, Cruickshanks KJ, Klein BE et al: The impact of hearing loss on quality of life in older adults, *Gerontologist* 43(5):661-668, 2003.

Dickerson SS, Stone VI, Panchura C et al: The meaning of communication: experiences with augmentative communication devices, *Rehabil Nurs* 27(6):215-220, 2002.

Elderkin-Thompson V, Silver R, Waitzkin H: When nurses double as interpreters: a study of Spanish-speaking patients in a US primary care setting, *Soc Sci Med* 52(9):1343-1358, 2001.

Frazier-Rios D, Zembrzuski C: Try this: best practices in nursing care for hospitalized older adults with dementia. Communication difficulties: assessment and interventions, *Dermatol Nurs* 17(4):319-320, 2005.

Galanti G: *Caring for patients from different cultures: case studies from American hospitals,* ed 2, Philadelphia, 1997, University of Pennsylvania Press.

Giger J, Davidhizar R: Communication in Giger and Davidhizar's *Transcultural nursing: assessment and intervention.* St. Louis, 2004, Mosby.

Greenbaum M, Flores G: Lost in translation. Professional interpreters needed to help hospitals treat immigrant patients, *Mod Healthc* 34(18):21, 2004.

Greener J, Enderby P, Whurr R: Speech and language therapy for aphasia following stroke, *Cochrane Database Syst Rev* (1): CD000425, 2006.

Gregg MF: Values in clinical nursing practice and caring, *Japan J Nurs Sci* 1(1):11-18, 2004.

Hagens C, Beaman A, Ryan **EB:** Reminiscing, poetry writing, and remembering boxes: personhood-centered communication with cognitively impaired older adults, *Activ Adapt Aging,* 27(3/4):97-112, 2003.

Halle J, Brady NC, Drasgow E: Enhancing socially adaptive communicative repairs of beginning communicators with disabilities, *Am J Speech Lang Pathol* 13(1):43-54, 2004.

Happ MB, Roesch TK, Garrett K: Electronic voice-output communication aids for temporarily nonspeaking patients in a medical intensive care unit: a feasibility study, *Heart Lung* 33(2):92-101, 2004.

Happ MB, Roesch TK, Kagan SH: Patient communication following head and neck cancer surgery: a pilot study using electronic speech generating devices, *Oncol Nurs Forum* 32(6):1179-87, 2005.

Harris J: Silent voices: meeting the communication needs of older African Americans *Top Lang Disorder* 19(4):23, 1997.

Hickson L, Worrall L, Donaldson-Scarinci N: Expanding speech pathology services for older people with hearing impairment, *Adv Speech Lang Pathol* 7(4):203-210, 2005.

Iezonni LI, O'Day BL, Killeen M et al: Communicating about health care: observations from persons who are deaf and hard of hearing, *Ann Int Med* 140(5):356-362, 2004.

Kelley J: Cultural and ethnic considerations. In Frisch NC, Frisch LE, editors: *Psychiatric mental health nursing,* Albany, NY, 1998, Delmar.

Kettunen T, Poskiparta M, Karhila P: Speech practices that facilitate patient participation in health counseling—a way to empowerment? *Health Educ J* 62(4):326-340, 2003.

Kreuter MW, Skinner CS, Steger-May K et al: Responses to behaviorally vs. culturally tailored cancer communication among African American women, *Am J Health Behav* 28(3):195-207, 2004.

Larsby B, Hallgren M, Lyxell B et al: Cognitive performance and perceived effort in speech processing tasks: effects of different noise backgrounds in normal-hearing and hearing-impaired subjects, *Int J Audiol* 44(3):131-143, 2005.

Law J, Garrett Z, Nye C: Speech and language therapy interventions for children with primary speech and language delay or disorder, *Cochrane Database Syst Rev* (3):CD004110, 2003.

Leininger MM, McFarland MR: *Transcultural nursing: concepts, theories, research and practices,* ed 3, New York, McGraw-Hill, 2002.

Milstein D, Weinstein BE: Effects of information sharing on follow-up after hearing screening for older adults, *J Acad Rehabil Audiol* 35:43-58, 2002.

Pope C: Addressing limited English proficiency and disparities for Hispanic postpartum women, *J Obstet Gynecol Neonatal Nurs* 34(4):512-520, 2005.

Roth EJ: Grand rounds. A set of observational measures for rating support and participation in conversation between adults with aphasia and their conversation partners, *Top Stroke Rehabil* 11(1):67-83, 2004.

Rudolfsson G, Hallberg LRM, Ringsberg KC et al: The nurse has time for me: the perioperative dialogue from the perspective of patients, *J Adv Perioperative Care* 1(3):77-84, 2003.

Sanders N, Davidhizar R: American Eskimos: The Yup'ik and Inupiat. *Transcultural nursing: assessment and intervention,* St. Louis, 2004, Mosby.

Schneider B, Scissons H, Arney L et al: Communication between people with schizophrenia and their medical professionals: a participatory research project, *Qual Health Res* 14(4):562-577, 2004.

Seideman RY, Jacobson S, Primeaux M et al: Assessing American Indian families, *MCN Am J Matern Child Nurs* 21(6):274-279, 1996.

Shattell M, Hogan B: Facilitating communication: how to truly understand what patients mean, *J Psychosoc Nurs Ment Health Serv* 43(10):29-32, 2005.

Sigafoos J, Drasgow E, Reichle J et al: Tutorial: teaching communicative rejecting to children with severe disabilities, *Am J Speech Lang Pathol* 13(1):31-42, 2004.

Stokes SA, Gordon SE: Common stressors experienced by the well elderly. Clinical implications, *J Gerontol Nurs* 29(5):38-46, 2003.

Sullivan M, Gaebler C, Beukelman D et al: Impact of palatal prosthodontic intervention on communication performance of patients' maxillectomy defects: a multilevel outcome study, *Head Neck* 24(6):530-538, 2002.

Summers LC: Mutual timing: an essential component of provider/patient communication, *J Am Acad Nurse Pract* 14(1):19, 2002.

Taylor SL, Lurie N: The role of culturally competent communication in reducing ethnic and racial healthcare disparities, *Am J Manag Care* 10:SP1-4, 2004.

Tsai JL, Simeonova DI, Watanabe JT: Somatic and social: Chinese Americans talk about emotion, *Pers Soc Psychol Bull* 30(9): 1226-1238, 2004.

van den Boogaard M, van Grunsven A: A new communication aid for mechanically ventilated patients, *Connect: The World of Critical Care Nursing* 3(1):20-23, 2004.

Williams K, Kemper S, Hummert L: Enhancing communication with older adults: overcoming elderspeak, *J Gerontol Nurs* 30(10):17-25, 2004.

Yeo S: Language barriers and access to care, *Ann Rev Nurs Res* 22:59-73, 2004.

Zwakhalen SMG, van Dongen KAJ, Hamers JPH et al: Pain assessment in intellectually disabled people: non-verbal indicators, *J Adv Nurs* 45(3):236-245, 2004.

Readiness for enhanced Communication

Gail B. Ladwig, MSN, CHTP, RN, and Stacey Carroll, PHD, RN

NANDA Definition

A pattern of exchanging information and ideas with others that is sufficient for meeting one's needs and life's goals and can be strengthened

Defining Characteristics

Able to speak a language; able to write a language; expresses feelings; expresses satisfaction with ability to share ideas with others; expresses satisfaction with ability to share information with others; expresses thoughts; expresses willingness to enhance communication; forms phrases; forms sentences; forms words; interprets nonverbal cues appropriately; uses nonverbal cues appropriately

• = Independent; ▲ = Collaborative; EBN = Evidence-Based Nursing; EB = Evidence-Based

C

Suggested NOC Outcomes

Communication, Communication: Expressive, Receptive

Example NOC Outcome with Indicators
Communication as evidenced by the following indicators: Use of spoken language/Use of written language/Acknowledgment of messages received/Exchanges messages accurately with others (Rate the outcome and indicators of **Communication:** 1 = severely compromised, 2 = substantially compromised, 3 = moderately compromised, 4 = mildly compromised, 5 = not compromised [see Section I].)

Client Outcomes

Client Will (Specify Time Frame):

- Express willingness to enhance communication
- Demonstrate ability to speak or write a language
- Form words, phrases, and language
- Express thoughts and feelings
- Use and interpret nonverbal cues appropriately
- Express satisfaction with ability to share information and ideas with others

Suggested NIC Interventions

Active Listening, Communication Enhancement: Hearing Deficit, Communication Enhancement: Speech Deficit

Example NIC Activities—Communication Enhancement: Hearing Deficit
Listen attentively; Validate understanding of messages by asking client to repeat what was said

Nursing Interventions and *Rationales*

- Establish a therapeutic nurse-client relationship: provide appropriate education for the client, demonstrate caring by being present to the client. **EB:** *A good nurse-client relationship is essential to meet the clinical, psychological, and social needs of the client to optimize treatment in clients with renal disease (Jenkins et al, 2002).* **EBN:** *Clients who were nonvocal and ventilated appreciated nursing care that was delivered in an individualized, caring manner (Carroll, 2004).*
- Carefully assess the client's readiness to communicate, using an individualized approach. Avoid making assumptions regarding the client's preferred communication method. **EBN:** *Best practice with regard to communication in palliative care was achieved by using a sensitive assessment of how each client chooses to cope with his or her situation rather than a uniform approach to care (Dean, 2002).*
- Assess the client's literacy level. **EB:** *Health literacy is increasingly recognized as a critical factor affecting communication across the continuum of cancer care. About one in five American adults may lack the necessary literacy skills to function adequately in our society (Davis et al, 2002).*
- Listen attentively and provide a comfortable environment for communicating; use these practical guidelines to assist in communication: Slow down and listen to the client's story; use augmentative and alternative communication methods (such as lip-reading, communication boards, writing, body language, and computer/electronic communication devices) as appropriate; repeat instructions if necessary; limit the amount of information given; have the client "teach back" to confirm understanding; avoid asking, "Do you understand?"; be respectful, caring, and sensitive. **EB:** *Practical communication aids can help bridge the communication gap in clients with cancer (Davis*

et al, 2002). **EBN:** *Listening to the client, considering the client's feelings, and having a connected relationship with the client conveyed caring (Gregg, 2004).*

▲ Provide communication with specialty nurses who have knowledge about the client's situation. **EBN:** *Clients supported by a nurse specialist are well informed and have a high degree of satisfaction (Greenhill, Betts & Pickard, 2002).*

▲ Refer couples in maladjusted relationships for psychosocial intervention and social support to strengthen communication; consider nurse specialists. **EB:** *Being part of a strong dyad may serve as a buffering factor; there is a need for psychosocial intervention for couples in maladjusted relationships (Banthia et al, 2003).* **EBN:** *Social support intervention may be most useful when delivered by clinical nurse specialists who have additional education, training in communication, and teaching and consulting skills (Daugherty et al, 2002).*

• Consider using music to enhance communication between client who is dying and his/ her family. **EB:** *Music therapy is described as a way to ease communication and sharing between dying clients and their loved ones (Krout, 2003).*

• See care plan for **Impaired verbal Communication.**

Pediatric

▲ All individuals involved in the care and everyday life of children with learning difficulties need to have a collaborate approach to communication. **EBN:** *Collaboration has the potential to enable health professionals to adopt methods of communication that are familiar to the child, such as those used in the school setting (Kerzman & Smith, 2004).*

• See care plan for **Impaired verbal Communication.**

Geriatric

▲ Assess for hearing and vision impairments and make appropriate referrals for hearing aids. **EB:** *Each client's vision and conversational performance along with hearing thresholds should be assessed before considering directions for rehabilitation. During face-to-face interaction, many people with adequate vision can compensate for a high-frequency hearing loss through lip reading, which may preclude the need for hearing aids; many people with poor vision cannot compensate for a high-frequency hearing loss through lip reading and may require hearing aids (Erber, 2002).*

• Use touch if culturally acceptable when communicating with older clients and their families. **EBN:** *The use of touch by the nurse conveys caring to the client (Gregg, 2004).*

• Caregivers may sing when delivering care and instructions for clients with dementia. **EBN:** *During caregiver singing, the client with dementia communicated with an increased understanding of the situation, both verbally and behaviorally (Gotell, Brown & Ekman, 2002).*

• See care plan for **Impaired verbal Communication.**

Multicultural

• See care plan for **Impaired verbal Communication.**

Home Care and Client/Family Teaching

• The interventions described previously may be used in home care.
• See care plan for **Impaired verbal Communication.**

evolve   See the EVOLVE website for World Wide Web resources for client education.

REFERENCES

Banthia R, Malcarne VL, Varni JW et al: The effects of dyadic strength and coping styles on psychological distress in couples faced with prostate cancer, *J Behav Med* 26(1):31-52, 2003.

Carroll SM: Nonvocal ventilated patients' perceptions of being understood, *West J Nurs Res* 26(1): 85-103, 2004.

Daugherty J, Saarmann L, Riegel B et al: Can we talk? Developing a social support nursing intervention for couples, *Clin Nurse Spec* 16(4):211-218, 2002.

Davis TC, Williams MV, Marin E et al: Health literacy and cancer communication, *CA Cancer J Clin* 52(3):130-149, 2002.

Dean A: Talking to dying clients of their hopes and needs, *Nurs Times* 98(43):34-35, 2002.

Erber NP: Hearing, vision, communication, and older people, *Semin Hear* 23(1):35-42, 2002.

Greenhill L, Betts T, Pickard N: The epilepsy nurse specialist— expendable handmaiden or essential colleague? *Seizure* 11(suppl A):615-620, 2002.

• = Independent;   ▲ = Collaborative;   EBN = Evidence-Based Nursing;   EB = Evidence-Based

Gregg, MF: Values in clinical nursing practice and caring, *Japan J Nurs Sci* 1(1):11-18, 2004.

Gotell E, Brown S, Ekman SL: Caregiver singing and background music in dementia care, *West J Nurs Res* 24(2):195-216, 2002.

Jenkins K, Bennett L, Lancaster L et al: Improving the nurse-patient relationship: a multi-faceted approach, *EDTNA ERCA J* 28(3):145-150, 2002.

Kerzman B, Smith P: Lessons from special education: enhancing communication between health professionals and children with learning difficulties, *Nurse Educ Pract* 4(4): 230-235, 2004.

Krout RE: Music therapy with imminently dying hospice patients and their families: facilitating release near the time of death, *Am J Hosp Palliat Care* 20(2):129-134, 2003.

Decisional Conflict (specify)   *Lisa Burkhart, MPH, PHD, RN, and Beverly Kopala, PHD, RN*

NANDA   Definition

Uncertainty about course of action to be taken when choice among competing actions involves risk, loss, or challenge to values and beliefs

Defining Characteristics

Delayed decision making; physical signs of distress or tension (e.g., increased heart rate, increased muscle tension, restlessness); questioning moral principles while attempting a decision; questioning moral rules while attempting a decision; questioning moral values while attempting a decision; questioning personal beliefs while attempting a decision; questioning personal values while attempting a decision; self-focusing; vacillation among alternative choices; verbalizes feeling of distress while attempting a decision; verbalizes uncertainty about choices; verbalizes undesired consequences of alternative actions being considered

Related Factors (r/t)

Divergent sources of information; interference with decision making; lack of experience with decision making; lack of relevant information; moral obligations require performing action; moral obligations require not performing action; moral principles support courses of action; moral rules support mutually inconsistent courses of action; moral values support mutually inconsistent courses of action; multiple sources of information; perceived threat to value system; support system deficit; unclear personal beliefs; unclear personal values

NOC   Outcomes (Nursing Outcomes Classification)

Suggested NOC Outcomes

Decision Making, Information Processing, Participation in Healthcare Decisions

Example NOC Outcome with Indicators
Decision-Making as evidenced by the following indicators: Identifies relevant information/Identifies alternatives/ Identifies potential consequences of each alternative/Identifies resources necessary to support each alternative (Rate the outcome and indicators of **Decision-Making:** 1 = severely compromised, 2 = substantially compromised, 3 = moderately compromised, 4 = mildly compromised, 5 = not compromised [see Section I].)

Client Outcomes

Client Will (Specify Time Frame):

• State the advantages and disadvantages of choices
• Share fears and concerns regarding choices and responses of others
• Seek resources and information necessary for making an informed choice
• Make an informed choice

| NIC | Interventions (Nursing Interventions Classification) |

Suggested NIC Intervention

Decision-Making Support

Example NIC Activities—Decision-Making Support
Inform patient of alternative views or solutions in a clear and supportive manner

Nursing Interventions and *Rationales*

- Observe for factors causing or contributing to conflict (e.g., value conflicts, fear of outcome, poor problem-solving skills). **EB:** *Among clients facing a real treatment decision, interventions to inform clients about hypertension and to clarify clients' values concerning outcomes of treatment are effective in reducing decisional conflict and increasing client knowledge (Montgomery, Fahey & Peters, 2003).*
- Work with and allow the client to make decisions in a way that is comfortable for the client, such as deferring (allowing others to decide), delaying (choosing an alternative that meets basic requirements), or deliberating (looking at all alternatives). **EB:** *Clients can be more involved in treatment decisions, and risks and benefits of treatment options can be explained in more detail, without adversely affecting client-based outcomes (Edwards et al, 2004).*
- Give the client time and permission to express feelings associated with decision making. **EB:** *The physician should take time to explore the client's values, concerns, and emotional and social needs (Whitney, McGuire & McCullough, 2004).* **EBN:** *Ethical conflict is resolved by educating the client or family to take action, through team/family discussions, or resolution by ethics committee (Redman & Fry, 1998).*
- Demonstrate reassurance with unconditional respect for and acceptance of the client's values, spiritual beliefs, and cultural norms. **EB:** *Trust in the client's physician is important in shared decision making. Supporting the client's autonomy is important (Kraetschmer et al, 2004).*
- ▲ Use decision aids or computer-based decision aid to assist clients in making decisions. **EB:** *An interactive computer program was more effective than standard genetic counseling for increasing knowledge of breast cancer and genetic testing among women at low risk of carrying a BRCA1 or BRCA2 mutation (Green et al, 2004a). In women at high risk for ovarian cancer, the group who received a decision aid package reported a significant decrease in decisional conflict compared to the group that received a pamphlet (Tiller et al, 2006). A study of pregnant women who received a decision-aid booklet had significantly improved decisional conflict scores (Shorten et al, 2005).*
- ▲ Initiate health teaching and referrals when needed. **EB:** *In this national survey 86% of ethics committees engage in ongoing clinical decision making via clinical ethics consultations, and 94% of those who engage in case consultation allow family members and clients to request an ethics consultation (McGee et al, 2001).*
- ▲ Facilitate communication between the client and family members regarding the final decision; offer support to the person actually making the decision. **EB:** *Formulation of an advance proxy plan is important to ensure that the client's previous wishes or best interests are considered when decisions about treatment strategies are made (Volicer, 2001). In this study of certified rehabilitation registered nurses, 29% of the respondents were able to resolve the ethical conflict through team/family discussions and educating the client or family to take action (Redman & Fry, 1998).*
- ▲ Provide detailed information on benefits and risks using functional terms and probabilities tailored to clinical risk, plus steps for considering the issues and means for making a decision, including values clarification and decision aids, when clients are faced with difficult treatment choices. **EB:** *Informed choices require information that is relevant, valid, and accessible (Oxman, 2004).*
- Encourage client to communicate values, beliefs, goals, and life plans and the ultimate decision with other healthcare providers, as appropriate. **EB:** *Clients who participated in an interactive workshop with feedback and point-of-care reminder had significantly similar decisional conflict scores than prior to attending the program (Légaré et al, 2006).*

C

Geriatric

- Carefully assess clients with dementia regarding ability to make decisions. *In evaluating reasoning it may be helpful to take the person through the reasoning process. Check if information is excluded because it was not remembered or because it was not important to the individual.* **EB:** *Most adults with mild dementia can participate in medical decision making as defined by legal standards. In dementia, assessments of reasoning about treatment options should focus on whether a person can describe salient reasons for a specific choice (Moye et al, 2004).*

- If end-of-life discussions are being avoided, nurses are in a better position than any other health team member to facilitate discussions of healthcare choices among older adults and their family members. **EBN:** *The literature indicates moderate to high stability of healthcare preferences into older adulthood. One study indicated that the majority of participants had living wills, medical power of attorney, or do-not-resuscitate (DNR) directives in place. Renewing advance directives periodically may not be critical for certain groups of individuals (Martin & Roberto, 2006).*

- ▲ Discuss the purpose of a living will and advance directives. **EBN:** *Elderly clients and their significant others need to know how to legally make end-of-life decisions. (*NOTE: *Laws differ in each state.) The presence of an advance directive can be very helpful in decreasing family stress when end-of-life decisions need to be made (Tilden et al, 2001).*

- ▲ Discuss choices or changes to be made (e.g., moving in with children, into a nursing home, or into an adult foster care home). *Caregivers need to provide support when the client and family are facing difficult decisions (Hurley & Volicer, 2002). Advanced practice nurses as case managers can make a positive contribution toward individualizing care for the elderly (Mick & Ackerman, 2002).*

Multicultural

- Assess for the influence of cultural beliefs, norms, and values on the client's decision-making conflict. **EBN:** *Cultural influences may interfere with the client's decision-making process (Wong & Anderson, 2003). Individuals of Chinese and Korean descent, as well as individuals of the Muslim religion, may accept the health provider's decision regarding medical needs rather than assert their own wishes (Valle, 2001). African-American women may use fatalistic and destiny beliefs to guide their health decisions (Green et al, 2004b).*

- Identify who will be involved in the decision-making process. **EBN:** *In a group of frail elderly clients, ethnic variations were found with regard to the family member identified as the decision maker (Hornung et al, 1998). Contrary to expectations, Latinas will often make decisions related to prenatal care and services (Browner, Preloran & Cox, 1999). Korean-American clients and other Asian clients may consider some decisions to be a family affair (D'Avanzo et al, 2001). Elders may play a key role in decision making in some Asian populations (Davis, 2000). Some Native-American societies are matriarchal in structure, and the matriarch's approval and support may be required for compliance with a treatment plan (Cesario, 2001). Other studies have shown that the role of family and physician's recommendations were highly valued in the decision-making process by Hispanic women (Ellington et al, 2003).*

- Use cross-cultural decision aids whenever possible to enhance an informed decision-making process. **EBN:** *Consumer-based cross-cultural decision aids inform clients of potential risks and benefits so that they can make value- and evidence-integrated decisions (Lawrence et al, 2000). Latinas' assessment of risk and uncertainty with procedures was associated with decisions to refuse certain procedures (Browner, Preloran & Cox, 1999). African-American women underwent immediate breast reconstruction at significantly lower rates compared with Caucasian, Hispanic, and Asian women. The decision pathways found that African-American women were less likely to be offered referrals for reconstruction, were less likely to accept offered referrals, were less likely to be offered reconstruction, and were less likely to elect reconstruction if it was offered (Tseng et al, 2004).*

- Provide support for client's decision making. **EB:** *Intervention efforts designed to promote repeat human immunodeficiency (HIV) test acceptance among low-income, African-American women should focus on changing perceptions of barriers and enhancing supportive factors to enhance decision making (Bonney, Crosby & Odenat, 2004).*

Home Care

- The interventions described previously may be adapted for home care use.
- ▲ Before providing any home care, assess the client plan for advance directives (living will and power of attorney). If a plan exists, place a copy in the client file. If no plan exists, offer information on advance directives according to agency policy. Refer for assistance in completing advance directives as necessary. Do not witness a living will. *This is a legal requirement of the Consolidated Omnibus Budget Reconciliation Act (COBRA, 2007).*
- Assess the client and family for consensus (or lack thereof) regarding the issue in conflict. When the conflict involves end-of-life decisions, work to shift the client's and family's expectations from curative to palliative. **EBN:** *Clients and families at the end of life should focus on changing expectations from unrealistic (curative) to realistic (palliative) (Norton & Bowers, 2001).*
- Refer to the care plan for **Anxiety** as indicated.

Client/Family Teaching

- ▲ Instruct the client and family members to provide advance directives in the following areas:
  - Person to contact in an emergency
  - Preference (if any) to die at home or in the hospital
  - Desire to sign a living will
  - Desire to donate an organ
  - Funeral arrangements (i.e., burial, cremation)

  EB: *A large discrepancy exists between the wishes of dying clients and their actual end-of-life care. Early advance care planning can markedly reduce this discrepancy (Schwartz et al, 2002).*
- ▲ Inform the family of treatment options; encourage and defend self-determination. **EBN:** *The Patient Self-Determination Act, effective since December 1991, has changed the importance of introducing life support options to clients (Beland & Froman, 1995).*
- Identify reasons for family decisions regarding care. Explore ways in which family decisions can be respected. **EBN:** *The need for increased client and family involvement in decision making is a common theme in discharge planning studies (Naylor, 2002).*
- Recognize and allow the client to discuss the selection of complementary therapies available, such as spiritual support, relaxation, imagery, exercise, lifestyle changes, diet (e.g., macrobiotic, vegetarian), and nutritional supplementation. **EBN:** *Cancer clients believed that complementary therapies helped to improve their quality of life (Sparber et al, 2000).* **EB:** *The use of complementary/alternative medicine for cancer care is widespread (Lewith, Broomfield & Prescott, 2002).*
- ▲ Provide the Physician Orders for Life-Sustaining Treatment (POLST) form for clients and families faced with end-of-life choices across the healthcare continuum. **EBN:** *The POLST form ensures end-of-life choices can be implemented in all settings, from the home through the healthcare continuum. The POLST form was congruent with residents' existing advance directives for health care (Meyers et al, 2004).*

 See the EVOLVE website for World Wide Web resources for client education.

REFERENCES

Beland K, Froman R: Preliminary validation of a measure of life support preferences, *Image J Nurs Sch* 27:307, 1995.

Bonney EA, Crosby R, Odenat L: Repeat HIV testing among low-income minority women: a descriptive analysis of factors influencing decisional balance, *Ethn Dis* 14(3):330-335, 2004.

Browner CH, Preloran HM, Cox SJ: Ethnicity, bioethics, and prenatal diagnosis: the amniocentesis decisions of Mexican-origin women and their partners, *Am J Public Health* 89(11):1658-1666, 1999.

Cesario S: Care of the Native American woman: strategies for practice, education, and research, *J Obstet Gynecol Neonatal Nurs* 30(1):13-19, 2001.

COBRA The Consolidated Omnibus Budget Reconciliation Act, available at http://www.dol.gov/dol/topic/health-plans/cobra.htm. Accessed on February 24, 2007.

D'Avanzo CE et al: Developing culturally informed strategies for substance-related interventions. In Naegle MA, D'Avanzo CE, editors: *Addictions and substance abuse: strategies for advanced practice nursing,* St Louis, 2001, Mosby.

Davis RE: The convergence of health and family in the Vietnamese culture, *J Fam Nurs* 6:136-156, 2000.

Edwards A, Elwyn G, Hood K et al: Patient-based outcome results from a cluster randomized trial of shared decision making skill development and use of risk communication aids in general practice, *Fam Pract* 21(4):347-354, 2004.

Ellington L, Wahab S, Sahami S et al: Decision-making issues for randomized clinical trial participation among Hispanics, *Cancer Control* 10(5 Suppl):84-86, 2003.

C

Green BL, Lewis RK, Wang MQ et al: Powerlessness, destiny, and control: the influence on health behaviors of African Americans, *J Community Health* 29(1):15-27, 2004b.

Green MJ, Peterson SK, Baker MW et al: Effect of a computer-based decision aid on knowledge, perceptions, and intentions about genetic testing for breast cancer susceptibility: a randomized controlled trial, *JAMA* 292(4):442-452, 2004a.

Hornung CA, Eleazer GP, Strothers HS 3rd et al: Ethnicity and decision makers in a group of frail elderly, *J Am Geriatr Soc* 46(3):280-286, 1998.

Hurley AC, Volicer L: Alzheimer disease: "It's okay, Mama, if you want to go, it's okay," *JAMA* 288(18):2324-2331, 2002.

Kraetschmer N, Sharpe N, Urowitz S et al: How does trust affect patient preferences for participation in decision-making? *Health Expect* 7(4):317-326, 2004.

Lawrence VA, Streiner D, Hazuda HP et al: A cross-cultural consumer based decision aid for screening mammography, *Prev Med* 30(3):200-208, 2000.

Légaré F, O'Connor AM, Graham ID et al: Impact of the Ottawa decision support framework on the agreement and the difference between patients' and physicians' decisional conflict, *Med Decis Making* 26(4)373-390, 2006.

Lewith GT, Broomfield J, Prescott P: Complementary cancer care in Southampton: a survey of staff and patients, *Complement Ther Med* 10(2):100-106, 2002.

Martin V, Roberto K: Assessing the stability of values and health care preferences of older adults: a long term comparison, *J Gerontol Nurs* 32(11):23-30, 2006.

McGee G, Spanogle JP, Caplan AL et al: A national study of ethics committees. *Am J Bioeth* 1(4):60-64, 2001.

Meyers JL, Moore C, McGrory A et al: Physician orders for life-sustaining treatment form: honoring end-of-life directives for nursing home residents, *J Gerontol Nurs* 30(9):37-46, 2004.

Mick DJ, Ackerman MH: New perspectives on advanced practice nursing case management for aging patients, *Crit Care Nurs Clin North Am* 14(3):281-291, 2002.

Montgomery AA, Fahey T, Peters TJ: A factorial randomised controlled trial of decision analysis and an information video plus leaflet for newly diagnosed hypertensive patients, *Br J Gen Pract* 53(491):446-453, 2003.

Moye J, Karel MJ, Azar AR et al: Capacity to consent to treatment: empirical comparison of three instruments in older adults with and without dementia, *Gerontologist* 44(2):166-175, 2004.

Naylor MD: Transitional care of older adults, *Annu Rev Nurs Res* 20:127-147, 2002.

Norton SA, Bowers BJ: Working toward consensus: providers' strategies to shift patients from curative to palliative treatment choices, *Res Nurs Health* 24:258-269, 2001.

Oxman AD: You cannot make informed choices without information, *J Rehabil Med* (43 Suppl):5-7, 2004.

Redman BK, Fry ST: Ethical conflicts reported by certified registered rehabilitation nurses, *Rehabil Nurs*, 23(4):179-184, 1998.

Schwartz CE, Wheeler HB, Hammes B et al: Early intervention in planning end-of-life care with ambulatory geriatric patients: results of a pilot trial, *Arch Intern Med* 162(14):1611-1618, 2002.

Shorten A, Shorten B, Keogh J et al: Making choices for childbirth: a randomized controlled trial of a decision-aid for informed birth after cesarean, *Birth* 32(4):252-261, 2005.

Sparber A, Bauer L, Curt G et al: Use of complementary medicine by adult patients participating in cancer clinical trials, *Oncol Nurs Forum* 27(4):623-630, 2000.

Tilden VP, Tolle SW, Nelson CA et al: Family decision making to withdraw life-sustaining treatments from hospitalized patients, *Nurs Res* 50(2):105-115, 2001.

Tiller K, Meiser B, Gaff C et al: A randomized controlled trial of a decision aid for women at increased risk of ovarian cancer, *Med Decis Making* 26(4):360-372, 2006.

Tseng JF, Kronowitz SJ, Sun CC et al: The effect of ethnicity on immediate reconstruction rates after mastectomy for breast cancer, *Cancer* 101(7):1514-1523, 2004.

Valle R: Cultural assessment in bioethical advocacy—toward cultural competency and bioethical practice, *Bioethics Forum* 17(1):15-26, 2001.

Volicer L: Management of severe Alzheimer's disease and end-of-life issues, *Clin Geriatr Med* 17(2):377-391, 2001.

Whitney SN, McGuire AL, McCullough LB: A typology of shared decision making, informed consent, and simple consent, *Ann Intern Med* 140(1):54-59, 2004.

Wong FW, Anderson SM: Team approach in cross-cultural ethical decision making: a case study, *Prog Transplant* 13(1):38-41, 2003.

Parental role Conflict   Gail B. Ladwig, MSN, CHTP, RN

NANDA   Definition

Parent's experience of role confusion and conflict in response to crisis

Defining Characteristics

Anxiety; demonstrated disruption in caretaking routines; expresses concern about perceived loss of control over decisions relating to their child; fear; parent(s) express(es) concern(s) about changes in parental role; parent(s) express(es) concern(s) about family (e.g., functioning, communication, health); parent(s) express(es) concerns(s) of inadequacy to provide for child's needs (e.g., physical, emotional); parent(s) express(es) feeling(s) of inadequacy to provide for child's needs (e.g., physical, emotional); reluctant to participate in usual caretaking activities even with encouragement and support; verbalizes feelings of frustration; verbalizes feelings of guilt

Related Factors (r/t)

Change in marital status; home care of a child with special needs; interruptions of family life due to home care regimen (e.g., treatments, caregivers, lack of respite); intimidation with invasive modali-

• = Independent;   ▲ = Collaborative;   EBN = Evidence-Based Nursing;   EB = Evidence-Based

ties (e.g., intubation); intimidation with restrictive modalities (e.g., isolation); separation from child due to chronic illness; specialized care center

NOC   Outcomes (Nursing Outcomes Classification)

Suggested NOC Outcomes

Caregiver Lifestyle Disruption, Coping, Parenting Performance, Family Coping

Example NOC Outcome with Indicators
Family Coping as evidenced by the following indicators: Demonstrates role flexibility/Manages family problems/ Uses family-centered stress reduction activities (Rate the outcome and indicators of **Family Coping:** 1 = never demonstrated, 2 = rarely demonstrated, 3 = sometimes demonstrated, 4 = often demonstrated, 5 = consistently demonstrated [see Section I].)

Client Outcomes

Client Will (Specify Time Frame):

- Express feelings and perceptions regarding impacts of illness, disability, and/or hospitalization on parental role
- Participate in hospital and home care as much as able given the availability of resources and support systems
- Exhibit assertiveness and responsibility in active family decision making regarding care of the child
- Describe and select available resources to support parental management of the child's and family's needs

NIC   Interventions (Nursing Interventions Classification)

Suggested NIC Interventions

Caregiver Support, Counseling, Decision-Making Support, Family Process Maintenance, Family Therapy, Role Enhancement

Example NIC Activities—Role Enhancement
Teach new behaviors needed by patient/parent to fulfill a role; Serve as role model for learning new behaviors as appropriate

Nursing Interventions and *Rationales*

- Assess and support parents' previous coping behaviors. **EB:** *Active coping strategies of parents are associated with fewer distress indices and thus if inculcated may improve the ability to bear the burden of the illness (Rao, Pradhan & Shah, 2004).* **EBN:** *Support and caring can go a long way to ease the burden of parents caring for children with chronic illness (Coffey, 2006).*
- Explore parent/family sources of stress, usual methods of coping, and perceptions of illness/condition. Capitalize on the strengths identified. **EB:** *Caregivers of children with disabilities experience stress that should be addressed by therapists to maximize compliance with home programs (Rone-Adams, Stern & Walker, 2004).*
- Evaluate the family's perceived strength of its social support system. Encourage the family to use social support to increase its resiliency and to moderate stress. **EBN:** *Perceived social support is a factor influencing resiliency and ability to cope with stress (Tak & McCubbin, 2002).* **EBN:** *Parental support had the strongest direct effect on mothers' quality of life (Sgarbossa & Ford-Gilboe, 2004).*
- Determine the older-than-average mother's support systems and self-expectations for motherhood. **EB:** *Early maternal role attainment in women over 30 failed to reflect on the challenges of raising a child to adulthood. The importance of these challenges was identified. (Dobrzykowski & Noerager Stern, 2003).*

• = Independent;   ▲ = Collaborative;   EBN = Evidence-Based Nursing;   EB = Evidence-Based

C

- Consider the use of family theory as a framework to help guide interventions (e.g., family stress theory, role theory, social exchange theory). **EBN:** *Use of a family assessment tool is an effective way of appraising families and addressing suffering (Hogan & Logan, 2004).*
- Be available to discuss concerns and be a good listener. **EBN:** *In this study of pediatric oncology, clients' supportive care that focuses on informational and emotional support appears to be most important from diagnosis to treatment (Kerr et al, 2004).*
- ▲ Sustain parental involvement in shared decision making with regard to care by using the following steps: Incorporate parents' information concerning the child's typical routines, behaviors, fears, likes, and dislikes; provide clear and direct firsthand information concerning the child's condition and progress; normalize the home/hospital environment as much as possible; collaborate in care by providing choices when possible. **EB:** *The physician should take time to explore the client's values, concerns, and emotional and social needs; educate the client and the family about the problem; and outline the available choices (Whitney, McGuire & McCullough, 2004).*
- Seek and support parental participation in care. **EBN:** *Family-centered caregiving is important. More open hours for parents and siblings to be with their baby, less punitive and restrictive language, and a move toward viewing parents as participants in their baby's care rather than as visitors should be part of the intensive care unit (ICU) environment (Browne et al, 2004).*
- Provide support for each parent's primary coping strategies. **EBN:** *Mothers may require additional support in their role in caring for chronically ill children. Mothers exhibit greater efforts than fathers in coping patterns, including strategies to acquire social support outside the family, increase self-worth, and decrease psychological tensions (Brazil & Krueger, 2002).*
- ▲ Offer respite care to assist parents in maintaining sufficient energy and personal resources to continue caregiving responsibilities. **EBN:** *Caregivers of a child with a tracheostomy and gastrostomy believed there was disruption of social interactions within and outside the family because of the child's condition. There is a need for developing home care plans that include respite services (Montagnino & Mauricio, 2004).*
- Encourage the parent to meet his or her own needs for rest, nutrition, and hygiene. Provide facilities so that the parent may stay with the sick child (e.g., cot, reclining chair). **EBN:** *Nursing care in neonatal units should focus on interventions for parents and other family members in addition to providing the necessary care of newborns (do Vale, de Souza & Carmona, 2005).*
- Provide family-centered care. Demonstrate safe places where the parent may touch or stroke the child. Encourage the parent to talk or sing to the child. Adjust equipment so that the parent is able to hold the child, and provide a comfortable chair, preferably a rocking chair. Provide opportunities and offer praise for successful caregiving. **EBN:** *The family-centered care model can be successfully implemented in the clinical pediatric unit in a large hospital setting. The children are happier. The families openly and continuously communicate with the nurses, being confident in caring for the children and satisfied with nursing care (Attharos et al, 2004).*
- ▲ Refer parents to available telephone counseling services. **EB:** *Phone interviews are a reliable method of interviewing for use in assessing clients for post-traumatic stress disorder and major depressive disorder (Aziz & Kenford, 2004).*
- Support young grandmothers of teen mothers in areas of mother-daughter conflict such as child-rearing decisions, time with friends, household chores, and teens' choices/priorities with appropriate community referrals. **EBN:** *Community- and home-based multigenerational parent support interventions for young grandmothers of teen mothers may address some of these grandmothers' concerns (Sadler & Clemmens, 2004).*

Multicultural

- Acknowledge racial/ethnic differences at the onset of care. **EBN:** *Acknowledgment of race/ethnicity issues will enhance communication, establish rapport, and promote treatment outcomes (Giger & Davidhizar, 2004).*
- Assess for the influence of cultural beliefs, norms, and values on the client's perceptions of the parental role. **EBN:** *What the client considers a normal or abnormal parental role may be based on cultural perceptions (Leininger & McFarland, 2002;). Some Mexican-American families may engage in an intergenerational family ritual called La Cuarentena, which lasts for 40 days after birth and involves prescriptions for maternal food, clothing, and paternal role (Niska, Snyder & Lia-Hoagberg, 1998).*

• = Independent;   ▲ = Collaborative;   EBN = Evidence-Based Nursing;   EB = Evidence-Based

- Acknowledge that value conflicts arising from acculturation stresses may contribute to increased anxiety and significant conflict with the parental role. **EBN:** *This study indicates that helping family members retain traditional values may be protective for family functioning. Family conflict is particularly deleterious for youth, regardless of acculturation level. Thus, clinical intervention efforts geared toward preventing and reducing conflict relations among family members appears key to promoting adolescents' well-being (Pasch et al, 2006).*
- Promote the female parenting role by providing a treatment environment that is culturally based and woman-centered. **EBN:** *Pregnant and postpartum Asian and Pacific Islander women in substance abuse treatment identified provisions for the newborn, infant health care, parent education, and infant-mother bonding as conducive to their treatment (Morelli, Fong & Oliveria, 2001). African-American mothers of medically fragile infants reported the sights and sounds of the hospital environment as an additional stress (Miles et al, 2002).*
- Support the client's parenting role in their usual setting via social exchange. **EBN:** *Social exchange is a useful theory in support of the nurse-client relationship and is useful in accomplishing client outcomes (Byrd, 2006).*

Home Care

- The interventions described previously may be adapted for home care use.
- Assess family adjustment prenatally and postpartum; assist new parents to renegotiate behavior around issues such as amount of time spent together, sexual relationship, resolution of disagreements, and provision of sufficient time for leisure/recreational activities. Encourage the father to take an active role in infant care. **EBN:** *Declining satisfaction in family function indicates a need for supportive nursing intervention. Less decline was evident when fathers were involved in infant care and household tasks (Knauth, 2000).*
- ▲ Assess interference with family functioning. Refer for family counseling as indicated. Parental role conflict can influence all areas of family life, creating additional stress and family dysfunction. Family therapy or counseling provides an opportunity to address stressors and improve family functioning.

Client/Family Teaching

- Furnish clear explanations and answer questions about condition, disease or disability, associated treatments, and prognosis. **EB:** *Improved communication with families may significantly increase their satisfaction with the care of their hospitalized child (Maisels & Kring, 2005).*
- For parents with medically fragile and developmentally disabled children, support the family's way of coping in addition to "normalization." **EB:** *Families with severe disabilities organized and managed their lives to have a "good life" that was not necessarily normal by usual standards (Rehm & Bradley, 2005).*
- ▲ Refer parents of children with behavioral problems to parenting programs. **EB:** *Parenting programs significantly reduced child behavior problems and improved mental health. At immediate and 6-month follow-ups, parents reported gains in confidence and feeling less stressed (Stewart-Brown et al, 2004).*
- ▲ Involve parents in formal and/or informal social support situations, such as internet support groups. **EBN:** *The majority of participants in an internet support group (IPSG) not only obtained what they sought, but found more than expected in terms of insight and people to trust. The strongest outcome factor related to satisfaction was an improved caregiver-children with special needs (CSHCN) relationship (Baum, 2004).*
- ▲ Teach the client about available community resources (e.g., therapists, ministers, counselors, self-help groups). **EBN:** *Families need assistance in coping with health changes. The nurse is often perceived as the individual who can help them obtain necessary social support (Tak & McCubbin, 2002; Northouse et al, 2002).*
- ▲ Encourage parents with human immunodeficiency virus/acquired immune deficiency syndrome (HIV/AIDS) to implement custody plans for their children. **EB:** *Parents living with HIV/AIDS in New York City indicate that an increasing number of children are likely to lose one or both of their parents to HIV disease. Interventions are needed to help affected families develop viable custody plans (Lightfoot & Rotheram-Borus, 2004).*

 See the EVOLVE website for World Wide Web resources for client education.

• = Independent;   ▲ = Collaborative;   EBN = Evidence-Based Nursing;   EB = Evidence-Based

C

REFERENCES

Attharos T, Khampalikit S, Phuphaibul R et al: Development of a family-centered care model for children with cancer in a pediatric cancer unit, *Thai J Nurs Res* 8(1):52-63, 2004.

Aziz MA, Kenford S: Comparability of telephone and face-to-face interviews in assessing patients with posttraumatic stress disorder, *J Psychiatr Pract* 10(5):307-313, 2004.

Baum LS: Internet parent support groups for primary caregivers of a child with special health care needs, *Pediatr Nurs* 30(5):381-388, 401, 389-390, 2004.

Brazil K, Krueger P: Patterns of family adaptation to childhood asthma, *J Pediatr Nurs* 17(3):167-173, 2002.

Browne JV, Sanchz E, Langlois A et al: From visitation policies to family participation guidelines in the NICU: the experience of the Colorado Consortium of Intensive Care Nurseries, *J Neonat Paediatr Child Health Nurs* 7(2):16-23, 2004.

Byrd ME: Social exchange as a framework for client-nurse interaction during public health nursing maternal-child home visits, *Public Health Nurs*, 23(3):271-276, 2006.

Coffey JS: Parenting a child with chronic illness: a metasynthesis, *Pediatr Nurs* 32(1):51-9, 2006.

Dobrzykowski TM, Noerager Stern P: Out of sync: a generation of first-time mothers over 30, *Health Care Women Int* 24(3):242-253, 2003.

do Vale IN, de Souza SR, Carmona EV: Nursing diagnoses identified during parent group meetings in a neonatal intensive care unit, *Int J Nurs Terminol Classif* 16(3-4):65-73, 2005.

Giger J, Davidhizar R: Social organization. In Giger and Davidhizar's *Transcultural nursing: assessment and intervention*, St. Louis, 2004, Mosby.

Hogan DL, Logan J: The Ottawa Model of Research Use: a guide to clinical innovation in the NICU, *Clin Nurse Spec* 18(5):255-261, 2004.

Kerr LMJ, Harrison MB, Medves J et al: Supportive care needs of parents of children with cancer: transition from diagnosis to treatment, *Oncol Nurs Forum* 31(6):E116-126, 2004.

Knauth DG: Predictors of parental sense of competence for the couple during the transition to parenthood, *Res Nurs Health* 23: 496-509, 2000.

Leininger MM, McFarland MR: *Transcultural nursing: concepts, theories, research and practices*, ed 3, New York, McGraw-Hill, 2002.

Lightfoot M, Rotheram-Borus MJ: Predictors of child custody plans for children whose parents are living with AIDS in New York City, *Social Work* 49(3):461-469, 2004.

Maisels MJ, Kring EA: A simple approach to improving patient satisfaction, *Clin Pediatr (Phila)* 44(9):797-800, 2005.

Miles MS, Burchinal P, Holditch-Davis D et al: Perceptions of stress, worry, and support in black and white mothers of hospitalized, medically fragile infants, *J Pediatr Nurs* 17(2):82-88, 2002.

Montagnino BA, Mauricio RV: The child with a tracheostomy and gastrostomy: parental stress and coping in the home—a pilot study, *Pediatr Nurs* 30(5):373-380, 389-390, 401, 2004.

Morelli PT, Fong R, Oliveria J: Culturally competent substance abuse treatment for Asian/Pacific Islander women, *J Hum Behav Soc Environ* 3(3/4):263, 2001.

Niska K, Snyder M, Lia-Hoagberg B: Family ritual facilitates adaptation to parenthood, *Public Health Nurs* 15(5):329-337, 1998.

Northouse LL, Mood D, Kershaw T et al: Quality of life of women with recurrent breast cancer and their family members, *J Clin Oncol* 20(19):4050-4064, 2002.

Pasch LA, Deardorff J, Tschann JM et al: Acculturation, parent-adolescent conflict, and adolescent adjustment in Mexican American families, *Fam Process* 45(1):75-86, 2006.

Rao P, Pradhan PV, Shah H: Psychopathology and coping in parents of chronically ill children, *Indian J Pediatr* 71(8):695-699, 2004.

Rehm R, Bradley J: Normalization in families raising a child who is medically fragile/technology dependent and developmentally delayed, *Qual Health Res* 15(6):807-820, 2005.

Rone-Adams SA, Stern DF, Walker V: Stress and compliance with a home exercise program among caregivers of children with disabilities, *Pediatr Phys Ther* 16(3):140-148, 2004.

Sadler LS, Clemmens DA: Ambivalent grandmothers raising teen daughters and their babies, *J Fam Nurs* 10(2):211-231, 2004.

Sgarbossa D, Ford-Gilboe M: Mother's friendship quality, parental support, quality of life, and family health work in families led by adolescent mothers with preschool children, *J Fam Nurs* 10(2):232-261, 2004.

Stewart-Brown S, Patterson J, Mockford C et al: Impact of a general practice based group parenting programme: quantitative and qualitative results from a controlled trial at 12 months, *Arch Dis Child* 89(6):519-525, 2004.

Tak YR, McCubbin M: Family stress, perceived social support and coping following the diagnosis of a child's congenital heart disease, *J Adv Nurs* 39(2):190-198, 2002.

Whitney SN, McGuire AL, McCullough LB: A typology of shared decision making, informed consent, and simple consent, *Ann Intern Med* 140(1):54-59, 2004.

Acute Confusion   *Betty Ackley, MSN, EdS, RN*

NANDA   ### Definition

Abrupt onset of reversible disturbances of consciousness attention, cognition, and perception that develop over a short period of time

Defining Characteristics

Fluctuation in cognition; level of consciousness; psychomotor activity; hallucinations; increased agitation; increased restlessness; lack of motivation to follow through with goal-directed behavior; lack of motivation to follow through with purposeful behavior; lack of motivation to initiate goal-directed behavior; lack of motivation to initiate purposeful behavior; misperceptions

Related Factors (r/t)

Alcohol abuse; delirium; dementia; drug abuse; fluctuation in sleep-wake cycle; over 60 years of age; polypharmacy

NOC   (Nursing Outcomes Classification)

Suggested NOC Outcomes

Cognition, Distorted Thought Self-Control, Information Processing, Memory

Example NOC Outcome with Indicators
Cognition as evidenced by the following indicators: Communicates clearly for age and ability/Comprehends the meaning of events and situations/Attentiveness/Concentration (Rate the outcome and indicators of **Cognition:** 1 = severely compromised, 2 = substantially compromised, 3 = moderately compromised, 4 = mildly compromised, 5 = not compromised [see Section I].)

Client Outcomes

Client Will (Specify Time Frame):

- Demonstrate restoration of cognitive status to baseline
- Obtain adequate amount of sleep
- Demonstrate appropriate motor behavior
- Maintain functional capacity
- Optimize hydration and nutrition

NIC   Interventions (Nursing Interventions Classification)

Suggested NIC Interventions

Delirium Management, Delusion Management

Example NIC Activities—Delirium Management
Inform patient of person, place, and time, as needed; Provide new information slowly and in small doses, with frequent rest periods

Nursing Interventions and *Rationales*

- Assess the client's behavior and cognition systematically and continually throughout the day and night, as appropriate. **EB:** *Rapid onset and fluctuating course are hallmarks of delirium (Murphy, 2000; Inouye, 2006). The Confusion Assessment Method (CAM) is sensitive, specific, reliable, and easy to use. Another tool to consider is the Mini-Mental State Examination (Inouye, 2006). It is necessary to pay attention to behavioral changes because recent research has shown that there may be a prodromal phase of delirium in which sudden disorientation and urgent calls for attention may precede the onset of delirium (Duppils & Wikblad, 2004).*
- Perform an accurate mental status examination that includes the following:
  - Overall appearance, manner, and attitude
  - Behavior characteristics and level of psychomotor behavior
  - Mood and affect (presence of suicidal or homicidal ideation as observed by others and reported by the client)
  - Insight and judgment
  - Cognition as evidenced by level of consciousness, orientation (to time, place, and person), thought process, and content (perceptual disturbances such as illusions and hallucinations, paranoia, delusions, abstract thinking)
  - Level of attention
  New onset of delirium in adults warrants a thorough examination to determine cause and treatment (Cole, Williams & Williams, 2006). **EB:** *Early intervention in the case of delirium may decrease the*

• = Independent;   ▲ = Collaborative;   EBN = Evidence-Based Nursing;   EB = Evidence-Based

C

severity and length of the delirious episode (Milisen et al, 2001). Clients discharged from the hospital with delirium had a high rate of institutionalization and mortality over a 1-year follow-up (McAvay et al, 2006).

▲ Assess for and report possible physiological alterations (e.g., sepsis, hypoglycemia, hypoxia, hypotension, infection, changes in temperature, fluid and electrolyte imbalance, use of medications with known cognitive and psychotropic side effects). *Early attention to these risk factors may prevent delirium or shorten the length of the delirium episode (Inouye, 2006).*

▲ Treat the underlying causes of delirium in collaboration with the healthcare team: Establish/ maintain normal fluid and electrolyte balance; establish/maintain normal nutrition, normal body temperature, normal oxygenation (if the client experiences low oxygen saturation, deliver supplemental oxygen), normal blood glucose levels, normal blood pressure. **EB:** *Dehydration is a significant risk factor for delirium and should be addressed aggressively (Inouye, 2000).*

▲ Communicate client status, cognition, and behavioral manifestations to all necessary providers.
   ■ Monitor for any trends occurring in these manifestations of delirium.
   EB: *Recognize that the client's fluctuating cognition and behavior are the hallmark of delirium and are not to be construed as client preference for certain caregivers (Inouye, van Dyck & Alessi, 1990).*
   EB: *Careful monitoring is needed to identify the potential etiologic factors for delirium (Milisen, 2004).*

▲ Laboratory results should be closely monitored and physiological support given as appropriate. **EBN:** *Once acute confusion has been identified, it is vital to recognize and treat the associated underlying causes (Rapp & Iowa Veterans Affairs Nursing Research Consortium, 1997).*

• Establish or maintain elimination patterns. **EBN and EB:** *Disruption in elimination may be a cause of confusion (Rapp & Iowa Veterans Affairs Nursing Research Consortium, 1997). Urinary retention or a urinary tract infection resulting in urosepsis, as well as constipation, may lead to delirium (Inouye, 2006).*

• Plan care that allows for an appropriate sleep-wake cycle. **EB:** *Disruptions in usual sleep and activity patterns should be minimized because those clients with nocturnal exacerbations experience more complications from delirium (Inouye, 2000).*

▲ Conduct a medication review. *Medication use is one of the most important modifiable factors that can cause or worsen delirium, especially the use of anticholinergics, benzodiazepines, and hypnotics (Inouye, 2006).*

• Modulate sensory exposure and establish a calm environment. **EBN:** *Extraneous lights and noise can give rise to agitation, especially if misperceived. Sensory overload or sensory deprivation can result in increased confusion (Rosen, 1994).* **EB:** *Clients with a hyperactive form of delirium often have increased irritability and startle responses and may be acutely sensitive to light and sound (Casey et al, 1996).*

• Provide reality orientation, including identifying self by name at each contact with the client; calling the client by their preferred name; using orientation techniques; providing familiar objects from home such as an afghan; providing clocks, calendars; and gently correcting misperceptions. **EBN:** *Use of reality orientation can help improve cognition in dementia clients (Forbes, 2007 in press).*

• Avoid use of validation therapy with the confused client, other than to validate the feelings the client may be expressing. **EB:** *A Cochrane review demonstrated that there is no evidence that validation therapy is helpful for clients with cognitive impairment (Neal & Briggs, 2003).*

• Use appropriate communication techniques for clients at risk for confusion including communicating clearly and providing simple explanations as needed (Inouye, 2000; Foreman, 2004).

• Provide supportive nursing care including meeting of basic needs such as feeding, toileting, and hydration. **EBN:** *Delirious clients are unable to care for themselves due to their confusion. Their care and safety needs must be anticipated by the nurse (Foreman et al, 1999).*

▲ Identify, evaluate, and treat pain quickly (see care plans for **Acute Pain** or **Chronic Pain**). **EB and EBN:** *Untreated pain is a potential cause of delirium (Inouye, 2000; Milisen et al, 2001).*

▲ Facilitate appropriate sensory input by having clients use aids (e.g., glasses, hearing aids) as needed. *Sensory impairment contributes to misinterpretation of the environment and significantly contributes to delirium (Inouye, 2006).*

▲ Recognize that delirium is frequently treated with an antipsychotic medication. Watch for side

---

• = Independent;   ▲ = Collaborative;   EBN = Evidence-Based Nursing;   EB = Evidence-Based

effects of the medications. **EB:** *Be aware of paradoxical effects and side effects such as extrapyramidal symptoms, agitation, sedation, and arrhythmias, because these may exacerbate the delirium (Schwartz & Masand, 2002).*

Geriatric

- Mobilize the client as soon as possible; provide active and passive range of motion. **EB:** *Older clients who had a low level of physical activity before injury are at particular risk for acute confusion (Inouye, 2000).*
- ▲ Evaluate all medications for potential to cause or exacerbate delirium. Review the Beers Criteria for Potentially Inappropriate Medication Use in Elderly. *The elderly are very prone to medication side effects, which can include confusion. Polypharmacy is a frequent cause of delirium in the elderly (Fick & Mion, 2005).*
- ▲ Provide sufficient medication to relieve pain. **EBN:** *Older clients may give inaccurate pain histories, underreport symptoms, not want to bother the nurse, or exhibit restlessness, agitation, or increased confusion (Matthiesen et al, 1994).*
- Explain hospital routines and procedures slowly and in simple terms; repeat information as necessary. **EBN:** *Anxiety and sensory impairment decrease the older client's ability to integrate new information (Matthiesen et al, 1994).*
- Provide continuity of care when possible (e.g., provide the same caregivers, avoid room changes) (Foreman, 2004). **EBN:** *Continuity of care helps decrease the disorienting effects of hospitalization (Matthiesen et al, 1994).*
- If clients know that they are not thinking clearly, acknowledge the concern. Fear is frequently experienced by people with delirium. **EBN and EB:** *Confusion is very frightening, and the memory of the delirium can be equally frightening (Breitbart, Gibson & Tremblay, 2002; Matthiesen et al, 1994).*
- Keep the client's sleep-wake cycle as normal as possible (e.g., avoid letting the client take daytime naps, avoid waking the client at night, give sedatives but not diuretics at bedtime, provide pain relief and back rubs). **EB and EBN:** *Acute confusion is accompanied by disruption of the sleep-wake cycle (Inouye, 2000; Matthiesen et al, 1994).*
- Maintain normal sleep-wake patterns (treat with bright light for 2 hours in the early evening). **EBN:** *Light treatment facilitates normal sleep-wake patterns (Rapp & Iowa Veterans Affairs Nursing Research Consortium, 1997).*

Home Care

- Some of the interventions described previously may be adapted for home care use.
- Assess and monitor for acute changes in cognition and behavior. *An acute change in cognition and behavior is the classic presentation of delirium. It should be considered a medical emergency.*
- Recognize that delirium is reversible but can become chronic if untreated. The client may be discharged from the hospital to home care in a state of undiagnosed delirium. **EBN:** *Staff should receive training in the assessment of acute confusion; assessment may be complicated by the presence of periods of lucidity (Mentes et al, 1999).* **EB:** *In a study of delirium among clients in a convalescent hospital following an acute care hospital stay for a variety of precipitating factors, 22% presented with delirium, and 93% of these had developed the delirium prior to convalescent home admission. Multiple precipitating factors were frequently present (Pi-Figueras et al, 2004).*
- Assess for treatable causes of changes in cognition and behavior. The mnemonic DEMENTIA can be used to remember potential causes of acute or chronic confusion (Smith, 2002):
  - **D:** Drugs and alcohol—including over-the-counter drugs
  - **E:** Eyes and ears—disorientation due to visual/auditory distortion
  - **M:** Medical disorders—e.g., diabetes, hypothyroidism
  - **E:** Emotional and psychological disturbances—e.g., mood or paranoid disorders
  - **N:** Neurological disorders—e.g., multi-infarct dementia
  - **T:** Tumors and trauma
  - **I:** Infections—e.g., urinary tract or upper respiratory tract
  - **A:** Arteriosclerosis—leading to heart failure, insufficient blood supply to heart and brain, confusion

---

• = Independent;   ▲ = Collaborative;   EBN = Evidence-Based Nursing;   EB = Evidence-Based

C

- Assess fluid intake, dementia status, and occurrence of a fall within the past 30 days in evaluating confusion. **EBN:** *Confusion may be explained by inadequate fluid intake, dementia, or a fall. In the last case, it is unclear if falls are a precipitating event or indicative of frailty (Mentes et al, 1999).*
- Avoid preconceptions about the source of acute confusion; assess each occurrence on the basis of available evidence. *Delirium may not be readily recognized, in part because of its varying presentations and in part because preconceptions interfere with accurate assessment. For example, although delirium may occur in advanced cancer clients prior to death, it also may arise in response to reversible causes that should be identified and treated, depending on the goals of care (Lawlor, 2001).*
- ▲ Institute case management of frail elderly clients to support continued independent living, if possible, once delirium has resolved.

Client/Family Teaching

- ▲ Teach the family to recognize signs of early confusion and seek medical help. **EBN:** *Early intervention can help prevent long-term complications (Rapp & Iowa Veterans Affairs Nursing Research Consortium, 1997).*
- Counsel the client and family regarding the management of delirium and its sequelae. **EB:** *Families experience a high degree of distress when observing a loved one in delirium. Families should be told that symptoms of delirium may persist for months following a delirious episode so that appropriate plans can be made for continuing care (Marcantonio et al, 2003).*

REFERENCES

Breitbart W, Gibson C, Tremblay A: The delirium experience: delirium recall and delirium related distress in hospitalized patients with cancer, their spouses/caregivers, and their nurses, *Psychosomatics* 43(3):183-194, 2002.

Casey DA, DeFazio JV Jr, Vansickle K et al: Delirium: quick recognition, careful evaluation, and appropriate treatment, *Postgrad Med* 100(1):121-124, 1996.

Cole CS, Williams, ER, Williams, RD: Assessment and discharge planning for hospitalized older adults with delirium, *Medsurg Nurs* 15(2):71-77, 2006.

Duppils GS, Wikblad K: Delirium: behavioural changes before and during prodromal phase, *J Clin Nurs* 13(5):609-616, 2004.

Fick D, Mion L: Assessing and managing delirium in persons with dementia. Try this: best practices in nursing care for hospitalized older adults, *The John A. Hartford Institute for Geriatric Nursing and the Alzheimer's Association,* 1(8):1-2, 2005.

Forbes D: Reality orientation. In Ackley B, Ladwig G, Swan B et al: *Evidence-based nursing guidelines: medical surgical interventions,* Philadelphia, 2007, Mosby (in press).

Foreman MD, Mion LC, Tryostad L et al: Standard of practice protocol: acute confusion/delirium, NICHE Faculty, *Geriatr Nurs* 20(3):147-152, 1999.

Inouye SK: Current concepts: delirium in older persons, *N Engl J Med* 354(11):1157-1165, 1217-1220, 2006.

Inouye SK: Prevention of delirium in hospitalized older patients: risk factors and targeted intervention strategies, *Ann Med* 32(4):257, 2000.

Inouye SK, van Dyck CH, Alessi CA et al: Clarifying confusion: the confusion assessment method: a new method for detection of delirium, *Ann Intern Med* 113(12):941-948, 1990.

Lawlor PG: Assessment of delirium in patients with advanced cancer, *Home Health Care Consult* 8(9):10, 2001.

Marcantonio ER, Simon SE, Bergmann MA et al: Delirium symptoms in post-acute care: prevalent, persistent, and associated with poor recovery, *J Am Geriatr Soc* 51(1):4-9, 2003.

Matthiesen V, Sivertsen L, Foreman MD et al: Acute confusion: nursing interventions in older patients, *Orthop Nurs* 13:25, 1994.

McAvay GJ, Van Ness PH, Bogardus ST Jr et al: Older adults discharged from the hospital with delirium: 1-year outcomes, *J Am Geriatr Soc,* 54(8):1245-1250, 2006.

Mentes J, Culp K, Maas M et al: Acute confusion indicators: risk factors and prevalence using MDS data, *Res Nurs Health* 22(2):95-105, 1999.

Milisen K et al: Early detection and prevention of delirium in older patients with cancer, *Eur J Cancer Care* 13(5):494-500, 2004.

Milisen K, Foreman MD, Abraham IL et al: A nurse-led interdisciplinary intervention program for delirium in elderly hip fracture patients, *J Am Geriatr Soc* 49(5):523-532, 2001.

Murphy BA: Delirium, *Emerg Med Clin North Am* 18:243, 2000.

Pi-Figueras M, Aguilera A, Arellano M et al: Prevalence of delirium in a geriatric convalescent hospital unit: patient's clinical characteristics and risk precipitating factor analysis, *Arch Gerontol Geriatr* (Suppl 9):333, 2004.

Neal M, Briggs M: Validation therapy for dementia, *Cochrane Database Syst Rev* (3):CD001394, 2003.

Rapp C, Iowa Veterans Affairs Nursing Research Consortium: *Acute confusion/delirium,* Iowa City, 1997, The Consortium.

Rosen SL: Managing delirious older adults in the hospital, *MedSurg Nurs* 3(3):181, 1994.

Schwartz TL, Masand PS: The role of atypical antipsychotics in the treatment of delirium, *Psychosomatics* 43:171, 2002.

Smith GB: Case management guideline: Alzheimer disease and other dementias, *Lippincotts Case Manag* 7(2):77-84, 2002.

Chronic Confusion   *Rebecca Davis, PhD, RN*

NANDA   Definition

Irreversible, long-standing, and/or progressive deterioration of intellect and personality character-ized by decreased ability to interpret environmental stimuli; decreased capacity for intellectual thought processes; and manifested by disturbances of memory, orientation, and behavior

Defining Characteristics

Altered interpretation; altered personality; altered response to stimuli; clinical evidence of organic impairment; impaired long-term memory; impaired short-term memory; impaired socialization; long-standing cognitive impairment; no change in level of consciousness; progressive cognitive impairment

Related Factors (r/t)

Alzheimer's disease; cerebral vascular attack; head injury; Korsakoff's psychosis; multi-infarct dementia

NOC   Outcomes (Nursing Outcomes Classification)

Suggested NOC Outcomes

Cognition, Cognitive Orientation, Distorted Thought Self-Control

Example NOC Outcome with Indicators
Cognition as evidenced by the following indicators: Communicates clearly for age and ability/Comprehends the meaning of events and situations/Attentiveness/Concentration (Rate the outcome and indicators of **Cognition:** 1 = severely compromised, 2 = substantially compromised, 3 = moderately compromised, 4 = mildly compromised, 5 = not compromised [see Section I].)

Client Outcomes

Client Will (Specify Time Frame):

* Remain content and free from harm
* Function at maximal cognitive level
* Participate in activities of daily living at the maximum of functional ability
* Have minimal episodes of agitation since agitation occurs in up to 70% of patients with dementia

NIC   Interventions (Nursing Interventions Classification)

Suggested NIC Interventions

Dementia Management, Environmental Management, Surveillance: Safety

Example NIC Activities—Dementia Management
Use distraction rather than confrontation to manage behavior; Give one simple direction at a time

Nursing Interventions and *Rationales*

* Determine the client's cognitive level using a screening tool such as the Mini-Mental State Exam (MMSE). The Mini-Cog is also a useful screening tool to be used in a busy setting. **EB:** *Use of a standard evaluation tool such as the MMSE can help determine the client's abilities and assist in planning appropriate nursing interventions (Borson & Scanlan, 2006; Borson et al, 2005; Wilber et al, 2005).*

C

- Gather information about the client's predementia cognitive functioning. **EBN and EB:** *Individuals with a history of cognitive dysfunction are at higher risk for acute confusion (i.e., sundowner's syndrome) during acute illness (Fick et al, 2005; Voyer et al, 2006).*
- Assess the client for signs of depression: insomnia, poor appetite, flat affect, and withdrawn behavior. **EB:** *Up to 95% of individuals with dementia have some neuropsychiatric problems, with the most common being depression (Aalten et al, 2005; Steinberg et al, 2006).*
- Determine client's normal routines and attempt to maintain them. **EB:** *Activities that are designed to be consistent with past routines were effective at providing engagement and interest and enhancing quality of life (Cohen-Mansfield & Jensen, 2006).*
- Begin each interaction with the client by identifying yourself and calling the client by name. Approach the client with a caring, loving, and accepting attitude, and speak calmly and slowly. **EBN and EB:** *Dementia causes a loss of the ability to learn new things and remember people and places (episodic memory)—thus clients will need reassurance and frequent reminding of the identity of caregivers (Golby et al, 2005; Son, Therrien & Whall, 2002).*
- Use a calm approach in interactions and use reminiscence therapy and validation (validating what the clients say is real instead of correcting them). **EB:** *Emotion-centered care, including validation therapy, reminiscence, and emotional support can help reduce anxiety and improve client satisfaction (Finnema et al, 2005).*
- Provide scheduled activities that are matched to the client's abilities and personality. **EBN:** *Activities that are individualized to the client's abilities and personality can reduce agitation and improve quality of life (Cohen-Mansfield & Jensen, 2006).*
- Provide periods of rest along with periods of activities. **EB:** *Balancing times of rest during non-arousal states and times of stimulation during arousal states can decrease agitation in those with dementia (Kovach et al, 2004).*
- Give one simple direction at a time and repeat it as necessary. Use verbal and physical prompts, and model the desired action if needed and possible. **EB:** *There are a variety of communication problems in dementia, but with time and prompting people with dementia can make their needs known (Bayles et al, 2006).*
- Break down self-care tasks into simple steps (e.g., instead of saying, "Take a shower," say to the client, "Please follow me. Sit down on the bed. Take off your shoes. Now take off your socks."). **EB:** *Verbal prompts, assistance with steps of a process, and cueing activities in sequential order can help those with dementia be more independent in activities of daily living (ADLs) (Bourgeois et al, 2003).*
- Engage the client in communication by individualizing the nurse's interactions to maximize client interaction and response. **EBN and EB:** *Individualized communication strategies that involve the client's interest have been shown to improve communication abilities in those with dementia above the level that would be expected from their cognitive abilities (Perry et al, 2005; van Weert et al, 2005).*
- For anxious clients who are having problems relaxing enough to eat, try having them listen to music during meals. **EB:** *Clients who listen to music have been shown to have less agitation and consumed more foods (Hicks-Moore, 2005).*
- Assess the cause of and consequences of wandering before attempting to control the wandering. **EBN:** *Wandering may be an adaptive response and not need an intervention. Other related problems, such as elopement or falls should be assessed (Algase, 1999; Lai & Arthur, 2003).*
- For individuals who have wandering behavior, individualize interventions such as those that provide a safe environment with physical barriers to exits, safe walking paths, and a daily schedule of activities. **EBN:** *Although studies are inconclusive, modifying the environment and providing daily activities have been shown to decrease some types of wandering (Siders et al, 2004).*
- Use symbols rather than words to identify areas such as the bathroom or kitchen. Utilize environmental cues such as clocks and a sign with mealtimes to decrease common mealtime questions and thus decrease agitation around mealtimes. **EBN:** *The results of a study in which a large clock and a sign with large lettering that identified mealtimes were hung in the dining area suggest cues can reduce repetitive questions commonly exhibited by individuals with dementia (Nolan & Mathews, 2004).*
- Set up scheduled quiet periods in a recliner or room. Use afghans and environmental cues to define rest periods. **EB:** *Sleep disorders are very common in those with dementia, and a lack of sleep has been shown to be related to poorer memory. One study showed that naps in older people can*

improve sleep amounts without decreasing nighttime sleep and improve cognitive and psychomotor performance (Eeles et all, 2006; Hatfield, Herbert & Someren, 2004; Mograss, Godbout & Guillem, 2006).

- Provide structured social and physical activities that are individualized for the client. **EB:** *Social activities and exercise have been shown to improve sleep quality, which is often impaired in individuals with dementia (Eggermont & Scherder, 2006; Montgomery & Dennis, 2003; Richards et al, 2005).*
- Provide quiet activities such as listening to music of the client's preference or introduce other cues that promote relaxation in the afternoon or early evening. **EB and EBN:** *Calming activities such as listening to preferred music can reduce agitation (Siders et al, 2004; Sung, 2005).*
- Provide simple activities for the client, such as folding washcloths and sorting or stacking activities or other hobbies the individual enjoyed prior to the onset of dementia. **EBN and EB:** *Activities such as folding washcloths, cooking, and gardening involve implicit memory and are thus something that the older adult can become engaged in, which can provide distraction and a sense of accomplishment (Golby et al, 2005; Son, Therrien & Whall, 2002).*
- Use cues, such as picture boards denoting day, time, and location, to help client with orientation. **EBN and EB:** *Reality orientation, used not when clients are agitated, but as overall reminders of orientation, can help some clients remain more oriented (Spector et al, 2000).*
- Use reminiscence and life review therapeutic interventions; ask questions about the client's work, children, or time spent in military service. Ask questions such as, "What was really important to you as you look back?" to engage the client in storytelling. **EB:** *Reminiscence and life review can help an older person reframe and accept life events and provide social engagement (Herrmann, 2005; Kim et al, 2006; Woods et al, 2005).*
- ▲ If the client becomes increasingly confused and agitated, perform the following steps:
  - ■ Assess the client for physiological causes, including acute hypoxia, pain, medication effects, malnutrition, infections such as urinary tract infection, fatigue, electrolyte disturbances, and constipation. *An acute change in behavior is a medical emergency and should be evaluated. A change in behavior may be due to physical causes, which should be ruled out before behavioral interventions are initiated (Volicer & Hurley, 2003).*
  - ■ Assess for psychological causes, including changes in the environment, caregiver, and routine; demands to perform beyond capacity; or multiple competing stimuli, including discomfort. **EBN:** *Agitated behaviors can be an expression of a need that is not being met (Kolanowski, Litaker & Buettner, 2005; Kovach et al, 2005).*
  - ■ In clients with agitated behaviors, rather than confronting the client, provide diversional behaviors such as singing, games, and the provision of textured items to handle. **EBN:** *Diversional activities that are individualized can be effective at reducing agitated behaviors (Colling & Buettner, 2002; Kolanowski, Richards & Sullivan, 2002).*
- Decrease stimuli in the environment (e.g., turn off the television, take the client to a quiet place). Institute activities associated with pleasant emotions, such as playing soft music the client likes, looking through a photo album, providing favorite food, or using simulated presence therapy. **EB and EBN:** *Decreasing stimuli can decrease agitation (Tilly & Reed, 2005).*
- If clients with dementia become more agitated, assess for pain. **EB and EBN:** *A change in behavior may indicate pain, and pain is often undertreated in those with dementia. Treating pain can improve social interaction, engagement, and decrease agitation (Chibnall et al, 2005; Cohen-Mansfield & Creedon, 2002).*
- Avoid using restraints if at all possible. **EB:** *Restraints have been shown to cause decline in cognition, socialization, and depression in nursing home residents (Castle, 2006).*
- ▲ Use PRN or low-dose regular dosing of psychotropic or antianxiety drugs only as a last resort. They can be effective in managing symptoms of psychosis and aggressive behavior, but have undesirable side effects. Start with the lowest possible dose. **EB and EBN:** *Psychotropic medication use is variable in those with dementia and has many side effects, including sleep disturbances and medication interactions. Effective nursing interventions can reduce psychotropic medication usage (Coker, 2006; Kim & Whall, 2006; Lonergan et al, 2002; Simpson et al, 2006).*
- ▲ Avoid the use of anticholinergic medications such as Benadryl. *Anticholinergic medications have a high side effect profile that includes disorientation, urinary retention, and excessive drowsiness (Han et al, 2001). The anticholinergic side effects outweigh the antihistaminic effects.*

C

- For predictable difficult times, such as during bathing and grooming, try the following:
  - Massage the client's hands lovingly or use therapeutic touch to relax the client. **EBN:** *Hand massage and therapeutic touch have been shown to induce relaxation that may allow care activities to take place without difficulty (Remington, 2002; Viggo Hansen, Jorgensen & Ortenblad, 2006).*
  - When bathing a client with dementia, minimize the client's discomfort by using the Bag Bath (if available). *Bathtime is an opportunity to emphasize person-centered nursing.* **EBN:** *Bathing is known to be stressful for clients with dementia as evidenced by the frequently seen agitation that occurs during this activity. The Bag Bath decreases discomfort during bathing, and the person-centered approach maintains self-esteem and a sense of control for the client (Somboontanont et al, 2004).*
  - Approach the client in a client-centered framework as this offers a sense of control and promotes self-esteem.
  - Involve family in care of the client. **EBN:** *Involving family in care of clients with dementia improved cognitive abilities (Jablonski, Reed & Maas, 2005).*
- For care of early dementia clients with primarily symptoms of memory loss, see the care plan for **Impaired Memory.**
- For care of clients with self-care deficits, see the appropriate care plan **(Feeding Self-care deficit; Dressing/grooming Self-care deficit;** and **Toileting Self-care deficit).**

Geriatric

NOTE: All interventions are appropriate with geriatric clients.

Multicultural

- Assess for the influence of cultural beliefs, norms, and values on the family's or caregiver's understanding of chronic confusion or dementia. **EBN:** *What the family considers normal and abnormal health behavior may be based on cultural perceptions (Leininger & McFarland 2002; Giger & Davidhizar, 2004). Research indicates that Caucasian older adults are significantly more knowledgeable about Alzheimer's disease (AD) than African-American, Asian, and Latino older adults (Ayalon & Arean, 2004). Another study showed African-Americans showed less awareness of facts about AD, reported fewer sources of information, and indicated less perceived threat of the disorder (Roberts et al, 2003).*
- Inform the client's family or caregiver of the meaning of and reasons for common behavior observed in clients with dementia. **EBN:** *An understanding of dementia behavior will enable the client's family or caregiver to provide the client with a safe environment. Black and Latino community-dwelling clients with moderate to severe dementia have a higher prevalence of dementia-related behaviors than whites (Sink et al, 2004).*
- Assist the family or caregiver in identifying barriers that would prevent the use of social services or other supportive services that could help reduce the impact of caregiving. **EBN:** *Expectations of discrimination, lack of knowledge about services, expectations embedded in familism, lack of sense of prevention, lack of health insurance, preference for traditional remedies, and neglect or abuse were barriers identified by researchers studying the low utilization of skilled home care nursing services by elderly Hispanic clients (Crist, 2002). Language may present another barrier to the access of supportive services (McGrath, Vun & McLeod, 2001). The lack of health insurance and financial resources for a substantial proportion of Mexican-American people means many do not receive medical care, so their Alzheimer's disease remains undiagnosed and untreated (Briones et al, 2002).*
- Assess the client for the presence of an instrumental activity of daily living (IADL) disability and chronic health conditions. **EBN:** *African-American clients with cognitive impairments had higher IADL disability, poorer self-rated health, higher cognitive errors, and more chronic health conditions (Chumbler et al, 2001).*
- ▲ Refer the family to social services or other supportive services to assist in meeting the demands of caregiving for the client with dementia. **EBN:** *African-American caregivers of dementia clients may evidence less desire than others to institutionalize their family members and are more likely to report unmet service needs (Hinrichsen & Ramirez, 1992). Families of dementia clients may report restricted social activity (Haley et al, 1995). Korean families reported waiting 3 to 4 years before seeking help for their family member with dementia. Help was sought when memory decline was accompanied by other problems (Watari & Gatz, 2004).*

• = Independent;   ▲ = Collaborative;   EBN = Evidence-Based Nursing;   EB = Evidence-Based

▲ Encourage the family to make use of support groups or other service programs. **EBN:** *Studies indicate that some minority families of clients with dementia may use few support programs even though these programs could have a positive impact on caregiver well-being (Cox, 1999).*

• Validate the family members' feelings with regard to the impact of the client's behavior on family lifestyle. **EBN:** *Validation lets family members know that the nurse has heard and understood what was said, and it promotes the relationship between the nurse and family members (Heineken, 1998).*

NOTE: Black and Latino community-dwelling clients with moderate to severe dementia have a higher prevalence of dementia-related behaviors than Caucasian clients. Therefore, as the aging minority population grows, it will be especially important to target caregiver education, in-home support, and resources to minority communities (Sink et al, 2004).

 Home Care

NOTE: Keeping the client as independent as possible is important. Because community-based care is usually less structured than institutional care; however, in the home setting the goal of maintaining safety for the client takes on primary importance.

• The interventions described previously may be adapted for home care use.

▲ Provide information to the family and home care client regarding advanced directives. This is a legal requirement of the Consolidated Omnibus Budget Reconciliation Act (COBRA). *The ability of the client to plan advance directives legally depends on the stage of dementia, the degree of certainty of the client's wishes for end-of-life care, and the degree of distress experienced by the client with dementia. Successful completion of advance directives by clients with mild to moderate dementia has been reported (Rempusheski & Hurley, 2000).*

• Assess the client's memory and executive function deficits before assuming the inability to make any medical decisions. **EB:** *A review of existing research on the decision-making competence of cognitively impaired older adults concluded that many persons with dementia are capable of decision making and that, at least in the early stages of dementia, interventions may improve decisional abilities (Kim, Karlawish & Caine, 2002).*

▲ Assess the home for safety features and client needs for assistive devices. Refer to the interventions for **Feeding Self-care deficit, Dressing Self-care deficit, Bathing Self-care deficit** as needed.

• Elements of reality orientation therapy may be applied in the home, incorporating person-centered respect, reminiscence, validation, and sensory-motor stimulation. **EB:** *In one study, participants with dementia were led in ecological exercises (e.g., a game around using money); personal, spatial, and social orientation; verbal and visual memory; verbal fluency; categorization; and auditory and visual attention. Improvement in cognition, language, memory, and affective function were noted (Savorani et al, 2004).*

▲ Provide education and support to the family of the client with a chronic and disabling condition; be prepared to offer support and information to family members who live at a distance as well. **EB:** *Increased self-efficacy for caregiving has been related to decreased caregiver stress and burden (Gonyea et al, 2005; Hepburn, Lewis & Narayan, 2005).*

• Use familiar aspects of the environment (smells, music, foods, pictures) to cue the client, capitalizing on habit to remind the client of activities in which the client can participate (e.g., cooperating with medication administration). **EBN:** *While clients with dementia are probably unable to learn new activities because of deteriorated explicit memory, preserved implicit memory or habit may be useful in maximizing functional ability (Son, Therrien & Whall, 2002).*

• Instruct the caregiver to provide a balanced activity schedule that does not stress the client nor deprive him or her of stimulation; avoid sustained low- or high-stimulation activity. **EBN:** *In one study, imbalances in the pacing of sensory stimulation and sensory calming (i.e., sustained low- and high-stimulation activity) contributed to agitation and functional decline (Kovach & Wells, 2002).*

▲ If the client will require extensive supervision on an ongoing basis, evaluate the client for day care programs. Refer the family to medical social services to assist with this process if necessary. *Day care programs provide safe, structured care for the client and respite for the family.* **EB:** *Adult Day programs have been shown to reduce stress associated with work, leisure, and family needs (Schacke & Zank, 2006; Baumgarten et al, 2002).*

• Encourage the family to include the client in family activities when possible. Reinforce the use of therapeutic communication guidelines (see Client/Family Teaching) and sensitivity to the

C

number of people present. *These steps help the client maintain dignity and lead to familial socialization of the client.*

- Assess family caregivers for caregiver stress, loneliness, and depression. **EBN:** *Caregiving is associated with poorer mental health. Increased burden (behavioral and health problems) is associated with more mental health problems in the caregiver (Willette-Murphy, Todero & Yeaworth, 2006).*
- Refer to the care plan for **Caregiver role strain.**
- ▲ Refer the client to medical social services as necessary to evaluate financial resources and initiate benefits or access to providers. *Limited resources serve as barriers to effective outcomes in addressing dementia (Smith, 2002).*
- ▲ Institute case management for frail elderly clients to support continued independent living.

Client/Family Teaching

- In the early stages of confusion (e.g., initial period following stroke), provide the caregiver with information on illness processes, needed care, and likely trajectory of progress. **EBN:** *In one study, family caregivers of stroke survivors felt abandoned by staff. Caregivers wanted information to ensure that they felt competent, confident, and able to provide care safely; they wanted to understand likely future demands (Brereton & Nolan, 2002; Kuhn & Fulton, 2004).*
- Teach the family how to converse with a memory-impaired person. Individuals with dementia have a variety of communication difficulties. *Good assessment and individualized interventions are necessary to improve communication (Frazier-Rios & Zembrzuski, 2005).*
- Teach the family how to provide physical care for the client (bathing, feeding, and ADLs). **EBN:** *Improved self-efficacy regarding how to care for loved ones has been shown to decrease caregiver burden (Gonyea et al, 2005).*
- Instruct the family and care providers that faith, humor, patience, and contact with friends and family have been identified as positive approaches in keeping a client with dementia engaged in their care. **EBN:** *This has been found to work in keeping a client with dementia from displaying passive behaviors (Colling, 2004).*
- Discuss with the family what to expect as the dementia progresses.
- ▲ Counsel the family about resources available regarding end-of-life decisions and legal concerns.
- ▲ Inform the family that as dementia progresses, hospice care may be available in the home in the terminal stages to help the caregiver. **EBN:** *Hospice services in the late stages of dementia can help support the family with nursing services and visitation by the primary care provider, home health aides, social services personnel, volunteer visitors, and a spiritual counselor if desired as the client is dying (Boyd & Vernon, 1998).*

NOTE: The nursing diagnoses **Impaired Environmental interpretation syndrome** and **Chronic Confusion** are very similar in definition and interventions. **Impaired Environmental interpretation syndrome** must be interpreted as a syndrome when other nursing diagnoses would also apply. **Chronic Confusion** may be interpreted as the human response to a situation or situations that require a level of cognition of which the individual is no longer capable. Further research is underway to make this distinction clear to the practicing nurse.

evolve See the EVOLVE website for World Wide Web resources for client education.

REFERENCES

Aalten P, de Vugt M, Jaspers N et al: The course of neuropsychiatric symptoms in dementia. Part I: findings from the two-year longitudinal Maasbed study, *Int J Geriatr Psychiatry* 20(6):523-530, 2005.

Algase D: Wandering: a dementia-compromised behavior, *J Gerontol Nurs* 25(9):10, 1999.

Ayalon L, Arean PA: Knowledge of Alzheimer's disease in four ethnic groups of older adults, *Int J Geriatr Psychiatry* 19(1):51-57, 2004.

Baumgarten M, Lebel P, Laprise H et al: Adult day care for the frail elderly: outcomes, satisfaction, and cost, *J Aging Health* 14(2):237-259, 2002.

Bayles K, Kim E, Chapman S et al: Evidence-based practice recommendations for working with individuals with dementia: simulated presence therapy, *J Med Speech-Lang Pathol* 14:13-21, 2006.

Borson S, Scanlan J: The accuracy of the mini-cog in screening low-educated elderly for dementia, *J Am Geriatr Soc* 54(2):376-378, 2006.

Borson S, Scanlan J, Watanabe J et al: Simplifying detection of cognitive impairment: comparison of the Mini-Cog and Mini-Mental State Examination in a multiethnic sample, *J Am Geriatr Soc* 53(5):871-874, 2005.

Bourgeois M, Camp C, Rose M et al: A comparison of training strategies to enhance use of external aids by persons with dementia, *J Commun Disord* 36(5):361-378, 2003.

Boyd CO, Vernon GM: Primary care of the older adult with end-stage Alzheimer's disease, *Nurs Pract* 23(4):63, 1998.

Brereton L, Nolan M: "Seeking": a key activity for new family carers of stroke survivors, *J Clin Nurs* 11(1):22-31, 2002.

Briones DF, Ramirez AL, Guerrero M et al: Determining cultural and psychosocial factors in Alzheimer disease among Hispanic populations, *Alzheimer Dis Assoc Disord* 16(Suppl 2):S86-88, 2002.

Castle N: Mental health outcomes and physical restraint among nursing homes, *Adm Policy Ment Health* 33(6)696-704, 2006.

Chibnall JT, Tait RC, Harman B et al: Effect of acetaminophen on behavior, well-being, and psychotropic medication use in nursing home residents with moderate-to-severe dementia, *J Am Geriatr Soc* 53(11):1921-1929, 2005.

Chumbler NR, Hartmann DJ, Cody M et al: Differences by race in the health status of rural cognitively impaired Arkansans, *Clin Gerontol* 24(1/2):103-121, 2001.

Cohen-Mansfield J, Creedon M: Nursing staff members' perceptions of pain indicators in persons with severe dementia, *Clin J Pain* 18(1):64-73, 2002.

Cohen-Mansfield J, Jensen B: Do interventions bringing current self-care practices into greater correspondence with those performed premorbidly benefit the person with dementia? A pilot study, *Am J Alzheimers Dis Other Demen* 21(5):312-317, 2006.

Coker E: Training and support for nursing home staff reduced neuroleptic drug use and did not increase aggression in residents with dementia, *Evid Based Nurs* 9(4):122, 2006.

Colling KB: Caregiver interventions for passive behaviors in dementia: links to the NDB model, *Aging Ment Health* 8(2):117-125, 2004.

Colling KB, Buettner LL: Simple pleasures: interventions from the need-driven Dementia-Compromised Behavior model, *J Gerontol Nurs* 28(10):16-20, 2002.

Cox C: Race and caregiving: patterns of service use by African-American and white caregivers of persons with Alzheimer's, *J Gerontol Soc Work* 32(2):5, 1999.

Crist JD: Mexican American elders' use of skilled home care nursing services, *Public Health Nurs* 19(5):366-376, 2002.

Eeles EM, Stephens M, Benedict C et al: Sleep in dementia assessment may require a multidisciplinary approach, *Am J Geriatr Psychiatry* 14(11):986-987, 2006.

Eggermont L, Scherder E: Physical activity and behaviour in dementia: a review of the literature and implications for psychosocial intervention in primary care, *Dementia* 5:411-428, 2006.

Fick D, Kolanowski A, Waller J et al: Delirium superimposed on dementia in a community-dwelling managed care population: a 3-year retrospective study of occurrence, costs, and utilization, *J Gerontol A Biol Sci Med Sci* 60(6):748-753, 2005.

Finnema E, Dröes RM, Ettema T et al: The effect of integrated emotion-oriented care versus usual care on elderly persons with dementia in the nursing home and on nursing assistants: a randomized clinical trial, *Int J Geriatr Psychiatry* 20(4):330-343, 2005.

Frazier-Rios D, Zembrzuski C: Try this: best practices in nursing care for hospitalized older adults with dementia. Communication difficulties: assessment and interventions, *Dermatol Nurs* 17:319-320, 2005.

Giger J, Davidhizar R: *Transcultural nursing: assessment and intervention*, St. Louis, 2004, Mosby.

Golby A, Silverberg G, Race E et al: Memory encoding in Alzheimer's disease: an fMRI study of explicit and implicit memory, *Brain* 128(Pt 4)773-787, 2005.

Gonyea J, O'Connor M, Carruth A et al: Subjective appraisal of Alzheimer's disease caregiving: the role of self-efficacy and depressive symptoms in the experience of burden, *Am J Alzheimers Dis Other Demen* 20:273-280, 2005.

Haley WE, West CA, Wadley VG et al: Psychological, social, and health impact of caregiving: a comparison of black and white dementia family caregivers and noncaregivers, *Psychol Aging* 10(4):540, 1995.

Han et al: Use of medications with anticholinergic effects predicts clinical symptoms of delirium intensity in older medical patients, *Arch Intern Med* 161(8):1099-1105, 2001.

Hatfield CF, Herbert J, Someren EJ: Disrupted daily activity/rest cycles in relation to daily cortisol rhythms of home-dwelling patients with early Alzheimer's dementia, *Brain* 127(Pt 5):1061-1074, 2004.

Heineken J: Patient silence is not necessarily client satisfaction: communication in home care nursing, *Home Helathc Nurs* 16(2):115, 1998.

Hepburn K, Lewis M, Narayan S: Partners in caregiving: a psychoeducation program affecting dementia family caregivers' distress and caregiving outlook, *Clin Gerontol* 29:53-69, 2005.

Herrmann N: Some psychosocial therapies may reduce depression, aggression, or apathy in people with dementia, *Evid Based Ment Health* 8(4):104, 2005.

Hicks-Moore SL: Relaxing music at mealtime in nursing homes: effect on agitated patients with dementia, *J Gerontol Nurs* 31(12):26-32, 2005.

Hinrichsen GA, Ramirez M: Black and white dementia caregivers: a comparison of their adaptation, *Gerontologist* 32(3):375, 1992.

Jablonski R, Reed D, Maas M: Care intervention for older adults with Alzheimer's disease and related dementias: effect of family involvement on cognitive and functional outcomes in nursing homes, *J Gerontol Nurs* 31(6):38-48, 2005.

Kim E, Cleary S, Hopper T et al: Evidence-based practice recommendations for working with individuals with dementia: group reminiscence therapy, *J Med Speech-Lang Pathol* 14, 23-24, 2006.

Kim H, Whall A: Factors associated with psychotropic drug usage among nursing home residents with dementia, *Nurs Res* 55(4):252-8, 2006.

Kim SY, Karlawish JH, Caine ED: Current state of research on decision-making competence of cognitively impaired elderly persons, *Am J Geriatr Psychiatry* 10(2):151-165, 2002.

Kolanowski AM, Litaker M, Buettner L: Efficacy of theory-based activities for behavioral symptoms of dementia, *Nurs Res* 54(4):219-228, 2005.

Kolanowski AM, Richards KC, Sullivan SC: Derivation of an intervention for need-driven behavior: activity preferences of persons with dementia, *J Gerontol Nurs* 28(10):12-15, 2002.

Kovach C, Noonan PE, Schlidt AM et al: A model of consequences of need-driven, dementia-compromised behavior, *J Nurs Scholarsh* 37(2):134-140, 2005.

Kovach C, Taneli Y, Dohearty P et al: Effect of the BACE intervention on agitation of people with dementia, *Gerontologist* 44(6):797-806, 2004.

Kovach CR, Wells T: Pacing of activity as a predictor of agitation for persons with dementia in acute care, *J Gerontol Nurs* 28(1):28-35, 2002.

Kuhn D, Fulton BR: Efficacy of an educational program for relatives of persons in the early stages of Alzheimer's disease, *J Gerontol Soc Work* 42(3/4):109-130, 2004.

Lai CK, Arthur DG: Wandering behaviour in people with dementia, *J Adv Nurs* 44(2):173-182, 2003.

Leininger MM, McFarland MR: *Transcultural nursing: concepts, theories, research and practices*, ed 3, New York, 2002, McGraw-Hill.

Lonergan E, Luxenberg J, Colford J: Haloperidol for agitation in dementia, *Cochrane Database Syst Rev* (2): CD002852, 2002.

McGrath P, Vun M, McLeod L: Needs and experiences of non-English-speaking hospice patients and families in an English-speaking country, *Am J Hosp Palliat Care* 18(5):305, 2001.

C

Mograss M, Godbout R, Guillem F: The ERP old-new effect: a useful indicator in studying the effects of sleep on memory retrieval processes, *Sleep* 29(11):1491-1500, 2006.

Montgomery P, Dennis J: Cognitive behavioural interventions for sleep problems in adults aged 601 Cochrane Database Syst Rev (1): CD003161, 2003.

Nolan BAD, Mathews RM: Facilitating resident information seeking regarding meals in a special care unit: an environmental design intervention, *J Gerontol Nurs* 30(10):12-16, 55-56, 2004.

Perry J, Galloway S, Bottorff J et al: Nurse-patient communication in dementia: improving the odds, *J Gerontol Nurs* 31(4):43-52, 2005.

Remington R: Calming music and hand massage with agitated elderly, *Nurs Res* 51(5):317-323, 2002.

Rempusheski V, Hurley A: Advance directives and dementia, *J Gerontol Nurs* 26(10):27-34, 2000.

Richards K, Beck C, O'Sullivan P et al: Effect of individualized social activity on sleep in nursing home residents with dementia, *J Am Geriatr Soc* 53(9):1510-1517, 2005.

Roberts JS, Connell CM, Cisewski D et al: Differences between African Americans and whites in their perceptions of Alzheimer disease, *Alzheimer Dis Assoc Disord* 17(1):19-26, 2003.

Savorani G, Chattat R, Capelli E et al: Immediate effectiveness of the "new identity" reality orientation therapy (ROT) for people with dementia in a geriatric day hospital, *Arch Gerontol Geriatr Suppl* (9):359-364, 2004.

Schacke C, Zank S: Measuring the effectiveness of adult day care as a facility to support family caregivers of dementia patients, *J Appl Gerontol* 25:65-81, 2006.

Siders C, Nelson A, Brown LM et al: Evidence for implementing nonpharmacological interventions for wandering, *Rehabil Nurs* 29(6):195-206, 2004.

Simpson K, Richards K, Enderlin C et al: Medications and sleep in nursing home residents with dementia, *J Am Psychiatr Nurses Assoc* 12:279-285, 2006.

Sink KM, Covinsky KE, Newcomer R et al: Ethnic differences in the prevalence and pattern of dementia-related behaviors, *J Am Geriatr Soc* 52(8):1277-1283, 2004.

Smith G: Case management guideline: Alzheimer disease and other dementias, *Lippincotts Case Manag* 7(2):77-84, 2002.

Somboontanont W, Sloane P, Floyd F et al: Assaultive behavior in Alzheimer's disease: identifying immediate antecedents during bathing, *J Gerontol Nurs* 30(9):22-29, 2004.

Son G, Therrien B, Whall A: Implicit memory and familiarity among elders with dementia, *J Nurs Scholarsh* 34(3):263-267, 2002.

Spector A, Orrell M, Davies S et al: Reality orientation for dementia, *Cochrane Database Syst Rev* (3):CD001119, 2000.

Steinberg M, Corcoran C, Tschanz J et al: Risk factors for neuropsychiatric symptoms in dementia: the Cache County Study, *Int J Geriatr Psychiatry* 21(9):824-830, 2006.

Sung HC: Use of preferred music to decrease agitated behaviours in older people with dementia: a review of the literature, *J Clin Nurs* 14(9):1133-1140, 2005.

Tilly J, Reed P: Interventions that optimize quality dementia care: a comprehensive literature search selects the best evidence-based interventions to improve quality dementia care in LTC facilities. *Can Nurs Home* 16:13-21, 2005.

van Weert J, van Dulmen A, Spreeuwenberg P et al: Effects of snoezelen, integrated in 24h dementia care, on nurse-patient communication during morning care, *Patient Educ Couns* 58(3):312-326, 2005.

Viggo Hansen N, Jorgensen T, Ortenblad L: Massage and touch for dementia, *CochraneDatabase Syst Rev* (4):CD004989, 2006.

Volicer L, Hurley A: Management of behavioral symptoms in progressive degenerative dementias, *J Gerontol A Biol Sci Med Sci* 58(9):M837-845, 2003.

Voyer P, Cole M, McCusker J et al: Prevalence and symptoms of delirium superimposed on dementia, *Clin Nurs Res* 15(1):46-66, 2006.

Watari KF, Gatz M: Pathways to care for Alzheimer's disease among Korean Americans, *Cultur Divers Ethnic Minor Psychol* 1(1):23-28, 2004.

Wilber S, Lofgren S, Mager T et al: An evaluation of two screening tools for cognitive impairment in older emergency department patients, *Acad Emerg Med* 12(7):612-616, 2005.

Willette-Murphy K, Todero C, Yeaworth R: Mental health and sleep of older wife caregivers for spouses with Alzheimer's disease and related disorders, *Issues Ment Health Nurs* 27(8):837-852, 2006.

Woods B, Spector A, Jones C et al: Reminiscence therapy for dementia, *Cochrane Database Syst Rev* (2):CD001120, 2005.

Risk for acute Confusion   Betty Ackley, MSN, EdS, RN

NANDA   Definition

At risk for reversible disturbances of consciousness, attention, cognition, and perception that develop over a short period of time

Risk Factors

Alcohol use; decreased mobility; decreased restraints; dementia; fluctuation in sleep-wake cycle; history of stroke; impaired cognition; infection; male gender; medication/drugs: anesthesia, anticholinergics, diphenhydramine, multiple medications, opioids, psychoactive drugs; metabolic abnormalities: azotemia, decreased hemoglobin, dehydration, electrolyte imbalances, increased BUN/creatine; malnutrition; over 60 years of age; pain; sensory deprivation; substance abuse; urinary retention

NOC   Outcomes (Nursing Outcomes Classification)

Suggested NOC Outcomes

Cognition, Distorted Thought Self-Control, Information Processing, Memory, Neurological Status: Consciousness, Sleep

• = Independent;   ▲ = Collaborative;   EBN = Evidence-Based Nursing;   EB = Evidence-Based

Client Outcomes

Client Will (Specify Time Frame):

- Demonstrate restoration of cognitive status to baseline
- Obtain adequate amount of sleep
- Demonstrate appropriate motor behavior
- Maintain functional capacity
- Optimize hydration and nutrition

NIC Interventions (Nursing Interventions Classification)

Suggested NIC Interventions

Delirium Management, Delusion Management

Example NIC Activities—Delirium Management
Inform patient of person, place, and time, as needed; Provide new information slowly and in small doses, with frequent rest periods

Nursing Interventions and *Rationales*

See the nursing interventions and rationales for **Acute Confusion.**

Constipation   *Marilee Schmelzer, PhD, RN, and Betty Ackley, EdS, MSN, RN*

NANDA   Definition

Decrease in normal frequency of defecation, accompanied by difficult or incomplete passage of stool and/or passage of excessively hard, dry stool

Defining Characteristics

Abdominal pain; abdominal tenderness with palpable muscle resistance; abdominal tenderness without palpable muscle resistance; anorexia; atypical presentations in older adults (e.g., change in mental status, urinary incontinence, unexplained falls, elevated body temperature); borborygmi; bright red blood with stool; change in bowel pattern; decreased frequency; decreased volume of stool; distended abdomen; feeling of rectal fullness; feeling of rectal pressure; generalized fatigue; hard; formed stool; headache; hyperactive bowel sounds; hypoactive bowel sounds; increased abdominal pressure; indigestion; nausea; oozing liquid stool; palpable abdominal mass; palpable rectal mass; presence of soft; paste-like stool in rectum; percussed abdominal dullness; pain with defecation; severe flatus; straining with defecation; unable to pass stool; vomiting

Related Factors (r/t)

Functional

Abdominal muscle weakness; habitual denial; habitual ignoring of urge to defecate; inadequate toileting (e.g., timeliness, positioning for defecation, privacy); irregular defecation habits; insufficient physical activity; recent environmental changes

• = Independent;   ▲ = Collaborative;   EBN = Evidence-Based Nursing;   EB = Evidence-Based

C

Psychological

Depression; emotional stress; mental confusion

Pharmacological

Aluminum containing antiacids; anticholinergics; anticonvulsants; antidepressants; antilipemic agents; bismuth salts; calcium carbonate; calcium channel blockers; diuretics; iron salts; laxative overuse use; nonsteroidal anti-inflammatory drugs; opiates; phenothiazines; sedatives; sympathomimetics

Mechanical

Electrolyte imbalance; hemorrhoids; Hirschsprung's disease; neurological impairment; obesity; post-surgical obstruction; pregnancy; prostate enlargement; rectal abscess; rectal anal fissures; rectal anal stricture; rectal prolapse; rectal ulcer; rectocele; tumors

Physiological

Change in eating patterns; change in usual foods; decreased motility of gastrointestinal tract; dehydration; inadequate dentition; inadequate oral hygiene; insufficient fiber intake; insufficient fluid intake; poor eating habits

NOC Outcomes (Nursing Outcomes Classification)

Suggested NOC Outcomes

Bowel Elimination, Hydration

Example NOC Outcome with Indicators
Bowel Elimination as evidenced by the following indicators: Elimination pattern/Stool soft and formed/Passage of stool without aids/Ease of stool passage (Rate the outcome and indicators of **Bowel Elimination:** 1 = severely compromised, 2 = substantially compromised, 3 = moderately compromised, 4 = mildly compromised, 5 = not compromised [see Section I].)

Client Outcomes

Client Will (Specify Time Frame):

- Maintain passage of soft, formed stool every 1 to 3 days without straining
- State relief from discomfort of constipation
- Identify measures that prevent or treat constipation

NIC Interventions (Nursing Interventions Classification)

Suggested NIC Intervention

Constipation/Impaction Management

Example NIC Activities—Constipation/Impaction Management
Identify factors (e.g., medications, bed rest, and diet) that may cause or contribute to constipation/impaction

Nursing Interventions and *Rationales*

- Assess usual pattern of defecation, including time of day, amount and frequency of stool, consistency of stool; history of bowel habits or laxative use; diet, including fiber and fluid intake; exercise patterns; personal remedies for constipation; obstetrical/gynecological history; surgeries; diseases that affect bowel motility; alterations in perianal sensation; present bowel regimen. *There often are multiple reasons for constipation; the first step is assessment of the usual patterns of bowel elimination.*

• = Independent;   ▲ = Collaborative;   EBN = Evidence-Based Nursing;   EB = Evidence-Based

C

- Have the client or family keep a diary of bowel habits using a Management of Constipation Assessment Inventory, including information such as time of day; usual stimulus; consistency, amount, and frequency of stool; fluid consumption; and use of any aids to defecation. **EBN:** *A diary of bowel habits is valuable in treatment of constipation; the use of a diary has proven to be more accurate than client recall in determining the presence of constipation (Karam & Nies, 1994; Hinrichs et al, 2001).*
- ▲ Review the client's current medications. **EB:** *Many medications are associated with chronic constipation including opiates, antidepressants, antispasmodics, diuretics, anticonvulsants, and antacids containing aluminum (Talley et al, 2003).*
- ▲ If the client is receiving temporary opioids (e.g., for acute postoperative pain), request an order for routine stool softeners from the primary care practitioner, monitor bowel movements, and request a laxative if the client develops constipation. If the client is receiving round-the-clock opiates (e.g., for palliative care), request an order for Senokot-S and institute a bowel regimen. *Opioids lead to constipation because they decrease propulsive movement in the colon and enhance sphincter tone, making it difficult to defecate. Senokot-S is recommended to prevent constipation when opioids are given round the clock (Robinson et al, 2000).*
- If new onset of constipation, determine if the client has recently stopped smoking. **EB:** *Constipation happens in one in six people who stop smoking and in some people can be very severe (Hajek, Gillison & McRobbie, 2003).*
- Palpate for abdominal distention, percuss for dullness, and auscultate bowel sounds. *In clients with constipation the abdomen is often distended and tender, and stool in the colon produces a dull percussion sound. Bowel sounds will be present (Hinrichs et al, 2001).*
- ▲ Check for impaction; if present, perform digital removal per physician's order. *An impaction is hard stool that is too large to move through the sphincter. Manual removal is necessary before a bowel routine can be instituted (Hinrichs et al, 2001).*
- ▲ If the client is uncomfortable or in pain due to constipation or has acute or chronic constipation that does not respond to increased fiber, fluid, activity, and appropriate toileting, refer the client to the primary care practitioner for an evaluation of bowel function and health status. *There can be multiple causes of constipation, such as hypothyroidism, depression, somatization, bowel obstruction, and Hirschsprung's disease (Arce, Ermocilla & Costa, 2002).*
- Encourage fiber intake of 20 g/day (for adults), ensuring that the fiber is palatable to the individual and that fluid intake is adequate. Add fiber gradually to decrease bloating and flatus. *Larger stools move through the colon faster than smaller stools, and dietary fiber makes stools bigger because it is undigested in the upper intestinal tract. Fiber fermentation by bacteria in the colon produces gas.* **EB:** *Analysis of survey data from a subset of women (N = 62,036) in the Nurses' Health Study Women found that those with a median fiber intake of 20 g/day were less likely to experience constipation than those with a median intake of 7 g/day (Dukas, Willett & Giovannucci, 2003).* **EBN:** *A study protocol that included high-fiber foods that had been tested for palatability and 1500 ml of fluid daily reduced constipation from 59% to 9%; reduced laxative use from 59% to 8%; and eliminated impactions in a group of hospitalized, immobilized, vascular clients (Hall et al, 1995).* **EB:** *Researchers found that rye bread shortened intestinal transit time, softened the feces, and eased defecation of 59 women with constipation, and that yogurt lessened the bloating and flatulence resulting from rye bread (Hongisto et al, 2006).*
- Use a mixture of bran cereal, applesauce, and prune juice; begin administration in small amounts and gradually increase amount. Keep refrigerated. Always check with the primary care practitioner before initiating this intervention. It is important that the client also ingest sufficient fluids. **EBN:** *This bran mixture has been shown to be effective even with short-term use in elderly clients recovering from acute conditions.* NOTE: *Giving fiber without sufficient fluid has resulted in worsening of constipation (Muller-Lissner et al, 2005).* **Additional Research:** *(Howard, West & Ossip-Klein, 2000, Gibson et al, 1995; Beverley & Travis, 1992; Neal, 1995).*
- Provide prunes or prune juice daily. *The laxative effect of prunes and prune juice is widely accepted because of conventional wisdom and common experience (Stacewicz-Sapuntzakis et al, 2001).*
- ▲ If client would prefer to increase fiber intake using a pill, recommend that client use a tablet that contains methylcellulose. See fluid intake below.
- Encourage a fluid intake of 1.5 to 2 L/day (six to eight glasses of liquids per day), unless contra-

C

indicated because of renal insufficiency. *Cereal fibers such as wheat bran add additional bulk by attracting water to the fiber, so adequate fluid intake is essential. Increasing fluid intake to 1.5 to 2 L/day while maintaining a fiber intake of 25 g can significantly increase the frequency of stools in clients with constipation (Weeks, Hubbartt & Michaels, 2000; Anti, 1998).* **EB:** *Increasing fluid intake is not helpful if the person is already well hydrated (Muller-Lissner et al, 2005).*

- Encourage clients to resume walking and activities of daily living as soon as possible if their mobility has been restricted. Encourage turning and changing positions in bed, lifting the hips off the bed, performing range-of-motion exercises, alternately lifting each knee to the chest, doing wheelchair lifts, doing waist twists, stretching the arms away from the body, and pulling in the abdomen while taking deep breaths. *Bed rest and decreased mobility lead to constipation, but additional exercise does not help the constipated person who is already mobile. When the client has diminished mobility, even minimal activity increases peristalsis, which is necessary to prevent constipation (Weeks, Hubbartt & Michaels, 2000).* **EB:** *Twelve weeks of physical activity significantly decreased symptoms of constipation and difficulty defecating in sedentary clients with chronic constipation, but transit time decreased only in subjects who had abnormally long transit time before starting the exercise program (DeSchryver et al, 2005).*

- Ask clients when they normally have a bowel movement and assist them to the bathroom at that same time every day to establish regular elimination. An optimal time for many individuals is 30 minutes after breakfast because of the gastrocolic reflex. **EBN:** *When 30 clients followed a bowel program that included adequate hydration, dietary fiber, and regular toileting, 26 resumed normal bowel elimination patterns without laxatives, and the other 4 subjects required fewer laxatives (Benton et al, 1997). When subjects who had suffered a stroke were randomly scheduled for morning or evening defecation, those defecating in the morning after breakfast returned to regular elimination patterns significantly faster. Subjects whose defecation was scheduled for the same time of day as their normal, pre-stroke patterns also resumed normal elimination patterns significantly faster (Venn, 1992).*

- Provide privacy for defecation. If not contraindicated, help the client to the bathroom and close the door. *Bowel elimination is a private act in Western cultures, and a lack of privacy can hinder the defecation urge, thus contributing to constipation (Weeks, Hubbartt & Michaels, 2000).*

- Help clients onto a bedside commode or toilet so they can either squat or lean forward while sitting. **EB:** *An experimental study of 10 healthy young men found that flexing the hip to 90 degrees or more straightens the angle between the anus and the rectum and pulls the anal canal open, to decrease the resistance to the movement of feces from the rectum and the amount of pressure needed to empty the rectum. Hip flexion is greatest when squatting or when leaning forward while sitting (Tagart, 1966). Sitting upright also allows gravity to aid defecation (Weeks, Hubbartt & Michaels, 2000).*

- Teach clients to respond promptly to the defecation urge. **EB:** *A study of 12 healthy male volunteers determined that the defecation urge can be delayed and that delaying defecation decreased bowel movement frequency, stool weight, and transit time (Klauser et al, 1990).*

▲ Provide laxatives, suppositories, and enemas only as needed if other more natural interventions are not effective, and as ordered only; establish a client goal of eliminating their use. *Use of stimulant laxatives should be avoided because they result in laxative dependence and loss of normal bowel function (Merli & Graham, 2003). Laxatives and enemas also damage the surface epithelium of the colon (Schmelzer et al, 2004).*

- When giving large-volume enema solutions (e.g., soapsuds or tap water enemas), measure the amount of fluid given and the amount expelled, especially when giving repeated enemas. Use a low concentration of Castile soap in the soapsuds enema. *Enema fluid can be retained, and this retained fluid can be harmful for the client prone to fluid overload.* **EBN:** *In studies comparing the effectiveness of soapsuds enemas in preoperative liver transplant clients (Schmelzer et al, 2000), and in healthy subjects (Schmelzer et al, 2004), the amount of enema solution given was often larger than the amount of returns, and some subjects retained large amounts of solution. Biopsies taken immediately after soapsuds and tap water enemas demonstrated damage to the surface epithelium of the colon (Schmelzer et al, 2004).*

Geriatric

- Explain the importance of adequate fiber intake, fluid intake, activity, and established toileting routines to ensure soft, formed stool. **EB:** *Increasing activity has been shown to be helpful for the*

• = Independent;   ▲ = Collaborative;   EBN = Evidence-Based Nursing;   EB = Evidence-Based

elderly with constipation (Muller-Lissner et al, 2005). **EBN:** *A study involving institutionalized elderly men with chronic constipation demonstrated that, with use of a bran mixture, clients were able to discontinue use of oral laxatives (Howard, West & Ossip-Klein, 2000).*

- Determine the client's perception of normal bowel elimination; promote adherence to a regular schedule. *Misconceptions regarding the frequency of bowel movements can lead to anxiety and overuse of laxatives.*
- Explain Valsalva maneuver and the reason it should be avoided. *Valsalva maneuver can cause bradycardia and even death in cardiac clients.*
- Respond quickly to the client's call for help with toileting.
- Avoid regular use of enemas in the elderly. *Enemas can cause fluid and electrolyte imbalances, damage to the colonic mucosa, and sometimes fecal incontinence (Schmelzer et al, 2004; Ostaszkiewicz, 2006).*
- ▲ Use opioids cautiously. If they are ordered, use stool softeners and bran mixtures to prevent constipation. *Use of opioids can cause constipation (Kurz & Sessler, 2003).*
- Position the client on the toilet or commode and place a small footstool under the feet. *Placing a small footstool under the feet increases intraabdominal pressure and makes defecation easier for an elderly client with weak abdominal muscles.*

 ### Home Care

- The interventions described previously may be adapted for home care use.
- Take complaints seriously and evaluate claims of constipation in a matter-of-fact manner. *Continued constipation can lead to bowel obstruction, a medical emergency. Use of a matter-of-fact manner will limit positive reinforcement of the behavior if actual constipation does not exist.* Refer to the care plan for **Perceived Constipation.**
- Assess the self-care management activities the client is already using. **EBN:** *Many older adults seek solutions to constipation, with laxative use a frequent remedy that creates its own problems (Annells & Koch, 2002).*
- The following treatment recommendations have been offered (Annells & Koch, 2002):
  - Acknowledge the client's lifelong experience of bowel function; respect beliefs, attitudes, and preferences, and avoid patronizing responses.
  - Make available comprehensive, useful written information about constipation and possible solutions.
  - Make available empathetic and accessible professional care to provide treatment and advice; a multidisciplinary approach (including physician, nurse, and pharmacist) should be used.
  - Institute a bowel management program.
  - Consider affordability when suggesting solutions to constipation; discuss cost-saving strategies.
  - Discuss a range of solutions to constipation and allow the client to choose the preferred options.
- ▲ Have orders in place for a suppository and enema as the need may occur. *As part of a bowel management program, suppositories or enemas may become necessary (Annels & Koch, 2002).*
- Although the use of a bedside commode may be necessitated by the client's condition, allow the client to use the toilet in the bathroom when possible and provide assistance. *Bowel elimination is a very private act, and a lack of privacy can contribute to constipation (Weeks, Hubbartt & Michaels, 2000).*
- In older clients, routinely advise consumption of fluids, fruits, and vegetables as part of the diet, and ambulation if the client is able. Introduce a bowel management program at the first sign of constipation. *Constipation is a major problem for terminally ill or hospice clients, who may need very high doses of opioids for pain management (Miller & Miller, 2002).*
- ▲ Refer for consideration of the use of polyethylene glycol 3350 (PEG-3350) for constipation. **EBN:** *In a study of PEG-3350 use for idiopathic constipation, researchers concluded that it appeared to be safe and efficacious when dietary and lifestyle changes were ineffective. Clients reported increased perceived bowel control, with reduced complaints of straining, stool hardness, bloating, and gas (Stolz et al, 2001).* **EB:** *There is good evidence to support the use of PEG for chronic constipation (Ramkumar & Rao, 2005).*

• = Independent;   ▲ = Collaborative;   EBN = Evidence-Based Nursing;   EB = Evidence-Based

C

- Advise the client against attempting to remove impacted feces on his or her own. *Older or confused clients in particular may attempt to remove feces and cause rectal damage.*
- When using a bowel program, establish a pattern that is very regular and allows the client to be part of the family unit. *Regularity of the program promotes psychological and/or physiological readiness to evacuate stool. Families of home care clients often cannot proceed with normal daily activities until bowel programs are complete.*

Client/Family Teaching

- Instruct the client on normal bowel function and the need for adequate fluid and fiber intake, activity, and a defined toileting pattern in a bowel program.
- Encourage the client to heed defecation warning signs and develop a regular schedule of defecation by using a stimulus such as a warm drink or prune juice. *Most cases of constipation are mechanical and result from habitual neglect of impulses that signal the appropriate time for defecation. The reflex that causes the urge to defecate diminishes after a few minutes and may remain quiet for several hours; as a result, the stool becomes hardened and more difficult to expel (American Academy of Family Physicians, 2005).*
- Encourage the client to avoid long-term use of laxatives and enemas and to gradually withdraw from their use if they are used regularly. *Use of stimulant laxatives should be avoided; long-term use can result in dependence on laxative for defecation (American Academy of Family Physicians, 2005).*
- If not contraindicated, teach the client how to do bent-leg sit-ups to increase abdominal tone; also encourage the client to contract the abdominal muscles frequently throughout the day. Help the client develop a daily exercise program to increase peristalsis.

evolve   See the EVOLVE website for World Wide Web resources for client education.

REFERENCES

American Academy of Family Physicians: Information from your family doctor: constipation, *Am Fam Physician* 71(3):539-540, 2005.

Annells M, Koch T: Older people seeking solutions to constipation: the laxative mire, *J Clin Nurs* 11:603, 2002.

Anti M: Water supplementation enhances the effect of high-fiber diet on stool frequency and laxative consumption in adult patients with functional constipation, *Hepatogastroenterology* 45(21):727, 1998.

Arce DA, Ermocilla CA, Costa H: Evaluation of constipation, *Am Fam Physician* 65:11, 2002.

Benton JM, O'Hara PA, Chen H et al: Changing bowel hygiene practice successfully: a program to reduce laxative use in a chronic care hospital. *Geriatric Nursing,* 18(1), 12-17, 1997.

Beverley L, Travis I: Constipation: proposed natural laxative mixtures, *J Gerontol Nurs* 18(10):5, 1992.

DeSchryver AM, Keulemans YC, Peters HP et al: Effects of regular physical activity on defecation pattern in middle-aged patients complaining of chronic constipation, *Scan J Gastroenterol* 40:422-429, 2005.

Dukas L, Willett WC, Giovannucci EL: Association between physical activity, fiber intake, and other lifestyle variables and constipation in a study of women, *Am Gastroenterol* 98(8):1790-1796, 2003.

Gibson CJ, Opalka PC, Moore CA et al: Effectiveness of bran supplement on the bowel management of elderly rehabilitation patients, *J Gerontol Nurs* 21(10):21, 1995.

Hajek P, Gillison F, McRobbie H: Stopping smoking can cause constipation, *Addiction* 98(11):1563, 2003.

Hall GR, Karstens M, Rakel B et al: Managing constipation using a research-based protocol, *Medsurg Nursing* 4(1):11-20, 1995.

Hinrichs M, Huseboe J, Tang JH et al: Research-based protocol. Management of constipation, *J Gerontol Nurs* 27(2):17, 2001.

Hongisto SM, Paajanen L, Saxelin M et al: A combination of fibre-rich rye bread and yoghurt containing *Lactobacillus GG* improves bowel function in women with self-reported constipation, *Eur J Clin Nutr* 60:319-324, 2006.

Howard LV, West D, Ossip-Klein DJ: Chronic constipation management for institutionalized older adults, *Geriatr Nurs* 21(2):78, 2000.

Karam SE, Nies DM: Student/staff collaboration: a pilot bowel management program, *J Gerontol Nurs* 20:3, 1994.

Klauser AG, Voderholzer WA, Heinrich C et al: Behavioral modification of colonic function. Can constipation be learned? *Dig Dis Sci* 35(10):1271-1275, 1990.

Kurz A, Sessler DI: Opioid-induced bowel dysfunction: pathophysiology and potential new therapies, *Drugs* 63:7, 2003.

Merli GJ, Graham MG: Three steps to better management of constipation, *Patient Care* 37:6, 2003.

Miller KE, Miller M: Managing common gastrointestinal symptoms at the end of life, *J Hosp Palliat Nurs* 4:1, 2002.

Muller-Lissner SA, Kamm MA, Scarpignato C et al: Myths and misconceptions about constipation, *AM J Gastroenterol* 100(1):232-242, 2005.

Neal LJ: "Power pudding": natural laxative therapy for the elderly who are homebound, *Home Healthcare Nurse* 13(3):66, 1995.

Ostaszkiewicz J: A clinical nursing leadership model for enhancing continence care for older adults in a subacute inpatient care setting, *J Wound Ostomy Continence Nurs* 33(6):624-629, 2006.

Ramkumar D, Rao SS: Efficacy and safety of traditional medical therapies for chronic constipation: systematic review, *Am J Gastroenterol* 100(4):936-971, 2005.

Robinson CB, Fritch M, Hullett et al: Development of a protocol to prevent opioid-induced constipation in patients with cancer: a research utilization project, *C J Oncol Nurs* 4(2):79-84, 2000.

Schmelzer M, Case P, Chappell SM et al: Colonic cleansing, fluid absorption, and discomfort following tap water and soapsuds enemas, *Appl Nurs Res* 13(2):83, 2000.

Schmelzer M, Schiller LR, Meyer R et al: Safety and effectiveness of large-volume enema solutions, *Appl Nurs Res* 17(4):265-274, 2004.

Stacewicz-Sapuntzakis M, Bowen PE, Hussain EA et al: Chemical composition and potential health effects of prunes: a functional food? *Crit Rev Food Sci Nutr* 41(4):251-286, 2001.

Stolz R, Weiss LM, Merkin DH et al: An efficacy and consumer preference study of polyethylene glycol 3350 for the treatment of constipation in regular laxative users, *Home Healthc Consult* 8(2):21, 2001.

Tagart REB: The anal canal and rectum: their varying relationship and its effect on anal continence, *Dis Colon Rectum* 9(6):449-452, 1966.

Talley NJ, Jones M, Nuyts G et al: Risk factors for chronic constipation based on a general practice sample, *Am J Gastroenterol* 98(5):1107, 2003.

Venn MR: The influence of timing and suppository use on efficiency and effectiveness of bowel training after a stroke, *Rehabil Nurs* 17(3):116-121, 1992.

Weeks SK, Hubbartt E, Michaels TK: Keys to bowel success, *Rehabil Nurs* 25(2):66, 2000.

Perceived Constipation   *Marilee Schmelzer, PhD, RN, and Betty Ackley, MSN, EdS, RN*

NANDA   Definition

Self-diagnosis of constipation and abuse of laxatives, enemas, and suppositories to ensure a daily bowel movement

Defining Characteristics

Expectation of a daily bowel movement; expectation of passage of stool at same time every day; overuse of laxatives; overuse of enemas; overuse of suppositories

Related Factors (r/t)

Cultural health beliefs; family health beliefs; faulty appraisals; impaired thought processes

NOC   Outcomes (Nursing Outcomes Classification)

Suggested NOC Outcomes

Bowel Elimination, Health Beliefs, Health Beliefs: Perceived Threat

Example NOC Outcome with Indicators
Bowel Elimination as evidenced by the following indicators: Elimination pattern/Stool soft and formed/Passage of stool without aids/Ease of stool passage (Rate the outcome and indicators of **Bowel Elimination:** 1 = severely compromised, 2 = substantially compromised, 3 = moderately compromised, 4 = mildly compromised, 5 = not compromised [see Section I].)

Client Outcomes

Client Will (Specify Time Frame):

• Regularly defecate soft, formed stool without using any aids
• Explain the need to decrease or eliminate the use of stimulant laxatives, suppositories, and enemas
• Identify alternatives to stimulant laxatives, enemas, and suppositories for ensuring defecation
• Explain that defecation does not have to occur every day

NIC   Interventions (Nursing Interventions Classification)

Suggested NIC Interventions

Bowel Management, Medication Management

Example NIC Activities—Bowel Management
Note preexistent bowel problems, bowel routine, and use of laxatives

• = Independent;   ▲ = Collaborative;   EBN = Evidence-Based Nursing;   EB = Evidence-Based

C

Nursing Interventions and *Rationales*

- Have the client keep a diary of bowel habits using a Management of Constipation Assessment Inventory, including information such as time of day; usual stimulus; consistency, amount, and frequency of stool; fluid consumption; and use of any aids to defecation. **EBN:** *A diary of bowel habits is valuable in the treatment of constipation; the use of a diary has proven to be more accurate than client recall in determining the presence of constipation (Hinrichs et al, 2001; Karam & Nies, 1994).*

- Determine the client's perception of an appropriate defecation pattern. *The client may need to be taught that one bowel movement every 1 to 3 days is normal (American Academy of Family Physicians, 2005).*

- Monitor the use of laxatives, suppositories, or enemas and suggest replacing them with increased fiber intake along with increased fluids to 2 L/day. *Long-term use of laxatives may result in a cathartic colon, with the inability to have a bowel movement without use of laxatives (Hinrichs et al, 2001). An increase in fiber intake to 20 to 30 g/day along with an increase in fluid intake can help clients with chronic constipation (Candelli et al, 2001).*

- Encourage fiber intake of 20 g/day (for adults), ensuring that the fiber is palatable to the individual and that fluid intake is adequate. Add fiber gradually to decrease bloating and flatus. *Larger stools move through the colon faster than smaller stools, and dietary fiber makes stools bigger because it is undigested in the upper intestinal tract. Fiber fermentation by bacteria in the colon produces gas (Wanitschke, Goerg & Loew, 2003).* **EB:** *Analysis of survey data from a subset of women (N = 62,036) in the Nurses' Health Study Women found that those with a median fiber intake of 20 g/day were less likely to experience constipation than those with a median intake of 7 g/day (Dukas, Willett & Giovannucci, 2003).* **EBN:** *A study protocol that included high-fiber foods that had been tested for palatability and 1500 ml of fluid daily reduced constipation from 59% to 9%; reduced laxative use from 59% to 8%; and eliminated impactions in a group of hospitalized, immobilized, vascular clients (Hall et al, 1995).* **EB:** *Researchers found that rye bread shortened intestinal transit time, softened the feces, and eased defecation of 59 women with constipation, and that yogurt lessened the bloating and flatulence resulting from rye bread (Hongisto et al, 2006).*

- Use a mixture of bran cereal, applesauce, and prune juice; begin administration in small amounts and gradually increase amount. Keep refrigerated. Always check with the primary care practitioner before initiating this intervention. It is important that the client also ingest sufficient fluids. **EBN:** *This bran mixture has been shown to be effective even with short-term use in elderly clients recovering from acute conditions.* NOTE: *Giving fiber without sufficient fluid has resulted in worsening of constipation (Muller-Lissner et al, 2005). Additional Research: (Howard, West & Ossip-Klein, 2000; Gibson et al, 1995; Beverley & Travis, 1992; Neal, 1995).*

- Teach clients to respond promptly to the defecation urge. **EB:** *A study of 12 healthy male volunteers determined that the defecation urge can be delayed and that delaying defecation decreased bowel movement frequency, stool weight, and transit time (Klauser et al, 1990). The defecation urge diminishes after a few minutes and may remain quiet for several hours; as a result, the stool becomes hardened and more difficult to expel (Folden, 2002).*

- If the client is uncomfortable or in pain due to constipation or has chronic constipation that does not respond to increased fiber and fluid intake, activity, and appropriate toileting, refer the client to a gastroenterologist for an evaluation of bowel function and health status. *The multiple causes of constipation include hypothyroidism, depression, somatization, bowel obstruction, and Hirschsprung's disease (Arce, Ermocilla & Costa, 2002).*

- ▲ Obtain a dietary referral for analysis of the client's diet and input on how to improve the diet to ensure adequate fiber intake and nutrition.

- ▲ Assess for signs of depression, other psychological disorders, and a history of physical or sexual abuse. *These factors are prevalent in people with chronic constipation, but the pathophysiology is unclear (Candelli et al, 2001).*

- Encourage the client to increase activity, walking for at least 30 minutes at least 5 days a week as tolerated. *Increased activity increases bowel motility, which decreases constipation (Hinrichs et al, 2001). Not being active predisposes to constipation (American Academy of Family Physicians, 2005).* **EB:** *Twelve weeks of physical activity significantly decreased symptoms of constipation and difficulty* *defecating in sedentary clients with chronic constipation, but transit time decreased only in subjects whose transit time was increased before starting the exercise program (De Schryver et al, 2005).*

▲ Observe for the presence of an eating disorder or the use of laxatives to control or decrease weight; refer for counseling if needed. **EB:** *Laxative abuse is found in clients with both anorexia and bulimia nervosa, and may be associated with worsening of the eating disorder as a form of self-harm (Tozzi et al, 2006).*

Home Care

- The interventions described previously may be adapted for home care use.
- Take complaints seriously and evaluate claims of constipation in a matter-of-fact manner. *Continued constipation can lead to bowel obstruction, a medical emergency. Presence of a pattern of perceived constipation does not mean actual constipation cannot occur. However, use of a matter-of-fact manner will limit positive reinforcement of the behavior.*
- Obtain family and client histories of bowel or other patterned behavior problems. *History may reveal a psychological cause for the constipation (e.g., withholding).*
- Observe family cultural patterns related to eating and bowel habits. *Cultural patterns may control bowel habits.*
- Encourage a mindset and program of self-care management. Elicit from the client the self-talk he or she uses to describe body perceptions; correct fatalistic interpretations.
- Instruct the client in a healthy lifestyle that supports normal bowel function (e.g., activity, fluid intake, diet) and encourage progressive inclusion of these elements into daily activities. *A study of cognitive patterns in individuals with somatization syndrome showed that body perceptions were assumed to be a sign of catastrophic occurrence (e.g., "physical complaints are always signs of disease") and concepts of health were very restrictive. Somatizing individuals were acutely aware of bodily sensations that would normally be considered automatic and would seek help immediately to obtain medications or other solutions. They did not participate in other types of health-seeking behavior (Rief, Hiller & Margraf, 1998).*
- Discuss the client's self-image. Help the client to reframe the self-concept as capable. *Somatizing individuals tend to see themselves as weak and therefore avoid exercise (Rief, Hiller & Margraf, 1998). Developing the ability to see themselves as capable of self-care management may take time, as will making lifestyle changes.*
- Instruct the client and family in appropriate expectations for having bowel movements.
- Offer instruction and reassurance regarding explanations for variation from the previous pattern of bowel movements. *The client may have unrealistic expectations regarding the frequency or type of bowel movements and may assume that constipation exists when there is a reasonable explanation for deviation from the past pattern. The client may resort to the use of laxatives inappropriately.*
- Contract with the client and/or a responsible family member regarding the use of laxatives. Have the client maintain a bowel pattern diary. Observe for diarrhea or frequent evacuation. *Intermittent care does not allow for 24-hour supervision. Contracting allows guided control of care by the client in partnership with the nurse, and the diary promotes more accurate reporting.*
- ▲ Teach the family to carry out the bowel program per the physician's orders.
- ▲ Refer for home health aide services to assist with personal care, including the bowel program, if appropriate.
- Identify a contingency plan for bowel care if the client is dependent on outside persons for such care.

Client/Family Teaching

- Explain normal bowel function and the necessary ingredients for a regular bowel regimen (e.g., fluid, fiber, activity, and regular schedule for defecation).
- Work with the client and family to develop a diet that fits the client's lifestyle and includes increased fiber.
- Teach the client that it is not necessary to have daily bowel movements and that the passage of anywhere from three stools each day to three stools each week is considered normal.
- Explain to the client the harmful effects of the continual use of defecation aids such as laxatives and enemas.

C

- Encourage the client to gradually decrease the use of the usual laxatives and/or enemas, and recognize it may take months for the process to do it gradually (American Academy of Family Physicians, 2005).
- Determine a method of increasing the client's fluid intake and fit this practice into the client's lifestyle.
- Explain what Valsalva maneuver is and why it should be avoided.
- Work with the client and family to design a bowel-training routine that is based on previous patterns (before laxative or enema abuse) and incorporates the consumption of warm fluids, increased fiber, and increased fluids; privacy; and a predictable routine.

Additional Nursing Interventions and *Rationales,* Client/Family Teaching

See care plan for **Constipation.**

evolve See the EVOLVE website for World Wide Web resources for client education.

REFERENCES

American Academy of Family Physicians: Information from your family doctor: constipation, *Am Fam Physician* 71(3):539-540, 2005.

Arce DA, Ermocilla CA, Costa H: Evaluation of constipation, *Am Fam Physician* 65:11, 2002.

Beverley L, Travis I: Constipation: proposed natural laxative mixtures, *J Gerontol Nurs* 18(10):5, 1992.

Candelli M, Nista EC, Zocco MA et al: Idiopathic chronic constipation: pathophysiology, diagnosis and treatment, *Hepatogastroenterology* 48(40):1050-1057, 2001.

De Schryver AM, Keulemans YC, Peters HP et al: Effects of regular physical activity on defecation pattern in middle-aged patients complaining of chronic constipation, *Scand J Gastroenterol* 40(4):422-429, 2005.

Dukas L, Willett WC, Giovannucci EL: Association between physical activity, fiber intake, and other lifestyle variables and constipation in a study of women, *Am J Gastroenterol* 98(8):1790-1796, 2003.

Folden SL: Practice guidelines for the management of constipation in adults, *Rehabil Nurs* 27(5):169, 2002.

Gibson CJ, Opalka PC, Moore CA et al: Effectiveness of bran supplement on the bowel management of elderly rehabilitation patients, *J Gerontol Nurs* 21(10):21, 1995.

Hall GR, Karstens M, Rakel B et al: Managing constipation using a research-based protocol, *Medsurg Nursing,* 4(1):11-20, 1995.

Hinrichs M, Huseboe J, Tang JH et al: Research-based protocol. Management of constipation, *J Gerontol Nurs* 27(2):17, 2001.

Hongisto SM, Paajanen L, Saxelin M et al: A combination of fibre-rich rye bread and yoghurt containing *Lactobacillus GG* improves bowel function in women with self-reported constipation, *Eur J Clin Nutr* 60(3):319-324, 2006.

Howard LV, West D, Ossip-Klein DJ: Chronic constipation management for institutionalized older adults, *Geriatr Nurs* 21(2):78, 2000.

Karam SE, Nies DM: Student/staff collaboration: a pilot bowel management program, *J Gerontol Nurs* 20(3):32, 1994.

Klauser AG, Voderholzer WA, Heinrich C et al: Behavioral modification of colonic function. Can constipation be learned? *Dig Dis Sci* 35(10):1271-1275, 1990.

Muller-Lissner SA, Kamm MA, Scarpignato C et al: Myths and misconceptions about constipation, *Am J Gastroenterol* 100(1): 232-242, 2005.

Neal LJ: "Power pudding": natural laxative therapy for the elderly who are homebound, *Home Healthc Nurse* 13(3):66, 1995.

Rief W, Hiller W, Margraf J: Cognitive aspects of hypochondriasis and somatization syndrome, *J Abnorm Psychol* 107:587, 1998.

Tozzi F, Thornton LM, Mitchell J et al: Features associated with laxative abuse in individuals with eating disorders, *Psychosom Med* 68(3):470-477, 2006.

Wanitschke R, Goerg KJ, Loew D Differential therapy of constipation—a review, *Int J Clin Pharmacol Ther* 41(1):14-21, 2003.

Risk for Constipation *Betty J. Ackley, MSN, EdS, RN*

NANDA Definition

At risk for a decrease in normal frequency of defecation accompanied by difficult or incomplete passage of stool and/or passage of excessively hard, dry stool

Related Factors (r/t)

Functional

Habitual denial/ignoring urge to defecate; recent environmental changes; inadequate toileting (e.g., timeliness, positioning for defecation, privacy); irregular defecation habits; insufficient physical activity; abdominal muscle weakness

• = Independent; ▲ = Collaborative; EBN = Evidence-Based Nursing; EB = Evidence-Based

Psychological

Depression; emotional stress; mental confusion

Physiological

Change in usual eating patterns; change in usual foods; decreased motility of gastrointestinal tract; dehydration; inadequate dentition; inadequate oral hygiene; insufficient fiber intake; insufficient fluid intake; poor eating habits

Pharmacological

Aluminum containing antiacids; anticholinergics; anticonvulsants; antidepressants; antilipemic agents; bismuth salts; calcium carbonate; calcium channel blockers; diuretics; iron salts; laxative overuse use; nonsteroidal anti-inflammatory drugs; opiates; phenothiazines; sedatives; and sympathomimetics

Mechanical

Electrolyte imbalance; hemorrhoids; Hirschsprung's disease; neurological impairment; obesity; post-surgical obstruction; pregnancy; prostate enlargement; rectal abscess; rectal anal fissures; rectal anal stricture; rectal prolapse; rectal ulcer; rectocele; tumors

NOC   Outcomes (Nursing Outcomes Classification)

Suggested NOC Outcome

Bowel Elimination

Example NOC Outcome with Indicators
Bowel Elimination as evidenced by the following indicators: Elimination pattern/Stool soft and formed/Passage of stool without aids/Ease of stool passage (Rate the outcome and indicators of **Bowel Elimination:** 1 = severely compromised, 2 = substantially compromised, 3 = moderately compromised, 4 = mildly compromised, 5 = not compromised [see Section I].)

Client Outcomes

Client Will (Specify Time Frame):

- Maintain passage of soft, formed stool every 1 to 3 days without straining
- Identify measures that prevent constipation
- Explain rationale for not using laxatives and enemas

NIC   Interventions (Nursing Interventions Classification)

Suggested NIC Intervention

Constipation/Impaction Management

Example NIC Activities—Constipation/Impaction Management
Identify factors (e.g., medications, bed rest, and diet) that may cause or contribute to constipation/impaction

Nursing Interventions and *Rationales* and Client/Family Teaching

See care plan for **Constipation.**

Contamination   *Laura Polk, DNSc, RN*

NANDA   Definition

Exposure to environmental contaminants in doses sufficient to cause adverse health effects

Defining Characteristics

Pesticides, Chemicals, Biologicals

Cardiovascular: Cardiac dysrhythmia; hypertension; hypotension
Gastrointestinal: Stomachache; diarrhea; cramping; nausea; vomiting
Neuromuscular: Muscle weaknesses; joint and muscle aches; hallucinations; confusion; seizures; decreased level of consciousness; pupil changes; blurred vision
Respiratory: difficulty breathing; cough; flu symptoms; labored breathing; cyanosis
Skin: skin lesions (rash, pustules, scabs)

Radiation

History of exposure to radiation; pregnancies resulting in birth defects; weakness; fatigue; paresthesia; confusion; lethargy; changes to level of consciousness; skin irritation; itching; blistering; burns; erythema; dry or moist desquamation; ulceration; nausea; abdominal pain; diarrhea; visual changes; cataracts; irregular heartbeat; changes in the electrocardiogram; hypertension; labored breathing; cough; presence of skin cancer; thyroid cancer; leukemia; bone marrow suppression

Symptoms of radiation sickness: Weakness; hair loss; changes in blood chemistries; hemorrhage; diminished organ function

Waste

Nausea; abdominal cramps; anorexia; diarrhea; weight loss; jaundice; weakness; fever

Pollution

Difficulty breathing; lung irritation; chest pain; headaches; eye irritation; wheezing; shortness of breath; pulmonary or nasal congestion; developmental delay

Community

Measurement of contaminants exceeding acceptable levels; clusters of patients seeking care for similar signs or symptoms; large numbers of patients with rapidly fatal illnesses; presence of sick, dying, or dead animals or fish; absence of insects; unusual liquids, sprays, or vapors at work or home; anger over loss of security and safety; confusion related to trying to understand highly technical information; community conflict

Related Factors

Presence of bacteria, viruses, toxins, vectors; exposure to heavy metals or chemicals, atmospheric pollutants, radiation; concomitant or previous exposures; nutritional factors or dietary practices; pre-existing disease states; gender, occupation, history of smoking; developmental characteristics; gestational age during exposure; recent vaccinations; insufficient or absent use of decontamination protocol; no use of or inappropriate use of protective clothing; bioterrorism; flooding, earthquakes, or other natural disasters; sewer line leaks; contamination of aquifers by septic tanks; intentional/accidental contamination of food and water supply; industrial plant emissions; discharge of contaminants by industries or businesses; physical factors: climactic conditions such as temperature, wind, geographic area; social factors: crowding, sanitation, poverty, personal and household hygiene practices, lack of access to health care; use of environmental contaminants in the home; playing in outdoor areas where environmental contaminants are present; community dynamics

• = Independent;   ▲ = Collaborative;   EBN = Evidence-Based Nursing;   EB = Evidence-Based

NOC   Outcomes (Nursing Outcomes Classification)

Suggested NOC Outcomes

Community Health Status, Family Physical Environment, Anxiety Level, Fear Level

Example NOC Outcome with Indicators
Community Health Status as evidenced by the following indicators: Evidence of health protection measures/ Compliance with environmental health standards (Rate the outcome and indicators of **Community Health Status:** 1 = poor, 2 = fair, 3 = good, 4 = very good, 5 = excellent.)

C

Client Outcomes

Client Will (Specify Time Frame):

- Have minimal health effects associated with contamination
- Cooperate with appropriate decontamination protocol
- Participate in appropriate isolation precautions

Community Will (Specify Time Frame):

- Utilize health surveillance data system to monitor for contamination incidents
- Utilize disaster plan to evacuate and triage affected members
- Have minimal health effects associated with contamination

NIC   Interventions (Nursing Intervention Classification)

Suggested NIC Interventions

Triage: Disaster, Infection Control, Anxiety Reduction, Crisis Intervention, Health Education

Example NIC Activities—Triage: Disaster
Initiate appropriate emergency measures, as indicated; Monitor for and treat life-threatening injuries or acute needs

Nursing Interventions and *Rationales*

- Help individuals cope with contamination incident by doing the following:
  - use groups that have survived terrorist attacks as useful resource for victims
  - provide accurate information on risks involved, preventive measures, use of antibiotics, and vaccines
  - assist to deal with feelings of fear, vulnerability, and grief
  - encourage individuals to talk to others about their fears
  - assist victims to think positively and to move toward the future
  EB: *Interventions aimed at supporting an individual's coping help the person deal with feelings of fear, helplessness, and loss of control that are normal reactions in a crisis situation (Boscarino et al, 2006; Lazarus & Folkman, 1984).*
- Triage, stabilize, transport, and treat affected community members. **EB:** *Accurate triage and early treatment provides the best chance of survival to affected persons (Murdoch & Cymet, 2006).*
- Utilize approved procedures for decontamination of persons, clothing, and equipment. *Victims may first require decontamination prior to entering health facility to receive care in order to prevent the spread of contamination (U.S. Army Medical Research Institute of Infectious Diseases, 2004).*
- Utilize appropriate isolation precautions: universal, airborne, droplet, and contact isolation. *Proper use of isolation precautions prevents cross-contamination by contaminating agents (US Army Medical Research Institute of Infectious Diseases, 2004).*

C

- Monitor individual for therapeutic effects, side effects, and compliance with postexposure drug therapy. *Drug therapy may extend over a long period of time and will require monitoring for compliance as well as therapeutic and side effects (Veenema, 2002).*
▲ Collaborate with other agencies (local health department, emergency medical service [EMS], state and federal agencies). *Communication among agencies increases ability to handle crisis efficiently and correctly (McKenna et al, 2003).*

Geriatric

- Help the client identify age-related factors that may affect response to contamination incidents.
- Encourage family members to acknowledge and validate the client's concerns. *Validation alleviates anxiety and increases client's ability to cope.*

Pediatric

- Provide environmental health hazard information. *Developing children are more vulnerable to environmental toxicants due to greater and longer exposure and particular susceptibility windows (Tamborlini, von Ehrenstein & Bertolini, 2002).*

Home Care

- Assess current environmental stressors and identify community resources. *Accessing resources decreases stress and increases ability to cope (Boscarino et al, 2006).*

Client/Family Teaching

- Provide truthful information to the person or family affected
- Discuss signs and symptoms of contamination
- Explain decontamination protocols
- Explain need for isolation procedures

Well-managed efforts at communication of contamination information ensures that messages are correctly formulated, transmitted, and received and that they result in meaningful actions (ATSDR, 2006).

REFERENCES

Agency for Toxic Substances and Disease Registry (ATSDR): *A primer on health risk communication: principles and practices. Overview of issues and guiding principles,* 2006, available at http://www.atsdr.cdc.gov/risk/riskprimer/vision.html. Accessed November 12, 2006.

Boscarino J, Adams R, Figley C et al: Fear of terrorism and preparedness in New York City 2 years after the attacks: implications for disaster planning and research, *J Public Health Manag Pract* 12(6):505-513, 2006.

Lazarus RS, Folkman S: *Stress, appraisal and coping.* New York, 1984, Springer.

McKenna VB, Gunn JE, Auerbach J et al: Local collaborations: development and implementation of Boston's bioterrorism surveillance system, *J Public Health Manag Pract* 9(5):384-393, 2003.

Murdoch S, Cymet TC: Treating victims after disaster: physical and psychological effects, *Compr Ther* 32(1):39-42, 2006.

Tamborlini G, von Ehrenstein OS, Bertolini R: *Children's health and environment: a review of evidence,* Rome, 2002, WHO European Center for Environment and Health, available at http://www.euro.who.int/document/e75518.pdf. Retrieved: Nov 12, 2006.

U.S. Army Medical Research Institute of Infectious Diseases: *USAMRIID's medical management of biological casualties handbook,* ed 5, Fort Detrick, MD, 2004, Author.

Veenema TG: Chemical and biological terrorism, *Nurs Educ Persp* 23(2):62-71, 2002.

Risk for Contamination   *Laura Polk, DNSc, RN*

NANDA   ### Definition

Accentuated risk of exposure to environmental contaminants in doses sufficient to cause adverse health effects

Risk Factors

Presence of bacteria, viruses, toxins, vectors; exposure to heavy metals or chemicals, atmospheric pollutants, radiation; concomitant or previous exposures; nutritional factors or dietary practices; pre-existing disease states; gender, occupation, history of smoking; developmental characteristics; gestational age during exposure; recent vaccinations; insufficient or absent use of decontamination protocol; no use of or inappropriate use of protective clothing; bioterrorism; flooding, earthquakes, or other natural disasters; sewer line leaks or contamination of aquifers by septic tanks; intentional/accidental contamination of food and water supply; industrial plant emissions; discharge of contaminants by industries or businesses

Physical factors: Climactic conditions such as temperature, wind; geographic area

Social factors: Crowding, sanitation, poverty, personal and household hygiene practices, lack of access to health care; use of environmental contaminants in the home; playing in outdoor areas where environmental contaminants are present; community dynamics

NOC   ### Outcomes (Nursing Outcomes Classification)

Suggested NOC Outcomes

Risk Control, Health Beliefs: Perceived Threat, Knowledge: Health Resources, Knowledge: Health Behavior, Community Disaster Readiness, Community Health Status

See **Contamination** for other possible NOC outcomes

Example NOC Outcome with Indicators
Risk Control as evidenced by the following indicators: Monitors environmental risk factors/Avoids exposure to health threats/Follows selected risk control strategies (Rate the outcome and indicators of **Risk Control:** 1 = never demonstrated, 2 = rarely demonstrated, 3 = sometimes demonstrated, 4 = often demonstrated, 5 = consistently demonstrated.)

Client Outcomes

Client Will (Specify Time Frame):

• Remain free of adverse effects of contamination

Community Will (Specify Time Frame):

• Utilize health surveillance data system to monitor for contamination incidents
• Participate in mass casualty and disaster readiness drills
• Remain free of contamination-related health effects
• Minimize exposure to contaminants

NIC   ### Interventions (Nursing Intervention Classification)

Suggested NIC Interventions

Environmental Risk Protection, Bioterrorism Preparedness, Environmental Management: Safety, Health Education, Health Screening, Immunization/Vaccination Management, Risk Identification, Surveillance: Safety, Community, Communicable Disease Management, Community Disaster Preparedness, Health Policy Monitoring

C

Example NIC Activities—Environmental Risk Protection

Assess environment for potential and actual risk; Monitor incidents of illness and injury related to environmental hazards; Collaborate with other agencies to improve environmental safety

Nursing Interventions and *Rationales*

▲ Conduct surveillance for environmental contamination. Notify agencies authorized to protect the environment of contaminants in the area. *Early surveillance and detection are critical components of preparation (McKenna, Gunn & Auerbach, 2003).*

• Assist individuals to modify the environment to minimize risk or assist in relocating to safer environment. *Modification of the environment will decrease the risk of actual contamination occurring (Ashford et al, 2003).*

• Schedule mass casualty and disaster readiness drills. *Practice in handling contamination occurrences will decrease the risk of exposure during actual contamination events (Chung & Shannon, 2005).*

• Provide accurate information on risks involved, preventive measures, use of antibiotics, and vaccines. *Well-managed efforts at communication of contamination information ensure that messages are correctly formulated, transmitted, and received, and that they result in meaningful actions (ATSDR, 2006).*

• Assist to deal with feelings of fear and vulnerability. **EB:** *Interventions aimed at supporting an individual's coping help the person deal with feelings of fear, helplessness, and loss of control that are normal reactions in a crisis situation (Boscarino et al, 2006; Lazarus & Folkman, 1984).*

• Assist with decontamination of persons, clothing, and equipment using approved procedure. *Victims may first require decontamination prior to entering health facility to receive care in order to prevent the spread of contamination (U.S. Army Medical Research Institute of Infectious Diseases, 2004).*

• Utilize appropriate isolation precautions: universal, airborne, droplet, and contact isolation. *Proper use of isolation precautions prevents cross-contamination by contaminating agent (U.S. Army Medical Research Institute of Infectious Diseases, 2004).*

• Monitor individual for therapeutic effects, side effects, and compliance with postexposure drug therapy. *Drug therapy may extend over a long period of time and will require monitoring for compliance as well as therapeutic and side effects (Veenema, 2002).*

▲ Collaborate with other agencies (local health department, emergency medical service [EMS], state and federal agencies. *Communication among agencies increases ability to handle crisis efficiently and correctly (McKenna et al, 2003).*

Geriatric

• Help the client identify age-related factors that may affect response to contamination incidents.

• Encourage family members to acknowledge and validate the client's concerns. *Validation alleviates anxiety and increases client's ability to cope.*

Pediatric

• Provide environmental health hazard information relevant to children. *Developing children are more vulnerable to environmental toxicants due to greater and longer exposure and particular susceptibility windows (Tamborlini, von Ehrenstein & Bertolini, 2002).*

Home Care

• Assess current environmental stressors and identify community resources. *Accessing resources decreases stress and increases ability to cope (Boscarino et al, 2006).*

Client/Family Teaching

• Provide truthful information to the person or family

• Discuss signs and symptoms of contamination

- Explain decontamination protocols
- Explain need for isolation procedures
  Well-managed efforts at communication of contamination information ensure that messages are correctly formulated, transmitted, and received, and that they result in meaningful actions (ATSDR, 2006).

REFERENCES

Agency for Toxic Substances and Disease Registry (ATSDR): *A primer on health risk communication: principles and practices. Overview of issues and guiding principles,* 2006, available at http://www.atsdr.cdc.gov/risk/riskprimer/vision.html. Accessed November 12, 2006.

Ashford DA, Kaiser RM, Bales ME et al: Planning against biological terrorism: lessons from outbreak investigations, *Emerg Infect Dis* 9(5):515-519, 2003, available at http://origin.cdc.gov/ncidod/EID/vol9no5/02-0388.htm. Accessed July 20, 2006.

Boscarino J, Adams R, Figley C et al: Fear of terrorism and preparedness in New York City 2 years after the attacks: implications for disaster planning and research, *J Public Health Manag Pract* 12(6):505-513, 2006.

Chung S, Shannon M: Hospital planning for acts of terrorism and other public health emergencies involving children, *Arch Dis Child* 90(12):1300-1307, 2005.

Lazarus RS, Folkman S: *Stress, appraisal and coping,* New York, 1984, Springer.

McKenna VB, Gunn JE, Auerbach J: Local collaborations: development and implementation of Boston's bioterrorism surveillance system, *J Public Health Manag Pract* 9(5):384-393, 2003.

Tamborlini G, von Ehrenstein OS, Bertolini R: *Children's health and environment: a review of evidence,* Rome, 2002, WHO European Center for Environment and Health, available at http://www.euro.who.int/document/e75518.pdf. Accessed November 12, 2006.

U.S. Army Medical Research Institute of Infectious Diseases: *USAMRIID's medical management of biological casualties handbook,* ed 5, Fort Detrick, MD, 2004, Author.

Veenema TG: Chemical and biological terrorism, *Nurs Educ Perspect* 23(2):62-71, 2002.

Compromised family Coping   *Katherina A. Nikzad, ABD, and Joseph E. Gaugler, PhD*

NANDA   Definition

Usually supportive primary person (family member or close friend) provides insufficient, ineffective, or compromised support, comfort, assistance, or encouragement that may be needed by the client to manage or master adaptive tasks related to his/her health challenge

Defining Characteristics

Objective

Significant person attempts assistive behaviors with unsatisfactory results; significant person attempts supportive behaviors with unsatisfactory results; significant person displays protective behavior disproportionate to client's abilities; significant person displays protective behavior disproportionate to client's need for autonomy; significant person enters into limited personal communication with client; significant person withdraws from client.

Subjective

Client expresses a complaint about significant other's response to health problem; client expresses a concern about significant other's response to health problem; significant person expresses an inadequate knowledge base, which interferes with effective supportive behaviors; significant person expresses an inadequate understanding, which interferes with supportive behaviors; significant person describes preoccupation with personal reaction (e.g., fear, anticipatory grief, guilt, anxiety) to client's need.

Related Factors (r/t)

Coexisting situations affecting the significant person; developmental crises the significant person may be facing; exhaustion of supportive capacity of significant people; inadequate information by a primary person; inadequate understanding of information by a primary person; incorrect information by a primary person; lack of reciprocal support; little support provided by client, in turn, for primary person; prolonged disease that exhausts supportive capacity of significant people; situational crises the significant person may be facing; temporary family disorganization; temporary family role changes; temporary preoccupation by a significant person

C

NOC   Outcomes (Nursing Outcomes Classification)

Suggested NOC Outcomes

Family Coping, Family Participation in Professional Care, Family Support during Treatment

Example NOC Outcome with Indicators
Family Coping as evidenced by the following indicators: Confronts family problems/Manages family problems/Seeks family assistance when appropriate (Rate the outcome and indicators of **Family Coping:** 1 = never demonstrated, 2 = rarely demonstrated, 3 = sometimes demonstrated, 4 = often demonstrated, 5 = consistently demonstrated [see Section I].)

Client Outcomes

Family/Significant Person Will (Specify Time Frame):

- Verbalize internal resources to help deal with the situation
- Verbalize knowledge and understanding of illness, disability, or disease
- Provide support and assistance as needed
- Identify need for and seek outside support

NIC   Interventions (Nursing Interventions Classification)

Suggested NIC Interventions

Coping Enhancement, Family Involvement Promotion, Family Support, Mutual Goal Setting

Example NIC Activities—Family Support
Appraise family's emotional reaction to patient's condition; Promote trusting relationship with family

Nursing Interventions and *Rationales*

- Assess the strengths and deficiencies of the family system. **EBN:** *Assessments allow for anticipatory care and guidance to help members acquire and maintain supports and coping strategies (Thomas & King, 2000).* **EB:** *Active coping strategies are associated with fewer distress indices and may improve the ability to bear the burden of the illness without becoming themselves affected by psychiatric illnesses (Rao, Pradhan & Shah, 2004).*
- Assess how family members interact with each other; observe verbal and nonverbal communication and individual and group responses to stress. **EBN:** *Understanding how families cope with stress is important (Weiss & Chen, 2002).*
- Establish rapport with families by providing accurate communication. **EBN:** *Families in psychiatric settings indicated that family care can be improved by focusing on building rapport and communicating problems and concerns between families and health professionals (Rose, Mallinson & Walton-Moss, 2004; Watson, Kieckhefer & Olshansky, 2006).*
- Consider the use of family theory as a framework to help guide interventions (e.g., family stress theory, role theory, social exchange theory, family systems theory). **EBN:** *Use of a family assessment tool is an effective way of appraising families and addressing suffering (Hogan & Logan, 2004).*
- Help family members recognize the need for help and teach them how to ask for it. **EBN:** *Recognizing the need for help and knowing how to ask for it enables family members to maintain control (Szabo & Strang, 1999).*
- Encourage expression of positive thoughts and emotions. **EB:** *Positive emotions initiate upward spirals toward enhanced emotional well-being (Fredrickson & Joiner, 2002).* **EBN:** *This study shows that clients believe that coping is important to their well-being (Watts & Edgar, 2004).*
- Encourage family members to verbalize feelings. Spend time with them, sit down and make eye contact, and offer coffee and other nourishment. **EBN:** *The expression of feelings helps family care-*

• = Independent;   ▲ = Collaborative;   EBN = Evidence-Based Nursing;   EB = Evidence-Based

givers to regain and maintain control (Hynan, 2005). Acceptance of nourishment indicates a beginning acceptance of the situation.

- Provide opportunities for families to discuss spirituality. **EB:** *This research provided by survivors of hematological malignancies gives insight into factors impacting their need to talk about spiritual issues (McGrath & Clarke, 2003).*
- Mothers may require additional support in their role of caring for chronically ill children. **EBN:** *Mothers exhibit greater efforts than fathers in coping patterns, including strategies to acquire social support outside the family, increase self-worth, and decrease psychological tensions (Brazil & Krueger, 2002).*
- Provide privacy during family visits. If possible, maintain flexible visiting hours to accommodate more frequent family visits. If possible, arrange staff assignments so the same staff members have contact with the family. Familiarize other staff members with the situation in the absence of the usual staff member. *Providing privacy, maintaining flexible hours, and arranging consistent staff assignments will reduce stress, enhance communication, and facilitate the building of trust.*
- Determine whether the family is suffering from additional stressors (e.g., child care issues, financial problems). **EBN:** *Mothers of low-birth-weight infants, the presence of other life stressors, and the family's use of internally focused coping strategies contributed to worse mental health outcomes for the mother (Weiss & Chen, 2002).*
- ▲ Refer the family with ill family members to appropriate resources for assistance as indicated (e.g., counseling, psychotherapy, financial assistance, or spiritual support). **EBN:** *The most important predictors of family health were family structural factors. It was found that the better the family structure and relationships were, the better the family health was (Astedt-Kurki et al, 2004).*

Pediatric

- Assess the adolescent's perception of support from family and friends during crisis. **EBN:** *Some teens find parents and friends burdensome during a time of grief, whereas others find their support critical for coping with crises. Recognition of individual perception can assist families in negotiating times of crisis (Rask, Kaunonen & Paunonen-Ilmonen, 2002).*
- Provide educational interventions and psychosocial interventions such as coping skills training in treatment for families and their adolescents who have type 1 diabetes. **EB:** *Psychosocial interventions such as coping skills training and behavioral family systems therapy have demonstrated improvements in metabolic control, self-efficacy, diabetes stress, quality of life, and parent-adolescent conflict. Family interventions are emerging as a positive way to improve interpersonal relations and assist the adolescent in transitioning from family-management toward self-management of their diabetes (Urban, Berry & Gray, 2004).*
- Encourage the use of family rituals such as connection, spirituality, love, recreation, and celebration, especially in single-parent families. **EBN:** *Data from this study indicated that these rituals were used by single-parent families as a way to facilitate family cohesion and instill family values (Moriarty & Wagner, 2004).*
- Encourage laughing, playing, singing, talking, and praying with seriously injured children. **EBN:** *Practices that help critically burned children to heal holistically are everyday practices identified as maintaining or reestablishing harmony of a child's mind, body, and spirit (Zengerle-Levy, 2004).*
- Staff should involve the family in decision-making processes, especially during hospital discharge planning. **EBN:** *Increasing parental involvement in caregiving procedures and including them in hospital discharge processes has been identified as an effective way to increase feelings of competence and confidence in family caregivers (Griffin & Abraham, 2006).*
- ▲ Link trained volunteers with "vulnerable" first-time parents. Provide social support and information related to age-appropriate expectations of infants. **EBN:** *This descriptive comparative design demonstrated participants' satisfaction with the program and improvement in family functioning. The program could be appropriate for all parents (Kelleher & Johnson, 2004).*

Geriatric

- Perform a holistic assessment of all needs of informal spousal caregivers. **EBN:** *The role of informal spousal caregivers has increased as the population ages (Cassells & Watt, 2003).*

• = Independent;   ▲ = Collaborative;   EBN = Evidence-Based Nursing;   EB = Evidence-Based

C

- Help caregivers establish one's priorities and concentrate on them, believe in themselves and their ability to handle the situation, taking life 1 day at a time, looking for positive things in each situation, and relying on their own individual expertise and experience. **EBN:** *Helpful coping strategies were identified in this major international research project on caregivers' work and coping in four countries (Kuuppelomaki et al, 2004).*
- ▲ Refer caregivers of clients with Alzheimer's disease to a monthly psychoeducational support group (i.e., the Alzheimer's Association). **EB:** *Nonpharmacologic interventions can be used for the management of clients with Alzheimer's disease (Cohen-Mansfield & Mintzer, 2006). This support group intervention has been well accepted by clients, families, and physicians in this study (Guerriero Austrom et al, 2004).*
- ▲ Consider the use of telephone support for caregivers of family members with dementia. **EBN:** *Family caregivers can be helped through a variety of social support mechanisms including telephone support (Chang et al, 2004).*
- Assist in finding transportation to enable family members to visit or arrange alternate ways of maintaining contact. *If a family member is homebound and unable to visit, encourage alternative contact (e.g., telephone, cards and letters, e-mail) to provide ongoing scheduled progress reports. Reducing loneliness and isolation has many positive psychosocial and physical health benefits (Drentea et al, 2006; Mittelman, 2005; Collins & Benedict, 2006).*

Multicultural

- Assess for the influence of cultural beliefs, norms, and values on the family's perceptions of coping. **EBN:** *What the family considers normal and abnormal coping behavior may be based on cultural perceptions (Giger & Davidhizar, 2004).* **EBN:** *The nurse should be cognizant of the fact that families provide more than just the physical necessities but meet needs according to developmental level of the members (Giger & Davidhizar, 2004).*
- Understand the importance of cultural beliefs and values the family may hold. **EBN:** *There are differences in some cultures regarding health beliefs, practices, and values (Camphinha-Bacote & Narayan, 2000).*
- Acknowledge racial/ethnic differences at the onset of care. **EBN:** *Acknowledgment of race/ethnicity issues will enhance communication, establish rapport, and promote treatment outcomes (D'Avanzo et al, 2001).* **EBN:** *In Hispanic families it is common to encounter a compadrazgo or godparent who provides important support to the child and family. Allowing this assistance can reduce fear and anxiety and enhance adjustment to the healthcare facility and the caregivers (Giger & Davidhizar, 2004).*
- Validate the family's feelings regarding the impact of the client's illness on the family's lifestyle. **EBN:** *Validation lets family members know that the nurse has heard and understood what was said, and it promotes the relationship between nurse and family members (Spiers, 2002).*
- Approach families of color with respect, warmth, and professional courtesy. **EB:** *Instances of disrespect and lack of caring have special significance for families of color (D'Avanzo et al, 2001). Latina mothers of developmentally disabled adults reported their relationship with the educational and service delivery systems to be characterized by poor communication, low effort in providing services, negative attitudes of professionals toward client-children, and negative treatment of parents by professionals (Shapiro et al, 2004).*
- Provide rationale when assessing families with regard to sensitive issues. **EBN:** *African-Americans and other people of color may expect Caucasian caregivers to hold negative and preconceived ideas about them. Providing a rationale for questions asked will help reduce this perception (D'Avanzo et al, 2001). Topics such as smoking in the household, financial difficulties, and emotional support available to the parent were more likely to be asked of parents of African-American and Hispanic children (Kogan et al, 2004).*
- Use a family-centered approach when working with Latino, Asian, African-American, and Native-American clients. **EBN:** *Latinos may perceive the family as a source of support, solver of problems, and source of pride. Asian-Americans may regard the family as the primary decision maker and influence on individual family members (D'Avanzo et al, 2001). Elders may play a key role in decision making for some Asian populations (Davis, 2000). Among Native-Americans, family connectedness and family support have been identified as important factors in maintaining physical and cultural survival, and preventing physical and emotional health complications within families (Teufel-Shone et al, 2005). Use of a family-based intervention among American-Indian families resulted in higher levels of*

child prosocial behavior and lowered drug use (Boyd-Ball, 2003). Among Mexican Americans with type 2 diabetes, higher levels of perceived family support and greater self-efficacy were associated with higher reported levels of diet and exercise self-care (Wen, Shepherd & Parchman, 2004).

Home Care

- The interventions described previously may be adapted for home care use.
- Assess the reason behind the breakdown of family coping. *Knowledge of the reasons behind compromised coping will assist in identification of appropriate interventions.* Refer to the care plan for **Caregiver role strain.**
- ▲ Assess the needs of the caregiver in the home. Intervene to meet needs as appropriate, and explore all available resources that may be used to provide adequate home care (e.g., parish nursing as an effective adjunct, home health aide services to relieve the caregiver's fatigue). *Meeting the needs of caregivers supports their ability to meet the needs of the client. Assess the client and caregiver separately and in interaction.* **EBN:** *The highest level of distress in heart transplantation clients was related to effects on their ability to work, while spouses felt higher levels of psychological distress (Bohachick et al, 2001).*
- During the time of compromised coping, increase visits to ensure the safety of the client, support of the family, and assistance with coping strategies. Provide reassurance regarding expectations for prognosis as appropriate. **EBN:** *The spouses of heart transplantation clients need support (Bohachick et al, 2001).*
- With a cancer client, encourage family discussion of stressors (including the meaning of the illness, fear of recurrence, the client's employment status) and resources (family social support). **EBN:** *Stressors and resources have been shown to play an important role in determining family quality of life among cancer survivors (Woodgate, 2006).*
- ▲ When a terminal illness is the precipitating factor for ineffective coping, offer hospice services and support groups as possible resources. **EB:** *Research has indicated that hospice care has the potential to mediate both the effects of burden caused by caregiving and the rate of mortality following the death of a spouse (Ahrens, 2005).*
- ▲ If compromised family coping interferes with the ability to support the client's treatment plan, refer for psychiatric home healthcare services for family counseling and implementation of a therapeutic regimen. **EBN:** *Psychiatric home care nurses can address issues related to family members' ability to adjust to changes in the client's health status. Behavioral interventions in the home can help the family to participate more effectively in the treatment plan (Logsdon, McCurry & Teri, 2005; Oneal et al, 2006).*

Client/Family Teaching

- Provide truthful information and support for the family and significant people regarding the client's specific illness or condition. **EBN:** *Attention needs to be given to methods of providing information and support to couples coping with prostate cancer. Both clients and partners need to be included in discussions about the effect of the illness and treatments so that both can feel more prepared to manage them (Harden et al, 2002).*
- ▲ Refer women with recurrent breast cancer and their family caregivers to a FOCUS Program (family involvement, optimistic attitude, coping effectiveness, uncertainty reduction, and symptom management), a family-based program of care. **EBN:** *Clients with recurrent breast cancer and their family members reported high satisfaction with the FOCUS Program (Northouse et al, 2002).*
- Promote individual and family relaxation and stress-reduction strategies. *The immune system weakens in response to stress; relaxation elicits the opposite, healthful response (Cass, 2006).*
- ▲ Provide a parent support and education group to provide opportunities for parents to access support, learn new parenting skills, and, ultimately, optimize their relationships with their children in families of children in residential care. **EB:** *Working with the families of children in residential care is critical to the success of the placement. A parent support and education group was designed and implemented. The responses of both parents and staff to this program were favorable (Modlin, 2003).*

 See the EVOLVE website for World Wide Web resources for client education.

• = Independent;   ▲ = Collaborative;   EBN = Evidence-Based Nursing;   EB = Evidence-Based

C

REFERENCES

Ahrens J: Research briefs: the positive impact of hospice care on the surviving spouse, *Home Healthc Nurse* 23(1):53-55, 2005.

Astedt-Kurki P, Lehti K, Tarkka M et al: Determinants of perceived health in families of patients with heart disease, *J Adv Nurs* 48(2):115-123, 2004.

Bohachick P, Reeder S, Taylor MV et al: Psychosocial impact of heart transplantation on spouses, *Clin Nurs Res* 10:6, 2001.

Boyd-Ball AJ: A culturally responsive, family intervention model, *Alcohol Clin Exp Res* 27(8):1356-1360, 2003.

Brazil K, Krueger P: Patterns of family adaptation to childhood asthma, *J Pediatr Nurs* 17(3):167, 2002.

Camphinha-Bacote J, Narayan M: Culturally competent health care at home, *Home Care Provid* 5(6):213, 2000.

Cass H: Stress and the immune system, *Total Health* 27(6):24-25, 2006.

Cassells C, Watt E: The impact of incontinence on older spousal caregivers, *J Adv Nurs* 42(6): 607-616, 2003.

Chang BL, Nitta S, Carter PA et al: Technology innovations. Perceived helpfulness of telephone calls: providing support for care-givers of family members with dementia, *J Gerontol Nurs* 30(9):14-21, 2004.

Cohen-Mansfield J, Mintzer JE: Time for change: the role of nonpharmacological interventions in treating behavior problems in nursing home residents with dementia, *Alzheimer Dis Assoc Disord* 19(1):37-40, 2006.

Collins C, Benedict J: Evaluation of a community based health promotion program for the elderly, *Am J Health Promotion* 21(1):45-48, 2006.

D'Avanzo CE et al: Developing culturally informed strategies for substance-related interventions. In Naegle MA, D'Avanzo CE, editors: *Addictions and substance abuse: strategies for advanced practice nursing.* St Louis, 2001, Mosby.

Davis RE: The convergence of health and family in the Vietnamese culture, *J Fam Nurs* 6(2):136, 2000.

Drentea P, Clay O, Roth D et al: Predictors of improvement in social support: five-year effects of a structured intervention for caregivers of spouses with Alzheimer's disease, *Soc Sci Med* 63(4):957-967, 2006.

Fredrickson BL, Joiner T: Positive emotions trigger upward spirals toward emotional well-being, *Psychol Sci* 13(2):172, 2002.

Giger J, Davidhizar R: *Transcultural nursing: assessment and intervention,* St. Louis, 2004, Mosby Year Book.

Griffin T, Abraham M: Transition to home from the newborn intensive care unit: applying the principles of family-centered care to the discharge process, *J Perinat Neonatal Nurs* 20(3):243-249, 2006.

Guerriero Austrom M, Damush TM, Hartwell CW et al: Development and implementation of nonpharmacologic protocols for the management of patients with Alzheimer's disease and their families in a multiracial primary care setting, *Gerontologist* 44(4):548-553, 2004.

Harden J, Schafenacker A, Northouse L et al: Couples' experiences with prostate cancer: focus group research, *Oncol Nurs Forum* 29(4):701-709, 2002.

Hogan DL, Logan J: The Ottawa Model of Research Use: a guide to clinical innovation in the NICU, *Clin Nurse Spec* 18(5):255-261, 2004.

Hynan MT: Supporting fathers during stressful times in the nursery: an evidence-based review, *Newborn Infant Nurs Rev* 5(2):87-92, 2005.

Kelleher L, Johnson M: An evaluation of a volunteer-support program for families at risk, *Pub Health Nurs* 21(4):297-305, 2004.

Kogan MD, Schuster MA, Yu SM et al: Routine assessment of family and community health risks: parent views and what they receive, *Pediatrics* 113(6 Suppl):1934-1943, 2004.

Kuuppelomaki M, Sasaki A, Yamada K et al: Coping strategies of family carers for older relatives in Finland, *J Clin Nurs* 13(6):697-706, 2004.

Logsdon R, McCurry S, Teri L: A home health care approach to exercise for persons with Alzheimer's disease, *Care Manag J* 6(2):90-97, 2005.

McGrath P, Clarke H: Creating the space for spiritual talk: insights from survivors of hematological malignancies, *Aust Health Rev* 26(3):16-132, 2003.

Mittelman M: Taking care of the caregivers, *Curr Opin Psychiatry* 18(6):633-639, 2005.

Modlin H: The development of a parent support group as a means of initiating family involvement in a residential program, *Child Youth Serv Rev* 25(1/2):169-189, 2003.

Moriarty PH, Wagner LD: Family rituals that provide meaning for single-parent families, *J Fam Nurs* 10(2):190-210, 2004.

Northouse LL, Walker J, Schafenacker A. et al: A family-based program of care for women with recurrent breast cancer and their family members, *Oncol Nurs Forum* 29(10):1411-1419, 2002.

Oneal B, Reeb R, Korte J et al: Assessment of home-based behavior modification programs for autistic children: reliability and validity of the behavioral summarized evaluation, *Prev Interv Community* 32(1-2):25-39, 2006.

Rao P, Pradhan PV, Shah H: Psychopathology and coping in parents of chronically ill children, *Indian J Pediatr* 71(8):695-699, 2004.

Rask K, Kaunonen MM, Paunonen-Ilmonen M: Adolescent coping with grief after the death of a loved one, *Int J Nurs Pract* 8(3):137, 2002.

Rose LE, Mallinson RK, Walton-Moss B: Barriers to family care in psychiatric settings, *J Nurs Scholarsh* 36(1):39-47, 2004.

Shapiro J, Monzo LD, Rueda R et al: Alienated advocacy: perspectives of Latina mothers of young adults with developmental disabilities on service systems, *Ment Retard* 42(1):37-54, 2004.

Spiers J: The interpersonal contexts of negotiating care in home care nurse-patient interactions, *Qual Health Res* 12(8):1033-1057, 2002.

Szabo V, Strang V: Experiencing control in caregiving, *Image J Nurs Scholarsh* 31(1):71, 1999.

Teufel-Shone N, Staten L, Irwin S et al: Family cohesion and conflict in an American Indian community, *Am J Health Behav* 29(5):413-422, 2005.

Thomas DJ, King MA: Parish nursing assessment—what should you know? *Home Healthc Nurs Manag* 4(5):11-13, 2000.

Urban AD, Berry D, Grey M: Optimizing outcomes in adolescents with type 1 diabetes and their families, *J Clin Outcomes Manag* 11(5): 299-306, 2004.

Watson K, Kieckhefer G, Olshansky E: Striving for therapeutic relationships: parent-provider communication in the developmental treatment setting, *Qual Health Res* 16(5):647-663, 2006.

Watts S, Edgar L: Nucare, a coping skills training intervention for oncology patients and families: participants' motivations and expectations, *Can Oncol Nurs J* 14(2):84-95, 2004.

Weiss S, Chen J: Factors influencing maternal mental health and family functioning during the low birthweight infant's first year of life, *J Pediatr Nurs* 17(2):114, 2002.

Wen LK, Shepherd MD, Parchman ML: Family support, diet, and exercise among older Mexican Americans with type 2 diabetes, *Diabetes Educ* 30(6):980-993, 2004.

Woodgate R: The importance of being there: perspectives of social support by adolescents with cancer, *J Pediatr Oncol Nurs* 23(3):122-134, 2006.

Zengerle-Levy K: Practices that facilitate critically burned children's holistic healing, *Qual Health Res* 14(9):1255-1275, 2004.

Defensive Coping   *Gail Ladwig, MSN, CHTP, RN*

NANDA   Definition

Repeated projection of falsely positive self-evaluation based on a self-protective pattern that defends against underlying perceived threats to positive self-regard

Defining Characteristics

Denial of obvious problems; denial of obvious weaknesses; difficulty establishing relationships; difficulty maintaining relationships; difficulty in perception of reality; difficulty in perception of reality testing; grandiosity; hostile laughter; hypersensitivity of criticism; hypersensitivity to slight; lack of follow-through in therapy; lack of follow-through in treatment; lack of participation in therapy; lack of participation in treatment; projection of blame; projection of responsibility; rationalization of failures; ridicule of others; superior attitude toward others

NOC   Outcomes (Nursing Outcomes Classification)

Suggested NOC Outcomes

Coping, Decision Making, Impulse Self-Control, Information Processing

Example NOC Outcome with Indicators
Coping as evidenced by the following indicators: Identifies effective and ineffective coping patterns/Modifies lifestyle as needed (Rate the outcome and indicators of **Coping**: 1 = never demonstrated, 2 = rarely demonstrated, 3 = sometimes demonstrated, 4 = often demonstrated, 5 = consistently demonstrated [see Section I].)

Client Outcomes

Client Will (Specify Time Frame):

- Acknowledge need for change in coping style
- Accept responsibility for own behavior
- Establish realistic goals with validation from caregivers
- Solicit caregiver validation in decision making

NIC   Interventions (Nursing Interventions Classification)

Suggested NIC Intervention

Self-Awareness Enhancement

Example NIC Activities—Self-Awareness Enhancement
Encourage patient to recognize and discuss thoughts and feelings; Assist patient in identifying behaviors that are self-destructive

Nursing Interventions and *Rationales*

- Assess for the presence of denial as a coping mechanism. **EB:** *A thorough assessment for behaviors indicating the presence of denial is necessary in order to address issues of nonadherence in persons with human immunodeficiency virus (HIV) (Power et al, 2003).*
- Do not confront denial if its consequences are not a significant threat to health. **EBN:** *A period of denial may be necessary for the client to develop a construct within which the given information has meaning and can be appraised as not being a threat to survival (Norris & Spelic, 2002). Denial may be protective (Stephenson, 2004).*
- Ask appropriate questions to assess whether denial (defensive coping) is being used in association with alcoholism. **EB:** *Alcohol abuse is a major problem in the United States, but individuals are*

C

not getting treatment. In this survey, denial or refusal to admit severity and fear of social embarrass-ment were the top two reasons for not seeking help (To & Vega, 2006).

- Develop a trusting, therapeutic relationship with the client and family. *The interview process itself can be therapeutic (Overcash, 2004).*
- Determine whether the client has a positive or negative overall appraisal of a given event. **EB:** *Adolescent cannabis abusers present with a variety of challenges in outpatient treatment. Accurate as-sessment is necessary for successful outcome (Tims et al, 2002).*
- Determine the client's perception of the problem and then provide reality-based examples of the true situation (e.g., witnesses to an accident, blood alcohol levels, problems caused by alcohol). **EBN:** *Psychological manifestations of defensive coping can be understood only after a thorough inquiry into the client's framework for appraisal (Dudley-Brown, 2002).*
- Help the client identify patterns of response in life that may be maladaptive. *A clear, honest re-counting of life incidents and their consequences in a trusting relationship may provide the motivation necessary to seek a change in behavior (Faltz & Skinner, 2002).*
- ▲ Promote the client's feelings of self-worth by using group or individual therapy, role playing, one-to-one interactions, and role modeling. **EBN:** *A variety of methods may be used to assist clients in their attempts to assimilate the implications of a health status change (Whittemore et al, 2002).*
- Support strengths and normal observations with "I note that" or "I want you to notice." Tell clients when they do something well. **EBN:** *Nurses effectively support adaptation to a change in health status by actively listening to the client at all stages and encouraging reflection and self-understanding throughout the process (Whittemore et al, 2002).*
- Teach the client to use positive thinking by blocking negative thoughts with the word "Stop!" and inserting positive thoughts (e.g., "I'm a good [person, friend, student]"). *Interventions that encourage the cognitive reframing of a change in health status within a more positive framework support adaptation to a change in health status (Dudley-Brown, 2002).*
- Provide feedback regarding others' perceptions of the client's behavior through group or milieu therapy or one-to-one interactions. **EBN:** *Group therapy is an effective component of treatment in women with a dual diagnosis (Moser, Sowell & Phillips, 2001).*
- Encourage the client to use "I" statements and to accept responsibility for and consequences of actions. **EB:** *Interventions that support self-efficacy and a building of the sense of self as an individual who can control his or her own response facilitate the client's meeting of his or her goals (Brun & Rapp, 2001).*
- Refer to the care plans for **Readiness for enhanced Coping, Ineffective Denial** and **Dysfunctional Family processes: alcoholism.**

Geriatric

- Assess the client for anger and identify previous outlets for anger. *Nurses can help individuals to cope effectively with a change in health status by teaching them alternative methods of coping (Reynaud & Meeker, 2002).*
- Assess the client for dementia or depression. *A thorough assessment must be conducted to determine if the aberrant behavior has an organic origin (Green, 2002). Clients may not readily admit to psycho-logical or substance abuse symptoms (Boyd & Stanley, 2002).*
- ▲ It is essential to identify problems with alcohol in the elderly with the appropriate tools and make appropriate referrals. *Tools such as the Alcohol Use Disorders Identification Test (AUDIT), Michigan Alcohol Screening Test-Geriatric Version (MAST-G), and the Alcohol-Related Problems Survey (ARPS) may have additional use in this population. Brief interventions have been shown to be effective in producing sustained abstinence or reducing levels of consumption, thereby decreasing hazard-ous and harmful drinking (Culberson, 2006).*
- ▲ Encourage exercise for positive coping. **EBN:** *After a 10-week period, the elderly participants in this exercise group reported significant improvements in stress, mood, and several quality-of-life indices (Starkweather, 2007).*
- If a traumatic event has occurred, support positive religious coping behaviors. **EBN:** *Religious coping behaviors, when positive, can facilitate a more constructive health outcome (Bell Meisenhelder, 2002). Women with cancer who are involved in religious activities and groups report a more positive adaptation (Ferrell et al, 2003).*

• = Independent;   ▲ = Collaborative;   EBN = Evidence-Based Nursing;   EB = Evidence-Based

Multicultural

- Assess for the influence of cultural beliefs, norms, and values on the client's feelings of defensiveness. **EBN:** *The "denial" perceived by the nurse may be an expected behavior within the culture of the client (Lindenberg et al, 2002).*
- Acknowledge racial/ethnic differences at the onset of care. **EBN:** *Acknowledgment of race/ethnicity issues will enhance communication, establish rapport, and promote treatment outcomes (D'Avanzo et al, 2001). African-American parents who denied experiences of racism reported higher rates of behavior problems in their children, in contrast to African-American parents who actively coped with racism and reported lower levels of behavior problems in their children (Caughy, O'Campo & Muntaner, 2004).*
- Use therapeutic communication techniques that emphasize acceptance, offer the self, validate the client's concerns, and convey respect. **EBN:** *Care needs to be taken to incorporate the concept of health and healing prevalent in the client's culture (Chen & Rankin, 2002). The therapeutic use of dichos (Spanish language proverbs and sayings) decreased defensiveness in a repopulation of Hispanic/Latino psychiatric inpatients (Aviera, 1996).*

Home Care

- The interventions described previously may be adapted for home care use.
- Observe family dynamics for dysfunctional and supportive communication. **EBN:** *An understanding of the family structure, patterns of communication, healthcare history, and cultural influences will facilitate effective interventions on the part of the nurse. In the context of some family patterns of communication, defensive coping may be a learned behavior (Hellemann, Lee & Kury, 2002).*
- ▲ Refer to a mental health professional for possible psychodrama therapy, especially if the client experiences difficulty in coping with a traumatic event. **EB:** *Psychodrama has been shown to help people begin to reframe their feelings of victimization as feelings of survival and begin to see the future as hopeful (Carbonell & Parteleno-Barehmi, 1999).*
- ▲ If medical diagnoses coexist with defensive coping, confirm and validate the client's mental health plan and progress. **EBN:** *The nurse is often perceived as the "constant" in a client's relationship with the healthcare system and as such can help bridge the gap between the client and available resources (Northouse et al, 2002; Tak & McCubbin, 2002).*

Client/Family Teaching

- ▲ Teach the client the actions and side effects of medications and the importance of taking them as prescribed, even when the client is feeling good. **EBN:** *Education about the desired effects and potential side effects increases the knowledge and effective decision-making ability of the client (Moser, Sowell & Phillips, 2001).*
- ▲ Work with the client's support group to identify harmful behaviors and to seek help for the client if he or she is unable to control behavior. **EBN:** *Families need assistance in identifying resources and therapeutic responses as they adapt to the individual client's behaviors (Faltz & Skinner, 2002).*
- Support family efforts using religious coping behaviors. **EBN:** *Interventions to enhance positive religious coping facilitate recovery (Bell Meisenhelder, 2002; Newlin, Knafi & Meldus, 2002).*

evolve See the EVOLVE website for World Wide Web resources for client education.

REFERENCES

*Refer to **ineffective Coping** for additional references.*

Aviera A: "Dichos" therapy group: a therapeutic use of Spanish language proverbs with hospitalized Spanish-speaking psychiatric patients, *Cult Divers Ment Health* 2(2):73-87, 1996.

Bell Meisenhelder J: Terrorism, posttraumatic stress, and religious coping, *Issues Ment Health Nurs* 23(8):771, 2002.

Boyd MA, Stanley M: Mental health assessment of the elderly. In Boyd MA, editor: *Psychiatric nursing in contemporary practice,* ed 2, Philadelphia, 2002, Lippincott.

Brun C, Rapp RC: Strengths-based case management: individual's perspectives on strengths and the case manager relationship, *Soc Work* 46(3):278, 2001.

Carbonell DM, Parteleno-Barehmi C: Psychodrama groups for girls coping with trauma, *Int J Group Psychother* 49(3):285-306, 1999.

Caughy MO, O'Campo PJ, Muntaner C: Experiences of racism among African American parents and the mental health of their preschool-aged children, *Am J Public Health* 94(12):2118-2124, 2004.

Chen JL, Rankin SH: Using the resiliency model to deliver culturally sensitive care to Chinese families, *J Pediatr Nurs* 17(3):157, 2002.

Culberson JW: Alcohol use in the elderly: beyond the CAGE. Part 2: Screening instruments and treatment strategies, *Geriatrics*, 61(11):20-26, 2006.

D'Avanzo CE et al: Developing culturally informed strategies for substance-related interventions. In Naegle MA, D'Avanzo CE, editors: *Addictions and substance abuse: strategies for advanced practice nursing*, St Louis, 2001, Mosby.

Dudley-Brown S: Prevention of psychological distress in persons with inflammatory bowel disease, *Issues Ment Health Nurs* 23:403, 2002.

Faltz BG, Skinner MK: Substance abuse disorders. In Boyd MA, editor: *Psychiatric nursing in contemporary practice,* ed 2, Philadelphia, 2002, Lippincott.

Ferrell BR, Smith SL, Juarez G et al: Meaning of illness and spirituality in ovarian cancer survivors, *Oncol Nurs Forum* 30(2):249, 2003.

Green GC: Guidelines for assessing and diagnosing acute psychosis: a primer, *J Emerg Nurs* 28:S1, 2002.

Hellemann MV, Lee KA, Kury FS: Strengths and vulnerabilities of women of Mexican descent in relation to depressive symptoms, *Nurs Res* 51(3):175, 2002.

Lindenberg CS, Solorzano RM, Bear D et al: Reducing substance use and risky sexual behavior among young, low-income, Mexican-American women: comparison of two interventions, *Appl Nurs Res* 16(2):137-148, 2002.

Moser KM, Sowell RL, Phillips KD: Issues of women dually diagnosed with HIV infection and substance use problems in the Carolinas, *Issues Ment Health Nurs* 22:23, 2001.

Newlin K, Knafl K, Meldus GD: African-American spirituality: a concept analysis, *ANS Adv Nurs Sci* 25(2):57, 2002.

Norris J, Spelic SS: Supporting adaptation to body image disruption, *Rehabil Nurs* 27(1):8, 2002.

Northouse L, Walker J, Schafenacker A et al: A family-based program of care for women with recurrent breast cancer and their family members, *Oncol Nurs Forum* 29(10):1411-1419, 2002.

Overcash JA: Using narrative research to understand the quality of life of older women with breast cancer, *Oncol Nurs Forum* 31(6):1153, 2004.

Power R, Koopman C, Volk J et al: Social support, substance use, and denial in relationship to antiretroviral treatment adherence among HIV-infected persons, *Aids Patient Care* 17(5):245, 2003.

Reynaud SN, Meeker BJ: Coping styles of older adults with ostomies, *J Gerontol Nurs* 28(5):30, 2002.

Starkweather AR: The effects of exercise on perceived stress and IL-6 levels among older adults, *Biol Res Nurs* 8(3):186-194, 2007.

Stephenson PS: Understanding denial, *Oncol Nurs Forum* 31(5):985, 2004.

Tak YR, McCubbin M: Family stress, perceived social support and coping following the diagnosis of a child's congenital heart disease, *J Adv Nurs* 39(2):190-198, 2002.

Tims FM, Dennis ML, Hamilton N et al: Characteristics and problems of 600 adolescent cannabis abusers in outpatient treatment, *Addiction* 97(Suppl 1):46, 2002.

To SE, Vega CP: Alcoholism and pathways to recovery: new survey results on views and treatment options, *MedGenMed* 8(1):2, 2006.

Whittemore R, Chase SK, Mandle CL et al: Lifestyle change in type 2 diabetes, *Nurs Res* 51(1):18, 2002.

Disabled family Coping   Gail B. Ladwig, MSN, CHTP, RN

NANDA   Definition

Behavior of significant person (family member or other primary person) that disables his/her capacity and the client's capacity to effectively address tasks essential to either person's adaptation to the health challenge

Defining Characteristics

Abandonment; aggression; agitation; carrying on usual routines without regard for client's needs; client's development of dependence; depression; desertion; disregarding client's needs; distortion of reality regarding client's health problem; family behaviors that are detrimental to well-being; hostility; impaired individualization; impaired restructuring of a meaningful life for self; intolerance; neglectful care of client in regard to basic human needs; neglectful care of client in regard to illness treatment; neglectful relationships with other family members; prolonged overconcern for client; psychosomaticism; rejection; taking on illness signs of client

Related Factors (r/t)

Arbitrary handling of family's resistance to treatment; dissonant coping styles for dealing with adaptive tasks by the significant person and client; dissonant coping styles among significant people; highly ambivalent family relationships; significant person with pressed feelings (e.g., guilt, anxiety, hostility, despair)

NOC   Outcomes (Nursing Outcomes Classification)

Suggested NOC Outcomes

Caregiver Well-Being, Family Coping, Caregiver Emotional Health, Coping

• = Independent;   ▲ = Collaborative;   EBN = Evidence-Based Nursing;   EB = Evidence-Based

Example NOC Outcome with Indicators

Coping as evidenced by the following indicators: Identifies effective coping patterns/Verbalizes sense of control/Seeks information concerning illness and treatment/Uses available social support/Identifies multiple coping strategies (Rate the outcome and indicators of **Coping:** 1 = never demonstrated, 2 = rarely demonstrated, 3 = sometimes demonstrated, 4 = often demonstrated, 5 = consistently demonstrated [see Section I].)

Client Outcomes

Family/Significant Person Will (Specify Time Frame):

- Express realistic understanding and expectations of the client
- Participate positively in the client's care within the limits of his or her abilities
- Identify responses that are harmful
- Acknowledge and accept the need for assistance with circumstances
- Express feelings openly, honestly, and appropriately

NIC   Interventions (Nursing Interventions Classification)

Suggested NIC Interventions

Family Support, Family Therapy, Coping Enhancement, Counseling, Family Integrity Promotion, Family Involvement Promotion, Mutual Goal Setting

Example NIC Activities—Family Therapy

Identify family strengths/resources; Facilitate family discussion

Nursing Interventions and *Rationales*

Refer to care plan **Compromised family Coping** for additional interventions

- Identify current behaviors of family members, such as withdrawal (e.g., not visiting, briefly visiting, ignoring client when visiting), anger and hostility toward the client and others, or expression of guilt. **EBN:** *Family cohesion, presence of a partner, emotional support, and a mother's satisfaction with her family all contributed to her better mental health in a research study focusing on mothers of low-birth-weight infants (Weiss & Chen, 2002).*
- Note other stressors in the family (e.g., financial, job-related). **EBN:** *In mothers of low-birth-weight infants, the presence of other life stressors and the family's use of internally focused coping strategies contributed to worse mental health outcomes for the mother (Weiss & Chen, 2002).*
- ▲ Evaluate the family's perceived strength of its social support system. Encourage the family to use social support to increase its resiliency and to moderate stress. *Perceived social support is a factor influencing resiliency and ability to cope with stress (Tak & McCubbin, 2002).*
- ▲ Observe for any symptoms of elder or child abuse or neglect. Prompt reporting of abuse according to local and state law is necessary. **EB:** *Elders need to be assessed for signs of abuse and neglect. Types of elder abuse existing in our society include physical, sexual, emotional, psychological, and exploitation (Roman, 2004). Physical child abuse is a significant social and medical problem (Bull, 2006).*
- Encourage family members to spend time with the client and to assist in care when possible. Support thoughts for positive outcome when possible. *This study of spouses of clients in the intensive care unit (ICU) demonstrated that preferences for closeness and helpfulness were strongly related, and together with optimism, predicted spouses' mood at some point of the course of the illness (Eldredge, 2004).*
- ▲ Encourage family members to participate in appropriate support programs (e.g., chronic obstructive pulmonary disease [COPD] support groups, Arthritis I Can Cope groups, Alzheimer's support groups, Art making groups, telesupport). **EBN:** *The stress of caregivers of clients with cancer was reduced when they attended an art-making class (Walsh et al, 2007).* **EB:** *Older caregivers in telesupport groups reported lower depression than control group caregivers (Winter & Gitlin, 2007).*

Geriatric

▲ If actual or potential abuse or neglect is an issue, report it to the appropriate agency. *All who provide care to an elder must be aware of the potential signs of abuse and the remedies available (Birke, 2004).*

▲ Refer the family to appropriate senior community resources (e.g., senior centers, Medicare assistance, meal programs, parish nursing services, charitable organizations). *This study demonstrates the importance of social support among visually impaired elders (Lee & Brennan, 2006).*

• Work with the family to manage common challenges related to normal aging. **EB:** *Maltreatment of elders is less likely when caregivers are trained to cope with the stress of caregiving of elders and potentially abusive elders (Nadien, 2006).*

▲ Provide support for family caregivers of persons with dementia and related disorders: Encourage pleasant event therapies (i.e., interventions that teach caregivers to identify and pursue experiences that give them pleasure on a regular basis). Provide dietary and physical activity interventions. Screen for signs of depression. *Collaborative care models are essential for treating physical and psychiatric conditions in caregivers. Such models should be adapted to caregivers' needs (Vitaliano & Katon, 2006).*

Multicultural

• Work to provide caregivers who understand the importance of cultural beliefs and values the family may hold. **EBN:** *Cultures can differ with regard to health beliefs, practices, and values (Campinha-Bacote & Narayan, 2000; Vitaliano & Katon, 2006). There is a stigma to having a family member with mental illness in China (Chang & Horrocks, 2006).*

▲ Develop programs to prevent injury from abuse and suffocation for the African-American community. **EB:** *This study demonstrated that African-American infants have 3.5 times increased risk of death from preventable injuries compared to white infants (Falcone, Brown & Garcia, 2007).*

Home Care

• The interventions described previously may be adapted for home care use.

▲ If disabled family coping interferes with the family member's ability to support the client's treatment plan, refer for psychiatric home healthcare services for family and client counseling and implementation of a therapeutic regimen. **EBN:** *Psychiatric home care nurses can address issues related to family members' ability to adjust to changes in the client's health status. Behavioral interventions in the home can help the family to participate more effectively in the treatment plan (Logsdon, McCurry & Teri, 2005; Oneal, Reeb & Korte, 2006).*

Client/Family Teaching

• Involve the client and family in the planning of care as often as possible; mutual goal setting is now considered part of "client safety." *Major changes in the fifth annual issuance of National Patient Safety Goals include Home Care, Assisted Living, and Disease-Specific Care programs in 2006. An expectation is to "Encourage patients' active involvement in their own care as a patient safety strategy" (Patient Safety, 2006).*

• Discuss with the family appropriate ways to demonstrate feelings such as reminiscence. *This study demonstrated the positive effects of reminiscence therapy among student nurses and older adults (Shellman, 2006).*

▲ Refer combat service members and their families for mental health treatment before and during deployment. **EB:** *Combat duty is associated with traumatic events, deprivation, and exposure to war atrocities that may result in acute, delayed, or chronic psychosocial issues during and after returning from deployment. Early identification and treatment of mental health problems may decrease the psychosocial impact of combat and thus prevent progression to more chronic and severe psychopathology such as depression and post-traumatic stress disorder (PTSD) (Gaylord, 2006).*

 See the EVOLVE website for World Wide Web resources for client education.

REFERENCES

Refer to **compromised family Coping** *for additional references.*

Birke MG: Elder law, Medicare, and legal issues in older patients, *Semin Oncol* 31(2): 282-292, 2004.

Bull L: Children's non-accidental injuries at an accident and emergency department: does the age of the child and the type of injury matter? *Accid Emerg Nurs* 14(3):155-159, 2006.

Campinha-Bacote J, Narayan M: Culturally competent health care at home, *Home Care Provid* 5(6):213-219, 2000.

Chang KH, Horrocks S: Lived experiences of family caregivers of mentally ill relatives, *J Adv Nurs* 53(4):435-443, 2006.

Eldredge D: Helping at the bedside: spouses' preferences for helping critically ill patients, *Res Nurs Health* 27(5):307-321, 2004.

Falcone RA, Brown RL, Garcia VF, The epidemiology of infant injuries and alarming health disparities, *J Pediatr Surg* 42(1):172-176, 2007.

Gaylord KM: The psychosocial effects of combat: the frequently unseen injury, *Crit Care Nurs Clin North Am* 18(3):349-357, 2006.

Lee EK, Brennan M: Stress constellations and coping styles of older adults with age-related visual impairment, *Health Soc Work* 31(4):289-298, 2006.

Logsdon RG, McCurry SM, Teri L: A home health care approach to exercise for persons with Alzheimer's disease, *Care Manag J* 6(2):90-97, 2005.

Nadien MB: Factors that influence abusive interactions between aging women and their caregivers, *Ann N Y Acad Sce* 1087:158-169, 2006.

Oneal BJ, Reeb RN, Korte JR et al: Assessment of home-based behavior modification programs for autistic children: reliability and validity of the behavioral summarized evaluation, *J Prev Interv Community* 32(1-2):25-39, 2006.

Patient Safety: Joint Commission announces 2007 national patient safety goals, *Obesity, Fitness & Wellness Week*, Jul 8, 2006, p. 1956.

Roman M: Elder Abuse, *Medsurg Matters*, 13(3):10-12, 2004.

Shellman J: "Making a connection": BSN students' perceptions of their reminiscence experiences with older adults, *J Nurs Educ* 45(12):497-503, 2006.

Tak YR, McCubbin M: Family stress, perceived social support and coping following the diagnosis of a child's congenital heart disease, *J Adv Nurs* 39(2):190, 2002.

Vitaliano PP, Katon WJ: Effects of stress on family caregivers: recognition and management, *Psychiatr Times*, 23(7):24, 2006.

Walsh S, Radcliffe RS, Castillo L et al: A pilot study to test the effects of art-making classes for family caregivers of patients with cancer, *Oncol Nurs Forum* 34(1):E9-E16, 2007.

Weiss S, Chen J: Factors influencing maternal mental health and family functioning during the low birthweight infant's first year of life, *J Pediatr Nurs* 17(2):114, 2002.

Winter L, Gitlin LN: Evaluation of a telephone-based support group intervention for female caregivers of community-dwelling individuals with dementia, *Am J Alzheimers Dis Other Demen* 21(6):391-397, 2007.

Ineffective Coping   Arlene Farren, RN, MA, AOCN

NANDA   Definition

Inability to form a valid appraisal of the stressors, inadequate choices of practiced responses, and/or inability to use available resources

Defining Characteristics

Abuse of chemical agents; change in usual communication patterns; decreased use of social support; destructive behavior toward others; destructive behavior toward self; fatigue; high illness rate; inability to meet basic needs; inability to meet role expectations; inadequate problem solving; lack of goal-directed behavior/resolution of problem, including inability to attend to and difficulty organizing information; poor concentration; risk taking; sleep disturbance; use of forms of coping that impede adaptive behavior; verbalization of inability to ask for help; verbalization of inability to cope

Related Factors

Disturbance in pattern of appraisal of threat; disturbance in pattern of tension release; gender differences in coping strategies; high degree of threat; inability to conserve adaptive energies; inadequate level of confidence in ability to cope; inadequate level of perception of control; inadequate opportunity to prepare for stressor; inadequate resources available; inadequate social support created by characteristics of relationships; maturational crisis; situational crisis; uncertainty

NOC   Outcomes (Nursing Outcomes Classification)

Suggested NOC Outcomes

Coping, Decision Making, Impulse Self-Control, Information Processing

• = Independent;   ▲ = Collaborative;   EBN = Evidence-Based Nursing;   EB = Evidence-Based

C

Client Outcomes

Client Will (Specify Time Frame):

- Use effective coping strategies
- Use behaviors to decrease stress
- Remain free of destructive behavior toward self or others
- Report decrease in physical symptoms of stress
- Report increase in psychological comfort
- Seek help from a healthcare professional as appropriate

NIC   Interventions (Nursing Interventions Classification)

Suggested NIC Interventions

Coping Enhancement, Decision-Making Support

Example NIC Activities—Coping Enhancement
Assist the patient in developing an objective appraisal of the event; Explore with the client previous methods of dealing with life problems

Nursing Interventions and *Rationales*

- Monitor the client's risk of harming self or others and intervene appropriately. See care plan for **Risk for Suicide. EBN:** *Hopelessness associated with depression is an indicator of a higher risk of suicidal behavior (Szanto et al, 2003). Adolescents may use self-harming behaviors as a means of communication or way of coping (Murray & Wright, 2006).*
- Observe for contributing factors of ineffective coping such as poor self-concept, grief, lack of problem-solving skills, lack of support, recent change in life situation, or gender differences in coping strategies. **EBN:** *Psychological manifestations of ineffective coping can be understood only after a thorough inquiry into the client's framework for appraisal (Dudley-Brown, 2002; Valente, 2005).* **EB:** *Males and females differ in appraisal of health and lifestyle choices and use of coping behavior (Dawson et al, 2007; Goodwin, 2006).*
- Use verbal and nonverbal therapeutic communication approaches including empathy, active listening, and confrontation to encourage the client and family to express emotions such as sadness, guilt, and anger (within appropriate limits); verbalize fears and concerns; and set goals. **EBN:** *Contributes to the development of a trusting relationship and feelings of connectedness, facilitates expression of feelings, and encourages the formulation of a plan (Dearing, 2004; Lin & Bauer-Wu, 2003; Overcash, 2004).*
- Collaborate with the client to identify strengths such as the ability to relate the facts and to recognize the source of stressors. **EBN:** *Successful adaptation requires a coordination of efforts to fit the nursing interventions to the client's perception of the threat, personal values and beliefs, and recognition of personal strengths (Evans, Crogan & Schultz, 2004; Raak, Hurtig & Wahren, 2003).*
- Encourage the client to describe previous stressors and the coping mechanisms used. **EBN:** *Recounting previous experiences perceived by the client as having been dealt with successfully strengthens effective coping and helps eliminate ineffective coping mechanisms (Northouse, Walker & Schafenacker et al, 2002). Evaluation of pessimism and optimism in family members of Parkinson's clients can help identify those who are at greater risk for negative health consequences (Lyons, Stewart & Archbold et al, 2004).*

C

- Be supportive of coping behaviors; allow the client time to relax. **EBN:** *Sharing of innermost cares and concerns requires that nurses provide opportunities for clients to feel safe enough to share (Richer & Ezer, 2002). The relationship the nurse has with the client has a positive effect on the coping of individuals with nonhealing ulcers (Hopkins, 2004).*
- Provide opportunities for the client to discuss the meaning the situation might have for the client. **EBN:** *Participants in this study shared the importance of framing the illness experience in ways that enabled a sense of normalcy. Clinicians should offer support as clients search for meanings (Houldin & Lewis, 2006). In this study, findings suggest that the meaning-making intervention significantly improved self-esteem and sense of security in facing uncertainty (Lee et al, 2006).*
- Assist the client to set realistic goals and identify personal skills and knowledge. **EBN:** *Efforts to educate regarding possible and/or potential effects of a specific diagnosis and the resources available to assist with coping are positive factors in successful adaptation (Brooks, 2003; Stevens & Sin, 2005).*
- Provide information regarding care before care is given. **EBN:** *In women who have had breast cancer, lymphedema information is necessary for informed choice with highest potential for a good outcome (Radina et al, 2004).* **EB:** *Before psychiatric clients can make decisions regarding treatment, they must have appropriate information (Linhorst et al, 2002). Epilepsy-related knowledge has been shown to assist clients and families to cope with the disease (May & Pfafflin, 2005).*
- Discuss changes with the client before making them. **EBN:** *Nurses are identified by clients as necessary in coordinating all aspects of their care (Hodgkinson & Lester, 2002).* **EBN:** *The nurse's ongoing interaction with individuals with nonhealing ulcers involved honest assessment and communication (Hopkins, 2004).*
- Encourage the client to make choices (as appropriate) and participate in planning care and scheduled activities. **EBN:** *The inclusion of consumer consultants in preparing discharge planning programs would increase client satisfaction (Cleary, Horsfall & Hunt, 2003). Collaborative triadic decision-making processes result in greater effectiveness of care (Dalton, 2003).*
- Provide mental and physical activities within the client's ability (e.g., reading, television, radio, crafts, outings, movies, dinners out, social gatherings, exercise, sports, games). **EBN:** *Nurses working with individuals with nonhealing ulcers helped them find ways to normalize their experience and positively impacted the individuals' adjustment (Hopkins, 2004). Distraction has been demonstrated to be effective in coping with pain of older people (Blomquist & Edberg, 2002).* **Additional relevant research:** *Goodwin, 2006; Schneider et al, 2004.*
- Encourage moderate aerobic exercise (as appropriate). **EBN:** *People with human immunodeficiency virus (HIV) reported using physical activity to effectively cope with depressive symptoms (Eller et al, 2005).* **EB:** *Exercise was found to improve quality of life in female cardiac clients (Tyni-Lenne et al, 2002) and decrease the likelihood for depressive feelings when used as a positive coping strategy for school-age children with angry feelings (Goodwin, 2006).*
- Discuss the client's and family's power to change a situation or the need to accept a situation. **EBN:** *An honest assessment of a particular situation as shared by the nurse is important to the family's sense of what is expected of them in adapting to a healthcare change (Weiss & Chen, 2002). A basic process of coping for significant others of persons living with HIV includes facing the change and dealing with it (Kylmä, 2005/2006).*
- Offer instruction regarding alternative coping strategies. **EBN:** *Humor has been shown to positively affect the immune system, improve pain thresholds, elevate natural killer cell activity, and produce biochemical changes that improve physical stress response and increase well-being (Christie & Moore, 2005). Relaxation training has been demonstrated to improve overall coping ability (Tyni-Lenne et al, 2002).* **EB:** *Meditative approaches have multifaceted effects on psychologic and biologic functions via the psychoneuroendocrine/immune and autonomic nervous system pathway and are efficacious and safe (Mindfulness Meditation, Relaxation Response, Yoga, etc.) (Arias et al, 2006). A pre-post intervention study of women with heart disease revealed that a mindfulness meditation intervention decreased anxiety, improved emotional control, and decreased reactive style coping (Tacón et al, 2003).*
- Encourage use of spiritual resources as desired. **EBN:** *Clients with enhanced psycho-spiritual well-being are thought to cope more effectively with the process of terminal illness and find meaning in the experience (Lin & Bauer-Wu, 2003). The strength to cope was identified as a major theme reflecting what spirituality provided African-American breast cancer survivors (Gibson & Hendricks, 2006).*

C

HeartTouch technique (HRTT) is an internal method for changing thoughts and feelings through centered awareness, loving connections with others, and connecting to a higher power; the experimental group of nurses using HRTT statistically significantly increased spiritual well-being (Walker, 2006).
- Encourage use of social support resources. **EBN:** *Good relationships with spouse/partner and other sources of social support have been found to be protective and enhance coping (Lin & Bauer-Wu, 2003). In a study of family caregivers in hospice care, support from the hospice team was associated with the use of fewer coping strategies that clients found effective (Raleigh et al, 2006).* **EB:** *Better adjustment in children of a parent with multiple sclerosis was related to higher levels of social support and approach coping strategies (Pakenham & Bursnall, 2006).*
▲ Refer for additional or more intensive therapies as needed. **EBN:** *Nurses are perceived as the bridge between the client and all other resources needed to manage an adaptive response to a healthcare change (Hodgkinson & Lester, 2002).*

Geriatric

▲ Assess and report possible physiological alterations (e.g., sepsis, hypoglycemia, hypotension, infection, changes in temperature, fluid and electrolyte imbalances, and use of medications with known cognitive and psychotropic side effects).
- Screen for elder neglect or other forms of elder mistreatment.
- Target selected coping mechanisms for older persons based on client features, use, and preferences. **EBN:** *Health, routine tasks, family issues, financial management, and living conditions are thought to improve support measures (Ark et al, 2006). Elders with arthritis reported cognitive efforts, diversional activities, and assertive actions were useful in dealing with daily stress (Tak, 2006). Additional Relevant Research: Boerner, Reinhardt & Horowitz 2006; Nokes, Chew & Altman, 2003; Tryssenaar, Chui & Finch, 2003.*
▲ Increase and mobilize support available to older persons by encouraging a variety of mechanisms involving family, friends, peers, and healthcare providers. **EBN:** *Relationships are pivotal in supporting coping in older adults. Social support was thought to be one of the dynamics in a peer-counseling program that was successful in terms of improving perceived health status, level of depression, and personal growth (Ho, 2007). Mobilizing religious coping styles has been found to be one way to measure health service use and length of stay for older persons (Ark et al, 2006). While limitations to telephone support groups for older HIV-positive persons may be difficult, it was found to facilitate connections with others and decrease geographical and logistical isolation (Nokes et al, 2003).*
- Actively listen to complaints and concerns. **EBN:** *The quality of care provided to elderly chronic pain clients living at home could be improved by active listening (Blomquist & Edberg, 2002).*
- Engage the client in reminiscence. **EBN:** *Life review as an intervention had a significant effect of lowering depression in individuals with cerebral vascular accident (Davis, 2004).* **EB:** *Reminiscence activates positive memories and evokes well-being (Puentes, 2002).*

Multicultural

- Assess for the influence of cultural beliefs, norms, and values on the client's perceptions of effective coping. *"Healthcare providers must recognize, respect, and integrate clients' cultural beliefs and practices into health prescriptions" (Purnell & Paulanka 2005).* **EBN:** *The client's coping behavior may be based on cultural perceptions of normal and abnormal coping behavior (Sterling & Peterson, 2003).* **EBN:** *Chinese women may be less likely to seek mental health services for postnatal depression (Chan et al, 2002). Gender and age mediate a woman's response to signs and symptoms of cardiac disease (Lefler & Bondy, 2004). For Mexican-American adolescents, positive reinterpretation, focusing and venting emotions, instrumental social support, active coping, religious, restraint, emotional support, acceptance, and planning were all forms of coping and were all associated with positive psychological and physical health (Vaughn & Roesch, 2003).*
- Assess the influence of fatalism on the client's coping behavior. **EBN:** *Fatalistic perspectives, which involve the belief that one cannot control one's own fate, may influence health behaviors in some Asian-American, African-American, and Latino populations (Chen, 2001).* **EBN:** *Clients with non–small cell lung cancer in Taiwan yielded that one response was to accept the outcome as fate (Kuo & Ma, 2002).*
- Assess the influence of cultural conflicts that may affect coping abilities. **EBN:** *It may be necessary*

---

to help the client to identify and find coping strategies that do not conflict with cultural expectations (Shibusawa & Mui, 2001).

- Assess for intergenerational family problems that can overwhelm coping abilities. **EBN:** *Family assessment is integral to nursing care of clients (Northouse et al, 2002).*
- Encourage spirituality as a source of support for coping. **EBN:** *Many African-Americans and Latinos identify spirituality, religiousness, prayer, and church-based approaches as coping resources (Abrums, 2004; Coon et al, 2004; Weaver & Flannelly, 2004). A sense of faith is an important component of psychosocial well-being in individuals with advanced cancer (Lin & Bauer-Wu, 2003). Spirituality has a positive effect on coping (Kelly, 2004).*
- Negotiate with the client with regard to the aspects of coping behavior that will need to be modified. **EBN:** *As a part of the assessment of coping behaviors, alternate methods may be introduced and offered to the client as a possible choice in new coping strategies (Wassem, Beckham & Dudley, 2001).*
- Identify which family members the client can count on for support. **EBN:** *In a variety of different cultures family members are relied on to cope with stress (Donnelly, 2002; Gleeson-Kreig, Bernal & Woolley, 2002; White et al, 2002).*
- Support the inner resources that clients use for coping. **EBN:** *African-American women in one study used inner resources to develop self-help strategies to cope with reactions following involuntary pregnancy loss (Van & Meleis, 2003).*
- Use an empowerment framework to redefine coping strategies. **EB:** *Empowerment strategies are important for people with severe mental illness (Linhorst et al, 2002).*

 ### Home Care

- The interventions described previously may be adapted for home care use.
- ▲ Assess for suicidal tendencies. Refer for mental health care immediately if indicated.
- Identify an emergency plan should the client become suicidal. *Ineffective coping can occur in a crisis situation and can lead to suicidal ideation if the client sees no hope for a solution. A suicidal client is not safe in the home environment unless supported by professional help.* Refer to the care plan for **Risk for Suicide.**
- Observe the family for coping behavior patterns. Obtain family and client history as possible. **EBN:** *Family assessment is necessary to guide interventions (Weiss & Chen, 2002; Northouse et al, 2002).* **EBN:** *The assessment of caregivers' coping and information styles is an important part of nursing care of women with advanced cancer (Nikoletti et al, 2003).*
- ▲ Assess for effective symptoms after cerebrovascular accident (CVA) in the elderly, particularly emotional lability and depression. Refer for evaluation and treatment as indicated. **EB:** *Elderly with first-ever stroke showed evidence of depression (Piamarta et al, 2004).*
- Encourage the client to use self-care management to increase the experience of personal control. Identify with the client all available supports and sense of attachment to others. Refer to the care plan for **Powerlessness. EBN:** *In a study of heart transplantation clients, personal control was positively associated with optimism, well-being, and satisfaction with life, and was negatively associated with anger and depression (Bohachick et al, 2002). Clients experiencing cancer-related fatigue report feeling loss of control, which can lead to helplessness (Potter, 2004).*
- ▲ Refer to medical social services for evaluation and counseling, which will promote adequate coping as part of the medical plan of care. If no primary medical diagnosis has been made, request medical social services to assist with community support contacts. *These nurses are frequently requested to monitor medication use and therefore need to know the plan of care.*
- ▲ Refer the client and family to support groups. **EBN:** *Support groups provide an essential resource to clients and their families when adapting to health status change (Fung & Chien, 2002). Support groups have a positive effect on individuals receiving chemotherapy (Ekman et al, 2004). An HIV self-care symptom management program implemented with African-American mothers produced positive outcomes in mental and physical health measures (Miles et al, 2003).*
- ▲ If monitoring medication use, contract with the client or solicit assistance from a responsible caregiver. *Elders with arthritis identified taking medications as an assertive action coping strategy (Tak, 2006).*
- ▲ Institute case management for frail elderly clients to support continued independent living. **EBN:** *Coping assistance (a cluster of nursing interventions) provided by nurse case managers to frail*

C

older persons resulted in a demonstrated increase in instrumental activity of daily living functioning (Schein et al, 2005).

▲ If the client is homebound, refer for psychiatric home healthcare services for client reassurance and implementation of a therapeutic regimen. **EB:** *Elderly stroke clients receiving home care were shown to have lower depression scores and lower rates of admission to nursing homes (Ricauda et al, 2004). An intervention study of a peer-based and regular case management for community-dwelling adults with severe mental illness demonstrated that improved positive regard at 6 months predicted and sustained treatment motivation for psychiatric, alcohol, and drug use problems and attendance at Alcoholics and Narcotics Anonymous meetings (Sells et al, 2006).*

Client/Family Teaching

- Teach the client to problem solve. Have the client define the problem and cause, and list the advantages and disadvantages of the options. **EBN:** *Cognitive behavioral therapy is a useful intervention when working on issues of hope (Collins & Cutcliffe, 2003).* **EB:** *Results of this study illustrate the value of positive coping in a rehabilitation setting (Greenglass et al, 2005).*
- Provide the seriously ill client and his or her family with needed information regarding the condition and treatment. **EBN:** *Middle-aged and older HIV-positive adults need concrete information regarding symptoms, medications, and treatments (Nokes et al, 2003).* **EB:** *Clients and families benefit from a sense of trust in healthcare providers that is based on honest communication regarding their condition and options (Fallowfield, Jenkins & Beveridge, 2002).*
- Teach relaxation techniques. **EBN:** *Relaxation training such as Mindfulness Meditation (MBSR) has demonstrated effectiveness in reducing anxiety and chronic pain, improving mood, and reducing stress. In a pilot study of MBSR in women with heart disease, women in the intervention group had improvements in anxiety at the end of the 8-week training (Tacón et al, 2003).*
- Work closely with the client to develop appropriate educational tools that address individualized needs. **EBN:** *Educational level may affect the client's level of concern and ability to process information (Miles et al, 2002). Caregiver and client coping patterns may vary (Kershaw, Northouse & Kritpacha, 2004).*
- ▲ Teach the client about available community resources (e.g., therapists, ministers, counselors, self-help groups). **EBN:** *Families need assistance in coping with health changes (Northouse et al, 2002; Tak & McCubbin, 2002). The degree of economic impact of the illness on a family will affect their ability to seek out and accept help from community resources (Montagnino & Mauricio, 2004).*

evolve See the EVOLVE website for World Wide Web resources for client education.

REFERENCES

Abrums M: Faith and feminism: how African American women from a storefront church resist oppression in healthcare, *ANS Adv Nurs Sci* 27(3):187-201, 2004.

Arias AJ, Steinberg K, Banga A et al: Systematic review of the efficacy of meditation techniques as treatments for medical illness, *J Alt Comp Med* 12(8):817-832, 2006.

Ark PD, Hull PC, Husaini BA et al: Religiosity, religious coping styles, and health service use, *J Geront Nurs* 32(8):20-9, 2006.

Blomquist K, Edberg AK: Living with persistent pain: experiences of older people receiving home care, *J Adv Nurs* 40(3):297-306, 2002.

Boerner K, Reinhardt JP, Horowitz A: The effect of rehabilitation service use on coping patterns over time among older adults with age-related vision loss, *Clin Rehab* 20(6):478-487, 2006.

Bohachick P, Taylor MV, Sereika S et al: Social support, personal control, and psychological recovery following heart transplant, *Clin Nurs Res* 11:34-51, 2002.

Brooks MV: Health-related hardiness and chronic illness: a synthesis of current research, *Nurs Forum* 38(3):11-20, 2003.

Chan SW, Levy V, Chung TK et al: A qualitative study of a group of Hong Kong Chinese women diagnosed with postnatal depression, *J Adv Nurs* 39(6):571-579, 2002.

Chen YC: Chinese values, health, and nursing, *J Adv Nurs* 36(2):270-273, 2001.

Christie W, Moore C: The impact of humor on patients with cancer, *Clin J Oncol Nurs* 9(2):211-218, 2005.

Cleary M, Horsfall J, Hunt GE: Consumer feedback on nursing care and discharge planning, *J Adv Nurs* 42(3):269-277, 2003.

Collins S, Cutcliffe JR: Addressing hopelessness in people with suicidal ideation: building upon the therapeutic relationship utilizing a cognitive behavioural approach, *J Psychiatr Ment Health Nurs,* 10(2):175-185, Apr 2003.

Coon DW, Rubert M, Solano N et al: Well-being, appraisal, and coping in Latina and Caucasian female dementia caregivers: findings from the REACH study, *Aging Ment Health* 8(4):330-345, 2004.

Dalton JM: Development and testing of the theory of collaborative decision-making in nursing practice for triads, *J Adv Nurs* 41(1):22-33, 2003.

Davis MC: Life review therapy as an intervention to manage depression and enhance life satisfaction in individuals with right hemisphere cerebral vascular accidents, *Issues Ment Health Nurs* 25(5):503-515, 2004.

Dawson KA, Schneider MA, Fletcher PC et al: Examining gender differences in the health behaviors of Canadian university students, *J R Soc Health* 127(1):38-44, 2007.

Dearing KS: Getting it, together: how the nurse patient relationship influences treatment compliance for patients with schizophrenia, *Arch Psychiatr Nurs* 18(5):155-163, 2004.

Donnelly TT: Contextual analysis of coping: implications for immigrants' mental health care, *Issues Ment Health Nurs* 23:715-32, 2002.

Dudley-Brown S: Prevention of psychological distress in persons with inflammatory bowel disease, *Issues Ment Health Nurs* 23:403-422, 2002.

Ekman I, Bergbom I, Ekman T et al: Maintaining normality and support are central issues when receiving chemotherapy for ovarian cancer, *Cancer Nurs* 27(3):177-182, 2004.

Eller LS, Corless I, Bunch EH et al: Self-care strategies for depressive symptoms in people with HIV disease, *J Adv Nurs* 51(2):119-130, 2005.

Evans BC, Crogan NL, Shultz JA: Resident coping strategies in the nursing home: an indicator of the need for dietary services change, *Appl Nurs Res* 17(2): 109-115, 2004.

Fallowfield LJ, Jenkins VA, Beveridge HA: Truth may hurt but deceit hurts more: communication in palliative care, *Palliat Med* 16(4):297-303, 2002.

Fung WY, Chien WT: The effectiveness of a mutual support group for family caregivers of a relative with dementia, *Arch Psychiatr Nurs* 26(3):134-144, 2002.

Gibson LM, Hendricks CS: Integrative review of spirituality in African American breast cancer survivors, *ABNF J* 17(2):67-72, 2006.

Gleeson-Kreig J, Bernal H, Woolley S: The role of social support in the self-management of diabetes mellitus among a Hispanic population, *Public Health Nurs* 19(3):215-222, 2002.

Goodwin RD: Association between coping with anger and feelings of depression among youths, *AM J Publ Health* 96(4): 664-669, 2006.

Greenglass ER, Marques S, deRidder M et al: Positive coping and mastery in a rehabilitation setting, *Int J Rehabil Res* 28(4):331-339, 2005.

Ho APY: A peer counseling program for the elderly with depression living in the community, *Aging Ment Health* 11(1):69-74, 2007.

Hodgkinson R, Lester H: Stresses and coping strategies of mothers living with a child with cystic fibrosis: implications for nursing professionals, *J Adv Nurs* 39(4):377-383, 2002.

Hopkins A: Disrupted lives: investigating coping strategies for non-healing leg ulcers, *Br J Nurs* 13(9): 556-563, May 13-26, 2004.

Houldin AD, Lewis FM: Salvaging their normal lives: a qualitative study of patients with recently diagnosed advanced colorectal cancer, *Oncol Nurs Forum* 33(4):719-725, 2006.

Kershaw T, Northouse L, Kritpracha C: Coping strategies and quality of life in women with advanced breast cancer and their family caregivers, *Psychol Health* 19(2):139-155, 2004.

Kelly J: Spirituality as a coping mechanism, *Dimen Crit Care Nurs* 23(4):162-168, 2004.

Kuo TT, Ma FC: Symptoms distresses and coping strategies in patients with non-small cell lung cancer, *Cancer Nurs* 25(4): 309-317, 2002.

Kylmä J: Hope, despair and hopelessness in significant others of adult persons living with HIV, *J Theory Construct Test* 9(2):49-54, 2005/2006.

Lee V, Cohen SR, Edgar L et al: Meaning-making and psychological adjustment to cancer: development of an intervention and pilot results, *Oncol Nurs Forum* 33(2):291-302, 2006.

Lefler L, Bondy KN: Women's delay in seeking treatment with myocardial infarction: a meta-synthesis, *J Cardiovasc Nurs* 19(4):251-268, 2004.

Lin HR, Bauer-Wu SM: Psycho-spiritual well-being in patients with advanced cancer: an integrative review of the literature, *J Adv Nurs* 44(1):69-80, 2003.

Linhorst DM, Hamilton G, Young E et al: Opportunities and barriers to empowering people with severe mental illness through participation in treatment planning, *Soc Work* 47(4):425-434, 2002.

Lyons KS, Stewart BJ, Archbold PG et al: Pessimism and optimism as early warning signs for compromised health for caregivers of patients with Parkinson's disease, *Nurs Res* 53(6):354-362, 2004.

May TW, Pfafflin M: Psychoeducational programs for patients with epilepsy, *Dis Manage Health Outcomes* 12(3):185-199, 2005.

Miles MS, Burchinal P, Holditch-Davis D et al: Perceptions of stress, worry, and support in black and white mothers of hospitalized, medically fragile infants, *J Pediatr Nurs* 17(2):82-88, 2002.

Miles MS, Holditch-Davis D, Eron A et al: An HIV self-care symptom management intervention for African American mothers, *Nurs Res* 52(6):350-360, 2003.

Montagnino BA, Mauricio RV: The child with a tracheostomy and gastrostomy: parental stress and coping in the home—a pilot study, *Pediatr Nurs* 30(5):373-401, 2004.

Murray BL, Wright K: Integration of a suicide risk assessment and intervention approach: the perspective of youth, *J Psychiatr Ment Health Nurs* 13(2):157-164, 2006.

Nikoletti S, Kristjanson LJ, Tataryn D et al: Information needs and coping styles of primary family caregivers of women following breast cancer surgery, *Oncol Nurs Forum* 30(6):987-996, 2003.

Nokes KM, Chew L, Altman C: Using a telephone support group for HIV-positive persons aged 50+ to increase social support and health-related knowledge, *AIDS Patient Care STDS* 17(7):345-351, 2003.

Northouse L, Walker J, Schafenacker A et al: A family-based program of care for women with recurrent breast cancer and their family members, *Oncol Nurs Forum* 29(10):1411-1419, 2002.

Overcash JA: Using narrative research to understand the quality of life of older women with breast cancer, *Oncol Nurs Forum* 31(6):1153-1159, 2004.

Pakenham KI, Bursnall S: Relations between social support, appraisal, and coping and both positive and negative outcomes for children of a parent with multiple sclerosis and comparisons with children of healthy parents, *Clin Rehab* 20(8):709-723, 2006.

Piamarta F, Iurlaro S, Isella V et al: Unconventional affective symptoms and executive functions after stroke in the elderly, *Arch Gerontol Geriatr Suppl* (9):315-323, 2004.

Potter, J: Fatigue experience in advanced cancer: A phenomenological approach, *Int J Palliat Nurs* 10(1):15-22, 2004.

Puentes WJ: Simple reminiscence: a stress-adaptation model of the phenomenon, *Issues Ment Health Nurs* 23(5):497-511, 2002.

Purnell LD, Paulanka BJ: *Guide to culturally competent health care,* Philadelphia, 2005, FA Davis Company.

Raak R, Hurtig I, Wahren LK: Coping strategies and life satisfaction in subgrouped fibromyalgia patients, *Bio Res Nurs* 4(3):193-202, 2003.

Radina ME, Armer JM, Culbertson SC et al: Post-breast cancer lymphedema: understanding women's knowledge of their condition, *Oncol Nurs Forum* 31(1):97-104, 2004.

Raleigh EDH, Robinson JH, Marold K et al: Family caregiver perception of hospice support, *J Hospice Palliat Nurs* 8(1):25-33, 2006.

Ricauda NA, Bo M, Molaschi M et al: Home hospitalization service for acute uncomplicated first ischemic stroke in elderly patients: a randomized trial, *J Am Geriatr Soc* 52:278-283, 2004.

Richer MC, Ezer H: Living in it, living with it, and moving on: dimensions of meaning during chemotherapy, *Oncol Nurs Forum* 29(1):113-119, 2002.

Schein C, Gagnon AJ, Chan L et al: The association between specific nurse case management interventions and elder health, *J Am Geriatr Soc* 53(4):597-602, 2005.

Schneider SM, Prince-Paul M, Allen JJ et al: Virtual reality as a distraction intervention for women receiving chemotherapy, *Oncol Nurs Forum* 31(1):81-88, 2004.

Sells D, Davidson L, Jewell C et al: The treatment relationship in peer-based and regular case management for clients with severe mental illness, *Psychiatr Serv* 57(8):1179-1184, 2006.

Shibusawa T, Mui AC: Stress, coping and depression among Japanese American elders, *J Gerontol Soc Work* 36(1/2):63, 2001.

Sterling YM, Peterson JW: Characteristics of African American women caregivers of children with asthma, *MCN Am J Matern Child Nurs* 28(1):32-38, 2003.

Stevens S, Sin J: Practice development: implementing a self-management model of relapse prevention for psychosis into routine clinical practice, *J Psychiatr Ment Health Nurs* 12(4):495-501, 2005.

Szanto K, Mulsant BH, Houck P et al: Occurrence and course of suicidality during short-term treatment of late-life depression, *Arch Gen Psychiatry* 60(6):610-617, 2003.

Tacón AM, McComb J, Caldera Y et al: Mindfulness meditation, anxiety reduction, and heart disease: a pilot study, *Fam Community Health* 26(1):25-33, 2003.

Tak SH: An insider perspective of daily stress and coping in elders with arthritis, *Orthop Nurs* 25(2): 27-32, 2006.

Tak YR, McCubbin M: Family stress, perceived social support and coping following the diagnosis of a child's congenital heart disease, *J Adv Nurs* 39(2):190-198, 2002.

Tryssenaar J, Chui A, Finch L: Growing older: the lived experience of older persons with serious mental illness, *Can J Community Ment Health* 22(1):21-36, 2003.

Tyni-Lenne R, Stryjan S, Eriksson B et al: Beneficial therapeutic effects of physical training and relaxation therapy in women with coronary syndrome X, *Physiother Res Int* 7(1):35-43, 2002.

Valente SM: Sexual abuse of boys, *J Child Adolesc Psychiatr Nurs* 18(1):10-16, 2005.

Van P, Meleis AI: Coping with grief after involuntary pregnancy loss: perspectives of African American women, *J Obstet Gynecol Neonatal Nurs* 32(1):28-39, 2003.

Vaughn AA, Roesch SC: Psychological and physical health correlates of coping in minority adolescents, *J Health Psychol* 8(6): 671-683, 2003.

Walker MJ: The effects of nurses' practicing of the HeathTouch Technique on perceived stress, spiritual well-being, and hardiness, *J Holistic Nurs* 24(3):164-175, 2006.

Wassem R, Beckham N, Dudley W: Test of a nursing intervention to promote adjustment to fibromyalgia, *Orthop Nurs* 20(3):33-45, 2001.

Weaver AJ, Flannelly KJ: The role of religion/spirituality for cancer patients and their caregivers, *South Med J* 97(12):1210-1214, 2004.

Weiss SJ, Chen JL: Factors influencing maternal mental health and family functioning during the low birth-weight infant's first year of life, *J Pediatr Nurs* 17(2):114-125, 2002.

White N, Bichter J, Koeckeritz J et al: A cross-cultural comparison of family resiliency in hemodialysis clients, *J Transcult Nurs* 13(3):218-227, 2002.

Ineffective community Coping

Margaret Lunney, RN, PhD, and Dawn Fairlie, MS, ANP, FNP, GNP, CDE

NANDA   Definition

Pattern of community activities for adaptation and problem solving that is unsatisfactory for meeting the demands or needs of the community

Defining Characteristics

Community does not meet its own expectations; deficits in community participation; excessive community conflicts; expressed community powerlessness; expressed vulnerability; high illness rates; increased social problems (e.g., homicides, vandalism, arson, terrorism, robbery, infanticide, abuse, divorce, unemployment, poverty, militancy, mental illness); stressors perceived as excessive

Related Factors (r/t)

Deficits in community social support services; deficits in community social support resources; natural disasters; man-made disasters; inadequate resources for problem solving; ineffective community systems (e.g., lack of emergency medical system, transportation system, or disaster planning systems); nonexistent community systems

NOC   Outcomes (Nursing Outcomes Classification)

Suggested NOC Outcomes

Community Competence, Community Health Status, Community Violence Level

• = Independent;   ▲ = Collaborative;   EBN = Evidence-Based Nursing;   EB = Evidence-Based

C

Community Outcomes

A Broad Range of Community Members Will (Specify Time Frame):

- Participate in community actions to improve power resources
- Develop improved communication among community members
- Participate in problem solving
- Demonstrate cohesiveness in problem solving
- Develop new strategies for problem solving
- Express power to deal with change and manage problems

NIC   Interventions (Nursing Interventions Classification)

Suggested NIC Interventions

Community Health Development, Program Development
NIC Interventions developed for use with individuals can be adapted for use with communities:
Coping Enhancement, Culture Brokerage, Mutual Goal Setting, Support System Enhancement

Nursing Interventions and *Rationales*

NOTE: The diagnosis of **Ineffective Coping** does not apply and should not be used when stress is being imposed by external sources or circumstance. If the community is a victim of circumstances, using the nursing diagnosis **Ineffective Coping** is equivalent to blaming the victim. See the care plans for **Ineffective community Therapeutic regimen management** and **Readiness for enhanced community Coping.**

- Establish a collaborative partnership with the community (see the care plan for **Ineffective community Therapeutic regimen management** for additional references). **EB:** *In a study conducted by Mt. Sinai researchers and clinicians with community leaders of east and central Harlem, the collaborative partnerships of researchers, clinicians, and community leaders were key assets to accomplishing community health goals (Horowitz et al, 2004). Community participation with health providers is an essential aspect of health and development (Sule, 2004).*
- Assist the community with team building. **EB:** *After completing a survey of 105 counties in Kansas, the researcher concluded that "encouraging a team-building approach during coalition development, emphasizing key exercises for coalition cohesion" and so forth may have helped to address some of the limitations reported by communities (Curtis, 2002). A nurse-community health advocate team successfully contributed to the health of urban immigrants (McElmurry, Park & Buseh, 2003).*
- Participate with community members in the identification of stressors and assessment of distress; for example, observe and participate in faith-based organizations that want to improve community stress management. **EBN:** *Health programs in faith-based organizations made a significant difference in health outcomes (DeHaven et al, 2004).*
- Identify community strengths with community members. **EBN:** *In an ethnographic study of health,*

C

environment, culture, and poverty, it was found that community members can describe their strengths and goals for future health-related activities (Bent, 2003).

- Assist community members to articulate the local perspective based on years of experience with the issue or concern. **EB:** *Scientific information may be used to resolve intractable conflicts, but the local experience is also very important but needs to be adequately described (Ozawa, 2006).*

▲ Identify the health services and information resources that are currently available in the community. **EBN:** *Helping a community to cope requires an understanding of the contextual nature of coping, including social, cultural, political, economic, and historical conditions and resources (Donnelly, 2002).*

▲ Consult with community mediation services, for example, the National Association of Community Mediation. **EB:** *In a review of community mediation research, it was shown that using community mediation services effectively resolves conflicts, and many of the resolutions are durable and cost efficient (Hedeen, 2004).*

- Work with community members to increase awareness of ineffective coping behaviors (e.g., conflicts that prevent community members from working together, anger and hate that paralyze the community, health risk behaviors of adolescents). **EBN:** *Problem solving is essential for effective coping. Community members in partnership with providers can modify behaviors that interfere with problem solving (Anderson & McFarlane, 2006; Chinn, 2004).* **EB:** *In a study of 319 college-age students, health risk behaviors were significantly higher for students who were exposed to community violence (Brady, 2006).*

- Provide support to the community and help community members to identify and mobilize additional supports. **EBN:** *In a 13-month three-group randomized clinical trial involving 125 women diagnosed with early-stage breast cancer, women in the two groups that received regular social support reported more positive outcomes, such as less mood disturbance and less loneliness, in the three phases of data collection (Samarel, Tulman & Fawcett, 2002). Often people need help in mobilizing supports that are available (Pender, Murdaugh & Parsons, 2006).*

- Use focus group methods to evaluate and strengthen interventions. **EBN:** *Focus group methodology strengthened population interventions in a Medicaid managed care population in Nebraska (Kaiser, Barry & Kaiser, 2002).*

- Use mentoring strategies for community members. **EBN:** *In a focus group study of 43 African-American teens and adults on the community problem of teenage pregnancy, the participants selected mentoring as a strategy to teach, counsel, and provide information (Tabi, 2002).*

- Advocate for the community in multiple arenas (e.g., television, newspapers, and governmental agencies). **EBN:** *Advocacy is a specific form of caring that enhances power resources for community coping (Anderson & McFarlane, 2006).* **EB:** *Increased state level support could help communities who did not complete health assessments (Curtis, 2002).*

- Work with community groups to improve the economic status and reduce unemployment. **EB:** *Analysis of population and labor force data from 1992 to 2002 indicated a strong significant correlation of penetrating trauma/crime indices and economic conditions, including unemployment (Cinat et al, 2004).*

- Write grant proposals to help community members obtain funds for programs that reduce stress or improve coping. (See Coley & Scheinberg, 2007, for program proposal-writing methods.) **EBN:** *The programs that are necessary may be expensive, and often funds may not be available without the assistance of public or privately funded grants (Anderson & McFarland, 2006).*

- Work with members of the community to identify and develop coping strategies that promote a sense of power (e.g., obtaining sources for funding, collaborating with other communities). **EBN:** *In a study of 39 blind subjects, those experiencing power as defined by Barrett's theory of power (power is being aware of what one is choosing to do, feeling free to do it, and doing it intentionally) reported better emotional and general health than individuals lacking power (Leksell et al, 2001). A first step in power enhancement is for the community to identify and develop its own coping strategies (Anderson & McFarlane, 2006).*

- Obtain police support for community partnerships aimed at healthy coping. **EB:** *Police programs have led to innovative programs that contribute to community health (Frommer & Papouchado, 2000).*

- Engage emotions during conflict mediation. **EB:** *An experienced mediator recommended that specific strategies can be used to engage the emotions that are present in conflict. Suggested strategies in the realm of art, rituals, and joking help to create a space in which new understandings can develop (Maiese, 2006).*

• = Independent;   ▲ = Collaborative;   EBN = Evidence-Based Nursing;   EB = Evidence-Based

- Protect children from exposure to community conflicts. **EB:** *Children exposed to community conflict have permanent negative effects from exposure to community conflicts, including increased health risk behaviors (Brady, 2006), increased physical symptoms (Wilson, Rosenthal & Austin, 2005), and psychological distress (Rosenthal & Wilson, 2003).*

 ### Multicultural

- Acknowledge the stressors unique to racial/ethnic communities. **EBN:** *Targeted alcohol and tobacco marketing, high levels of unemployment, lack of health insurance, and racism are stressors unique to culturally diverse communities (D'Avanzo et al, 2001).* **EBN:** *Socioeconomic status, geographical location, and risks associated with health seeking behavior all influence the likelihood that clients will seek health care and be compliant with a regimen they are given (Appel, Giger & Davidhizar, 2005).*
- Work with members of the community to prioritize and target health goals specific to the community. **EB:** *Such prioritization and targeting will increase feelings of control over and sense of ownership of programs (Anderson & McFarlane, 2006; Chinn, 2004; National Institutes of Health, 1998).*
- Approach community leaders and members of color with respect, warmth, and professional courtesy. **EBN:** *Instances of disrespect and lack of caring have special significance for individuals of color (D'Avanzo et al, 2001).*
- Establish and sustain partnerships with key individuals within communities when developing and implementing programs. **EBN:** *Local leaders are excellent sources of information and their participation will enhance the credibility of programs (National Institutes of Health, 1998).*
- Use community church settings as a forum for advocacy, teaching, and program implementation. **EBN:** *Evaluation of a faith-based program supplied to 125 people from 18 congregations showed an increase in health promotion knowledge, rise in consumer satisfaction, and improvement in health (Kotecki, 2002). A literature review of church-based health promotion programs showed that they are successful in helping people to adopt health-promoting behaviors (Peterson, Atwood & Yates, 2002). Church-based programs are especially effective in communities of color.*
- Ask political leaders to become part of the partnership process. **EB:** *The Carnegie Commission on Preventing Deadly Conflict established the importance of political leaders' working to prevent community conflicts and violence (Hamburg, George & Ballentine, 1999).*

 ### Community Teaching

- Teach strategies for stress management.
- Explain the relationship between enhancing power resources and coping.

evolve See the EVOLVE website for World Wide Web resources for client education.

REFERENCES

Anderson ET, McFarlane J: *Community as partner: theory and practice in nursing,* ed 5, Philadelphia, 2006, Lippincott Williams & Wilkins.

Appel SJ, Giger JN, Davidhizar RE: Opportunity cost: the impact of contextual risk factors on the cardiovascular health of low-income rural southern African-American women, *J Cardiovasc Nurs* 20:315-324, 2005.

Bent KN: "The people know what they want": an empowerment process of sustainable, ecological community health, *Adv Nurs Science* 26(3):215-226, 2003.

Brady SS: Lifetime community violence exposure and health risk behavior among young adults in college, *J Adolesc Health* 39:610-613, 2006.

Chinn PL: *Peace and power: creative leadership for building community,* ed 6, Boston, 2004, Jones & Bartlett.

Cinat ME, Wilson SE, Lush S et al: Significant correlation of trauma epidemiology with economic conditions of a community, *Arch Surg* 139(12):1350-1355, 2004.

Coley SM, Scheinberg CA: *Proposal writing,* ed 3, Thousand Oaks, CA, 2007, Sage.

Curtis DC: Evaluation of community health assessment in Kansas, *J Public Health Manag Pract* 8(4):20-25, 2002.

D'Avanzo CE et al: Developing culturally informed strategies for substance-related interventions. In Naegle MA, D'Avanzo CE, editors: *Addictions and substance abuse: strategies for advanced practice nursing,* St Louis, 2001, Mosby.

DeHaven MJ, Hunter IB, Wilder L et al: Health programs in faith-based organizations: are they effective? *Am J Pubic Health* 94:1030-1036, 2004.

Donnelly TT: Contextual analysis of coping: implications for immigrants' mental health care, *Issues Ment Health Nurs* 23(7):715, 2002.

Frommer P, Papouchado K: Police as contributors to healthy communities: Aiken, South Carolina, *Public Health Rep* 115(2-3):249, 2000.

Hamburg DA, George A, Ballentine K: Preventing deadly conflict: the critical role of leadership, *Arch Gen Psychiatry* 56(11):971, 1999.

Hedeen T: The evolution and evaluation of community mediation: limited research suggests unlimited progress, *Conflict Resolut Q* 22(1/2):101-113, 2004.

Horowitz CR, Arniella A, James S et al: Using community-based participatory research to reduce health disparities in East and Central Harlem, *Mt Sinai J Med* 71(6):368-374, 2004.

Kaiser MM, Barry TL, Kaiser KL: Using focus groups to evaluate and strengthen public health nursing population-focused interventions, *J Transcult Nurs* 13(4):303, 2002.

Kotecki CN: Developing a health promotion program for faith-based communities, *Holist Nurs Pract* 16(3):61, 2002.

Leksell JK, Johansson I, Wibell LB et al: Power and self-perceived health in blind diabetic and nondiabetic individuals, *J Adv Nurs* 34(4):511-519, 2001.

Maiese M: Engaging the emotions in conflict intervention, *Conflict Resolut Q* 24(2):187-195, 2006.

McElmurry BJ, Park CG, Buseh AG: The nurse-community health advocate team for urban immigrant primary health care, *J Nurs Schol* 35(3):275-281, 2003.

National Institutes of Health: *Salud para su corazon: bringing heart health to Latinos: a guide for building community programs,* DHHS Pub No 98-3796, Washington, DC, 1998, US Government Printing Office.

Ozawa CP: Science and intractable conflict, *Conflict Resolut Q* 24:197-205, 2006.

Pender NJ, Murdaugh CL, Parsons MA: *Health promotion in nursing practice,* ed 5, Upper Saddle River, NJ, 2006, Prentice Hall.

Peterson J, Atwood JR, Yates B: Key elements for church-based health promotion programs: outcome-based literature review, *Public Health Nurs* 19(6):401, 2002.

Rosenthal BS, Wilson WC: The association of ecological variables and psychological distress with exposure to community violence among adolescents, *Adolescence* 38(151):459-479, 2003.

Samarel N, Tulman L, Fawcett J: Effects of two types of social support and education on adaptation to early-stage breast cancer, *Res Nurs Health* 25(6):459, 2002.

Sule SS: Community participation in health and development, *Niger J Med* 13:276-281, 2004.

Tabi MM: Community perspective on a model to reduce teenage pregnancy, *J Adv Nurs* 40(3):275, 2002.

Wilson WC, Rosenthal BS, Austin S: Exposure to community violence and upper respiratory illness in older adolescents, *J Adolesc Health* 36:313-319, 2005.

Readiness for enhanced Coping   Gail B. Ladwig, MSN, CHTP, RN

NANDA   Definition

Pattern of cognitive and behavioral efforts to manage demands that is sufficient for well-being and can be strengthened

Defining Characteristics

Acknowledges power; aware of possible environmental changes; defines stressors as manageable; seeks knowledge of new strategies; seeks social support; uses a broad range of emotion-oriented strategies; uses a broad range of strategies; uses spiritual resources

NOC   Outcomes (Nursing Outcomes Classification)

Suggested NOC Outcomes

Coping, Personal Well-Being, Social Interaction Skills, Quality of life

Example NOC Outcome with Indicators
Coping as evidenced by the following indicator: Identifies effective coping patterns/Uses effective coping strategies (Rate the outcome and indicators of **Coping:** 1 = never demonstrated, 2 = rarely demonstrated, 3 = sometimes demonstrated, 4 = often demonstrated, 5 = consistently demonstrated [see Section I].)

Client Outcomes

Client Will (Specify Time Frame):

- Verbalize ability to cope and ask for help when needed
- Demonstrate ability to solve problems related to current needs
- Communicate needs and negotiate with others to meet needs
- State that stressors are manageable
- Demonstrate new effective coping strategies
- Seek social support for problems associated with coping
- Seek spiritual support of personal choice

NIC   Interventions (Nursing Interventions Classification)

Suggested NIC Interventions

Coping Enhancement, Decision-Making Support

Example NIC Activities—Coping Enhancement
Assist patient in developing an objective appraisal of the event; Explore with client previous methods of dealing with life problems

Nursing Interventions and *Rationales*

- Observe for strengths such as the ability to relate the facts and to recognize the source of stressors. **EBN:** *Successful adaptation requires a coordination of efforts to fit the nursing interventions to the client's perception of the threat, personal values and beliefs, and recognition of personal strengths (Norris & Spelic, 2002).*
- Use empathetic communication and encourage the client and family to verbalize fears, express emotions, and set goals. Be present for clients physically or by telephone. **EBN:** *This study of social support by telephone demonstrated that therapeutic presence facilitated Outcomes that include problem solving, adaptive behavior change, and diminished distress (Finfgeld-Connett, 2005). Presence involves knowing the uniqueness of the person, listening intently, and mutually defining changes in the provision of confident caring (Caldwell et al, 2005).*
- Help the client set realistic goals and identify personal skills and knowledge. **EBN and EB:** *Efforts to educate the client regarding possible and/or potential effects of a specific diagnosis and the resources available to assist with coping are a positive factor in successful adaptation (Wassem, Beckham & Dudley, 2001).*
- Encourage expression of positive thoughts and emotions. **EB:** *Positive emotions initiate upward spirals toward enhanced emotional well-being (Fredrickson & Joiner, 2002).* **EBN:** *This study shows that clients believe that coping is important to their well-being (Edgar & Watt, 2004).*
- Encourage the use of cognitive behavioral relaxation (e.g., music therapy, guided imagery). **EBN:** *Relaxation training has been demonstrated to improve overall coping ability (Tyni-Lenne et al, 2002).*
- ▲ Refer for cognitive behavioral therapy. **EBN:** *A cognitive behavioral nursing program was effective in increasing adjustment to fibromyalgia (Wassem et al, 2001).*
- Encourage the client to use spiritual coping mechanisms such as faith and prayer. **EBN:** *Prayer is a powerful way of coping and is practiced by all Western religions and several Eastern traditions (Mohr, 2006).*
- Help the client with depression to maintain social support networks or assist in building new ones. **EBN:** *An important task for the nurse is to support the client in maintaining the client's existing social network or in building a new one (Skarsater et al, 2003).*
- ▲ Consider a workplace stress management program to enhance coping skills. **EB:** *A work site program that focuses on stress, anxiety, and coping measurement along with small group educational intervention can significantly reduce illness and health care use (Rahe et al, 2002).*
- ▲ Refer the client with breast cancer to a psychosocial group intervention for coping skills training, stress management, relaxation exercises, and psychosocial support. **EB:** *In women with primary breast carcinoma, a psychosocial group intervention reduced psychological distress and enhanced coping (Schulz, 2001).*
- Refer to the care plans for **Readiness for enhanced Communication** and **Readiness for enhanced Spiritual well-being.**

Pediatric

- Encourage exercise for children and adolescents to promote positive self-esteem, to enhance coping, and to prevent behavioral and psychological problems. **EBN:** *Exercise has positive short-term effects on self-esteem in children and young people (Ekeland et al, 2004).*

Geriatric

- Consider the use of telephone support for caregivers of family members with dementia. **EBN and EB:** *Family caregivers can be helped through a variety of social support mechanisms including telephone support (Chang et al, 2004; Belle et al, 2006).*
- ▲ Refer the client with Alzheimer's disease who is terminally ill to hospice. **EBN:** *Home care and hospice nurses can provide invaluable care in helping families cope with this disease and end-of-life issues (Head, 2003).*
- ▲ Refer the widowed older client to self-help support groups. **EBN:** *Bereaved older clients who attended face-to-face support groups for 20 weeks reported increased hope, improved skills in developing social relationships, enhanced coping, new role identities, and less loneliness (Stewart et al, 2001).*

Multicultural

- Encourage spirituality as a source of support for coping. **EBN:** *Many African-Americans and Latinos identify spirituality, religiousness, prayer, and church-based approaches as coping resources (Abrums, 2004; Coon et al, 2004; Weaver & Flannelly, 2004).*
- Refer to care plans for **Ineffective Coping**

Home Care

- The interventions described previously may be adapted for home care use.
- Observe the family for coping behavior patterns. Obtain family and client history as possible. **EBN:** *Family assessment is necessary to guide interventions (Weiss & Chen, 2002; Northouse et al, 2002).*
- Encourage the client to use self-care management to increase the experience of personal control. Identify with the client all available supports and sense of attachment to others. **EBN:** *In heart transplantation clients, personal control was positively associated with optimism, well-being, and satisfaction with life, and was negatively associated with anger and depression (Bohachick et al, 2002).*
- ▲ Refer the client and family to support groups. **EBN:** *Support groups provide an essential resource to clients and their families when adapting to health status change (Fung & Chien, 2002).*
- ▲ Refer the client for a behavioral program that teaches coping skills via "Lifeskills" workshop and/ or video. **EB:** *This study demonstrated that a commercially available, facilitator- or self-administered behavioral training product can have significant beneficial effects on psychosocial well-being in a healthy community sample (Kirby et al, 2006).*
- ▲ Refer combat veterans and service members directly involved in combat as well as those providing support to combatants, including nurses for mental health services. **EBN:** *Early identification and treatment of mental health problems may decrease the psychosocial impact of combat and thus prevent progression to more chronic and severe psychopathology such as depression and post-traumatic stress disorder (PTSD) (Gaylord, 2006).* **EB:** *Combat duty in Iraq was associated with high utilization of mental health services and attrition from military service after deployment (Hoge, Auchterlonie & Milliken, 2006).*

Client/Family Teaching

- Teach relaxation techniques. **EBN:** *Relaxation training has been demonstrated to improve self-efficacy in family caregivers of clients with Alzheimer's disease (Fisher & Laschinger, 2001).*
- ▲ Teach the client about available community resources (e.g., therapists, ministers, counselors, self-help groups). **EBN:** *Families need assistance in coping with health changes. The nurse is often perceived as the individual who can help them obtain necessary social support (Tak & McCubbin, 2002; Northouse et al, 2002).*

 See the EVOLVE website for World Wide Web resources for client education.

REFERENCES

Refer to **ineffective Coping** for additional references.

Abrums M: Faith and feminism: how African American women from a storefront church resist oppression in healthcare, *Adv Nurs Science* 27(3):187-201, 2004.

Belle S, Burgio L, Burns R et al: Enhancing the quality of life of dementia caregivers from different ethnic or racial groups: a randomized, controlled trial, *Ann Intern Med* 145(10):727-738, 2006.

Bohachick P, Taylor MV, Sereika S et al: Social support, personal control, and psychological recovery following heart transplant, *Clin Nurs Res* 11(1):34-51, 2002.

Caldwell B, Dolye M, Morris M et al: Presencing: channeling therapeutic effectiveness with the mentally ill in a state psychiatric hospital, *Issues Ment Health Nurs* 26:853-871, 2005.

Chang BL, Nitta S, Carter PA et al: Technology innovations. Perceived helpfulness of telephone calls: providing support for care-givers of family members with dementia, *J Gerontol Nurs* 30(9):14-21, 2004.

Coon DW, Rubert M, Solano N et al: Well-being, appraisal, and coping in Latina and Caucasian female dementia caregivers: findings from the REACH study, *Aging Ment Health* 8(4):330-345, 2004.

Edgar L, Watt S: Nucare, a coping skills training intervention for oncology patients and families: participants' motivations and expectations, *Can Oncol Nurs J* 14(2):84-95, 2004.

Ekeland E, Heian F, Hagen KB et al: Exercise to improve self-esteem in children and young people, *Cochrane Database Syst Rev* (1): CD003683, 2004.

Finfgeld-Connett D: Telephone social support or nursing presence? Analysis of a nursing intervention, *Qual Health Res* 15(1):19-29, 2005.

Fisher PA, Laschinger HS: A relaxation training program to increase self-efficacy for anxiety control in Alzheimer family caregivers, *Holist Nurs Pract* 15(2):47, 2001.

Fredrickson BL, Joiner T: Positive emotions trigger upward spirals toward emotional well-being, *Psychol Sci* 13(2):172, 2002.

Fung WY, Chien WT: The effectiveness of a mutual support group for family caregivers of a relative with dementia, *Arch Psychiatr Nurs* 26(3):134, 2002.

Gaylord KM: The psychosocial effects of combat: the frequently unseen injury, *Crit Care Nurs Clin North Am* 18(3):349-357, 2006.

Head G: Palliative care for persons with dementia, *Home Healthc Nurse* 21(1):53, 2003.

Hoge CW, Auchterlonie JL, Milliken CS: Mental health problems, use of mental health services, and attrition from military service after returning from deployment to Iraq or Afghanistan, *JAMA* 295(9):1023-1032, 2006.

Kirby ED, Williams VP, Hocking MC et al: Psychosocial benefits of three formats of a standardized behavioral stress management program, *Psychosom Med* 68(6):816-823, 2006.

Mohr WK: Spiritual issues in psychiatric care, *Perspect Psychiatr Care* 42(3)174-183, 2006.

Norris J, Spelic SS: Supporting adaptation to body image disruption, *Rehabil Nurs* 27(1):8, 2002.

Northouse LL, Mood D, Kershaw T et al: Quality of life of women with recurrent breast cancer and their family members, *J Clin Oncol* 20(19):4050-4064, 2002.

Rahe RH, Taylor CB, Tolles RL et al: A novel stress and coping workplace program reduces illness and healthcare utilization, *Psychosom Med* 64(2):278-286, 2002.

Schulz K: A psychosocial group intervention reduced psychological distress and enhanced coping in primary breast cancer, *Evid Based Ment Health* 4(1):15, 2001.

Skarsater I, Dencker K, Haggstrom L et al: A salutogenetic perspective on how men cope with major depression in daily life, with the help of professional and lay support, *Int J Nurs Stud* 40(2):153, 2003.

Stewart M, Craig D, MacPherson K et al: Promoting positive affect and diminishing loneliness of widowed seniors through a support intervention, *Public Health Nurs* 18(1):54, 2001.

Tak YR, McCubbin M: Family stress, perceived social support and coping following the diagnosis of a child's congenital heart disease, *J Adv Nurs* 39(2):190, 2002.

Tyni-Lenne R, Stryjan S, Eriksson B et al: Beneficial therapeutic effects of physical training and relaxation therapy in women with coronary syndrome X, *Physiother Res Int* 7(1):35-43, 2002.

Wassem R, Beckham N, Dudley W: Test of a nursing intervention to promote adjustment to fibromyalgia, *Orthop Nurs* 20(3):33-45, 2001.

Weaver AJ, Flannelly KJ: The role of religion/spirituality for cancer patients and their caregivers, *South Med J* 97(12):1210-1214, 2004.

Weiss SJ, Chen JL: Factors influencing maternal mental health and family functioning during the low birth-weight infant's first year of life, *J Pediatr Nurs* 17(2):114, 2002.

Readiness for enhanced community Coping

Margaret Lunney, RN, PhD, and Dawn Fairlie, MS, ANP, FNP, GNP, CDE

NANDA   Definition

Pattern of community activities for adaptation and problem solving that is satisfactory for meeting the demands or needs of the community but that can be improved for management of current and future problems/stressors

Defining Characteristics

One or more characteristics that indicate effective coping: Active planning by community for predicted stressors; active problem solving by community when faced with issues; agreement that community is responsible for stress management; positive communication among community members;

C

positive communication between community/aggregates and larger community; programs available for recreation; programs available for relaxation; resources sufficient for managing stressors

Related Factors (r/t)

Community has sense of power to manage stressors; resources available for problem solving; social supports available

NOC   Outcomes (Nursing Outcomes Classification)

Suggested NOC Outcomes

Community Competence, Community Health Status

Example NOC Outcome with Indicators
Community Health Status as evidenced by the following indicators: Prevalence of health promotion programs/Health status of infants, children, adolescents, adults, elders/Attendance at programs for healthy states (Rate the outcome and indicators of **Community Health Status:** 1 = poor, 2 = fair, 3 = good, 4 = very good, 5 = excellent [see Section I].)

Community Outcomes

Community Will (Specify Time Frame):

- Develop enhanced coping strategies
- Maintain effective coping strategies for management of stress

NIC   Interventions (Nursing Interventions Classification)

Suggested NIC Interventions

Environmental Management: Community, Health Policy Monitoring
NIC Interventions developed for use with individuals can be adapted for use with communities: Coping Enhancement, Culture Brokerage, Mutual Goal Setting, Support System Enhancement

Example NIC Activities—Coping Enhancement
Explore with community members previous methods of dealing with life problems; Assist the community to solve problems in a constructive manner

Nursing Interventions and *Rationales*

NOTE: Interventions depend on the specific aspects of community coping that can be enhanced (e.g., planning for stress management, communication, development of community power, community perceptions of stress, community coping strategies). Nursing interventions are conducted in collaboration with key members of the community, community/public health nurses, and members of other disciplines (Anderson & McFarlane, 2006).

- Describe the roles of community/public health nurses in working with healthy communities. **EBN:** *Nurses at general and specialists' levels (bachelor's and master's degrees) have significant roles in helping communities to achieve optimum health, including coping with stress (Chinn, 2004; Logan, 2005; Stanhope & Lancaster, 2006).*
- Help the community to obtain funds for additional programs. (See Coley & Scheinberg, 2007, for proposal-writing methods.) **EBN:** *Healthy communities may need additional funding sources to strengthen community resources (Anderson & McFarlane, 2006; Chinn, 2004).*
- Encourage positive attitudes toward the community through the media and other sources. **EB:** *Negative attitudes or stigmas create additional stress and deficits in social support (Anderson & McFarlane, 2006; Chinn, 2004; Stanhope & Lancaster, 2006).*

- Help community members to collaborate with one another for power enhancement and coping skills. **EBN:** *Community members may not have sufficient skills to collaborate for enhanced coping. Healthcare providers can promote effective collaboration skills (Anderson & McFarlane, 2006; Chinn, 2004).*
- Assist community members with cognitive skills and habits of mind for problem solving. **EBN:** *The cognitive skills and habits of mind of critical thinking support problem-solving ability (Rubenfeld & Scheffer, 2006).*
- Demonstrate optimum use of the power resources. **EBN:** *Optimum use of power resources and working for community empowerment supports coping (Bent, 2003; Chinn, 2004).*
- Reduce poverty whenever possible. **EB:** *Public health studies in most countries of the world show that poverty is an important predictor of health status in all categories (Wagstaff et al, 2004). Socioeconomic inequalities are most likely relevant to the health of people in all age groups.*
- ▲ Collaborate with community members to improve educational levels within the community. **EBN:** *In many population level studies, educational levels were associated with stress, health disparities, and increased illness (Park et al, 2006). For example, in an analysis of mortality data in Wisconsin from 1990-2000, there was a graded associated between education and premature mortality (Reither et al, 2006).*

Multicultural

Refer to care plan **Ineffective community Coping**

Community Teaching

- Review coping skills, power for coping, and the use of power resources.

evolve   See the EVOLVE website for World Wide Web resources for client education.

REFERENCES

Refer to Coping, Community, ineffective for additional references.

Anderson ET, McFarlane J: *Community as partner: theory and practice in nursing,* ed 4, Philadelphia, 2006, Lippincott Williams & Wilkins.

Bent KN: "The people know what they want": an empowerment process of sustainable ecological community health, *Adv Nurs Sci* 26(3):215-226, 2003.

Chinn PL: *Peace and power: creative leadership for building community,* ed 6, Boston: 2004, Jones and Bartlett.

Coley SM, Scheinberg CA: *Proposal writing,* ed 3, Thousand Oaks, CA, 2007, Sage.

Logan L: The practice of certified community health CNSs, *Clin Nurse Spec* 19(1):43-48, 2005.

Park MJ, Yun KE, Lee GE, Cho HJ, Park HS: A cross-sectional study of socioeconomic status and the metabolic syndrome in Korean adults. *Ann Epidemiol Feb 12,* epub. 20076

Reither EN, Peppard PE, Remington PL, Kindig DA: Increasing educational disparities in premature adult mortality, Wisconsin, 1990-2000. *WMJ* 105(7), 38-41, 2006.

Rubenfeld MG, Scheffer BK: *Critical thinking TACTICS for nurses,* Boston, 2006, Jones and Bartlett.

Stanhope M, Lancaster J: *Foundations of nursing in the community: community-oriented approach,* ed 2, St. Louis, 2006, Mosby.

Wagstaff A, Bustreo F, Bryce J et al: Child health: reaching the poor, *Am J Public Health* 94(5):726-736, 2004.

Readiness for enhanced family Coping   *Keith A. Anderson, MSW, and Joseph E. Gaugler, PhD*

NANDA   Definition

Effective management of adaptive tasks by family member involved with client's health challenge, who now exhibits desire and readiness for enhanced health and growth with regard to self and in relation to client

Defining Characteristics

Individual expresses interest in making contact with others who have experienced a similar situation; family member attempts to describe growth impact of crisis; family member moves in direction of enriching lifestyle; family member moves in direction of health promotion; chooses experiences that optimize wellness

Related Factors (r/t)

Adaptive tasks effectively addressed to enable goals of self-actualization to surface; needs sufficiently gratified to enable goals of self-actualization to surface

NOC   Outcomes (Nursing Outcomes Classification)

Suggested NOC Outcomes

Family Coping, Health-Seeking Behavior, Participation in Healthcare Decisions

Example NOC Outcome with Indicators
Coping as evidenced by the following indicators: Shares responsibility for family tasks/Manages family problems/Seeks family assistance when appropriate (Rate the outcome and indicators of Family **Coping:** 1 = never demonstrated; 2 = rarely demonstrated; 3 = sometimes demonstrated; 4 = often demonstrated; 5 = constantly demonstrated [see Section I].)

Client Outcomes

Family Will (Specify Time Frame):

• State a plan for growth
• Perform tasks needed for change
• State positive effects of changes made

NIC   Interventions (Nursing Interventions Classification)

Suggested NIC Interventions

Family Integration Promotion, Family Involvement Promotion, Family Support, Mutual Goal Setting

Example NIC Activities—Family Support
Facilitate communication of concerns and feelings between clients and family or among family members; Identify and respect family's coping mechanisms

Nursing Interventions and *Rationales*

Refer to **Compromised family Coping,** for additional interventions

• Assess the structure, resources, and coping abilities of families. **EBN:** *The utilization of established assessment instruments (e.g., Calgary Family Assessment Model) can provide insight into family dynamics and the coping styles and resources of family systems (Wright & Leahey, 2005).*
• Establish rapport with families through effective and accurate communication. **EBN:** *Rapport and working relationships with families can be established and enhanced by providing timely and accurate information via functional communication patterns, thereby empowering families through knowledge (Rose, Mallinson & Walton-Moss, 2004).*
▲ Encourage family caregivers to become involved with mutual support groups. **EBN:** *Mutual support groups for family caregivers have been found to be associated with decreased levels of caregiver burden and increased family functioning by providing interactions and support from other families in similar situations (Chien, Norman & Thompson, 2004).*
▲ Develop and encourage the use of counseling services for family caregivers. **EBN:** *Counseling and specialist educational services for family caregivers may be effective in improving the emotional state and quality of life for caregivers and increasing satisfaction with care and caregiver knowledge through the provision of expert services (Visser-Meily et al, 2005).*
• Provide family-focused education to family caregivers to encourage adherence to medical care plans. **EBN:** *Family education and support interventions for clients and their family caregivers have been found to increase the adherence of clients to medical care plans (Dunbar et al, 2005).*

• = Independent;   ▲ = Collaborative;   EBN = Evidence-Based Nursing;   EB = Evidence-Based

C

- Acknowledge the importance of cultural influences and ensure assessment tools are culturally appropriate. **EBN:** *Culture may impact the psychometric properties of assessment tools and should be considered when employing nursing assessments of families (Chen et al, 2003; Friedemann et al, 2003).*
- Develop and implement psycho-educational interventions for family members and clients to improve overall functioning, coping, and health outcomes. **EBN:** *Comprehensive psycho-educational interventions for clients and their partner/spouses that build knowledge and lend support have been associated with higher levels of well-being, better couple communication, higher self-efficacy, and improved mental health status (Karlson et al, 2004).*
- Increase the use of technology in providing supportive and educational services to family members. **EB:** *Web-based psycho-educational intervention for clients and their families may be effective in lowering perceived stress in clients and improving perceived social support by providing enhanced access to information and alternative avenues of communication (Rotondi et al, 2005).*
- ▲ Identify and refer to support groups that discuss problems and concerns similar to those faced by the family (e.g., Alzheimer's Association; MUMS – National Parent to Parent Network; OncoChat–Online cancer support for clients, families, and friends). *Participation with such groups can provide families with a venue to discuss the issues and concerns faced by others in similar situations.*

Pediatric

- Provide expecting parents with educational resources and support to encourage the use of prenatal health services. **EBN:** *Comprehensive parenting education programs (incorporating interventions such as home visits and hospital-based group sessions) for expecting mothers that emphasize the importance of prenatal care have been related to increased infant wellness care and an increased adherence to age-appropriate immunizations (El-Mohandes et al, 2003).*
- Implement developmentally supportive family-centered services for infants and their caregivers. **EBN:** *Developmentally supportive family care interventions that are individualized to the specific needs of families have been found to be associated with lower levels of stress in infants and less use of sedatives/narcotics and vasopressors (Byers et al, 2006).*
- Empower parental caregivers through educational and behavioral enhancement programs. **EBN:** *Preventative, educational-behavioral programs for parental caregivers of critically ill children have been associated with improvements in maternal functioning and emotional coping outcomes, as well as fewer child adjustment problems (Melnyk et al, 2004).*
- Employ family support programs that deliver services in multiple formats to maximize potential efficacy. **EB:** *Multi-format support interventions for children with chronic illness and their mothers have been found to have positive effects in promoting mental health and adjustment in children through the incorporation of multiple formats (e.g., telephone, face-to-face meetings, group events) (Chernoff et al, 2002).*

Geriatric

- Encourage family caregivers to participate in supportive counseling programs. **EB:** *Supportive counseling interventions for family caregivers of clients with Alzheimer's disease have been found to be related to sustained reduction in depressive symptoms in caregivers (Mittelman et al, 2004).*
- Encourage family caregivers to become involved with mutual support groups. **EBN:** *Participation in mutual support groups for family caregivers of relatives with dementia has been associated with decreased stress levels and higher quality of life for caregivers by providing family members with peer support and informal information networks (Fung & Chien, 2002).*
- ▲ Provide psychosocial services to family caregivers that focus on skill-building, information, and support. **EBN:** *Caregiver interventions that focus on skill-building and supportive-educational programs can be effective in lowering depressive symptoms in caregivers of older adult family members with dementia (Farran et al, 2004).*
- Older adults living in residential facilities should be provided with companion animals and plants and frequent visits with children. *In this study these interventions helped to reduce loneliness, helplessness, and boredom. Family involvement should be encouraged (Robinson & Rosher, 2006).*
- Enhance the coping abilities of family caregivers of relatives living in long-term care settings.

D

EBN: *Participation in empowerment intervention programs for family caregivers of residents with dementia living in long-term care has been associated with greater competence in dealing with nursing home staff members and addressing the challenges of the caregiver role (Ducharme et al, 2005).*

- Provide psycho-educational support for family members providing end-of-life care in the home setting. **EBN:** *Psycho-educational interventions for family caregivers providing palliative care to clients dying at home found that participation was associated with more positive experiences and rewards in the caregiver role (Hudson, Aranda & Hayman-White, 2005).*

Multicultural, Home Care, and Client/Family Teaching

Refer to **Family coping, compromised** for additional interventions

evolve   See the EVOLVE website for World Wide Web resources for client education.

REFERENCES

Byers JF, Lowman LB, Francis J et al: A quasi-experimental trial on individualized, developmentally supportive family-centered care, *J Obstet Gynecol Neonatal Nurs* 35(1):105-115, 2006.

Chen JL, Kennedy C, Kools S et al: Culturally appropriate family assessment: analysis of the Family Assessment Device in a pediatric Chinese population, *J Nurs Measure* 11(1):41-59, 2003.

Chernoff RG, Ireys HT, DeVet KA et al: A randomized, controlled trial of a community-based support program for families of children with chronic illness: pediatric outcomes, *Arch Pediatr Adolesc Med* 15(6):533-539, 2002.

Chien WT, Norman I, Thompson DR: A randomized controlled trial of a mutual support group for family caregivers of patients with schizophrenia, *Int J Nurs Stud* 41:637-649, 2004.

Ducharme F, Levesque L, Lachance L et al: "Taking care of myself": efficacy of an intervention programme for caregivers of a relative with dementia living in a long-term care setting, *Dementia* 4(1):23-47, 2005.

Dunbar SB, Clark PC, Deaton C et al: Family education and support interventions in heart failure, *Nurs Res* 54(3):158-166, 2005.

El-Mohandes AAE, Katz KS, El-Khorazaty MN et al: The effect of a parenting education program on the use of preventative pediatric health care services among low-income, minority mothers: a randomized, controlled study, *Pediatrics* 111(6):1324-1332, 2003.

Farran CJ, Gilley DW, McCann JJ et al: Psychosocial interventions to reduce depressive symptoms of dementia caregivers: a randomized clinical trial comparing two approaches, *J Mental Health Aging* 10(4):337-350, 2004.

Friedemann ML, Astedt-Kurki P, Paavilainen E: Development of a family assessment instrument for transcultural use, *J Transcult Nurs* 14(2):90-99, 2003.

Fung WY, Chien WT: The effectiveness of a mutual support group for family caregivers of a relative with dementia, *Arch Psychiatr Nurs* 16(3):134-144, 2002.

Hudson PL, Aranda S, Hayman-White K: A psycho-educational intervention for family caregivers of patients receiving palliative care: a randomized controlled trial, *J Pain Sympt Manag* 30(4):329-341, 2005.

Karlson EW, Liang MH, Eaton H et al: A randomized clinical trial of a psychoeducational intervention to improve outcomes in systemic lupus erythematosus, *Arthritis Rheum* 50(6):1832-1841, 2004.

Melnyk BM, Alpert-Gillis L, Feinstein NF et al: Creating opportunities for parent empowerment: program effects on the mental health/coping outcomes of critically ill young children and their mothers, *Pediatrics* 113(6Suppl):e597-607, 2004.

Mittelman MS, Roth DL, Coon DW et al: Sustained benefit of supportive intervention for depressive symptoms in caregivers of patients with Alzheimer's disease, *Am J Psychiatry* 161(5):850-856, 2004.

Robinson S, Rosher R: Tangling with the barriers to culture change, *J Gerontol Nurs* 32(10):19-26, 2006.

Rose LE, Mallinson RK, Walton-Moss B: Barriers to family care in psychiatric settings, *J Nurs Scholarsh* 36(1):39-47, 2004.

Rotondi AJ, Haas JL, Anderson CM et al: A clinical trial to test the feasibility of a telehealth psychoeducational intervention for persons with schizophrenia and their families: intervention and 3-month findings, *Rehab Psychol* 50(4):325-336, 2005.

Visser-Meily A, van Heugten C, Post M et al: Intervention studies for caregivers of stroke survivors: a critical review, *Patient Educ Couns* 56(3):257-267, 2005.

Wright LM, Leahey M: *Nurses and families: a guide to family assessment and intervention,* ed 4, Philadelphia, 2005, FA Davis.

Risk For sudden infant Death syndrome
Mary Stahle, MSN-NEdu, CEN, RN, and Betty J. Ackley, MSN, EdS, RN

NANDA   Definition

Presence of risk factors for sudden death of an infant under 1 year of age

Risk Factors

Modifiable: Delayed prenatal care; infant overheating; infant overwrapping; infants placed to sleep in the prone position; infants placed to sleep in the side-lying position; lack of prenatal care; postnatal infant smoke exposure; prenatal infant smoke exposure; soft underlayment (loose articles in the sleep environment)

• = Independent;   ▲ = Collaborative;   EBN = Evidence-Based Nursing;   EB = Evidence-Based

Potentially Modifiable: Low birth weight, prematurity, young maternal age
Nonmodifiable: Ethnicity (e.g., African American or Native American), male gender, seasonality of SIDS deaths (e.g., winter and fall months), infant age of 2-4 months, identified genetic component

NOC   Outcomes (Nursing Outcomes Classification)

Suggested NOC Outcomes

Knowledge: Child Physical Safety, Parenting Performance, Safe Home Environment

Example NOC Outcome with Indicators
Knowledge: Child Physical Safety as evidenced by the following indicators: Description of methods to prevent SIDS/Description of first aid techniques (Rate the outcome and indicators of **Knowledge: Child Physical Safety:** 1 = none, 2 = limited, 3 = moderate, 4 = substantial, 5 = extensive [see Section I].)

Client Outcomes

Client Will (Specify Time Frame):

- Explain appropriate measures to prevent SIDS
- Demonstrate correct techniques for positioning the infant, protecting the infant from harm

NIC   Interventions (Nursing Interventions Classification)

Suggested NIC Interventions

Infant Care, Teaching: Infant Safety 0-3 months

Example NIC Activities—Teaching: Infant Safety
Instruct parent/caregiver to place infant on back to sleep and keep loose bedding, pillows, and toys out of crib; Avoid holding infant while smoking or drinking hot liquids

Nursing Interventions and *Rationales*

- Position infant on back to sleep, do not position in the prone position. **EB:** *The prone position for sleeping infants is a risk factor for SIDS (Li et al, 2003; Malloy & Freeman, 2004). There is a striking trend in decreased incidence of SIDS since parents have been taught not to place infants in the prone position (Ponsonby, Dwyer & Cochrane, 2002). Side sleeping is not as safe as supine sleeping and is not advised (American Academy of Pediatrics, 2005).*
- Avoid use of loose bedding, such as blankets and sheets for sleeping. If blankets are used, they should be tucked in around the crib mattress so the infant's face is less likely to become covered by bedding. *"One strategy is to make up the bedding so that the infant's feet are able to reach the foot of the crib with the blankets tucked in around the crib mattress and reaching only the level of the infant's chest" (American Academy of Pediatrics, 2000).* **EB:** *Soft surfaces are a significant risk factor for SIDS, especially when these items are placed under the sleeping infant (Mitchell et al, 1998; Ponsonby et al, 1998).*
- To avoid overbundling and overheating the infant, lightly clothe the child for sleep. The infant should not feel hot to touch. **EB:** *Overheating the infant has been associated with increased risk of SIDS (Gilbert et al, 1992; Ponsonby et al, 1992).*
- Provide the infant a certain amount of time in prone position, or "tummy time," while the infant is awake and observed. *A period on the tummy is recommended for developmental reasons and to help prevent flat spots on the back of the head (American Academy of Pediatrics, 2000).*
- Consider offering the infant a pacifier during sleep times. **EB:** *A pacifier given at bedtime enhances the infant's ability to maintain a more adequate oral airflow (Cozzi et al, 2002). The reduced risk of SIDS associated with pacifier use during sleep is compelling, and the evidence that pacifier use inhibits breastfeeding or causes later dental complications is not (American Academy of Pediatrics, 2005).*

• = Independent;   ▲ = Collaborative;   EBN = Evidence-Based Nursing;   EB = Evidence-Based

▲ Use electronic respiratory or cardiac monitors to detect cardiorespiratory arrest only if ordered. **EB:** *There is no evidence that infants prone to SIDS can be identified by monitoring of respiratory or cardiac function in the hospital (Malloy & Hoffman, 1996; Committee on Fetus & Newborn, 2003). There is no evidence that use of such home monitors decreases the incidence of SIDS (American Academy of Pediatrics, 2005).*

Home Care

- Most of the interventions above are relevant to home care.
- Evaluate home for potential safety hazards, such as inappropriate cribs, cradles, or strollers.
- Determine where and how the child sleeps, and provide instructions on safe sleeping positions and environments as needed.

Multicultural

- Discuss cultural norms with families to provide care that is appropriate for promoting safety for the infant in sleeping arrangements and care. **EBN:** *Misinterpretation of parenting behaviors can occur when the nurse and parent are from different cultures (Guarnaccia, 1998).*
- Encourage American-Indian mothers to avoid drinking alcoholic beverages and to avoid wrapping infants in excessive blankets or clothing. **EB:** *In the American-Indian population, an association has been shown between binge drinking during pregnancy and having two or more layers of clothing on the infant (Iyasu et al, 2002).*
- Encourage African-American mothers to find alternatives to bed sharing and to avoid placing pillows, soft toys, and soft bedding in the sleep environment. **EB:** *A higher incidence of SIDS occurs in African-American infants. The infants that died are commonly found in the supine position, but are more likely to be sharing a bed with another person (Unger et al, 2003). The greatest impact for SIDS reduction in the African-American population is the need to change behaviors regarding sleep locations by reducing the instances of placing infants for sleep on adult beds, sofas, or cots (Rasinski et al, 2003; Hauck et al, 2003).*

Client/Family Teaching

- Teach families to position infants to sleep on their back rather than in the prone position. **EB:** *The prone position for sleeping infants is a risk factor for SIDS (Li et al, 2003; Malloy & Freeman, 2004).*
- Teach the parents to place the infant supine to sleep with the head rotated to one side for a week, and then to the other side for the next week. Parents should also change the orientation of the crib at intervals, so the infant turns the head in alternate directions. *This is necessary to prevent the infant from developing a flat area on the back of the head (American Academy of Pediatrics, 2000; Persing et al, 2003).*
- Recommend the following infant care practices to parents:
  - Infants should not be put to sleep on soft surfaces such as waterbeds, sofas, or soft mattresses.
  - Avoid placing soft materials in the infant's sleeping environment such as pillows, quilts, and comforters. Do not use sheepskins under a sleeping infant.
  - Avoid the use of loose bedding, such as blankets and sheets.

  EB: *Placing an infant to sleep on a soft surface is a strong independent risk factor for SIDS (Hauck et al, 2003).*
- Teach parents the need to obtain a crib that conforms to the safety standards of the Consumer Product Safety Commission. *Although many cradles and bassinets also may provide safe sleeping enclosures, safety standards have not been established for these items (American Academy of Pediatrics, 2000).*
- Teach parents not to place the infant in an adult bed to sleep, or a sofa or chair. Infants should sleep in a crib. *Sleep surfaces designed for adults have the risk of trapping the baby between the mattress and the structure of the bed (e.g., the headboard, footboard, side rails, and frame), the wall, or adjacent furniture, as well as between railings in the headboard or footboard (American Academy of Pediatrics, 2000).* **EB:** *Over half of the infants who have died from SIDS were sleeping in the same bed as an adult, which suggests that some of the deaths were due to unintentional suffocation from the adult or from compressible bedding (Person et al, 2002). The risk of suffocation increases by two times when infants are placed to sleep in an adult bed rather than in a crib (Scheers, Rutherford & Kemp, 2003).*

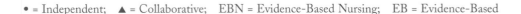

- Teach parents not to sleep with an infant, especially if alcohol or medications/illicit drugs are used by the parents. **EB:** *Parents under the influence of alcohol or illicit drugs or who smoke are more likely to have a SIDS result (James, Klenka & Manning, 2003). Mothers who consume three or more alcoholic drinks in the past 24 hours increase the risk of SIDS when bed sharing with an infant (Carpenter et al, 2004).*
- Recommend an alternative to sleeping with an infant; parents might consider placing the infant's crib near their bed to allow for more convenient breastfeeding and parent contact. *The safety of mother–infant sleeping is debated in the research literature, because results of studies vary (Mesich, 2005).*
- Teach parents to avoid overbundling and overheating the infant by lightly clothing the child for sleep. The infant should not feel hot to touch. The bedroom temperature should be comfortable for an adult wearing light bedclothing. **EB:** *Overheating the infant has been associated with an increased risk of SIDS (Gilbert et al, 1992; Ponsonby et al, 1992).*
- Question parents regarding following recommendations for the prevention of SIDS at each well-baby visit or visit with healthcare practitioner for illness. Strongly encourage compliance with precautions to prevent SIDS. **EB:** *Although a majority of British mothers knew the precautions, 25% of mothers were not following the recommended practice (Roberts & Upton, 2000).*
- Teach the need to stop smoking during pregnancy and to not smoke around the infant, because smoking is a risk factor for SIDS. **EBN:** *Newborns whose mothers smoke have a limited ability to maximize and vary their heart rate, which can result in the infant being unable to maximize cardiac output during stress. This increases the infant's risk for morbidity and possibly mortality (Sherman et al, 2002).* **EB:** *Smoke in the environment after birth is considered a risk factor for SIDS (Mitchell et al, 2000; Schoendorf & Kiely, 1992; U.S. Department of Health and Human Services, 2004).*
- Recommend that parents with infants in child care make it very clear to the employees that the infant must always be placed in the supine position to sleep, not prone or in a side-lying position. **EB:** *Only 14.3% of licensed child care facilities are in compliance with the recommendation that infants be placed in the supine position to sleep (Ford & Linker, 2002). Temporary caretakers who change an infant's usual sleeping position increase the risk of SIDS, because infant sleep physiology differs when they are sleeping in the prone position rather than the supine position (Li et al, 2003).*
- ▲ Suggest speaking with a physician about genetic counseling. *In light of recent genetic research, it is reasonable to suggest that families that have lost an infant to SIDS or who have a family history of other unexplained deaths, fainting episodes, or seizures seek consultation (Mayo Clinic, 2006).*
- Teach child care employees how best to position infants for sleeping and the dangers of a too soft environment. **EB:** *A 60-minute educational experience designed for child care providers may be effective in increasing the compliance with guidelines and increasing the number of written sleep position policies at the child care centers (Moon & Oden, 2003).*
- Teach parents living in deprived areas of precautions to prevent SIDS. **EB:** *SIDS is more common in infants living in deprived areas, although SIDS can occur in infants living in any situation (Mitchell et al, 2000).*
- ▲ Involve family members in learning and practicing rescue techniques, including treatment of choking, breathing, and cardiopulmonary resuscitation (CPR). Initiate referral to formal training classes. *Family members need adequate preparation to deal with emergency situations and should take part in the AHA Basic Lifesaving Course or the American Red Cross Infant/Child CPR Course (CDC, 2002).* **EBN:** *Learning CPR does not reduce anxiety in the parents regarding SIDS but does increase their confidence in dealing with emergencies (Clarke, 1998).*

evolve   See the EVOLVE website for World Wide Web resources for client education.

REFERENCES

American Academy of Pediatrics Task Force on Infant Sleep Position and Sudden Infant Death Syndrome: Changing concepts of sudden infant death syndrome: implications for infant sleeping environment and sleep position, *Pediatrics* 105(3 Pt 1):650-656, 2000.

American Academy of Pediatrics Task Force on Sudden Infant Death Syndrome: The changing concept of sudden infant death syndrome: diagnostic coding shifts, controversies regarding the sleeping environment, and new variables to consider in reducing risk, *Pediatrics* 116(5):1245-1255, 2005.

Carpenter RG, Irgens LM, Blair PS et al: Sudden unexplained infant death in 20 regions in Europe: case control study, *Lancet* 363(9404):185-191, 2004.

• = Independent;   ▲ = Collaborative;   EBN = Evidence-Based Nursing;   EB = Evidence-Based

D

Centers for Disease Control and Prevention (CDC): Nonfatal choking-related episodes among children—United States, 2001, *MMWR Morb Mortal Wkly Rep* 51(42):945-948, 2002.

Clarke K: Research. Infant CPR: the effect on parental anxiety regarding SIDS, *Br J Midwifery* 6(11):710, 1998.

Committee on Fetus and Newborn. American Academy of Pediatrics: Apnea, sudden infant death syndrome, and home monitoring, *Pediatrics* 111(4 Pt 1):914-917, 2003.

Cozzi F, Morini F, Tozzi C et al: Effect of pacifier use on oral breathing in healthy newborn infants, *Pediatr Pulmonol* 33(5):368-373, 2002.

Ford KM, Linker LA: Compliance of licensed child care centers with the American Academy of Pediatrics' recommendations for infant sleep positions, *J Community Health Nurs* 19(2):83-91, 2002.

Gilbert R, Rudd P, Berry PJ et al: Combined effect of infection and heavy wrapping on the risk of sudden unexpected infant death, *Arch Dis Child* 67(2):171-177, 1992.

Guarnaccia P: Multicultural experiences of family caregiving: a study of African American, European American, and Hispanic American families, *New Dir Ment Health Serv* 77:45-61, 1998.

Hauck FR, Herman SM, Donovan M et al: Sleep environment and the risk of sudden infant death syndrome in an urban population: the Chicago infant mortality study, *Pediatrics* 111(5 Part 2):1207-1214, 2003.

Iyasu S, Randall LL, Welty TK et al: Risk factors for sudden infant death syndrome among northern plains Indians, *JAMA* 288(21):2717-2723, 2002.

James C, Klenka H, Manning D: Sudden infant death syndrome: bed sharing with mothers who smoke, *Arch Dis Child* 88(2):112-113, 2003.

Li DK, Petitti DB, Willinger M et al: Infant sleeping position and the risk of sudden infant death syndrome in California, 1997-2000, *Am J Epidemiol* 157(5):446-455, 2003.

Malloy MH, Freeman DH: Age at death, season, and day of death as indicators of the effect of the back to sleep program on sudden infant death syndrome in the United States, 1992-1999, *Arch Pediatr Adolesc Med* 158(4):359-365, 2004.

Malloy MH, Hoffman H: Home apnea monitoring and sudden infant death syndrome, *Prev Med* 25:645-649, 1996.

Mayo Clinic in Rochester: *Researchers link two more genes to sudden infant death syndrome*, Rochester, MN, 2006, Mayo Clinic. Retrieved January, 6, 2007 from http://www.mayoclinic.org/news2006-rst/3408.html.

Mesich HM: Mother-infant co-sleeping: understanding the debate and maximizing infant safety, *MCN Am J Matern Child Nurs* 30(1):30-37, 2005.

Mitchell EA, Stewart AW, Crampton P et al: Deprivation and sudden infant death syndrome, *Soc Sci Med* 51(1):147-150, 2000.

Mitchell EA, Thompson JM, Ford R et al: Sheepskin bedding and the sudden infant death syndrome. New Zealand Cot Death Study Group, *J Pediatr* 133(5):701-704, 1998.

Moon RY, Oden RP: Back to sleep: can we influence child care providers? *Pediatrics* 112(4):878-882, 2003.

Persing J, James H, Swanson J et al: Prevention and management of positional skull deformities in infants, *Pediatrics* 112(1 Pt 1):199-202, 2003.

Person TL, Lavezzi WA, Wolf BC: Cosleeping and sudden unexpected death in infancy, *Arch Pathol Lab Med* 126(3):343-345, 2002.

Ponsonby A, Dwyer T, Cochrane J: Population trends in sudden infant death syndrome, *Semin Perinatol* 26(4):296-305, 2002.

Ponsonby AL, Dwyer T, Gibbons LE et al: Thermal environment and sudden infant death syndrome: case-control study, *BMJ* 304(6822):277-282, 1992.

Ponsonby AL, Dwyer T, Couper D et al: Association between use of a quilt and sudden infant death syndrome: case-control study, *BMJ* 316(7126):195-196, 1998.

Rasinski KA, Kuby A, Bzdusek SA et al: Effect of a sudden infant death syndrome risk reduction education program on risk factor compliance and information sources in primarily black urban communities, *Pediatrics* 111(4 Pt 1):E347-E354, 2003.

Roberts H, Upton D: Research. New mother's knowledge of sudden infant death syndrome, *Br J Midwifery* 8(3):147, 2000.

Scheers NJ, Rutherford GW, Kemp JS: Where should infants sleep? A comparison of risk for suffocation of infants sleeping in cribs, adult beds, and other sleeping locations, *Pediatrics* 112(4):883-889, 2003.

Schoendorf KC, Kiely JL: Relationship of sudden infant death syndrome to maternal smoking during and after pregnancy, *Pediatrics* 90:905-908, 1992.

Sherman J, Young A, Sherman MP et al: Prenatal smoking and alterations in newborn heart rate during transition, *J Obstet Gynecol Neonatal Nurs* 31(6):680-687, 2002.

Unger B, Kemp JS, Wilkins D et al: Racial disparity and modifiable risk factors among infants dying suddenly and unexpectedly, *Pediatrics* 111(2):E127-E131, 2003.

US Department of Health and Human Services: *The health consequences of smoking: a report of the Surgeon General*, U.S. Department of Health and Human Services, CDC, 2004.

Readiness for enhanced Decision-making   *Margaret Lunney, RN, PhD, and Marie Giordano, MS, RN*

NANDA   Definition

A pattern of choosing courses of action that is sufficient for meeting short and long term health-related goals and can be strengthened

Defining Characteristics

Expresses desire to enhance decision making; expresses desire to congruency of decisions with personal values and goals; expresses desire to congruency of decisions with sociocultural values and goals; expresses desire to risk benefit analysis of decisions; expresses desire to understand choices for decision making; expresses desire to enhance understanding of the meaning of choices; expresses desire to enhance use of reliable evidence for decisions

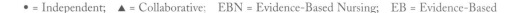

• = Independent;   ▲ = Collaborative;   EBN = Evidence-Based Nursing;   EB = Evidence-Based

NOC   Outcomes (Nursing Outcomes Classification)

Suggested NOC Outcomes

Decision Making, Information Processing, Participation in Healthcare Decisions, Personal Autonomy

> **Example NOC Outcome with Indicators**
>
> **Participation in Healthcare Decisions** as evidenced by the following indicators: Claims decision making responsibility/Demonstrates self direction in decision making/Seeks relevant information/Specifies health outcome preferences (Rate the outcome and indicators of **Participation in Healthcare Decisions:** 1 = never demonstrated, 2 = rarely demonstrated, 3 = sometimes demonstrated, 4 = often demonstrated, 5 = consistently demonstrated [see Section I].)

Client Outcomes

Client Will (Specify Time Frame):

- Review treatment options with providers
- Ask questions about the benefits and risks of treatment options
- Communicate decisions about treatment options to providers in relation to personal preferences, values, and goals

 NIC   Interventions (Nursing Interventions Classification)

Suggested NIC Interventions

Decision Making Support, Mutual Goal Setting, Self Awareness Enhancement, Support System Enhancement, Values Clarification

> **Example NIC Activities—Decision Making Support**
>
> Help patient identify the advantages and disadvantages of each alternative; Facilitate collaborative decision making; Help patient explain decisions to others, as needed

Nursing Interventions and *Rationales*

- Support and encourage clients and their representatives to engage in healthcare decisions. **EB:** *"A number of research studies have concluded that there is a positive link between the practice of client-centered healthcare in clinical settings and positive outcomes." The positive health outcomes of client-centered care include "patient satisfaction, emotional health, symptom resolution, function, physiological measures, quality of life" (Harkness, 2005).* **EB:** *Weinfurt (2003) found that reduced anxiety and uncertainty were associated with clients' involvement in decision making.*
- Respect personal preferences, values, needs, and rights. **EB:** *Only the client and family for whom treatment is intended can know how the treatment will affect them (Harkness, 2005; O'Connor et al, 1998).*
- Determine the degree of participation desired by the client. **EBN:** *Nurses are not always aware of their clients' perspectives and may tend to overestimate the clients' willingness to participate (Florin et al, 2006).*
- Provide access to healthcare services as needed. One type of access to consider is interactive Internet-based decision supports. **EB:** *Decision making related to healthcare services is directly affected by access to such services (Harkness, 2005).* **EB:** *Traditional formats, such as verbal instructions and reading materials with intense amounts of information, often do not work. The internet can offer clients a range of opportunities to ask complex questions related to health and illness (Evans, Elwyn & Edwards, 2004).*

• = Independent;   ▲ = Collaborative;   EBN = Evidence-Based Nursing;   EB = Evidence-Based

D

- Provide information that is appropriate, relevant, and timely. **EB:** *Information sharing "enables patients [and their representatives] to make informed decisions and to take effective action to improve their health" (Harkness, 2005).*
- Tailor information to the specific needs of individual clients, according to principles of health literacy. **EB:** *The format of relevant information should be adapted in consideration of the individual's condition, language, age, understanding, abilities, and culture (Harkness, 2005).*
- Motivate clients to be as independent as possible in decision making. **EB:** *Clients should be the leaders in their own healthcare decisions (Harkness, 2005).*
- Identify the client's level of choice in decision making. **EB:** *Some clients want to be completely involved in all decisions; other clients prefer to have less involvement (Harkness, 2005).* **EBN:** *Clients prefer to share decision making with their providers (O'Connor et al, 1998).*
- Focus on the positive aspects of decision making, rather than decisional conflicts. **EBN:** *Promotion differs from prevention and requires a positive rather than negative approach (Pender, Murdaugh & Parsons, 2006).*
- Use existing decision aids for particular types of decisions, or develop decision aids as indicated. **EBN:** *Decision aids can promote optimum decision making. Over 200 decision aids are identified (O'Connor et al, 2003a).* **EBN:** *In a study that examined the effects of a decision aid to help women decide about hormone replacement therapy (n = 94) on decisional conflict, knowledge and expectations, and change in value congruence with decisions, use of the decision aid had significantly positive effects on these variables (O'Connor et al, 1998).* **EBN:** *A decision-making tree developed by Wu et al (2005) predicted 13 criteria that Taiwanese women use to make decisions about hysterectomy.*
- Design educational interventions for decision support. **EBN:** *The analyses of decision supports show that decisional supports are available that should be shared with consumers (O'Connor et al. 1998, 2003a, 2003b).*
- Provide clients with the benefits of decisions at the same time you help them to identify strategies to reduce the barriers for healthful decisions. **EBN:** *In a study of 88 clinic clients who had previously had myocardial infarction (MI), knowing the benefits of exercise was insufficient for decision making; it was also necessary to reduce the barriers (Al-Hassan & Wierenga, 2000). The interaction of benefits and barriers significantly predicted stress for 48 participants who did not exercise after an MI.*
- Acknowledge the complexity of everyday self-care decisions related to self-management of chronic illnesses. **EBN:** *Providers need to recognize that everyday self-care decisions with chronic illnesses are personally constructed, unique, constantly changing, and require the authoritative knowledge that comes with living with the illness (Paterson, Russell & Thorne, 2001).* **EBN:** *Seniors are resourceful with respect to self-care decision making related to musculoskeletal pain (Ross et al, 2001).* **EBN:** *65% of Canadian adults reported making complex health-related decisions (O'Connor et al, 2003b).*
- Determine the health literacy of clients and their representatives before helping with decision making. **EB:** *Canadian adults with less formal education reported more difficulties making decisions and relied more on health providers for decision making. Decision support interventions tailored to clients' health literacy contribute to informed decision making (O'Connor et al, 2003b).*
- Reframe professional image, role, and values to incorporate a vision of clients as the experts in their own care. **EBN:** *In a phenomenological study of the experiences of eight nurses who had been using an agency supported client-centered model of care for a year, Brown, William & Ward-Griffin (2006) found that the "nurses persistently described themselves as the experts who knew best."*

 Home Care

- The previously mentioned interventions should be adapted for home care use.
- Develop clinical practice guidelines that include shared decision making. **EBN:** *Clinical practice guidelines that focus on client autonomy and shared decision making are effective in helping older adults to improve their use of assistive devices (Roelands et al, 2004).*
- Contribute to home care policy making that supports the adequacy of home care services. **EBN:** *In a pilot study in Canada of the decision-making needs of 20 women at the end of life, most of the women indicated that home was the preferred location (Murray et al, 2003). Home care services are not always adequate, however, for women in need of palliative and other types of care.*

• = Independent;   ▲ = Collaborative;   EBN = Evidence-Based Nursing;   EB = Evidence-Based

Client/Family Teaching

- Before teaching, identify client preferences in involvement with decision making. **EBN:** *Healthcare providers cannot know client preferences unless they ask them (Munhall, 1993).*

evolve See the EVOLVE website for World Wide Web resources for client education.

REFERENCES

Al-Hassan M, Wierenga M: Exercise participation decisions of Jordanian myocardial infarction patients: application of the decisional conflict theory, *Int J Nurs Stud* 37:119-136, 2000.

Brown D, William C, Ward-Griffin C: Client-centred empowering partnering in nursing. *J Adv Nurs* 53(2):160-168, 2006.

Evans R, Elwyn G, Edwards A: Making interactive decision support for patients a reality, *Inform Prim Care* 12:109-113, 2004.

Florin J, Ehrenberg A, Ehnfors M: Patient participation in clinical decision-making in nursing: a comparative study of nurses' and patients' perceptions, *J Clin Nurs* 15(12):1498-1508, 2006.

Harkness J: Patient involvement: a vital principle for patient-centered health care, *World Hosp Health Serv* 41(2):12-16, 2005.

Munhall PL: "Unknowing": toward another pattern of knowing in nursing. *Nurs Outlook* 41:125-128, 1993.

Murray MA, O'Connor AM, Fiset V et al: Women's decision making needs regarding place of care at end of life, *J Palliat Care* 19(3):176-184, 2003.

O'Connor AM, Drake ER, Wells GA et al: A survey of the decision-making need of Canadians faced with complex health decisions, *Health Expect* 6:97-109, 2003b.

O'Connor AM, Stacey D, Entwistle V et al: Decision aids for people facing health treatment or screening decisions, *Cochrane Database Syst Rev* (1):CD001431, 2003a.

O'Connor AM, Tugwell P, Wells GA et al: A decision aid for women considering hormone therapy after menopause: decision support framework and evaluation, *Patient Educ Couns* 33:267-279, 1998.

Paterson BL, Russell C, Thorne S: Critical analysis of everyday self-care decision making in chronic illness, *J Adv Nurs* 35(3):335-341, 2001.

Pender NJ, Murdaugh CL, Parsons MA: *Health promotion in nursing practice*, ed 5, Upper Saddle River, NJ, 2006, Pearson Prentice Hall.

Roelands M, Van Oost P, Stevens V et al: Clinical practice guidelines to improve shared decision-making about assistive device use in home care: a pilot interventions study, *Patient Educ Couns* 55:252-264, 2004.

Ross MM, Carswell A, Hing M et al: Seniors decision making about pain management, *J Adv Nurs* 35(3):442-451, 2001.

Weinfurt KP: Outcomes research related to patient decision making in oncology, *Clin Ther* 25(2):671-683, 2003.

Wu SM, Yu YMC, Yang CF et al: Decision-making tree for women considering hysterectomy, *J Adv Nurs* 51(4):361-368, 2005.

Ineffective Denial   *Gail Ladwig, MSN, CHTP, RN*

NANDA   Definition

The conscious or unconscious attempt to disavow the knowledge or meaning of an event to reduce anxiety/fear, but leading to the detriment of health

Defining Characteristics

Delays seeking healthcare attention to the detriment of health; displaces fear of impact of the condition; displaces source of symptoms to other organs; displays inappropriate affect; does not admit fear of death; does not admit fear of invalidism; does not perceive personal relevance of danger; does not perceive personal relevance of symptoms; makes dismissive comments when speaking of distressing events; minimizes symptoms; refuses healthcare attention to the detriment of health; unable to admit impact of disease on life pattern; uses self-treatment

Related Factors (r/t)

Anxiety; fear of death; fear of loss of autonomy; fear of separation; lack of competency in using effective coping mechanisms; lack of control of life situation; lack of emotional support from others; overwhelming stress; threat of inadequacy in dealing with strong emotions; threat of unpleasant reality

NOC   Outcomes (Nursing Outcomes Classification)

Suggested NOC Outcomes

Acceptance: Health Status, Anxiety Self-Control, Health Beliefs: Perceived Threat, Symptom Control

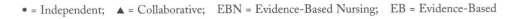

• = Independent;   ▲ = Collaborative;   EBN = Evidence-Based Nursing;   EB = Evidence-Based

D

Client Outcomes

Client Will (Specify Time Frame):

- Seek out appropriate healthcare attention when needed
- Use home remedies only when appropriate
- Display appropriate affect and verbalize fears
- Remain substance free
- Actively engage in treatment program related to identified "substance" of abuse
- Demonstrate alternate adaptive coping mechanism

NIC   Interventions (Nursing Interventions Classification)

Suggested NIC Intervention

Anxiety Reduction

Example NIC Activities—Anxiety Reduction
Use a calm, reassuring approach; Stay with the patient to promote safety and reduce fear

Nursing Interventions and *Rationales*

- Assess the client's understanding of symptoms and illness. **EBN:** *Negative responses to a need for behavioral change related to altered health status can only be understood following a thorough assessment of the client's appraisal framework (Dudley-Brown, 2002).*
- Spend time with the client, and allow time for responses. *Nursing presence and one-on-one interaction support the nurse-client relationship. Nurses must understand that presence provides meaning; engenders feelings of comfort and peacefulness; diminishes anxiety, loneliness, and vulnerability; and reassures when no words exist (Stanley, 2006).*
- Assess whether the use of denial is helping or hindering the client's care. Provide support for clients who are using denial as a way of coping. **EBN:** *Denial may be used as an adaptive mechanism during times of illness and stress. Patience, understanding, and self-awareness are crucial for providing a safe, trusting environment for clients who are experiencing denial (Stephenson, 2004).*
- Allow the client to express and use denial as a coping mechanism. **EBN:** *This period of denial may be necessary for the client to develop a construct within which the information has meaning and can be appraised as not a threat to survival (Norris & Spelic, 2002).*
- Assess for subtle signs of denial (e.g., unrealistic display of optimism, downplaying of symptoms, inability to admit one's own fear). *Minimization and denial are part of the alcoholism pathophysiology (Becker & Walton-Moss, 2001).*
- Avoid confrontation. *Rather than direct confrontation, informing the client of the reality of consequences of a specific behavior may be more therapeutically assimilated into the client's appraisal framework. Assess individual spiritual coping style (Faltz & Skinner, 2002).*
- Support the client's spiritual coping measures. **EBN:** *Most religious coping is considered positive (Meisenhelder, 2002). Physical and mental health is interrelated with spiritual health (Taylor, 2002).*
- Develop a trusting, therapeutic relationship with the client/family. **EBN:** *Nurses who develop trusting relationships demonstrate a holistic approach to caring; show their understanding of clients' suffering; are aware of their unvoiced needs; provide comfort without actually being asked; and are reliable, proficient, competent, and dedicated in their care (Mok & Chui, 2004).*
- Encourage individual family members to share their concerns and worries. **EBN:** *This communi-*

• = Independent;   ▲ = Collaborative;   EBN = Evidence-Based Nursing;   EB = Evidence-Based

cation may help reframe the experience in a way that is acceptable, and allows the nurse to identify possible misperceptions and/or questions (Mellon, 2002).

- Sit at eye level. *Honest caring behaviors on the part of the nurse facilitate acceptance of reality by the client (Faltz & Skinner, 2002).*
- Use touch if appropriate and with permission. Touch the client's hand or arm. *Appropriate expression of caring on the part of the nurse facilitates therapeutic client response (Faltz & Skinner, 2002).*
- Explain signs and symptoms of illness; as necessary, reinforce use of the prescribed treatment plan. *A straightforward education on the effects of an abused substance is integral to the client's motivation (Becker & Walton-Moss, 2001).*
- Have the client make choices regarding treatment and actively involve him or her in the decision-making process. **EB:** *"Forced retention" is not linked to positive results for drug addicted offenders (Brochu et al, 2006).*
- Help the client recognize existing and additional sources of support; allow time for adjustment. *The influence of environment on a positive adaptation is significant (Moser et al, 2001).*
- Refer to care plans **Defensive Coping** and **Dysfunctional Family processes: alcoholism**

Geriatric

- Identify recent losses of the client, because grieving may prolong denial. Encourage the client to take one day at a time. *Older adult clients often have experienced significant, multiple losses in a variety of domains. This may complicate adaptation to an individual change in health status, because the resources formerly used for successful adaptation are no longer available (Boyd & Stanley, 2002).*
- Encourage the client to verbalize feelings. **EBN:** *Bereaved individuals benefit from individual, family and group therapy to discuss losses (Douglas, 2004).*
- Encourage communication among family members. *Communication problems within families are pivotal in the development of family adjustment to a change in health status and/or adaptation to a life change (Hanson et al, 2002).*
- Recognize denial. **EB:** *Older adults selected more avoidance-denial strategies than young adults when solving interpersonal problems (Blanchard-Fields et al, 2007).*
- Use reality-focusing techniques. Wherever possible, provide realistic feedback, allowing the client to validate his or her perceptions. *Providing validation of actual stressors and available resources aids in a positive adaptation (Pakenham, 2001).*

Multicultural

- Assess for the influence of cultural beliefs, norms, and values on the client's understanding of and ability to acknowledge health status. **EBN:** *Willingness to acknowledge health status may be based on cultural perceptions (Giger & Davidhizar, 2004).*
- Discuss with the client those aspects of his or her health behavior/lifestyle that will remain unchanged by health status. **EBN:** *Aspects of the client's life that are meaningful and valuable to him or her should be understood and preserved without change (Leininger & McFarland, 2002).*
- Negotiate with the client regarding the aspects of health behavior that will need to be modified as a result of health status. **EBN:** *Give and take with the client will lead to culturally congruent care (Leininger & McFarland, 2002).*
- Assess the role of fatalism on the client's ability to acknowledge health status. **EBN:** *Fatalistic perspectives, which involve the belief that you cannot control your own fate, may influence health behaviors in some Asian, African-American, and Latino populations (Chen, 2001; Harmon et al, 1996; Phillips et al, 1999). A culturally appropriate way to deal with fatalistic views is to communicate to the family that it is also fate that the best care is available (Munet-Vilaro, 2004).*
- Validate the client's feelings of anxiety and fear related to health status. **EBN:** *Validation lets family members know that the nurse has heard and understood what was said, and it promotes the relationship between nurse and family members (Spiers, 2002).*

Home Care

- Previously mentioned interventions may be adapted for home care use.
- Observe family interaction and roles. Assess whether denial is being used to meet the needs of

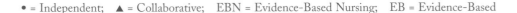

D

another family member. *Communication problems within families are pivotal in the development of family adjustment to a change in health status and/or adaptation to a life change (Hanson, 2002).* Refer the client/family for follow-up if prolonged denial is a risk. *Family therapy has been demonstrated to enhance treatment adherence and facilitate implementation and monitoring of contingency contracts with opioid-dependent clients (Work Group on Substance Use Disorders, 2006).*

- Encourage communication between family members, particularly when dealing with the loss of a significant person. **EBN:** *An understanding of the family structure, patterns of communication, healthcare history, and cultural influences will facilitate effective nursing interventions. In the context of some family patterns of communication, defensive coping may be a learned behavior (Hellemann et al, 2002).*

Client/Family Teaching

- Teach signs and symptoms of illness and appropriate responses (e.g., taking medication, going to the emergency department, calling the physician). Provide a list of names and numbers. *Family members should be involved at all points of care to ensure that the necessary care will be provided in a safe, accurate manner (Harmon, 2001).*
- Teach family members that denial may continue throughout the adjustment to treatment and they should not be confrontational. *These individuals often are in denial of their substance abuse problem—a normal part of their disease—and require behavioral modification therapy for effective treatment (Spolarich, 2006).*
- ▲ If the problem is substance abuse, refer to an appropriate community agency (e.g., Alcoholics Anonymous). **EBN:** *Families need assistance in coping with health changes. The nurse is often perceived as the individual who can help them obtain necessary social support (Northouse et al, 2002; Tak & McCubbin, 2002).*
- Teach families of clients with brain injuries that denial has been associated with damage to the right hemisphere. *The client may exhibit inappropriate affect and anxiety.*
- Inform family of available community support resources. *Mutual support groups can have a positive effect not only in Western cultures but also in Eastern cultures (Fung & Chien, 2002).*

evolve See the EVOLVE website for World Wide Web resources for client education.

REFERENCES

*See **Defensive Coping** for additional references.*

Becker KL, Walton-Moss B: Detecting and addressing alcohol abuse in women, *Nurse Pract* 26(10):13, 2001.

Blanchard-Fields F, Mienaltowski A, Seay RB: Age differences in everyday problem-solving effectiveness: older adults select more effective strategies for interpersonal problems, *J Gerontol B Psychol Sci Soc Sci* 62(1):P61-P64, 2007.

Boyd MA, Stanley M: Mental health assessment of the elderly. In Boyd MA, editor: *Psychiatric nursing in contemporary practice*, ed 2, Philadelphia, 2002, Lippincott.

Brochu S, Cournoyer LG, Tremblay J et al: Understanding treatment impact on drug-addicted offenders, *Subst Use Misuse* 41(14):1937-1949, 2006.

Chen YC: Chinese values, health and nursing, *J Adv Nurs* 36(2):270, 2001.

Douglas DH: The lived experience of loss: a phenomenological study, *J Am Psychiatr Nurses Assoc* 10(1):24-32, 2004.

Dudley-Brown S: Prevention of psychological distress in persons with inflammatory bowel disease, *Issues Ment Health Nurs* 23(4):403-422, 2002.

Faltz BG, Skinner MK: Substance abuse disorders. In Boyd MA, editor: *Psychiatric nursing in contemporary practice*, ed 2, Philadelphia, 2002, Lippincott.

Fung WY, Chien WT: The effectiveness of a mutual support group for family caregivers of a relative with dementia, *Arch Psychiatr Nurs* 16(3):134, 2002.

Giger J, Davidhizar R: *Transcultural nursing: assessment and intervention*, ed 4, St Louis, 2004, Mosby.

Hanson E, Andersson BA, Magnusson L et al: Information Center: responding to needs of older people and carers, *Br J Nurs* 11(14):935-940, 2002.

Harmon MP, Castro FG, Coe K: Acculturation and cervical cancer: knowledge, beliefs, and behaviors of Hispanic women, *Women Health* 24(3):37, 1996.

Harmon SMH: *Family health care nursing*, Philadelphia, 2001, FA Davis.

Hellemann MS V, Lee KA, Kary FS: Strengths and vulnerabilities of women of Mexican descent in relation to depressive symptoms, *Nurs Res* 51(3):175, 2002.

Leininger MM, McFarland MR: *Transcultural nursing: concepts, theories, research and practices,* ed 3, New York, 2002, McGraw-Hill.

Meisenhelder JB: Terrorism, posttraumatic stress, and religious coping, *Issues Ment Health Nurs* 23:771, 2002.

Mellon S: Comparisons between cancer survivors and family members on meaning of the illness and family quality of life, *Oncol Nurs Forum* 29(7):1117, 2002.

Mok E, Chui PC: Nurse-patient relationships in palliative care, *J Adv Nurs* 48(5):475-483, 2004.

Moser KM, Sowell RL, Phillips KD: Issues of women dually diagnosed with HIV infection and substance abuse problems in the Carolinas, *Issues Ment Health Nurs* 22:23, 2001.

Munet-Vilaro F: Delivery of culturally competent care to children with cancer and their families—the Latino experience, *J Pediatr Oncol Nurs* 21(3):155-159, 2004.

Norris J, Spelic SS: Supporting adaptation to body image disruption, *Rehabil Nurs* 27(1):8, 2002.

Northouse LL, Walker J, Schafenacker A et al: A family-based program of care for women with recurrent breast cancer and their family members, *Oncol Nurs Forum* 29(10):1411-1419, 2002.

Pakenham KI: Application of a stress and coping model to caregiving in multiple sclerosis, *Psychol Health Med* 6(1):13, 2001.

Phillips JM, Cohen MZ, Moses G: Breast cancer screening and African American women: fear, fatalism, and silence, *Oncol Nurs Forum* 26(3):561, 1999.

Spiers J: The interpersonal contexts of negotiating care in home care nurse-patient interactions, *Qual Health Res* 12(8):1033-1057, 2002.

Spolarich A: Addressing addiction, *Mod Hyg* 2(9):22-25, 2006.

Stanley K: The healing power of presence: respite from the fear of abandonment, *Oncol Nurs Forum* 33(4):J935-J942, 2006.

Stephenson PS: Understanding denial, *Oncol Nurs Forum* 31(5):985-988, 2004.

Tak YR, McCubbin M: Family stress, perceived social support and coping following the diagnosis of a child's congenital heart disease, *J Adv Nurs* 39(2):190-198, 2002.

Taylor EJ: *Spiritual care: nursing theory, research and practice,* Upper Saddle River, NJ, 2002, Prentice-Hall.

Work Group on Substance Use Disorders: Treatment of patients with substance use disorders, second edition. American Psychiatric Association, *Am J Psychiatry* 163(suppl 8):5-82, 2006.

Impaired Dentition   *Betty J. Ackley, MSN, EdS, RN*

NANDA   Definition

Disruption in tooth development/eruption patterns or structural integrity of individual teeth

Defining Characteristics

Abraded teeth, absence of teeth; asymmetrical facial expression; crow caries; erosion of enamel; excessive calculus; excessive plaque; halitosis; incomplete eruption for age (may be primary or permanent teeth); loose teeth; malocclusion; missing teeth; premature loss of primary teeth; root caries; tooth enamel discoloration; tooth fracture(s); tooth misalignment; toothache; worn down teeth

Related Factors (r/t)

Barriers to self-care; bruxism; chronic use of coffee; chronic use of tea; chronic use of red wine; chronic use of tobacco; chronic vomiting; deficient knowledge regarding dental health; dietary habits; economic barriers to professional care; excessive use of abrasive cleaning agents; excessive intake of fluorides; genetic predisposition; ineffective oral hygiene; lack of access to professional care; nutritional deficits; selected prescription medications; sensitivity to cold; sensitivity to heat

NOC   Outcomes (Nursing Outcomes Classification)

Suggested NOC Outcomes

Oral Hygiene, Self-Care: Oral Hygiene

Example NOC Outcome with Indicators
Oral Hygiene as evidenced by the following indicators: Cleanliness of teeth/Cleanliness of gums/Cleanliness of dentures/Tongue integrity/Gum integrity (Rate the outcome and indicators of **Oral Hygiene:** 1 = severely compromised, 2 = substantially compromised, 3 = moderately compromised, 4 = mildly compromised, 5 = not compromised [see Section I].)

Client Outcomes

Client Will (Specify Time Frame):

• Have clean teeth, gums healthy pink color, mouth with pleasant odor
• Demonstrate ability to masticate foods without difficulty
• State no pain originating from teeth
• Demonstrate measures can take to improve dental hygiene

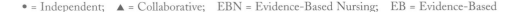

NIC   Interventions (Nursing Interventions Classification)

Suggested NIC Interventions

Oral Health Maintenance, Oral Health Promotion, Oral Health Restoration

Example NIC Activities—Oral Health Maintenance
Establish a mouth care routine; Arrange for dental checkups, as needed

D

Nursing Interventions and *Rationales*

▲ Inspect oral cavity/teeth at least once daily and note any discoloration; presence of debris; amount of plaque buildup; presence of lesions, edema, or bleeding; and intactness of teeth. Refer to a dentist or periodontist as appropriate. *Systematic inspection can identify impending problems.*

• If the client is free of bleeding disorders and is able to swallow, encourage the client to brush teeth with a soft toothbrush, using fluoride-containing toothpaste at least twice daily and to floss teeth daily. **EB:** *The benefits of fluoride toothpaste in preventing caries in children and adolescents has been firmly established (Marinho et al, 2003). Flossing daily decreased plaque and gingivitis, as compared to brushing teeth alone (Schiff et al, 2006).* **EBN:** *The toothbrush is the most important tool for oral care; toothbrushing is the most effective method of reducing plaque and controlling periodontal disease (Stiefel et al, 2000; Pearson & Hutton, 2002).*

• Use a powered sonic toothbrush for removal of dental plaque and prevention of gingivitis. **EB:** *Use of powered toothbrushes with a rotation oscillation reduced plaque and incidence of gingivitis versus a manual toothbrush (Robinson et al, 2005). Power toothbrushes were more effective in removing plaque and reducing papillary bleeding than the manual toothbrush (Zimmer et al, 2005). The amount of interproximal plaque is lowest with sonic brushing (Sjogren et al, 2004).*

• If the client is unable to brush his or her teeth, follow this procedure:
  1. Position the client upright or on side.
  2. Use a soft bristle baby toothbrush.
  3. Use fluoride toothpaste and tap water or saline as a solution.
  4. Brush teeth in an up-and-down manner.
  5. Suction as needed.

• Avoid using foam sticks to clean teeth; use them only to swab out the oral cavity. *Use of this nursing protocol improved oral hygiene in a vulnerable population (Stiefel et al, 2000).* **EBN:** *Foam sticks are not as effective as the toothbrush for removing plaque (Pearson & Hutton, 2002).*

• Monitor the client's nutritional and fluid status to determine if adequate. Recommend the client eat a balanced diet and limit between meal snacks. *Poor nutrition predisposes clients to dental disease (ADA, 2007).*

• Recommend the client decrease or preferably stop intake of soft drinks. *Sugar-containing soft drinks can cause cavities, and the low pH of the drink can cause erosion in teeth (ADA, 2007).* **EB:** *Persons who consumed sugared soft drinks three or more times daily had 17%-62% higher rate of dental caries than those who consumed no soft drinks (Heller, Burt & Eklund, 2001).*

• If client has halitosis, review good oral care with the client, including brushing teeth, using floss, and brushing the tongue. *Halitosis can be an early sign of gingivitis, and can be eradicated by a good program of dental hygiene (Obesity, 2006).*

▲ Assess the client for underlying an medical condition that may be causing halitosis. *Causes of halitosis can be associated with the mouth or upper respiratory tract, or it may occur from systemic diseases (Tangerman, 2002).* **EB:** *Clients who believe they have oral malodor often have a dry mouth condition instead (Kleinberg, Wolff & Codipilly, 2002).*

• Determine the client's mental status and manual dexterity; if the client is unable to care for self, nursing personnel must provide dental hygiene. The nursing diagnosis **Bathing/hygiene Self-Care deficit** is then applicable.

• Determine the client's usual method of oral care. Whenever possible, build on the client's existing knowledge and current practices to develop an individualized plan of care.

• = Independent;   ▲ = Collaborative;   EBN = Evidence-Based Nursing;   EB = Evidence-Based

- Tell the client to direct the toothbrush vertically toward the tooth surfaces. **EB:** *Brushing with the toothbrush bristles perpendicular to the surface of the teeth has a high efficacy of plaque removal and maintains good gingival condition (Sasahara & Kawamura, 2000).*
- Instruct the client to clean the tongue when performing oral hygiene. Brush tongue with tongue scraper and follow with a mouth rinse. *Tongue brushing and mouth rinsing are basic treatment measures for halitosis (Yaegaki et al, 2002; Krespi, 2006).* **EB:** *Tongue cleaning is effective for short-term control of halitosis (Outhouse et al, 2006).*
- Use tap water or saline only for a mouth rinse. Avoid the use of hydrogen peroxide, lemon-glycerin swabs, or alcohol-based mouthwashes. **EBN:** *Hydrogen peroxide can cause mucosal damage and is extremely foul tasting to clients (Tombes & Gallucci, 1993). Lemon-glycerin swabs can result in decreased salivary amylase and oral moisture, as well as erosion of tooth enamel (Foss-Durant & McAffee, 1997; Poland, 1987).*
- If the client does not have a bleeding disorder, encourage the client to floss daily with approximately 18 inches of floss, using a gentle up-and-down rubbing motion. *Floss is useful for removing plaque buildup between the teeth (Brown & Yoder, 2002; ADA, 2007).*
- ▲ Recommend client see a dentist at prescribed intervals, generally two times per year if teeth are in satisfactory condition. *It is important to see a dentist at regular intervals for preventative dental care (ADA, 2007).*
- ▲ If there are any signs of bleeding when the teeth are brushed, refer the client to a dentist; or if there are obvious signs of inflamed gums, refer the client to a periodontist. *Bleeding along with halitosis is associated with gingivitis (Obesity, 2006).*
- If platelet numbers are decreased, or if the client is edentulous, use moistened toothettes or a specially made, very soft toothbrush for oral care. *A toothbrush can cause soft tissue injury and bleeding in clients with low platelet counts.*
- Provide scrupulous dental care to critically ill clients. *Cultures of the teeth of critically ill clients have yielded significant bacterial colonization, which can cause nosocomial pneumonia (Scannapieco, Stewart & Mylotte, 1992).*
- If teeth are nonfunctional for chewing, modification of oral intake (e.g., edentulous diet, soft diet) may be necessary. The nursing diagnosis **Imbalanced Nutrition: less than body requirements** may apply.
- If the client is unable to swallow, keep suction nearby when providing oral care.
- See care plan for **Impaired Oral mucous membrane.**

Pregnant Client

- Encourage the expectant mother to eat a healthy, balanced diet that is rich in calcium. *The teeth usually start to form in the gums during the second trimester of pregnancy. To encourage the development of good, strong teeth, expectant mothers should eat a healthy, balanced diet that is rich in calcium (Koop, 2007).*

Infant Oral Hygiene

- Gently wipe baby's gums with a washcloth or sterile gauze at least once a day. *Wiping gums prevents bacterial buildup in the mouth.* **EB:** *Infants of breastfeeding mothers need early and consistent mouth care when the teeth erupt (Valaitis et al, 2000).*
- Never allow child to fall asleep with a bottle containing milk, formula, fruit juice, or sweetened liquid, or give child a pacifier dipped in any sweet liquid. Avoid filling a child's bottle with such liquids as sugar water and soft drinks. *Decay occurs when sweetened liquids are given and are left clinging to an infant's teeth for long periods. Decay in infants and children most often occurs in the upper front teeth, but other teeth may also be affected. Many sweet liquids cause problems, including milk, formula, and fruit juice (ADA, 2007).*
- When multiple teeth appear, brush with a small toothbrush with a small (pea-size) amount of fluoride toothpaste. Recommend that the child use either a fluoride gel or fluoride varnish. *Use of topical fluoride (mouth rinses, gels, or varnishes) in addition to toothpaste containing fluoride resulted in a modest reduction of cavity formation versus use of fluoride toothpaste only (Marinho et al, 2003).*

D

Older Children

▲ Encourage the family to talk with the dentist about dental sealants, which can help prevent cavities in permanent teeth. **EB:** *Sealants should be available to all children regardless of socioeconomic status. Children of low socioeconomic status have a higher rate of caries in primary and permanent teeth than children of higher socioeconomic status (Gillcrist et al, 2001).*

▲ Recommend the child use dental floss to help prevent gum disease. The dentist will give guidelines on when to start using floss.

• Recommend to parents that they not permit the child to smoke or chew tobacco, and stress the importance of setting a good example by not using tobacco products themselves.

• Recommend the child drink fluoridated water when possible. **EB:** *Drinking-water fluoridation is associated with an increase in the percentage of 5-year-old children with no experience of tooth decay (Gray & Davies-Slowik, 2001).*

• If a child has halitosis, consider the presence of parasites in the gastrointestinal system as a cause. **EB:** *18 of 28 children with evidence of parasites in stool were treated with mebendazole and recovered from halitosis (Ermis, 2002).*

Geriatric

▲ Provide dentists with accurate medication history to avoid drug interaction (Little et al, 2002).

• Carefully observe oral cavity and lips for abnormal lesions when providing dental care. **EB:** *Oral lesions may be found in clients with pemphigus vulgaris, cicatricial pemphigoid, leukemia, lichen planus, lupus, neutropenia, anemia, salivary gland tumors, cancer, and a host of other conditions (Little et al, 2002).*

▲ Consider professional oral health care for older adults in nursing homes. **EB:** *Professional oral health care administered by dental hygienists to a group of elderly clients needing daily nursing care was associated with a reduction in prevalence of fever and fatal pneumonia (Adachi, 2002).*

• Ensure that dentures are removed and cleaned regularly, preferably after every meal and before bedtime; select appropriate adhesives to improve breath. *Dentures left in the mouth at night impede circulation to the palate and predispose the client to oral lesions.* **EB:** *Fixodent denture adhesives provide the denture wearer with a noticeable improvement in breath odor (Myatt et al, 2002).*

• Support other care givers providing oral hygiene. **EBN:** *Physical and cognitive impairment in older adults can interfere with the client's ability to perform oral hygiene. In many cases care givers take over these procedures. If no care giver is available, the client is prone to dental problems (Little, 2002).*

▲ The medication profile should be reviewed to determine if an older adult is taking anticoagulants. If so, the International Normalized Ration (INR) should be reviewed before providing dental care. **EB:** *Clients with an INR greater than 3.5 should have their dosage of Coumadin reduced by their physician 3-5 days before any dental procedures (Little, 2002).*

Multicultural

• Assess for the influence of cultural beliefs, norms, and values on the client's understanding of dental care. **EBN:** *What the client considers normal and abnormal dental care may be based on cultural perceptions (Leininger & McFarland, 2002; Giger & Davidhizar, 2004).*

• Assess for barriers to access to dental care, such as lack of insurance. *Children from racial minority groups may have significantly more difficulty in accessing dental care (Savage et al, 2004).* **EBN:** *Poverty and lack of dental care insurance may prevent the obtainment of dental care (Woolfolk et al, 1999). African Americans and persons of lower socioeconomic status reported more new dental symptoms, were less likely to obtain dental care, and reported more tooth loss (Gilbert, Duncan & Shelton, 2003).*

• Instruct mothers on the danger of feeding infants bottles filled with soda, juice, or milk when the infant goes to sleep. **EBN:** *Navajo, African-American, Latino, and some other cultural groups engage in this feeding practice, which is known to cause dental caries in children (Andrews, 2003).*

• Assess for dental anxiety. **EBN:** *Anxiety is a major reason for infrequent dental checkups (Woolfolk et al, 1999).*

▲ Introduce the dental home concept to improve families' access to dental care. **EB:** *The dental home is a locus for preventive oral health supervision and emergency care. When culture and ethnicity*

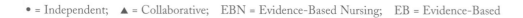

• = Independent;   ▲ = Collaborative;   EBN = Evidence-Based Nursing;   EB = Evidence-Based

are barriers to care, the dental home offers a site adapted to care delivery and sensitive to family values (Nowak & Casamassimo, 2002).

Home Care

- Assess client patterns for daily and professional dental care and related patterns (e.g., smoking, nail biting). Assess for environmental influences on dental status (e.g., fluoride). **EB:** *Many dental problems are preventable with good dental hygiene and care. Behaviors to preserve oral health in old age are essential (Barmes, 2000).*
- Assess client facilities and financial resources for providing dental care. *Lack of appropriate facilities or financial resources is a barrier to positive dental care patterns. Provision for dental care may be missing from healthcare plans or unavailable to the uninsured.*
- Request a dietary log from the client, adding columns for type of food (i.e., soft, pureed, regular).
- Observe a typical meal to assess the impact of impaired dentition on nutrition. *Clients, especially older adults, are often hesitant to admit nutritional changes that may be embarrassing.*
- Identify mechanical needs for food preparation and ease of ingestion/digestion to meet the client's dental/nutritional needs.
- Assist the client with accessing financial or other resources to support optimum dental and nutritional status.

Client/Family Teaching

- Teach how to inspect the oral cavity and monitor for problems with the teeth and gums.
- Teach how to implement a personal plan of dental hygiene, including appropriate brushing of teeth and tongue and using dental floss.
- Teach the client the value of having an optimal fluoride concentration in drinking water and of brushing teeth twice daily with fluoride toothpaste.
- Teach clients of all ages the need to decrease intake of sugary foods and to brush teeth regularly.
- Suggest chewing gum with sugar to reduce oral malodor. *Sugarless chewing gum increased methyl mercaptan, one of the principal components of oral malodor (Yaegaki, 2002).*
- Inform individuals who are considering tongue piercing of the potential complications, such as chipping and cracking of teeth and possible trauma to the gingiva. If piercing is done, teach the client how to care for the wound and prevent complications. **EB:** *Complications identified in the literature from tongue piercing include postoperative swelling, infection, and bleeding; damage to the teeth; and trauma to the soft tissues (Knox, 2002).*

evolve See the EVOLVE website for World Wide Web resources for client education.

REFERENCES

Adachi M, Ishihara K, Abe S et al: Effect of professional oral health care on the elderly living in nursing homes, *Oral Surg Oral Med Oral Pathol Oral Radiol Endod* 94(2):191-195, 2002.

American Dental Association (ADA): Oral health topics A-Z. Available at http://www.ada.org/public/index.asp, accessed on February 21, 2007.

Andrews MM: Transcultural perspectives in the nursing care of children. In Andrews MM, Boyle J, editors: *Transcultural concepts in nursing practice*, Philadelphia, 2003, JB Lippincott.

Barmes DE: Public policy on oral health and old age: a global view, *J Public Health Dent* 60(4):335, 2000.

Brown CG, Yoder LH: Stomatitis: an overview, *Am J Nurs* 102(suppl 4):20, 2002.

Ermis B, Aslan T, Beder L et al: A randomized placebo-controlled trial of mebendazole for halitosis, *Arch Pediatr Adolesc Med* 156(10):995-998, 2002.

Foss-Durant AM, McAffee A: A comparison of three oral care products commonly used in practice, *Clin Nurs Res* 6:1, 1997.

Giger J, Davidhizar R: *Transcultural nursing: assessment and intervention*, ed 4, St Louis, 2004, Mosby Year Book.

Gilbert GH, Duncan RP, Shelton BJ: Social determinants of tooth loss, *Health Serv Res* 38(6 Pt 2), 2003.

Gillcrist JA, Brumley DE, Blackford JU: Community socioeconomic status and children's dental health, *J Am Dent Assoc* 132(2): 216, 2001.

Gray MM, Davies-Slowik J: Changes in the percentage of 5-year-old children with no experience of decay in Dudley towns since the implementation of fluoridation schemes in 1987, *Br Dent J* 190(1):30, 2001.

Heller K, Burt BA, Eklund SA: Sugared soda consumption and dental caries in the United States, *J Dent Res* 80(10):1949, 2001.

Kleinberg I, Wolff MS, Codipilly DM: Role of saliva in oral dryness, oral feel and oral malodour, *Int Dent J* 52(suppl 3):236, 2002.

Knox KT: The potential complications of intra-oral and peri-oral piercing, *Dent Health* 41:3, 2002.

Koop CE: Kids' dental health. Available at www.drkoop.com/template.asp?page = newsdetailandap = 93andid = 508508, accessed on March 12, 2007.

Krespi YP Shrime MG, Kacker A: The relationship between oral malodor and volatile sulfur compound-producing bacteria, *Otolaryngol Head Neck Surg,* 135(5):671-676, 2006.

Leininger MM, McFarland MR: *Transcultural nursing: concepts, theories, research and practices,* ed 3, New York, 2002, McGraw-Hill.

Little J, Falace D, Miller C et al: *Dental management of the medically compromised patient,* ed 6, St Louis, 2002, Mosby.

Marinho VC, Higgins JP, Logan S et al: Topical fluoride (toothpastes, mouthrinses, gels or varnishes) for preventing dental caries in children and adolescents, *Cochrane Database Syst Rev* (4):CD002278, 2003.

Myatt GJ, Hunt SA, Barlow AP et al: A clinical study to assess the breath protection efficacy of denture adhesive, *J Contemp Dent Pract* 3(4):1-9, 2002.

Nowak AJ, Casamassimo PS: The dental home: a primary care oral health concept, *J Am Dent Assoc* 133(1):93-98, 2002.

Obesity, Fitness & Wellness Week: Dental research; Gingival bleeding and halitosis are greatly reduced after a two-week oral hygiene program, August 26, 2006:843.

Outhouse TL, Fedorowicz Z, Keenan JV et al: A Cochrane systematic review finds tongue scrapers have short-term efficacy in controlling halitosis, *Gen Dent* 54(5):352-360, 367-368, 2006.

Pearson LS, Hutton JL: A controlled trial to compare the ability of foam swabs and toothbrushes to remove dental plaque, *J Adv Nurs* 39(5):480, 2002.

Poland JM: Comparing Moi-Stir to lemon-glycerin swabs, *Am J Nurs* 87(4):422, 1987.

Robinson PG, Deacon SA, Deery C et al: Manual versus powered toothbrushing for oral health, *Cochrane Database Syst Rev* (2): CD002281, 2005.

Sasahara H, Kawamura M: Behavioral dental science: the relationship between tooth-brushing angle and plaque removal at the lingual surfaces of the posterior teeth in the mandible, *J Oral Sci* 42(2):79, 2000.

Savage MF, Lee JY, Kotch JB et al: Early preventive dental visits: effects on subsequent utilization and costs, *Pediatrics* 114(4): e418-423, 2004.

Scannapieco FA, Stewart EM, Mylotte JM: Colonization of dental plaque by respiratory pathogens in medical intensive care patients, *Crit Care Med* 20:740, 1992.

Schiff T, Proskin HM, Zhang YP et al A clinical investigation of the efficacy of three different treatment regimens for the control of plaque and gingivitis, *J Clin Dent* 17(5):138-144, 2006.

Sjogren K, Lundberg AB, Birkhed D et al: Interproximal plaque mass and fluoride retention after brushing and flossing—a comparative study of powered toothbrushing, manual toothbrushing and flossing, *Oral Health Prev Dent* 2(2):119-124, 2004.

Stiefel KA, Damron S, Sowers NJ et al: Improving oral hygiene for the seriously ill patient: implementing research-based practice, *Medsurg Nurs* 9(1):40-43, 2000.

Tangerman A: Halitosis in medicine: a review, *Int Dent J* 52(suppl 3):201-206, 2002.

Tombes MB, Gallucci B: The effects of hydrogen peroxide rinses on the normal oral mucosa, *Nurs Res* 42:332, 1993.

Valaitis R, Hesch R, Passarelli C et al: A systematic review of the relationship between breastfeeding and early childhood caries, *Can J Public Health* 91(6):411-417, 2000.

Woolfolk MW, Lang WP, Borgnakke WS et al: Determining dental checkup frequency, *J Am Dental Assoc* 130(5):715, 1999.

Yaegaki K, Coil JM, Kamemizu T et al: Tongue brushing and mouth rinsing as basic treatment measures for halitosis, *Int Dent J* 52(suppl 3):192-196, 2002.

Zimmer S, Strauss J, Bizhang M et al: Efficacy of the Cybersonic in comparison with the Braun 3D Excel and a manual toothbrush, *J Clin Periodontol* 32(4):360-363, 2005.

Risk for delayed Development   *Gail B. Ladwig, MSN, CHTP, RN*

NANDA **Definition**

At risk for delay of 25% or more in one or more of the areas of social or self-regulatory behavior or cognitive, language, gross, or fine motor skills

Risk Factors

Prenatal

Endocrine disorders; genetic disorders; illiteracy; inadequate nutrition; infections; lack of prenatal care; late prenatal care; maternal age <15 years; maternal age >35 years; poor prenatal care; poverty; substance abuse; unplanned pregnancy; unwanted pregnancy

Individual

Adopted child; behavior disorders; brain damage (e.g., hemorrhage in postnatal period, shaken baby, abuse, accident); chemotherapy; chronic illness; congenital disorders; failure to thrive; foster child; frequent otitis media; genetic disorders; hearing impairment; inadequate nutrition; lead poisoning; natural disasters; positive drug screen(s); prematurity; radiation therapy; seizures; substance abuse; technology-dependent; vision impairment

Environmental

Poverty; violence

• = Independent;   ▲ = Collaborative;   EBN = Evidence-Based Nursing;   EB = Evidence-Based

Caregiver

Abuse; mental illness; mental retardation or severe learning disability

Outcomes (Nursing Outcomes Classification)

Suggested NOC Outcomes

Child Development: 1 Month, 2 Months, 4 Months, 6 Months, 12 Months, 2 Years, 3 Years, 4 Years, Preschool, Middle Childhood, Adolescence, Growth, Neglect Recovery, Knowledge: Infant Care, Parenting

Example NOC Outcome with Indicators
Child Development as evidenced by the following indicators: Appropriate milestones of physical, cognitive, and psychosocial age appropriate progression (Rate the outcome and indicators of **Child Development:** 1 = never demonstrated, 2 = rarely demonstrated, 3 = sometimes demonstrated, 4 = often demonstrated, 5 = consistently demonstrated [see Section I].)

Client Outcomes

Client/Parents/Primary Caregiver Will (Specify Time Frame):

- Describe realistic, age-appropriate patterns of development
- Promote activities and interactions that support age-related developmental tasks

NIC Interventions (Nursing Interventions Classification)

Suggested NIC Interventions

Active Listening, Developmental Enhancement: Child, Emotional Support, Kangaroo Care, Self-Care Assistance, Self-Responsibility Facilitation

Example NIC Activities—Developmental Enhancement: Child
Teach caregivers about normal developmental milestones and associated behaviors; Establish one-on-one interaction with child

Nursing Interventions and *Rationales*

- Refer to care plan for **Delayed Growth and development.**

Preconception/Pregnancy

- Males and females should avoid exposure to organic solvents before and during pregnancy. **EB:** *Exposure in utero to organic solvents is associated with poorer performance on some specific subtle measures of neurocognitive function, language, and behavior (Laslo-Baker et al, 2004). There is some indication of an increased risk of functional developmental disorders in offspring among painters with intermediate and high model predicted exposures (Hooiveld et al, 2006).*
- Avoid exposure to heavy metals, pesticides, herbicides, sterilants, anesthetic gases, and anticancer drugs used in health care. **EB:** *Many toxicants with unambiguous reproductive and developmental effects are still in regular commercial or therapeutic use and thus present exposure potential to workers. Caregivers must be aware of their clients' potential environmental and workplace exposures (McDiarmid & Gehle, 2006). Increased maternal lead concentration at third trimester of pregnancy, especially around week 28, was associated with decreased intellectual child development (Schnaas et al, 2006).*

 Multicultural

Parents

- Assess for the influence of cultural beliefs, norms, and values on the client's perceptions of child development. **EBN:** *Latino mothers of children with developmental disabilities viewed their child as*

D

not being responsible for the behavior problem (Chavira et al, 2000). Latino mothers of developmentally disabled adults reported their relationship with the educational and service delivery systems to be characterized by poor communication, low effort in providing services, negative attitudes of professionals toward the client/children, and negative treatment of parents by professionals (Shapiro et al, 2004).

Infants

- Carefully assess Pakistani and Bangladeshi infants for developmental milestones, and supply appropriate preventive interventions, such as adequate nutrition. *Deprivation among these groups must be addressed to reduce the likelihood of developmental delay and possible longer term behavioral and cognitive problems and consequent opportunities throughout life (Kelly et al, 2006).*

 ### Home Care

- Teach the parents to provide toys and books and read aloud to young children in the home. *Reading aloud and providing toys are associated with better child cognitive and language development (Tomopoulos et al, 2006).*

 ### Client/Family Teaching

- ▲ Encourage mothers to abstain from alcohol and cocaine use during pregnancy; refer them to treatment programs for substance abuse. **EB:** *Prenatal exposures to both cocaine and opiates were strongly associated with elevated risk of central nervous system/autonomic nervous system (CNS/ANS) manifestations (Das, Poole & Bada, 2004). Smoking during pregnancy is a well-established determinant of fetal growth and risk of low birth weight. Maternal smoking in pregnancy may influence the development of the fetal respiratory system (Jaakkola & Gissler, 2004).*
- Encourage adequate antepartum and postpartum care for both mother and child. *Access to prenatal and postnatal health care promotes optimal growth and development (Bland et al, 2000).*
- Counsel parents, siblings, and caregivers about the importance of smoking cessation and the necessity of eliminating all secondhand smoke exposure. *Smoking affects development not only during intrauterine life but also during the early stage of extrauterine life (Bottini et al, 2004).*
- Teach caregivers of children appropriate developmental interactions; use anticipatory guidance to facilitate preparation for developmental milestones. **EB:** *Two postnatal factors—home environment and caregiver-child interaction—were associated with full-scale IQ scores of 90 or higher. These potentially malleable postnatal factors can be targeted for change to improve cognitive outcome of inner-city children (Hurt et al, 1998).*
- Provide developmental care interventions to preterm infants to improve neurodevelopmental outcomes. **EB:** *Developmental care is effective to improve outcomes (Symington & Pinelli, 2002).*
- ▲ Provide information on support groups and education on human immunodeficiency virus (HIV) and caring for infants with this diagnosis. *Developmental delay has been well documented in infants with HIV (Potterton & Eales, 2001).*

evolve See the EVOLVE website for World Wide Web resources for client education.

REFERENCES

Bland M, Vermillion ST, Soper DE et al: Late third trimester treatment of rectovaginal group B streptococci with benzathine penicillin G, *Am J Obstet Gynecol* 183(2):372, 2000.

Bottini N, Gloria-Bottini F, Magrini A et al: Maternal cigarette smoking, metabolic enzyme polymorphism, and developmental events in the early stages of extrauterine life, *Hum Biol* 76(2):289-297, 2004.

Chavira V, Lopez SR, Blacher J et al: Latina mothers' attributions, emotions, and reactions to the problem behaviors of their children with developmental disabilities, *J Child Psychol Psychiatry* 41(2):245-252, 2000.

Das A, Poole WK, Bada HS: Repeated measures approach for simultaneous modeling of multiple neurobehavioral outcomes in newborns exposed to cocaine in utero, *Am J Epidemiol* 159(9):891-899, 2004.

Hooiveld M, Haveman W, Roskes K et al: Adverse reproductive outcomes among male painters with occupational exposure to organic solvents, *Occup Environ Med* 63(8):538-544, 2006.

Hurt H, Malmud E, Braitman LE et al: Inner-city achievers: who are they? *Arch Pediatr Adolesc Med* 152(10):993-997, 1998.

Jaakkola JJ, Gissler M: Maternal smoking in pregnancy, fetal development, and childhood asthma, *Am J Public Health* 94(1):136-140, 2004.

Kelly Y, Sacker A, Schoon I et al: Ethnic differences in achievement of developmental milestones by 9 months of age: the Millennium Cohort Study, *Dev Med Child Neurol* 48(10):825-830, 2006.

Laslo-Baker D, Barrera M, Knittel-Keren D et al: Child neurodevelopmental outcome and maternal occupational exposure to solvents, *Arch Pediatr Adolesc Med* 158(10):956-961, 2004.

McDiarmid MA, Gehle K: Preconception brief: occupational/environmental exposures, *Matern Child Health J* 10(suppl 5):123-128, 2006.

Potterton J, Eales C: Prevalence of developmental delay in infants who are HIV positive, *S Afr J Physiother* 57(3):11, 2001.

Schnaas L, Rothenberg S, Flores M et al: Reduced intellectual development in children with prenatal lead exposure, *Environ Health Perspect* 114(5):791-797, 2006.

Shapiro J, Monzo LD, Rueda R et al: Alienated advocacy: perspectives of Latina mothers of young adults with developmental disabilities on service systems, *Ment Retard* 42(1):37-54, 2004.

Symington A, Pinelli J: Developmental care for promoting development and preventing morbidity in preterm infants, *Cochrane Database Syst Rev* (3):CD001814, 2002.

Tomopoulos S, Dreyer BP, Tamis-LeMonda C et al: Books, toys, parent-child interaction, and development in young Latino children, *Ambul Pediatr* 6(2):72-78, 2006.

Diarrhea   *Betty J. Ackley, MSN, EdS, RN*

NANDA   Definition

Passage of loose, unformed stools

Defining Characteristics

Abdominal pain; at least 3 loose liquid stools per day; cramping; hyperactive bowel sounds; urgency

Related Factors (r/t)

Psychological

Anxiety; high stress levels

Situational

Adverse effects of medications; alcohol abuse; contaminants; travel; laxative abuse; radiation; toxins; tube feedings

Physiological

Infectious processes; inflammation; irritation; malabsorption; parasites

NOC   Outcomes (Nursing Outcomes Classification)

Suggested NOC Outcomes

Bowel Elimination, Electrolyte and Acid-Base Balance, Fluid Balance, Hydration, Treatment Behavior: Illness or Injury

> **Example NOC Outcome with Indicators**
>
> **Bowel Elimination** as evidenced by the following indicators: Elimination pattern/Stool soft and formed/Diarrhea not present/Control of bowel movements/Comfort of stool passage/Pain with passage of stool not present (Rate the outcome and indicators of **Bowel Elimination:** 1 = severely compromised, 2 = substantially compromised, 3 = moderately compromised, 4 = mildly compromised, 5 = not compromised [see Section I].)

Client Outcomes

Client Will (Specify Time Frame):

- Defecate formed, soft stool every day to every third day
- Maintain a rectal area free of irritation
- State relief from cramping and less or no diarrhea
- Explain cause of diarrhea and rationale for treatment
- Maintain good skin turgor and weight at usual level
- Contain stool appropriately (if previously incontinent)

• = Independent;   ▲ = Collaborative;   EBN = Evidence-Based Nursing;   EB = Evidence-Based

D

Suggested NIC Intervention

Diarrhea Management

Example NIC Activities—Diarrhea Management
Evaluate medication profile for gastrointestinal side effects; Suggest trial elimination of foods containing lactose

Nursing Interventions and *Rationales*

- Assess pattern of defecation, or have the client keep a diary that includes the following: time of day defecation occurs; usual stimulus for defecation; consistency, amount, and frequency of stool; type of, amount of, and time food consumed; fluid intake; history of bowel habits and laxative use; diet; exercise patterns; obstetrical/gynecological, medical, and surgical histories; medications; alterations in perianal sensations; and present bowel regimen. *Assessment of defecation pattern will help direct treatment.*
- Assess stool consistency and its influence on risk for stool loss. Several classification systems for stool have been promulgated. **EBN:** *A study of stool consistency found good reliability when evaluated by professional nurses, student nurses, and clients. Word-only descriptors yielded equivocal consistency when assessed by subjects as did tools that combined words with illustrations of various stool consistencies (Bliss et al, 2001).*
- ▲ Identify cause of diarrhea if possible based on history (e.g., rotavirus or norovirus exposure; HIV infection; food poisoning; medication effect; radiation therapy; protein malnutrition; laxative abuse; stress). See Related Factors (r/t). *Identification of the underlying cause is important, because the treatment often depends on it (Thielman & Guerrant, 2004).*
- ▲ If the client has watery diarrhea, a low-grade fever, abdominal cramps, and a history of antibiotic therapy, consider possibility of *Clostridium difficile* infection. C. difficile *infection and pseudomembranous colitis have become increasingly common because of the frequent use of broad-spectrum antibiotics (Thielman & Guerrant, 2004).* **EB:** *No specific antibiotic or combination of antibiotics account for the difference in the clients with* C. difficile*–positive stool compared to a control group of clients with diarrhea. However, the clients with* C. difficile*–positive stools are more severely ill, as rated on a severity of illness scale (Vesta et al, 2005).*
- ▲ Obtain stool specimens as ordered, to either rule out or diagnose an infectious process (e.g., ova and parasites, *C. difficile* infection, bacterial cultures).
- ▲ Use standard precautions when caring for clients with diarrhea to prevent spread of infectious diarrhea; use gloves and hand washing. C. difficile *and viruses causing diarrhea have been shown to be contagious.* C. difficile *is difficult to eradicate because of spore formation (Poutanen & Simor, 2004).* **EBN and EB:** *A nursing review of the most recent development in client care related to* C. difficile *summarizes care to include: contact isolation, soap and water hand washing, use of disposable equipment, and intensive housekeeping using hypochlorite-based products for disinfection (Todd, 2006). Bacterial spores, such as* C. difficile, *are not destroyed by alcohol, chlorhexidine, or triclosan products. Even vigorous hand washing is minimally effective. Vegetative cells of* C. difficile *can survive for at least 24 hours on inanimate surfaces, and spores can survive up to five months (Kampf & Kramer, 2004).*
- ▲ If the client has diarrhea associated with antibiotic therapy, consult with the primary care practitioner regarding the use of probiotics, such as yogurt, with active cultures to treat diarrhea (Van Niel et al, 2002), or also use probiotics to prevent diarrhea when first beginning antibiotic therapy. **EB:** *Probiotics have been shown to be helpful to prevent antibiotic-associated diarrhea (D'Souza et al, 2002; Teitelbaum & Walker, 2002). Probiotics are a useful adjunct to rehydration therapy in treating acute infectious diarrhea in both adults and children (Bricker et al, 2005).*
- Ask the client to examine intake of high fructose corn syrup and fructose sweeteners in relation to onset of diarrhea symptoms. If diarrhea is associated with fructose ingestion, intake should be limited or eliminated. **EB:** *High fructose corn syrup or fructose sweeteners from fruit juices can cause*

gastrointestinal (GI) symptoms of bloating, rumbling, flatulence, and diarrhea at amounts of 25-50 g. Malabsorption is demonstrated in clients after 25 g fructose, and most clients develop symptoms with 50 g fructose (Beyer, Caviar & McCallum, 2005).

- If the client has infectious diarrhea, avoid using medications that slow peristalsis. *If an infectious process is occurring, such as* C. difficile *infection or food poisoning, medication to slow down peristalsis should generally not be given (Bliss et al, 2000). The increase in gut motility helps eliminate the causative factor, and use of antidiarrheal medication could result in a toxic megacolon (Sunenshine & McDonald, 2006).*

- Inspect, palpate, percuss, and auscultate abdomen; note whether bowel sounds are frequent.

- Assess for dehydration by observing skin turgor over sternum and inspecting for longitudinal furrows of the tongue. Watch for excessive thirst, fever, dizziness, lightheadedness, palpitations, excessive cramping, bloody stools, hypotension, and symptoms of shock. *Severe diarrhea can cause deficient fluid volume with extreme weakness (Mentes, 2006).*

- Observe for symptoms of sodium and potassium loss (e.g., weakness, abdominal or leg cramping, dysrhythmia). Note results of electrolyte laboratory studies. *Stool contains electrolytes; excessive diarrhea causes electrolyte abnormalities that can be especially harmful to clients with existing medical conditions.*

- Monitor and record intake and output; note oliguria and dark, concentrated urine.

- Measure specific gravity of urine if possible. *Dark, concentrated urine, along with a high specific gravity of urine, is an indication of deficient fluid volume.*

- Weigh the client daily and note decreased weight. *An accurate daily weight is an important indicator of fluid balance in the body (Metheny, 2000).*

- Give dilute clear fluids as tolerated (e.g., clear soda, gelatin dessert), serving at lukewarm temperature.

▲ If the client has chronic diarrhea causing fecal incontinence at intervals, consider suggesting use of dietary fiber from psyllium or gum arabic after consultation with primary practitioner. **EBN and EB:** *Use of a fiber supplement decreases the number of incontinent stools and improves stool consistency (Bliss et al, 2001). The use of soluble dietary fiber is useful for controlling diarrhea and normalizing the intestinal flora (Nakao et al, 2002).*

▲ If diarrhea is chronic and there is evidence of malnutrition, consult with primary care practitioner for a dietary consult and possible use of a hydrolyzed formula (a clear liquid supplement containing increased protein) to maintain nutrition while the gastrointestinal system heals. *A hydrolyzed formula contains protein that is partially broken down to amino acids for people who cannot digest nutrients (Lutz & Przytulski, 2005).*

- Encourage the client to eat small, frequent meals, to consume foods that are easy to digest (e.g., bananas, crackers, pretzels, rice, potatoes, clear soups, applesauce), and to avoid milk products, foods high in fiber, and caffeine (dark sodas, tea, coffee, chocolate). *The use of a BRAT diet (bananas, rice, applesauce, and toast) with avoidance of milk products (since a transient lactase deficiency may occur) is commonly recommended, although limited data supports this (Thielman & Guerrant, 2004).*

- Provide a readily available bedpan, commode, or bathroom.

- If the client has diarrhea and incontinence, consider use of a Perineal Assessment Tool to measure the risk for perineal skin injury. **EBN:** *The Perineal Assessment Tool has been developed to determine the risk of perineal skin injury. The initial results of the study are encouraging, and further studies are needed (Nix, 2002).*

- Thoroughly cleanse and dry the perianal and perineal skin daily and as needed (PRN) using a cleanser capable of stool removal. Select a product with a slightly acidic pH designed to preserve the skin's acid mantle, and designed to remove irritants from the skin with minimal physical force. Avoid vigorous scrubbing with water, soap, and a washcloth. Consider selection of a product with a moisturizer. *Traditional soaps tend to be alkaline, interfering with the natural acid mantle of the integument and increasing its susceptibility to irritant dermatitis and secondary infection. Brisk scrubbing may exacerbate skin erosion and further increase the risk of irritation and infection (Gray, 2004; Gray, Ratliff & Donovan, 2002).*

▲ If the client is receiving a tube feeding, note rate of infusion, and prevent contamination of

---

• = Independent;   ▲ = Collaborative;   EBN = Evidence-Based Nursing;   EB = Evidence-Based

D

feeding by rinsing container every 8 hours and replacing it every 24 hours. *Rapid administration of tube feeding and contaminated feedings have been associated with diarrhea.*

▲ If the client is receiving a tube feeding, suggest formulas that contain a bulking agent, such as Jevity, or add soluble dietary fiber to the feeding per physician's/dietitian's order. **EB:** *Bulking agents including soluble fiber are useful in tube feedings to prevent or treat diarrhea in the tube-fed client (Nakao et al, 2002).*

Pediatric

▲ Recommend the parents give the child oral rehydration fluids to drink in the amounts specified by the physician, especially during the first 4 to 6 hours to replace lost fluid. Once the child is rehydrated, an orally administered maintenance solution should be used along with food. **EB:** *Treatment with oral rehydration fluids for children are generally as effective as intravenous (IV) fluids; IV fluids do not shorten the duration of gastroenteritis and are more likely to cause adverse effects than oral rehydration therapy (Banks & Meadows, 2005).*

• Recommend the mother resume breastfeeding as soon as possible.

• Recommend parents not give the child decarbonated soda, fruit juices, gelatin dessert, or instant fruit drink. *These fluids have a high osmolality from carbohydrate contents and can exacerbate diarrhea. In addition they have low sodium concentrations that can aggravate existing hyponatremia (Behrman, Kliegman & Jenson, 2004).*

• Recommend parents give children foods with complex carbohydrates, such as potatoes, rice, bread, cereal, yogurt, fruits, and vegetables. The BRAT diet is often advocated. Avoid fatty foods and foods high in simple sugars (Behrman, Kliegman & Jenson, 2004). *When a child has diarrhea, dietary modification includes avoiding dairy products, because viral or bacterial infections can cause a transient lactase deficiency. Easily digested food, such as bananas, rice, applesauce, and toast, are also recommended (Amerine & Keirsy, 2004).*

Geriatric

▲ Evaluate medications the client is taking. Recognize that many medications can result in diarrhea, including digitalis, propranolol, angiotensin-converting enzyme (ACE) inhibitors, histamine-receptor antagonists, nonsteroidal antiinflammatory drugs (NSAIDs), anticholinergic agents, oral hypoglycemia agents, antibiotics, and others. *A drug-associated cause should always be considered when treating diarrhea in the older person; many drugs can result in diarrhea (Ratnaike, 2000).*

▲ Monitor the client closely to detect whether an impaction is causing diarrhea; remove impaction as ordered. *Clients with fecal impaction commonly experience leakage of mucus or liquid stool from rectal irritation, distention, and impaired anal sensation (Butcher, 2004).*

▲ Seek medical attention if diarrhea is severe or persists for more than 24 hours, or if the client has history of dehydration or electrolyte disturbances, such as lassitude, weakness, or prostration. *Older adult clients can dehydrate rapidly; especially serious is development of hypokalemia with dysrhythmias.* C. difficile *is a common cause of diarrhea in older adult clients when they have been subjected to long-term antibiotic therapy. Proper infection control practices should be maintained within the home to avoid cross contamination.*

• Provide emotional support for clients who are having trouble controlling unpredictable episodes of diarrhea. *Diarrhea can be a great source of embarrassment to older clients and can lead to social isolation and a feeling of powerlessness.*

Home Care

• Previously mentioned interventions may be adapted for home care use.

• Assess the home for general sanitation and methods of food preparation. Reinforce principles of sanitation for food handling. *Poor sanitation or mishandling of food may cause bacterial infection or transmission of dangerous organisms from utensils to food.*

▲ Assess for methods of handling soiled laundry if the client is bed bound or has been incontinent. Instruct or reinforce Universal Precautions with family and blood-borne pathogen precautions with agency caregivers. *The Bloodborne Pathogen Regulations of the Occupational Safety and Health Administration (OSHA) identify legal guidelines for caregivers.*

▲ When assessing medication history, include over-the-counter (OTC) drugs, both general and those currently being used to treat the diarrhea. Instruct clients not to mix OTC medications when self-treating. *Mixing OTC medications can further irritate the gastrointestinal system, intensifying the diarrhea or causing nausea and vomiting.*

▲ Evaluate current medications for indication that specific interventions are warranted. *Blood levels of medications may increase during prolonged episodes of diarrhea, indicating the need for close monitoring of the client or direct intervention.*

▲ Consult with physician regarding need for blood work or stool specimens. *Laboratory tests may be needed to identify presence of a bacterial pathogen or assess for electrolyte imbalance.*

▲ Evaluate need for home health aide or homemaker service referral. *Caregiver may need support for maintaining client cleanliness to prevent skin breakdown.*

▲ Evaluate need for durable medical equipment in the home. *The client may need bedside commode, call bell, or raised toilet seat to facilitate prompt toileting.*

Client/Family Teaching

- Encourage avoidance of coffee, spices, milk products, and foods that irritate or stimulate the gastrointestinal tract.
- Teach appropriate method of taking ordered antidiarrheal medications; explain side effects.
- Explain how to prevent the spread of infectious diarrhea (e.g., careful hand washing, appropriate handling and storage of food).
- Help the client to determine stressors and set up an appropriate stress reduction plan.
- Teach signs and symptoms of dehydration and electrolyte imbalance.
- Teach perirectal skin care.

 See the EVOLVE website for World Wide Web resources for client education.

REFERENCES

Amerine E, Keirsy M: Managing acute diarrhea, *Nursing* 3(9):64, 2004.

Banks JB, Meadows S: Intravenous fluids for children with gastroenteritis, *Am Fam Physician* 71(1):121, 2005.

Behrman RE, Kliegman RM, Jenson HB: *Nelson textbook of pediatrics,* ed 17, Philadelphia, 2004, Saunders.

Beyer PL, Caviar EM, McCallum RW: Fructose intake at current levels in the United States may cause gastrointestinal distress in normal adults, *J Am Diet Assoc* 105(10):1559-1566, 2005.

Bliss DZ, Johnson S, Savik K et al: Fecal incontinence in hospitalized patients who are acutely ill, *Nurs Res* 49(2):101, 2000.

Bliss DZ, Jung HJ, Savik K et al: Supplementation with dietary fiber improves fecal incontinence, *Nurs Res* 50(4):203, 2001.

Bricker E, Garg R, Nelson R et al: Antibiotic treatment for *Clostridium difficile*–associated diarrhea in adults, *Cochrane Database Syst Rev* (1):CD004610, 2005.

Butcher L: Clinical skills: nursing considerations in patients with faecal incontinence, *Br J Nurs* 13(13):760, 2004.

D'Souza AL, Rajkumar C, Cooke J et al: Probiotics in prevention of antibiotic associated diarrhea: meta-analysis, *BMJ* 324(7350):1361, 2002.

Gray M: Preventing and managing perineal dermatitis: a shared goal for wound and continence care, *J Wound Ostomy Continence Nurs* 31(suppl 1):S2-S9, 2004.

Gray M, Ratliff C, Donovan A: Perineal skin care for the incontinent patient, *Adv Skin Wound Care* 15:170, 2002.

Kampf G, Kramer A: Epidemiologic background of hand hygiene and evaluation of the most important agents for scrubs and rubs, *Clin Microbiol Rev* 17(4):863-893, 2004.

Lutz C, Przytulski K: *Nutrition and diet therapy,* Philadelphia, 2005, FA Davis.

Mentes J: Oral hydration in older adults: greater awareness is needed in preventing, recognizing, and treating dehydration, *Am J Nurs* 106(6):40-49, 2006.

Metheny N: *Fluid and electrolyte balance: nursing considerations,* ed 4, Philadelphia, 2000, Lippincott Williams & Wilkins.

Nakao M, Ogura Y, Satake S et al: Usefulness of soluble dietary fiber for the treatment of diarrhea during general nutrition in elderly patients, *Nutrition* 18(1):35, 2002.

Nix DH: Validity and reliability of the Perineal Assessment Tool, *Ostomy Wound Manage* 48:2, 2002.

Poutanen SM, Simor AE: *Clostridium difficile*-associated diarrhea in adults, *CMAJ* 171(1):51, 2004.

Ratnaike RN: Drug-induced diarrhea in older persons, *Clin Geriatr* 8(1):67, 2000.

Sunenshine RH, McDonald LC: Clostridium difficile-associated disease: new challenges from an established pathogen, *Cleve Clin J Med* 73(2):187-197, 2006.

Teitelbaum JE, Walker WA: Nutritional impact of pre- and probiotics as protective gastrointestinal organisms, *Annu Rev Nutr* 22:107, 2002.

Thielman NM, Guerrant RL: Clinical practice. Acute infectious diarrhea, *N Engl J Med* 350(1):38, 2004.

Todd B: *Clostridium difficile:* familiar pathogen, changing epidemiology: a virulent strain has been appearing more often, even in patients not taking antibiotics, *Am J Nurs* 106(5):33-36, 2006.

Van Niel CW, Feudtner C, Garrison MM et al: Lactobacillus therapy for acute infectious diarrhea in children: a meta-analysis, *Pediatrics* 109(4):678, 2002.

Vesta KS, Wells PG, Gentry CA et al: Specific risk factors for *Clostridium difficile*-associated diarrhea: a prospective, multicenter, case control evaluation, *Am J Infect Control* 33(8):469-472, 2005.

• = Independent;   ▲ = Collaborative;   EBN = Evidence-Based Nursing;   EB = Evidence-Based

Risk for compromised Human Dignity

Susan Rosenberg, MSN, RN, CHI, and Betty Ackley, MSN, EdS, RN

NANDA   Definition

At risk for perceived loss of respect and honor

Risk Factors

Cultural incongruity; disclosure of confidential information; exposure of the body; inadequate participation in decision making; loss of control of body functions; perceived dehumanizing treatment; perceived humiliation; perceived intrusion by clinicians; perceived invasion of privacy; stigmatizing label; use of undefined medical terms

NOC   Outcomes (Nursing Outcomes Classification)

Suggested NOC Outcomes

Health beliefs: perceived control, Decision-Making, Spiritual control

Example NOC Outcome with Indicators
Health Beliefs: Perceived Control as evidenced by the following indicators: Perceived responsibility for health decisions/Requested involvement in health decisions/Efforts at gathering information/Belief that own decisions control health outcomes/Willingness to designate surrogate decision maker (Rate the outcome and indicators of **Health Beliefs: Perceived Control:** 1 = very weak, 2 = weak, 3 = moderate, 4 = strong, 5 = very strong [see Section I].)

Client Outcomes

Client Will (Specify Time Frame):
- Perceive that dignity is maintained throughout hospitalization
- Consistently be called by name of choice
- Have privacy maintained at all times

NIC   Interventions (Nursing Interventions Classification)

Suggested NIC Interventions

Presence, Decision-Making Support, Spiritual Support, Hope Instillation

Example NIC Activities—Presence
Demonstrate accepting attitude; Listen to patient's concerns

Nursing Interventions and *Rationales*

- Be authentically present when with the client, try to limit extraneous thoughts of self or others, concentrate on the well being of the client. *Helping the client feel important is a core value in the nursing profession. Respect for human dignity includes self-worth, autonomy, self-determination, individuality, and client rights (DiBartolo, 2006; Coventry, 2006). The nurse attempts to enter into and stay within the other's frame of reference to connect with the inner life world of meaning and spirit of the other; together they join in a mutual search for meaning and wholeness of being and becoming to potentiate comfort measures, pain control, a sense of well-being, wholeness, or even spiritual transcendence of suffering (Chantal, 2003).*
- Accept the client as is, with unconditional positive regard. *The person is viewed as whole and complete, regardless of illness, or social situation. Dignity is an inherent characteristic of being human (DiBartolo, 2006). Being treated with unconditional love is a healing experience in itself.*

• = Independent;   ▲ = Collaborative;   EBN = Evidence-Based Nursing;   EB = Evidence-Based

- Use loving appropriate touch based on client's culture. When first meeting the client, shake hands with younger clients, touch the arm or shoulder of older clients. *Ideally the caring relationship with client and family begins on hospital admission and is carried through to discharge and into the home if possible.* **EB:** *Touch can lower anxiety (Moon & Cho, 2001). Touch can help build interpersonal relationships (Edvarsson, Sandman & Rasmussen, 2003; Salzmann-Erikson & Eriksson, 2005).*
- Determine the client's perspective about their health. Example questions include: "Tell me about your health." "What is it like to be in your situation?" "Tell me how you perceive yourself in this situation." "What meaning are you giving to this situation?" "Tell me about your health priorities." "Tell me about the harmony you wish to reach." *Such questions usually contribute to helping people find meaning to the crisis in their life (Watson, 2007, in press).*
- Create a loving, healing environment for the client to help meet physical, psychological, and spiritual needs as possible. *The goal is to develop a healing environment in which wholeness, beauty, comfort, dignity, and peace are potentiated (Watson & Foster, 2003).*
- Determine the client's preferences for when and how nursing care is needed and follow the client's guidelines if at all possible. *The client's autonomy must be recognized as part of dignified nursing care (Coventry, 2006).*
- Include the client in all decision making. If the client does not chose to be part of the decision, or is no longer capable of making a decision, use the named surrogate decision maker.
- Encourage the client to share his/her feelings, both positive and negative as appropriate and as the client is willing. *Being present to and supportive of the expression of positive and negative feelings is a connection with deeper spirit of self and the one-being-cared-for (Watson, 2007).*
- Ask the client what they would like to be called and use that name consistently.
- Maintain privacy at all times.
- Avoid authoritative care where the nurse knows what should be done, and the client is powerless. *Authoritative practice does not acknowledge the rights and dignity of others; those who have power must constrain themselves and use caution in applying care based on own judgments (Matiti & Cotrel-Gibbons, 2006).*
- Sit down when talking to clients in the bed, establish appropriate eye contact. *Towering over a client makes communication difficult; the nurse is displaying power behaviors that make the client uncomfortable and decrease communication.*
- Actively listen to what the client is saying both verbally and non-verbally.
- Encourage the client to share thoughts about spirituality as desires. *The care of the soul remains the most powerful aspect of the art of caring in nursing. The caring occasion becomes "transpersonal" when "it allows for the presence of the spirit of both—then the event of the moment expands the limits of openness and has the ability to expand human capabilities" (Watson, 2007, in press).*
- Utilize interventions to instill increased hope; see the care plan **Readiness for enhanced Hope.**
- For further interventions on spirituality, see the care plan for **Readiness for enhanced Spiritual well-being.**

Geriatrics

- Avoid calling elderly clients "sweetie," "honey," "Gramps," or other terms that can be demeaning unless this is acceptable in the client's culture or requested by the client. *Appropriate forms of address must be used with the elderly to maintain dignity (Woolhead et al, 2006).*
- Treat the elderly client with the utmost respect, even if delirium or dementia is present with confusion. *Confused clients respond positively to caregivers who approach gently, with positive regard, and treat the confused client with respect and dignity.*
- Avoid use of restraints. *The paternalistic use of physical restraints is morally unjustified and a violation of the client's autonomy. Dignity is not maintained (Cheung & Yam, 2005).*

Multicultural

- Assess for the influence of cultural beliefs, norms, and values on the client's way of communicating, and follow the client's lead in communicating in matters of eye contact, amount of personal space, voice tones, and amount of touching. *What the client considers normal and appropriate com-*

munication that maintains and facilitates dignity is based on cultural perceptions (Leininger & Mc-Farland, 2002; Giger & Davidhizar, 2004).

Home Care

- Most of the interventions described previously may be adapted for home care use.
- Recognize that the client with the caregiver have complete autonomy in the home. *The nurse's role is to provide the care needed and desired. The client and caregiver determine if the care offered is acceptable.*

Client/Family Teaching

- Teach family and caregivers the need for the dignity of the client to be maintained at all times. NOTE: Caring is integral to maintaining dignity. According to Jean Watson, a caring occasion is the moment (focal point in space and time) when the nurse and another person come together in such a way that an occasion for human caring is created. Both the one cared-for and the one caring can be influenced by the caring moment through the choices and actions decided within the relationship, thereby, influencing and becoming part of their own life history (Watson, 2007 in press).

REFERENCES

Chantal C: A pragmatic view of Jean Watson's caring theory, *Int J Hum Caring* 7(3):51-61, 2003.

Cheung PP, Yam BM: Patient autonomy in physical restraint, *J Clin Nurs* 14 (Suppl 1):34-40, 2005.

Coventry ML: Care with dignity: a concept analysis, *J Gerontol Nurs* 32(5):42-49, 2006.

DiBartolo MC: Respect and dignity: enduring concepts, enduring challenges, *J Gerontol Nurs* 32(5):12, 2006.

Edvardsson JD, Sandman PO, Rasmussen BH: Meanings of giving touch in the care of older patients: becoming a valuable person and professional, *J Clin Nurs* 12(4):601-609, 2003.

Giger J, Davidhizar R: Transcultural nursing: assessment and intervention, St. Louis, 2004, Mosby.

Leininger MM, McFarland MR: Transcultural nursing: concepts, theories, research and practices, ed 3, New York, 2002, McGraw-Hill.

Matiti M, Cotrel-Gibbons L: Patient dignity—promoting good practice, *Dev Pract Improv Care* 3(5):1-4, 2006.

Moon JS, Cho KS: The effects of handholding on anxiety in cataract surgery patients under local anaesthesia, *J Adv Nurs* 35(3):407-415, 2001.

Salzmann-Erikson M, Eriksson H: Encouraging touch: a path to affinity in psychiatric care, *Issues Ment Health Nurs* 26:843-852, 2005.

Watson J: *Nursing. The philosophy and science of caring*, revised and updated edition, Boulder, 2007, University Press of Colorado (in press).

Watson, J: The June Watson Human Caring Web Site, at http://www2.uchsc.edu/son/caring/content/evolution.asp. Accessed March 30, 2007.

Watson J, Foster R: The attending nurse caring model: integrating theory, evidence and advanced caring-healing therapeutics for transforming professional practice, *J Clin Nurs* 12(3):360-365, 2003.

Woolhead G, Tadd W, Boix-Ferrer JA et al: "Tu" or "Vous?" A European qualitative study of dignity and communication with older people in health and social care settings, *Patient Educ Couns* 61(3):363-371, 2006.

Moral Distress   *Beverly Kopala, PhD, RN, and Lisa Burkhart, PhD, MPH, RN*

NANDA   Definition

Response to the inability to carry out one's chosen ethical/moral decision/action

Defining Characteristics

Patient/family expresses anguish (e.g., powerlessness, guilt, frustration, anxiety, self-doubt, fear) over difficulty acting on one's moral choice

Related Factors

End-of-life decisions; treatment decisions; time constraints for decision making; conflicting information guiding moral/ethical decision-making; conflict among decision makers; physical distance of decision maker; loss of autonomy; cultural conflicts (Kopala, Burkhart, 2004)

NOC   Outcomes (Nursing Outcomes Classification)

Suggested NOC Outcomes

Personal Autonomy, Client Satisfaction: Protection of Rights

• = Independent;   ▲ = Collaborative;   EBN = Evidence-Based Nursing;   EB = Evidence-Based

Client Outcomes

Client Will (Specify Time Frame):

- Be able to act in accordance with values, goals, and beliefs
- Regain confidence in the ability to make decision and/or act in accord with values, goals, and beliefs
- Expresses satisfaction with the ability to make decisions consistent with values, goals, and beliefs
- Have choices respected

 Interventions (Nursing Interventions Classification)

Suggested NIC Interventions

Patient Rights Protection, Multidisciplinary Care Conference

Example NIC Activities—Patient Rights Protection
Provide environment conducive for private conversations between patient, family, and healthcare professionals

Nursing Interventions and *Rationales*

- Examine the source of moral distress. *Rushton's model of "4 A's to Rise Above Moral Distress" states that the first step is to determine the exact nature of the problem (Rushton, 2006).*
- Affirm and validate the client's feelings and perceptions of others. *The second phase of Rushton's model is to affirm distress, commitment, feelings, perceptions of others, and obligations (Rushton, 2006).*
- ▲ Provide adequate information and emotional and psychological support to assist in coping and making collaborative decisions with the healthcare team. *Provide accurate information and discuss decisions throughout hospitalization (Gutierrez, 2005).*
- Assist client in evaluating the situation. *In a study of certified rehabilitation registered nurses (n = 91), survey research found 22% of the respondents were able to resolve the ethical conflict through team/family discussions (Redman & Fry, 1998a). In another study, Redman & Fry (1998b) surveyed 147 registered nurse/certified diabetes educators and found that 3% resolved ethical conflicts through team/family discussions. At an ethics session at a national oncology conference, 136 participants evaluated three ethics case studies and found the nurses' role was to provide the client with treatment options/alternatives, explore and clarify the client's decision, and identify values that are in conflict (Ferrell & Rivera, 1995).*
- Assess personal source of distress to contemplate ability to act. *The third phase of Rushton's model is to identify source and severity of distress and readiness to act on the distress (Rushton, 2006). At an ethics session at a national oncology conference, 136 participants evaluated three ethics case studies and found the nurses' role was examine the client's fears (Ferrell & Rivera, 1995).*
- Implement strategies to initiate changes to resolve moral distress. *The fourth phase of Rushton's model is to take action on the moral distress (Rushton, 2006).*
- Confront the barrier. *In a study of certified rehabilitation registered nurses (n = 91), survey research found 50% of the respondents were able to resolve the ethical conflict through team/family discussions, taking action to protect the client, educating the client or family to take action, or referral to ethics committee (Redman & Fry, 1998a).*
- ▲ Improve communication and collaboration among client, family, and healthcare team. *Expert opinion recommends ethics rounds to discuss moral issues and related client treatment goals to resolve or prevent conflicts (Gutierrez, 2005). A study of 118 certified pediatric nurse practitioners found that 34% of the conflicts involved child/parent/practitioner relationships (Butz, Redman & Fry, 1998). At an ethics session at a national oncology conference, 136 participants evaluated three ethics case studies*

D

and found the nurses' role was to explore client-physician relationships, minimize distress for family, provide support to client and family, and help family cope with decision (Ferrell & Rivera, 1995).

- Advocate for the client (Ferrell, 2006). *Develop a forum for ethical discussions. Expert opinion encourages the nurse to voice moral distress issues regularly in an established forum (Gutierrez, 2005).*

- Teach the client how to take action. *In a study of certified rehabilitation registered nurses (n = 108), survey research found 7% of the respondents were able to resolve the ethical conflict by educating the client or family to take action. (Redman & Fry, 1998a). In another study, Redman & Fry (1998b) surveyed 147 registered nurse/certified diabetes educators and found that 11% resolved ethical conflicts by educating client/family to take action.*

- Empower the client to eliminate the barrier. *In a study of certified rehabilitation registered nurses (n = 108), survey research found 50% of the respondents were able to resolve the ethical conflict through team/family discussions, action taken to protect the client, education of the client or family to take action, or referral to ethics committee (Redman & Fry, 1998a). In another study, Redman & Fry (1998b) surveyed 147 registered nurse/certified diabetes educators and found that 29% resolved ethical conflicts by empowering the client to change the practice.*

- ▲ Consult with other healthcare providers that may include the family. *In a study of certified rehabilitation registered nurses (n = 108), survey research found 35% of the respondents were able to resolve the ethical conflict by educating the client or family to take action, through team/family discussions, or resolution by ethics committee (Redman & Fry, 1998a). In another study, Redman & Fry (1998b) surveyed 147 registered nurse/certified diabetes educators and found that 13% sought resolution through confrontation/discussion with physician/administration.*

- ▲ Contact an ethicist or the ethics committee to ensure the client's rights are protected. *In a study of certified rehabilitation registered nurses (n = 108), survey research found 2% of the respondents referred the conflict to the ethics committee or a consultant (Redman & Fry, 1998a). In another study, Redman & Fry (1998b) surveyed 147 registered nurse/certified diabetes educators and found that 1% referred ethical conflicts to ethics committee or consultant.*

Pediatric

- Consider the developmental age of children when evaluating decisions and conflict. *This study of children's emotional consequences of desire fulfillment versus desire inhibition demonstrated differences in psychological, deontic, and future-oriented reasoning about emotions as well as the development of self-control (Lagattuta, 2005).*

Multicultural

- Acknowledge and understand that cultural differences may influence a client's moral choices. *In this study it was demonstrated that African Americans and Caucasians differ in beliefs about genetic testing and the basis for moral decision making (Zimmerman et al, 2006). Our beliefs about morality are culturally embedded in social, religious, and political ideologies that influence individuals and communities. Attention to the meaning of concepts and their cultural contexts is crucial in fostering mutual respect and understanding for different cultural frames of reference (Andersson, Mendes & Trevizan, 2002).*

REFERENCES

Andersson M, Mendes IA, Trevizan MA: Universal and culturally dependent issues in health care ethics, *Med Law* 21(1):77-85, 2002.

Butz AM, Redman BK, Fry ST: Ethical conflicts experienced by certified pediatric nurse practitioners in ambulatory settings, *J Ped Health Care* 12:176-182, 1998.

Ferrell BR: Understanding the moral distress of nurses witnessing medically futile care, *Oncol Nurs Forum* 33(5):922-930, 2006.

Ferrell BR, Rivera LM: Ethical decision making in oncology, *Cancer Pract* 3:94-99, 1995.

Gutierrez KM: Critical care nurses' perception of responses to moral distress, *Dimens Crit Care Nurs* 24(5):229-241, 2005.

Kopala B, Burkhart L: Ethical dilemma and moral distress: proposed new NANDA diagnoses, *Int J Nurs Terminol Classif* 16(1):3-13, 2004.

Lagattuta KH: When you shouldn't do what you want to do: young children's understanding of desires, rules, and emotions, *Child Dev* 76(3):713-733, 2005.

Redman BK, Fry ST: Ethical conflicts reported by certified registered rehabilitation nurses. *Rehabil Nurs* 23:179-184, 1998a.

Redman, BK, Fry ST: Ethical conflicts reported by registered nurses certified diabetes educators: a replication, *J Adv Nurs* 28:1320-1325, 1998b.

Rushton CH: Defining and addressing moral distress: tools for critical care nursing leaders, *AACN Adv Crit Care* 17(2):161-168, 2006.

Zimmerman RK, Tabbarah M, Nowalk MP et al: Racial differences in beliefs about genetic screening among patients at inner-city neighborhood health centers, *J Natl Med Assoc* 98(3):370-377, 2006.

Risk for Disuse syndrome   *Betty J. Ackley, MSN, EdS, RN*

NANDA   Definition

At risk for a deterioration of body systems as the result of prescribed or unavoidable musculoskeletal inactivity

Risk Factors

Altered level of consciousness; mechanical immobilization; paralysis; prescribed immobilization; severe pain (*NOTE:* Complications from immobility can include pressure ulcer, constipation, stasis of pulmonary secretions, thrombosis, urinary tract infection and/or retention, decreased strength or endurance, orthostatic hypotension, decreased range of joint motion, disorientation, disturbed body image, and powerlessness.)

NOC   Outcomes (Nursing Outcomes Classification)

Suggested NOC Outcomes

Endurance, Immobility Consequences: Physiological, Mobility, Neurological Status: Consciousness, Pain Level

Example NOC Outcome with Indicators
Immobility Consequences: Physiological as evidenced by the following indicators: Pressure sores/Constipation/Compromised nutrition status/Urinary calculi/Compromised muscle strength (Rate the outcome and indicators of **Immobility Consequences: Physiological:** 1 = severe, 2 = substantial, 3 = moderate, 4 = mild, 5 = none [see Section I].)

Client Outcomes

Client Will (Specify Time Frame):

- Maintain full range of motion in joints
- Maintain intact skin, good peripheral blood flow, and normal pulmonary function
- Maintain normal bowel and bladder function
- Express feelings about imposed immobility
- Explain methods to prevent complications of immobility

NIC   Interventions (Nursing Interventions Classification)

Suggested NIC Interventions

Energy Management, Exercise Therapy: Joint Mobility, Muscle Control

Example NIC Activities—Energy Management
Access patient's physiologic status for deficits resulting in fatigue within the context of age and development; Determine the patient/significant other's perception of causes of fatigue

Nursing Interventions and *Rationales*

- Use a functional assessment instrument to evaluate abilities, including such instruments as the Barthel Index, the Katz Index of Activities of Daily Living, or the FIM instrument. *There are many instruments available to measure client function, and a baseline measurement of function should be done to determine appropriate level of care and services (Quigly, 2001).*
- ▲ Have the client do exercises in bed if not contraindicated (e.g., flexing and extending feet and quadriceps, performing gluteal and abdominal sitting exercises, lifting small weights to maintain muscle strength). *A person who is immobilized for 3 weeks may lose half of his or her muscle strength*

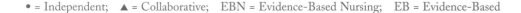

• = Independent;   ▲ = Collaborative;   EBN = Evidence-Based Nursing;   EB = Evidence-Based

D

(Fried & Fried, 2001). In-bed exercises help maintain muscle strength and tone *(Kasper & Talbor, 2002).* **EB:** *Strength improvement in response to resistance exercises is possible even in very old adults and extremely sedentary clients with multiple chronic diseases and functional disabilities (Connelly, 2000).*

▲ If not contraindicated by the client's condition, obtain referral to physical therapy for use of tilt table to provide weight bearing on long bones. *The upright position helps maintain bone strength, increase circulation, and prevent postural hypotension (Kasper et al, 2005).*

• Perform range of motion exercises for all possible joints at least twice daily; perform passive or active range of motion exercises as appropriate. *If not used, muscles weaken and shorten; contractures begin forming after 8 hours of immobility (Fletcher, 2005).*

▲ Use high-top sneakers or specialized boots from the occupational therapy department to prevent foot drop; remove shoes twice daily to provide foot care. *Sneakers or boots help keep the foot in normal anatomical alignment; foot drop can make it difficult or impossible to walk after bed rest.*

• Position the client so that joints are in normal anatomical alignment at all times. *Improper positioning can damage peripheral nerves and blood vessels and cause joint deformities (Fried & Fried, 2001).*

• When positioning clients on the side, tilt clients 30° or less while lying on their side. *Full (versus tilt) side-lying position places high pressure on the trochanter (Hoeman, 2002).*

• If client is immobile, consider use of a transfer chair, which is a chair that becomes a stretcher. *Using a transfer chair, where the client is pulled onto a flat surface and then helped to sit up in the chair, can help previously immobile clients get out of bed (Nelson et al, 2003).*

• Assess skin condition at least daily and more frequently if needed. Refer to care plan of **risk for impaired Skin integrity.**

• Turn clients at high risk for pressure/shear/friction frequently (Salcido, 2004). *Turn clients **at least** every 2-4 hours on pressure-reducing mattress or every 2 hours on standard foam mattress (WOCN Society, 2003).* **EBN:** *When they used a prevention model (Lyder et al, 2004), staff improved their ability to identify clients at high risk for pressure ulcers and the need for repositioning bed-bound clients.*

• Provide the client with a pressure-relieving horizontal support surface. For further interventions on skin care, refer to the care plan for **impaired Skin integrity.**

• Assist the client to walk as soon as medically possible. **EB:** *Almost all clients can get out of bed now with use of the stretcher-chair, which converts from a stretcher to a chair. Bed rest is almost always harmful to clients; early mobilization is better than bed rest for most health conditions (Allen, Glasziou & Del Mar, 1999).*

▲ Recognize that the client who has been in an intensive care environment may develop a neuromuscular disorder resulting in extreme weakness. The client may need a workup to determine the cause before satisfactory ambulation can begin. *Critical care clients can develop such disorders as critical illness myopathy or a polyneuropathy due to ischemia, pressure, prolonged recumbency, compartment syndrome, or hematomas (Maramattom & Wijdicks, 2006).*

▲ Consider use of a continuous lateral rotation therapy bed. **EBN:** *Implementing kinetic therapy in the intensive care unit (ICU) resulted in improved oxygenation and decreased length of stay for clients with pulmonary disorders (Powers & Daniels, 2004).*

▲ If at all possible, help the client begin a walking program, using a physical therapist as needed. **EB:** *Early mobilization has been shown to improve the outcome for clients after treatment of medical conditions and procedures (Allen, Glasziou & Del Mar, 1999).*

• Be very careful when helping the client into a chair and when transferring. Be sure to lock beds and wheelchairs. Recognize that there is a high probability for falls. **EB:** *Nonambulatory clients have a substantially greater number of serious falls than their ambulatory peers (Thapa et al, 1996).*

• Minimize cardiovascular deconditioning by positioning clients as close to upright as possible, several times daily. *Decondition of the cardiovascular system occurs within days and involves fluid shifts, fluid loss, decreased cardiac output, decreased peak oxygen uptake, and increased resting heart rate (Fletcher, 2005; Kasper et al, 2005).*

• When getting the client up after bed rest, do so slowly and watch for signs of postural hypotension, tachycardia, nausea, diaphoresis, or syncope. Take the blood pressure lying, sitting, and

• = Independent;   ▲ = Collaborative;   EBN = Evidence-Based Nursing;   EB = Evidence-Based

standing, waiting 2 minutes between each reading. *Sitting or standing after 3 or 4 days of bed rest results in postural hypotension because of cardiovascular reflex dysfunction (Fletcher, 2005).*

▲ Obtain assistive devices, such as braces, crutches, or canes, to help the client reach and maintain as much mobility as possible.

▲ Request a physical therapy referral to help the client learn how to move self in bed, including bridging, and also how to transfer out of bed (Fried & Fried, 2001).

▲ Apply graduated compression stockings as ordered. Ensure proper fit by measuring, remove at least twice, in the morning with bath and in the evening to assess condition of extremity, then reapply. **EBN and EB:** *Graduated compression stockings reduced the incidence of deep venous thrombosis (DVT) in a high-risk orthopedic surgical population, and additional antithrombotic measures combined with stockings decreased the incidence even further (Joanna Briggs Institute, 2001). Graduated compression stockings, alone or used in conjunction with other prevention modalities, prevents DVT in hospitalized clients (Amarigiri & Lees, 2000).*

• Monitor peripheral circulation and especially note color, pulse, and calf or thigh swelling; check Homans' sign, but recognize that it is an unreliable sign of DVT. *Because of venous stasis, pressure of mattress against veins, and hypercoagulability of blood, bed rest predisposes the client to DVT (Fried & Fried, 2001).*

• Have the client cough and take deep breaths or use incentive spirometry every 2 hours while he or she is awake. *Bed rest compromises breathing, because of decreased chest expansion, decreased cilia activity, and pooling of mucous (Fletcher, 2005).*

• Monitor respiratory functions, noting breath sounds and respiratory rate. Percuss for new onset of dullness in lungs. *Immobility results in hypoventilation, which predisposes the client to atelectasis, which is the pooling of respiratory secretions, and thus pneumonia (Fried & Fried, 2001; Fletcher, 2005).*

• Note bowel function daily. Provide increased fluids, fiber, and natural laxatives, such as prune juice, as needed. *Constipation is common in immobilized clients because of decreased activity and fluid and food intake.*

• Increase fluid intake to 2000 mL/day within the client's cardiac and renal reserve. *Adequate fluids help prevent kidney stones and constipation and help counteract dehydration associated with bed rest (Rubin, 1988).*

• Encourage intake of a balanced diet with adequate amounts of fiber and protein. *Reduced muscular activity and lowered metabolism generally reduce the appetite of a client on bed rest (Fletcher, 2005).*

Geriatrics

• Help the mostly immobile client achieve mobility as soon as possible, depending on physical condition. *In older adults, mobility impairment can predict increased mortality and dependence; however, this can be prevented by physical exercise (Fletcher, 2005; Hirvensalo, Rantanen & Heikkinen, 2000).*

• Use the Outcome Expectation for Exercise Scale to determine client's self-efficacy expectations and outcomes expectations toward exercise. **EBN:** *The client's self-efficacy expectations and outcome expectations for exercise will greatly influence his or her willingness to exercise. If the individual has a low outcome, interventions can be implemented to strengthen the expectations and hopefully improve exercise behavior (Resnick, Zimmerman & Orwig, 2001).*

• If client is frail, ensure good nutrition, appropriate medications, attention to vision and hearing deficits, and increase social support along with exercise. *Frailty in older adults can be multifactorial and often can be ameliorated or reversed (Storey & Thomas, 2004).*

• If the client is mostly immobile, encourage him or her to attend a low-intensity aerobic chair exercise class that includes stretching and strengthening chair exercises. **EBN:** *Chair exercises have been shown to increase flexibility and balance (Mills, 1994).*

▲ Refer the client to physical therapy for resistance exercise training as able, including abdominal crunch, leg press, leg extension, leg curl, calf press, and more. **EB:** *Clients in an extended care facility started a strength, balance, and endurance training program; the clients' balance and mobility improved significantly (Rydwik, Kerstin & Akner, 2005). Progressive resistance training is effective in increasing strength in older people (Latham et al, 2003).*

▲ If the client is elderly and scheduled for an elective surgery that will result in admission into ICU and immobility such as recovering from a knee replacement, initiate a prehabilitation program that includes a warm-up, aerobic strength, flexibility, and functional task work. **EBN:** *By increasing the functional capacity of the individual before the stressor of inactivity, the predictable declines in physical activity can be prevented or alleviated (Topp, Ditmyer & King, 2002). Clients who performed strength activities preoperatively walked significantly greater distances postoperatively after total hip replacement (Whitney & Parkman, 2002).*

• Monitor for signs of depression: flat affect, poor appetite, insomnia, many somatic complaints. *Depression commonly accompanies decreased mobility and function in older adults (Fletcher, 2005; Resnick, 1998).*

• Keep careful track of bowel function in elderly clients, and do not allow them to become constipated. *Older adults can easily develop impactions as a result of immobility.*

Home Care

• Some of the previously mentioned interventions may be adapted for home care use.

▲ Begin discharge planning as soon as possible with case manager or social worker to assess need for home support systems and community or home health services.

▲ Become oriented to all programs of care for the client before discharge from institutional care.

▲ Confirm the immediate availability of all necessary assistive devices for home.

• Perform complete physical assessment and recent history at initial visit.

▲ Refer to physical and occupational therapies for immediate evaluations of the client's potential for independence and functioning in the home setting and for follow-up care.

• Allow the client to have as much input and control of the plan of care as possible. *Client perception of control increases self-esteem and motivation to follow medical plan of care.*

• Assess knowledge of all care with caregivers. Review as necessary. *Having the necessary knowledge and skills to perform care decreases caregiver role strain and supports safety of the client.*

▲ Support the family of the client in assuming caregiver activities. Refer for home health aide services for assistance and respite as appropriate. Refer to medical social services as appropriate.

▲ Institute case management of frail older adults to support continued independent living if possible in the home environment.

Client/Family Teaching

• Teach how to perform range of motion exercises in bed if not contraindicated.

• Teach the family how to turn and position the client and provide all care necessary.

NOTE: Nursing diagnoses that are commonly relevant when the client is on bed rest include **Constipation, risk for impaired Skin integrity, disturbed Sensory perception, disturbed Sleep pattern, adult Failure to thrive,** and **Powerlessness.**

evolve See the EVOLVE website for World Wide Web resources for client education.

REFERENCES

Allen C, Glasziou P, Del Mar C: Bed rest: a potentially harmful treatment needing more careful attention, *Lancet* 354(9186):1229, 1999.

Amarigiri SV, Lees TA: Elastic compression stockings for prevention of deep vein thrombosis, *Cochrane Database Syst Rev* (3): CD001484, 2000.

Connelly DM: Resisted exercise training of institutionalized older adults for improved strength and functional mobility: a review, *Top Geriatr Rehabil* 15(3):6, 2000.

Fletcher K: Immobility: geriatric self-learning module, *Medsurg Nurs* 14(1):35, 2005.

Fried KM, Fried GW: Immobility. In Derstine JB, Hargrove SD, editors: *Comprehensive rehabilitation nursing,* Philadelphia, 2001, WB Saunders.

Hirvensalo M, Rantanen T, Heikkinen E: Mobility difficulties and physical activity as predictors of mortality and loss of independence in the community-living older population, *J Am Geriatr Soc* 48(5):493, 2000.

Hoeman SP: Movement, functional mobility, and activities of daily living. In Hoeman SP, editor: *Rehabilitation nursing: process, application, and outcomes,* ed 3, St Louis, 2002, Mosby.

Joanna Briggs Institute: Best practice: graduated compression stockings for the prevention of post-operative venous thromboembolism, *Evidenced Based Practice Information Sheets for Health Professions* 5:2, 2001.

Kasper CE, Talbor LA: Skeletal muscle damage and recovery, *AACN Clin Issues* 13(2):237, 2002.

Kasper DL, Braunwald E, Fauci A et al: *Harrison's principles of internal medicine,* ed 16, New York, 2005, McGraw-Hill.

Latham N, Anderson C, Bennett D et al: Progressive resistance strength training for physical disability in older people, *Cochrane Database Syst Rev* (2):CD002759, 2003.

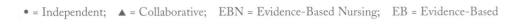

Lyder CH, Grady J, Mathur D et al: Preventing pressure ulcers in Connecticut hospitals by using the plan-do-study-act model of quality improvement, *Jt Comm J Qual Saf* 30(4):205-214, 2004.

Maramattom BV, Wijdicks EF: Acute neuromuscular weakness in the intensive care unit, *Crit Care Med* 34(11):2835-2841, 2006.

Mills EM: The effect of low-intensity aerobic exercise on muscle strength, flexibility, and balance among sedentary elderly persons, *Nurs Res* 43:207, 1994.

Nelson A, Owen B, Lloyd JD et al: Safe patient handling and movement, *Am J Nurs* 103(3):32-43, 2003.

Powers J, Daniels D: Turning points: implementing kinetic therapy in the ICU, *Nurs Manage* 35(5):1, 2004.

Quigley P: Functional assessment. In Derstine JB, Hargrove SD, editors: *Comprehensive rehabilitation nursing,* Philadelphia, 2001, WB Saunders.

Resnick B, Zimmerman S, Orwig D: Model testing for reliability and validity of the outcome expectations for exercise scale, *Nurs Res* 50(5):293, 2001.

Resnick N: *Geriatric medicine in current medical diagnosis and treatment,* ed 37, Stamford, Conn, 1998, Appleton and Lange.

Rubin M: The physiology of bed rest, *Am J Nurs* 88:50, 1988.

Rydwik E, Kerstin F, Akner G: Physical training in institutionalized elderly people with multiple diagnoses—a controlled pilot study, *Arch Gerontol Geriatr* 40(1):29, 2005.

Salcido R: Patient turning schedules: why and how often? *Adv Skin Wound Care* 17(4 pt 1):156, 2004.

Story E, Thomas RL: Understanding and ameliorating frailty in the elderly, *Top Geriatr Rehabil* 20(1):86, 2004.

Thapa PB, Brockman KG, Gideon P et al: Injurious falls in nonambulatory nursing home residents: a comparative study of circumstances, incidence, and risk factors, *J Am Geriatr Soc* 44:273, 1996.

Topp R, Ditmyer M, King K: The effect of bedrest and potential of prehabilitation on patients in the intensive care unit, *AACN Clin Issues* 13(2):263, 2002.

Whitney JA, Parkman S: Preoperative physical activity, anesthesia, and analgesia: effects on early postoperative walking after total hip replacement, *Appl Nurs Res* 15(1):19, 2002.

Wound, Ostomy, and Continence Nurses Society (WOCN): *Guideline for prevention and management of pressure ulcers,* Glenview, Ill, 2003, The Society.

D

Deficient Diversional activity   *Betty J. Ackley, MSN, EdS, RN*

NANDA   Definition

Decreased stimulation from (or interest or engagement in) recreational or leisure activities

Defining Characteristics

Patient's statements regarding boredom (e.g., wish there was something to do, to read, etc.); usual hobbies cannot be undertaken in hospital

Related Factor (r/t)

Environmental lack of diversional activity

NOC   Outcomes (Nursing Outcomes Classification)

Suggested NOC Outcomes

Leisure Participation, Play Participation, Social Involvement

Example NOC Outcome with Indicators
Leisure Participation as evidenced by the following indicators: Expresses satisfaction with leisure activities/Feels relaxed from leisure activities/Enjoys leisure activities (Rate the outcome and indicators of **Leisure Participation:** 1 = never demonstrated, 2 = rarely demonstrated, 3 = sometimes demonstrated, 4 = often demonstrated, 5 = consistently demonstrated [see Section I].)

Client Outcome

Client Will (Specify Time Frame):

• Engage in personally satisfying diversional activities

NIC   Interventions (Nursing Interventions Classification)

Suggested NIC Interventions

Recreation Therapy, Self-Responsibility Facilitation

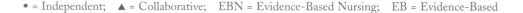

• = Independent;   ▲ = Collaborative;   EBN = Evidence-Based Nursing;   EB = Evidence-Based

D

Example NIC Activities—Recreation Therapy
Assist patient to identify meaningful recreational activities; Provide safe recreational equipment

Nursing Interventions and *Rationales*

- Observe for signs of deficient diversional activity: restlessness, unhappy facial expression, and statements of boredom and discontent.
- Observe ability to engage in activities that require good vision and use of hands. *Diversional activities must be tailored to the client's capabilities.*
- Discuss activities with clients that are interesting and feasible in the present environment.
- Encourage the client to share feelings about situation of inactivity away from usual life activities. *Work and hobbies provide structure and continuity to life; the client can feel a sense of loss when unable to engage in usual activities.* **EB:** *Spinal cord injury clients who experienced increased frequency of recreational experiences had increased levels of well-being (Lee & McCormick, 2004).*
- Encourage a mix of physical and mental activities if possible (e.g., crafts, videotapes).
- Provide videos and/or DVDs of movies for recreation and distraction.
- Provide magazines and/or books of interest.
- Set up a puzzle in a community space, or provide individual puzzles as desired.
- Provide access to a portable computer so that the client can access e-mail and the Internet. Give client a list of interesting websites, including games and directions on how to use a search engine (e.g., Google) if desired.
- Help client find a support group for the appropriate condition on the internet if interested, and if support group is available.
- Use "bread therapy" in long term units—clients/staff bake bread with a bread maker as desired. *Assembling the ingredients is a group activity and can be therapeutic. The smell of bread baking gives a homelike, loving atmosphere to a healthcare environment.*
- ▲ Arrange animal-assisted therapy if desired, with a dog, cat, or bird for the client to interact with and if possible care for. **EB and EBN:** *Increased feelings of self-worth, reduce anxiety, reduce blood pressure and triglycerides, and increase relaxation and social functioning in clients involved in animal-assisted therapy (Stanley-Hermanns & Miller, 2002; Gagnon et al, 2004). Clients receiving a canary had decreased symptoms of depression and increased perception of quality of life (Colombo et al, 2006).*
- Encourage the client to schedule visitors so that they are not all present at once or at inconvenient times. *A schedule prevents the client from becoming exhausted from frequent company.*
- Provide reading material, television, radio, and books on tape.
- If clients are able to write, help them keep journals; if clients are unable to write, have them record thoughts on tape or on videotape. *Writing is personal freedom. It frees people as an individual apart from the masses. Writing helps people survive as individuals (Quindlen, 2007).*
- ▲ Request recreational or art therapist to assist with providing diversional activities. *Recreational therapists specialize in helping people have fun. Art therapy can be effective for helping people express emotions, as well as providing diversion (Shaw & Wilkinson, 1996).*
- Provide a change in scenery; get the client out of the room if possible. *A lack of sensory stimulation has significant adverse effects on clients.*
- Help the client experience nature by looking at a nature scene from a window, or walking through a garden if possible. **EBN:** *Exposure to a natural environment can be helpful to promote relaxation, stress recovery, and mental restoration (Jones & Haight, 2002). Listening to birds and feeling the sun on their faces can be a wonderful experience for long-term clients (Fioravanti, 2004).*
- Structure the environment as needed to promote optimal comfort and sensory diversity (e.g., have family bring in posters, banners, or a sound system; change lighting; change direction bed faces). *Modification of the environment is sometimes necessary for the well-being of the client.*
- Work with family to provide music that is enjoyable to the client. **EBN:** *Music can help decrease anxiety in hospitalized clients (Evans, 2002; Smolen, Topp & Singer, 2002).*
- Structure the client's schedule around personal wishes for time of care, relaxation, and participation in fun activities. *Increased client control fosters increased client self-esteem.*

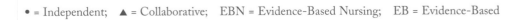

• = Independent;   ▲ = Collaborative;   EBN = Evidence-Based Nursing;   EB = Evidence-Based

- Spend time with the client when possible or arrange for a friendly visitor. *Presence involves knowing the uniqueness of the person, listening intently, involving the person, mobilizing resources, and mutually defining changes in the provision of confident caring (Caldwell et al, 2005).*

Pediatric

▲ Request an order for a child life specialist or, if not available, a play therapist for children.
- Provide activities, such as video projects and access to computer-based support groups for children (e.g., Starbright World: a computer network where children interact virtually, sharing their experiences and escaping hospital routines; http://www.starbrightworld.org). **EB:** *Starbright World was shown to significantly reduce loneliness and withdrawn behavior in chronically ill children (Battles et al, 2002).*
- Provide computer games and virtual reality experiences for children, which can be used as distraction techniques during venipuncture or other procedures. *Virtual reality experiences as a distraction technique can be effective and result in positive clinical outcomes (Schneider & Workman, 2000).*

Geriatrics

- If the client is able, arrange attendance with senior citizen group activities. **EBN:** *Participation in social behavior improved performance of older adults in activities of daily living. Social behaviors included communication, concentration skills, and occupational tasks (Patton, 2006).*
- Encourage involvement in senior citizen activities (e.g., AARP, YMCA, church groups). Arrange transportation to activities as needed.
- Encourage clients to use their ability to help others by volunteering. *Assisting others can help the client grow as a generative human being.*
- Provide an environment that promotes activity (e.g., one that has adequate lighting for crafts, large-print books); allow periods of solitude and privacy. *Periods of solitude are important for emotional well-being in older adult clients.*
- ▲ Use reminiscence therapy in conjunction with the expression of emotions. Refer to a reminiscence group if available. **EBN and EB:** *Participation in a reminiscence group reduced symptoms of depression (Zauszniewski et al, 2004; Jones & Beck-Little, 2002). Reminiscence therapy can also increase social interaction, self-esteem, and well-being (Jonsdottir et al, 2001).*
- ▲ Use the Eden Alternative with the elderly; bring in appropriate plants for the elderly client to care for; animals, such as birds, fish, dogs, and cats, as appropriate for the client; and children to visit. *The Eden Alternative offers a more natural human habitat where the quality of life is improved and loneliness, helplessness, and boredom are decreased (Barba, Tesh & Courts, 2002).* **EBN:** *An animal-assisted therapy program for clients with dementia resulted in decreased agitation behavior and increased social interactions (Richeson, 2003). The heart rate and systolic blood pressure decreased significantly in older adult women who were interacting with small dogs (Luptak & Nuzzo, 2004).*
- For clients who love gardening, bring in seeds, soil, and pots for indoor gardening. Use seeds, such as sunflower, pumpkin, and zinnia, that grow rapidly. *Nursing home residents who participated in a weekly gardening experience demonstrated increased socialization and increased physical functioning (Brown et al, 2004).*
- For clients in assisted living facilities, provide leisure educational programs. **EB:** *Participation in leisure education programs resulted in increased perception of quality of life (Janssen, 2004).*
- ▲ Provide recreational therapy exercises in the morning for clients with dementia in the extended care facility. **EB:** *Morning recreational exercises resulted in decreased agitation and passivity and also increased strength and flexibility (Buetttner & Fitzsimmons, 2004).*

Multicultural

- Assess for the influence of cultural beliefs, norms, and values on the client's leisure activity interests. **EBN:** *Leisure interests or hobbies may be based on cultural preferences (Leininger & McFarland, 2002; Giger & Davidhizar, 2004).*
- Validate the client's feelings and concerns related to lack of stimulation or interest in leisure activities.

D

 Home Care

Note: Many of the previously listed interventions should be administered in the home setting.

- Explore previous interests with the client; consider related activities that are within the client's capabilities.
- ▲ Assess the client for depression. Refer for mental health services as indicated. *Lack of interest in previously enjoyed activities is part of the syndrome of depression.*
- Assess the family's ability to respond to the client's psychosocial needs for stimulation. Assist as able.
- ▲ Refer to occupational therapy to assist the client and family with identifying diversional activities within the capability of the client and family.
- ▲ Introduce (or continue) friendly volunteer visitors if the client is willing and able to have the company. If transportation is an issue or if the client does not want visitors in the home, consider alternatives (e.g., telephone contacts, computer messaging).
- For clients who are interested and capable, suggest involvement in a community gardening experience through the senior center. *A community elder gardening experience in ambulatory people decreased depression and increased level of functioning (Austin, Johnson & Morgan, 2006).*
- ▲ In the presence of a psychiatric disorder, refer for psychiatric home healthcare services for client reassurance and implementation of therapeutic regimen.
- If the client is dying, and is interested, assist in making a videotape, audiotape or memory book for family members with treasured stories, memoirs, pictures, and video clips. *"Wouldn't all of us love to have a journal, a memoir, a letter, from those we have loved and lost? Shouldn't all of us leave a bit of that behind?" (Quindlen, 2007)*

 Client/Family Teaching

- Work with the client and family on learning diversional activities that the client is interested in (e.g., knitting, hooking rugs, writing memoirs).
- If the client is in isolation, give the client complete information on why isolation is needed and how it should be accomplished, especially guidelines for visitors. **EBN:** *Clients who were in isolation identified their greatest needs, which were for more information about the isolation regulations and the need for guidelines for visitors so that visitors would be comfortable and continue to visit (Ward, 2000).*

 See the EVOLVE website for World Wide Web resources for client education.

REFERENCES

Austin EN, Johnson YAM, Morgan LL: Community gardening in a senior center: a therapeutic intervention to improve the health of older adults, *Ther Recreation J* 40(1):48-56, 2006.

Barba BE, Tesh AS, Courts NF: Promoting thriving in nursing homes, the Eden alternative, *J Gerontol Nurs* 28(3):7, 2002.

Battles HB, Weiner LS: Effects of an electronic network on the social environment of children with life-threatening illness, *Child Health Care* 31(1):47-68, 2002.

Brown VM, Allen AC, Dwozan M et al: Indoor gardening and older adults: effects on socialization, activities of daily living, and loneliness, *J Gerontol Nurs* 30(10):34-42, 2004.

Buettner LL, Fitzsimmons S: Recreational therapy exercise on the special care unit: impact on behaviors, *Am J Recreation Ther* 3(4):8-24, 2004.

Caldwell B, Dolye M, Morris et al: Presencing: channeling therapeutic effectiveness with the mentally ill in a state psychiatric hospital, *Issues Men Health Nurs* 26:853-871, 2005.

Colombo G, Buono MD, Smania K et al: Pet therapy and institutionalized elderly: a study on 144 cognitively unimpaired subjects, *Arch Gerontol Geriatr* 42(2):207-216, 2006.

Evans D: The effectiveness of music as an intervention for hospital patients: a systematic review, *J Adv Nurs* 37(1):8, 2002.

Fioravanti MA: Helping patients break the boredom, *RN* 67(1):46-49, 2004.

Gagnon J, Bouchard F, Landry M et al: Implementing a hospital-based animal therapy program for children with cancer: a descriptive study, *Can Oncol Nurs J* 14(4):210-222, 2004.

Giger J, Davidhizar R: *Transcultural nursing: assessment and intervention*, St Louis, 2004, Mosby Year Book.

Janssen MA: The use of leisure education in assisted living facilities, *Am J Recreation Ther* 3(4):25-30, 2004.

Jones ED, Beck-Little R: The use of reminiscence therapy for the treatment of depression in rural-dwelling older adults, *Issues Ment Health Nurs* 23:3, 2002.

Jones MM, Haight BK: Environmental transformations: an integrative review, *J Gerontol Nurs* 28(3):23, 2002.

Jonsdottir H, Jonsdottir G, Steingrimsdottir E et al: Group reminiscence among people with end-stage chronic lung diseases, *J Adv Nurs* 35(1):79-87, 2001.

Lee Y, McCormick B: Subjective well-being of people with spinal cord injury: does leisure contribute? *J Rehabil* 70(3):5-12, 2004.

Leininger MM, McFarland MR: *Transcultural nursing: concepts, theories, research and practices*, ed 3, New York, 2002, McGraw-Hill.

Luptak JE, Nuzzo NA: The effects of small dogs on vital signs in elderly women: a pilot study, *Cardiopulm Phys Ther J* 15(1), 2004.

Patton D: The value of reality orientation with older adults. *J Gerontol Nurs* 32(12):6-13, 2006.

Quindlen A: The last word, *Newsweek,* 149(3):74, 2007.

Richeson NE: Effects of animal–assisted therapy on agitated behaviors and social interactions of older adults with dementia, *Am J Alzheimers Dis Other Demen* 18(6):353-358, 2003.

Schneider SM, Workman ML: Virtual reality as a distraction intervention for older children receiving chemotherapy, *Pediatr Nurs* 26(6):593, 2000.

Shaw R, Wilkinson W: Therapy and rehabilitation: building the pyramids—palliative care patients' perceptions of making art, *Int J Palliat Nurs* 2(4):217-219, 1996.

Smolen D, Topp R, Singer L: The effect of self-selected music during colonoscopy on anxiety, heart rate, and blood pressure, *Appl Nurs Res* 15(3):126, 2002.

Stanley-Hermanns M, Miller J: Animal-assisted therapy, *Am J Nurs* 102(10):69, 2002.

Ward D: Infection control: reducing the psychological effects of isolation, *Br J Nurs* 9(3):162, 2000.

Zauszniewski JA, Eggenschwiler K, Preechawong S et al: Focused reflection reminiscence group for elders: implementation and evaluation, *Appl Gerontol* 23(4):429-442, 2004.

E

Disturbed Energy field   *Gail B. Ladwig, MSN, CHTP, RN, and Diane Wind Wardell, PhD, RNC*

NANDA   Definition

Disruption of the flow of energy surrounding a person's being results in disharmony of the body, mind, and/or spirit

Defining Characteristics

Perceptions of changes in patterns of energy flow, such as movement (wave, spike, tingling, density, flowing); sounds (tone, words); temperature change (warmth, coolness); visual changes (image, color); disruption of the field (deficit, hole, spike, bulge, obstruction, congestion, diminished flow in energy field)

Related Factors

Slowing or blocking of energy flows secondary to: maturational factors: age-related developmental crisis or difficulties; pathophysiologic factors: illness, injury, pregnancy; situational factors: anxiety, fear, grieving, pain; treatment-related factors: chemotherapy, immobility, labor and delivery, perioperative experience

NOC   Outcomes (Nursing Outcomes Classification)

Suggested NOC Outcomes

Personal Well-Being, Comfort Level, Spiritual Health

Example NOC Outcome with Indicators
Personal Well-Being as evidenced by the following indicators: Psychological health/Spiritual life/Ability to relax/ Level of happiness (Rate the outcome and indicators of **Personal Well-Being:** 1 = not all satisfied, 2 = somewhat satisfied, 3 = moderately satisfied, 4 = very satisfied, 5 = completely satisfied [see Section I].)

Client Outcomes

Client Will (Specify Time Frame):

- State sense of well-being
- State feeling of relaxation
- State decreased pain
- State decreased tension
- Demonstrate evidence of physical relaxation (e.g., decreased blood pressure, pulse, respiration rate, muscle tension)

NIC Interventions (Nursing Interventions Classification)

Suggested NIC Intervention

Therapeutic Touch

Example NIC Activities—Therapeutic Touch
Focus awareness on the inner self; Focus on the intention to facilitate wholeness and healing at all levels of consciousness

Nursing Interventions and *Rationales*

- Refer to care plans for **Anxiety, Acute Pain,** and **Chronic Pain.**
- Consider using Therapeutic Touch (TT) and/or Healing Touch (HT) for clients with anxiety, tension, pain, or other conditions that indicate a disruption in the flow of energy. **EBN:** *TT and HT, when provided in the clinical setting, promote comfort, calmness, and well-being among hospitalized clients (Newshan & Schuller-Civitella, 2003; Seskevich et al, 2004).* **EBN:** *TT and HT may be effective treatments for relieving pain and improving quality of life in this specific population of persons with fibromyalgia syndrome (Denison, 2004). Gentle touch used with clients with cancer showed significant improvements in psychological and physical functioning, quality of life, stress and relaxation, severe pain/discomfort, and depression/anxiety (Weze et al, 2004). HT has been used in a variety of cancer studies showing improved quality of life, decreased pain and anxiety, and better symptom management (Cook et al, 2004; Post-White et al, 2003; Wardell & Weymouth, 2004).*
- Consider HT treatments for clients with psychological depression. **EBN:** *HT can be a complementary approach to help in the reconnection process to self and others (Van Aken, 2004).*
- Administer TT and/or HT as described in the following discussion (may also include Reiki practice). **EBN:** *TT has a positive, medium effect on physiological and psychological variables (Peters, 1999).* **EBN:** *HT may reduce stress, anxiety, and pain; facilitate healing; have some improvement in biochemical and physiological markers; and a greater sense of well-being. Nurses may provide safe, noninvasive care to promote healing with HT (Wardell & Weymouth, 2004).*

Guidelines for Therapeutic Touch and Healing Touch

- TT and HT may be practiced by anyone with the requisite preparation, desire, and commitment. *TT requires preparation is the completion of a minimum 12–contact hour basic workshop by a TT practitioner who meets the criteria as a Nurse Healer–Professional Associates International, Inc. HT requires preparation at the minimum of a 16–contact hour level 1 workshop (out of five levels needed for program completion) by a Certified HT Instructor (Hover-Kramer, 2001).*
- Those who are not licensed healthcare professionals may practice TT and HT within their families and religious or spiritual community and on friends.
- NOTE: Nurses who are not trained in TT or HT should consider spending quiet time with clients listening to their concerns. **EBN:** *Nurses who are not trained in the administration of TT may use quiet time and dialogue to enhance feelings of calmness and relaxation in clients with breast cancer (Kelly et al, 2004).*
- TT is conducted according to the standards for its practice developed by Dolores Krieger (1997) and Dora Kunz (2004). *It is used in accordance with guidelines provided by the Nurse Healers Professional Associates (NH-PAI, Inc., 2006).*
- HT is conducted according to the code of ethics and standards of practice developed by Healing Touch International, Inc. *(Healing Touch International, Inc., 2006).*
- Administer TT and HT according to the guidelines established by the prospective therapies and programs. *A description of HT is found at Healing Touch International (2006) and for TT at Therapeutic Touch (2007).*

Pediatric

- Consider using TT or HT for pediatric clients with adjunct therapies to decrease stress, anxiety, and pain. **EBN:** *HT and TT are unique touch techniques. They are widely available in pediatric hos-*

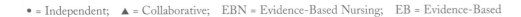

pitals. Practitioners, as well as clients, may notice improved sense of well-being during and after treatments. These therapies are safe and readily available (Kemper & Kelly, 2004).

- Teach that when working with the very young, old, or ill, or in the head area, TT should be gentle and used only for short periods. *Exercise caution when using TT with clients who may exhibit an extreme sensitivity to the process (e.g., premature infants, frail elderly, psychotic clients) (Sayer-Adams, 1994).*

Geriatric

- Consider TT and HT for agitated clients with Alzheimer's disease. **EBN:** *TT and HT may be an effective technique to alleviate agitation in people with Alzheimer's disease (Hawranik, Deatrich & Johnston, 2004; Wang & Hermann, 2006).*

Multicultural

- Assess for the influence of cultural beliefs, norms, and values on the client's sense of disharmony of mind and spirit. **EBN:** *The client's sense of disharmony may have cultural roots (Leininger & McFarland, 2002; Giger & Davidhizar, 2004). Nurses can increase their knowledge about other health systems through assessment and incorporate these into the plan of care for clients as needed (Snyder & Niska, 2003).*
- Assess for the presence of specific culture-bound syndromes that may manifest as disturbances in energy or spirit. **EBN:** *Voodoo death, evil eye, and trance dissociation are some of the culture-bound syndromes that have symptoms of disharmony of mind and spirit (Arnault, 1998).*
- Validate the client's feelings and concerns related to sense of disharmony or energy disturbance. **EBN:** *Validation lets family members know that the nurse has heard and understood what was said, and it promotes the relationship between nurse and family members (Spiers, 2002).*

Home Care

- See Guidelines for TT and HT.
- Help the client and family accept TT and HT as healing interventions. *Consultation and collaboration with a specialist may be the best approach to nursing care. Numerous studies have reported positive outcomes of HT as a noninvasive complementary therapy (Umbreit, 2000). HT has been used in the home care setting for chronic pain clients and for hospice care (Wardell et al, 2006; Ziembroski et al, 2003).*
- Assist the family with providing an appropriate space in which TT and or HT can be administered.
- ▲ Assess clients with bipolar disorder for the occurrence of social rhythm disruption, particularly during periods of stressful life events. Refer for mental health treatment. *Stressful life events, particularly those involving social rhythm disruption, appear to play a role in initiating manic episodes (Malkoff-Schwartz et al, 2000).*
- ▲ In the presence of a psychiatric disorder, refer for psychiatric home healthcare services for client reassurance and implementation of therapeutic regimen. **EBN:** *Psychiatric home care nurses can address issues relating to the client's bipolar disorder and its interference with ability to adjust to changes in health status. Behavioral interventions in the home can assist the client to participate more effectively in treatment plan (Patusky, Rodning & Martinez-Kratz, 1996).*

Client/Family Teaching

- Teach the TT and/or specific HT technique process to clients and family members. **EBN:** *Helping clients while using touch therapy related to Ki (a Korean type of energy therapy) was found to be a dynamic process with each participant actively engaged in increasing the activating, potential power of the human being (Chang, 2003). HT was taught to caregivers of veterans experiencing chronic pain from spinal cord injury (Wardell et al, 2006).*
- Teach that when working with the very young, old, or ill, or in the head area, TT should be gentle and used only for short periods. *Exercise caution when using TT with clients who may exhibit an extreme sensitivity to the process (e.g., premature infants, frail elderly, psychotic clients) (Sayer-Adams, 1994).*
- Teach the client how to use guided imagery. *The nurse can facilitate healing by helping the client re-*

contact and reclaim parts of the self (resolve energy disturbance) through guided imagery (Rancour, 1994).

- Teach the client to use deep breathing to relax. Ask the client to create an image of the disease, affected organ, or symptom. After the image has been identified, ask the client to speak with the image to address an unresolved issue. *By describing a previously unacknowledged part of the self, liberated energy can transform resistance, defenses, and disease into self-acceptance, peace, and wholeness (Remen, 1994).*

evolve   See the EVOLVE website for World Wide Web resources for client education.

REFERENCES

Arnault DS: Framework for culturally relevant psychiatric nursing. In Varcarolis EM, editor: *Foundations of psychiatric mental health nursing*, ed 3, Philadelphia, 1998, W.B. Saunders.

Chang SO: The nature of touch therapy related to Ki: practitioners' perspective, *Nurs Health Sci* 5(2):103-114, 2003.

Cook CAL, Guerrerio JF, Slater VE: Healing touch and quality of life in women receiving radiation treatment for cancer: a randomized controlled trial, *Alt Ther Health Med* 10(3):24-41, 2004.

Denison B: Touch the pain away: new research on therapeutic touch and persons with fibromyalgia syndrome, *Holist Nurs Pract* 18(3):142-151, 2004.

Giger JN, Davidhizar RE: *Transcultural nursing: assessment and intervention*, ed 4, St Louis, 2004, Mosby.

Hawranik P, Deatrich J, Johnston P: Therapeutic touch: another approach for the management of agitation, *Can Nurs Home* 15(1):46-48, 2004.

Healing Touch International, Inc, 2006, at http://wwwl.healingtouchinternational.org. Accessed April 19, 2007.

Hover-Kramer D: *Healing touch: a guidebook for practitioners*, Albany, NY, 2001, Delmar Publishers.

Kelly AE, Sullivan P, Fawcett J et al: Therapeutic touch, quiet time, and dialogue: perceptions of women with breast cancer, *Oncol Nurs Forum* 31(3):625-631, 2004.

Kemper KJ, Kelly EA: Treating children with therapeutic and healing touch, *Pediatr Ann* 33(4):248-252, 2004.

Krieger D: *Therapeutic touch inner workbook*, Santa Fe, NM, 1997, Bear and Company.

Kuntz D, Keriger D: *The spiritual dimension of therapeutic work*, 2004, Inner Traditions International, Limited.

Leininger MM, McFarland MR: *Transcultural nursing: concepts, theories, research and practices*, ed 3, New York, 2002, McGraw-Hill.

Malkoff-Schwartz S, Frank E, Anderson BP et al: Social rhythm disruption and stressful life events in the onset of bipolar and unipolar episodes, *Psychol Med* 30:1005, 2000.

Newshan G, Schuller-Civitella D: Large clinical study shows value of therapeutic touch program, *Holist Nurs Pract* 17(4):189-192, 2003.

Nurse Healers-Professional Associates International: *Guidelines of recommended standards and scope of practice for therapeutic touch*, www.therapeutic-touch.org/content/guidelines.asp, accessed March 15, 2006.

Patusky KL, Rodning C, Martinez-Kratz M: Clinical lessons in psychiatric home care: a case study approach, *J Home Healthcare Manage* 9:18, 1996.

Peters RM: The effectiveness of therapeutic touch: a meta-analytic review, *Nurs Sci Q* 12(1):52, 1999.

Post-White J, Kinney ME, Savik K et al: Therapeutic massage and healing touch improve symptoms in cancer, *Integr Cancer Ther* 2(4):332-344, 2003.

Rancour P: Interactive guided imagery with oncology patients, *J Holist Nurs* 12:149, 1994.

Remen N: Psychosynthesis and healing, *J Holist Nurs* 12:150, 1994.

Sayer-Adams J: Complementary therapies: therapeutic touch nursing function, *Nurs Stand* 8:25, 1994.

Seskevich JE, Crater SW, Lane JD et al: Beneficial effects of noetic therapies on mood before percutaneous intervention for unstable coronary syndromes, *Nurs Res* 53(2):116-121, 2004.

Snyder M, Niska K: Cultural related complementary therapies: their use in critical care units, *Crit Care Nurs Clin North Am* 15(3):341-346, 2003.

Spiers J: The interpersonal contexts of negotiating care in home care nurse-patient interactions, *Qual Health Res* 12(8):1033-1057, 2002.

Umbreit AW: Healing touch: applications in the acute care setting, *AACN Clin Issues* 11(1):105, 2000.

Van Aken R: *The experiential process of healing touch for people with moderate depression*, Lismore, NSW, Australia, 2004, Southern Cross University.

Wang K, Hermann C: Pilot study to test the effectiveness of healing touch on agitation levels in people with dementia, *Geriatr Nurs* 27(1):34-40, 2006.

Wardell D, Rintala D, Tan G et al: Pilot study of healing touch and progressive relaxation for chronic neuropathic pain in persons with spinal cord injury, *J Holist Nurs* 24(4):231-240, 2006.

Wardell DW, Weymouth KF: Review of studies of healing touch, *J Nurs Scholarship* 36(2):147-154, 2004.

Weze C, Leathard HL, Grange J: Evaluation of healing by gentle touch in 35 clients with cancer, *Eur J Oncol Nurs* 8(1):40-49, 2004.

Ziembroski J, Gilbert N, Bossarte R et al: Healing touch and hospice care: examining outcomes at the end of life, *Altern Complement Ther* 9(3):146-151, 2004.

Impaired Environmental interpretation syndrome *Betty J. Ackley, MSN, EdS, RN*

NANDA   Definition

Consistent lack of orientation to person, place, time, or circumstances for more than 3 to 6 months, necessitating a protective environment

Defining Characteristics

Chronic confusional states; consistent disorientation; inability to concentrate; inability to follow simple directions; inability to reason; loss of occupation; loss of social functioning; slow in responding to questions

Related Factors (r/t)

Dementia; depression; Huntington's disease

NOC   Outcomes (Nursing Outcomes Classification)

Suggested NOC Outcomes

Cognitive Orientation, Concentration, Information Processing, Memory, Neurological Status: Consciousness

Example NOC Outcome with Indicators
Concentration as evidenced by the following indicators: Maintains focus without being distracted/Responds appropriately to visual cues/Responds appropriately to language cues/Draws a circle (on command)/Draws a pentagon (on command) (Rate the outcome and indicators of **Concentration:** 1 = severely compromised, 2 = substantially compromised, 3 = moderately compromised, 4 = mildly compromised, 5 = not compromised [see Section I].)

Client Outcomes

Client Will (Specify Time Frame):

- Remain content and free from harm
- Function at maximal cognitive level
- Participate in activities of daily living (ADLs) at the maximum of functional ability

NIC   Interventions (Nursing Interventions Classification)

Suggested NIC Interventions

Dementia Management, Environmental Management, Reality Orientation, Surveillance: Safety

Example NIC Activities—Dementia Management
Identify usual patterns of behavior for such activities as sleep, medication use, elimination, food intake, and self-care

Nursing Interventions and *Rationales* Client/Family Teaching

Refer to care plan for **Chronic Confusion.**

F

Adult Failure to thrive   *Gail B. Ladwig, MSN, CHTP, RN*

NANDA   Definition

Progressive functional deterioration of a physical and cognitive nature. The individual's ability to live with multisystem diseases, cope with ensuing problems, and manage his or her care are remarkably diminished.

Defining Characteristics

Altered mood state; anorexia; apathy; cognitive decline: problems with responding to environmental stimuli; demonstrated difficulty in concentration; demonstrated difficulty in decision making; demonstrated difficulty in judgment; demonstrated difficulty in memory; demonstrated difficulty in reasoning; decreased perception; consumption of minimal to no food at most meals (i.e., consumes <75% of normal requirements); decreased participation in activities of daily living; decreased social skills; expresses loss of interest in pleasurable outlets; frequent exacerbations of chronic health problems; inadequate nutritional intake; neglect of home environment; neglect of financial responsibilities; physical decline (e.g., fatigue, dehydration, incontinence of bowel and bladder); self-care deficit; social withdrawal; unintentional weight loss (e.g., 5% in 1 month, 10% in 6 months); verbalizes desire for death

Related Factor (r/t)

Depression

NOC   Outcomes (Nursing Outcomes Classification)

Suggested NOC Outcomes

Physical Aging, Psychosocial Adjustment: Life Change, Will to Live

Example NOC Outcome with Indicators
Will to Live as evidenced by the following indicators: Expression of determination to live/Expression of hope/Use of strategies to compensate for problems associated with disease (Rate the outcome and indicators of **Will to Live:** 1 = severely compromised, 2 = substantially compromised, 3 = moderately compromised, 4 = mildly compromised, 5 = not compromised [see Section I].)

Client Outcomes

Client Will (Specify Time Frame):

- Resume highest level of functioning possible
- Express feelings
- Participate in ADLs
- Participate in social interactions
- Consume adequate dietary intake for weight and height
- Maintain usual weight
- Have adequate fluid intake with no signs of dehydration
- Maintain clean personal and home environment

NIC   Interventions (Nursing Interventions Classification)

Suggested NIC Interventions

Hope Inspiration, Mood Management, Self-Care Assistance

Example NIC Activities—Hope Installation
Assist patient/family identify areas of hope in life; Involve the patient actively in own care

• = Independent;   ▲ = Collaborative;   EBN = Evidence-Based Nursing;   EB = Evidence-Based

Nursing Interventions and *Rationales*
Psychosocial

- Elderly clients who have failure to thrive (FTT) should be evaluated by review of their ADLs, cognitive function, and mood; a targeted history and physical examination; and selected laboratory studies. **EB:** *A mental status examination is crucial in the diagnosis of delirium. It is precipitated by medial illness, substance intoxication/withdrawal or medication effect and is a leading presenting symptom of illness in the elderly (Nassisi et al, 2006).* **Adult Failure to thrive** *is characterized by lower-than-expected physical function and needs to be identified and treated early to enhance a positive outcome (Higgins & Daly, 2005).*

- Assess for depression with a geriatric depression scale. Be alert for depression in clients newly admitted to nursing homes. **EBN:** *Depression was identified in 52% of the homebound elderly adults according to the Geriatric Depression Scale (Loughlin, 2004).* **EB:** *Clients discharged to a nursing home from a medical rehabilitation unit reported higher levels of depressive symptoms than those discharged to live alone (Loeher, Bank & MacNeill, 2004).*

- Screen for depression in persons with adult macular degeneration and low vision or vision loss. **EB:** *Elderly macular degeneration clients met DSM-IV criteria for syndromal depression, and visual acuity was the only variable significantly associated with vision-specific function. Both psychotherapy and antidepressants are efficacious and may indirectly improve function among older people with vision loss (Casten, Rovner & Edmonds, 2002).*

- ▲ Carefully assess for elder abuse and refer for treatment. **EB:** *Elderly men and women of all socioeconomic and ethnic backgrounds are vulnerable to mistreatment, and most often it goes undetected (Kahan & Paris, 2003).*

- Provide reality orientation for clients with mild dementia. **EBN:** *Reality orientation is effective in improving cognitive ability (Bates, Boote & Beverly, 2004).*

- Instill hope and encourage the expression of positive thoughts. **EB:** *Positive emotions can protect older disabled women against adverse health outcomes (Penninx et al, 2000).* **EB:** *Hopefulness appears to be central to a family's coping with the impact of mental illness (Bland & Darlington, 2002).*

- Provide music for clients with dementia. **EBN:** *When using music therapy in clients with senile dementia, their scores for "irritability" decreased significantly (Suzukie et al, 2004).*

- ▲ Consider the use of light therapy. **EB:** *Bright light treatment may be effective among institutionalized older adults, providing nonpharmacological intervention in the treatment of depression (Sumaya et al, 2001).*

- ▲ Provide opportunities for visitation from animals. **EBN:** *Animal visitation programs have been used in a wide variety of clinical settings with predominantly positive outcomes reported anecdotally (Smith & Buckwalter, 2006). In cognitively intact residents of a nursing home the group that received a canary had fewer depressed symptoms and an increased perception of quality of life (Colombo et al, 2005).*

- Encourage clients to reminiscence and share and compile life histories. **EBN:** *Reminiscence can improve well-being (Reichman et al, 2004; McKee et al, 2003).*

- Encourage clients to pray if they wish. **EB:** *Prayer can be used as a coping strategy (Ai et al, 2004).*

- Encourage elderly clients to take part in activities and social relationships according to their capacity and wishes. **EBN:** *Thriving is related to helping elderly persons concentrate on activities that they are still able to do (Bergland & Kirkevold, 2001).*

- Help clients participate in activities by assessing motivation and helping them identify reasons to participate, such as better mobility, more independence, and feelings of well-being. **EBN:** *Motivation has been identified as an important factor in the older adult's ability to perform functional activities (Resnick, 2002).*

- Provide physical touch for clients. Touch the client's hand or arm when speaking with him or her; offer hugs with permission. **EBN:** *Appropriate use of touch by nurses has the potential to significantly improve the health status of older adults (Bush, 2001; Edvardsson, Sandman & Rasmussen, 2003).*

- Administer TT. **EBN:** *TT can improve overall well-being, provide pain relief, reduce stress and anxiety, and decrease and prevent disruptive behavior for aged residents in an aged care environment (Gregory & Verdouw, 2005). TT may be an effective technique to alleviate agitation in people with Alzheimer's disease (Hawranik et al, 2004).*

F

• = Independent;   ▲ = Collaborative;   EBN = Evidence-Based Nursing;   EB = Evidence-Based

F

Physiological

▲ Assess possible causes for adult FTT and treat any underlying problems such as malnutrition, diarrhea, renal failure, and illnesses caused by physical and cognitive changes. **EBN:** *Weight loss is one of the most important indicators of malnutrition. Both low body weight and weight loss are highly predictive of morbidity and death in elderly persons (Levinson et al, 2005; Hickson, 2006).* **EB:** *Physicians who care for elderly clients should be alert to the possible presence of diarrhea and malabsorption if there is unexplained weight loss and FTT. Older clients may not admit to having chronic diarrhea, particularly if they also are incontinent (Holt, 2001).* **EB:** *The elderly client with renal failure is more often admitted for failure to thrive (Van den Noortgate et al, 2001).*

▲ Assess for signs of fatigue and sensory changes that may indicate an infection is present that may be related to undetected diabetes mellitus, human immunodeficiency virus (HIV), or *Staphylococcus aureus* bacteremia. **EB:** *A substantial proportion of group care home residents not known to have diabetes and able to undergo testing had undetected diabetes based on a 2-hour postglucose load (Sinclair et al 2001).* **EB:** *Many older adults are sexually active and often demonstrate risky sexual behavior, such as dispensing with the use of condoms, and the isolation that frequently accompanies old age can lead to alcoholism and injectable drug use (Lieberman, 2000).* S. aureus *bacteremia should be suspected in elderly adults with previous hospitalization (3 months), residence in a long-term care facility, and altered mental status (Bader, 2006).*

• Monitor weight loss, leaving 25% or more of food uneaten at most meals, psychiatric/mood diagnoses, and deteriorated ability to participate in activities of daily living. **EBN:** *The above criteria are significant predictors of protein calorie malnutrition (Higgins & Daly, 2005). Diagnosis and intervention of malnutrition can prevent loss of function and independence and decrease morbidity and mortality in the elderly (Ennis, Saffel-Shrier & Verson, 2001).*

• Assess for signs of dehydration. **EBN:** *Dehydration is the most common fluid and electrolyte imbalance in older adults (Hodgkinson, Evans & Wood, 2003; Mentes, 2006).*

• Play soothing music during mealtimes to increase the amount of food eaten and promote decreased agitation. **EBN:** *Soothing music selections have beneficial effects on relaxation in community-residing elderly people (Lai, 2004). Relaxing music played during the evening meal may reduce the overall level of agitation among nursing home residents with severe cognitive impairment (Hicks-Moore, 2005).*

• Decrease noise and increase lighting in the dining area. **EB:** *Lighting enhancement and noise reduction may further improve dietary intake, which, in turn, may promote improved nutritional status (McDaniel et al, 2001; Dorner, 2005).*

• Serve "family-style" meals. **EBN:** *Family-style meals may result in modest increases in mealtime participation and communication of residents with dementia (Altus, Engelman & Mathews, 2002).*

▲ Refer to a dietician for individualized nutrition therapy. **EB:** *For the obese older person, modest weight reduction can possibly result in health benefits. For the undernourished older person, early recognition of inadequate nutrition and declining weight with timely intervention is critical (Callahan & Jensen, 2004).*

• Refer to care plan **Readiness for enhanced Nutrition** for additional interventions.

• Assess how often the frail elder living at home goes outdoors. (Ask, "How often do you go outside the house?" Examples include shopping, taking a walk, working in the garden.) Encourage outside activities. **EB:** *Frail elders living at home in Japan who went outdoors less than once a week were part of a high-risk group for functional decline, intellectual activity, and self-efficacy. This question may be a useful and simple indicator to predict these changes (Kono et al, 2004).*

• Provide opportunities for interaction with the natural environment. **EB:** *Interaction with the natural world is a vital part of biopsychosocial-spiritual well-being (Irvine & Warber, 2002).*

• Assess grip strength. **EB:** *Grip strength may prove a more useful single marker of frailty for older people of similar age than chronological age alone. (Syddall, Cooper & Martin, 2003).*

• Frail elderly clients should also participate in carefully supervised group exercise as well as balance and gait programs accompanied by music. **EB:** *Exercise preserves lean body mass and energy intake and helps improve or maintain physical fitness and functioning vital for independent living (De Jong & Franklin, 2004).* **EB:** *In long-term care residents with dementia using wheelchair bicycle riding, depression levels were significantly reduced. Improvements were also found in sleep and levels of* *activity engagement (Buettner & Fitzsimmons, 2002).* **EBN:** *Residents reported significantly enhanced mood while exercising to music (Van de Winckel et al, 2004).* **EB:** *Balance exercises led to improvements in static balance function and gait exercises resulted in improvements to dynamic balance and gait functions in the very frail elderly (Shimada, Uchiyama & Kakurai, 2003).*

▲ Refer for possible pharmacological intervention. **EB:** *A client with multiple myeloma with FTT was successfully treated with modafinil and mirtazapine. By using combination pharmacotherapy, immediate results were achieved in a gravely ill client (Schillerstrom & Seaman, 2002).*

• Refer to care plans for **Imbalanced Nutrition: less than body requirements, Hopelessness,** and **Disturbed Energy field.**

Multicultural

• Assess for the influence of cultural beliefs, norms, and values on the family's or caregiver's understanding of FTT. **EBN:** *What the family considers normal and abnormal health behavior may be based on cultural perceptions (Leininger & McFarland, 2002).*

• Actively listen and be sensitive to how communication is shared culturally. Some cultures communication with eye contact and some avoid eye contact. **EBN:** *The nurse who actively listens encourages sharing of thoughts and feelings, communicates respect, and provides clients with feedback about things they might not be aware of. Finally, active listening involves attention to cultural bias (Davidhizar, 2004).*

▲ Refer culturally diverse clients to appropriate social, medical, mental health, and long-term care services. **EB:** *In a system providing access to and coordination of comprehensive medical and long-term care services for frail older people, black clients showed a lower mortality rate than white clients (Tan, Lui & Eng, 2003). Being black was associated with moderately high and very high levels of nutritional risk (Sharkey & Schoenberg, 2002).*

Home Care

• The above interventions may be adapted for home care use.

• If FTT is attributable to a dementing illness, refer to care plan for **Chronic Confusion.**

▲ Institute case management and refer for care housing of frail elderly to support continued independent living. *With the number of people needing long-term care services, the car housing model is needed for people until they are restored and discharged to a less costly level of care and a more productive quality of life. The case management systems automatically trigger standard interventions for their standard needs and customize interventions for their special needs using templates for personalizing them into a problem-driven action plan (Rhoades, 2007; Newcomer et al, 2004).*

▲ Refer for individualized care management for home healthcare services such as homemaker or psychiatric home healthcare services for respite, client reassurance, and implementation of therapeutic regimen. **EB:** *There is a need for individualized care management assessment and service planning (Akema, Reyes & Wilber, 2006).*

Client/Family Teaching

▲ Consider use of a nurse-managed telehealth system with clients who have been discharged early from the hospital to monitor symptoms, provide education, and make referrals if necessary. *This system helps the client/family manage their own care, reinforces change, and moves clients toward optimum functioning (Martin & Coyle, 2006).*

▲ Refer for medical evaluation when cognitive changes are noticed. **EB:** *The combination of functional imaging and neuropsychological tests can diagnose with high sensitivity and specificity if a client is suffering cognitive impairment in its early stages and may aid in predicting the risk of developing dementia (Cabranes et al, 2004).*

• Encourage family to provide social interaction with the client. **EBN:** *The importance of family involvement may be effective in enhancing the lives of frail elders (Gosline, 2003).*

• Instruct the family to monitor the elder person's weight. **EBN:** *Monitoring the elder's weight regularly is a surveillance measure of nutritional status (Cowan, Roberts & Fitzpatrick, 2004).*

▲ Provide referral for evaluation of hearing and appropriate hearing aids. **EB:** *Residents older than 65 years (mean age, 79 years) living in nursing homes demonstrated that hearing loss affects the communication, sociability, and psychological aspects of quality of life (Tsuruoka et al, 2001).*

• = Independent;   ▲ = Collaborative;   EBN = Evidence-Based Nursing;   EB = Evidence-Based

▲ Refer for psychotherapy and possible medication if the etiology is depression. *Geriatric depression is a common but frequently unrecognized or inadequately treated condition in the elderly population. Nonpharmacological and pharmacological treatment options for managing depression are available (Lapid & Rummans, 2003).*

▲ Refer for possible medication therapy when the diagnosis is dementia. **EB:** *Residents with dementia in nursing homes showed that Tacrine was associated with lower mortality (Ott & Lapane, 2002).*

evolve See the EVOLVE website for World Wide Web resources for client education.

REFERENCES

Ai AL, Peterson C, Tice TN et al: Faith-based and secular pathways to hope and optimism subconstructs in middle-aged and older cardiac patients, *J Health Psychol* 9(3):435-450, 2004.

Alkema G, Reyes J, Wilber K: Characteristics associated with home- and community-based service utilization for Medicare managed care consumers, *Gerontologist* 46(2):173-183, 2006.

Altus DE, Engelman KK, Mathews RM: Using family-style meals to increase participation and communication in persons with dementia, *J Gerontol Nurs* 28(9):47-53, 2002.

Bader MS: *Staphylococcus aureus* bacteremia in older adults: predictors of 7-day mortality and infection with a methicillin-resistant strain, *Infect Control Hosp Epidemiol* 27(11):219-225, 2006.

Bates J, Boote J, Beverley C: Psychosocial interventions for people with a milder dementing illness: a systematic review, *J Adv Nurs* 45(6):644-658, 2004.

Bergland A, Kirkevold M: Thriving—a useful theoretical perspective to capture the experience of well-being among frail elderly in nursing homes? *J Adv Nurs* 36(3):426-432, 2001.

Bland R, Darlington Y: The nature and sources of hope: perspectives of family caregivers of people with serious mental illness, *Perspect Psychiatr Care* 38(2):61, 2002.

Buettner LL, Fitzsimmons S: AD-venture program: therapeutic biking for the treatment of depression in long-term care residents with dementia, *Am J Alzheimers Dis Other Demen* 17(2):121-127, 2002.

Bush E: The use of human touch to improve the well-being of older adults: a holistic nursing intervention, *J Holist Nurs* 19(3):256-270, 2001.

Cabranes JA, De Juan R, Encinas M et al: Relevance of functional neuroimaging in the progression of mild cognitive impairment, *Neurol Res* 26(5):496-501, 2004.

Callahan E, Jensen G: Weight issues in later years, *Generations* 28(3):39-45, 2004.

Casten RJ, Rovner BW, Edmonds SE: The impact of depression in older adults with age-related macular degeneration, *J Vis Impair Blindness* 96(6):399, 2002.

Colombo G, Buono MD, Smania K et al: Pet therapy and institutionalized elderly: a study on 144 cognitively unimpaired subjects, *Arch Gerontol Geriatr* 42:207-216, 2005.

Cowan DT, Roberts JD, Fitzpatrick JM: Nutritional status of older people in long term care settings: current status and future directions, *Int J Nurs Stud* (3):225-237, 2004.

Davidhizar R: Listening: a nursing strategy to transcend culture, *J Pract Nurs* 54(2):22, 2004.

De Jong AA, Franklin BA: Prescribing exercise for the elderly: current research and recommendations, *Curr Sports Med Rep* 3(6):337-343, 2004.

Dorner B: Nutrition for the dementia resident, *Nursing Homes* 54(5):29-31, 2005.

Edvardsson JD, Sandman P, Rasmussen RH: Meanings of giving touch in the care of older patients: becoming a valuable person and professional, *J Clin Nurs* 12(4):601-609, 2003.

Ennis BW, Saffel-Shrier S, Verson H: Diagnosing malnutrition in the elderly, *Nurse Pract* 26(3):52, 2001.

Gosline MB: Client participation to enhance socialization for frail elders, *Geriatr Nurs* 24(5):286-289, 2003.

Gregory S, Verdouw J: Therapeutic touch: its application for residents in aged care, *Aus Nurs J* 12(7):23-26, 2005.

Hawranik P, Deatrich J, Johnston P: Therapeutic touch: another approach for the management of agitation, *Can Nurs Home* 15(1):46-48, 2004.

Hicks-Moore SL: Relaxing music at mealtime in nursing homes, *J Gerontol Nurs* 31(12):26-33, 2005.

Hickson M: Malnutrition and aging, *Postgrad Med J* 82(963):2-8, 2006.

Higgins P, Daly B: Adult failure to thrive in the older rehabilitation patient, *Rehab Nurs* 30(4):152-160, 2005.

Hodgkinson B, Evans D, Wood J: Maintaining oral hydration in older adults: a systematic review, *Int J Nurs Pract* 9(3):S19-S28, 2003.

Holt PR: Diarrhea and malabsorption in the elderly, *Gastroenterol Clin North Am* 30(2):427, 2001.

Irvine KN, Warber SL: Greening healthcare: practicing as if the natural environment really mattered, *Altern Ther Health Med* 8(5):76, 2002.

Kahan FS, Paris BE: Why elder abuse continues to elude the health care system, *Mt Sinai J Med* 70(1):62, 2003.

Kono A, Kai I, Sakato C et al: Frequency of going outdoors: a predictor of functional and psychosocial change among ambulatory frail elders living at home, *J Gerontol A Biol Sci Med Sci* 59(3):275-280, 2004.

Lai H: Music preference and relaxation in Taiwanese elderly people, *Geriatr Nurs* 25(5):286-291, 2004.

Lapid MI, Rummans TA: Evaluation and management of geriatric depression in primary care, *Mayo Clin Proc* 78(11):1423-1429, 2003.

Leininger MM, McFarland MR: *Transcultural nursing: concepts, theories, research and practices,* ed 3, New York, 2002, McGraw-Hill.

Levinson Y, Dwolatzky T, Epstein A et al: Is it possible to increase weight and maintain the protein status of debilitated elderly residents of nursing homes? *J Gerontol A Biol Sci Med Sci* 60(7):878-881, 2005.

Lieberman R: HIV in older Americans: an epidemiologic perspective, *J Midwifery Womens Health* 45(2):176, 2000.

Loeher KE, Bank AL, MacNeill SE: Nursing home transition and depressive symptoms in older medical rehabilitation patients, *Clin Gerontol* 27(1/2):59-70, 2004.

Loughlin A: Depression and social support: effective treatments for homebound elderly adults, *J Gerontol Nurs* 30(5):11-15, 2004.

Martin E, Coyle M: Nursing protocol for telephonic supervision of clients, *Rehab Nurs* 31(2):54-59, 2006.

McDaniel JH et al: Impact of dining room environment on nutritional intake of Alzheimer's residents: a case study, *Am J Alzheimers Dis Other Demen* 16(5):297, 2001.

McKee KJ, Wilson F, Elford H et al: Reminiscence: is living in the past good for wellbeing? *Nurs Residential Care* 5(10):489-491, 2003.

Mentes J: Oral hydration in older adults: greater awareness is needed in preventing, recognizing, and treating dehydration, *Am J Nurs* 106(6):40-49, 2006.

Nassisi D, Korc B, Hahn S et al: The evaluation and management of the acutely agitated elderly patient, *Mt Sinai J Med* 73(7):976-984, 2006.

Newcomer R, Maravilla V, Faculijak P et al: Outcomes of preventive case management among high-risk elderly in three medical groups: a randomized clinical trial, *Eva Health Prof* 27(4):323, 2004.

Ott BR, Lapane KL: Tacrine therapy is associated with reduced mortality in nursing home residents with dementia, *J Am Geriatr Soc* 50(1):35, 2002.

Penninx BW, Guralnik JM, Bandeen-Roche K et al: The protective effect of emotional vitality on adverse health outcomes in disabled older women, *J Am Geriatr Soc* 48(11):1359-1366, 2000.

Resnick B: Geriatric rehabilitation: the influence of efficacy beliefs and motivation, *Rehab Nurs* 27(4):152-161, 2002.

Reichman S, Leonard C, Mintz T et al: Compiling life history resources for older adults in institutions: development of a guide, *J Gerontol Nurs* 30(2):20, 2004.

Rhoades J: Cultural dysfunction, *Nurs Homes* 56(1):10-11, 2007.

Schillerstrom JE, Seaman JS: Modafinil augmentation of mirtazapine in a failure-to-thrive geriatric inpatient, *Int J Psychiatry Med* 32(4):405-410, 2002.

Sharkey JR, Schoenberg NE: Variations in nutritional risk among black and white women who receive home-delivered meals, *J Women Aging* 14(3-4):99-119, 2002.

Shimada H, Uchiyama Y, Kakurai S: Specific effects of balance and gait exercises on physical function among the frail elderly, *Clin Rehabil* 17(5):472-479, 2003.

Sinclair AJ, Gadsby R, Penfold S et al: Prevalence of diabetes in care home residents, *Diabetes Care* 24(6):1066-1068, 2001.

Smith M, Buckwalter K: Behaviors associated with dementia, *Clin J Oncol Nurs* 10(2):183-192, 2006.

Sumaya IC, Rienzi BM, Deegan JF II et al: Bright light treatment decreases depression in institutionalized older adults: a placebo-controlled crossover study, *J Gerontol A Biol Sci Med Sci* 56(6): M356-M360, 2001.

Suzuki M, Kanamori M, Watanabe M et al: Behavioral and endocrinological evaluation of music therapy for elderly patients with dementia, *Nurs Health Sci* 6(1):11-18, 2004.

Syddall H, Cooper C, Martin F: Is grip strength a useful single marker of frailty? *Age Ageing* 32(6):650-656, 2003.

Tan EJ, Lui LY, Eng C: Differences in mortality of black and white patients enrolled in the program of all-inclusive care for the elderly, *J Am Geriatr Soc* 51(2):246-251, 2003.

Tsuruoka H, Masuda S, Ukai K et al: Hearing impairment and quality of life for the elderly in nursing homes, *Auris Nasus Larynx* 28(1):45-54, 2001.

Van de Winckel A, Feys H, De Weerdt W et al: Cognitive and behavioural effects of music-based exercises in patients with dementia, *Clin Rehabil* 18(3):253-260, 2004.

Van den Noortgate NJ, Janssens WH, Afschrift MB et al: Renal function in the oldest-old on an acute geriatric ward, *Int Urol Nephrol* 32(4):531-537, 2001.

Risk for Falls   *Sherry A. Greenberg, MSN, APRN, BC, GNP*

NANDA   **Definition**

Increased susceptibility to falling that may cause physical harm

Risk Factors (Intrinsic and Extrinsic)

Adults

Age 65 or older; history of falls; lives alone; lower limb prosthesis; use of assistive devices (e.g., walker, cane); wheelchair use

Children

Less than 2 years of age; bed located near window; lack of auto restraints; lack of gate on stairs; lack of window guard; lack of parental supervision; male gender when less than one year of age; unattended infant on elevated surface (e.g., bed/changing table)

Cognitive

Diminished mental status

Environment

Cluttered environment; dimly lit room; no antislip material in bath or shower; restraints; throw rugs; unfamiliar room; weather conditions (e.g., wet floors, ice)

Medications

ACE inhibitors; alcohol use; antianxiety agents; antihypertensive agents; diuretics; hypnotics; narcotics; tranquilizers; tricyclic antidepressants

• = Independent;   ▲ = Collaborative;   EBN = Evidence-Based Nursing;   EB = Evidence-Based

Physiological

Anemias; arthritis; diarrhea; decreased lower extremity strength; difficult with gait; faintness when extending neck; faintness when turning neck; foot problems; hearing difficulties; impaired balance; impaired physical mobility; incontinence; neoplasms (i.e., fatigue/limited mobility); neuropathy; orthostatic hypotension; postoperative conditions; postprandial blood sugar changes; presence of acute illness; proprioceptive deficits; sleeplessness; urgency; vascular disease; visual difficulties

NOC   Outcomes (Nursing Outcomes Classification)

Suggested NOC Outcomes

Fall Prevention Behavior, Knowledge: Child Physical Safety

Example NOC Outcome with Indicators
Fall Prevention Behavior as evidenced by the following indicators: Uses assistive devices correctly/Eliminates clutter, spills, glare from floors/Uses safe transfer procedure (Rate the outcome and indicators of **Fall Prevention Behavior:** 1 = never demonstrated, 2 = rarely demonstrated, 3 = sometimes demonstrated, 4 = often demonstrated, 5 = consistently demonstrated [see Section I].)

Client Outcomes

Client Will (Specify Time Frame):

- Remain free of falls
- Change environment to minimize the incidence of falls
- Explain methods to prevent injury

NIC   Interventions (Nursing Interventions Classification)

Suggested NIC Interventions

Dementia Management, Fall Prevention, Post-Fall Assessment, Surveillance: Safety

Example NIC Activities—Fall Prevention
Assist unsteady individual with ambulation; Monitor gait, balance, and fatigue level with ambulation

Nursing Interventions and *Rationales*

- Determine risk of falling by using an evaluation tool such as the Fall Risk Assessment (Gray-Miceli, 2006; Farmer, 2000), The Conley Scale (Conley, Schultz & Selvin, 1999), or the FRAINT Tool for fall risk assessment (Parker, 2000). *Risk factors for falling include recent history of falls, confusion, depression, altered elimination patterns, cardiovascular/respiratory disease impairing perfusion or oxygenation, postural hypotension, dizziness or vertigo, primary cancer diagnosis, and altered mobility (Farmer, 2000; Hendrich et al, 1995). Predictors of fall risk in the community included atrial fibrillation, neurological problems, living alone, and not adhering to a regular exercise program (Resnick, 1999).*
- Complete a fall risk assessment for older adults in acute care using a valid and reliable tool such as The Hendrich II Model. *It is quick to administer and provides a determination of risk for falling based on gender, mental and emotional status, symptoms of dizziness, and known categories of medications increasing risk (Hendrich, Bender & Nyhuis, 2003). This tool screens for primary prevention of falls and is integral in a post-fall assessment for the secondary prevention of falls (Gray-Miceli, 2006).*
- Screen all clients for balance and mobility skills (supine to sit, sitting supported and unsupported, sit to stand, standing, walking and turning around, transferring, stooping to floor and recovering, and sitting down). Use tools such as the Balance Scale by Tinetti or the Get Up and Go Scale by Mathais. *It is helpful to determine the client's functional abilities and then plan for ways to improve problem areas or determine methods to ensure safety (Tinetti, 2003).*

• = Independent;   ▲ = Collaborative;   EBN = Evidence-Based Nursing;   EB = Evidence-Based

- Recognize that when people attend to another task while walking, such as carrying a cup of water, clothing, or supplies, they are more likely to fall. **EB:** *When patients were given a carrying task in addition to walking, there was a higher risk for subsequent falls (Lundin-Olsson, Nysberg & Gustafson, 1998).*
- Be careful when getting a mostly immobile client up. Be sure to lock the bed and wheelchair and have sufficient personnel to protect the client from falls. When the client is rising from a lying position, have the client change positions slowly, dangle legs, and stand next to the bed before walking to prevent orthostatic hypotension. *A very important preventive measure to reduce the risk of injurious falls for nonambulatory residents involves increasing safety measures while transferring, including careful locking of equipment such as wheelchairs and beds before moves. These immobile clients can sustain the most serious injuries when they fall.*
- Identify clients likely to fall by placing a "fall precautions" sign on the doorway and by keying the Kardex and chart. Use a "high-risk fall" armband and room sign to alert staff for increased vigilance and mobility assistance. *These steps alert the nursing staff of the increased risk of falls (McCarter-Bayer, Bayer & Hall, 2005).*
- ▲ Evaluate the client's medications to determine whether they increase the risk of falling; consult physician regarding the client's need for medication if appropriate. *Polypharmacy has been associated with increased falls. Medications such as benzodiazepines, antipsychotics, and antidepressants given to promote sleep increase the rate of falls (Capezuti et al, 1999; Wooten & Galavis, 2005).* **EB:** *Use of selective serotonin reuptake inhibitors and tricyclic antidepressants resulted in increased incidences of falls (Liu et al, 1998; Thapa et al, 1998).*
- Thoroughly orient the client to the environment. Place the call light within reach and show how to call for assistance; answer call light promptly.
- Use one-quarter- to one-half-length side rails only and maintain bed in a low position. Ensure that wheels are locked on bed and commode. Keep dim light in room at night. *Use of full side rails can result in the client climbing over the rails, leading with the head, and sustaining a head injury. Side rails with widely spaced vertical bars and side rails not situated flush with the mattress have been associated with asphyxiation deaths because of rail and in-bed entrapment and should not be used (Capezuti, 2004).*
- Routinely assist the client with toileting on his or her own schedule. *Always take the client to bathroom on awakening, before bedtime, and before administering sedatives (McCarter-Bayer, Bayer & Hall, 2005). Keep the path to the bathroom clear, label the bathroom, and leave the door open. The majority of falls are related to toileting. It is more acceptable to fall than to "wet yourself." Falls are often linked to the need to eliminate in a hurry (Wilson, 1998).*
- ▲ Avoid restraints if at all possible. Obtain a physician's order if restraints are necessary, and use the least restrictive device. *The use of restraints has been associated with serious injuries, including rhabdomyolysis, brachial plexus injury, neuropathy, dysrhythmias, strangulation, asphyxiation, traumatic brain injuries, and all the consequences of immobility (Capezuti, 2004).* **EBN and EB:** *There was no increase in falls or injuries in a group of clients in a nursing home who were not restrained versus a similar group that was restrained (Capezuti et al, 1999). Restrained elderly clients often have an increased number of falls, possibly as a result of muscle deconditioning or loss of coordination (Tinetti, Liu & Ginter, 1992).* **EB:** *When restraints were not used in two acute care hospitals there was no increase in client falls, injuries, or therapy disruptions (Mion et al, 2001).*
- In place of restraints, use the following:
  - Well-staffed and educated nursing personnel with frequent client contact with careful consideration during shift changes
  - Nursing units designed to care for clients with cognitive or functional impairments
  - Nonskid footwear, sneakers preferable
  - Adequate lighting, night light in bathroom
  - Frequent toileting
  - Frequent assessment of the need for invasive devices, tubes, intravenous (IV) lines
  - Tubes hidden with bandages to prevent pulling of tubes
  - Alternative IV placement site to prevent client from pulling it out
  - Alarm systems with ankle, above-the-knee, or wrist sensors
  - Bed or wheelchair alarms
  - Wedge cushions on chairs to prevent slipping

F

- Increased observation of the client
- Locked doors to unit
- Low or very low height beds
- Border-defining pillow or mattress to remind the client to stay in bed
  These alternatives to restraints can be helpful to prevent falls (McCarter-Bayer, Bayer & Hall, 2005; Capezuti, 2004; Cotter & Evans, 2006).
- If the client has an acute change in mental status (delirium), recognize that the cause is usually physiological and is a medical emergency. Provide reality orientation when interacting. Have family bring in familiar items, clocks, and watches from home to maintain orientation. *Reality orientation can help prevent or decrease the confusion that increases risk of falling for clients with delirium.* See interventions for **Acute Confusion.**
- If the client has chronic confusion with dementia, use validation therapy that reinforces feelings but does not confront reality. *Validation therapy is effective for clients with dementia (Fine & Rouse-Bane, 1995).* See interventions for **Chronic Confusion.**
- Ask family to stay with the client to assist with ADLs and prevent the client from accidentally falling or pulling out tubes.
▲ If the client is unsteady on feet, have two nursing staff members alongside when walking the client. Consider referral to physical therapy for gait training and strengthening. *The client can walk independently, but the nurse can rapidly ensure safety if the knees buckle. Interdisciplinary care is most comprehensive and beneficial to the client.*
- Place a fall-prone client in a room that is near the nurses' station. *Such placement allows more frequent observation of the client.*
- Help clients sit in a stable chair with arm rests. Avoid use of wheelchairs and "geri-chairs" except for transportation as needed. *Clients are likely to fall when left in a wheelchair or "geri-chair" because they may stand up without locking the wheels or removing the footrests. Wheelchairs do not increase mobility; people sit in them the majority of the time (Simmons et al, 1995).*
- Ensure that the chair or wheelchair fits the build, abilities, and needs of the client to ensure propulsion with legs or arms and ability to reach the floor, eliminating footrests and minimizing problems with shearing. *The seating system should fit the needs of the client so that the client can move the wheels, stand up from the chair without falling, and not be harmed by the chair. Footrests can cause skin tears and bruising as well as postural alignment and sitting posture problems (Nelson, 2004).*
- Avoid use of wheelchairs as much as possible because they can serve as a restraint device. Most people in wheelchairs do not move. *Wheelchairs unfortunately serve as a restraint device.* **EB:** *A study has shown that only 4% of residents in wheelchairs were observed to propel them independently and only 45% could propel them, even with cues and prompts. Another study showed that no residents could unlock wheelchairs without help, the wheelchairs were not fitted to residents, and residents were not trained in propulsion (Simmons et al, 1995). Another study performed on rehabilitation clients found that two variables predicted falls: use of a wheelchair and risk-taking behavior in stroke clients and orthopedic rehabilitation clients (Aizen, Shugaey & Lenger, 2007).*
▲ Refer to physical therapy for strengthening exercises, gait training, and help with balance to increase mobility. **EB:** *Balance, gait training, and strengthening exercises in physical therapy have been shown to be effective for preventing falls (Gillespie, Gillespie & Robertson, 2005; Robertson et al, 2001).*

Geriatric

- Assess ability to move using the Get Up and Go test. Ask the client to rise from a sitting position, walk 10 feet, turn, and return to the chair to sit. *Performance on this screening exam demonstrates the client's mobility and ability to leave the house safely. If the client completes the test in less than 20 seconds, he or she usually can live independently. If completing the test takes longer than 30 seconds, clients are more likely to be dependant on others, and more likely to sustain a fall (Robertson & Montagnini, 2004).*
- Complete a fall risk assessment for older adults in acute care using a valid and reliable tool such as The Hendrich II Model. *It is quick to administer and provides a determination of risk for falling based on gender, mental and emotional status, symptoms of dizziness, and known categories of medications increasing risk (Hendrich et al, 2003). This tool screens for primary prevention of falls and is integral in a post-fall assessment for the secondary prevention of falls (Gray-Miceli, 2006).*

▲ If new onset of falling, assess for laboratory abnormalities and signs and symptoms of infection and dehydration. Check blood pressure and pulse rate supine, sitting, and standing for orthostatic hypotension. *If orthostatic hypotension is present and there is minimal change in the heart rate, most likely the baroreceptors are not working to maintain blood pressure on rising. This is common in the elderly and can be from cardiovascular disease, neurological disease, or a medication effect (Sclater & Kannayiram, 2004).*

• Encourage the client to wear glasses and use walking aids when ambulating.

• Help the client obtain and wear a specially designed hip protector when ambulating. Hip protectors are worn in a specially designed stretchy undergarment containing a pocket on each side for placement of the protector. **EB:** *Hip protectors are only somewhat effective for vulnerable clients in institutions because of resistance to wearing them (Parker, Gillespie & Gillespie, 2005). The use of external hip protectors could reduce hip fractures among older adults at risk (Heikinheimo et al, 2004).*

• If the client experiences dizziness when getting up because of orthostatic hypotension, teach methods to decrease dizziness such as rising slowly, remaining seated several minutes before standing, flexing feet upward several times while sitting, sitting down immediately if feeling dizzy, and having someone present when standing. *Always have the client dangle at the bedside before trying to stand to evaluate for postural hypotension. Watch the client closely for dizziness during increased activity. Postural hypotension can be detected in up to 30% of elderly clients. These methods can help prevent falls (Tinetti, 2003).*

▲ If the client has syncope, determine symptoms that occur before syncope and note medications that the client is taking. Refer for medical care. The circumstances surrounding syncope often suggest the cause. *Use of many medications, including diuretics, antihypertensives, digoxin, beta-blockers, and calcium channel blockers, can cause syncope. Use of the tilt table can be diagnostic in incidences of syncope (Cox, 2000).*

▲ Observe client for signs of anemia, and refer to primary care practitioner for testing if appropriate. **EB:** *Elderly clients with mild anemia had three times the incidence of falls (Dharmarajan & Norkus, 2004).*

▲ Evaluate client for chronic alcohol intake as well as mental health and neurologic function. **EBN:** *Age, gender, neurological disease, mental health, and regular use of alcohol significantly influence the rate of falls (Resnick & Junlapeeya, 2004).*

▲ Refer to physical therapy for strength training with free weights or machines. *Strength improvement in response to resisted exercise is possible even in the very elderly, extremely sedentary client with multiple chronic diseases and functional disabilities. Increased strength can help prevent falls (Connelly, 2000).* **EBN:** *One such program, Walking for Wellness, identified that screening procedures often identify which clients would benefit from physical therapy (Tucker, Molsberger & Clark, 2004).*

▲ If an elderly woman has symptoms of urge incontinence, refer to a urologist for evaluation and ensure the path to the bathroom is well lit and free of obstructions. *Urge urinary incontinence was associated with an increased incidence of falls in older women (Brown et al, 2000).*

 Home Care

• Some of the above interventions may be adapted for home care use.

• If the client was identified as a fall risk in the hospital, recognize that there is a high incidence of falls after discharge and use all measures possible to reduce the incidence of falls. **EBN:** *The rate of falls is substantially increased in the geriatric client who has been recently hospitalized, especially during the first month after discharge (Mahoney et al, 2000).*

• Assess and monitor for acute changes in cognition and behavior. *An acute and fluctuating change in cognition and behavior is the classic presentation of delirium.* **EBN:** *Falls may be a precipitating event or an indication of frailty consistent with acute confusion (Mentes et al, 1999).*

• Assess for cause of delirium and/or falls with an interdisciplinary team.

• Assess for additional factors leading to risk for falls. **EB:** *Risk factors include medical history (neurological and cardiovascular impairments), medication use (antipsychotic and tricyclic antidepressant medications), and fall history (fall recurrence during the preceding 3 months) (Lewis et al, 2004).*

• Assess home environment for threats to safety including clutter, slippery floors, scatter rugs, and other potential hazards. Additionally, assess external environment (e.g., uneven pavement, unleveled stairs or steps). *Clients with impaired mobility, impaired visual acuity, and neurological dys-*

F

function, including dementia and other cognitive functional deficits, are all at risk for injury from common hazards. These recommendations were shown to be effective to reduce falls (Tinetti, 2003).

▲ Institute a home-based, nurse-delivered exercise program to reduce falls or refer to physical therapy services for client and family education of safe transfers and ambulation and for strengthening exercises for the client. *A home-based, nurse-delivered exercise program was effective in reducing the number of falls, especially in clients older than 80 years (Robertson et al, 2001).* **EBN:** *There was a 4% reduction in the rate of falls in individuals who received fall prevention programs (Hill-Westmoreland, Soeken & Spellbring, 2002).*

▲ Instruct the client and family or caregivers on how to correct identified hazards. Refer to physical and occupational therapy services for assistance if needed. **EB:** *Home visits by a health professional to assess and modify the home environment have been shown to be effective to reduce the number of falls (Gillespie et al, 2005).*

• Use a multifactorial assessment along with interventions targeted to the identified risk factors. Key components of the interventions include evaluating need for all medications, balance, gait and strength training, use of strategies to deal with postural hypotension if present, home safety evaluation with needed modifications, and any needed cardiovascular treatment. **EB:** *The use of a multifactorial assessment along with interventions identified have been shown to be very effective in reducing the number of falls (Close et al, 1999; Tinetti et al, 1994).*

• Encourage the client to eat a balanced diet, with particular inclusion of vitamin D and calcium. *Hypovitaminosis D and hypocalcemia are common in older adults, contributing to falls, musculoskeletal symptoms, and functional and mobility deficits (Dharmarajan, Ahmed & Russell, 2001; Currie, 2006).*

• If the client lives alone or spends a lot of time alone, teach the client what to do if he or she falls and cannot get up, and make sure he or she has a personal emergency response system or a cellular phone that is available from the floor (Tinetti, 2003).

• If the client is at risk for falls, use a gait belt and additional persons when ambulating. *Gait belts decrease the risk of falls during ambulation.* **EBN:** *Be aware that clients may react ambivalently to a personal emergency response system. While the system alleviates some anxiety about ability to receive help, the clients may show concern about being shocked by hearing strangers enter the home (Porter, 2003).*

• Ensure appropriate nonglare lighting in the home. Ask the client to install indoor strip or "runway" type of lighting to baseboards to help clients balance. Install motion-sensitive lighting that turns on automatically when the client gets out of bed to go to the bathroom. *Up to 79% of the elderly have inadequate lighting in their homes, predisposing them to falls (Slay, 2002). The disorientation of waking in the dark could affect the client's balance. Caregiver may be alerted by light that the client is awake and out of bed.*

• Have the client wear supportive low-heeled shoes with good traction when ambulating. *Supportive shoes provide better balance and protect the client from instability on uneven surfaces.*

• Avoid use of slip-on footwear (e.g., clogs, slip-on slippers or sneakers). *Rubber-soled and enclosed footwear prevents falls and minimizes injury.*

• Consider the use of external hip protectors for clients at risk of falls. **EB:** *A study suggested that the use of external hip protectors could reduce hip fractures among older adults at risk (Heikinheimo et al, 2004).*

▲ Refer to physical therapy services for the client and family education of safe transfers and ambulation and for strengthening/balance exercises for the client for ambulation and transfers. **EB:** *A program of muscle strengthening and balance training taught by a professional has been shown effective to reduce falls (Gillespie et al, 2005).*

• Provide a signaling device for clients who wander or are at risk for falls. *Orienting a vulnerable client to a safety net relieves anxiety of the client and caregiver and allows rapid response to a crisis situation.*

• Provide a medical identification bracelet for clients at risk for injury from dementia, diabetes, seizures, or other medical disorders.

• Suggest a tai chi class designed for the elderly to selected clients who have sufficient balance to participate. *Functional balance can be improved by tai chi (Geriatrics, 2005).* **EB:** *Elderly who participate in a tai chi class have half the number of falls as elderly clients who do not (Wolf et al, 1996).*

• = Independent; ▲ = Collaborative; EBN = Evidence-Based Nursing; EB = Evidence-Based

Client/Family Teaching

- Teach the client how to ambulate safely at home, including using safety measures such as hand rails in bathroom and the need to avoid carrying things or performing other tasks while walking. *In the frail elderly, multitasking results in decreased motor performance and may lead to falls (Hauer, Marburger & Oster, 2002).*
- Teach the client the importance of maintaining a regular exercise program such as walking. If the client is afraid of falling while walking outside during cold or wet weather, suggest walking the length of a local mall. *Lack of a consistent exercise program was one of the variables associated with a higher incidence of falls (Resnick, 1999).*

REFERENCES

Aizen E, Shugaey I, Lenger R: Risk factors and characteristics of falls during inpatient rehabilitation of elderly patients, *Arch Gerontol Geriatr* 44(1):1-12, 2007.

Brown JS, Vittinghoff E, Wyman JF et al: Urinary incontinence: does it increase risk for falls and fractures? Study of Osteoporotic Fractures Research Group, *J Am Geriatr Soc* 48(7):721, 2000.

Capezuti E: Minimizing the use of restrictive devices in dementia patients at risk for falling, *Nurs Clin North Am* 39:625, 2004.

Capezuti E, Strumpf N, Evans I et al: Outcomes of nighttime physical restraint removal for severely impaired nursing home residents, *Am J Alzheimers Dis Other Demen* 14(3):157, 1999.

Close J, Ellis M, Hooper R et al: Prevention of falls in the elderly trial (PROFET): a randomized controlled trial, *Lancet* 353:93, 1999.

Conley D, Schultz AA, Selvin R: The challenge of predicting patients at risk for falling: development of the Conley Scale, *Medsurg Nurs* 8(6):348, 1999.

Connelly DM: Resisted exercise training of institutionalized older adults for improved strength and functional mobility: a review, *Top Geriatr Rehabil* 15(3):6, 2000.

Cotter VT, Evans L: *Best practices in nursing care to older adults from The John A. Hartford Institute for Geriatric Nursing and the Alzheimer's Association. Avoiding restraints in older adults with dementia,* www.hartfordign.org/publications/trythis/dementia.pdf, accessed November 26, 2006.

Cox MM: Uncovering the cause of syncope, *Patient Care* 30:39, 2000.

Currie LM: Fall and injury prevention, *Ann Rev Nurs Res* 24:39-74, 2006.

Dharmarajan TS, Ahmed S, Russell RO: Recurrent falls from hypocalcemia due to vitamin D deficiency: a preventable problem in home care, *Home Healthcare Consult* 8(8):8, 2001.

Dharmarajan TS, Norkus EP: Mild anemia and the risk of falls in older adults from nursing homes and the community, *J Am Med Dir Assoc* 5(6):395, 2004.

Farmer BC: Try this: fall risk assessment, *J Gerontol Nurs* 26(7):6, 2000.

Fine JI, Rouse-Bane S: Using validating techniques to improve communication with cognitively impaired older adults, *J Gerontol Nurs* 21:39, 1995.

Functional balance can be improved by tai chi, *Geriatrics* 60(2), 2005.

Gillespie LD, Gillespie WJ, Robertson MC et al: Interventions for preventing falls in elderly people, *Cochrane Database Syst Rev* (3): CD000340, 2005.

Gray-Miceli D: *Try this: best practices in nursing care to older adults from The John A. Hartford Institute for Geriatric Nursing. Fall risk assessment in older adults: the Hendrich II model,* www.hartfordign.org/publications/trythis/issue08.pdf, accessed November 26, 2006.

Hauer K, Marburger C, Oster P: Motor performance deteriorates with simultaneously performed cognitive tasks in geriatric patients, *Arch Phys Med Rehabil* 83(2):217, 2002.

Heikinheimo R, Jalonen-Mannikko A, Asumaniemi H et al: External hip protectors in home-dwelling older persons, *Aging Clin Exp Res* 16:41, 2004.

Hendrich AL, Bender PS, Nyhuis A: Validation of the Hendrich II Fall Risk Model: a large concurrent CASE/control study of hospitalized patients, *Appl Nurs Res* 16(1):9-21, 2003.

Hendrich A, Nyhuuis A, Kippenbrock T et al: Hospital falls: development of a predictive model for clinical practice, *Appl Nurs Res* 8:129-139, 1995.

Hill-Westmoreland EE, Soeken K, Spellbring AM: A meta-analysis of fall prevention programs for the elderly: how effective are they? *Nurs Res* 51(1):1, 2002.

Lewis CL, Moutoux M, Slaughter M et al: Characteristics of individuals who fell while receiving home health services, *Phys Ther* 84(1):23, 2004.

Liu B, Anderson G, Mittmann N et al: Use of selective serotonin-reuptake inhibitors of tricyclic antidepressants and risk for hip fractures in elderly people, *Lancet* 351(9112):1303, 1998.

Lundin-Olsson L, Nysberg L, Gustafson Y: Attention, frailty, and falls: the effect of a manual task on basic mobility, *J Am Geriatr Soc* 46:758, 1998.

Mahoney JE, Palta M, Johnson J et al: Temporal association between hospitalization and rate of falls after discharge, *Arch Intern Med* 160(18):2788, 2000.

McCarter-Bayer A, Bayer F, Hall K: Preventing falls in acute care: an innovative approach, *J Gerontol Nurs* 31(3):25, 2005.

Mentes J, Culp K, Maas M et al: Acute confusion indicators: risk factors and prevalence using MDS data, *Res Nurs Health* 22:95, 1999.

Mion LC, Fogel J, Sandhu S et al: Outcomes following physical restraint reduction programs in two acute care hospitals, *Jt Comm J Qual Improv* 27(11):605-618, 2001.

Nelson A: Technology to promote safe mobility in the elderly, *Nurs Clin North Am* 39:649, 2004.

Parker MJ, Gillespie LD, Gillespie WJ: Hip protectors for preventing hip fractures in the elderly, *Cochrane Database Syst Rev* (3): CD001255, 2005.

Parker R: Assessing the risk of falls among older inpatients, *Prof Nurse* 15(8):511, 2000.

Porter EJ: Moments of apprehension in the midst of a certainty: some frail older widows' lives with a personal emergency response system, *Qual Health Res* 13(9):1311, 2003.

Resnick B: Falls in a community of older adults, *Clin Nurs Res* 8(3):251, 1999.

Resnick B, Junlapeeya P: Falls in a community of older adults: findings and implications for practice, *Appl Nurs Res* 17(2):81, 2004.

Robertson MC, Devlin N, Gardner MM et al: Effectiveness and economic evaluation of a nurse delivered home exercise programme to prevent falls. 1: Randomised controlled trial, *BMJ* 322(7288):697, 2001.

Robertson RG, Montagnini M: Geriatric failure to thrive, *Am Fam Physician* 70(2):343, 2004.

Sclater A, Kannayiram A: Orthostatic hypotension: a primary care primer for assessment and treatment, *Geriatrics* 59(8), 2004.

Simmons SF, Schnelle JF, MacRae PG et al: Wheelchairs as mobility restraints: predictors of wheelchair activity in nonambulatory nursing home residents, *J Am Geriatr Soc* 43:384, 1995.

Slay DH: Home-based environmental lighting assessments for people who are visually impaired: developing techniques and tools, *J Vis Impair Blindness* 96(2):109, 2002.

Thapa PB, Gideon P, Cost TW et al: Antidepressants and the risk of falls among nursing home residents, *N Engl J Med* 339(13):875, 1998.

Tinetti ME: Preventing falls in elderly persons, *N Engl J Med* 348(1):42, 2003.

Tinetti ME, Baker DI, McAvay G et al: A multifactorial intervention to reduce the risk of falling among elderly persons living in the community, *N Engl J Med* 331:821, 1994.

Tinetti ME, Liu WL, Ginter SF: Mechanical restraint use and fall-related injuries among residents of skilled nursing facilities, *Ann Intern Med* 116:369, 1992.

Tucker D, Molsberger S, Clark A: Walking for wellness: a collaborative program to maintain mobility in hospitalized older adults, *Geriatr Nurs* 25(4):242-245, 2004.

Wilson EB: Preventing patient falls, *AACN Clin Issues* 9(1):100, 1998.

Wolf SL, Barnhart HX, Kutner NG et al: Reducing frailty and falls in older persons: an investigation of tai chi and computerized balance training, *J Am Geriatr Soc* 44:489, 1996.

Wooten J, Galavis J: Polypharmacy. Keeping the elderly safe, *RN* 68(8):45-51, 2005.

Dysfunctional Family processes: alcoholism   *Gail B. Ladwig, MSN, CHTP, RN*

NANDA   Definition

Psychosocial, spiritual, and physiological functions of the family unit are chronically disorganized, which leads to conflict, denial of problems, resistance to change, ineffective problem solving, and a series of self-perpetuating crises.

Defining Characteristics

Behavioral

Alcohol abuse; agitation; blaming; broken promises; chaos; contradictory communication; controlling communication; criticizing; deficient knowledge about alcoholism; denial of problems; dependency; difficulty having fun; difficulty with intimate relationships; difficulty with life cycle transitions; diminished physical contact; disturbances in academic performance in children; disturbances in concentration; enabling to maintain alcoholic drinking pattern; escalating conflict; failure to accomplish developmental tasks; family special occasions are alcohol centered; harsh self-judgment; immaturity; impaired communication; inability to accept health; inability to accept help; inability to accept a wide range of feelings; inability to meet emotional needs of its members; inability to meet security needs of its members; inability to meet spiritual needs of its members; inability to receive help appropriately; inadequate understanding of alcoholism; inappropriate expression of anger; ineffective problem-solving skills; isolation; lack of dealing with conflict; lack of reliability; lying; manipulation; nicotine addiction; orientation toward tension relief rather than achievement of goals; paradoxical communication; power struggles; rationalization; refusal to get help; seeking affirmation; seeking approval; self-blaming; stress-related physical illnesses; substance abuse other than alcohol; unresolved grief; verbal abuse of children; verbal abuse of parent; verbal abuse of spouse

Feelings

Abandonment; anger; anxiety; being different from other people; being unloved; confused love and pity; confusion; decreased self-esteem; depression; dissatisfaction; distress; embarrassment; emotional control by others; emotional isolation; failure; fear; frustration; guilt; hopelessness; hostility; hurt; insecurity; lack of identity; lingering resentment; loneliness; loss; mistrust; misunderstand; moodiness; powerlessness; rejection; repressed emotions; responsibility for alcoholic's behavior; suppressed rage; shame; tension; unhappiness; vulnerability; worthlessness

Roles and Relationships

Altered role function; chronic family problems; closed communication systems; deterioration in family relationships/disturbed family dynamics; disrupted family rituals; disrupted family roles; economic problems; family does not demonstrated respect for autonomy of its members; family does not demonstrate respect for individuality of its members; inconsistent parenting; ineffective spouse communication; intimacy dysfunction; lack of cohesiveness; lack of skills necessary for relationships; low perception of parental support; marital problems; neglected obligations; pattern of rejection; reduced ability of family members to relate to each other for mutual growth and maturation; triangulating family relationships

Related Factors (r/t)

Abuse of alcohol; addictive personality; biochemical influences; family history of alcoholism; family history of resistance to treatment; genetic predisposition; inadequate coping skills; lack of problem-solving skills

NOC   Outcomes (Nursing Outcomes Classification)

Suggested NOC Outcomes

Family Coping, Family Functioning, Family Health Status, Substance Addiction Consequences

Example NOC Outcome with Indicators
Family Coping as evidenced by the following indicators: Confronts/manages family problems/Seeks family assistance when appropriate (Rate the outcome and indicators of **Family Coping:** 1 = never demonstrated, 2 = rarely demonstrated, 3 = sometimes demonstrated, 4 = often demonstrated, 5 = consistently demonstrated [see Section I].)

Client Outcomes

Family/Client Will (Specify Time Frame):

- Develop relationship with nurse that demonstrates at least minimal level of trust
- Demonstrate an understanding of alcoholism as a family illness and the severity of the threat to emotional and physical health of family members
- Develop and state a belief in feasibility and effectiveness of efforts to address alcoholism
- Demonstrate change from dysfunctional patterns by moving from inappropriate to appropriate role relationships, improving cohesion among family members, decreasing conflict and social isolation, and improving coping behaviors
- Maintain improvements

NIC   Interventions (Nursing Interventions Classification)

Suggested NIC Interventions

Family Process Maintenance, Substance Use Treatment

Example Activities—Family Process Maintenance
Identify effects of role changes on family process; Assist family members to use existing support mechanisms

Nursing Interventions and *Rationales*

- Refer to care plans for **Ineffective Denial** and **Defensive Coping** for additional interventions.
- When completing a family assessment, assess behaviors of alcohol abuse, loss of control of drinking, denial, nicotine addiction, impaired communication, inappropriate expression of anger, and enabling behaviors. **EB:** *A set of standard measures is available for helping assess the needs of concerned and affected family members, derived from an explicit model of the family in relation to excessive drinking, drug taking, or gambling (Orford et al, 2005).*
- Screen clients for at-risk drinking during routine primary care visits. **EB:** *Researchers from the United States and the United Kingdom believe the Alcohol Use Disorders Identification Test (AUDIT) is now one of the most effective and cost-efficient means for identifying hazardous and harmful drinkers in the primary care setting. AUDIT is a 10-item questionnaire specifically developed for use as a short*

screening instrument for the identification of hazardous, harmful, or dependent alcohol users (Drugs and Alcohol Today, 2006).

- Provide brief (5-10 minute) advice and counseling as a routine part of primary care. *This practice, along with alcohol screening, can reduce alcohol consumption by high-risk drinkers (Reiff-Heffing et al, 2005).*
- Instill hope and encourage the expression of positive thoughts. **EB:** *Hopefulness appears to be central to a family's coping with the impact of mental illness. Nurses should be mindful of their capacity to sustain or diminish the hopes of family members (Bland & Darlington, 2002).*
- Stress early treatment and brief intervention to resolve the problem. **EBN:** *This study demonstrated cost-effectiveness of the early treatment model (project TrEAT; Trial for Early Alcohol Treatment) (Mundt, 2006).*
- Assist with stabilization and maintenance of positive change in the family. Instruct the alcoholic's family members before the client's discharge to give verbal messages that convey concern about the alcoholic's problem drinking, their observations of the alcoholic's past episodes of drinking, and wishes and support for abstinence. **EB:** *This intervention method can help the alcoholic face the reality of his or her drinking problem and alcohol dependence and thus remain longer in long-term rehabilitation programs, which is a prerequisite for successful recovery from alcohol dependence (Ino & Hayasida, 2000).*
- Provide activities that are physical in nature, such as adventure therapy and therapeutic camping, as part of a substance abuse treatment program. **EBN:** *Mental health promotion is considered a strategy to promote health (Epstein, 2004).*
- ▲ Consider alternative therapies such as acupuncture. *Acupuncture may be helpful in detoxification and is valuable when used in combination with counseling (Serrano, 2003).*
- ▲ Refer for possible use of medications such as naltrexone and acamprosate to control problem drinking. **EB:** *Pharmacotherapeutic strategies are effective in the relapse prevention of alcoholism (Kiefer et al, 2003).*

Pediatric

- Educate family members about available educational and support programs and encourage limited alcohol use in the home. **EBN:** *The family remains a strong factor in moderating adolescent substance use (Kingon & O'Sullivan, 2001). Both individual and multiperson interventions exert an influential role in family-based therapy for treatment of adolescent drug abuse (Hoque et al, 2006).*
- Use closed-ended questions when questioning adolescents about drinking behavior. *Student reports of specific beverage type use were higher when using closed-ended questions compared with open-ended question. The adolescent drinking amount self-reports seem reasonably reliable and valid both on a population and individual level (Lintonen, Ahlstro & Metso, 2004).*
- ▲ Provide a brief motivational interviewing and cognitive/behavioral-based alcohol intervention group program for young people at risk of developing a problem with alcohol. **EB:** *Participants showed an increase in readiness to reduce their alcohol consumption and a reduction in their frequency of drinking at posttreatment and the first follow-up assessment (Bailey et al, 2004).*
- Encourage parent involvement with adolescents for both supervision and emotional support. *The results of this study indicate that inadequate parent involvement may be a form of neglect, which leads to adolescent alcohol involvement. Neglected adolescents were more likely to develop alcohol use disorders (Duncan et al, 2003).*
- Work at strengthening adolescents' relationships in and out of the home. *Prevention interventions focusing on increasing socially conforming attitudes and on strengthening relationships both in and out of the home during adolescence are likely to be effective in reducing aspects of alcohol involvement for women in the general community (Locke & Newcomb, 2004).*
- ▲ Provide school-based prevention programs using peer leaders at an early age. **EB:** *Targeting middle school–aged children and designing programs that can be delivered primarily by peer leaders will increase the effectiveness of school-based substance use prevention programs (Gottfredson & Wilson, 2003).*
- ▲ Provide a school-based drug-prevention program to junior high students. **EB:** *Students who received the drug prevention program during junior high school were less likely to have violations and points on their driving records (Griffin, Botvin & Nichols, 2004; Warner, White & Johnston, 2007).*

Geriatric

- Include assessment of possible alcohol abuse when assessing elderly family members. **EB:** *Alcohol abuse and alcoholism are common but underrecognized problems among older adults (Rigler, 2000).* **EB:** *Alcohol abuse and dependence in older people are important problems that frequently remain undetected by health services (Beullens & Aertgeerts, 2004). The majority of elderly alcoholics are married, have low education levels, and do not belong to high social classes (Shahpesandy et al, 2006).*
- ▲ Provide alcohol treatment programs for geriatric clients in primary care settings. **EB:** *Older primary care clients were more likely to accept collaborative mental health treatment within primary care than in mental health/substance abuse clinics. These results suggest that integrated service arrangements improve access to mental health and substance abuse services for older adults who underuse these services (Bartels et al, 2004).*

Multicultural

- Acknowledge racial/ethnic differences at the onset of care. **EBN:** *Acknowledgment of race/ethnicity issues will enhance communication, establish rapport, and promote treatment outcomes (D'Avanzo et al, 2001; Giger & Davidhizar, 2004).*
- Approach families of color with respect, warmth, and professional courtesy. **EBN:** *Instances of disrespect and lack of caring have special significance for families of color (D'Avanzo et al, 2001; Vontress & Epp, 1997).*
- Give rationale when assessing black families about alcohol use and misuse. **EBN:** *Many blacks may expect white caregivers to hold negative and preconceived ideas. Giving a rationale for questions asked will help alleviate this perception (D'Avanzo et al, 2001; Vontress & Epp, 1997).*
- Use a family-centered approach when working with Latino, Asian-American, African-American, and Native-American clients. **EBN:** *Latinos may perceive family as a source of support, solver of problems, and source of pride. Asian Americans may regard the family as the primary decision maker and influence on individual family members (D'Avanzo et al, 2001). Native-American families may be extended structures that could exert powerful influences over functioning (Seideman et al, 1996). Family therapy is important in addressing the needs of Hispanic families with adolescent substance abusers (Santisteban et al, 2006).*
- When working with Asian-American clients, provide opportunities for the family to save face. **EBN:** *This will allow the family to not have to own the shame of the alcohol problem. Asian-American families may avoid situations that bring shame on the family unit (Chen, 2001; D'Avanzo et al, 2001).*
- Some less-acculturated Latino families may be unwilling to discuss family issues with healthcare providers until they perceive a close personal relationship with the provider. **EBN:** *Some Latino families may believe that personal problems should be kept private and may not respond to the healthcare provider until there is an established personal relationship (Galanti, 2003).*
- Use family strengthening interventions such as behavioral parent training, family skills training, in-home family support, brief family therapy, and family education when working with culturally diverse families. **EB:** *Comprehensive prevention programs combining multiple approaches produced large positive effects when used with different cultural groups and with different ages of children (Kumpfer, Alvarado & Whiteside, 2003). Increased alcohol use is strongly related to increased separation from family and increased family conflict in both Mexican-American and African-American adolescents (Bray et al, 2001).*
- Work with families in a way that incorporates cultural elements. **EB:** *Activities such as tundra walks and time with elders supported in treatment were used successfully for substance abuse treatment with Yup'ik and Cup'ik Eskimos (Mills, 2003).*

Home Care

NOTE: In the community setting, alcoholism as cause of dysfunctional family processes must be considered in two categories (1) when the client suffers personally from the illness and (2) when a significant other suffers from the illness, that is, the client is not the active alcoholic but may depend on the alcoholic for caregiving. The following considerations apply to both situations with appropriate adaptation for the circumstances.

- The previous interventions may be adapted for home care use.

F

- Identify client and family expectations of the home care nurse and nurse expectations of the client and family by use of a well-defined contract. Be specific and realistic. Adjust the contract only with clear consent and understanding of the client and family. *A well-defined contract supports success in meeting goals and encourages positive family dynamics.*
- Work with family members to support a sense of valued fit on their part; include them in treatment planning and identify the importance of their roles in the client's care. At the same time, encourage their pursuit of positive outside activities that enhance their sense of belonging. **EBN:** *Sense of belonging (valued fit) has been identified as a buffer to depression among both depressed and nondepressed individuals with a family history of alcoholism. A buffering effect was not found for individuals with a family history of drug abuse (Sargent et al, 2002).*
- ▲ Establish well-defined contingency and emergency plans for the care of the client. **EB:** *Safety of the client between visits is a primary goal of the home care nurse (Stanhope & Lancaster, 1996).*
- Request concrete, measurable tasks of the client and family for caregiving and provide concrete, nonjudgmental instruction to the client and family regarding the interactions of alcohol use with medications and the therapeutic regimen. *Clear information, delivered without judgment of the person, may provide the client and family with motivation to modify, if not discontinue, alcohol use.*
- ▲ Observe for abuse of other medications. Notify physician of problems noted. *Cross addiction is a concern. Clients may substitute the use of other psychoactive medications for alcohol or may already be addicted to hypnotics and/or pain medications. The presence of other addictions may raise issues regarding withdrawal and synergistic effects.*
- ▲ If the client is a recovering alcoholic, extreme care must be taken in the use of psychoactive or pain medications. Notify physician if inappropriate medications have been inadvertently ordered. *Addiction to alcohol increases the potential for readdiction, especially if strong pain medications are introduced. In many instances, it is policy to prescribe nothing stronger than extra-strength acetaminophen for recovering alcoholics in need of pain medication. Sleep medications should be avoided.*
- ▲ Refer for medical social work services at the outset of care. *The social worker can help identify, set the structure for, and guide appropriate client/family and client/family/nurse interactions that will promote the plan of care throughout the length of stay.*
- ▲ Provide information regarding available substance use treatment programs and support groups. *A variety of program types are available, from Alcoholics Anonymous (AA) to intensive inpatient treatment, with specialty units available in some areas for older adults.*
- Acknowledge without judging when resolution of alcoholism is not a goal of care. *It is usually not appropriate for terminally ill or hospice clients or their families to change family life patterns. Recognizing this fact nonjudgmentally helps the client or family use remaining energy to complete other end-of-life work.*
- ▲ Refer for psychiatric home healthcare services for client reassurance and implementation of therapeutic regimen. **EBN:** *Psychiatric home care nurses can address issues relating to the client's or family member's alcoholism and its interference with ability to adjust to changes in health status. Behavioral interventions in the home can help the client participate more effectively in the treatment plan (Patusky et al, 1996).*

 Client Family Teaching

- Suggest the client complete a confidential Internet self-screening test for identification of problems and suggestions for treatment if a problem with alcohol is suspected. Many tools are available. *The website www.AlcoholScreening.org helps individuals assess their own alcohol consumption patterns to determine if their drinking is likely harming their health or increasing their risk for future harm. Through education and referral, the site urges those whose drinking is harmful or hazardous to take positive action and informs all adults who consume alcohol about guidelines and caveats for lower risk drinking (Boston University School of Public Health, 2005).*

evolve See the EVOLVE website for World Wide Web resources for client education.

• = Independent;   ▲ = Collaborative;   EBN = Evidence-Based Nursing;   EB = Evidence-Based

REFERENCES

Bailey KA, Baker AL, Webster RA et al: Pilot randomized controlled trial of a brief alcohol intervention group for adolescents, *Drug Alcohol Rev* 23(2):157-166, 2004.

Bartels SJ, Coakley EH, Zubritsky C et al: Improving access to geriatric mental health services: a randomized trial comparing treatment engagement with integrated versus enhanced referral care for depression, anxiety, and at-risk alcohol use, *Am J Psychiatry* 161(8):1455-1462, 2004.

Beullens J, Aertgeerts B: Screening for alcohol abuse and dependence in older people using DSM criteria: a review, *Aging Ment Health* 8(1):76-82, 2004.

Bland R, Darlington Y: The nature and sources of hope: perspectives of family caregivers of people with serious mental illness, *Perspect Psychiatr Care* 38(2):61, 2002.

Boston University School of Public Health: *How much is too much?* www.alcoholscreening.org, accessed January 18, 2005.

Bray JH, Adams GJ, Getz JG et al: Developmental, family, and ethnic influences on adolescent alcohol usage: a growth curve approach, *J Fam Psychol* 15(2):301-314, 2001.

Chen YC: Chinese values, health and nursing, *J Adv Nurs* 36(2):270, 2001.

D'Avanzo CE et al: Developing culturally informed strategies for substance-related interventions. In Naegle MA, D'Avanzo CE, editors: *Addictions and substance abuse: strategies for advanced practice nursing,* St Louis, 2001, Mosby.

Duncan SC, Duncan TE, Stryker LA: Family influences on youth alcohol use: a multiple-sample analysis by ethnicity and gender, *J Ethn Subst Abuse* 2(2):17-33, 2003.

Epstein I: Adventure therapy: a mental health promotion strategy in pediatric oncology, *J Pediatr Oncol Nurs* 21(2):103-110, 2004.

Galanti GA: The Hispanic family and male-female relationships: an overview, *J Transcult Nurs* 14(3):180-185, 2003.

Giger J, Davidhizar R: *Transcultural nursing: assessment and intervention,* ed 4, St. Louis, 2004, Mosby.

Gottfredson DC, Wilson DB: Characteristics of effective school-based substance abuse prevention, *Prev Sci* 4(1):27, 2003.

Griffin KW, Botvin GJ, Nichols TR: Long-term follow-up effects of a school-based drug abuse prevention program on adolescent risky driving, *Prev Sci* 5(3):207-212, 2004.

Hoque A, Dauber S, Samuolis J et al: Treatment techniques and outcomes in multidimensional family therapy for adolescent behaviour problems, *J Fam Psychol* 20(4):535-543, 2006.

Ino A, Hayasida M: Before-discharge intervention method in the treatment of alcohol dependence, *Alcohol Clin Exp Res* 24(3):373, 2000.

Kiefer F, Jahn H, Tarnaske T et al: Comparing and combining naltrexone and acamprosate in relapse prevention of alcoholism: a double-blind, placebo-controlled study, *Arch Gen Psychiatry* 60(1):92-99, 2003.

Kingon YS, O'Sullivan AL: The family as a protective asset in adolescent development, *J Holist Nurs* 19(2):102-121, 2001.

Kumpfer KL, Alvarado R, Whiteside HO: Family-based interventions for substance use and misuse prevention, *Subst Use Misuse* 38(11-13):1759-1787, 2003.

Lintonen T, Ahlstro MS, Metso L: The reliability of self-reported drinking in adolescence, *Alcohol Alcohol* 39(4):362-368, 2004.

Locke TF, Newcomb MD: Adolescent predictors of young adult and adult alcohol involvement and dysphoria in a prospective community sample of women, *Prev Sci* 5(3):151-168, 2004.

Mills PA: Incorporating Yup'ik and Cup'ik Eskimo traditions into behavioral health treatment, *J Psychoactive Drugs* 35(1):85-88, 2003.

Mundt M: Analyzing the costs and benefits of brief intervention, *Alcohol Res Health* 29(1):34-36, 2006.

Orford J, Templeton L, Velleman R et al: Family members of relatives with alcohol, drug and gambling problems: a set of standardized questionnaires for assessing stress, coping and strain, *Addiction* 100(11):1611-1624, 2005.

Patusky KL, Rodning C, Martinez-Kratz M: Clinical lessons in psychiatric home care: a case study approach, *J Home Healthcare Manag* 9:188, 1996.

Reiff-Hekking S, Ockene JK, Hurley TG et al: Brief physician and nurse practitioner-delivered counseling for high-risk drinking. Results at 12-month follow-up, *J Gen Intern Med* 20(1):96-97, 2005.

Rigler SK: Alcoholism in the elderly, *Am Fam Physician* 61(6):1710, 2000.

Santisteban DA, Suarez-Morales L, Robbins MS et al: Brief strategic family therapy: lessons learned in efficacy research and challenges to blending research and practice, *Fam Process* 45(2):259-271, 2006.

Sargent J, Williams RA, Hagerty B et al: Sense of belonging as a buffer against depressive symptoms, *J Am Psychiatr Nurs Assoc* 8(4):120-129, 2002.

Seideman RY, Jacobson S, Primeaux M et al: Assessing American Indian families, *MCN Am J Matern Child Nurs* 21(6):274, 1996.

Serrano R: *Solution focused addictions counseling, acupuncture treatment for substance abuse,* www.holisticwebs.com/solution/sfac4.html, accessed January 18, 2003.

Shahpesandy H, Pristasova J, Janikova Z et al: Alcoholism in the elderly: a study of elderly alcoholics compared with healthy elderly and young alcoholics, *Neuro Endocrinol Lett* 27(5):651-657, 2006.

Simple test for alcoholism proves hit with GPs, *Drugs Alcohol Today* 6(3):11-1, 2006.

Stanhope M, Lancaster J, editors: *Community health nursing: promoting health of aggregates, families, and individuals,* ed 4, St Louis, 1996, Mosby.

Vontress CE, Epp LR: Historical hostility in the African American client: implications for counseling, *J Multicult Counseling Dev* 25:170, 1997.

Warner LA, White HR, Johnson V: Alcohol initiation experiences and family history of alcoholism as predictors of problem-drinking trajectories, *J Stud Alcohol* 68(1):56-65, 2007.

Interrupted Family processes   *Gail B. Ladwig, MSN, CHTP, RN*

NANDA   Definition

Change in family relationships and/or functioning

Defining Characteristics

Changes in assigned tasks; changes in availability for affective responsiveness; changes in availability for emotional support; changes in communication patterns; changes in effectiveness in completing assigned tasks; changes in expressions of conflict with community resources; changes in expressions of

• = Independent;   ▲ = Collaborative;   EBN = Evidence-Based Nursing;   EB = Evidence-Based

isolation from community resources; changes in expressions of conflict within family; changes in intimacy; changes in mutual support; changes in patterns; changes in participation in problem solving; changes in participation in decision making; changes in power alliances; changes in rituals; changes in satisfaction with family; changes in somatic complaints; changes in stress-reduction behaviors

Related Factors (r/t)

Developmental crises; developmental transition; family roles shift; interaction with community; modification in family finances; modification in family social status; power shift of family members; shift in health status of a family member; situation transition; situational crises

NOC   Outcomes (Nursing Outcomes Classification)

Suggested NOC Outcomes

Family Coping, Family Social Climate, Family Functioning, Family Normalization, Parenting Performance, Psychosocial Adjustment: Life Change, Role Performance

---

Example NOC Outcome with Indicators

Family Coping as evidenced by the following indicators: Confronts/manages family problems/Involves family members in decision making (Rate the outcome and indicators of **Family Coping:** 1 = never demonstrated, 2 = rarely demonstrated, 3 = sometimes demonstrated, 4 = often demonstrated, 5 = consistently demonstrated [see Section I].)

Client Outcomes

Family/Client Will (Specify Time Frame):

- Express feelings (family)
- Identify ways to cope effectively and use appropriate support systems (family)
- Treat impaired family member as normally as possible to avoid overdependence (family)
- Meet physical, psychosocial, and spiritual needs of members or seek appropriate assistance (family)
- Demonstrate knowledge of illness or injury, treatment modalities, and prognosis (family)
- Participate in the development of the plan of care to the best of ability (significant person)

NIC   Interventions (Nursing Interventions Classification)

Suggested NIC Interventions

Family Integrity Promotion, Family Process Maintenance, Family Therapy, Normalization Promotion, Role Enhancement, Support System Enhancement

---

Example NIC Activities—Family Integrity Promotion

Collaborate with family in problem solving and decision making; Counsel family members on additional effective coping skills for their own use

---

Nursing Interventions and *Rationales*

Refer to the care plan **Readiness for enhanced Family processes** for additional interventions.
- Establish rapport with families by providing accurate communication. **EBN:** *Family care can be improved by focusing on building rapport and communicating problems and concerns between families and health professionals (Rose, Mallinson & Walton-Moss, 2004).*
- Acknowledge the range of emotions and feelings that may be experienced when the health status of a family member changes; counsel family members that it is normal to be angry and afraid. **EBN:** *The experiences of the family members after death of clients in the Intensive Care Unit resembled a vortex: a downward spiral of prognoses, difficult decisions, feelings of inadequacy, and eventual loss despite the members' best efforts, and perhaps no goodbyes (Kirchhoff et al, 2002).*

- Encourage family members to list their personal strengths. *A list of strengths provides information that family members can refer to for positive feedback.*
- Involve family members in the care, information, and client teaching sessions with the client. *Family-focused activities can help families cope better with the hospital experience (Worthington, 1995).*
- Encourage family to visit the client; adjust visiting hours to accommodate family's schedule (e.g., schedule around work, school, babysitting needs). Assist with sleeping arrangements if family is spending the night; provide a place to lie down, pillows, and blankets.
- Allow and encourage family to assist in the client's care. Allow family presence during invasive procedures and resuscitation. **EBN:** *Families in critical care units play a significant role in the client's care (Johnson, 2004).*
- ▲ Consider use of video home training as a method of early support in problems of family life control. **EBN:** *Video home training helped the families gain better control over their family life (Haggman-Laitila et al, 2003).*

Pediatric

- ▲ Carefully assess potential for reunifying children placed in foster care with their birth parents. **EB:** *Reunifying children placed in foster care with their birth parents is a primary goal of the child welfare system (Wulczyn, 2004).*
- Allow and encourage family to assist in the client's care. **EBN:** *Parents need to be able to negotiate with health staff what this participation will involve and negotiate new roles for themselves in sharing care of their sick child. Parents should be involved in the decision-making process (Corlett & Twycross, 2006).*
- ▲ Refer children and mothers exposed to violence in the home to theraplay: an attachment-based intervention that uses the four core elements of nurturing, engagement, structure, and challenge in interactions between mother and her child. **EBN:** *This family connections program improves the quality of life for mothers and children during a short shelter stay;. it has potential to improve quality of life long term (Bennett, Shriner & Ryan, 2006)*

Geriatric

- Encourage family members to be involved in the care of relatives who are in residential care settings. **EB:** *Family involvement in residential long-term care is important (Gaugler et al, 2004). If family satisfaction is to be achieved, family presence in a nursing home needs to give caregivers a sense of positive involvement and influence over the care of their relative (Tornatore & Grant, 2004).*
- Support group problem solving among family members and include the older member. *Problem solving is an effective method to manage stressors for family members of all ages.*
- ▲ Refer family for counseling with a psychotherapist who is knowledgeable about gerontology.
- Refer to care plan for **Readiness for enhanced Family processes** for additional interventions.

Multicultural

- Refer to the care plan **Readiness for enhanced Family process** for additional interventions.

Home Care

- The nursing interventions described in the care plan for **Compromised family Coping** should be used in the home environment with adaptations as necessary.
- Request help from the family when communicating with clients with advanced stages of cancer who are no longer able to communicate their illness and symptom needs. **EBN:** *Next of kin play an integral role in fostering optimal quality of life in symptomatic clients who are coping with cancer in the home setting (Lobchuk & Degner, 2002).*

Client/Family Teaching

- Refer to Client/Family Teaching in **Compromised family Coping** and **Readiness for enhanced family Coping** for suggestions that may be used with minor adaptations.

 See the EVOLVE website for World Wide Web resources for client education.

• = Independent;   ▲ = Collaborative;   EBN = Evidence-Based Nursing;   EB = Evidence-Based

REFERENCES

Bennett L, Shiner S, Ryan S: Using Theraplay in shelter setting with mothers and children who have experienced violence in the home, *J Psychosoc Nurs Ment Health Serv* 44(10):38-48, 2006.

Corlett J, Twycross A: Negotiation of parental roles within family-centred care: a review of the research, *J Clin Nurs* 15(10):1308-1316, 2006.

Gaugler JE, Anderson KA, Zarit SH et al: Family involvement in nursing homes: effects on stress and well-being, *Aging Ment Health* 8(1):65-75, 2004.

Haggman-Laitila A, Pietila AM, Friis L et al: Video home training as a method of supporting family life control, *J Clin Nurs* 12(1):93, 2003.

Johnson P: Reclaiming the everyday world: how long-term ventilated patients in critical care seek to gain aspects of power and control over their environment, *Intens Crit Care Nurs* 20(4):190-199, 2004.

Kirchhoff KT, Walker L, Hutton A et al: The vortex: families' experiences with death in the intensive care unit, *Am J Crit Care* 11(3):200, 2002.

Lobchuk MM, Degner LF: Patients with cancer and next-of-kin response comparability on physical and psychological symptom well-being: trends and measurement issues, *Cancer Nurs* 25(5):358, 2002.

Rose LE: Mallinson RK, Walton-Moss B: Barriers to family care in psychiatric settings, *J Nurs Sch* 36(1):39-47, 2004.

Tornatore JB, Grant LA: Family caregiver satisfaction with the nursing home after placement of a relative with dementia, *J Gerontol B Psychol Sci Soc Sci* 59(2):S80-S88, 2004.

Worthington R: Effective transitions for families: life beyond the hospital, *Pediatr Nurs* 21:8, 1995.

Wulczyn F: Family reunification, *Future Child* 14(1):94-113, 2004.

F

Readiness for enhanced Family processes   *Gail B. Ladwig, MSN, CHTP, RN*

NANDA   Definition

A pattern of family functioning that is sufficient to support the well-being of family members and can be strengthened.

Defining Characteristics

Activities support the growth of family members; activities support the safety of family members; balance exists between autonomy and cohesiveness; boundaries of family members are maintained; communication is adequate; energy level of family supports activities of daily living; expresses willingness to enhance family dynamics; family adapts to change; family functioning meets needs of family members; family resilience is evident; family roles are appropriate for developmental stages; family roles are flexible for developmental stages; family tasks are accomplished; interdependent with community; relationships are generally positive; respect for family members is evident

NOC   Outcomes (Nursing Outcomes Classification)

Suggested NOC Outcomes

Family Coping, Family Physical Environment, Health Orientation, Health-Promoting Behavior, Health-Seeking Behavior, Leisure Participation, Parent-Infant Attachment, Parenting Performance, Psychosocial Adjustment: Life Change, Risk Control, Role Performance, Social Support, Spiritual Health

Example NOC Outcome with Indicators
Family Coping as evidenced by the following indicators: Confronts/manages family problems/Involves family members in decision making (Rate the outcome and indicators of **Family Coping:** 1 = never demonstrated, 2 = rarely demonstrated, 3 = sometimes demonstrated, 4 = often demonstrated, 5 = consistently demonstrated [see Section I].)

Client Outcomes

Family/Client Will (Specify Time Frame):

• Identify ways to cope effectively and use appropriate support systems (family)
• Meet physical, psychosocial, and spiritual needs of members or seek appropriate assistance (family)

• = Independent;   ▲ = Collaborative;   EBN = Evidence-Based Nursing;   EB = Evidence-Based

- Demonstrate knowledge of potential environmental, lifestyle, and genetic risks to health and use appropriate measures to decrease possibility of risk (family)
- Focus on wellness, disease prevention, and maintenance (family and individual)
- Seek balance among exercise, work, leisure, rest, and nutrition (family and individual)

NIC   Interventions (Nursing Interventions Classification)

Suggested NIC Interventions

Active Listening, Anticipatory Guidance, Attachment Promotion, Coping Enhancement, Decision-Making Support, Environmental Management: Attachment Process, Exercise Promotion, Family Integrity Promotion, Family Involvement Promotion, Family Mobilization, Family Process Maintenance, Health Screening, Mutual Goal Setting, Parent Education: Adolescent, Childrearing Family, Risk Identification, Role Enhancement

Example NIC Activities—Risk Identification
Determine community support systems; Determine presence and quality of family support

Nursing Interventions and *Rationales*

- Assess the family's stress level and coping abilities during the initial nursing assessment. **EBN:** *Nurses need to assess the family's baseline stress level and effectiveness of coping responses and assist the family as a whole, as well as individual members, in meeting their varying needs (Rutledge, Donaldson & Pravikoff, 2000).*
- Consider the use of family theory as a framework to help guide interventions (e.g., family stress theory, role theory, social exchange theory). **EBN:** *A family assessment tool is an effective way of appraising families and addressing suffering (Hogan & Logan, 2004).*
- Use family-centered care and role modeling for holistic care of families. **EBN:** *Specific techniques of role modeling and reflective practice are suggested as effective approaches to teach family sensitive care in clinical settings in which families are part of the care environment (Tomlinson et al, 2002).*
- Discuss with family members how they have handled previous crises. *Such a discussion gives the nurse clues and information that can help in the plan of care (Coleman & Taylor, 1995).*
- Support family empowerment; strength, and resourcefulness. **EBN:** *The family can empower itself, but it is also possible to empower the family from the outside, such as in child health clinics (Pilkonen & Hakulinen, 2002).*
- Spend time with family members; allow them to verbalize their feelings. **EBN:** *Interactions help the client and family feel relieved and allow anxiety levels to decrease. Critical care nurses can provide support for families after the death of a loved one (Coolican & Politoski, 1994).*
- Encourage family members to find meaning in a serious illness such as cancer. **EBN:** *The positive dimensions of survivorship in meaning of the illness and family quality of life were seen for clients and family members with cancer (Mellon, 2002).*
- ▲ Provide family-centered care to explore and use all available resources appropriate for the situation (e.g., counseling, social services, self-help groups, pastoral care). **EBN:** *Family-centered care has become a cornerstone of pediatric practice (Shields, Pratt & Hunter, 2006).*
- ▲ Consider referral for walk-in family therapy. **EB:** *This therapy modality is aimed at providing an immediately accessible, affordable, nonstigmatizing, single-session–focused resource (Miller & Slive, 2004).*

Pediatric

- Provide a parenting class series based on individual and couple changes in meaning and identity, roles, and relationships and interaction during the transition to parenthood. Address mother and father roles, infant communication abilities, and patterns of the first 3 months of life in a mutually enjoyable, possibility focused manner. **EBN:** *Interventions that enhance mutual parent-child interaction through increased sensitivity to cues and responsiveness to infant needs or signals are important avenues for facilitating secure attachment, father and mother involvement, optimal development, and prevention of child abuse and neglect (Bryan, 2000).*

• = Independent;   ▲ = Collaborative;   EBN = Evidence-Based Nursing;   EB = Evidence-Based

- Encourage families with adolescents to have family meals. *Eating family meals may enhance the health and well-being of adolescents. Public education on the benefits of family mealtime is recommended (Eisenberg et al, 2004).*
▲ Consider the use of adventure therapy for adolescents with cancer. **EBN:** *This mental health promotion is considered a strategy to promote health (Epstein, 2004).*

Geriatric

- Carefully listen to residents and family members in the long-term care facility. **EBN:** *Nurses can improve life and dignity for residents by listening to residents and family members (Iwasiw et al, 2003).*
- Support caregivers' awareness of the positive effects of their contribution to the well-being of parents. **EBN:** *Client-focused and family-focused care requires attention to design. One successful model is The Caring Model, which demonstrates the difference between direct caregivers and indirect caregivers within the family (Dossey, Keegan & Guzzetta, 2005).*
- Teach family members about the impact of developmental events (e.g., retirement, death, change in health status, and household composition). *Knowledge regarding normative developmental challenges of aging can reduce the stress such challenges place on families.*
- Encourage social networks; social integration; and social engagement with friends, children, and relatives of the elderly. **EB:** *A longitudinal study indicated that few social ties, poor integration, and social disengagement are risk factors for cognitive decline among community-dwelling elderly persons (Zunzunegui, 2003).*

Multicultural

- Assess for the influence of cultural beliefs, norms, and values on the family's perceptions of normal functioning. **EBN:** *What the family considers normal and abnormal family functioning may be based on cultural perceptions (Giger & Davidhizar, 2004). Latino families who express a higher degree of familism are characterized by positive interpersonal familial relationships, high family unity, social support, interdependence in the completion of daily activities, and close proximity with extended family members (Romero et al, 2004).* **EBN:** *Spiritual beliefs, the role of prayer, and the role of family in caregiving were predominant aspects in the end-of-life experience investigated in a sample of Mexican Americans (Gelfand et al, 2001).* **EBN:** *Depending on the culture, a decision about consent to treatment, receiving care or teaching, or whether to follow instructions may need to be made individually (Haddad, 2001).* **EBN:** *On the other hand, a client may not feel comfortable in making a healthcare decision without the spouse or family. In some situations the client may defer to the spouse for decision making (Davidhizar & Shearer, 2002).* **EBN:** *In still other situations, another individual or group such as a deacon or a church member may need to be involved (Schwartz, 2002).*
- Identify and acknowledge the stresses unique to racial/ethnic families. **EBN:** *Women in Turkey perceive themselves as wives sharing everything within the family; their decision-making rate was lower than that of men, except for selecting clothes (Erci, 2003). Access to care, financial means, and mistrust of the healthcare system are significant obstacles for low-income southern Black American women (Appel, Giger & Davidhizar, 2005).*
- Assess and support spiritual needs of families. **EBN:** *A study of African-American mothers demonstrated that spirituality helped them cope during the time of their infants' hospitalization for a serious illness (Wilson & Miles 2001).*
- With the client's consent, facilitate a group meeting for family members to discuss how the family is functioning. **EBN:** *A family meeting opens communication and lets each family member know it is okay to talk about what is happening (Rivera-Andino & Lopez, 2000). Focus groups with African Americans found that families could benefit from help with placement of family members in nursing homes and hospitals and the process of family decision making (Turner et al, 2004).*
- Facilitate modeling and role playing for the client and family regarding healthy ways to start a discussion about the client's prognosis. **EBN:** *It is helpful for families and the client to practice communication skills in a safe environment before trying them in a real-life situation (Rivera-Andino & Lopez, 2000).*
- Encourage family mealtimes. **EB:** *Frequency of family meals was inversely associated with tobacco, alcohol, and marijuana use; low grade point average; depressive symptoms; and suicide involvement of diverse adolescents (Eisenberg et al, 2004).*

Home Care

- The previous nursing interventions should be used in the home environment with adaptations as necessary.
- Provide a videophone network for peer support for frail elderly people living at home. **EB:** *A videophone network appears to be helpful for elderly people in their peer support relationships. It supports and improves the functional independence of frail elderly people at home (Ezumi et al, 2003).*
- Encourage families to help women caring for husbands with chronic obstructive pulmonary disease by providing respite care so the women may have recreation time. **EBN:** *Women caregivers of husbands with chronic obstructive pulmonary disease were dissatisfied with their lack of recreation as well as support from friends, families, and healthcare providers (Bergs, 2002).*

Client/Family Teaching

- Refer to Client/Family Teaching in **Readiness for enhanced family Coping** for suggestions that may be used with minor adaptations.

 See the EVOLVE website for World Wide Web resources for client education.

REFERENCES

Appel SJ, Giger JN, Davidhizar RE: Opportunity cost: the impact of contextual risk factors on the cardiovascular health of low-income rural southern African American women, *J Cardiovasc Nurs* 20:315-324, 2005.

Bergs D: "The hidden client"—women caring for husbands with COPD: their experience of quality of life, *J Clin Nurs* 11(5):613, 2002.

Bryan AA: Enhancing parent-child interaction with a prenatal couple intervention, *MCN Am J Matern Child Nurs* 25(3):139, 2000.

Coleman W, Taylor E: Family-focused pediatrics: issues, challenges, and clinical methods, *Pediatr Clin North Am* 42(1):119, 1995.

Coolican MB, Politoski G: Donor family programs, *Crit Care Nurs Clin North Am* 6(3):613, 1994.

Davidhizar R, Shearer R: Helping children cope with public disasters, *Am J Nurs* 102(3):26-33, 2002.

Dossey B, Keegan L, Guzzetta C: *Holistic nursing*, ed 4, Boston, 2005, Jones & Bartlett.

Eisenberg ME, Olson RE, Neumark-Sztainer D et al: Correlations between family meals and psychosocial well-being among adolescents, *Arch Pediatr Adolesc Med* 158(8):792-796, 2004.

Epstein I: Adventure therapy: a mental health promotion strategy in pediatric oncology, *J Pediatr Oncol Nurs* 21(2):103-110, 2004.

Erci B: Women's efficiency in decision making and their perception of their status in the family, *Public Health Nurs* 20(1):65, 2003.

Ezumi H, Ochiai N, Oda M et al: Peer support via video-telephony among frail elderly people living at home, *J Telemed Telecare* 9(1):30-34, 2003.

Gelfand D, Balcazar H, Parzuchowski J et al: Mexicans and care for the terminally ill: family, hospice and the church, *Am J Hospice Palliat Care* 18(6):391-396, 2001.

Giger JN, Davidhizar RE: *Transcultural nursing: assessment & intervention*, ed 4, St Louis, 2004, Mosby.

Haddad A: Ethics in action. A competent, elderly Chinese woman who needs immediate treatment says she can't give consent because she must wait for her family to arrive to give approval, *RN* 64(3):21-24, 2001.

Hogan DL, Logan J: The Ottawa Model of Research Use: a guide to clinical innovation in the NICU, *Clin Nurse Spec* 18(5):255-261, 2004.

Iwasiw C, Goldenberg D, Bol N et al: Resident and family perspectives: the first year in a long-term care facility, *J Gerontol Nurs* 29(1):45, 2003.

Mellon S: Comparisons between cancer survivors and family members on meaning of the illness and family quality of life, *Oncol Nurs Forum* 29(7):1117, 2002.

Miller JK, Slive A: Breaking down the barriers to clinical service delivery: walk-in family therapy, *J Marital Fam Ther* 30(1):95-103, 2004.

Pilkonen M, Hakulinen T: An empowerment model for family nursing [in Finnish], *Hoitotiede* 14(5):202, 2002.

Rivera-Andino J, Lopez L: When culture complicates care, *RN* 63(7):47, 2000.

Romero AJ, Robinson TN, Haydel KF et al: Associations among familism, language preference, and education in Mexican-American mothers and their children, *J Dev Behav Pediatr* 25(1):34-40, 2004.

Rutledge DN, Donaldson NE, Pravikoff DS: Caring for families of patients in acute or chronic health care settings: Part I—principles, *Online J Clin Innovat* 3(3):1, 2000.

Schwartz K: Breast cancer and health care beliefs, values, and practices of Amish women, *Diss Abstracts Int* 29(1):31-33, 2002.

Shields L, Pratt J, Hunter J: Family centred care: a review of qualitative studies, *J Clin Nurs* 15(10):1317-1323, 2006.

Tomlinson PS, Thomlinson E, Peden-McAlpine C et al: Clinical innovation for promoting family care in paediatric intensive care: demonstration, role modeling and reflective practice, *J Adv Nurs* 38(2):161, 2002.

Turner WL, Wallace BR, Anderson JR et al: The last mile of the way: understanding caregiving in African American families at the end-of-life, *J Marital Fam Ther* 30(4):427-438, 2004.

Wilson SM, Miles MS: Spirituality in African-American mothers coping with a seriously ill infant, *J Soc Pediatr Nurs* 6(3):116-122, 2001.

Zunzunegui MV, Alvarado BE, Del Ser T et al: Social networks, social integration, and social engagement determine cognitive decline in community-dwelling Spanish older adults, *Gerontol B Psychol Sci Soc Sci* 58(2):S93, 2003.

F

Fatigue Barbara Given, PhD, FAAN, RN, and Paula Sherwood, PhD, RN, CNRN *evolve*

NANDA Definition

An overwhelming, sustained sense of exhaustion and decreased capacity for physical and mental work at usual level.

Defining Characteristics

Compromised concentration; compromised libido; decreased performance; disinterest in surroundings; drowsy; feelings of guilt for not keeping up with responsibilities; inability to maintain usual level of physical activity; inability to maintain usual routines; inability to restore energy even after sleep; increase in physical complaints; increase in rest requirements; introspection; lack of energy; lethargic; listless; perceived need for additional energy to accomplish routine tasks; tired; verbalization of an unremitting lack of energy; verbalization of an overwhelming lack of energy

Related Factors (r/t)

Psychological

Anxiety; boring lifestyle; depression

Physiological

Anemia; disease states; increased physical exertion; malnutrition; poor physical condition; pregnancy; sleep deprivation

Environmental

Humidity; lights; noise; temperature

Situational

Negative life events; occupation

NOC Outcomes (Nursing Outcomes Classification)

Suggested NOC Outcomes

Concentration, Endurance, Energy Conservation, Nutritional Status, Energy, Vitality

Example NOC Outcome with Indicators
Endurance as evidenced by the following indicators: Performance of usual routine/Activity/Rested appearance/Blood oxygen level/Muscle endurance (Rate the outcome and indicators of **Endurance:** 1 = severely compromised, 2 = substantially compromised, 3 = moderately compromised, 4 = mildly compromised, 5 = not compromised [see Section I].)

Client Outcomes

Client Will (Specify Time Frame):

- Identify potential factors that aggravate and relieve fatigue
- Describe ways to assess and track patterns of fatigue
- Describe ways in which fatigue affects the ability to accomplish goals
- Verbalize increased energy and improved well-being
- Explain energy conservation plan to offset fatigue
- Explain energy restoration plan to offset fatigue

NIC Interventions (Nursing Interventions Classification)

Suggested NIC Intervention

Energy Management (including conservation and restoration)

• = Independent; ▲ = Collaborative; EBN = Evidence-Based Nursing; EB = Evidence-Based

Example NIC Activities—Energy Management
Assess patient's physiologic status for deficits resulting in fatigue within the context of age and development; Determine patient/significant other's perception of causes of fatigue

Nursing Interventions and *Rationales*

- Assess severity of fatigue on a scale of 0 to 10 (average fatigue, worst and best levels); assess frequency of fatigue (number of days per week and time of day), activities and symptoms associated with increased fatigue (e.g., pain), ability to perform ADLs and instrumental ADLs, interference with social and role function, times of increased energy, ability to concentrate, mood, and usual pattern of activity. Consider use of an instrument such as the Profile of Mood State Short Form Fatigue Subscale, the Multidimensional Assessment of Fatigue, the Lee Fatigue Scale, the Multidimensional Fatigue Inventory, the HIV-Related Fatigue Scale, the Brief Fatigue Inventory, or the Dutch Fatigue Scale to assess fatigue accurately. *These assessments have all been shown to have good internal reliability. The Profile of Mood State Short Form Fatigue Scale was the strongest performer in one study (Meek et al, 2000).* **EBN:** *The Dutch Fatigue Scale, which is based on NANDA-I defining characteristics, is a reliable and valid measurement tool for assessment of fatigue (Tiesinga et al, 2001). The HIV-Related Fatigue EBN Scale is valuable for measuring fatigue in HIV-positive clients (Barroso & Lynn, 2002). The Revised Schwartz Cancer Fatigue Scale and the M.D. Anderson Symptom Inventory are valuable for assessing fatigue in clients with cancer (Cleeland et al, 2000; Schwartz & Meek, 1999).*
- Evaluate adequacy of nutrition and sleep patterns (napping throughout the day, inability to fall asleep or stay asleep). Encourage the client to get adequate rest, limit naps (particularly in the late afternoon or evening), use a routine sleep/wake schedule, avoid caffeine in the late afternoon or evening, and eat a well-balanced diet with at least eight glasses of water a day. Refer to **Imbalanced Nutrition: less than body requirements** or **Sleep Deprivation** if appropriate. **EBN:** *A commonly suggested treatment for fatigue is rest, although excessive sleep can aggravate fatigue (Carpenter et al, 2004; Pigeon, Sateia & Ferguson, 2003). Inadequate nutrition can also contribute to fatigue.*
- ▲ Collaborate with the primary care practitioner to identify physiological and/or psychological causes of fatigue that could be treated, such as anemia, pain, electrolyte imbalance (e.g., altered potassium levels), hypothyroidism, depression, or medication effect. **EB:** *The presence of fatigue is associated with biological, psychological, social, and personal factors (Barsevick et al, 2004; Craig & Kakumanu, 2002; Forlenza et al, 2005; Ranjith, 2005). If an etiology for fatigue can be determined, the condition should be treated according to the underlying cause. Depression and anxiety have been significantly correlated with fatigue (Phillips et al, 2004).*
- ▲ Work with the primary care practitioner to determine if the client has chronic fatigue syndrome. *The Centers for Disease Control and Prevention define chronic fatigue syndrome as "Clinically evaluated, unexplained, persistent, or relapsing chronic fatigue (over 6 months' duration) that is of new or definite onset (has not been lifelong); is not the result of ongoing exertion; is not alleviated by rest; and results in substantial reduction in previous levels of occupational, educational, social, or personal activities. In addition, four or more the following symptoms must concurrently be present for over 6 months: impaired memory or concentration, sore throat, tender cervical or axial lymph nodes, muscle pain, multi-joint pain, new headaches, unrefreshing sleep, and postexertion malaise lasting more than 24 hours" (Walker, 1999).*
- Encourage the client to express feelings about fatigue, including potential causes of fatigue, and possible interventions to alleviate fatigue such as setting small, easily achieved short-term goals and developing energy management techniques; use active listening techniques and help identify sources of hope. **EBN and EB:** *Problem solving interventions have been shown to lower the incidence of fatigue (Given et al, 2002; Mathiowetz et al, 2005; Vanage, Gilbertson & Mathiowetz, 2003).*
- Encourage the client to keep a journal of activities, symptoms of fatigue, and feelings, including how fatigue affects the client's normal activities and roles. **EBN:** *The journal can increase the client's awareness of symptoms and sense of control and facilitate communication with healthcare practitioners (Schumacher et al, 2002).*

• = Independent;   ▲ = Collaborative;   EBN = Evidence-Based Nursing;   EB = Evidence-Based

- Help the client identify sources of support and essential and nonessential tasks to determine which tasks can be delegated to whom. Give the client permission to limit social and role demands if needed (e.g., switch to part-time employment, hire cleaning service). **EBN:** *The nurse can help the client problem solve to decrease the impact of fatigue on daily activities (Given et al, 2002).*
▲ Collaborate with the primary care practitioner regarding the appropriateness of referrals to physical therapy for carefully monitored aerobic exercise program and possible physical aids, such as a walker or cane. **EBN:** *Aerobic exercise and physical therapy can reduce fatigue in some cancer clients (Conn et al, 2006; Stone, 2002).* **EB:** *An exercise program for clients receiving chemotherapy or radiation treatments for breast cancer helped improve levels of fatigue (Mock et al, 2005). An exercise program can also be helpful to the client with other medical conditions, such as cardiac disease (Gary et al, 2004; Puetz, Beasman & O'Connor, 2006).* **EB:** *Supervised aerobic exercise training has beneficial effects on physical capacity and fibromyalgia symptoms (Busch et al, 2002).*
- Clients may desire multiple strategies to relieve fatigue rather than one single intervention, particularly when there are multiple potential etiologies present. **EB:** *Participants often used multiple strategies to alleviate their fatigue, possibly because of their tendency to attribute it to multiple causes (Seigal, Brown-Bradley & Lekas, 2004).*
▲ Refer the client to diagnosis-appropriate support groups such as National Chronic Fatigue Syndrome Association, Multiple Sclerosis Association, or cancer fatigue websites such as the Oncology Nurses Association *(www.ons.org).* **EB:** *Support groups can help clients legitimize their symptoms and cope with the frequent depression that accompanies fatigue (Friedberg, Leung & Quick, 2005).*
▲ For a cardiac client, recognize that fatigue is common after a myocardial infarction (Lee et al, 2000). Refer to cardiac rehabilitation for carefully prescribed and monitored exercise program. **EBN:** *Carefully monitored exercise is thought to decrease symptoms of fatigue in cardiac clients (Gary et al, 2004).*
- For fatigue associated with multiple sclerosis, encourage energy conservation, "recharging efforts," and excellent self-care; consider use of a cooling suit because fatigue increases in a warm environment. **EBN:** *Use of a cooling suit by individuals with multiple sclerosis may decrease their sense of fatigue (Flensner & Lindencrona, 2002).*
▲ Consider referring for cognitive therapy to help deal with symptoms of fatigue and help change negative thought patterns. **EB:** *Cognitive behavior therapy significantly benefits physical functioning in adult outpatients with chronic fatigue syndrome (Price & Couper, 2000).*
- If fatigue is associated with cancer or cancer-related treatment, assess for other symptoms that may enhance fatigue (e.g., pain or depression). **EBN:** *Clients with cancer who reported both pain and fatigue reported three times as many other symptoms as clients who reported neither pain nor fatigue; fatigue was linked to the presence of pain, multiple comorbid conditions, and site of cancer (Given et al, 2001).*
▲ Collaborate with primary care practitioners to identify attentional fatigue, which may manifest itself as the inability to direct attention necessary to perform usual activities. **EBN:** *Reduced performance in cognitive function was observed before treatment and found to persist over time in older women newly diagnosed with breast cancer (Cimprich & Ronis, 2003).*

Geriatric

- Review comorbid conditions that may contribute to fatigue, such as congestive heart failure, arthritis, and cancer.
- Identify recent losses; monitor for depression as a possible contributing factor to fatigue. **EBN:** *There is a high correlation between depression and fatigue (Suguhara et al, 2004).*
▲ Review medications for side effects. *Certain medications (e.g., antihistamines, pain medications, anticonvulsants, chemotherapeutic agents) may cause fatigue, particularly in the elderly.*

Home Care

- The above interventions may be adapted for home care use.
- Assess the client's history and current patterns of fatigue as they relate to the home environment and environmental and behavioral triggers of increased fatigue. **EBN and EB:** *Fatigue may be*

• = Independent; ▲ = Collaborative; EBN = Evidence-Based Nursing; EB = Evidence-Based

more pronounced in specific settings for physical, environmental (e.g., stairs required to reach bathroom, patterns of movement around home, cleaning activities that require high energy), or psychological (e.g., rooms associated with loss of loved ones) reasons (Gitlin et al, 2006; Suguhara et al, 2004).

▲ Refer to occupational and/or physical therapy if substantial intervention is needed to assist the client in adapting to home and daily patterns. **EB:** *Interventions in the elderly led by occupational and physical therapists have been associated with less difficulty in ADLs and instrumental ADLs, which may lead to lower levels of fatigue (Gitlin et al, 2006).*

• For clients receiving chemotherapy, intervene to:
  ■ Relieve symptom distress (negative mood, nausea, difficulty sleeping)
  ■ Encourage as much physical activity as possible
  ■ Support a positive attitude for the future
  ■ Support adequate recovery time between treatments

  EBN: *The above factors have been identified as contributing to fatigue, particularly during early stages of chemotherapy (Berger & Walker, 2001).*

▲ Refer cancer clients to a community-based pain and fatigue management program, such as the I Feel Better program, if available. **EB:** *A program such as I Feel Better was received with enthusiasm and rapid enrollment by cancer clients (Grant et al, 2000).*

• Teach the client and family the importance of and methods for setting priorities for activities, especially those with high energy demand (e.g., home or family events). Instruct in realistic expectations and behavioral pacing. **EBN:** *The client and/or family may assume a more rapid rate of energy recovery than actually occurs. Assistance may be needed to ensure accuracy of expectations for the client. Unrealistic expectations provoke guilt feelings in the client, leading to efforts that can exceed the client's energy capacity (Patusky, 2002).*

• Assess effect of fatigue on the client's relatedness; recognize that the client's fatigue affects the whole family. Initiate the following interventions:
  ■ Avoid dismissing reports of fatigue; validate the client's experience and foster hope for eventual treatment, if not resolution, of the fatigue.
  ■ Identify with the client ways in which he or she continues to be a valued part of his or her social environment.
  ■ Identify with the client ways in which he or she continues to participate in equitable exchange with others.
  ■ Encourage the client to maintain regular family routines (e.g., meals, sleep patterns) as much as possible.
  ■ Initiate cognitive restructuring to refute the client's guilt-producing and negative thought patterns.
  ■ Assess and intervene with family's and friends' contributions to guilt-inducing self-talk.
  ■ Work with the client to inoculate against the negative thinking of others.
  ■ Explore family life and demands to identify accommodations.
  ■ Support the client's efforts at limit setting on the demands of others.
  ■ Assist the client to move toward a state of parallelism by working to identify and relieve sources of physical or emotional discomfort. Degree of involvement, limited by fatigue, need not be changed.

  EBN: *Based on reports of fatigued women, the above interventions have been suggested as addressing problem areas. Parallelism is a state of comfortable noninvolvement and was described by some fatigued women as achievable and relatively positive state, given their fatigue (Patusky, 2002). Closeness and acceptance in relationships may decrease the psychological burden and modify the fatigue of chemotherapy recipients (Berger & Walker, 2001).*

▲ Refer for family therapy in the event the client's fatigue interferes with normal family functioning. **EBN:** *Family therapy may be necessary to address underlying problems that may be magnified by the influence of fatigue (Patusky, 2002).*

▲ If fatigue has affected the client's ability to participate in relationships effectively, refer for psychiatric home healthcare services for client reassurance and implementation of therapeutic regimen. **EBN:** *Psychiatric home care nurses can address issues relating to the client's ability to adjust to changes in health status. Behavioral interventions in the home can help the client participate more effectively in the treatment plan (Patusky, 2002).*

F

Client/Family Teaching

- Help client to reframe cognitively; share information about fatigue and how to live with it, including need for positive self-talk. **EBN:** *Cognitive behavioral approaches to managing fatigue enhance the client's sense of control over the symptom (Given et al, 2001).*
- Teach strategies for energy conservation (e.g., sitting instead of standing during showering, storing items at waist level). **EB:** *Energy conservation strategies can decrease the amount of energy used (Vanage, Gilbertson & Mathiowetz, 2003).*
- Teach the client to carry a pocket calendar, make lists of required activities, and post reminders around the house. **EBN:** *Fatigue is often associated with memory loss and sometimes difficulty thinking. Fatigue can also result in the inability to direct attention to a certain task, such as cooking or paying bills (i.e., attentional fatigue) (Cimprich & Ronis, 2003).*
- Teach the importance of following a healthy lifestyle with adequate nutrition fluids and rest, pain relief, insomnia correction, and appropriate exercise to decrease fatigue (i.e., energy restoration).
- See **Depression** care plan if appropriate. **EB:** *Depression is correlated with increased fatigue (Phillips et al, 2004).*

evolve See the EVOLVE website for World Wide Web resources for client education.

REFERENCES

Barroso J, Lynn MR: Psychometric properties of the HIV-Related Fatigue Scale, *J Assoc Nurses AIDS Care* 13(1):66, 2002.

Barsevick A, Dudley W, Beck S et al: A randomized clinical trial of energy conservation for patients with cancer-related fatigue, *Cancer* 100(6):1302, 2004.

Berger AM, Walker SN: An explanatory model of fatigue in women receiving adjuvant breast cancer chemotherapy, *Nurs Res* 50:42, 2001.

Busch A, Schachter CL, Peloso PM et al: Exercise for treating fibromyalgia syndrome, *Cochrane Database Syst Rev* (3):CD003786, 2002.

Carpenter J, Elan J, Ridner S et al: Sleep, fatigue, and depressive symptoms in breast cancer survivors and matched healthy women experiencing hot flashes, *Oncol Nurs Forum* 31(3):591, 2004.

Cimprich B, Ronis D: An environmental intervention to restore attention in women with newly diagnosed breast cancer, *Cancer Nurs* 26(4):284, 2003.

Cleeland CS, Mendoza TR, Wang XS et al: Assessing symptom distress in cancer patients: the MD Anderson Symptom Inventory, *Cancer* 89(7):1634, 2000.

Conn V, Hafdahl A, Porock D et al: A meta-analysis of exercise interventions among people treated for cancer, *Support Care Cancer* 14(7):699-712, 2006.

Craig T, Kakumanu S: Chronic fatigue syndrome: evaluation and treatment, *Am Fam Physician* 65(5):1083, 2002.

Flensner G, Lindencrona C: The cooling-suit: case studies of its influence on fatigue among eight individuals with multiple sclerosis, *J Adv Nurs* 37(6):541, 2002.

Forlenza MJ, Hall P, Lichtenstein P et al: Epidemiology of cancer-related fatigue in the Swedish twin registry, *Cancer* 104(9):2022-2031, 2005.

Friedberg F, Leung DW, Quick J: Do support groups help people with chronic fatigue syndrome and fibromyalgia? *J Rheumatol* 32(12):2416-2420, 2005.

Gary RA, Sueta CA, Dougherty M et al: Home-based exercise improves functional performance and quality of life in women with diastolic heart failure, *Heart Lung* 33(4):210-218, 2004.

Gitlin L, Winter L, Dennis M et al: A randomized trial of a multicomponent home intervention to reduce functional difficulties in older adults, *J Am Geriatr Soc* 54:809-816, 2006.

Given B, Given CW, McCorkle R et al: Pain and fatigue management: Results of a nursing randomized clinical trial, *Oncol Nurs Forum* 29(6):949-956, 2002.

Given C, Given B, Azzouz F et al: Predictors of pain and fatigue in the year following diagnosis among elderly cancer patients, *J Pain Symptom Manage* 21(6):456, 2001.

Grant M, Golant M, Rivera L et al: Developing a community program on cancer pain and fatigue, *Cancer Pract* 8(4):187, 2000.

Lee H, Kohlman GC, Lee K et al: Fatigue, mood, and hemodynamic patterns after myocardial infarction, *Appl Nurs Res* 13(2):60, 2000.

Mathiowetz V, Finlayson M, Matuska K et al: Randomized controlled trial of an energy conservation course for persons with multiple sclerosis, *Mult Scler* 11(5):592-601, 2005.

Meek PM, Nail LM, Barsevick A et al: Psychometric testing of fatigue instruments for use with cancer patients, *Nurs Res* 49(4):181, 2000.

Mock V, Frangakis C, Davidson NE et al: Exercise manages fatigue during breast cancer treatment: a randomized controlled trial, *Psychooncology* 14(6):464-477, 2005.

Patusky KL: Relatedness theory as a framework for the treatment of fatigued women, *Arch Psychiatr Nurs* 5:224, 2002.

Phillips K, Sowell R, Rojas M et al: Physiological and psychological correlates of fatigue in HIV disease, *Biol Res Nurs* 6(1):59, 2004.

Pigeon W, Sateia M, Ferguson R: Distinguishing between excessive daytime sleepiness and fatigue: toward improved detection and treatment, *J Psychosom Res* 54(1):61, 2003.

Price JR, Couper J: Cognitive behaviour therapy for adults with chronic fatigue syndrome, *Cochrane Database Syst Rev* (2): CD001027, 2000.

Puetz TW, Beasman KM, O'Connor PJ: The effect of cardiac rehabilitation exercise programs on feelings of energy and fatigue: a meta-analysis of research from 1945 to 2005, *Eur J Cardiovasc Prev Rehabil* 13(6):886-893, 2006.

Ranjith G: Epidemiology of chronic fatigue syndrome, *Occup Med* 55(1):13-19, 2005.

Schumacher A, Wewers D, Heinecke A et al: Fatigue as an important aspect of quality of life in patients with acute myeloid leukemia, *Leuk Res* 26(4):355, 2002.

Schwartz A, Meek P: Additional construct validity of the Schwartz Cancer Fatigue Scale, *J Nurs Meas* 7(1):35, 1999.

Seigel K, Brown-Bradley C, Lekas H: Strategies for coping with fatigue among HIV-positive individuals fifty years and older, *AIDS Patient Care* 18(5):275, 2004.

Stone P: The measurement, causes and effective management of cancer-related fatigue, *Int J Palliative Nurs* 8(3):120, 2002.

Sugahara H, Adamine M, Kondo T et al: Somatic symptoms most often associated with depression in an urban hospital medical setting in Japan, *Psychiatry Res* 128(3):305-311, 2004.

Tiesinga LJ et al: Sensitivity, specificity and usefulness of the Dutch Fatigue Scale, *Nurs Diagn* 12(3):93, 2001.

Vanage S, Gilbertson K, Mathiowetz V: Effects of an energy conservation course on fatigue impact for persons with progressive multiple sclerosis, *Am J Occup Ther* 57(3):315, 2003.

Walker TL: Chronic fatigue syndrome. Do you know what it means, *Am J Nurs* 99(3):70, 1999.

Fear   *Michele Walters, RN, MSN, ARNP*

F

NANDA   Definition

Response to perceived threat that is consciously recognized as a danger.

Defining Characteristics

Report of alarm; apprehension; being scared; increased tension; decreased self-assurance; dread; excitement; jitteriness; panic; terror

Cognitive

Diminished productivity; learning ability; problem-solving ability; identifies object of fear; stimulus believed to be a threat

Behaviors

Attack or avoidance behaviors; impulsiveness; increased alertness; narrowed focus on the source of fear

Physiological

Anorexia; diarrhea; dry mouth; dyspnea; fatigue; increased perspiration, pulse, respiratory rate, systolic blood pressure; muscle tightness; nausea; pallor; pupil dilation; vomiting

Related Factors (r/t)

Innate origin (e.g., sudden noise, height, pain, loss of physical support); innate releasers (neurotransmitters); language barrier; learned response (e.g., conditioning, modeling from or identification with others); phobic stimulus; sensory impairment; separation from support system in potentially stressful situation (e.g., hospitalization, hospital procedures); unfamiliarity with environmental experience(s)

NOC   Outcomes (Nursing Outcomes Classification)

Suggested NOC Outcome

Fear Self-Control

Example NOC Outcome with Indicators

Fear Self-Control as evidenced by the following indicators: Eliminates precursors of fear/Seeks information to reduce fear/Plans coping strategies for fearful situations (Rate the outcome and indicators of **Fear Self-Control:** 1 = never demonstrated, 2 = rarely demonstrated, 3 = sometimes demonstrated, 4 = often demonstrated, 5 = consistently demonstrated [see Section I].)

Client Outcomes

Client Will (Specify Time Frame):

- Verbalize known fears
- State accurate information about the situation

• = Independent;   ▲ = Collaborative;   EBN = Evidence-Based Nursing;   EB = Evidence-Based

- Identify, verbalize, and demonstrate those coping behaviors that reduce own fear
- Report and demonstrate reduced fear

NIC   Interventions (Nursing Interventions Classification)

Suggested NIC Interventions

Anxiety Reduction, Coping Enhancement, Security Enhancement

Example NIC Activities—Anxiety Reduction
Use a calm, reassuring approach; Stay with the patient to promote safety and reduce fear

Nursing Interventions and *Rationales*

- Assess source of fear with the client. **EB:** *The capacity to experience fear is adaptive, enabling rapid and energetic response to imminent threat or danger (Poulton & Menzies, 2002).*
- Assess for a history of anxiety. **EB:** *Participants in a study of stress responses who were found to have a higher level of anxiety reported higher levels of increased fears (Ronen, Rahav & Appel, 2003).*
- Have the client draw the object of his or her fear. **EBN:** *Drawing can be used as an assessment tool to better understand the experience of the client to facilitate better nursing and professional practice in valuing the experience of others (Locsin, Barnard & Matua, 2003).*
- Discuss the situation with the client and help distinguish between real and imagined threats to well-being. **EB:** *Fear activation occurs before conscious cognitive analysis of the stimulus can occur (Mineka & Ohman, 2002).*
- Encourage the client to explore underlying feelings that may be contributing to the fear. *Exploring underlying feelings may help the client confront unresolved conflicts and develop coping abilities (Townsend, 2003).*
- Stay with clients when they express fear; provide verbal and nonverbal (touch and hug with permission and if culturally acceptable) reassurances of safety if safety is within control. **EBN:** *Healing touch may reduce stress, anxiety, and pain and provide a greater sense of well-being (Wardell & Weymouth, 2004).*
- Explore coping skills previously used by the client to deal with fear; reinforce these skills and explore other outlets. **EBN:** *Recounting previous experiences that were perceived by the client as having been dealt with successfully strengthens effective coping and helps eliminate ineffective coping mechanisms (Northouse et al, 2002).*
- Provide backrubs and massage for clients to decrease anxiety. **EB:** *Massage is effective in reducing distress and pain (Taylor et al, 2003).*
- Use TT and HT techniques. **EBN:** *Nurses may offer TT, quiet time, or dialogue when feelings of calmness and relaxation are desired (Kelly et al, 2004).*
- ▲ Refer for cognitive behavior therapy. **EB:** *Individuals treated for fear of flying with cognitive-behavioral therapy can maintain treatment gains in the face of a catastrophic fear-related event (Anderson et al, 2006). Cognitive behavioral therapy has been shown to be effective in reducing symptoms and relapse rates in a wide variety of psychiatric disorders (Beck, 2005).*
- ▲ Animal-assisted therapy can be incorporated into the care of perioperative clients. **EB:** *Animal assisted-therapy may have a useful role in psychiatric and medical therapies in which the therapeutic procedure is inherently fear inducing or has a negative societal perception (Barker, Pandurangi & Best, 2003).*
- Encourage clients to express their fears in narrative form. **EB:** *One of the main ways in which people adjust to threats associated with serious illness is through the use of narrative, which helps make sense of illness (Crossley, 2003).*
- Refer to care plans for **Anxiety** and **Death Anxiety.**

Pediatric

- Use draw-and-tell conversations with children about fear. **EB:** *The draw-and-tell conversation as a child-centered and child-directed approach to data collection provides new insight into how children describe and experience fear (Driessnack, 2006).*

• = Independent;   ▲ = Collaborative;   EBN = Evidence-Based Nursing;   EB = Evidence-Based

- Explore coping skills previously used by the client to deal with fear. *Children generally rate their coping behaviors as helpful. A variety of coping behaviors reported were seeking support from parents, avoidance, distraction, trying to sleep, and clinging to stuffed animals (Muris et al, 2001).*
- Teach parents to use cognitive-behavioral strategies such as positive coping statements ("I am a brave girl [boy]. I can take care of myself in the dark.") and rewards of bravery tokens for appropriate behavior. *Cognitive-behavioral strategies appear to be effective interventions, but more research is indicated because of methodological limitations (Gordon & King, 2002).*
- Screen for depression in clients who report social or school fears. *Evidence corroborates a significant relation between depression and childhood social or school fears (Neal, Edelmann & Glachan, 2002).*
- Teach relaxation techniques to children to induce calmness. **EB:** *Relaxation training may reduce somatic or psychological symptoms and support children's ability to cope with emotional reactions (Lohaus & Klein-Hessling, 2003).*

Geriatric

- Establish a trusting relationship so that all fears can be identified. *An elderly client's response to a real fear may be immobilizing.*
- Monitor for dementia and use appropriate interventions. *Fear may be an early indicator of disorientation or impaired reality testing in elderly clients.*
- Provide a protective and safe environment, use consistent caregivers, and maintain the accustomed environmental structure. *Elderly clients tend to have more perceptual impairments and adapt to changes with more difficulty than younger clients, especially during an illness.*
- Observe for untoward changes if antianxiety drugs are taken. *Advancing age renders clients more sensitive to both the clinical and toxic effects of many agents.*
- Assess for fear of falls in hospitalized clients with hip fractures to determine risk of poor health outcomes. **EBN:** *Fear of falls correlated with poor health outcomes and has a major impact on function, especially with regard to walking (McKee et al, 2002).*
- Encourage exercises to improve physical skills and levels of mobility to decrease fear of falling. *Improving physical skills and levels of mobility counteract excessive fear during activity performance (Fuzhong et al, 2002).*
- Assist the client in identifying and reducing risk factors of falls, including environmental hazards in and out of the home, the importance of good nutrition and activity, proper footwear, and how to stand up after a fall. **EB:** *Clients receiving education focused on identifying and reducing risk factors for falls were found to have a significant reduction in their fear of falling (Brouwer et al, 2003).*

Multicultural

- Assess for the presence of culture-bound anxiety and fear states. **EBN:** *The context in which anxiety and fear is experienced, its meaning, and responses to it are culturally mediated (Emery, 2006; Kuipers, 2004).*
- Assess for the influence of cultural beliefs, norms, and values on the client's perspective of a stressful situation. **EBN:** *What the client considers stressful may be based on cultural perceptions (Leininger & McFarland, 2002).*
- Identify what triggers fear response. **EBN:** *Arab Muslim clients may express a high correlation between fear and pain (Sheets & El-Azhary, 1998).*
- Identify how the client expresses fear. **EBN:** *Research indicates that the expression of fear may be culturally mediated (Shore & Rapport, 1998).*
- Validate the client's feelings regarding fear. **EBN:** *Validation is a therapeutic communication technique that lets the client know that the nurse has heard and understands what was said, and it promotes the nurse-client relationship (Heineken, 1998).*
- Assess for fears of racism in culturally diverse clients. **EB:** *Findings suggest that, independent of the effects of gender, age, and household social class, being worried about being a victim of racial harassment could have an important impact on an individual's health experience (Karlsen & Nazroo, 2004).*

Home Care

- The previous interventions may be adapted for home care use.

• = Independent;   ▲ = Collaborative;   EBN = Evidence-Based Nursing;   EB = Evidence-Based

- Assess to differentiate the presence of fear versus anxiety.
- Refer to care plan for **Anxiety.**
- During initial assessment, determine whether current or previous episodes of fear relate to the home environment (e.g., perception of danger in the home or neighborhood or of relationships that have a history in the home). *Investigating the source of the fear allows the client to verbalize feelings and the nurse to determine appropriate interventions.*
- Identify with the client what steps may be taken to make the home a "safe" place to be. *Identifying a given area as a safe place reduces fear and anxiety when the client is in that area.*
- ▲ Encourage the client to seek or continue appropriate counseling to reduce fear associated with stress or resolve alterations in irrational thought processes. *Correcting mistaken beliefs reduces anxiety.*
- ▲ Encourage the client to have a trusted companion, family member, or caregiver present in the home for periods when fear is most prominent. Pending other medical diagnoses, a referral to homemaker or home health aide services may meet this need. *Creating periods when fear and anxiety can be reduced allows the client periods of rest and supports positive coping.*
- ▲ Offer to sit quietly with a terminally ill client as needed by the client or family, or provide hospice volunteers to do the same. *Terminally ill clients and their families often fear the dying process. The presence of a nurse or volunteer lets clients know they are not alone. Fears are reduced, and the dying process becomes more easily tolerated.*

Client/Family Teaching

- Teach the client the difference between warranted and excessive fear. *Different interventions are indicated for rational and irrational fears.*
- Teach clients to use guided imagery when they are fearful; have them use all senses to visualize a place that is "comfortable and safe" for them. *Imagery makes use of subjective symbolism bypassing the rational mind and making the areas "safe" that the client may otherwise be reluctant to face (Yip, 2003).*
- ▲ Teach use of appropriate community resources in emergency situations (e.g., hotlines, emergency departments, law enforcement, judicial systems). *Serious emergencies need immediate assistance to ensure the client's safety.*
- ▲ Encourage use of appropriate community resources in nonemergency situations (e.g., family, friends, neighbors, self-help and support groups, volunteer agencies, churches, recreation clubs and centers, seniors, youths, others with similar interests).
- ▲ If fear is associated with bioterrorism, provide accurate information and ensure that healthcare personnel have appropriate training and preparation. *Clear, consistent, accessible, reliable, and redundant information (received from trusted sources) will diminish public uncertainty about the cause of symptoms that might otherwise prompt persons to seek unnecessary treatment. Training for providers is essential (Benedek, Holloway & Becker, 2002).*

evolve See the EVOLVE website for World Wide Web resources for client education.

REFERENCES

Anderson P, Jacobs CH, Lindner GK et al: Cognitive behavior therapy for fear of flying: sustainability of treatment gains after September 11, *Behav Ther* 37(1):91-97, 2006.

Barker SB, Pandurangi AK, Best AM: Effects of animal-assisted therapy on patients' anxiety, fear, and depression before ECT, *J ECT* 19(1):38-44, 2003.

Beck AT: The current state of cognitive therapy: a 40-year retrospective, *Arch Gen Psychiatry* 62(9):953-959, 2005.

Benedek DM, Holloway HC, Becker SM: Emergency mental health management in bioterrorism events, *Emerg Med Clin North Am* 20(2):393, 2002.

Brouwer B, Walker C, Rydahl S et al: Reducing fear of falling in seniors through education and activity programs: a randomized trial, *J Am Geriatr Soc* 51:829-834, 2003.

Crossley ML: "Let me explain": narrative employment and one patient's experience of oral cancer, *Soc Sci Med* 56(3):439, 2003.

Driessnack M: Draw and tell conversations with children about fear, *Qual Health Res* 16(10):1414-1435, 2006.

Emery P: Building a new culture of aging: revolutionizing long-term care, *J Christ Nurs* 23(1):16-24, 2006.

Fuzhong L, McAuley E, Fisher KJ et al: Self-efficacy as a mediator between fear of falling and functional ability in the elderly, *J Aging Health* 14(4):452, 2002.

Gordon J, King N: Children's night-time fears: an overview, *Couns Psychol Q* 15(2):121, 2002.

Heineken J: Patient silence is not necessarily client satisfaction: communication in home care nursing, *Home Healthc Nurs* 16(2):115, 1998.

• = Independent; ▲ = Collaborative; EBN = Evidence-Based Nursing; EB = Evidence-Based

Karlsen S, Nazroo JY: Fear of racism and health, *J Epidemiol Community Health* 58(12):1017-1018, 2004.

Kelly A, Sullivan P, Fawcett J et al: Therapeutic touch, quiet time and dialogue: perceptions of women with breast cancer, *Oncol Nurs Forum* 31(3):645, 2004.

Kuipers J: Mexican Americans. In Giger J, Davidhizar R, editors, *Transcultural nursing: Assessment and intervention,* St Louis, 2004, Mosby.

Leininger MM, McFarland MR: *Transcultural nursing: concepts, theories, research and practices,* ed 3, New York, 2002, McGraw-Hill.

Locsin RC, Barnard A, Matua AG: Surviving Ebola: understanding experience through artistic expression, *Int Nurs Rev* 50:156-166, 2003.

Lohaus A, Klein-Hessling J: Relaxation in children: effects of extended and intensified training, *Psychol Health* 18(2):237-249, 2003.

McKee KJ, Orbell S, Austin CA et al: Fear of falling, falls efficacy, and health outcomes in older people following hip fracture, *Disabil Rehabil* 24(6):327, 2002.

Mineka S, Ohman A: Phobias and preparedness: the selective, automatic, and encapsulated nature of fear, *Biol Psychiatry* 15(52):10, 2002.

Muris P, Merckelbach H, Ollendick TH et al: Children's night-time fears: parent-child ratings of frequency, content, origins, coping behaviors and severity, *Behav Res Ther* 39(1):13-28, 2001.

Neal J, Edelmann R, Glachan M: Behavioural inhibition and symptoms of anxiety and depression: is there a specific relationship with social phobia? *Br J Clin Psychol* 41:361, 2002.

Northouse LL, Walker J, Schafenacker A et al: A family-based program of care for women with recurrent breast cancer and their family members, *Oncol Nurs Forum* 29(10):1411-1419, 2002.

Poulton R, Menzies RG: Non-associative fear acquisition: a review of the evidence from retrospective and longitudinal research, *Behav Res Ther* 40(2):127, 2002.

Ronen T, Rahav G, Appel N: Adolescent stress responses to a single acute stress and to continuous external stress: terrorist attacks, *J Loss Trauma* 8(4):261-282, 2003.

Sheets DL, El-Azhary RA: The Arab Muslim client: implications for anesthesia, *AANA J* 66(3):304, 1998.

Shore GN, Rapport MD: The fear survey schedule for children-revised (FSSC-HI): ethnocultural variations in children's fearfulness, *J Anxiety Disord* 2(5):437-461, 1998.

Taylor A, Galper D, Taylor P et al: Effects of adjunctive Swedish massage and vibration therapy on short-term postoperative outcomes: a randomized, controlled trial, *J Altern Complement Med* 9(1):77-89, 2003.

Townsend M: *Psychiatric mental health nursing: concepts of care,* ed 4, Philadelphia, 2003, F.A. Davis.

Wardell D, Weymouth K: Review of studies of healing touch, *J Nurs Scholarsh* 36(2):147-154, 2004.

Yip K: The relief of a caregiver's burden through guided imagery, role-playing, humor, and paradoxical intervention, *Am J Psychother* 57(1):109-122, 2003.

Readiness for enhanced Fluid balance   Betty J. Ackley, MSN, EdS, RN

NANDA   Definition

A pattern of equilibrium between fluid volume and chemical composition of body fluids that is sufficient for meeting physical needs and can be strengthened.

Defining Characteristics

Dehydration; expresses willingness to enhance fluid balance; good tissue turgor; intake adequate for daily needs; moist mucous membranes; no evidence of edema; no excessive thirst; specific gravity within normal limits; stable weight; straw-colored urine; urine output appropriate for intake

NOC   Outcomes (Nursing Outcomes Classification)

Suggested NOC Outcomes

Fluid Balance, Hydration, Nutritional Status: Food and Fluid Intake

Example NOC Outcome with Indicators

Fluid Balance as evidenced by the following indicators: Skin turgor/Moist mucous membranes/Orthostatic hypotension not present/24-hour intake and output balance/Urine specific gravity (Rate the outcome and indicators of **Fluid Balance:** 1 = severely compromised, 2 = substantially compromised, 3 = moderately compromised, 4 = mildly compromised, 5 = not compromised [see Section I].)

Client Outcomes

Client Will (Specify Time Frame):

- Maintain light-yellow urine output
- Maintain elastic skin turgor, moist tongue, and mucous membranes
- Explain measures that can be taken to improve fluid intake

• = Independent;   ▲ = Collaborative;   EBN = Evidence-Based Nursing;   EB = Evidence-Based

NIC Interventions (Nursing Interventions Classification)

Suggested NIC Intervention

Fluid Management

Example NIC Activities—Fluid Management
Monitor hydration status (e.g., moist mucous membranes, adequacy of pulses, and orthostatic blood pressure) as appropriate; Monitor food/fluid ingested and calculate daily caloric intake, as appropriate

F

Nursing Interventions and *Rationales*

- Discuss normal fluid requirements. *A guideline is 1 to 1.5 mL of fluid per each calorie needed, so an average intake would be between 2000 and 3000 mL/day, or at least 8 cups of fluid (Grodner, Long & DeYoung, 2004). The adequate intake recommendation is 3 L for the 19- to 30-year-old male and 2.2 L for the 19- to 30-year-old female. Water balance studies suggest that adult men require 2.5 L per day (Institute of Medicine, 2004).* **EB:** *Increased daily fluid intake by 1.5 L has no negative effect in healthy men aged 55 to 75 years. On average, intervention subjects increased daily intake by 1 L, with no significant changes in blood pressure, sodium level, glomerular filtration rate, or quality of life (Spigt et al, 2006).*
- Recommend intake of mainly water, but milk or fruit juice can also be effective in maintaining good fluid balance (Cataldo, DeBruyne & Whitney, 2003).
- Recommend the client decrease the use of alcoholic beverages and beverages containing caffeine to provide fluid to the body. *Both alcohol and caffeine act as a diuretic, causing increased loss of fluid in the urine. But drinking fluids with caffeine or alcohol is not associated with increased incidence of dehydration, and consumption of these fluids does contribute to the total body fluid needs of individuals (Institute of Medicine, 2004).*
- Recommend the client avoid intake of carbonated beverages; instead suggest the client drink water. *Most carbonated beverages contain large amounts of sugar (10 or more tsp), are a significant source of empty calories, and can cause significant damage to the teeth (American Dental Association, 2007).*

Geriatric

- Encourage the elderly client to develop a pattern of drinking water regularly. *Thirst sensations diminish with aging; dehydration can threaten elderly clients (Mentes, 2004).* **EB:** *Healthy men age 67 to 75 years are less thirsty and replace less fluid than young people during fluid deprivation (Philips et al, 1984). In a study of standards for calculating recommended fluid intake, the results closely support other recommendations of 1500 to 2000 mL fluid intake per day (Chidester & Spangler, 1997) In a study of 883 people with a mean age of 74 years, interviews and examinations revealed that most estimated their usual fluid intake as equal to or exceeded six glasses per day. Significant hypernatremia was not observed in the individuals ingesting less than this; hyponatremia was rare in this population. Encouraging a fluid intake of eight glasses (2 L) per day seems to serve little useful purpose (Lindeman et al, 2000).*
- See care plan for **Deficient Fluid volume** for interventions to increase fluid intake in the elderly.

Home Care

- Assess availability of clean drinking water in the home, or assess resources to acquire bottled water. *Willingness to maintain fluid balance may be compromised by a lack of available clean water.*
- ▲ Assess available and preferred fluids. Refer for social services if resources are needed to purchase adequate fluid. *Affordability of milk or juice may be an obstacle to availability of fluids. Assistance to obtain food stamps may be indicated.*

Client/Family Teaching

- Teach the client to drink water before and while engaging in activities that can quickly result in dehydration, such as distance running or gardening in hot weather. *Maintaining hydration before, during, and after training and competition helps reduce fluid loss; maintain performance; and reduce heat stress, heat exhaustion, and possible heat stroke (Von Duvillard et al, 2004).* **EB:** *There is a decrease in long-term memory when exercising in a hot environment and not replacing lost fluids (Cian* *et al, 2001). Drinking fluids earlier results in a faster rate of plasma and fluid balance restoration (Kovacs et al, 2002).*

- Caution the athlete client not to drink excessively during competition or training but to follow the dictates of thirst. *There have been at least seven deaths and 250 cases of hyponatremic encephalopathy since the advice of "drink the maximum amount that can be tolerated" (Noakes, 2003). Excessive hydration without adequate sodium intake may result in sodium depletion (Institute of Medicine, 2004; Von Duvillard et al, 2004).*

- Teach clients who work in hot environments or exercise in hot environments to increase intake of both water and electrolyte-carbohydrate beverages. *Sports drinks are needed when exercise exceeds 1 hour or during prolonged competitive games that require repeated intermittent activity (Welsh et al, 2002). Drinks containing low to moderate levels of electrolytes and carbohydrates may provide significant advantages in industrial situations (Clap et al, 2002).* **EB:** *Drinking flavored drinks during sports athletic activity compared with water enhances fluid balance (Minehan, Riley & Burke, 2002).*

- Ask the client to monitor the color of urine to tell if adequately hydrated. *In a hydrated person the urine should be light yellow—the color of lemonade. Urine the color of apple juice indicates slight dehydration (Cataldo et al, 2003).* **EBN:** *Urine color significantly correlates with urine osmolality, serum sodium, and blood urea nitrogen (BUN)/creatinine ratio (Wakefield et al, 2002).*

evolve   See the EVOLVE website for World Wide Web resources for client education.

REFERENCES

American Dental Association: *Oral health topics A-Z,* www.ada.org/public/topics, accessed March 3, 2007.

Cataldo CB, DeBruyne LK, Whitney EN: *Nutrition and diet therapy,* ed 6, Belmont, CA, 2003, Thomson Wadsworth.

Chidester JC, Spangler AA: Fluid intake in the institutionalized elderly, *J Am Diet Assoc* 97(1):23-28, 1997.

Cian C, Barraud PA, Melin B et al: Effects of fluid ingestion on cognitive function after heat stress or exercise-induced dehydration, *Int J Psychophysiol* 42(3):243, 2001.

Clap AJ, Bishop PA, Smith JF et al: A review of fluid replacement for workers in hot jobs, *AIHA J (Fairfax, Va)* 63(2):190-198, 2002.

Grodner M, Long S, DeYoung S: *Foundations and clinical applications of nutrition: a nursing approach,* ed 3, St Louis, 2004, Mosby.

Institute of Medicine: Applications of dietary reference intakes for electrolytes and water, *National Academy of Sciences,* 2004, National Academies Press.

Kovacs EM, Schmahl RM, Senden JM et al: Effect of high and low rates of fluid intake on post-exercise rehydration, *Int J Sport Nutr Exerc Metab* 12(1):14, 2002.

Lindeman RD, Romero LJ, Liang HC et al: Do elderly persons need to be encouraged to drink more fluids? *J Gerontol A Biol Sci Med Sci* 55(7):M361-M365, 2000.

Mentes JC: *Hydration management,* Iowa City, IA, 2004, University of Iowa Gerontological Nursing Interventions Research Center.

Minehan MR, Riley MD, Burke LM: Effect of flavor and awareness of kilojoule content of drinks on preference and fluid balance in team sports, *Int J Sport Nutr Exerc Metab* 12(1):81, 2002.

Noakes TD: Overconsumption of fluids by athletes, *BMJ* 327(7407):113, 2003.

Philips PA, Rolls BJ, Ledingham JG et al: Reduced thirst after water deprivation in healthy elderly men, *N Engl J Med* 311(12):753, 1984.

Spigt MG, Knottnerus JA, Westerterp KR et al: The effects of 6 months of increased water intake on blood sodium, glomerular filtration rate, blood pressure, and quality of life in elderly (aged 55-75) men, *J Am Geriatr Soc* 54(3):438-443, 2006.

Von Duvillard SP, Braun WA, Markofski M et al: Fluids and hydration in prolonged endurance performance. *Nutrition* 20(7-8):651, 2004.

Wakefield B, Mentes J, Diggelmann L et al: Monitoring hydration status in elderly veterans, *West J Nurs Res* 24(2):132, 2002.

Welsh RS, Davis JM, Burke JR et al: Carbohydrates and physical/mental performance during intermittent exercise to fatigue, *Med Sci Sports Exerc* 34(4):723, 2002.

Deficient Fluid volume   Betty J. Ackley, MSN, EdS, RN   **evolve**

NANDA   Definition

Decreased intravascular, interstitial, and/or intracellular fluid. This refers to dehydration, water loss alone without change in sodium level.

Defining Characteristics

Change in mental state; decreased blood pressure; decreased pulse pressure; decreased pulse volume; decreased skin turgor; decreased tongue turgor; decreased urine output; decreased venous filling; dry mucous membranes; dry skin; elevated hematocrit; increased body temperature; increased pulse rate; increased urine concentration; sudden weight loss (except in third spacing); thirst; weakness

● = Independent;   ▲ = Collaborative;   EBN = Evidence-Based Nursing;   EB = Evidence-Based

Related Factors (r/t)

Active fluid volume loss; failure of regulatory mechanisms

Suggested NOC Outcomes

Electrolyte and Acid-Base Balance, Fluid Balance, Hydration, Nutritional Status: Food and Fluid Intake

Example NOC Outcome with Indicators
Fluid Balance as evidenced by the following indicators: Skin turgor/Moist mucous membranes/Orthostatic hypotension not present/24-hour intake and output balance/Urine specific gravity (Rate the outcome and indicators of **Fluid Balance:** 1 = severely compromised, 2 = substantially compromised, 3 = moderately compromised, 4 = mildly compromised, 5 = not compromised [see Section I].)

Client Outcomes

Client Will (Specify Time Frame):

• Maintain urine output more than 1300 mL/day (or at least 30 mL/hr)
• Maintain normal blood pressure, pulse, and body temperature
• Maintain elastic skin turgor; moist tongue and mucous membranes; and orientation to person, place, and time
• Explain measures that can be taken to treat or prevent fluid volume loss
• Describe symptoms that indicate the need to consult with healthcare provider

Suggested NIC Interventions

Fluid Management, Hypovolemia Management, Shock Management: Volume

Example NIC Activities—Fluid Management
Monitor hydration status (e.g., moist mucous membranes, adequacy of pulses, and orthostatic blood pressure) as appropriate; Administer IV at room temperature

Nursing Interventions and *Rationales*

• Watch for early signs of hypovolemia, including restlessness, weakness, muscle cramps, headaches, inability to concentrate, and postural hypotension. *Late signs include oliguria, abdominal or chest pain, cyanosis, cold clammy skin, and confusion (Kasper et al, 2005).* **EB:** *A study of healthy volunteers who experienced a fluid restriction of up to 37 hours reported symptoms of headache, decreased alertness, and inability to concentrate (Shirreffs et al, 2004).*
• Monitor for the existence of factors causing deficient fluid volume (e.g., vomiting, diarrhea, difficulty maintaining oral intake, fever, uncontrolled type 2 diabetes, diuretic therapy). *Early identification of risk factors and early intervention can decrease the occurrence and severity of complications from deficient fluid volume. The gastrointestinal system is a common site of abnormal fluid loss (Metheny, 2000).*
• Monitor daily weight for sudden decreases, especially in the presence of decreasing urine output or active fluid loss. Weigh the client on the same scale with the same type of clothing at same time of day, preferably before breakfast. *Body weight changes reflect changes in body fluid volume (Kasper et al, 2005). Weight loss of 2.2 pounds is equal to fluid loss of 1 liter (Linton & Maebius, 2003).* **EB:** *A systematic review demonstrated that measurement of weight is a safe technique to assess hydration status, especially for dehydration that occurs over a period of 1 to 4 hours; less-frequent measurement may reflect changes in respiratory water loss or gain or loss of adipose tissue; thus weight changes may be a less-accurate indicator of hydration status (Armstrong, 2005).*

• = Independent;   ▲ = Collaborative;   EBN = Evidence-Based Nursing;   EB = Evidence-Based

- Monitor total fluid intake and output every 8 hours (or every hour for the unstable client). Recognize that urine output is not always an accurate indicator of fluid balance. *A urine output of less than 30 mL/hr is insufficient for normal renal function and indicates hypovolemia or onset of renal damage (Metheny, 2000). Urine output can be an unreliable indicator of fluid balance because if the client is hypothermic or elderly or has renal dysfunction, the client may be unable to concentrate urine, leading to falsely high urine output (Schulman, 2002).*
- Watch trends in output for 3 days; include all routes of intake and output and note color and specific gravity of urine. *Monitoring for trends for 2 to 3 days gives a more valid picture of the client's hydration status than monitoring for a shorter period (Metheny, 2000). Dark-colored urine with increasing specific gravity reflects increased urine concentration.*
- Monitor vital signs of clients with deficient fluid volume every 15 minutes to 1 hour for the unstable client (every 4 hours for the stable client). Observe for tachycardia, tachypnea, decreased pulse pressure first, then hypotension, decreased pulse volume, and increased or decreased body temperature. **EB:** *A systematic review demonstrated that hypotension and tachycardia, and occasionally fever, are clinical signs of dehydration (Ferry, 2005).*
- Check orthostatic blood pressures with the client lying, sitting, and standing. *A 20-mm Hg drop when upright or an increase of 15 beats/min in the pulse rate is seen with deficient fluid volume (Kasper et al, 2005). If the systolic blood pressure drops 20 mm Hg and the pulse rate does not change, the baroreceptors in the body are not working and the cause can be cardiovascular, neurologic, or a medication effect (Sclater & Kannayiram, 2004).* **EB:** *A systematic review demonstrated that in adults with suspected blood loss, the most helpful physical findings are either severe postural dizziness (preventing measurement of upright vital signs) or a postural pulse increment of 30 beats/min or more. The finding of mild postural dizziness has no proven value. In clients with vomiting, diarrhea, or decreased oral intake, the presence of a dry axilla supports the diagnosis of hypovolemia, and moist mucous membranes and a tongue without furrows argue against it.*
- Monitor for thirst, dry tongue and mucous membranes, longitudinal tongue furrows, speech difficulty, dry skin, sunken eyeballs, weakness (especially of upper body), headache, and confusion. *These are symptoms of decreased body fluids (Metheny, 2000).*
- Provide frequent oral hygiene, at least twice a day (if mouth is dry and painful, provide hourly while awake). *Oral hygiene decreases unpleasant tastes in the mouth and allows the client to respond to the sensation of thirst.*
- Provide fresh water and oral fluids preferred by the client (distribute over a period of 24 hours [e.g., 1200 mL on days, 800 mL on evenings, and 200 mL on nights]); provide prescribed diet; offer snacks (e.g., frequent drinks, fresh fruits, fruit juice); and instruct significant other to assist the client with feedings as appropriate. *The oral route is preferred for maintaining fluid balance (Metheny, 2000). Distributing the intake over the entire 24-hour period and providing snacks and preferred beverages increases the likelihood that the client will maintain the prescribed oral intake.*
- Provide free water with tube feedings as appropriate: 50 to 100 mL every 4 hours or 30 mL/kg of body weight (Suhayda & Walton, 2002). *This provides water for replacement of intravascular or intracellular volume as necessary. Tube feeding has been found to increase the risk for dehydration (Sheehy, Perry & Cromwell, 1999).*
- Institute measures to rest the bowel when the client is vomiting or has diarrhea (e.g., restrict food or fluid intake when appropriate, decrease intake of milk products).
- ▲ Provide oral replacement therapy as ordered and tolerated with a hypotonic glucose-electrolyte solution when the client has acute diarrhea or nausea and vomiting. Provide small, frequent quantities of slightly chilled solutions. *Maintenance of oral intake stabilizes the ability of the intestines to digest and absorb nutrients; glucose-electrolyte solutions increase net fluid absorption while correcting deficient fluid volume. Use diluted carbohydrate-electrolyte solutions such as sports replacement drinks, cola, and ginger ale, which are often tolerated better than other solutions, sometimes even with vomiting and diarrhea (Suhayda & Walton, 2002).* **EB:** *Decreasing the osmolality of standard glucose-electrolyte oral replacement solutions improves the absorption of water and stool volume (Farthing, 2002).*
- ▲ Administer antidiarrheals and antiemetics as appropriate. *The goal is to stop the fluid loss that results from vomiting or diarrhea.*
- ▲ Hydrate the client with ordered intravenous (IV) solutions if prescribed. *The most common cause*

of deficient fluid volume is gastrointestinal loss of fluid. At times it is preferable to allow the gastrointestinal system to rest before resuming oral intake. Hydration should be maintained. Refer to care plan for **Diarrhea** *or* **Nausea***.*

▲ If the client requires IV fluid replacement, maintain patent IV access, set an appropriate IV infusion flow rate, and administer at a constant flow rate as ordered. *Isotonic IV fluids such as 0.9% normal saline or Ringer's lactate allow replacement of intravascular volume (Kasper et al, 2005).*

• Assist with ambulation if the client has postural hypotension. *Postural hypotension can cause dizziness, which places the client at higher risk for injury.*

Critically Ill

• If a trauma client, check manual blood pressure until the systolic pressure is 110 mm Hg. Do not rely on automatic blood pressure measurements. Check vital signs frequently. **EB:** *Automatic blood pressure measurements are consistently higher than manual, and the manual blood pressures better represent the injury severity, degree of acidosis, and resuscitation volume needed (Davis et al, 2003).* **EB:** *Emergency and critical care treatment guidelines outline that mild hypovolemia (20% of the blood volume) can result in mild tachycardia but relatively few other signs. With moderate hypovolemia (20% to 40% of the blood volume) increasing tachycardia postural hypotension and anxiety may be seen. If hypovolemia is severe (40% of the blood volume), the classic signs of shock appear with hypotension, significant tachycardia, oliguria, and agitation or confusion. The transition from mild to severe hypovolemic shock can be insidious or extremely rapid (Harrison's Online, 2006; Kolecki and Menckhoff, 2007).*

• Monitor central venous pressure, right atrial pressure, and pulmonary wedge pressure for decreases. *Hemodynamic parameters are sensitive indicators of intravascular fluid volume, and hemodynamic measurements are especially needed in the client with cardiac or renal problems (Kasper et al, 2005).* **EB:** *Arterial cannulation, central venous pressure, and pulmonary artery catheterization provide an accurate measurement of intraarterial pressure to enable decisions about immediate therapy in critically ill clients (Alspach, 2006).*

• Monitor serum and urine osmolality, serum sodium, BUN/creatinine ratio, and hematocrit for elevations. *These are all measures of concentration and will be elevated with decreased intravascular volume (Kasper et al, 2005).*

• Use a sublingual capnometry device if available to determine level of tissue hypoxia caused by lack of fluid volume. *Recognizing decreased perfusion during resuscitation from blood loss can help avoid onset of multiple organ failure (Boswell & Scalea, 2003).*

▲ Insert a Foley catheter if ordered and measure urine output hourly. Notify physician if <30 mL/hour. *A decrease in urine output is seen with increasing severity of shock in the client with normal kidneys (Docherty & McIntyre, 2002).*

▲ When ordered, initiate a fluid challenge of crystalloids (0.9% normal saline or Ringer's lactate) for replacement of intravascular volume; monitor the client's response to prescribed fluid therapy and fluid challenge, especially noting central venous pressure and pulmonary capillary wedge pressure readings, vital signs, urine output, blood lactate concentrations, and lung sounds. *A fluid challenge can help the client with deficient fluid volume regain intravascular volume quickly, but the client must be carefully observed to ensure that he or she does not go into fluid volume overload (Kruse, Fink & Carlson, 2003).*

• Position the client flat with legs elevated when hypotensive, if not contraindicated. *This position enhances venous return, thus contributing to the maintenance of cardiac output.*

▲ Monitor trends in serum lactic acid levels and base deficit obtained from blood gases as ordered. *A trend of increasing lactic acid levels and increasing base deficit can help identify occult hypoperfusion, which results in decreased survival and increased incidence of organ failure (Schulman, 2002).*

▲ Consult physician if signs and symptoms of deficient fluid volume persist or worsen. *Prolonged deficient fluid volume increases the risk for development of complications, including shock, multiple organ failure, and death.*

Pediatric

• Monitor the child for signs of deficient fluid volume, including capillary refill time, skin turgor, and respiratory pattern along with other symptoms. **EB:** *These factors are more significant in iden-*

---

tifying dehydration, but are still imprecise and it is difficult to determine the exact degree of dehydration (Steiner, DeWalt & Byerley, 2004).

▲ Reinforce the physician's recommendation for the parents to give the child oral rehydration fluids to drink in the amounts specified, especially during the first 4 to 6 hours to replace fluid losses. Once the child is rehydrated, an orally administered maintenance solution should be used along with food. **EBN and EB:** *Oral rehydration therapy is effective for treating mild to moderate dehydration in children with diarrhea and may help prevent the need for hospitalization with administration of IV fluids (Larson, 2000).* **EB:** *Treatment with oral rehydration fluids for children were generally as effective as IV fluids, and IV fluids did not shorten the duration of gastroenteritis and are more likely to cause adverse effects than oral rehydration therapy (Banks & Meadows, 2005).*

• Recommend the mother initiate, continue, or resume breastfeeding as soon as possible. *One of the most common problems identified in the early newborn period is dehydration (Paul et al, 2004).*

• Recommend parents not give the child carbonated soda, fruit juices, gelatin dessert, or instant fruit drink mix. *These fluids have a high osmolality due to carbohydrate contents and can exacerbate diarrhea. In addition they have low sodium concentrations, which can aggravate existing hyponatremia (Behrman, Kliegman & Jenson, 2004).*

• Recommend parents give children foods with complex carbohydrates such as potatoes, rice, bread, cereal, yogurt, fruits, and vegetables. *The BRAT diet is often advocated: bananas, rice, applesauce, and toast. Avoid fatty foods and foods high in simple sugars (Behrman et al, 2004).*

Geriatric

• Monitor elderly clients for deficient fluid volume carefully, noting new onset of weakness, dizziness, or dry mouth with longitudinal furrows on the tongue. **EB:** *Older adults have a higher osmotic point for thirst sensation and a diminished sensitivity to thirst relative to younger adults (Kenney & Chiu, 2001). The elderly are predisposed to deficient fluid volume because of decreased fluid in body, decreased thirst sensation, and decreased ability to concentrate urine (Suhayda & Walton, 2002).*

• Evaluate the risk for dehydration using the Dehydration Risk Appraisal Checklist (Mentes, 2004).

• Check skin turgor of elderly clients on the forehead, sternum, or inner thigh; also look for the presence of longitudinal furrows on the tongue and dry mucous membranes. *Elderly people commonly have decreased skin turgor from normal age-related loss of elasticity; therefore checking skin turgor on the arm is not reflective of fluid volume (Suhayda & Walton, 2002). The presence of longitudinal furrows or dry mucous membranes is a good indication of dehydration in the elderly (Bennett, 2000).*

• Encourage fluid intake by offering fluids regularly to cognitively impaired clients. **EB:** *Dehydration by overnight fluid restriction in both young and older subjects results in impaired alertness; in older individuals it also results in slower psychomotor processing speed and impaired memory performance (Ritz & Berrut, 2005).*

• Incorporate regular hydration into daily routines (e.g., extra glass of fluid with medication or social activities). Consider use of a beverage cart and a hydration assistant to routinely offer increased beverages to clients in extended care. **EBN and EB:** *Institution of a beverage cart with a trained hydration assistant resulted in increased number of bowel movements, less use of laxatives, decreased number of falls, fewer urinary tract an respiratory infections, and less skin breakdown (Robinson & Rosher, 2002). Verbal prompting and offers of preference fluids resulted in increased fluid intake among nursing home residents (Simmons, Alessi & Schnelle, 2001).*

• If client is identified as having chronic dehydration, flag the food tray to indicate to caregivers they should finish 75% to 100% of their food and fluids (Mentes, 2004).

• Recognize that lower blood pressures and a higher BUN/creatinine ratio can be significant signs of dehydration in the elderly. **EBN:** *Dehydrated older adults have significantly lower systolic and diastolic blood pressures and significantly higher BUN levels but similar creatinine levels compared with nondehydrated adults (Bennett, Thomas & Riegel, 2004).*

• Note the color of urine and compare against a urine color chart to monitor adequate fluid intake. **EBN:** *A research study on elderly veterans demonstrated that urine color correlated significantly with urine osmolality, serum sodium, and BUN/creatinine ratio (Wakefield et al, 2002).*

F

- Monitor elderly clients for excess fluid volume during the treatment of deficient fluid volume: listen to lung sounds, watch for edema, and note vital signs. *The elderly client has a decreased ability to adapt to rapid increases in intravascular volume and can quickly develop fluid overload (Allison & Lobo, 2004).*

 Home Care

- Teach family members how to monitor output in the home (e.g., use of commode "hat" in the toilet, urinal, or bedpan or use of catheter and closed drainage). Instruct them to monitor both intake and output.
- When weighing the client, use the same scale each day. Be sure scale is on a flat, not cushioned, surface. Do not weigh the client with scale placed on any kind of rug. Use bed or chair scales for clients who are unable to stand.
- ▲ Teach family about complications of deficient fluid volume and when to call physician.
- ▲ If the client is receiving IV fluids, there must be a responsible caregiver in the home. Teach caregiver about administration of fluids, complications of IV administration (e.g., fluid volume overload, speed of medication reactions), and when to call for assistance. Assist caregiver with administration for as long as necessary to maintain client safety. *Administration of IV fluids in the home is a high-technology procedure and requires sufficient professional support to ensure safety of the client.*
- ▲ Identify an emergency plan, including when to call 911. *Some complications of deficient fluid volume cannot be reversed in the home and are life threatening. Clients progressing toward hypovolemic shock will need emergency care.*
- If the client is terminal, determine if it is appropriate to intervene for deficient fluid volume or allow the client to die comfortably without fluids as desired. *Deficient fluid volume may be a symptom of impending death in terminally ill clients. The deficit may result in a mild euphoria and a more comfortable death (Bennett, 2000).* **EB:** *A study of witnessed death by hospice nurses demonstrated that clients who voluntarily refused fluids and food usually die a "good" death within 2 weeks (Ganzini et al, 2003).*

 Client/Family Teaching

- Instruct the client to avoid rapid position changes, especially from supine to sitting or standing.
- Teach the client and family about appropriate diet and fluid intake.
- Teach the client and family how to measure and record intake and output accurately.
- Teach the client and family about measures instituted to treat hypovolemia and prevent or treat fluid volume loss.
- Instruct the client and family about signs of deficient fluid volume that indicate they should contact the healthcare provider.

  See the EVOLVE website for World Wide Web resources for client education.

REFERENCES

Allison SP, Lobo DN: Fluid and electrolytes in the elderly, *Curr Opin Clin Nutr Metab Care* 7(1):27, 2004.

Alspach JG, editor: *Core curriculum for critical care nursing,* ed 6, St Louis, 2006, W.B. Saunders.

Armstrong LE: Hydration assessment techniques, *Nutr Rev* 63(6 Pt 2): S40-S54, 2005.

Banks JB, Meadows S: Intravenous fluids for children with gastroenteritis, *Am Family Physician* 71(1):121, 2005.

Bennett JA: Dehydration: hazards and benefits, *Geriatr Nurs* 21(2):84, 2000.

Bennett JA, Thomas V, Riegel B: Unrecognized chronic dehydration in older adults: examining prevalence rate and risk factors, *J Gerontol Nurs* 30(11):22-28, 2004.

Behrman RE, Kliegman RM, Jenson HB: *Nelson textbook of pediatrics,* ed 17, Philadelphia, 2004, W.B. Saunders.

Boswell SA, Scalea TM: Sublingual capnometry: an alternative to gas-

tric tonometry for the management of shock resuscitation, *AACN Clin Issues* 14(2):176, 2003.

Davis JW, Davis IC, Bennink LD et al: Are automated blood pressure measurements accurate in trauma patients? *J Trauma* 55(5):860, 2003.

Docherty B, McIntyre L: Nursing considerations for fluid management in hypovolaemia, *Prof Nurse* 17(9):545, 2002.

Farthing MJ: Oral rehydration: an evolving solution, *J Pediatr Gastroenterol Nutr* 34(suppl 1):S64, 2002.

Ferry M: Strategies for ensuring good hydration in the elderly. *Nutr Rev* 63(6 pt 2):S22-S29, 2005.

Ganzini L, Goy ER, Miller LL et al: Nurses' experiences with hospice patients who refuse food and fluids to hasten death, *N Engl J Med* 349(4):359, 2003.

Harrison's Online: *Approach to the patient with shock,* www.harrisonsonline.com, Accessed February 27, 2006.

• = Independent;   ▲ = Collaborative;   EBN = Evidence-Based Nursing;   EB = Evidence-Based

Kasper DL et al, editors: *Harrison's principles of internal medicine,* ed 16, New York, 2005, McGraw-Hill.

Kenney WL, Chiu P: Influence of age on thirst and fluid intake, *Med Sci Sports Exerc* 33(9):1524-1532, 2001.

Kolecki P, Menckhoff CR: *Shock, hypovolemic,* www.emedicine.com/EMERG/topic532.htm, accessed February 27, 2007.

Kruse JA, Fink MP, Carlson RW: *Saunders manual of critical care,* Philadelphia, 2003, W.B. Saunders.

Larson CE: Evidence-based practice: safety and efficacy of oral rehydration therapy for the treatment of diarrhea and gastroenteritis in pediatrics, *Pediatr Nurs* 26(2):177, 2000.

Linton AD, Maebius NK: *Introduction to medical-surgical nursing,* ed 3, Philadelphia, 2003, Saunders.

Mentes JC: *Hydration management,* Iowa City, IA, 2004, University of Iowa Gerontological Nursing Interventions Research Center.

Metheny N: *Fluid and electrolyte balance: nursing considerations,* ed 4, Philadelphia, 2000, J.B. Lippincott.

Paul IM, Phillips TA, Widome MD et al: Cost-effectiveness of postnatal home nursing visits for prevention of hospital care for jaundice and dehydration, *Pediatrics* 114(4):1015-1022, 2004.

Ritz P, Berrut G: The importance of good hydration for day-to-day health, *Nutr Rev* 63(6 pt 2), S6-S13, 2005.

Robinson SB, Rosher RB: Can a beverage cart help improve hydration? *Geriatr Nurs* 23:4, 2002.

Schulman C: End points of resuscitation: choosing the right parameters to monitor, *Dimens Crit Care Nurs* 21(1):2, 2002.

Sclater A, Kannayiram A: Orthostatic hypotension: a primary care primer for assessment and treatment, *Geriatrics* 59(8):22, 2004.

Sheehy CM, Perry PA, Cromwell SL: Dehydration: biological considerations, age-related changes, and risk factors in older adults, *Biol Res Nurs* 1(1):30, 1999.

Shirreffs SM, Merson SJ, Fraser SM et al: The effects of fluid restriction on hydration status and subjective feelings in man, *Br J Nutr* 91(6):951, 2004.

Simmons SF, Alessi C, Schnelle JF: An intervention to increase fluid intake in nursing home residents: prompting and preference compliance, *J Am Geriatr Soc* 49(7):926, 2001.

Steiner MJ DeWalt DA, Byerley JS: Is this child dehydrated? *JAMA* 291(22):2764, 2004.

Suhayda R, Walton JC: Preventing and managing dehydration, *Medsurg Nurs* 11(6):267, 2002.

Wakefield B, Mentes J, Diggelmann L et al: Monitoring hydration status in elderly veterans, *West J Nurs Res* 24(2):132, 2002.

Excess Fluid volume   Betty J. Ackley, MSN, EdS, RN

NANDA   Definition

Increased isotonic fluid retention

Defining Characteristics

Adventitious breath sounds; altered electrolytes; anasarca; anxiety; azotemia; blood pressure changes; change in mental status; changes in respiratory pattern; decreased hematocrit; decreased hemoglobin; dyspnea; edema; increased central venous pressure; intake exceeds output; jugular vein distention; oliguria; orthopnea; pleural effusion; positive hepatojugular reflex; pulmonary artery pressure changes; pulmonary congestion; restlessness; specific gravity changes; S_3 heart sound; weight gain over short period of time

Related Factors (r/t)

Compromised regulatory mechanism; excess fluid intake; excess sodium intake

NOC   Outcomes (Nursing Outcomes Classification)

Suggested NOC Outcomes

Electrolyte and Acid-Base Balance, Fluid Balance, Hydration

Example NOC Outcome with Indicators
Fluid Balance as evidenced by the following indicators: Peripheral edema/Neck vein distention/Adventitious breath sounds/Orthostatic hypotension/Intake and output imbalance (Rate the outcome and indicators of **Fluid Balance:** I = severe, 2 = substantial, 3 = moderate, 4 = mild, 5 = none [see Section I].)

Client Outcomes

Client Will (Specify Time Frame):

- Remain free of edema, effusion, anasarca; weight appropriate for the client
- Maintain clear lung sounds, no evidence of dyspnea or orthopnea

• = Independent;   ▲ = Collaborative;   EBN = Evidence-Based Nursing;   EB = Evidence-Based

F

- Remain free of jugular vein distention, positive hepatojugular reflex, and gallop heart rhythm
- Maintain normal central venous pressure, pulmonary capillary wedge pressure, cardiac output, and vital signs
- Maintain urine output within 500 mL of intake with normal urine osmolality and specific gravity
- Explain measures that can be taken to treat or prevent excess fluid volume, especially fluid and dietary restrictions and medications
- Describe symptoms that indicate the need to consult with healthcare provider

NIC Interventions (Nursing Interventions Classification)

Suggested NIC Interventions

Fluid Management, Fluid Monitoring

Example NIC Activities—Fluid Monitoring
Monitor weight; Keep an accurate record of intake and output

Nursing Interventions and *Rationales*

- Monitor location and extent of edema; use a millimeter tape in the same area at the same time each day to measure edema in extremities. *Generalized edema (e.g., in the upper extremities and eyelids) is associated with decreased oncotic pressure often as a result of nephrotic syndrome. Measuring the extremity with a millimeter tape is more accurate than using the 1+ to 4+ scale (Metheny, 2000). Heart failure and renal failure are usually associated with dependent edema because of increased hydrostatic pressure; dependent edema causes swelling in the legs and feet of ambulatory clients and the presacral region of clients on bed rest.* **EBN:** *Dependent edema was found to demonstrate the greatest sensitivity as a defining characteristic for excess fluid volume (Rios et al, 1991).*
- Monitor daily weight for sudden increases; use same scale and type of clothing at same time each day, preferably before breakfast. **EB:** *Measurement of body weight change is a safe technique to assess hydration status (Armstrong, 2005).* **EB:** *Body weight could safely be used to monitor for fluid overload when administering hyperhydration with high-dose chemotherapy (Mank et al, 2003).*
- Monitor lung sounds for crackles, monitor respirations for effort, and determine the presence and severity of orthopnea. *Pulmonary edema results from excessive shifting of fluid from the vascular space into the pulmonary interstitial space and alveoli. Pulmonary edema can interfere with the oxygen/carbon dioxide exchange at the alveolar-capillary membrane (Metheny, 2000), resulting in dyspnea and orthopnea.*
- With head of bed elevated 30 to 45 degrees, monitor jugular veins for distention in the upright position; assess for positive hepatojugular reflex. *Increased intravascular volume results in jugular vein distention, even in a client in the upright position, and a positive hepatojugular reflex (Kasper et al, 2005).*
- ▲ Monitor central venous pressure, mean arterial pressure, pulmonary artery pressure, pulmonary capillary wedge pressure, and cardiac output; note and report trends indicating increasing pressures over time. *Increased vascular volume with decreased cardiac contractility increases intravascular pressures, which are reflected in hemodynamic parameters. Over time, this increased pressure can result in uncompensated heart failure (Kasper et al, 2005).*
- Monitor vital signs; note decreasing blood pressure, tachycardia, and tachypnea. Monitor for gallop rhythms. If signs of heart failure are present, see the care plan for **Decreased Cardiac output.** *Heart failure results in decreased cardiac output and decreased blood pressure. Tissue hypoxia stimulates increased heart and respiratory rates.*
- ▲ Monitor serum osmolality, serum sodium, BUN/creatinine ratio, and hematocrit for decreases. *These are all measures of concentration and will decrease (except in the presence of renal failure) with*

• = Independent;   ▲ = Collaborative;   EBN = Evidence-Based Nursing;   EB = Evidence-Based

increased intravascular volume. In clients with renal failure, BUN will increase because of decreased renal excretion (Kasper et al, 2005).

- Monitor intake and output; note trends reflecting decreasing urine output in relation to fluid intake. *Accurately measuring intake and output is vital for the client with fluid volume overload.*
- Monitor urine color for lighter colored urine as a sign of fluid overload in the client with functioning kidneys. **EBN:** *There is a positive association between urine color and urine specific gravity and urine osmolality, and between urine osmolality and serum sodium and BUN/creatinine ratio in hospitalized clients and residents of a short-term rehabilitation unit (Wakefield et al, 2002). Urine color significantly correlates with urine specific gravity in nursing home residents (Mentes, 2006).*
- Monitor the client's behavior for restlessness, anxiety, or confusion; use safety precautions if symptoms are present. *When excess fluid volume compromises cardiac output, the client may have cerebral tissue hypoxia and demonstrate restlessness and anxiety (Kasper et al, 2005). When the excess fluid volume results in hyponatremia, symptoms such as agitation, irritability, inappropriate behavior, confusion, and seizures may occur (Kasper et al, 2005; Kruse, Fink & Carlson, 2003).*
- Monitor for the development of conditions that increase the client's risk for excess fluid volume. *Common causes are heart failure, renal failure, and liver failure, all of which result in decreased glomerular filtration rate and fluid retention. Other causes are increased intake of oral or IV fluids in excess of the client's cardiac and renal reserve levels, increased levels of antidiuretic hormone, or movement of fluid from the interstitial space to the intravascular space (Kasper et al, 2005).*
- ▲ Assist with continuous renal replacement therapy as ordered if the client is critically ill and excessive fluid must be removed. *Continuous renal replacement therapy is indicated for severe volume overload, refractory heart failure, oliguric renal failure, metabolic acidosis, and azotemia with uremic symptoms (Kempher, 2003; Kruse et al, 2003).*
- ▲ Provide a restricted-sodium diet as appropriate if ordered. *Restricting the sodium in the diet will favor the renal excretion of excess fluid. Take care to avoid hyponatremia. Decreasing sodium can be just as important as restricting fluid intake with fluid overload (Kasper et al, 2005).*
- Monitor serum albumin level and provide protein intake as appropriate. *Serum albumin is the main contributor to serum oncotic pressure, which favors the movement of fluid from the interstitial space into the intravascular space. When serum albumin is low, peripheral edema may be severe.*
- ▲ Administer prescribed diuretics as appropriate; check blood pressure before administration to ensure it is adequate. If administering a diuretic IV, note and record urine output after the dose.
- Monitor for side effects of diuretic therapy: orthostatic hypotension (especially if the client is also receiving ACE inhibitors), hypovolemia and electrolyte imbalances (hypokalemia and hyponatremia). Observe for hyperkalemia in clients receiving a potassium-sparing diuretic, especially with the concurrent administration of an ACE inhibitor (Kasper et al, 2005).
- ▲ Implement fluid restriction as ordered, especially when serum sodium is low; include all routes of intake. Schedule fluids around the clock and include the type of fluids preferred by the client. *Fluid restriction may decrease intravascular volume and myocardial workload. Overzealous fluid restriction for cardiac clients should not be used because hypovolemia can worsen heart failure.*
- Calculate an appropriate daily fluid intake amount and work with client to establish a fluid intake goal. **EB:** *A cognitive-behavioral group effectively helps hemodialysis clients adhere to fluid restrictions (Sharp et al, 2005).*
- Maintain the rate of all IV infusions carefully with an IV pump. *This is done to prevent inadvertent exacerbation of excess fluid volume.*
- Turn clients with dependent edema frequently (i.e., at least every 2 hours). *Edematous tissue is vulnerable to ischemia and pressure ulcers (Casey, 2004).*
- Provide scheduled rest periods. *Bed rest can induce diuresis related to diminished peripheral venous pooling, resulting in increased intravascular volume and glomerular filtration rate (Metheny, 2000).*
- Promote a positive body image and good self-esteem. *Visible edema may alter the client's body image.* Refer to the care plan for **Disturbed Body image.**
- ▲ Consult physician if signs and symptoms of excess fluid volume persist or worsen. *Because excess*

• = Independent;   ▲ = Collaborative;   EBN = Evidence-Based Nursing;   EB = Evidence-Based

fluid volume can result in pulmonary edema, it must be treated promptly and aggressively (Kasper et al, 2005).

Geriatric

- Recognize that the presence of risk factors for excess fluid volume is particularly serious in the elderly. *Sodium and fluid overload is common in hospitalized elderly clients and can result in increased morbidity and mortality in surgical clients (Allison & Lobo, 2004).*

Home Care

- Assess client and family knowledge of disease process causing excess fluid volume.
- ▲ Teach about disease process and complications of excess fluid volume, including when to contact physician.
- Assess client and family knowledge and compliance with medical regimen, including medications, diet, rest, and exercise. Assist family with integrating restrictions into daily living. *Assistance with integration of cultural values, especially those related to foods, with medical regimen promotes compliance and decreased risk for complications.*
- ▲ Teach and reinforce knowledge of medications. Instruct the client not to use over-the-counter medications (e.g., diet medications) without first consulting the physician.
- ▲ Instruct the client to make primary physician aware of medications ordered by other physicians.
- Identify emergency plan for rapidly developing or critical levels of excess fluid volume when diuresing is not safe at home. *When out of control, excess fluid volume can be life threatening.*
- ▲ Teach about signs and symptoms of both excess and deficient fluid volume and when to call physician. *Fluid volume balance can change rapidly with aggressive treatment.*

Client/Family Teaching

- Describe signs and symptoms of excess fluid volume and actions to take if they occur.
- ▲ Teach client on diuretics to weigh self daily in the morning and notify the physician of a change in weight of 3 pounds or more (Karch, 2004).
- ▲ Teach the importance of fluid and sodium restrictions. Help the client and family devise a schedule for intake of fluids throughout the entire day. Refer to dietitian concerning implementation of low-sodium diet.
- ▲ Teach how to take diuretics correctly: take one dose in the morning and second dose (if taken) no later than 4 PM. Adjust potassium intake as appropriate for potassium-losing or potassium-sparing diuretics. Note the appearance of side effects such as weakness, dizziness, muscle cramps, numbness and tingling, confusion, hearing impairment, palpitations or irregular heartbeat, and postural hypotension.
- Caution the athlete client not to drink excessively during competition or training, but to follow the dictates of thirst. *Excessive hydration without adequate sodium intake may result in sodium depletion and can result in encephalopathy and death (Appel et al, 2004; Von Duvillard et al, 2004; Noakes, 2003).*
- For the client undergoing hemodialysis, spend time with the client to detect any factors that may interfere with the client's compliance with the fluid restriction or restrictive diet. **EBN:** *The nurse who knows the client well is able to develop individualized interventions to help the client adhere to the restriction (Morgan, 2001).*

 See the EVOLVE website for World Wide Web resources for client education.

REFERENCES

Allison SP, Lobo, DN: Fluid and electrolytes in the elderly, *Curr Opin Clin Nutr Metab Care* 7(1):27, 2004.

Appel L et al: Dietary intake levels for water, salt, potassium, chloride and sulfate, Institute of Medicine, 2004.

Armstrong LE: Hydration assessment techniques, *Nutr Rev* 63(6 pt 2), S40-S54, 2005.

Casey G: Edema: causes, physiology and nursing management, *Nur Stand* 18(51):45, 2004.

Karch AM: Practice errors. On the rebound: maintaining normal fluid intake is critical while on diuretics, *Am J Nurs* 104(10):73, 2004.

Kasper DL et al, editors: *Harrison's principles of internal medicine*, ed 16, New York, 2005, McGraw-Hill.

Kempher KJ: Continuous renal replacement therapy for management of overhydration in heart failure, *AACN Clin Issues* 14(4):512, 2003.

Kruse JA, Finnk MP, Carlson RW: *Saunders manual of critical care,* Philadelphia, 2003, W.B. Saunders.

Mank A, Semin-Goossens A, Lelie J et al: Monitoring hyperhydration during high-dose chemotherapy: body weight or fluid balance? *Acta Haematol* 109(4):163, 2003.

Mentes JC: A typology of oral hydration problems exhibited by frail nursing home residents, *J Gerontol Nurs* 32(1):13-19, 2006.

Metheny N: *Fluid and electrolyte balance: nursing considerations,* ed 4, Philadelphia, 2000, J.B. Lippincott.

Morgan L: A decade review: methods to improve adherence to the treatment among hemodialysis patients, *EDTNA, ERCA* 27(1):7-12, 2001.

Noakes T: Fluid replacement during marathon running, *Clin J Sport Med* 13(5):309-318, 2003.

Rios H, Delaney C, Kruckeberg T et al: Validation of defining characteristics of four nursing diagnoses using a computerized data base, *J Prof Nurs* 7:293, 1991.

Sharp J, Wild MR, Gumley AI et al: A cognitive behavioral group approach to enhance adherence to hemodialysis fluid restrictions: a randomized controlled trial, *Am J Kidney Dis* 45(6):1046-1057, 2005.

Von Duvillard SP, Braun WA, Markofski M et al: Fluids and hydration in prolonged endurance performance, *Nutrition* 20(7-8):651-656, 2004.

Wakefield B, Mentes J, Diggelmann L et al: Monitoring hydration status in elderly veterans, *West J Nurs Res* 24(2):132-142, 2002.

F

Risk for deficient Fluid volume   Betty J. Ackley, MSN, EdS, RN

NANDA   Definition

At risk for experiencing vascular, cellular, or intracellular dehydration

Risk Factors

Deviations affecting access of fluids; deviations affecting intake of fluids; deviations affecting absorption of fluids; excessive losses through normal routs (e.g., diarrhea); extremes of age; extremes of weight; factors influencing fluid needs (e.g., hypermetabolic state); loss of fluid through abnormal routes (e.g., indwelling tubes); knowledge deficiency; medication (e.g., diuretics)

NOC   Outcomes (Nursing Outcomes Classification)

Suggested NOC Outcomes

Fluid Balance, Hydration, Knowledge: Treatment Regimen

Example NOC Outcome with Indicators
Fluid Balance as evidenced by the following indicators: Skin turgor/Moist mucous membranes/Orthostatic hypotension not present/24-hour intake and output balance/Urine specific gravity (Rate the outcome and indicators of **Fluid Balance:** 1 = severely compromised, 2 = substantially compromised, 3 = moderately compromised, 4 = mildly compromised, 5 = not compromised [see Section I].)

Client Outcomes

Client Will (Specify Time Frame):

- Maintain urine output of more than 1300 mL/day (or at least 30 mL/hr)
- Maintain normal blood pressure, pulse, and body temperature
- Maintain elastic skin turgor; moist tongue and mucous membranes; and orientation to person, place, and time
- Explain measures that can be taken to treat or prevent fluid volume loss
- Describe symptoms that indicate the need to consult a healthcare provider

NIC   Interventions (Nursing Interventions Classification)

Suggested NIC Interventions

Fluid Management, Fluid Monitoring, Hypovolemia Management

• = Independent;   ▲ = Collaborative;   EBN = Evidence-Based Nursing;   EB = Evidence-Based

F

Example NIC Activities—Fluid Management
Monitor hydration status (e.g., moist mucous membranes, adequacy of pulses, and orthostatic blood pressure) as appropriate

Nursing Interventions and *Rationales*

- Watch for early signs of hypovolemia, including restlessness, weakness, muscle cramps, head-aches, inability to concentrate, and postural hypotension. *Late signs include oliguria, abdominal or chest pain, cyanosis, cold clammy skin, and confusion (Kasper et al, 2005).* **EB:** *A study of healthy volunteers who had fluid restriction of up to 37 hours reported symptoms of headache, decreased alertness, and inability to concentrate (Shirreffs et al, 2004).*
- Monitor for the existence of factors causing deficient fluid volume (e.g., vomiting, diarrhea, difficulty maintaining oral intake, fever, uncontrolled type 2 diabetes, diuretic therapy). *Early identification of risk factors and early intervention can decrease the occurrence and severity of complications from deficient fluid volume. The gastrointestinal system is a common site of abnormal fluid loss (Metheny, 2000).*
- Monitor daily weight for sudden decreases, especially in the presence of decreasing urine output or active fluid loss. Weigh the client on the same scale with the same type of clothing at same time of day, preferably before breakfast. *Body weight changes reflect changes in body fluid volume (Kasper et al, 2005; Suhayda & Walton, 2002).*
- Monitor total fluid intake and output every 8 hours (or every hour for the unstable client). Recognize that urine output is not always an accurate indicator of fluid balance. *A urine output of less than 30 mL/hr is insufficient for normal renal function and indicates hypovolemia or onset of renal damage (Metheny, 2000). Urine output can be an unreliable indicator of fluid balance because if the client is hypothermic or elderly or has renal dysfunction, the client may be unable to concentrate urine, leading to falsely high urine output (Schulman, 2002).*
- Check orthostatic blood pressures with the client lying, sitting, and standing. *A 20-mm Hg drop when upright or an increase of 15 beats/min in the pulse rate is seen with deficient fluid volume (Kasper et al, 2005). If the systolic blood pressure drops 20 mm Hg and the pulse rate does not change, the baroreceptors in the body are not working and the cause can be cardiovascular, neurologic, or a medication effect (Sclater & Kannayiram, 2004).*
- Monitor for inelastic skin turgor, thirst, dry tongue and mucous membranes, longitudinal tongue furrows, speech difficulty, dry skin, sunken eyeballs, weakness (especially of upper body), head-ache, and confusion. *These are symptoms of decreased body fluids (Metheny, 2000).*
- Use appropriate preoperative fasting guidelines as ordered: "allow the consumption of clear liquids up to two hours before elective surgery, a light breakfast (tea and toast, for example) 6 hours before the procedure, and a heavier meal 8 hours beforehand" (Crenshaw & Winslow, 2002). **EBN and EB:** *Pulmonary aspiration is a rare complication of anesthesia, and prolonged fasting before surgery can lead to dehydration, headache, and hypoglycemia (Smith, Vallance & Slater, 1997; Hung, 1992). Most clients received instructions of nothing by mouth after midnight for preoperative fasting, resulting in some clients with afternoon surgeries fasting up to 20 hours from liquids and 37 hours from solids (Crenshaw & Winslow, 2002). Dehydration by overnight fluid restriction in both young and older subjects results in impaired alertness; in older individuals it also resulted in slower psychomotor processing speed and impaired memory performance (Ritz & Berrut, 2005).*
- Refer to care plan for **Deficient Fluid volume.**

Home Care

- Assess availability of clean drinking water in the home or resources to acquire bottled water. *Willingness to maintain fluid balance may be compromised by a lack of available clean water.*
- ▲ Assess available and preferred fluids. Refer for social services if resources are needed to purchase adequate fluid. *Affordability of milk or juice may be an obstacle to availability of fluids. Assistance to obtain food stamps may be indicated.*

• = Independent;   ▲ = Collaborative;   EBN = Evidence-Based Nursing;   EB = Evidence-Based

Client/Family Teaching

- Teach clients who work in hot environments or exercise in hot environments to increase intake of both water and electrolyte-carbohydrate beverages. *A review of the literature demonstrated that drinks containing low to moderate levels of electrolytes and carbohydrates may provide significant advantages in industrial situations (Clap et al, 2002).*

evolve   See the EVOLVE website for World Wide Web resources for client education.

REFERENCES

Clap AJ, Bishop PA, Smith JF et al: A review of fluid replacement for workers in hot jobs, *AIHA J* 63(2):190, 2002.

Crenshaw JT, Winslow EH: Preoperative fasting: old habits die hard, *Am J Nurs* 102(5):36, 2002.

Hung P: Preoperative fasting, *Nurs Times* 88:48, 1992.

Kasper DL et al, editors: *Harrison's principles of internal medicine,* ed 16, New York, 2005, McGraw-Hill.

Metheny N: *Fluid and electrolyte balance: nursing considerations,* ed 4, Philadelphia, 2000, Lippincott.

Ritz P, Berrut G: The importance of good hydration for day-to-day health, *Nutr Rev* 63(6 pt 2):S6-S13, 2005.

Schulman C: End points of resuscitation: choosing the right parameters to monitor, *Dimens Crit Care Nurs* 21(1):2, 2002.

Sclater A, Kannayiram A: Orthostatic hypotension: a primary care primer for assessment and treatment, *Geriatrics* 59(8):22, 2004.

Shirreffs SM, Merson SJ, Fraser SM et al: The effects of fluid restriction on hydration status and subjective feelings in man, *Br J Nutr* 91(6):951, 2004.

Smith AF, Vallance H, Slater RM: Shorter preoperative fluid fasts reduce postoperative emesis, *BMJ* 314(7092):1486, 1997.

Suhayda R, Walton JC: Preventing and managing dehydration, *Medsurg Nurs* 11(6):267, 2002.

F

Risk for imbalanced Fluid volume   *Terri Foster, BSN, CNOR, RN, and Betty J. Ackley, MSN, EdS, RN*

NANDA   Definition

At risk for a decrease, increase, or rapid shift from one to the other of intravascular, interstitial, and/or intracellular fluid (refers to body fluid loss, gain, or both)

Risk Factor

Scheduled for major invasive procedures

NOC   Outcomes (Nursing Outcomes Classification)

Suggested NOC Labels

Fluid Balance, Electrolyte and Acid-Base Balance, Hydration

Example NOC Outcome with Indicators
Maintains **Fluid Balance** as evidenced by the following indicators: Blood pressure/Peripheral pulses palpable/Skin turgor/Moist mucous membranes/Serum electrolytes/Hematocrit/Peripheral edema/Neck vein distention/Stable body weight/24-hour intake and output balance/Urine specific gravity/Adventitious breath sounds (Rate the outcome and indicators of **Fluid Balance:** 1 = severely compromised, 2 = substantially compromised, 3 = moderately compromised, 4 = mildly compromised, 5 = not compromised [see Section I].)

Client Outcomes

- Lung sounds clear, respiratory rate 12 to 20, and free of dyspnea postoperatively
- Urine output greater than 30 mL/hr (Beyea, 2002)
- Blood pressure, pulse rate, temperature, and pulse oximetry within expected range (Beyea, 2002)
- Laboratory values within expected range (Beyea, 2002)
- Nonedematous extremities and dependent areas
- Mental orientation unchanged from preoperative status

• = Independent;   ▲ = Collaborative;   EBN = Evidence-Based Nursing;   EB = Evidence-Based

NIC   Interventions (Nursing Interventions Classification)

Suggested NIC Interventions

Acid-Base Management, Acid-Base Monitoring, Autotransfusion, Bleeding Precautions, Bleeding Reduction: Wound, Electrolyte Management, Fluid Management, Fluid Monitoring, Hemodynamic Regulation, Hypervolemia Management, Hypovolemia Management, Intravenous Therapy, Invasive Hemodynamic Monitoring, Shock Management: Volume

Example NIC Activities—Fluid Management

Maintain accurate intake and output record; Monitor vital signs, as appropriate

Nursing Interventions and *Rationales*

- Monitor vital signs of clients with deficient fluid volume every 15 minutes if unstable or every 4 hours if stable. Observe for tachycardia, tachypnea, and decreased pulse pressure, which will occur first, followed by hypotension, decreased pulse volume, and increased or decreased body temperature. *Decreased intravascular volume results in hypotension and decreased tissue oxygenation. A decrease in temperature is a result of decreased metabolism, and an increase in temperature is a result of presence of infection or hypernatremia (Metheny, 2000).*
- Check the client's orthostatic blood pressure. *A 20 mm Hg drop in systolic blood pressure when upright or an increase of 15 beats/min in pulse rate is seen with deficient fluid volume (Kasper et al, 2005).*
- Monitor for nonelastic skin turgor, thirst, dry tongue and mucous membranes, longitudinal tongue furrows, difficulty speaking, dry skin, sunken eyeballs, weakness (especially upper body), headache, and confusion, which are symptoms of decreased body fluids (Metheny, 2000). **EB:** *A study of healthy volunteers who had fluid restriction of up to 37 hours reported symptoms of headache, decreased alertness, and inability to concentrate (Shirreffs et al, 2004).*
- Provide frequent oral hygiene—at least twice daily. If the client's mouth is dry and painful, provide oral hygiene hourly while client is awake. *Oral hygiene decreases unpleasant tastes in the mouth and allows the client to respond to the sensation of thirst.*
- ▲ Initiate measures to rest the bowel when the client is vomiting or has diarrhea; that is, restrict food or fluid intake when appropriate, and decrease intake of milk products. Hydrate the client with any prescribed (ordered) IV solutions. *The most common cause of deficient fluid volume is gastrointestinal loss of fluid. At times it is preferable to allow the gastrointestinal system to rest before resuming oral intake. Hydration should be maintained.* Refer to care plan for **Diarrhea** or **Nausea.**
- ▲ Provide oral replacement therapy as ordered and tolerated, with a hypotonic glucose-electrolyte solution when the client has acute diarrhea or nausea and vomiting. Provide small, frequent qualities of slightly chilled solutions. *Use carbohydrate-electrolyte solutions such as sports replacement drinks, cola, and ginger ale, which are often tolerated better than other solutions when vomiting and diarrhea occur (Suhayda & Walton, 2002).* **EB:** *Decreasing the osmolality of standard glucose-electrolyte oral replacement solutions improves the absorption of water and stool volume (Farthing, 2002).*
- Maintain patent IV access if the client requires IV fluid replacement. *Isotonic IV fluids such as 0.9% normal saline or Ringer's lactate allow replacement of intravascular volume (Kasper et al, 2005).*
- Monitor for factors causing deficient fluid volume, such as vomiting, diarrhea, difficulty maintaining oral intake, fever, uncontrolled type 2 diabetes, diuretic therapy, and preoperative bowel preparation. *Early identification of risk factors and early intervention can decrease the occurrence and severity of complications caused by deficient fluid volume. The gastrointestinal system is a common site of abnormal fluid loss (Metheny, 2000).*
- ▲ When ordered, administer a fluid challenge, giving a specified amount of IV fluid, such as 0.9% normal saline rapidly IV, for replacement of intravascular volume and monitor the client's response by noting vital signs, lung sounds, urine output, and pulmonary capillary wedge pressure or central venous pressures if applicable. *A fluid challenge can help rapidly reverse deficient fluid volume, but the client must be carefully observed to ensure he or she does not go into fluid volume overload (Kruse et al, 2003).*

• = Independent;   ▲ = Collaborative;   EBN = Evidence-Based Nursing;   EB = Evidence-Based

- Keep all IV fluids on a volumetric pump. *This is done to decrease the risk of fluid overload and ensure that the client receives sufficient fluids.*
- Monitor intake and output. *Assessment, accurate documentation of intake and output, and management of fluid and electrolyte imbalances are crucial to prevent serious problems (Kasper, 2005).*
- ▲ Measure urine output hourly. If urine output is less than 30 mL/hr or 0.5 mL/kg/hr, notify the physician. *Urine output may not always be an accurate indicator of fluid balance. Urine output less than 30 mL/hr is insufficient for normal renal function and indicates hypovolemia or onset of renal damage (Metheny, 2000). Urine output can be an unreliable indicator of fluid balance because hypothermic clients, the elderly, and clients with renal dysfunction may not be able to concentrate urine, leading to a falsely high urine output (Schulman, 2002).*
- Observe for trends in output for 3 days; include all routes of intake and output and note color and specific gravity of urine. *Monitoring for trends for 2 to 3 days gives a more valid picture of the client's hydration status than monitoring over a shorter period (Metheny, 2000). Dark-colored urine with increasing specific gravity reflects increased urine concentration.*
- Monitor daily weight for sudden decreases, especially in the presence of decreasing urine output or active fluid loss. Weigh the client on the same scale, in the same type clothing, at the same time of day, preferably before breakfast. *Body weight changes reflect changes in body fluid volume (Suhayda & Walton, 2002). A 1-pound weight loss reflects a fluid loss of about 500 mL (Metheny, 2000).*
- ▲ Monitor trends in serum lactic acid levels and base deficit, obtained from blood gases as ordered. *A trend of increasing lactic acid levels and increasing base deficit can help identify occult hypoperfusion, which results in decreased survival and increased incidence of organ failure (Schulman, 2002).*

Surgical Clients

- ▲ Perform a preoperative assessment to identify clients with increased risk for hemorrhage or hypovolemia (e.g., recent traumatic injury, abnormal bleeding or clotting times; complicated renal or liver disease; diabetes; cardiovascular disease; major organ transplant; history of aspirin or nonsteroidal antiinflammatory drug use or anticoagulant therapy; or history of hemophilia, von Willebrand's disease, or disseminated intravascular coagulation). *Use of laxatives, preoperative dehydration, infection, abnormal drainage, and hemorrhage can lead to hypotension during anesthesia induction if not corrected preoperatively. Nothing-by-mouth status preoperatively can lead to dehydration and, when combined with the stress of undergoing surgery, can cause changes in the circulating volume and hydrostatic-oncotic pressure (Van Wissen & Breton, 2004). Assessment of the client's use of herbal products is important because some herbs act as anticoagulants and could cause increased blood loss, and some herbs have diuretic or laxative effects (Edlund, 2003). Preoperative hydration recommendations are not always evidence based. Recommendations in specific instances may obtain or show positive outcomes but may not be applicable in all instances. Weight of the client, fluid and electrolyte excess/deficit, insensible water loss, and gastrointestinal and renal loss are factors used to determine fluid replacement in clients undergoing a major surgical procedure (Hughes, 2004).* **EB:** *Intraoperative fluid replacement should not routinely contain glucose because plasma cortisol increases during surgery, which in turn causes hyperglycemia (van Wissen & Breton, 2004).*
- Monitor for signs of intraoperative hypovolemia (e.g., dry skin, dry mucous membranes, tachycardia, decreased urinary output, decreased central venous pressure, hypotension, increased pulse, and/or deep rapid respirations). *Hypovolemia can occur in the surgical client due to nothing-by-mouth status, hemorrhage, or third spacing (van Wissen & Breton, 2004). To ensure adequate hydration, it is important to provide replacement fluids during the postoperative period (Hughes, 2004). Elevating the hypovolemic client's legs can aid venous return and cardiac output unless the client also has severe oligemia (Phillips, 2004). Hypovolemic clients should be kept warm, but not overheated, because perspiration increases fluid loss (Phillips, 2004).* **EB:** *Goal-directed fluid administration leads to an earlier return of bowel function, a lower incidence of postoperative nausea and vomiting, and a decrease in length of postoperative hospital stay (Gan et al, 2002). Evidence shows that fluid lost should be replaced, that is, principles of restricted IV fluid therapy. Fluid overload should be avoided (Brandstrup, 2006).*
- Monitor for signs of intraoperative hypervolemia (dyspnea, coarse crackles, increased pulse and respirations, decreased urinary output), all of which could progress to pulmonary edema.

F

F

Surgical clients with preexisting chronic kidney or liver disease or congestive heart failure may be prone to hypervolemia. Increased fluid intake can potentially increase postoperative cardiac morbidity, predispose the client to pneumonia and respiratory failure, cause urinary retention from increased excretory demands on the kidney and resultant diuresis, inhibition of gastrointestinal motility resulting in prolonged postoperative ileus, decreased tissue oxygenation resulting in poor wound healing, and postoperative thrombosis formation from coagulation being enhanced (Holte, Sharrock & Kehlet, 2002).

- Monitor for signs of intraoperative third spacing. *Third spacing can occur as a result of surgery itself. It may be necessary to replace fluid intraoperatively (Holte et al, 2002). Fluid can shift to the surgical site and produce edema because of the surgically induced inflammatory response. This fluid is temporarily unavailable and requires replacement to prevent hypovolemic shock (Hughes, 2004).* **EB:** *Evidence shows that predetermined algorithms for replacement of fluid caused by third spacing and from diuresis are not necessary (Joshi, 2005).*

- In the critically ill surgical client with a pulmonary artery catheter, monitor pressures, especially wedge pressure. *Pulmonary artery pressures are helpful for determining fluid balance, especially in the cardiac or renal client, and can help guide fluid administration and administration of vasoactive IV drips such as dopamine.* **EB:** *Use of the Starling curve in combination with central venous pressures or esophageal Doppler cardiac output measurements "optimize" cardiac function by allowing better fluid regimens. Fluids must be individually titrated based on each client's changes in monitored variables (Mitchell et al, 2003).*

- Monitor clients undergoing laparoscopic or hysteroscopic procedures for the development of pulmonary edema when Dextran is used as the irrigation fluid (Gordon, 2003). *The manufacturer of Dextran recommends vigilance for pulmonary edema when laparoscopic and hysteroscopic procedures last longer than 45 minutes, when more than 250 mL of Dextran 70 is absorbed, when large areas of endometrium are resected, or when IV fluid administration is greater then maintenance rate (Cooper & Brady, 2000). Frequent monitoring of infusion/recovery rates (every 15 minutes) keeps the nurse cognizant of absorption rates (Cooper & Brady, 2000).* **EB:** *In a study of women who underwent a hysteroscopy, 5% had excessive hypotonic fluid absorption (Belloni, 2001).*

- Monitor intraoperative intake and output. **EB:** *Low molecular weight fluids can cause fluid overload; therefore it is mandatory that an accurate accounting of input and output be maintained (Gordon, 2003).* **EB:** *When a fluid deficit of 1000 mL occurs and the surgical procedure is halted, serious sequelae are rare (Belloni, 2001).*

- Monitor clients undergoing transurethral resection of the prostate (TURP) procedures for TURP syndrome symptoms: headache, visual changes, agitation, lethargy, vomiting, muscle twitching, bradycardia, diminished pupillary reflexes, hypertension, and respiratory distress (Metheny, 2000). *Considerable fluid absorption occurs during TURP procedures (Kukreja et al, 2002).*

- If the client is undergoing endometrial ablation under general anesthesia, watch for symptoms of decreased body temperature, decreased oxygen saturation, dilated pupils, and tremulousness (Metheny, 2000). *Serious fluid overload and dilutional hyponatremia can develop in surgeries such as transurethral resections of the prostate, transcervical resection of the endometrium, or a hysteroscopy as a result of the absorption of large amounts of irrigation solution in the circulation, which can cause permanent morbidity or death (Rose, 2001). Nonelectronic (saline cannot be used), isotonic irrigating solution must be used to ensure electrical current is transmitted and keep the area clear for visualization (Rothrock, 2003).*

- Monitor clients undergoing percutaneous nephrolithotomy procedures for excessive fluid absorption and volume overload. *Clients with borderline cardiorespiratory or renal status can have clinically significant volume overload during percutaneous nephrolithotomy procedures, especially if they also have excessive bleeding and large perforations. The volume of fluid absorbed has been shown to increase with the amount of irrigation fluid used and the length of the procedure (Kukreja et al, 2002).*

- Observe the surgical client for signs of hyperkalemia, that is, cardiac dysrhythmias, heart block, asystole, abdominal distention, and weakness. *Hyperkalemia can occur intraoperatively as a result of massive blood transfusions, tissue breakdown from surgery, shifting of potassium from the cells into the extracellular fluid, decreased potassium excretion caused by renal failure or hypovolemia, crush injuries, or burns (Rothrock, 2003).*

- Observe surgical clients closely for signs of hypokalemia. *Hypokalemia commonly causes dysrhythmias. Stress and/or gastrointestinal fluid loss in surgical clients makes them susceptible to hypokalemia.*

- Recognize that the surgical client may develop hyponatremia related to inappropriate antidiuretic hormone secretion, which can be caused by trauma, thrombosis, abscesses, hemorrhages, or hematomas. *Antidiuretic hormone, which acts on the kidneys to control water loss and retention, is an important factor in surgical clients under stress (Metheny, 2000).*
- Clients undergoing abdominal lavage should be monitored for hyperchloremic acidosis. **EB:** *Large amounts of irrigation fluid may possibly result in hyperchloremic acidosis (Scheingraber et al, 2004).*
- Monitor the surgical client for signs and symptoms of hyponatremia: nausea, confusion, disorientation, muscle twitching, seizures, hypovolemia, tachycardia, and/or hypotension. *Risk factors for hyponatremia include prolonged surgery, large tissue resection, and excessive height of the irrigation reservoir, which, in turn, causes the fluid to be introduced into the body under high pressure (Rose, 2001).* **EB:** *In a study of 12 clients who underwent surgical procedures lasting more than 4 hours, metabolic acidosis was found to occur in relation to chloride administration, which was probably from the normal saline IV, because there was no increase in plasma volume (Waters et al, 1999).*
- Accurately measure blood loss intraoperatively. *Weighing sponges is a reliable means of estimating blood loss and gauging replacement needs (Rothrock, 2003). Estimates of intraoperative blood loss can be inaccurate and lead to inappropriate fluid management (Kreimeier, 2000).* **EB:** *Maximizing cardiac output as a result of optimizing fluid management leads to improved surgical outcomes (McFall, Woods & Wakeling, 2004).*
- Provide appropriate supplies, instruments, and techniques to control hemorrhage (Beyea, 2002).
- Recognize that evidence-based procedure-specific protocols for administration of fluid postoperatively are unavailable (Kehlet & Dahl, 2003).
- Accurate postoperative assessment and fluid management should include traditional intake and output measurement as well as monitoring of the client's weight, laboratory values, and checks of peripheral pulses. *Measurement of intake and output may be of limited use for fluid balance determination because input could be much higher then output (van Wissen & Breton, 2004). Poor peripheral pulses are a good indication that blood volume is inadequate, and volume deficit is indicated when the extremities are cool and cyanosed and have poor capillary refill (van Wissen & Breton, 2004).* **EBN:** *To ensure adequate hydration of the client and safe nursing practice, it is necessary for postoperative fluid replacement to occur (Hughes, 2004).*

Geriatric

- Be especially vigilant when monitoring vital signs and fluids in elderly surgical clients. *Fluid intake in the geriatric client should be at least 1500 mL. Some geriatric clients limit fluid intake because of the fear of incontinence, inability to drink on their own, altered sensorium/cognition, or decreased thirst as a part of the aging process (Phillips, 2004). Because the aging process causes a decrease in thirst, once a geriatric client experiences thirst, he or she may have a severe water deficit (Ferry, 2005).* **EB:** *Geriatric clients have a higher risk of developing dehydration than younger clients (Ferry, 2005).*
- Assess preoperatively for symptoms of dehydration: weakness, dizziness, dry mouth, sunken eyes and cheeks, concentrated urine, and decreased skin turgor. *The elderly are predisposed to deficient fluid volume because of decreased fluid in the body, decreased thirst sensation, and decreased ability to concentrate urine (Suhayda & Walton, 2002; Bennett, 2000).* **EB:** *Dehydrated geriatric clients who are to undergo surgery should receive IV fluids preoperatively in an effort to prevent complications from dehydration (Phillips, 2004).*
- Ensure that when food intake is reduced or limited it is compensated with an increase in water/fluid intake. **EB:** *Food contains water, thus any reduction in food intake also involves a reduction in water intake (Ferry, 2005). Anorexia increases the risk of dehydration; the geriatric client is frequently anorexic (Ferry, 2005).*
- Check skin turgor of the elderly client on the forehead, sternum, or inner thigh; also look for the presence of longitudinal tongue furrows and dry mucous membranes. *Elderly people commonly have decreased skin turgor from normal age-related loss of elasticity; therefore checking skin turgor on the arm is not reflective of fluid volume (Suhayda & Walton, 2002).*
- Encourage fluid intake regularly to cognitively impaired clients. *The elderly have a decreased thirst sensation (Metheny, 2000), and short-term memory loss may impede the client's memory of fluid intake.*
- Incorporate regular hydration into daily routines, such as providing an extra glass of fluid with

F

medication or during social activities. Consider using a beverage cart and a hydration assistant to routinely offer beverages to clients in extended care facilities. **EBN and EB:** *Institution of a beverage cart with a trained hydration assistant resulted in an increased number of bowel movements and decreased laxative use, number of falls, urinary tract infections, respiratory infections, and skin breakdown (Robinson & Rosher, 2002). Verbal prompting and offering preferred fluids resulted in increased fluid intake among nursing home residents (Simmons, Alessi & Schnelle, 2001).*

- Note the color of urine and compare against a urine color chart to monitor adequate fluid intake. **EBN:** *Urine color significantly correlates with urine osmolality, serum sodium, and BUN/creatinine ratio (Wakefield, Mentes & Diggelman, 2002).*
- Monitor elderly clients for excess fluid volume during the treatment of deficient fluid volume: listen to lung sounds, watch for edema, and note vital signs. *The elderly client has a decreased ability to adapt to rapid increases in intravascular volume and can quickly develop fluid overload (Allison & Lobo, 2004).*

Pediatric

- Administer fluids preoperatively until NPO status must be initiated so that fluid deficit is decreased. **EB:** *Recommendations for pediatric NPO times have been revised to allow clear liquids up to 2 hours preoperatively for pediatric clients <6 months age and up to 3 hours preoperatively for pediatric clients 6 months and older (Aker, 2002).*

evolve   See the EVOLVE website for World Wide Web resources for client education.

REFERENCES

Aker J: Pediatric fluid management, *Curr Rev Pain* 24(7):73-84, 2002.

Allison SP, Lobo DN: Fluid and electrolytes in the elderly, *Curr Opin Clin Nutr Metab Care* 7(1):27, 2004.

Belloni C: Intraoperative complications of 697 consecutive operative hysteroscopies, *Minerva Ginecol* 53(1):13, 2001.

Bennett JA: Dehydration: hazards and benefits, *Geriatric Nursing* 21(2):84, 2000.

Beyea S: Fluid/electrolyte/acid-base balances. *Perioperative nursing data set: the perioperative nursing vocabulary*, ed 2, Denver, 2002, The Association of Perioperative Nursing.

Brandstrup B: Fluid therapy for the surgical patient, *Best Pract Res Clin Anaesthesiol* 20(2):265-283, 2006.

Cooper JM, Brady RM: Intraoperative and early postoperative complications of operative hysteroscopy, *Obstet Gynecol Clin North Am* 23(2):347-365, 2000.

Edlund BJ: Fluid and electrolyte imbalances, *The Learning Scope* 5(15):17, 2003.

Farthing MJ: Oral rehydrations: an evolving solution, *J Pediatr Gastroenterol Nutr* 34(suppl 1):S64, 2002.

Ferry M: Strategies for ensuring good hydration in the elderly, *Nutr Rev* 63(6):S22, 2005.

Gan TJ, Soppitt A, Maroof M et al: Goal-directed intraoperative fluid administration reduces length of hospital stay after major surgery, *Anesthesiology* 97(4):820, 2002.

Gordon AG: Complications of hysteroscopy. In *WHO Collaborating Centre in Education and Research in Human Reproduction*, Geneva Switzerland, 2003, The Foundation.

Holte K, Sharrock NE, Kehlet H: Pathophysiology and clinical implications of perioperative fluid excess, *Br J Anaesth* 89(4):622-632, 2002.

Hughes E: Principles of post-operative patient care, *Nurs Stand* 19(5):43-51, 2004.

Joshi GP: Intraoperative fluid restriction improves outcome after major elective gastrointestinal surgery, *Anesth Analg* 101(2):601-605, 2005.

Kasper DL, Braunwald E, Fauci AS et al: *Harrison's principles of internal medicine*, ed 16, Philadelphia, 2005, McGraw-Hill.

Kehlet H, Dahl JB: Anaesthesia, surgery, and challenges in postoperative recovery. *Lancet* 362(9399):1921-1928, 2003.

Kreimeier U: Pathophysiology of fluid imbalance, *Crit Care* 4(suppl 2):S3-S7, 2000.

Kruse JA, Mitchell P, Fine R et al: *Saunders manual of critical care*, St Louis, 2003, Saunders.

Kukreja RA, Desai MR, Sabnis RB et al: Fluid absorption during percutaneous nephrolithotomy: does it matter? *J Endourol* 16(4):221-224, 2002.

McFall MR, Woods GA, Wakeling HG: The use of oesophageal Doppler cardiac output measurement to optimize fluid management during colorectal surgery [letter], *Eur J Anaesthesiol* 21(7):581, 2004.

Metheny N: *Fluid and electrolyte balance: nursing considerations*, ed 4, Philadelphia, 2000, Lippincott.

Mitchell G, Hucker T, Venn R et al: Pathophysiology and clinical implications of perioperative fluid excess [letter], *Br J Anaesth* 90(3):395, 2003.

Phillips N: *Berry & Kohn's operating room technique*, ed 10, St Louis, 2004, Mosby.

Robinson SB, Rosher RB: Can a beverage cart help improve hydration? *Geriatr Nurs* 23(4):208-211, 2002.

Rose BD: *Hyponatremia following transurethral resection or laparoscopic irrigation*, www.uptodateonline.com, accessed October 2001.

Rothrock J: *Alexander's care of the patient in surgery*, ed 12, St Louis, 2003, Mosby.

Scheingraber S, Boehme J, Scharbert G et al: Monitoring of acid-base and regulating variables during abdominal lavage, *Anaesth Intensive Care* 32(5):637-643, 2004.

Schulman C: End points of resuscitation: choosing the right parameters to monitor, *Dimens Crit Care Nurs* 21:1, 2002.

Shirreffs SM, Merson SJ, Fraser SM et al: The effects of fluid restriction on hydration status and subjective feelings in man, *Br J Nutr* 91(6):951, 2004.

Simmons SF, Alessi C, Schnelle JF: An intervention to increase fluid intake in nursing home residents: prompting and preference compliance, *J Am Geriatr Soc* 49(7):926, 2001.

Suhayda R, Walton JC: Preventing and managing dehydration, *Medsurg Nurs* 11(6):267, 2002.

Van Wissen K, Breton C: Perioperative influences on fluid distribution. *Medsurg Nurs* 13(5):304-311, 2004.

Wakefield B, Mentes J, Diggelmann L et al: Monitoring hydration status in elderly veterans, *West J Nurs Res* 24(2):132, 2002.

Waters JH, Miller LR, Clack S et al: Cause of metabolic acidosis in prolonged surgery, *Crit Care Med* 27(10):2142, 1999.

Impaired Gas exchange   *Julie T. Sanford, PhD, RN, and Mike Jacobs, DNS, RN*

G

NANDA   Definition

Excess or deficit in oxygenation and/or carbon dioxide elimination at the alveolar-capillary membrane

Defining Characteristics

Abnormal arterial blood gases; abnormal arterial pH; abnormal breathing (e.g., rate, rhythm, depth); abnormal skin color (e.g., pale, dusky); confusion; cyanosis (in neonates only); decreased carbon dioxide; diaphoresis; dyspnea; headache upon awakening; hypercapnia; hypercarbia; hypoxemia; hypoxia; irritability; nasal flaring; restlessness; somnolence; tachycardia; visual disturbances

Related Factors (r/t)

Alveolar-capillary membrane changes; ventilation-perfusion imbalance

NOC   Outcomes (Nursing Outcomes Classification)

Suggested NOC Outcomes

Respiratory Status: Gas Exchange, Ventilation

Example NOC Outcome with Indicators
Achieves appropriate **Respiratory Status: Gas Exchange** as evidenced by the following indicators: Cognitive status/Partial pressure of oxygen/Partial pressure of carbon dioxide/Arterial pH/Oxygen saturation (Rate the outcome and indicators of **Respiratory Status:** 1 = severely compromised, 2 = substantially compromised, 3 = moderately compromised, 4 = mildly compromised, 5 = not compromised [see Section I].)

Client Outcomes

Client Will (Specify Time Frame):

- Demonstrate improved ventilation and adequate oxygenation as evidenced by blood gas levels within normal parameters for that client.
- Maintain clear lung fields and remain free of signs of respiratory distress.
- Verbalize understanding of oxygen supplementation and other therapeutic interventions.

NIC   Interventions (Nursing Interventions Classification)

Suggested NIC Interventions

Acid-Base Management, Airway Management

Example NIC Activities—Acid-Base Management
Monitor for symptoms of respiratory failure (e.g., low PaO_2 and elevated $PaCO_2$ levels and respiratory muscle fatigue); monitor determinants of tissue oxygen delivery (e.g., PaO_2, SaO_2, hemoglobin levels, and cardiac output) if available

• = Independent;   ▲ = Collaborative;   EBN = Evidence-Based Nursing;   EB = Evidence-Based

Nursing Interventions and *Rationales*

- Monitor respiratory rate, depth, and effort, including use of accessory muscles, nasal flaring, and abnormal breathing patterns. *Increased respiratory rate, use of accessory muscles, nasal flaring, abdominal breathing, and a look of panic in the client's eyes may be seen with hypoxia.*
- Auscultate breath sounds every 1 to 2 hours. The presence of crackles and wheezes may alert the nurse to airway obstruction, which may lead to or exacerbate existing hypoxia. *In severe exacerbations of chronic obstructive pulmonary disease (COPD), lung sounds may be diminished or distant with air trapping (Zampella, 2003).*
- Monitor the client's behavior and mental status for the onset of restlessness, agitation, confusion, and (in the late stages) extreme lethargy. *Changes in behavior and mental status can be early signs of impaired gas exchange (Simmons & Simmons, 2004). In the late stages the client becomes lethargic and somnolent.*
- Monitor oxygen saturation continuously by pulse oximetry. Note blood gas results as available. *An oxygen saturation of less than 90% (normal, 95% to 100%) or a PaO$_2$ of less than 80 mm Hg (normal, 80 to 100 mm Hg) indicates significant oxygenation problems (Clark, Giuliano & Chen, 2006). The goal of inpatient therapy for the client with COPD is to maintain the oxygen saturation greater than 90% and PaO$_2$ at or above 80 mm Hg to maintain cellular oxygenation (Celli, MacNee & ATS/ERS Task Force, 2004).*
- Observe for cyanosis of the skin; especially note color of the tongue and oral mucous membranes. *Central cyanosis of the tongue and oral mucosa is indicative of serious hypoxia and is a medical emergency. Peripheral cyanosis in the extremities may or may not be serious (Kasper, 2005).*
- Position clients in semi-Fowler's position, with an upright posture at 45 degrees if possible. **EB:** *Research done on clients on a ventilator demonstrated that being in a 45-degree upright position increased oxygenation and ventilation (Speelberg & Van Beers, 2003). In a mechanically ventilated client, there is a decreased incidence of pneumonia if the client is positioned at a 45-degree semirecumbent position as opposed to a supine position (Seckel, 2007).*
- If the client has unilateral lung disease, alternate semi-Fowler's position in an upright posture with a lateral position (with 10- to 15-degree elevation and "good lung down") for 60 to 90 minutes. This method is contraindicated for clients with pulmonary abscess, hemorrhage, or interstitial emphysema. *Gravity and hydrostatic pressure allow the dependent lung to become better ventilated and perfused, which increases oxygenation (Marklew, 2006).*
- If the client has bilateral lung disease, position the client in either semi-Fowler's or a side-lying position, which increases oxygenation as indicated by pulse oximetry (or, if the client has a pulmonary catheter, venous oxygen saturation).
- Turn the client every 2 hours. Monitor mixed venous oxygen saturation closely after turning. If it drops below 10% or fails to return to baseline promptly, return the client to the supine position and evaluate oxygen status. If the client does not tolerate turning, consider use of a kinetic bed that rotates the client from side to side in a turn of at least 40 degrees. **EBN:** *Use of the kinetic bed was shown to decrease development of atelectasis and ventilator-associated pneumonia in critically ill clients (Ahrens et al, 2004). Rotational therapy may decrease the incidence of pneumonia but has little affect on mortality rates, number of days on ventilator, or number of days in the intensive care unit (Goldhill et al, 2007).*
- If the client is obese or has ascites, consider positioning the client in reverse Trendelenburg position at 45 degrees for periods as tolerated. **EBN:** *Use of reverse Trendelenburg position at 45 degrees results in increased tidal volumes and decreased respiratory rates in a group of intubated clients with obesity, abdominal distention, and ascites (Burns et al, 1994).*
- ▲ If the client has adult respiratory distress syndrome or difficulty maintaining oxygenation, consider positioning the client prone with the upper thorax and pelvis supported, allowing the abdomen to protrude. Monitor oxygen saturation and turn back to supine position if desaturation occurs. **EBN and EB:** *Oxygenation levels have been shown to improve in the prone position, probably because of decreased shunting and better perfusion of the lungs (Curley, Thompson & Arnold, 2000; Mure, Martling & Lindahl, 1997; Michaels et al, 2002; Marklew, 2006).*
- If the client is acutely dyspneic, consider having the client lean forward over a bedside table if tolerated. *Leaning forward can help decrease dyspnea, possibly because gastric pressure allows better*

• = Independent;   ▲ = Collaborative;   EBN = Evidence-Based Nursing;   EB = Evidence-Based

contraction of the diaphragm (Celli, 1998). This is called the tripod position and is used during times of distress (Zampella, 2003).

- Help the client deep breathe and perform controlled coughing. Have the client inhale deeply, hold the breath for several seconds, and cough two or three times with the mouth open while tightening the upper abdominal muscles as tolerated. *Controlled coughing uses the diaphragmatic muscles, which makes the cough more forceful and effective.* NOTE: If the client has excessive fluid in the respiratory system, see the interventions for **ineffective Airway clearance.**

▲ Monitor the effects of sedation and analgesics on the client's respiratory pattern; use judiciously. *Both analgesics and medications that cause sedation can depress respiration at times. However, these medications can be helpful for decreasing the sympathetic nervous system discharge that accompanies hypoxia.*

- Schedule nursing care to provide rest and minimize fatigue. *The hypoxic client has limited reserves; inappropriate activity can increase hypoxia.*

▲ Administer humidified oxygen through an appropriate device (e.g., nasal cannula or Venturi mask per the physician's order); aim for an oxygen saturation level of 90%. Watch for onset of hypoventilation as evidenced by increased somnolence. *There is a fine line between ideal or excessive oxygen therapy; increasing somnolence is caused by retention of carbon dioxide (CO_2) leading to CO_2 narcosis (Simmons & Simmons, 2004).*

- Assess nutritional status, including serum albumin level and body mass index (BMI). *Weight loss in a client with COPD has a negative effect on the course of the disease; it can result in loss of muscle mass in the respiratory muscles, including the diaphragm, which can lead to respiratory failure (Berry & Baum, 2001; Celli et al, 2004).* **EB:** *Being underweight, with a BMI of less than 21, has been associated with increased mortality rate in clients with COPD (Schols et al, 1995).*

- Help the client eat frequent small meals and use dietary supplements as necessary. For some clients, drinking 30 mL of a supplement such as Ensure or Pulmocare every hour while awake can be helpful. **EB:** *Improved nutrition can help increase muscle aerobic capacity and exercise tolerance (Palange et al, 1995).* **EBN:** *Nutritional problems in clients with COPD can be visual; early identification of clients at risk is essential to maintaining BMI. Subjective reports of hunger, company at mealtimes, and time can decrease clients' nutritional intake. Assistance with meal preparation, from shopping to cooking and arranging Meals on Wheels, also results in improved nutritional status (Odencrants, Ehnfors & Grobe, 2005).*

- If the client is severely debilitated from chronic respiratory disease, consider the use of a wheeled walker to help in ambulation. **EB:** *Use of a wheeled walker has been shown to result in significant decrease in disability, hypoxemia, and breathlessness during a 6-minute walk test (Honeyman, Barr & Stubbing, 1996). A study found that clients with COPD should titrate their exercise to breathlessness to achieve a peak level of tolerance (Turner et al, 2004).*

▲ Watch for signs of psychological distress, including anxiety, agitation, and insomnia. Refer for counseling as needed. **EBN:** *There is a clear association between hospitalization for COPD and psychological distress (Andenaes, Kalfoss & Wahl, 2004).*

▲ Refer the client with COPD to a pulmonary rehabilitation program. **EB:** *Outpatient rehabilitation programs can achieve worthwhile benefits, including decreased perception of dyspnea, increased physical performance, and improved quality of life (Verrill et al, 2005). Pulmonary rehabilitation programs resulted in an improvement in depression, a decrease in symptoms, increase in ADLs, and an improvement in reports of dyspnea (Paz-Diaz et al, 2007).* NOTE: If the client becomes ventilator dependent, see the care plan for **Impaired spontaneous Ventilation.**

Geriatric

▲ Use central nervous system (CNS) depressants carefully to avoid decreasing respiration rate. *An elderly client is prone to respiratory depression.*

▲ Maintain low-flow oxygen therapy. *An elderly client is susceptible to oxygen-induced respiratory depression.*

Home Care

- Assess the home environment for irritants that impair gas exchange. Help the client adjust the home environment as necessary (e.g., install an air filter to decrease the level of dust).

• = Independent;   ▲ = Collaborative;   EBN = Evidence-Based Nursing;   EB = Evidence-Based

▲ Refer the client to occupational therapy as necessary to help the client adapt the home and environment and conserve energy.

• Help the client identify and avoid situations that exacerbate impairment of gas exchange (e.g., stress-related situations, exposure to pollution of any kind, proximity to noxious gas fumes such as chlorine bleach). *Irritants in the environment decrease the client's effectiveness in accessing oxygen during breathing.*

• Refer to GOLD and ACP-ASIM/ACCP guidelines for management of home care and indications of hospital admission criteria (Chojnowski, 2003).

• Instruct the client to keep the home temperature above 68° F (20° C) and avoid cold weather. *Cold air temperatures cause constriction of the blood vessels and increased moisture, which impairs the client's ability to absorb oxygen.*

• Instruct the client to limit exposure to persons with respiratory infections.

• Instruct the family in the complications of the disease and the importance of maintaining the medical regimen, including when to call a physician.

▲ Refer the client for home health aide services as necessary for assistance with activities of daily living. *Clients with decreased oxygenation have decreased energy to carry out personal and role-related activities.*

• When respiratory procedures are being implemented, explain equipment and procedures to family members and provide needed emotional support. *Family members assuming responsibility for respiratory monitoring often find this stressful. They may not have been able to assimilate fully any instructions provided by hospital staff (McNeal, 2000).*

• When electrically based equipment for respiratory support is being implemented, evaluate home environment for electrical safety, proper grounding, and so forth. Ensure that notification is sent to the local utility company, the emergency medical team, and police and fire departments. *Notification is important to provide priority service (McNeal, 2000).*

▲ Assess family role changes and coping ability. Refer the client to medical social services as appropriate for assistance in adjusting to chronic illness. *Inability to maintain the level of social involvement experienced before illness leads to frustration and anger in the client and may create a threat to the family unit.* **EBN:** *Clients with COPD reported that breathlessness was the most troublesome symptom, causing feelings of frustration and fatigue leading to loss of social activity, loss of the family role, and loss of intimacy in personal relationships (Barnett, 2005).*

• Support the family of the client with chronic illness. *Severely compromised respiratory functioning causes fear and anxiety in clients and their families. Reassurance from the nurse can be helpful.*

Client/Family Teaching

• Teach the client how to perform pursed-lip breathing, controlled diaphragmatic breathing, and how to use the tripod position. Have the client watch the pulse oximeter to note improvement in oxygenation with these breathing techniques. *The controlled breathing technique can help increase sputum clearance and decrease cough spasms (Donahue, 2002; Nursing2004, 2004). Controlled coughing uses the diaphragmatic muscles, making the cough more forceful and effective.* **EB:** *Pursed-lip breathing reduces end-expiratory volume and breathlessness (Bianchi et al, 2004).*

• Teach the client energy conservation techniques and the importance of alternating rest periods with activity. See nursing interventions for **Fatigue. EBN:** *Fatigue is a common symptom of COPD and needs to be assessed and managed (Theander & Unosson, 2004).*

▲ Teach the importance of not smoking:
  ▪ Be very clear in approach, and ask the client to set a date for smoking cessation.
  ▪ Recommend pharmacological support or else contraindicated (nicotine replacement therapy or antidepressant).
  ▪ Refer the client to smoking-cessation programs.
  ▪ Encourage clients who relapse to keep trying to quit.
  Clinicians need to address smoking cessation at every entry into the healthcare system (U.S. Public Health Service, 2003). **EB:** *Giving up smoking can slow the course of disease, and some clients may regain some lung function (Willemse et al, 2004). A combination of psychosocial and pharmacological interventions was more effective than either intervention alone to stop smoking behavior (van der Meer et al, 2003).*

▲ Instruct the family regarding home oxygen therapy if ordered (e.g., delivery system, liter flow, safety precautions). *Long-term oxygen therapy can improve survival, exercise ability, sleep, and ability to think in hypoxemic clients. Client education improves compliance with prescribed use of oxygen (Celli et al, 2004).*

• Teach the client the need to receive a yearly influenza vaccine (Centers for Disease Control and Prevention, 2006). **EB:** *Receiving the vaccine may reduce exacerbations of COPD (Miller, 2005).*

• Teach the client relaxation techniques to help reduce stress responses and panic attacks resulting from dyspnea. **EB:** *Relaxation therapy can help reduce dyspnea and anxiety (National Lung Health Education Program, 2007).*

• Teach the client to use music along with a rest period to decrease dyspnea and anxiety. **EBN:** *Use of music along with a resting period is effective in relieving anxiety and exercise-induced dyspnea in clients with COPD (Sidani et al, 2004).*

evolve   See the EVOLVE website for World Wide Web resources for client education.

REFERENCES

Ahrens T, Kollef M, Stewart J et al: Effect of kinetic therapy on pulmonary complications, *Am J Crit Care* 13(5):376-383, 2004.

Andenaes R, Kalfoss MH, Wahl A: Psychological distress and quality of life in hospitalized patients with chronic obstructive pulmonary disease, *J Adv Nurs* 46(5):523-530, 2004.

Barnett M: Chronic obstructive pulmonary disease: a phenomenological study of patients' experiences, *J Clin Nurs* 14(7):805-812, 2005.

Berry JK, Baum CL: Malnutrition in chronic obstructive pulmonary disease: adding insult to injury, *AACN Clin Issues* 12(2):210-219, 2001.

Bianchi R, Gigliotti F, Romagnoli I et al: Chest wall kinematics and breathlessness during pursed-lip breathing in patients with COPD, *Chest* 125(2):459-465, 2004.

Burns SM, Egloff MB, Ryan B et al: Effect of body position on spontaneous respiratory rate and tidal volume in patients with obesity, abdominal distention and ascites, *Am J Crit Care* 3(2):102-106, 1994.

Celli BR: Pulmonary rehabilitation for COPD. A practical approach for improving ventilatory conditioning, *Postgrad Med* 103(4):159, 1998.

Celli BR, MacNee W, ATS/ERS Task Force: Standards for the diagnosis and treatment of patients with COPD: a summary of the ATS/ERS position paper, *Eur Respir J* 23(6):932-946, 2004.

Centers for Disease Control and Prevention: Prevention and control of influenza: recommendations of the advisory committee on immunization practices, *MMWR Recommendations and Reports* 55(RR10):1, 2006.

Chojnowski D: "GOLD" standards for acute exacerbation in COPD, *Nurs Pract* 28(5):26, 2003.

Clark AP, Giuliano K, Chen HM: Pulse oximetry revisited: "but his O(2) sat was normal!" *Clin Nurs Spec* 20(6):268-272, 2006.

Curley MA, Thompson JE, Arnold JH: The effects of early and repeated prone positioning in pediatric patients with acute lung injury, *Chest* 118(1):156-163, 2000.

Donahue M: "Spare the cough, spoil the airway": back to the basics in airway clearance, *Pediatr Nurs* 28(2):107-111, 2002.

Goldhill DR, Imhoff M, McLean B et al: Rotational bed therapy to prevent and treat respiratory complications: a review and meta-analysis, *Am J Crit Care* 16(1):50-61, 2007.

Honeyman P, Barr P, Stubbing DG: Effect of a walking aid on disability, oxygenation, and breathlessness in patients with chronic airflow limitation, *J Cardiopulm Rehabil* 16(1):63-67, 1996.

Kasper DL: *Harrison's principles of internal medicine*, ed 16, New York, 2005, McGraw Hill.

Marklew A: Body positioning and its effect on oxygenation—a literature review, *Br Assoc Crit Care Nurs* 11(1):16-22, 2006.

McNeal GJ: *AACN guide to acute care procedures in the home*, Philadelphia, 2000, Lippincott.

Michaels AJ, Wanek SM, Dreifuss BA et al: A protocolized approach to pulmonary failure and the role of intermittent prone positioning, *J Trauma* 52(6):1037-1047, 2002.

Miller KE: Effectiveness of influenza vaccine in patients with COPD, *Am Fam Phys* 71(7):1412, 2005.

Mure M, Martling CR, Lindahl SG: Dramatic effect on oxygenation in patients with severe acute lung insufficiency treated in the prone position, *Crit Care Med* 25(9):1539-1544, 1997.

National Lung Health Education Program: A breath of fresh air, *Consum Rep Health* 19(2):3, 2007.

Odencrants S, Ehnfors M, Grobe SJ: Living with chronic obstructive pulmonary disease: part 1. Struggling with meal-related situations: experiences among persons with COPD, *Scand J Caring Sci* (19):230-239, 2005.

Palange P, Forte S, Felli A et al: Nutritional state and exercise tolerance in patients with COPD, *Chest* 107(5):1206-1212, 1995.

Paz-Diaz H, Montes de Oca M, Lopez JM et al: Pulmonary rehabilitation improves depression, anxiety, dyspnea and health status in patients with COPD, *Am J Phys Med Rehab* 86(1):30-36, 2007.

Respiratory challenge, *Nursing2004* 34(11):70, 2004.

Schols AM, Soeters PB, Mostert R et al: Physiologic effects of nutritional support and anabolic steroids in patients with chronic obstructive pulmonary disease. A placebo-controlled randomized trial, *Am J Respir Crit Care Med* 152(4 pt 1):1268-1274, 1995.

Seckel M: Implementing evidence-based practice guidelines to minimize ventilator-associated pneumonia, *AACN News* 24(1):8-10, 2007.

Sidani S et al: Evaluating the effects of music on dyspnea and anxiety on patients with COPD, *Int Nurs Perspect* 4(1):5-13, 2004.

Simmons P, Simmons M: Informed nursing practice: the administration of oxygen to patients with COPD, *Medsurg Nurs* 13(2):82-85, 2004.

Speelberg B, Van Beers F: Artificial ventilation in the semi-recumbent position improves oxygenation and gas exchange, *Chest* 124(4):203S, 2003.

Theander K, Unosson M: Fatigue in patients with chronic obstructive pulmonary disease, *J Adv Nurs* 45(2):172-177, 2004.

Turner SE, Eastwood PR, Cecins NM et al: Physiologic responses to incremental and self-paced exercise in COPD, *Chest* 126(3):766-773, 2004.

U.S. Public Health Service: *Treating tobacco use and dependence—clini-*

• = Independent;   ▲ = Collaborative;   EBN = Evidence-Based Nursing;   EB = Evidence-Based

cian's packet. A how-to guide for implementing the Public Health Service Clinical Practice Guideline, 2003, www.surgeongeneral.gov/tobacco/clinpack.html, accessed February 7, 2007.

van der Meer RM, Wagena EJ, Ostelo RW et al: Smoking cessation for chronic obstructive pulmonary disease, *Cochrane Database Syst Rev* (2):CD002999, 2003.

Verrill D, Barton C, Beasley W et al: The effects of short-term and long-term pulmonary rehabilitation on functional capacity, perceived dyspnea, and quality of life, *Chest* 128(2):673-683, 2005.

Willemse BW, ten Hacken NH, Rutgers B et al: Smoking cessation improves both direct and indirect airway hyperresponsiveness in COPD, *Eur Respir J* 24(3):391-436, 2004.

Zampella MA: COPD: managing flare-ups, *RN* 14:14, 2003.

Risk for unstable blood Glucose   *Paula D. Hopper, MSN, RN*

NANDA   Definition

Risk for variation of blood glucose/sugar levels from the normal range

Risk Factors

Deficient knowledge of diabetes management (e.g., action plan); developmental level; dietary intake; inadequate blood glucose monitoring; lack of acceptance of diagnosis; lack of adherence to diabetes management (e.g., action plan); lack of diabetes management (e.g., action plan); medication management; mental health status; physical activity level; physical health status; pregnancy; rapid growth periods; stress; weight gain; weight loss

NOC   Outcomes (Nursing Outcomes Classification)

Suggested NOC Outcome

Blood Glucose Level

Example NOC Outcome with Indicators
Blood Glucose Level as evidenced by the following indicators: Blood glucose/Glycosylated hemoglobin/Fructosamine/Urine glucose/Urine ketones (Rate the outcome and indicators of **Blood Glucose Level:** 1 = severe deviation from normal range, 2 = substantial deviation from normal range, 3 = moderate deviation from normal range, 4 = mild deviation from normal range, 5 = no deviation from normal range [see Section I].)

Client Outcomes

Client Will (Specify Time Frame):

- Maintain preprandial blood glucose level between 90 and 130 mg/dL (American Diabetes Association [ADA], 2007); consult primary care provider for client-specific goals
- Maintain postprandial glucose level less than 180 mg/dL (ADA, 2007)
- Maintain hemoglobin A1c level <7% (normal, 4%-6%) (ADA, 2007)
- Maintain blood glucose level as close as possible to 110 mg/dL if critically ill (ADA, 2007)
- In gestational diabetes, maintain fasting blood glucose level ≤105 mg/dL, 1-hour after the meal (pc) level ≤155 mg/dL, and 2-hour pc level ≤130 mg/dL (ADA, 2004)
- Demonstrate how to test blood glucose accurately
- Identify self-care actions to take if blood glucose level is too low or too high
- Demonstrate correct administration of prescribed medications

NIC   Interventions (Nursing Interventions Classification)

Suggested NIC Interventions

Hypoglycemia Management, Hyperglycemia Management

Example NIC Activities—Hypoglycemia Management
Monitor blood glucose levels, as indicated; Provide simple carbohydrates, as indicated

● = Independent;   ▲ = Collaborative;   EBN = Evidence-Based Nursing;   EB = Evidence-Based

Nursing Interventions and *Rationales*

- Monitor blood glucose before meals and at bedtime. *Clients using multiple insulin injections should perform self-monitoring of blood glucose three or more times daily. Self-monitoring of blood glucose is also useful for clients on less-intensive therapy to reach blood glucose goals (ADA, 2007).*
- Monitor blood glucose every 4 to 6 hours in clients with a nothing-by-mouth order or who are continuously fed. *Testing every 4 to 6 hours usually is sufficient for determining correction insulin doses (ADA, 2007).*
- Monitor blood glucose level hourly for clients on continuous insulin drips; may decrease to every 2 hours once stable. *Bedside monitoring can be done rapidly, where therapeutic decisions are made (ADA, 2007).*
- Evaluate hemoglobin A1c level for glucose control over the previous 2 to 3 months. *"All clients with diabetes admitted to the hospital should have an A1c obtained for discharge planning if the result of testing in the previous 2 to 3 months is not available" (ADA, 2007).*
- Monitor for signs and symptoms of hypoglycemia. Rapidly falling blood glucose level can cause sympathetic symptoms such as anxiety, dizziness, diaphoresis, tachycardia, headache, tremor, or hunger. *Confusion, irritability, lethargy, or behavior changes may signal low glucose level in the central nervous system, which can lead to coma if not treated. Early recognition and treatment of falling glucose level can prevent more severe hypoglycemia (Tomky, 2005).*
- Be alert to hypoglycemia in clients with heart failure, renal or liver disease, malignancy, infection, sepsis, sudden reduction of corticosteroids, altered ability to self-report symptoms, reduced nutritional intake, emesis, new nothing-by-mouth status, or altered consciousness. *Clients may develop hypoglycemia in relation to these conditions (ADA, 2007).*
- If a client is experiencing signs and symptoms of hypoglycemia, test glucose. If the result is below 70 mg/dL, administer 15 to 20 g glucose (½ cup fruit juice or regular [not diet] soda, 1 cup milk, 1 small piece of fruit, or 3 to 4 glucose tablets). Repeat test in 60 minutes or if symptoms recur. *"Ten grams oral glucose raise plasma glucose levels by about 40 mg/dL over 30 minutes, while 20 g oral glucose raises plasma glucose levels by about 60 mg/dL over 45 minutes. In each case, glucose levels often begin to fall about 60 minutes after ingestion. Adding protein to carbohydrate does not affect the glycemic response and does not prevent subsequent hypoglycemia" (ADA, 2007).*
- Administer intravenous 50% dextrose or intramuscular glucagon according to agency protocol if client is hypoglycemic and is unable to take oral carbohydrate. *Intravenous bolus of 50% dextrose or intramuscular glucagon is an alternative to oral carbohydrate (Tomky, 2005).*
- Monitor for signs and symptoms of hyperglycemia, such as polydipsia, polyuria, and polyphagia. *Early recognition and treatment of hyperglycemia can prevent progression to ketoacidosis or hyperosmolar hyperglycemia (ADA, 2004).*
- Test urine for ketones during acute illness or stress or when blood glucose levels are >300 mg/dL. *"The presence of ketones may indicate impending or even established ketoacidosis, a condition that requires immediate medical attention" (ADA, 2004).*
- Maintain tight glucose control in critically ill hospitalized clients. **EB:** *Maintenance of blood glucose levels of 80 to 110 m/dL reduced mortality, sepsis, renal failure, need for transfusion, and polyneuropathy in a study of critically ill clients (Garber et al, 2006). Maintain blood glucose levels as close to 110 mg/dL as possible to improve outcomes (ADA, 2007).*
- If client is acutely ill, continue insulin and oral hypoglycemic agents and frequent monitoring. Assure client is receiving adequate fluids and carbohydrates. **EB:** *"Acute illnesses can lead to the development of hyperglycemia and, in individuals with type 1 diabetes, ketoacidosis. During acute illnesses, with the usual increases in counterregulatory hormones, the need for insulin and oral glucose-lowering medications continues and often is increased. Testing plasma glucose and ketones, drinking adequate amounts of fluid, and ingesting carbohydrate, especially if plasma glucose is <100 mg/dL, are all important during acute illness. In adults, ingestion of 150 to 200 g carbohydrate daily (45 to 50 g every 3 to 4 hours) should be sufficient to prevent starvation ketosis" (ADA, 2007).*
- Prime tubing with 20 mL diluted intravenous insulin solution before initiating insulin drip. *Glucose adsorbs to intravenous tubing; priming with 20 mL is enough to minimize this effect (Goldberg et al, 2006).*

• = Independent;   ▲ = Collaborative;   EBN = Evidence-Based Nursing;   EB = Evidence-Based

- Evaluate the client's medication regimen for medications that can alter blood glucose. *Some antipsychotic agents, diuretics, and glucocorticoids, among others, can cause hyperglycemia. Alcohol, aspirin, and ß-blockers are among agents that can cause hypoglycemia (Bernstein, 2007).*
- Evaluate blood glucose level in hospitalized clients before administering oral hypoglycemic agents or insulin. *"Scheduled prandial (meal) insulin doses should be given in relation to meals and should be adjusted according to point-of-care glucose levels" (ADA, 2007).*
- ▲ Refer client to dietitian for carbohydrate counting instruction. **EB:** *"Monitoring carbohydrate, whether by carbohydrate counting, exchanges, or experience-based estimation, remains a key strategy in achieving glycemic control" (ADA, 2007).*
- ▲ Refer overweight clients to a dietitian for weight loss counseling. **EB:** *"In overweight and obese insulin-resistant individuals, modest weight loss has been shown to improve insulin resistance" (ADA, 2007).*

Geriatric

- Assess possible barriers to following nutrition recommendations: food preferences, ability to prepare meals, dentition, swallowing problems, decreased appetite or thirst sensation, use of taste-altering medications, limited finances, and social isolation. *An individual nutrition plan can minimize barriers in nutrition management and facilitate changes in eating behavior that will result in improved clinical outcomes, improved function, and enhanced quality of life (Suhl & Bonsignore, 2006).*
- Assess for age-related cognitive changes that can impair self-management of diabetes. **EB:** *Some studies suggest that deficits in cognitive functions are associated with poorer glycemic control (Awad, Gagnon & Messier, 2004).*
- Assess for vision and dexterity impairments that may affect the older client's ability to measure insulin doses accurately. *Medication therapy can present a challenge because of possible visual and dexterity impairments (Haas, 2006).*
- Teach client and family caregivers to recognize signs and symptoms of hyperosmolar hyperglycemia. *"Adequate supervision and help from staff or family may prevent many of the admissions for hyperosmolar hyperglycemia due to dehydration among elderly individuals who are unable to recognize or treat this evolving condition" (ADA, 2007).*
- Help client set up pill boxes or reminder system for taking medications. *Therapy may involve many medications and can become confusing (Haas, 2006).*

Pediatric

- Ensure that daycare or school personnel are trained in diabetes management and treatment of emergencies. *"Knowledgeable trained personnel are essential if the student is to avoid the immediate health risks of low blood glucose and to achieve the metabolic control required to decrease risks for later development of diabetes complications" (ADA, 2007).*
- Be aware that young children (<6 or 7 years) may not be aware of symptoms of hypoglycemia. *Counterregulatory mechanisms are immature and may not cause hypoglycemia symptoms; in addition, children may not recognize symptoms (ADA, 2007).*

Home Care

- Teach family how to use an emergency glucagon kit (if prescribed). *Severe hypoglycemia in which client is unable to take oral glucose should be treated with glucagon (ADA, 2007).*

Client Education

- Provide "survival skills" education for hospitalized clients, including information about (1) diabetes and its treatment, (2) medication administration, (3) nutrition therapy, (4) self-monitoring of blood glucose, (5) symptoms and treatment of hypoglycemia, (6) basic foot care, and (7) follow-up appointments for in-depth training. *Clients need enough information to be safely discharged and can then be followed up with outpatient instruction (Nettles, 2005).*
- Educate clients on self-monitoring of blood glucose. **EB:** *A systematic review found that self-monitoring of blood glucose is an effective tool in the self-management of glucose levels in clients using insulin therapy. Clients can use the glucose values to adjust their insulin doses. Clients with type 2 diabetes who are not using insulin can use glucose values to adjust diet and lifestyle (Welschen et al, 2005).*

• = Independent;   ▲ = Collaborative;   EBN = Evidence-Based Nursing;   EB = Evidence-Based

- Educate clients with type 2 diabetes to monitor blood glucose before meals and bedtime. *Intensive self-monitoring of blood glucose can improve glucose control for clients with type 2 diabetes (Murata et al, 2003).*
- ▲ Refer client to a diabetes treatment and teaching program for training in flexible intensive insulin therapy and dietary freedom. Most large hospitals or medical centers offer such programs. *Type 1 diabetes clients at risk for severe hypoglycemia or ketoacidosis had fewer incidents of severe hypoglycemia and ketoacidosis, fewer hospital days, and improved hemoglobin A1c levels after attending a diabetes treatment and teaching program (Samann et al, 2006).*
- ▲ Refer client for blood glucose awareness training for instruction in detection, anticipation, avoidance, and treatment of extremes in blood glucose levels. **EB:** *Blood glucose awareness training has been shown to reduce both hypoglycemia and hyperglycemia significantly (Cox et al, 2006).*
- Teach client to maintain a blood glucose diary. *A diary can help clients learn to associate symptoms with actual glucose readings as well as guide treatment (Cox et al, 2006).*
- Provide group-based training programs for instruction. **EB:** *Adults with type 2 diabetes who participate in group-based training programs have improved fasting blood glucose and hemoglobin A1c levels (Deakin et al, 2005).*
- Educate client about the benefits of smoking cessation. **EB:** *"Smoking has been linked to worsening diabetes control and insulin resistance and may even induce diabetes" (Capri, 2005). Refer to care plan* for **Health-seeking behaviors.**
- Teach client the benefits of regular adherence to prescribed exercise regimen. **EB:** *A systematic review found that "exercise significantly improves glycemic control and reduces visceral adipose tissue and plasma triglycerides, but not plasma cholesterol, in people with type 2 diabetes, even without weight loss" (Thomas, Elliott & Naughton, 2006). At least 150 minutes per week of moderate-intensity aerobic physical activity, and/or at least 90 minutes per week of vigorous aerobic exercise improves glycemic control, helps with weight maintenance, and reduces risk of cerebrovascular disease (ADA, 2007).*
- Teach clients who are treated with insulin that they may need to eat extra carbohydrates before exercise, depending on how exercise affects their blood glucose levels. *A dose of 40 g glucose taken 15 minutes before exercise can prevent hypoglycemia in a client engaging in 60 minutes of moderate exercise (Dube et al, 2005). In individuals taking insulin or oral medications that stimulate insulin secretion, physical activity can cause hypoglycemia if medication dose or carbohydrate consumption is not adjusted (Sigal et al, 2006).*
- Teach client that stopping insulin therapy can lead to hyperglycemic crisis (ketoacidosis or hyperosmolar hyperglycemia). Ensure client has resources to purchase insulin. *Stopping insulin is a common precipitant of diabetic ketoacidosis in African Americans (ADA, 2004).*

REFERENCES

American Diabetes Association: 2004 clinical practice recommendations *Diabetes Care* 27(1):53, 2004.

American Diabetes Association: 2007 clinical practice recommendations *Diabetes Care* 30(1):53, 2007.

Awad N, Gagnon M, Messier C: The relationship between impaired glucose tolerance, type 2 diabetes, and cognitive function, *J Clin Exp Neuropsychol* 26(8):1044-1080, 2004.

Bernstein RK: *Drugs that may affect blood glucose levels*, diabetesincontrol.com/issues/issue246/drugs.pdf, accessed March 17, 2007.

Capri GH et al: Smoking and the incidence of diabetes amongst US adults, *Diabetes Care* 28:2501-2507, 2005.

Cox DJ, Gonder-Frederick L, Ritterband L et al: Blood glucose awareness training: what is it, where is it, and where is it going? *Diabetes Spectr* 19(1):43-49, 2006.

Deakin T, McShane CE, Cade JE et al: Group based training for self-management strategies in people with type 2 diabetes mellitus, *Cochrane Database Systematic Rev* (2):CD003417, 2005.

Dube M, Weisnagel S, Prodhomme D et al: Exercise and newer insulins: how much glucose supplement to avoid hypoglycemia? *Med Sci Sports Exer* 37(8):1276-1282, 2005.

Garber AJ, Moghissi ES, Buonocore D et al: American College of Endocrinology and American Diabetes Association consensus statement on inpatient diabetes and glycemic control: a call to action, *Diabetes Care* 29(8):1955-1962, 2006.

Goldberg PA, Kedves A, Walter K et al: "Waste not, want not": determining the optimal priming volume for intravenous insulin infusions, *Diabetes Technol Ther* 8(5):598-601, 2006.

Haas L: Caring for community-dwelling older adults with diabetes: perspectives from health care providers and caregivers, *Diabetes Spectr* 19(4):240-244, 2006.

Murata GH, Shah JH, Hoffman RM et al: Intensified blood glucose monitoring improves glycemic control in stable, insulin-treated veterans with type 2 diabetes: the diabetes outcomes in veterans study (DOVES), *Diabetes Care* 26(6):1759-1763, 2003.

Nettles A: Patient education in the hospital, *Diabetes Spectr* 18(1):44-48, 2005.

Samann A, Muhlhauser I, Bender R et al: Flexible intensive insulin therapy in adults with type 1 diabetes and high risk for severe hypoglycemia and diabetic ketoacidosis, *Diabetes Care* 29(10):2196-2199, 2006.

Sigal RJ, Kenny GP, Wasserman DH et al: Physical activity/exercise and type 2 diabetes: a consensus statement from the American Diabetes Association, *Diabetes Care* 29(6):1433-1438, 2006.

Suhl E, Bonsignore P: Diabetes self-management education for older adults: general principles and practical application, *Diabetes Spectr* 19(4):234-250, 2006.

Thomas DE, Elliott EJ, Naughton GA: Exercise for type 2 diabetes mellitus, *Cochrane Database Syst Rev* (3):CD002968, 2006.

Tomky D: Detection, prevention, and treatment of hypoglycemia in the hospital, *Diabetes Spectr* 18(1):39-44, 2005.

Welschen LMC, Bloemendal E, Nijpels G et al: Self-monitoring of blood glucose in patients with type 2 diabetes mellitus who are not using insulin, *Cochrane Database Syst Rev* (2):CD005060, 2005.

Grieving   *T. Heather Herdman, RN, PhD*

NANDA   Definition

A normal, complex process that includes emotional, physical, spiritual, social, and intellectual responses and behaviors by which individuals, families, and communities incorporate a loss into their daily lives

Defining Characteristics

Alteration in activity level; alterations in immune function; alterations in neuroendocrine function; alteration in sleep patterns; alteration in dream patterns; anger; blame; detachment; despair; disorganization; experiencing relief; maintaining connection to the deceased; making meaning of the loss; pain; panic behavior; personal growth; psychological distress; suffering

Related Factors (r/t)

Anticipatory loss of significant object (e.g., possession, job, status, home, parts & processes of body); anticipatory loss of a significant other; death of a significant other; loss of significant object (e.g., possession, job, status, home, parts & processes of body)

NOC   Outcomes (Nursing Outcomes Classification)

Suggested NOC Outcomes

Family Resiliency, Dignified Life Closure, Grief Resolution, Hope, Mood Equilibrium, Personal Well-Being, Psychosocial Adjustment: Life Change

Example NOC Outcome with Indicators
Family Resiliency with plans to adapt and integrate the loss as evidenced by the following indicators: Mobilizes quickly following the loss/anticipated loss/Discusses meaning of crisis/loss/Supports members/Prepares for future challenges/Accepts respite from friends; Uses community groups for emotional support/(Rate the outcome and indicators of **Family Resiliency:** 1 = never demonstrated, 2 = rarely demonstrated, 3 = sometimes demonstrated, 4 = often demonstrated, 5 = consistently demonstrated [see Section I].)

Client/Family Outcomes

Client/Family Will (Specify Time Frame):

- Discuss meaning of the loss to his/her life and the functioning of the family
- Identify ways to support family members and articulate methods of support he or she requires from family and friends
- Utilize effective conflict management strategies
- Accept assistance in meeting the needs of the family from friends/extended family

NIC   Interventions (Nursing Interventions Classification)

Suggested NIC Interventions

Family Integrity Promotion, Dying Care, Emotional Support, Grief Work Facilitation, Grief Work Facilitation: Perinatal Death, Hope Installation, Support System Enhancement

• = Independent;   ▲ = Collaborative;   EBN = Evidence-Based Nursing;   EB = Evidence-Based

Example NIC Activities—Family Integrity Promotion

Determine family understanding of condition; Collaborate with family in problem solving and decision making; Identify typical family coping mechanisms; Refer family to support group of other families dealing with similar problems

Nursing Interventions and *Rationales*

- Concentrate on improving communication and providing an environment in which families can physically touch and care for their seriously ill loved one as much as possible. **EBN:** *Caregivers play an important role in the dying experience; these interventions have been identified in research studies as ways that improve the death experience for loved ones (Kruse, 2004).* **EB:** *Communication within the family has been shown to be a major predictor of grief because it is an important component in the ability to share grief and express feelings about the loss in a supportive environment (Traylor et al, 2003).*

- Focus on enhancing coping skills of the person's grieving to alleviate life problems and distressing symptoms such as anxiety and depression. Learning new coping strategies aimed at resuming former roles or assuming new roles is important over time. **EBN:** *Numerous bereavement studies indicate that different symptoms decline at different rates over time, with symptoms of depression being the most pervasive. Learning to live with the loss, development of a new relationship with the deceased, and establishment of a new life with attention refocusing away from self are important for successful resolution of grieving (Ott & Lueger, 2002).*

- Understand and support the family's expression of pain in its own way and in its own time. Encourage the family to create quiet and comfortable healing environments. **EBN:** *Especially when faced with traumatic grief, such as related to suicide or unexpected and/or violent death, intense emotional responses need to be accepted as appropriate and healthy responses to catastrophic loss (Kalischuk & Hayes, 2004).*

- Encourage the family to follow comforting grief rituals such as interacting with nature, lighting votive candles, saying a prayer, or whatever ritual brings spiritual comfort in dealing with the loss. *These traditional methods of grieving can help the family find meaning in the loss (Eisenhandler, 2004).*

- ▲ Refer the family members for spiritual counseling if desired. **EB:** *People who profess stronger spiritual beliefs seem to resolve their grief more rapidly and completely after the death of a close person than people with no spiritual beliefs (Walsh et al, 2002).*

- Help the family determine the best way and place to find social support. Encourage family members to continue to use supports for 1 to 2 years. **EB:** *Social support has been shown to help bereaved individuals as they reconstruct their lives and find new meaning in life (Hogan, Worden & Schmidt, 2004). Web memorials may be one method of enabling family support across distance and time (Nager & deVries, 2004).*

- ▲ Identify available community resources, including bereavement groups at local hospitals and hospice centers. Volunteers who provide bereavement support can also be effective. *Support groups can have positive effects on bereavement outcomes. Group counseling is an effective intervention because it addresses the issue of disenfranchised grief (Barlow & Morrison, 2002).*

 ### Pediatric/Parent

- Treat the child with respect, give him or her the opportunity to talk about concerns, and answer questions honestly. *Children know much more than many adults realize. They generally know if a parent or loved one is dying and/or the cause of death, even if they have not been told (Schuurman, 2002).*

- Listen to the child's expression of grief. *The best thing to help children is to listen to them with our ears, eyes, hearts, and souls and recognize that we do not have to have answers (Schuurman, 2002).*

- Consider giving the child a "memory bag" to have after experiencing a sudden death; contents include a teddy bear, a coloring book on working through grief for different ages, a journal for children to write in, and crayons. *The memory bags give children permission to grieve and feel the loss they experience so deeply (Foley, 2004).*

• = Independent;   ▲ = Collaborative;   EBN = Evidence-Based Nursing;   EB = Evidence-Based

G

- Help parents recognize that the child does not have to be "fixed," instead he or she needs support going through an experience of grieving just as adults do. *The role of the nurse, parent, and friends is to support and assist, not help a child "get over it" (Schuurman, 2002).*
- ▲ Refer grieving children and parents to a program to help facilitate grieving if desired, especially if the death was traumatic. **EB:** *Treatment for children and parents with grief associated with trauma helps decrease symptoms of posttraumatic stress disorder (PTSD) (Cohen, Mannarino & Knudsen, 2004).* **EBN:** *A program desired for grieving children involving riding horses was shown to increase self-confidence and self-esteem (Glazer, Clark & Stein, 2004).*
- Help the adolescent determine sources of support and how to use them effectively. **EBN:** *In a study of adolescents dealing with the death of a loved one, the most important factors that helped adolescents cope with the grief were self-help and support from parents, relatives, and friends (Rask, Kaunonen & Paunonen-Ilmonen, 2002).*
- ▲ Encourage parents to seek mental health services as needed, learn stress reduction, and take good care of their health. *The loss of a child for a mother results in an increased loss of life within 18 years either from disease or suicide (Lawson, 2003).* **EBN:** *A study analyzing the grief and coping of mothers who had lost children younger than 7 years found that the spouse, remaining children, grandparents, next of kin, friends, and colleagues were the main sources of support (Laakso & Paunonen-Ilmonen, 2002).*

Geriatric

- ▲ Monitor an older adult who has been treated for bereavement-related depression for relapse or recurrence. **EB:** *Loss of a significant other can trigger ineffective coping mechanisms that can require intervention from medication to hospitalization for behavior modification (Davies, 2001).*
- ▲ Use reminiscence therapy in conjunction with the expression of emotions. Refer to a reminiscence group if available. **EBN and EB:** *Two studies demonstrated that participation in a reminiscence group reduced symptoms of depression (Jones, 2003; Zauszniewski et al, 2004).*
- Provide support for the family when the loss is associated with dementia of the family member. *Psychosocial death is a significant dimension of the dementia of the Alzheimer's-type disease process. Grieving occurs throughout the illness of the parent (Furlini, 2001).*

Multicultural

- Assess the influence of cultural beliefs, norms, and values on the client's grief and mourning practices. **EBN:** *Grief and mourning practices may be based on cultural conventions (Clements et al, 2004).*
- Empathy may be especially important in caring for women with pregnancy loss who live in patrilineal cultures in which producing children is a critical role for women. *Use of narrative therapy may support in empowering mothers and assist them in moving forward (Hsu et al, 2003).*
- Validate the client's feelings regarding the loss. **EBN:** *Clients who were from an ethnic minority group were significantly more likely to report that interviews about death, dying, and bereavement were helpful (Emanuel et al, 2004). Storytelling was at the heart of every African-American widow's description of her bereavement experience (Rodgers, 2004).*
- Teach clients to recognize grief responses. **EBN:** *Recognition of grief patterns allows clients to manage their responses more effectively and may prevent adverse outcomes to their physical and mental health (Van & Meleis, 2003).*

Home Care

NOTE: **Grieving** may be encountered as the client comes to terms with his or her own loss or death, or as the family reacts to the client's death.
- The interventions previously described may be adapted for home care use.
- Actively listen as the client grieves for his or her own death or for real or perceived loss. Normalize the client's expressions of grief for himself or herself. Demonstrate a caring and hopeful approach. **EBN:** *Caring for and with the client and projecting hopefulness have been shown to inspire hope in bereavement counseling (Cutcliffe, 2004).*
- ▲ Refer the client to medical social services as necessary for losses not related to death. *Support is helpful to grief work for all types of losses. Social workers can help the client plan for financial changes as a result of job losses and help with community referrals as appropriate.*

▲ Refer the bereaved to hospice bereavement programs. *Relief of the suffering of clients and families (physical, emotional, and spiritual) is the goal of hospice care (Krisman-Scott & McCorkle, 2002).*

▲ Refer the bereaved spouse to an Internet self-help group if desired. *Palliative home care resources include a number of available websites (Smith-Stoner & Oliver, 2003). An Internet-based self-help group can assist the bereaved spouse in coping, receiving support, developing a sense of family, sharing information, and helping others (Bacon, Condon & Fernsler, 2000).*

• Assess caregiver reaction to bereavement issues and caregiver burden. Suggest preventive intervention for potential bereavement maladjustment if indicated. **EB:** *Bereavement maladjustment is more likely with caregivers who are older than 61 years, who perceive a substantial emotional burden, and who have been unable to continue working. Preventive interventions could reduce health and social costs (Rossi Ferrario et al, 2004).*

• Modify expectations of the family's response according to the degree of anticipation of the loved one's death. *If the loved one died at an old age or of a natural cause, the family most likely has anticipated the loss; the current reaction may be less than expected. If the loved one died of accidental or criminal causes, the grief reaction may be magnified. Grief may be prolonged, and a referral for supportive counseling is more likely to be needed.*

▲ After loss of a pregnancy, encourage the client and family to follow through on a counseling referral. **EBN and EB:** *Parents with a history of perinatal loss are at higher risk for depressive symptoms and pregnancy-specific anxiety during subsequent pregnancies, particularly before the third trimester. Nurses need to be alert to mothers' reactions during this trauma, as they often must overcome self-blame (Hsu et al, 2003; Armstrong, 2002).*

evolve See the EVOLVE website for World Wide Web resources for client education.

REFERENCES

Armstrong DS: Emotional distress and prenatal attachment in pregnancy after perinatal loss, *J Nurs Scholarsh* 34:339-345, 2002.

Bacon ES, Condon EH, Fernsler JI: Young widows' experience with an internet self-help group, *J Pshchosoc Nurs Ment Health Serv* 38(7):24-33, 2000.

Barlow CA, Morrison H: Survivors of suicide. Emerging counseling tragedies, *J Psychosoc Nurs Ment Health Serv* 40(1):28-39, 2002.

Clements PT, DeRanieri JT, Vigil GJ et al: Life after death: grief therapy after the sudden traumatic death of a family member, *Perspect Psychiatr Care* 40(4):149-154, 2004.

Cohen JA, Mannarino AP, Knudsen K: Treating childhood traumatic grief: a pilot study, *J Am Acad Child Adolesc Psychiatry* 43(10):1225-1233, 2004.

Cutcliffe JR: The inspiration of hope in bereavement counseling, *Issues Ment Health Nurs* 25(2):165-190, 2004.

Davies B: Supporting families in palliative care. In Ferrell BF, Coyle N, editors: *Textbook of palliative care nursing*, New York, 2001,Oxford University Press, pp. 712-716.

Eisenhandler SA: The arts of consolation: commemoration and folkways of faith, *Generations* 28(2):37, 2004.

Emanuel EJ, Fairclough DL, Wolfe P et al: Talking with terminally ill patients and their caregivers about death, dying, and bereavement: is it stressful? Is it helpful? *Arch Intern Med* 164(18):1999-2004, 2004.

Foley T: Encouraging the inclusion of children in grief after a sudden death: memory bags, *J Emerg Nurs* 30(4):341-342, 2004.

Furlini L: The parent they knew and the "new" parent: daughters' perceptions of dementia of the Alzheimer's type, *Home Health Care Serv Q* 20(1):21-38, 2001.

Glazer HR, Clark MD, Stein DS: The impact of hippotherapy on grieving children, *J Hospic Palliat Nurs* 6(3):171-175, 2004.

Hogan N, Worden JW, Schmidt L: An empirical study of the proposed complicated grief disorder criteria, *OMEGA* 48(3):263-277, 2004.

Hsu MT, Tseng YF, Banks J et al: Interpretations of stillbirth, *J Adv Nurs* 47(4):408-416, 2003.

Jones ED: Reminiscence therapy for older women with depression. Effects of nursing intervention classification in assisted-living long-term care, *J Gerontol Nurs* 29(7):26-33, 2003.

Kalischuk R, Hayes V: Grieving, mourning, and healing following youth suicide: a focus on health and well-being in families, *Omega* 48(1):45-67, 2004.

Krisman-Scott MA, McCorkle R: The tapestry of hospice, *Holist Nurs Pract* 16(2):32-39, 2002.

Kruse B: The meaning of letting go: the lived experience for caregivers of persons at the end of life, *J Hospice Palliat Nurs* 6(4):215-222, 2004.

Laakso H, Paunonen-Ilmonen M: Mothers' experience of social support following the death of a child, *J Clin Nurs* 11(2):176-185, 2002.

Lawson W: Grieving mothers suffer early deaths, *Psychology Today* 36(3):18, 2003.

Nager E, deVries B: Memorializing on the World Wide Web: patterns of grief and attachment in adult daughters of deceased mothers, *Death Stud* 49(1):43-56, 2004.

Ott C, Lueger R: Patterns of change in mental health status during the first two years of spousal bereavement, *Death Stud* 26:387-411, 2002.

Rask K, Kaunonen M, Paunonen-Ilmonen M: Adolescent coping with grief after the death of a loved one, *Int J Nurs Pract* 8(3):137-142, 2002.

Rodgers LS: Meaning of bereavement among older African American widows, *Geriatr Nurs* 25(1):10-16, 2004.

Rossi Ferrario S, Cardillo V, Vicario F et al: Advanced cancer at home: caregiving and bereavement, *Palliative Med* 18:129-136, 2004.

Schuurman DL: *The club no one wants to join: a dozen lessons I've learned from grieving children and adolescents,* Centre for Grief Education, 2002, www.grief.org.au/child_support.html, accessed March 7, 2005.

• = Independent; ▲ = Collaborative; EBN = Evidence-Based Nursing; EB = Evidence-Based

Smith-Stoner M, Oliver M: Ten palliative home care resources, *Home Healthc Nurs* 21(11):731-733, 2003.

Traylor E, Hayslip B, Kaminski P et al: Relationships between grief and family system characteristics: a cross lagged longitudinal analysis, *Death Stud* 27:575-601, 2003.

Van P, Meleis AI: Coping with grief after involuntary pregnancy loss: perspectives of African American women, *J Obstet Gynecol Neonatal Nurs* 32(1):28-39, 2003.

Walsh K, King M, Jones L et al: Spiritual beliefs may affect outcome of bereavement: prospective study, *BMJ* 324(7353):1551, 2002.

Zauszniewski JA, Eggenschwiler K, Preechawong S et al: Focused reflection reminiscence group for elders: implementation and evaluation, *Appl Gerontol* 23(4):429, 2004.

Complicated Grieving   *T. Heather Herdman, RN, PhD*

NANDA   Definition

A disorder that occurs after the death of a significant other in which the experience of distress accompanying bereavement fails to follow normative expectations and manifests in functional impairment.

Defining Characteristics

Decreased functioning in life roles; decreased sense of well-being; depression; experiencing somatic symptoms of the deceased; fatigue; grief avoidance; longing for the deceased; low levels of intimacy; persistent emotional distress; preoccupation with thoughts of the deceased; rumination; searching for the deceased; self-blame; separation distress; traumatic distress; verbalizes anxiety; verbalizes distressful feelings about the deceased; verbalizes feeling dazed; verbalizes feeling empty; verbalizes feeling in shock; verbalizes feeling stunned; verbalizes feelings of anger; verbalizes feelings of detachment from others; verbalizes feelings of disbelief; verbalizes feelings of mistrust; verbalizes lack of acceptance of the death; verbalizes persistent painful memories; verbalizes self-blame; yearning

Related Factors (r/t)

Death of a significant other; emotional instability; lack of social support; sudden death of a significant other

NOC   Outcomes (Nursing Outcomes Classification)

Suggested NOC Outcomes

Anxiety Level, Coping, Depression Self-Control, Grief Resolution, Hope, Immune Status, Mood Equilibrium, Personal Well-Being, Psychosocial Adjustment: Life Change, Sleep, Spiritual Health

> **Example NOC Outcome with Indicators**
>
> **Grief Resolution** with plans for a positive future as evidenced by the following indicators: Resolves feelings about loss/Verbalizes acceptance of loss/Reports absences of somatic distress/Reports decreased preoccupation with loss/ Discusses unresolved conflict(s)/Reports adequate nutritional intake (Rate the outcome and indicators of **Grief Resolution:** 1 = never demonstrated, 2 = rarely demonstrated, 3 = sometimes demonstrated, 4 = often demonstrated, 5 = consistently demonstrated [see Section I].)

Client Outcomes

Client Will (Specify Time Frame):

• Express appropriate feelings of guilt, fear, anger, or sadness
• Identify somatic distress associated with grief (e.g., anxiety, changes in appetite, insomnia, nightmares, loss of libido, decreased energy, altered activity levels)
• Seek support in dealing with grief-associated issues
• Identify personal strengths and effective coping strategies
• Function at a normal developmental level and begin to successfully and increasingly perform activities of daily living

NIC Interventions (Nursing Interventions Classification)

Suggested NIC Interventions

Grief Work Facilitation, Grief Work Facilitation: Perinatal Death, Guilt Work Facilitation, Hope Installation

Example NIC Activities—Grief Work Facilitation
Encourage the patient to verbalize memories of the loss, both past and current; Assist to identify personal coping strategies

Nursing Interventions and *Rationales*

- Assess the client's state of grieving. Use a tool such as the Texas Revised Inventory of Grief (TRIG), Pathological Grief Items (PGI), Impact of Events Scale (IES), Hogan Grief Reaction Checklist (HGRC), Beck Depression Inventory (BDI-II), Hamilton Rating Scale for Depression or Social Adjustment Scale – Self Report (SAS-SR). **EBN and EB:** *It is important to differentiate between depression and complicated grief because they can be easily confused (Ogrodniczuk et al, 2003; Hogan, Worden & Schmidt, 2004; Ott & Lueger, 2002; Matthews & Marwit, 2004). These standardized tools have been shown to measure grief symptoms effectively and may help differentiate depression from complicated grief (Ogrodniczuk et al, 2003; Hogan, Worden & Schmidt, 2004).*
- ▲ Determine whether the client is experiencing depression, suicidal tendencies, or other emotional disorders. Refer the client for counseling or therapy as appropriate. **EB:** *Counseling, including the use of relaxation therapy, desensitization, cognitive-behavioral therapy, biofeedback, and/or traditional psychotherapy, has been shown to be supportive (Matthews & Marwit, 2004). Cognitive-behavioral therapy can be helpful for traumatic grief (Matthews & Marwit, 2004; Jacobs & Prigerson, 2000).*
- Identify problems of eating and sleeping; ensure that basic human needs are being met. **EB:** *Bereaved individuals, regardless of whether they have counseling for grief resolution, have a moderate risk for poor nutrition (Johnson, 2002).*
- Develop a trusting relationship with the client by using presence and therapeutic communication techniques. **EB:** *Fathers who had lost infants before birth seek understanding from both the hospital personnel and their partners as well as from relatives. Being able to protect their partners and grieve in their own way is important to the fathers (Samuelsson, Radestad & Segesten, 2001).*
- Educate the client and his or her support systems that grief resolution is not a sequential process and that the positive outcome of grief resolution is the integration of the deceased into the ongoing life of the griever. **EB:** *Expectation that the griever will in some way "get over" or "get past" the grief is no longer seen as valid; continued involvement with the deceased regularly occurs (Matthews & Marwit, 2004).*
- Understand and support the client's expression of pain in his or her own way and in his or her own time. Encourage the client to create quiet and comfortable healing environments. **EBN:** *Especially when faced with traumatic grief, such as related to suicide or unexpected and/or violent death, intense emotional responses need to be accepted as appropriate and healthy responses to catastrophic loss (Kalischuk & Hayes, 2004).*
- ▲ Assess for spiritual distress; refer the client to an appropriate spiritual leader, if appropriate. **EB:** *Nurses need to assess and treat spiritual distress related to grieving. People who profess stronger spiritual beliefs seem to resolve their grief more rapidly and completely after the death of a close person than people with no spiritual beliefs (Walsh et al, 2002).*
- Focus on enhancing coping skills to alleviate life problems and distressing symptoms such as anxiety and depression. *Learning new coping strategies aimed at resuming former roles or assuming new roles is important over time.* **EBN:** *Different symptoms decline at different rates over time, with symptoms of depression being the most pervasive. Learning to live with the loss, development of a new relationship with the deceased, and establishment of a new life with attention refocusing away from self are important for successful resolution of grieving (Ott & Lueger, 2002).*
- Encourage the client to follow comforting grief rituals such as interacting with nature, lighting votive candles, saying a prayer, or whatever ritual brings spiritual comfort in dealing with the

G

G

loss. *These traditional methods of grieving can help the client find meaning in the loss (Eisenhandler, 2004).*

▲ Identify available community resources, including community and/or Web-based bereavement groups. Volunteers who provide bereavement support can also be effective. **EB and EBN:** *Social support has been shown to help bereaved individuals as they reconstruct their lives and find new meaning in life (Douglas, 2004; Hogan, Worden & Schmidt, 2004). Web memorials may be one method of enabling family support across distance and time (Nager & deVries, 2004).* **EBN:** *Psychoeducational group activity and self-assessment caused suicide rates to decrease among elderly women in a Japanese culturally sensitive intervention study (Oyama et al, 2005).*

Pediatric/Parent

• If client is an adolescent exposed to a peer's suicide, watch for symptoms of traumatic grief as well as PTSD, which include numbness, preoccupation with the deceased, functional impairment, and poor adjustment to the loss. **EB:** *Adolescents in this situation are at high risk for depression, anxiety disorder, substance abuse, conduct disorder, and attention deficit–hyperactivity disorder (Melhem et al, 2004).*

• See the interventions and rationales in the care plan for **Grieving.**

Geriatric

▲ Use reminiscence therapy in conjunction with the expression of emotions. Refer to a reminiscence group if available. **EBN and EB:** *Participation in a reminiscence group may reduce symptoms of depression (Zauszniewski et al, 2004; Jones, 2003).*

• Identify previous losses and assess the client for depression. *Losses and changes associated with aging often occur in rapid succession without adequate recovery time (Hegge & Fischer, 2000).* **EBN:** *Having more than two concurrent losses increases the incidence of unresolved grief (Herth, 1990). The grieving elderly widow may develop depression that results in poor nutrition, noncompliance with medication regimens, decreasing cognition, and multiple health problems (Fischer & Hegge, 2000).*

• Monitor an older adult who has been treated for bereavement-related depression for relapse or recurrence. **EB:** *Older adults treated for bereavement-related depression may experience relapse or recurrence (Pasternak et al, 1997).*

• Evaluate the social support system of the elderly client. If the support system is minimal, help the client determine how to increase available support. **EBN:** *The elderly who have poor grieving outcomes often do not live with family members and have a minimal support system. The support of family, especially children, and friends is a common way for elderly widows to cope with a loss (Hegge & Fischer, 2000).*

Multicultural

• See the interventions and rationales in the care plan for **Grieving.**

• Assess for the influence of cultural beliefs, norms, and values on the client's grief and mourning practices. **EBN:** *Cubans may observe a wake service the day after the announcement of the death. Extreme care is taken to notify relatives and significant others to announce the death. Finding out about the death later adds to a feeling of estrangement and defeat (Franco & Wilson, 2008, in press).* **EBN:** *When an Amish person is near death, it is extremely useful to have the client in a private room to allow as many visitors as can comfortably stand. The visitors sing softly to the client to make the journey to their God more peaceful. Death is not feared but is rather a solemn and profound event in the life of a person. Amish persons tend to prefer to die at home without the interference of institutional rules (Helmuth & Schwartz, 2008, in press).* **EBN:** *Many of the beliefs and practices about death are so woven into the fabric of Vietnamese life that it is difficult to separate them into either religious or cultural concepts. An important aspect of filial piety and family loyalty is an obligation that extends beyond death: observing the anniversary day of the death, gathering at the family home and altar, and cleaning the ancestral tombs. For Buddhists, there typically are special observances, usually with elaborate rites at 100 days, and 1 and 2 years after the death (Stauffer, 2008, in press).*

• Assess for the influence of cultural beliefs, norms, and values on the client's expressions of grief. **EBN:** *Cuban wake and funeral services are dictated by the religious identity and economic status of the deceased. Catholics traditionally have a priest present at the wake who provides a short prayer service.*

• = Independent;   ▲ = Collaborative;   EBN = Evidence-Based Nursing;   EB = Evidence-Based

Jewish practices depend on orthodox, conservative, or reformed traditions and are primarily solemn expressions of grief for 7 days, with burial in a wooden coffin the day after death (Franco & Wilson, 2008, in press).

- Encourage discussion of the grief process. **EBN:** *Clients who were from an ethnic minority group were significantly more likely to report that interviews about death, dying, and bereavement were helpful (Cherry & Giger, 2008, in press).* **EBN:** *While Afghans grieve expressively and strongly over the death of a loved one, death is seen as the beginning of a new and better life. Close family members gather together to mourn at specified intervals for 40 days or related to the number of children (Lipson, Askaryar & Omidian, 2008, in press).*
- Identify whether the client had been notified of the health status of the deceased and was able to be present during illness and death. **EBN:** *Not being present during terminal illness and death can disrupt the grieving process (Franco & Wilson, 2008, in press).*

 Home Care

- See the interventions and rationales in the care plan for **Grieving.**

 See the EVOLVE website for World Wide Web resources for client education.

REFERENCES

Cherry B, Giger J: African-Americans. In Giger J, Davidhizar RE: *Transcultural nursing: assessment and intervention,* ed 5, St Louis, 2008, Mosby. In press.

Douglas DH: The lived experience of loss: a phenomenological study, *J Am Psychiatr Nurses Assoc* 10(1):24, 2004.

Eisenhandler SA: The arts of consolation: commemoration and folkways of faith, *Generations* 28(2):37, 2004.

Fischer C, Hegge M: The elderly woman at risk, *Am J Nurs* 100(6):54, 2000.

Franco M, Wilson T: Cuban Americans. In Giger J, Davidhizar RE: *Transcultural nursing: assessment and intervention,* ed 5, St Louis, 2008, Mosby. In press.

Hegge M, Fischer C: Grief responses of senior and elderly widows: practice implications, *J Gerontol Nurs* 26(2):35, 2000.

Helmuth M, Schwartz K: Amish. In Giger J, Davidhizar RE: *Transcultural nursing: assessment and intervention,* ed 5, St Louis, 2008, Mosby. In press.

Herth K: Relationship of hope, coping styles, concurrent losses, and setting to grief resolution in the elderly widow(er), *Res Nurs Health* 13:109, 1990.

Hogan NS, Worden JW, Schmidt LA: An empirical study of the proposed complicated grief disorder criteria, *Omega* 48(3):263-277, 2004.

Jacobs S, Prigerson H: Psychotherapy of traumatic grief: a review of evidence for psychotherapeutic treatments, *Death Stud* 24:479, 2000.

Johnson CS: Nutritional considerations for bereavement and coping with grief, *J Nutr Health Aging* 6(3):171, 2002.

Jones ED: Reminiscence therapy for older women with depression: effects of nursing intervention classification in assisted-living long-term care, *J Gerontol Nurs* 29(7):26, 2003.

Kalischuk R, Hayes V: Grieving, mourning, and healing following youth suicide: a focus on health and well-being in families, *Omega* 48(1):45-67, 2004.

Lipson J, Askaryar R, Omidian P: Afghans and Afghan Americans. In Giger, Davidhizar RE: *Transcultural nursing: assessment and intervention,* ed 5, St Louis, 2008, Mosby. In press.

Matthews L, Marwit S: Complicated grief and the trend toward cognitive-behavioral therapy, *Death Stud* 28:849-863, 2004.

Melhem NM, Day N, Shear MK et al: Traumatic grief among adolescents exposed to a peer's suicide, *Am J Psychiatry* 161(8):1411, 2004.

Nager E, deVries B: Memorializing on the World Wide Web: patterns of grief and attachment in adult daughters of deceased mothers, *Death Stud* 49(1):43-56, 2004.

Ogrodniczuk J, Piper W, Joyce A et al: Differentiating symptoms of complicated grief and depression among psychiatric outpatients, *Can J Psychiatry* 48(2):87-93, 2003.

Ott C, Lueger R: Patterns of change in mental health status during the first two years of spousal bereavement, *Death Stud* 26:387-411, 2002.

Oyama H, Watanabe N, Ono Y et al: Community-based suicide prevention through group activity for the elderly successfully reduced the high suicide rate for females, *Psychiatr Clin Neurosci* 59(3):337-344, 2005.

Pasternak RE, Prigerson H, Hall M et al: The posttreatment illness course of depression in bereaved elders, *Am J Geriatr Psychiatry* 5:54, 1997.

Samuelsson M, Radestad I, Segesten K: A waste of life: fathers' experience of losing a child before birth, *Birth* 28(2):124, 2001.

Stauffer R: Vietnamese. In Giger, Davidhizar RE: *Transcultural nursing: assessment and intervention,* ed 5, St Louis, 2008, Mosby. In press.

Walsh K, King M, Jones L et al: Spiritual beliefs may affect outcome of bereavement: prospective study, *BMJ* 324(7353):1551, 2002.

Zauszniewski JA, Eggenschwiler K, Preechawong S et al: Focused reflection reminiscence group for elders: implementation and evaluation, *Appl Gerontol* 23(4):429, 2004.

• = Independent;   ▲ = Collaborative;   EBN = Evidence-Based Nursing;   EB = Evidence-Based

Risk for complicated Grieving   *T. Heather Herdman, RN, PhD*

NANDA   **Definition**

At risk for a disorder that occurs after the death of a significant other in which the experience of distress accompanying bereavement fails to follow normative expectations and manifests in functional impairment

Risk Factors

Death of a significant other; emotional instability; lack of social support

NOC   **Outcomes (Nursing Outcomes Classification)**

Suggested NOC Outcomes

Anxiety Level, Coping, Depression Self-Control, Grief Resolution, Hope, Immune Status, Mood Equilibrium, Personal Well-Being, Psychosocial Adjustment: Life Change, Sleep, Spiritual Health

Example NOC Outcome with Indicators
Grief Resolution with plans for a positive future as evidenced by the following indicators: Resolves feelings about loss/Verbalizes acceptance of loss/Reports absences of somatic distress/Reports decreased preoccupation with loss/Discusses unresolved conflict(s)/Reports adequate nutritional intake (Rate the outcome and indicators of **Grief Resolution:** 1 = never demonstrated, 2 = rarely demonstrated, 3 = sometimes demonstrated, 4 = often demonstrated, 5 = consistently demonstrated [see Section I].)

Client Outcomes

Client Will (Specify Time Frame):

- Express appropriate feelings of guilt, fear, anger, or sadness
- Identify somatic distress associated with grief (e.g., anxiety, changes in appetite, insomnia, nightmares, loss of libido, decreased energy, altered activity levels)
- Seek support in dealing with grief-associated issues
- Identify personal strengths and effective coping strategies
- Function at a normal developmental level and begin to successfully and increasingly perform activities of daily living

NIC   **Interventions (Nursing Interventions Classification)**

Suggested NIC Interventions

Grief Work Facilitation: Perinatal Death, Guilt Work Facilitation, Hope Installation

Example NIC Activities—Grief Work Facilitation
Encourage the patient to verbalize memories of the loss, both past and current; Assist to identify personal coping strategies

Nursing Interventions and *Rationales,* Client Teaching

- Refer to care plan for **Complicated Grieving.**

Delayed Growth and development   *Gail B. Ladwig, MSN, CHTP, RN*

NANDA   Definition

Deviations from age-group norms

Defining Characteristics

Altered physical growth; decreased response time; delay in performing skills typical of age group; difficulty in performing skills typical of age group; inability to perform self-care activities appropriate for age; inability to perform self-control activities appropriate for age; flat affect; listlessness

Related Factors (r/t)

Effects of physical disability; environmental deficiencies; inadequate caretaking; inconsistent responsiveness; indifference; multiple caretakers; prescribed dependence; separation from significant others; stimulation deficiencies

NOC   Outcomes (Nursing Outcomes Classification)

Suggested NOC Outcomes

Child Development: 2 Months, 4 Months, 6 Months, 12 Months, 2 Years, 3 Years, 4 Years, Preschool, Middle Childhood, Adolescence, Growth, Mobility, Neurological Status, Physical Maturation: Female, Male, Knowledge Parenting

Example NOC Outcome with Indicators
Growth as evidenced by the following indicators: Weight percentiles for age, sex, and height (Rate the outcome and indicators of **Growth:** 1 = severe deviation from normal range, 2 = substantial deviation from normal range, 3 = moderate deviation from normal range, 4 = mild deviation from normal range, 5 = no deviation from normal range [see Section I].)

Client Outcomes

Client/Parents/Primary Caregiver Will (Specify Time Frame):

- Describe realistic, age-appropriate patterns of growth and development
- Promote activities and interactions that support age-related developmental tasks
- Display consistent, sustained achievement of age-appropriate behaviors (social, interpersonal, and/or cognitive) and/or motor skills
- Achieve realistic developmental and/or growth milestones based on existing abilities, extent of disability, and functional age
- Exhibit limited temporary behavioral regression that reverses shortly after episode of illness or hospitalization
- Attain steady gains in growth patterns

NIC   Interventions (Nursing Interventions Classification)

Suggested NIC Interventions

Active Listening, Body Image Enhancement, Developmental Enhancement: Adolescent, Child, Emotional Support, Kangaroo Care, Nutrition Therapy, Nutritional Monitoring, Positioning, Self-Care Assistance, Self-Responsibility Facilitation

Example NIC Activities—Nutritional Monitoring
Monitor trends in weight loss and gain; Monitor food preferences and choices

Nursing Interventions and *Rationales*

- To determine risk for or actual deviations in normal development, consider the use of a screening tool. *Some tools are the Brigance Infant and Toddler Screens and the Pregnancy Risk Assessment Monitoring System (PRAMS).* **EB:** *The Brigance Infant and Toddler Screens are shown to be accurate, valid, and reliable tools that can be administered by a range of professionals using either parental interview, direct elicitation and observation, or both (Glascoe, 2002).* **EB:** *PRAMS collects state-specific, population-based data on maternal attitudes and experiences before, during, and immediately after pregnancy (Centers for Disease Control and Prevention, 2002).*
- Regularly compare height and weight measurements for the child or adolescent with established age-appropriate norms and previous measurements. **EB:** *The revised growth charts provide an improved tool for evaluating the growth of children in clinical and research settings (Centers for Disease Control and Prevention, 2007).*
- ▲ Identify coexisting health or medical conditions that may be contributing to the alteration in growth and/or development, and refer the client to a specialist in the appropriate healthcare discipline for management. **EB:** *A specific cause can be determined in the majority of children with global developmental delay. Certain routine screening tests are indicated and, depending on history and examination findings, additional specific testing may be performed (Shevell et al, 2003).*
- Provide skin-to-skin contact for newborns and moms. Place the naked baby prone on the mother's bare chest at birth or soon afterwards (<24 hours). **EBN:** *There are positive effects with early skin-to-skin contact on breastfeeding at 1 to 3 months after birth (Anderson et al, 2003).*
- Provide opportunities for mother-infant skin-to-skin contact (kangaroo care) for preterm infants. **EB:** *The neurodevelopmental profile was more mature for infants receiving kangaroo care. Results underscore the role of early skin-to-skin contact in the maturation of the autonomic and circadian systems in preterm infants (Feldman & Eidelman, 2003).*
- Provide neonatal positioning procedures for preterm infants to prevent extremity malalignment, skull deformities, and gross motor delay. *Alignment and shaping of the musculoskeletal system occur with each body position change in a neonatal intensive care unit; proper positioning strategies promote skeletal integrity, postural control, and sensorimotor organization (Sweeney & Gutierrez, 2002).*
- Provide developmental care interventions to preterm infants. *This improves neurodevelopmental outcomes (Symington & Pinelli, 2002).*
- Provide meaningful stimulation for hospitalized infants and children. *Stimulation is essential to the development of gross and fine motor adaptive skills, language, and personal-social functioning in infants and children. Hospitalized infants are often subjected to understimulation or an overabundance of meaningless stimulation (Slusher & McClure, 1995).*
- Provide support groups and education on human immunodeficiency virus (HIV) and caring for infants with this diagnosis. *Developmental delay has been well documented infants with HIV (Potterton & Eales, 2001).*
- ▲ Engage the child in appropriate play activities. Refer the child to a play or recreational therapist (if available) for supplemental strategies. **EB:** *Play is essential for learning in children. Toys should be safe, affordable, and developmentally appropriate. Children do not need expensive toys (Glassy & Romano, 2003).*
- Provide an environment that promotes additional sleep and rest opportunities. **EB:** *Reduced quality of sleep can have important implications for the developing child because it can impair growth, learning, and emotional development (Boyle & Copley, 2004).*

Multicultural

- Assess the influence of cultural beliefs, norms, and values on the client's perceptions of child development. **EBN:** *What the client considers normal and abnormal child development may be based on cultural perceptions (Leininger & McFarland, 2002: Giger & Davidhizar, 2004).*
- Assess and identify for possible environmental conditions, which may be a contributing factor to altered growth and development. **EB:** *Insecticide exposures were widespread among minority women in New York City during pregnancy, and high levels were associated with lower birth weight and length (Whyatt et al, 2004).*

- Acknowledge racial and ethnic differences at the onset of care. **EBN:** *Acknowledgment of race and ethnicity issues enhances communication, establishes rapport, and promotes treatment outcomes (D'Avanzo & Naegle, 2001; Ludwick & Silva, 2000).*
- Use a neutral, indirect style in addressing areas in which improvement is needed (such as a need for verbal stimulation) when working with Native American clients. **EBN:** *Indirect statements such as "Other mothers have tried…" or "I had a client who tried 'X' and it seemed to work very well," help avoid resentment of the parent (Seideman et al, 1996).*
- Provide information on the effects of environmental risk exposure on growth and development. **EB:** *Minority children with prenatal environmental tobacco smoke exposure were twice as likely to be classified as significantly cognitively delayed when compared with unexposed children (Rauh et al, 2004). Data suggest that environmental exposure may lead to delayed growth and pubertal development in African-American and Mexican-American girls (Shevell et al, 2003).*

Home Care

- The interventions previously described may be adapted for home care use.
- Assess whether exposure to community violence is contributing to developmental problems. **EBN:** *Exposure to community violence has been associated with increases in aggressive behavior and depression in children (Gorman-Smith & Tolan, 1998).*
- ▲ Refer maternal drug users to home intervention programs. **EB:** *Ongoing maternal drug use was associated with worse developmental outcomes among a group of drug-exposed infants. A home intervention led to higher scores on the Bayley Scales of Infant Development among drug-exposed infants (Schuler, Nair & Kettinger, 2003).*
- ▲ If possible, refer the family to a program of animal-assisted therapy. **EBN:** *Interactions with dogs may help clients with pervasive developmental disorders establish bonds with their social environment. Children with pervasive developmental disorders were more playful, more focused, and more aware of their social environment in the presence of a therapy dog than in the presence of a toy or a stuffed dog (Martin & Farnum, 2002).*

Client/Family Teaching

- ▲ Encourage parents to take infants and children for routine health visits to the family physician or pediatrician. *Family physicians play a major role in the early recognition and referral of children with developmental delays or mental retardation. Once the physician has recognized a possible developmental problem, she or he can help determine whether neurological, audiological, or ophthalmological evaluations or rehabilitative services are needed (Moeschler & Shevell, 2006).*
- Provide parents and/or caregivers realistic expectations for attainment of growth and development milestones. Clarify expectations and correct misconceptions. **EBN:** *Learning about the growth and developmental differences between children with congenital heart defect and normal children may help parents of the former to detect problems associated with delayed growth and development earlier (Chen, Li & Wang, 2004).*
- Have parents and/or caregivers rehearse coping strategies for approaching developmental milestones and acknowledge positive actions and behaviors. *Anticipating and preparing can strengthen their ability to deal with situations and enhance achievement (Reisch & Forsyth, 1992).*
- Teach methods of providing meaningful stimulation for infants and children. *Stimulation is essential to the development of gross and fine motor adaptive skills, language, and personal-social functioning in infants and children (Slusher & McClure, 1995).*
- Instruct the client regarding appropriate baby equipment. **EBN:** *The use of baby walkers is controversial. They may delay walking by 11 to 26 days. There was no support that they aided walking. Further work is required to determine if they are an independent causal factor in accidents (Burrows & Griffiths, 2002).*
- ▲ Elicit the involvement of parents and caregivers in social support groups and parenting classes. *Postnatal services that included parenting classes had a positive impact on children's health and supported developmental development (Miller, 2006).*
- ▲ Furnish information about community resources. *Support groups and other opportunities to obtain*

• = Independent;   ▲ = Collaborative;   EBN = Evidence-Based Nursing;   EB = Evidence-Based

guidance serve to empower parents and clarify and reinforce knowledge and parenting skills (Kinney, Mannetter & Carpenter, 1992; McCloskey & Bulechek, 1992).

evolve   See the EVOLVE website for World Wide Web resources for client education.

REFERENCES

Anderson GC, Moore E, Hepworth J et al: Early skin-to-skin contact for mothers and their healthy newborn infants, *Cochrane Database Syst Rev* (2):CD003519, 2003.

Boyle J, Copley M: Children's sleep: problems and solutions, *J Fam Health Care* 14(3):61-63, 2004.

Burrows P, Griffiths P: Do baby walkers delay onset of walking in young children? *Br J Community Nurs* 7(11):581, 2002.

Centers for Disease Control and Prevention: *Using surveillance to promote public health examples from the Pregnancy Risk Assessment Monitoring System (PRAMS),* 2002, www.cdc.gov/PRAMS/dataAct2002/prams.htm, accessed February 28, 2007.

Centers for Disease Control and Prevention: *National Center for Health Statistics clinical growth charts,* 2007, www.cdc.gov/nchs/about/major/nhanes/growthcharts/clinical_charts.htm, accessed February 28, 2007.

Chen C, Li C, Wang J: Growth and development of children with congenital heart disease, *J Adv Nurs* 47(3):260-269, 2004.

D'Avanzo CE, Naegle MA: Developing culturally informed strategies for substance-related interventions. In Naegle MA, D'Avanzo CE, editors: *Addictions and substance abuse: strategies for advanced practice nursing,* St Louis, 2001, Mosby.

Feldman R, Eidelman A: Skin-to-skin contact (kangaroo care) accelerates autonomic and neurobehavioural maturation in preterm infants, *Dev Med Child Neurol* 45(4):274, 2003.

Giger JN, Davidhizar RE: *Transcultural nursing: assessment and intervention,* ed 4, St Louis, 2004, Mosby.

Glascoe FP: The Brigance Infant and Toddler Screen: standardization and validation, *J Dev Behav Pediatr* 23(3):145, 2002.

Glassy D, Romano J: Selecting appropriate toys for young children: the pediatrician's role, *Pediatrics* 111(4 pt 1):911, 2003.

Gorman-Smith D, Tolan P: The role of exposure to community violence and developmental problems among inner city youth, *Dev Psychopathol* 10(1):101, 1998.

Kinney CK, Mannetter R, Carpenter MA: Support groups. In Bulechek GM, McCloskey JC, editors: *Nursing interventions: essential nursing treatment,* Philadelphia, 1992, W.B. Saunders.

Leininger MM, McFarland MR: *Transcultural nursing: concepts, theories, research and practices,* ed 3, New York, 2002, McGraw-Hill.

Ludwick R, Silva M: Nursing around the world: cultural values and ethical conflicts, *NursingWorld,* August 14, 2000, www.nursingworld.org/ojin/ethicol/ethics_4.htm, accessed June 19, 2003.

Martin F, Farnum J: Animal-assisted therapy for children with pervasive developmental disorders, *West J Nurs Res* 24:657, 2002.

McCloskey JC, Bulechek GM, editors: *Nursing interventions classification (NIC),* St Louis, 1992, Mosby.

Miller K: Interventions for child health and parenting practices, *Am Fam Physician* 74(12):2112-2113, 2006.

Moeschler J, Shevell M: American Academy of Pediatrics Committee on Genetics: Clinical genetic evaluation of the child with mental retardation or developmental delays, *Pediatrics* 117(6):2304-2316, 2006.

Potterton J, Eales C: Prevalence of developmental delay in infants who are HIV positive, *S Afr J Physiother* 57(3):11, 2001.

Rauh VA, Whyatt RM, Garfinkel R et al: Developmental effects of exposure to environmental tobacco smoke and material hardship among inner-city children, *Neurotoxicol Teratol* 26(3):373-385, 2004.

Reisch SK, Forsyth DM: Preparing to parent the adolescent: a theoretical overview, *J Child Adolesc Psychiatr Ment Health Nurs* 5:31, 1992.

Schuler ME, Nair P, Kettinger L: Drug-exposed infants and developmental outcome: effects of a home intervention and ongoing maternal drug use, *Arch Pediatr Adolesc Med* 157(2):133, 2003.

Seideman RY, Jacobson S, Primeaux M et al: Assessing American Indian families, *MCN Am J Matern Child Nurs* 21(6):274-279, 1996.

Shevell M, Ashwal S, Donley D et al: Practice parameter: evaluation of the child with global developmental delay: report of the Quality Standards Subcommittee of the American Academy of Neurology and The Practice Committee of the Child Neurology Society, *Neurology* 60(3):367-380, 2003.

Slusher IL, McClure MJ: Infant stimulation during hospitalization, *J Pediatr Nurs* 7:276, 1995.

Sweeney J, Gutierrez T: Musculoskeletal implications of preterm infant positioning in the NICU, *J Perinat Neonatal Nurs* 16(1):58, 2002.

Symington A, Pinelli J: Developmental care for promoting development and preventing morbidity in preterm infants, *Cochrane Database Syst Rev* (3):CD001814, 2002.

Whyatt RM, Rauh V, Barr DB et al: Prenatal insecticide exposures and birth weight and length among an urban minority cohort, *Environ Health Perspect* 112(10):1125, 2004.

Risk for disproportionate Growth   *Gail B. Ladwig, MSN, CHTP, RN*

NANDA   **Definition**

At risk for growth above the 97th percentile or below the third percentile for age, crossing two percentile channels

Risk Factors

Caregiver

Abuse; mental illness; mental retardation; or severe learning disability

Environmental

Deprivation; lead poisoning; natural disasters; poverty; teratogen; violence

---

• = Independent;   ▲ = Collaborative;   EBN = Evidence-Based Nursing;   EB = Evidence-Based

Individual

Anorexia; caregiver maladaptive feeding behaviors; chronic illness; individual maladaptive feeding behaviors; infection; insatiable appetite; prematurity; malnutrition; substance abuse

Prenatal

Congenital/genetic disorders; maternal infection; maternal nutrition; multiple gestation; teratogen exposure; substance use/abuse

NOC   Outcomes (Nursing Outcomes Classification)

Suggested NOC Outcomes

Body Image, Child Development: 2 Months, 4 Months, 6 Months, 12 Months, 2 Years, 3 Years, 4 Years, Preschool, Middle Childhood, Adolescence, Growth, Knowledge: Infant Care, Preconception Maternal Health, Pregnancy, Physical Maturation: Female, Male, Weight: Body Mass

Example NOC Outcome with Indicators
Growth as evidenced by the following indicators: Weight percentiles for age, sex, and height (Rate the outcome and indicators of **Growth:** 1 = severe deviation from normal range, 2 = substantial deviation from normal range, 3 = moderate deviation from normal range, 4 = mild deviation from normal range, 5 = no deviation from normal range [see Section I].)

Client Outcomes

Client/Parents/Primary Caregiver Will (Specify Time Frame):

- State information related to possible teratogenic agents
- State information related to adequate nutrition
- Seek help from appropriate professionals for nutritional needs

NIC   Interventions (Nursing Interventions Classification)

Suggested NIC Interventions

Behavior Modification, Counseling, Nutrition Therapy, Nutritional Monitoring, Teaching: Infant Nutrition, Toddler Nutrition, Parent Education: Child-Rearing Family

Example NIC Activities—Parent Education: Child-rearing Family
Review nutritional requirements for specific age-groups; Inform parents of community resources

Nursing Interventions and *Rationales*

Preconception/Pregnancy

- ▲ Assess and limit exposure to all drugs (prescription, "recreational," and over the counter) and give the mother information on known teratogenic agents. **EB:** *No drug can be considered safe during pregnancy. It should be emphasized that any drug has the potential to cause a birth defect, so no listing of known teratogens is ever complete (Florida Birth Defects Registry, 2007).* **EBN:** *The consumption of alcohol during pregnancy can irreparably harm the fetus. Preventive measures can be helpful in decreasing or stopping the use of alcohol during pregnancy. Alcohol is a definite teratogen (Eustace, Kang & Coombs, 2003).*
- All women of childbearing age who are capable of becoming pregnant should take 400 mcg of folic acid daily. **EB:** *Periconceptional use of folic acid reduces the incidence of neural tube defects. Up to 70% of neural tube defects could be prevented if all women who can become pregnant consumed 400 mcg of folic acid from at least 1 month before conception through the first trimester of pregnancy (Florida Birth Defects Registry, 2007).*

• = Independent;   ▲ = Collaborative;   EBN = Evidence-Based Nursing;   EB = Evidence-Based

G

▲ Women with phenylketonuria should be referred to a nutritionist experienced in the dietary implications of phenylalanine restriction. *Because 40% of all pregnancies are unplanned, women with phenylketonuria are urged to maintain phenylalanine restriction throughout their childbearing years.* **EB:** *Phenylalanine has been found to be one of the most potent teratogens. Dietary restriction of phenylalanine should thus be started before conception; and birth outcomes can be normal with such restriction. Initiation of phenylalanine restriction in the first trimester improves developmental outcome, but this is often too late to avoid structural birth defects and brain damage in the fetus (Florida Birth Defects Registry, 2007).*

▲ Promote a team approach toward preconception and pregnancy glucose control for women with diabetes. **EB:** *Offspring of women with diabetes mellitus type 1 or type 2 have a two- to fourfold increased risk of birth defects. Available data suggest that excellent preconception and first-trimester glucose control in the mother can greatly reduce, if not eliminate, this risk. Fetal morbidity may still be high in the second and third trimesters if gestational diabetes is not under good control. Programs with a team approach have been the most successful (Florida Birth Defects Registry, 2007).*

 Infants/Children

• Consider breast milk for extremely low birth weight infants in the neonatal intensive care unit. *Research demonstrated that there was a significant difference in mental development and psychomotor development in breastfed infants. The long-term benefit of breast milk has the potential to optimize cognitive potential and reduce the need for early intervention and special education services (Vohr et al, 2006). Counseling mothers of very low birth weight infants increases the incidence of lactation initiation and breast milk feeding without increasing maternal stress and anxiety (Sisk et al, 2006).*

▲ Provide tube feedings per physician's orders when appropriate for clients with neuromuscular impairment. **EB:** *Infants with isolated neonatal swallowing dysfunction have a good long-term prognosis. Nasogastric feedings followed by a gastrostomy is recommended in those without gastroesophageal reflux. Jejunal feedings are necessary in some. Although most infants improve over time, they may need nutritional support for 3 years or more (Heuschkel et al, 2003).*

▲ Reduce the risk of TORCH infections (*t*oxoplasmosis, *o*ther infections, *r*ubella, *c*ytomegalovirus infection, and *h*erpes simplex) as follows:
  ▪ Varicella-zoster and rubella viruses: vaccinate nonimmune women before conception
  ▪ Cytomegalovirus: practice meticulous handwashing and secretion control and limit exposure to large numbers of infants and children
  ▪ *Toxoplasma gondii:* avoid exposure to cat litter and avoid work in the garden or areas where cat feces may be present; do not feed undercooked meats to cats
  ▪ Parvovirus: limit contact with persons with known fifth disease
  ▪ Herpes virus: practice meticulous handwashing and secretion control, especially in contact with young infants

  EB: *Infection with any of the aforementioned agents can cause fetal harm and result in serious damage to the central nervous system and other organs (Florida Birth Defects Registry, 2007).*

• Provide for adequate nutrition and nutritional monitoring in clients with developmental disorders. **EB:** *When nutrition therapy is given in the early stages of diagnosis and treatment of cerebral palsy, growth delays may be prevented or remedied (Sanders et al, 1990). Nutrient needs may be altered as a result of long-term medication for conditions such as epilepsy, recurrent urinary or respiratory tract infections, chronic constipation, and behavioral problems (American Dietetic Association, 1997).*

▲ Adequate intake of vitamin D is set at 200 IU/day by the National Academy of Sciences. Because adequate sunlight exposure is difficult to determine, a supplement of 200 IU/day is recommended for the following groups to prevent rickets and vitamin D deficiency in healthy infants and children:
  ▪ All breastfed infants unless they are weaned to at least 500 mL/day of vitamin D–fortified formula or milk
  ▪ All non-breastfed infants who are ingesting less than 500 mL/day of vitamin D–fortified formula or milk
  ▪ Children and adolescents who do not receive regular sunlight exposure, do not ingest at least 500 mL/day of vitamin D–fortified milk, or do not take a daily multivitamin supplement containing at least 200 IU of vitamin D

EB: *Cases of rickets in infants attributable to inadequate vitamin D intake and decreased exposure to sunlight continue to be reported in the United States. Rickets is an example of extreme vitamin D deficiency. A state of deficiency occurs months before rickets is obvious on physical examination. The new recommendation by the National Academy of Sciences for adequate intake of vitamin D to prevent vitamin D deficiency in normal infants, children, and adolescents is 200 IU/day (Gartner and Greer, 2003).*

- Provide adequate nutrition to clients with active intestinal inflammation. **EB:** *Nutrition is clearly disturbed by active intestinal inflammation. Linear growth and pubertal development in children are notably retarded, body composition is altered, and significant psychosocial disturbance may be present. Increasing evidence shows that an aggressive nutritional program may in itself be sufficient to reduce the mucosal inflammatory response (Murch & Walker-Smith, 1998).*
- Provide for adequate nutrition for pediatric and adolescent clients on long-term oral glucocorticoid therapy (e.g., those treated for chronic severe asthma). **EB:** *Growth may be inhibited by long-term use of these agents; however, recent studies suggest that use of the inhaled form of such agents does not affect long-term growth (Agertoft & Pedersen, 2000).*
- Refer to the care plan for **Delayed Growth and development.**

Multicultural

- Assess the influence of cultural beliefs, norms, values, and expectations on parents' perceptions of normal growth and development. **EBN:** *One Mexican-American pediatrician reported that the primary complaint of his Mexican-American parents is that their children do not eat enough despite being obviously overweight (Garcia, 2004). Nutrition education efforts targeting Latino mothers of young children can be culturally reframed to identify positive eating behaviors rather than focusing on a child's weight (Crawford et al, 2004).*
- Assess for the influence of acculturation. **EB:** *Acculturation to the United States is a risk factor for obesity-related behaviors among Asian-American and Hispanic adolescents (Unger et al, 2004).*
- Assess whether the parents are concerned about the amount of food eaten. **EBN:** *Some cultures may add semisolid food within the first month of life because of concerns that the infant is not getting enough to eat and the perception that "big is healthy" (Bentley et al, 1999; Higgins, 2000).*
- Assess the influence of family support on patterns of nutritional intake. **EBN:** *Women are the keepers and transmitters of culture in families. Female family members can play a dominant role in how children and infants are fed (Cesario, 2001; Pillitteri, 1999).*
- Negotiate with clients regarding which aspects of healthy nutrition can be modified while still honoring cultural beliefs. **EBN:** *Give and take with clients will lead to culturally congruent care (Leininger & McFarland, 2002).*
- Encourage parental efforts at increasing physical activity and decreasing dietary fat for their children. **EB:** *Physical activity and dietary fat consumption were inversely related among African-American girls (Thompson et al, 2004). Interventions to increase physical activity among preadolescent African-American girls may benefit from a parental component to encourage support and self-efficacy for daughters' physical activity (Adkins et al, 2004).*
- Encourage limiting television viewing to <2 hours/day for children and discourage the consumption of sweetened soft drinks. **EB:** *Longer hours of child television viewing and higher soft drink intake was associated with the occurrence of overweight for Hispanic children (Ariza et al, 2004; Giammattei et al, 2003).*

Home Care

- The interventions previously described may be adapted for home care use.

Client/Family Teaching

- ▲ Provide prenatal counseling for women with unintended pregnancies to evaluate if they have been exposed to teratogenic agents. *Women with unintended pregnancies had a risk of being exposed to alcohol, medications, cigarette smoking, and radiographs during the first trimester (Han, Nava-Ocampo & Koren, 2005).*
- ▲ Refer clients to a registered dietitian for nutritional counseling. *Help from qualified professionals is often needed to meet the nutritional needs of clients with deviations in normal growth.*

- Teach families the importance of taking measures to prevent lead poisoning. *The child's exposure to ingested lead can be lowered by following the latest protocols (Kemper et al, 2003).*

evolve See the EVOLVE website for World Wide Web resources for client education.

REFERENCES

Adkins S, Sherwood NE, Story M et al: Physical activity among African-American girls: the role of parents and the home environment, *Obes Res* (suppl 12):38S-45S, 2004.

Agertoft L, Pedersen S: Effect of long-term treatment with inhaled budesonide on adult height in children with asthma, *N Engl J Med* 343(15):1064-1069, 2000.

American Dietetic Association: Position of the American Dietetic Association: nutrition in comprehensive program planning for persons with developmental disabilities, *J Am Diet Assoc* 97(2):189-193, 1997.

Ariza AJ, Chen EH, Binns HJ et al: Risk factors for overweight in five- to six-year-old Hispanic-American children: a pilot study, *J Urban Health* 81(1):150-161, 2004.

Bentley M, Gavin L, Black MM et al: Infant feeding practices of low-income, African-American, adolescent mothers: an ecological, multigenerational perspective, *Soc Sci Med* 49(8):1085-1100, 1999.

Cesario S: Care of the Native American woman: strategies for practice, education, and research, *J Gynecol Neonat Nurs* 30(1):13, 2001.

Crawford PB, Gosliner W, Anderson C et al: Counseling Latina mothers of preschool children about weight issues: suggestions for a new framework, *J Am Diet Assoc* 104(3):387-394, 2004.

Eustace LW, Kang DH, Coombs D: Fetal alcohol syndrome: a growing concern for health care professionals, *J Obstet Gynecol Neonatal Nurs* 32(2):215-221, 2003.

Florida Birth Defects Registry: *Prevention strategies index: strategies to prevent birth defects: limit all drug exposures (prescriptions, "recreational," and over-the-counter),* http://www.fbdr.org/2005/birthdefects/prevention/beforepregnancy.asp, http://www.fbdr.org/2005/birthdefects/prevention/duringpregnancy.asp. Accessed February 21, 2007.

Garcia RS: No come nada, *Health Aff* 23(2):215-219, 2004.

Gartner M, Greer F: Prevention of rickets and vitamin D deficiency: new guidelines for vitamin D intake, *Pediatrics* 111(4):908, 2003.

Giammattei J, Blix G, Marshak HH et al: Television watching and soft drink consumption: associations with obesity in 11- to 13-year-old schoolchildren, *Arch Pediatr Adolesc Med* 157(9):882-886, 2003.

Han JY, Nava-Ocampo AA, Koren G: Unintended pregnancies and exposure to potential human teratogens, *Birth Defects Res A Clin Mol Teratol* 73(4):245-248, 2005.

Heuschkel RB, Fletcher K, Hill A et al: Isolated neonatal swallowing dysfunction: a case series and review of the literature, *Dig Dis Sci* 48(1):30-35, 2003.

Higgins B: Puerto Rican cultural beliefs: influence on infant feeding practices in western New York, *J Transcult Nurs* 11(1):19, 2000.

Leininger MM, McFarland MR: *Transcultural nursing: concepts, theories, research and practices,* ed 3, New York, 2002, McGraw-Hill.

Kemper AR, Uren RL, Hudson, SR: Childhood lead poisoning prevention activities within Michigan local public health departments, *Pub Health Rep* 122(1):88-92, 2007.

Murch SH, Walker-Smith JA: Nutrition in inflammatory bowel disease, *Baillieres Clin Gastroenterol* 12(4):719, 1998.

Pillitteri A: Nutritional needs of the newborn. In Pillitteri A, editor: *Maternal and child health nursing: care of the childbearing and childrearing family,* Philadelphia, 1999, Lippincott Williams & Wilkins.

Sanders K, Cox K, Cannon R et al: Growth response to enteral feeding by children with cerebral palsy, *JPEN J Parenter Enteral Nutr* 14(1):23-26, 1990.

Sisk PM, Lovelady CA, Dillard RG et al: Lactation counseling for mothers of very low birth weight infants: effect on maternal anxiety and infant intake of human milk, *Pediatrics,* 117(5):1859-1860, 2006.

Thompson D, Jago R, Baranowski T et al: Covariability in diet and physical activity in African-American girls, *Obes Res* 12(suppl):46S-54S, 2004.

Unger JB, Reynolds K, Shakib S et al: Acculturation, physical activity, and fast-food consumption among Asian-American and Hispanic adolescents, *J Community Health* 29(6):467-481, 2004.

Vohr BR, Poindexter BB, Dusick AM et al: Beneficial effects of breast milk in the neonatal intensive care unit on the developmental outcome of extremely low birth weight infants at 18 months of age, *Pediatrics* 118(1):e115-e123, 2006.

Ineffective Health maintenance

Kathaleen C. Bloom, PhD, CNM, and Barbara J. Olinzock, EdD, MSN, RN

NANDA **Definition**

Inability to identify, manage, and/or seek out help to maintain health

Defining Characteristics

Demonstrated lack of adaptive behaviors to environmental changes; demonstrated lack of knowledge regarding basic health practices; lack of expressed interest in improving health behaviors; history of lack of health seeking behavior; inability to take responsibility for meeting basic health practices; impairment of personal support systems

• = Independent; ▲ = Collaborative;   EBN = Evidence-Based Nursing;   EB = Evidence-Based

Related Factors (r/t)

Cognitive impairment; complicated grieving; deficient communication skills; diminished fine motor skills; diminished gross motor skills; inability to make appropriate judgments; ineffective family coping; ineffective individual coping; insufficient resources (e.g., equipment finances); lack of fine motor skills; lack of gross motor skills; perceptual impairment; spiritual distress; unachieved developmental tasks

NOC   Outcomes (Nursing Outcomes Classification)

Suggested NOC Outcomes

Health Beliefs: Perceived Resources, Health-Promoting Behavior, Health-Seeking Behavior

Example NOC Outcome with Indicators
Health-Seeking Behavior as evidenced by the following indicators: Completes health-related tasks/Performs self-screening when indicated/Seeks assistance from health professionals when indicated (Rate the outcome and indicators of **Health-Seeking Behavior:** 1 = never demonstrated, 2 = rarely demonstrated, 3 = sometimes demonstrated, 4 = often demonstrated, 5 = consistently demonstrated [see Section I].)

H

Client Outcomes

Client Will (Specify Time Frame):

- Discuss fear of or blocks to implementing health regimen
- Follow mutually agreed on healthcare maintenance plan
- Meet goals for healthcare maintenance

NIC   Interventions (Nursing Interventions Classification)

Suggested NIC Interventions

Health Education, Health System Guidance, Support System Enhancement

Example NIC Activities—Health Education
Prioritize identified learner needs based on client preference, skills of nurse, resources available, and likelihood of successful goal attainment; Emphasize immediate or short-term positive health benefits to be received by positive lifestyle behaviors rather than long-term benefits or negative effects of noncompliance

Nursing Interventions and *Rationales*

- Assess the client's feelings, values, and reasons for not following the prescribed plan of care. See Related Factors. **EBN:** *Assessment of an individual's preferences for participation in decision-making will allow for enlisting involvement in decision-making at the preferred level (Florin, Ehrenberg & Ehnfor, 2006).*
- Assess for family patterns, economic issues, and cultural patterns that influence compliance with a given medical regimen. **EB:** *The family's reaction to the diagnosis has a significant influence on adherence to the treatment regimen (Sher et al, 2005). There are marked differences in use of healthcare services among different cultural groups (Uiters et al, 2006).*
- Help the client to choose a healthy lifestyle and to have appropriate diagnostic screening tests. **EBN:** *Healthy lifestyle measures, such as exercising regularly, maintaining a healthy weight, not smoking, and limiting alcohol intake, help reduce the risk of cancer and other chronic illnesses (Holmes, 2006).*
- Assist the client in reducing stress. **EB:** *Individuals with high perceived stress are significantly more likely to be nonadherent with treatment regimens. This happens with individuals with HIV/AIDS (French et al, 2005), clients who have experienced a cardiac event (Shemesh et al, 2004; Spindler & Pedersen, 2005), and clients who have had an organ transplant (Achille et al, 2006; Kerkar et al, 2006).*

• = Independent;   ▲ = Collaborative;   EBN = Evidence-Based Nursing;   EB = Evidence-Based

H

- Help the client determine how to manage complex medication schedules (e.g., HIV/AIDS regimens or polypharmacy). **EBN:** *Taking 12 or more doses of medication in a day is a strong predictor of adherence (Johnson et al, 2005). Simplifying treatment regimens and tailoring them to individual lifestyles encourages adherence to treatment (Battaglioli-Denero, 2007).* **EB:** *For individuals who are taking multiple medications or whose memory may be impaired, the use of a written medication schedule and daily containers increases adherence with the prescribed schedule (Carlson et al, 2005).*
- Identify complementary healing modalities, such as herbal remedies, acupuncture, healing touch, yoga, or cultural shamans, that the client uses in addition to or instead of the prescribed allopathic regimen. **EB:** *Use of complementary healing modalities among clients with chronic disease is relatively high, ranging from 41% in clients with diabetes to 59.6% in clients with arthritis. Less than 30% of users of complementary healing modalities share this information with their healthcare provider (Saydah & Eberhardt, 2006).*
- ▲ Refer the client to appropriate services as needed. **EBN:** *When appropriate referrals are missed, clients often experience poor outcomes, including complications, psychological distress, and hospital readmissions (Bowles, Foust & Naylor, 2003).*
- ▲ Refer the client to community agencies for appropriate follow-up care (e.g., day treatment or adult day health program). **EBN:** *Use of community-based services and conventional or web-based support groups appears to extend positive health effects promoting behavior change (Clark et al, 2005).*
- ▲ Identify support groups related to the disease process (e.g., Reach to Recovery for a woman who has had a mastectomy). **EBN:** *Individuals attend support groups to meet others with the same diagnosis and to gain more information about the diagnosis (Purk, 2004).*
- ▲ Ensure that follow-up appointments are scheduled before the client is discharged; discuss a way to ensure that appointments are kept. **EB:** *Compliance with recommended care is higher for people with scheduled follow-up appointments than for those who self-initiate follow-up (Ahluwalia et al, 2000).*

Geriatric

- ▲ Assess sensory deficits and psychomotor skills. Supply the appropriate assistive devices. **EB:** *Older individuals with disabilities view eyeglasses, canes, walkers, telephones, oxygen tanks, dentures, 3-in-1 commodes, computers, and wheelchairs as important for maintaining independence (Mann et al, 2002).*
- Recognize resistance to change in lifelong patterns of personal health care. **EB:** *Resistance to change in diet and physical activity is common in older adults; this resistance may be related to failure to value the health-related benefits of change (Afonso et al, 2001; de Almeida et al, 2001).*
- Discuss "symptoms of daily living" in addition to the major illness. **EB:** *Old age itself is perceived as the cause for decline in functional ability (Sarkisian et al, 2001).*
- Discuss with the client and support person realistic goals for changes in health maintenance. **EB:** *The importance of personalized goals and social support in designing health interventions for older adults is a unique predictor of health goal attainment (VonDras & Madey, 2004).*
- Educate the client about the symptoms of life-threatening illness, such as myocardial infarction (MI), and the need for timeliness in seeking care. **EBN:** *Women, especially those of advanced age, wait longer before seeking treatment for signs and symptoms of acute MI (Lefler & Bondy, 2004; Rosenfeld, 2004).*
- Consider the age of the client when suggesting screening for disease. **EB:** *The small benefit of screening in older adults may be outweighed by the harms, which include anxiety, additional testing, and unnecessary treatment (Rich & Black, 2000).*

Multicultural

- Assess influence of cultural beliefs, norms, and values on the client's ability to modify health behavior. **EBN:** *What the client considers normal and abnormal health behavior may be based on cultural perceptions (Leininger & McFarland, 2002).*
- Assess the effect of fatalism on the client's ability to modify health behavior. **EBN:** *Fatalistic perspectives, which involve the belief that one cannot control one's own fate, may influence health behaviors in some Asian, African-American, and Latino populations (Chen, 2001).*
- Assess access to health services. **EB:** *Compared with Caucasians, African-American women reported*

significantly less access to health services for bone mineral density testing and prescription and nonprescription osteoporosis therapy (Mudano et al, 2003).

• Discuss with the client those aspects of health behavior and lifestyle that will remain unchanged by health status. **EBN:** *Use of culturally-tailored teaching-learning strategies improves self-care management, decreases symptom distress, and improves quality of life (Wang & Chang, 2005; Brown et al, 2005).*

 ### Home Care

• The interventions described previously may be adapted for home care use.

▲ Include a health promotion focus for the client with disabilities, with the goals of reducing secondary conditions (e.g., obesity, hypertension, pressure sores), maintaining functional independence, providing opportunities for leisure and enjoyment, and enhancing overall quality of life. **EB:** *People with disabilities who participate in a planned health promotion program report improved self-efficacy, increased health behavior, reduced limitations from secondary conditions, decreased number of unhealthy days, and decreased need for health care (Ravesloot et al, 2006; Robinson-Whelen et al, 2006).*

• Encourage a regular routine for health-related behaviors. **EBN:** *Individuals who establish a regular routine for exercise are more likely to be compliant over time than those who use an ad hoc approach to exercise (Hines, Seng & Messer, 2007; Resnik, 2002).*

• Provide sufficient outside supports (e.g., written notices, calendars, planned ride shares) to assist with follow-through on the agreed-on actions. **EBN:** *Intervention strategies that include self-contract, reinforcement, and self-monitoring are effective in helping clients change behavior (Sagawa et al, 2003).*

• Assist client to develop confidence in ability to manage the health condition. **EB:** *Self-management education targeted at self-efficacy improves physiologic outcomes, enhances coping techniques, and reduces healthcare use (Wade, Michaud & Brown, 2006; Wolf et al, 2003).*

• Establish a written contract with the client to follow the agreed-upon healthcare regimen. Written agreements reinforce the verbal agreement and serve as a reference. **EB:** *Written agreement between healthcare providers and clients is an effective strategy for promoting adherence (Resnik, 2005).*

• Meet with the client following completion of the proposed actions to review the contract and determine the next course of action. Do this until the client is able to initiate and follow through independently. *Successful completion of contracts increases self-esteem and positive coping.*

• Using self-care management precepts, instruct the client about possible situations to which he or she may need to respond; include the use of role playing. Instruct in generating hypotheses from available evidence rather than solely from experience. **EBN:** *Interventions that focus on increasing self-awareness of cues relative to health increase the client's ability to recognize and respond to changes in symptoms and health status (Hernandez & Williamson, 2004).* **EB:** *Addition of self-awareness and response training to self-monitoring of blood glucose is highly effective in managing hypoglycemia (Cox et al, 2004).*

 ### Client/Family Teaching

• Provide the family with website addresses where information can be obtained from the Internet. (Most libraries have Internet access with printing capabilities.) **EBN:** *Internet/video-delivered interventions are successful in increasing physical activity and reducing dietary fat intake (Frenn et al, 2005).* **EB:** *One third of older adults perform online searches for information about their own health or health care (Flynn, Smith & Freese, 2006).*

▲ Develop collaborative multidisciplinary partnerships. **EBN:** *Multidisciplinary and multifactorial interventions are likely to be more effective in achieving desired outcomes (Gillespie et al, 2003; Goldstein et al, 2004; Whitlock et al, 2002).*

• Tailor both the information provided and the method of delivery of information to the specific client and/or family. **EB:** *Client-centered educational interventions that support client choice and self-management improve quality of life, confidence in coping ability, and satisfaction, and reduce the need for healthcare resources (Kennedy et al, 2004).*

• Obtain or design educational material that is appropriate for the client; use pictures if possible.

• = Independent;   ▲ = Collaborative;   EBN = Evidence-Based Nursing;   EB = Evidence-Based

H

EB: *The use of materials tailored to the individual has a stronger effect than the use of standard materials (Kroeze, Werkman & Brug, 2006; Lancaster & Stead, 2005). Inclusion of pictures in written materials increases attention, recall, and comprehension. Use of pictures can change adherence to health instructions, but emotional response to pictures affects whether they increase or decrease target behaviors (Houts et al, 2006).*

- Teach the client about the symptoms associated with discontinuation of medications, such as a selective serotonin reuptake inhibitor (SSRI). **EBN:** *Educate client about SSRI discontinuation syndrome, which may include lightheadedness, dizziness, headaches, GI disturbances, diaphoresis, lethargy, vivid dreams, and flu-like symptoms. A 3- to 4-week graded dosage tapering is encouraged with short-acting SSRIs to avoid this syndrome (Antai-Otong, 2003).*
- Explain nonthreatening aspects before introducing more anxiety-producing information regarding possible side effects of the disease or medical regimen. **EBN:** *Anxiety often interferes with concentration and the ability to understand (Stephenson, 2006).*
- Treat tobacco use as a chronic problem. Acknowledge the pleasure associated with smoking. Encourage the client to work towards a goal of permanent abstinence. Advise the client about possible relapse. **EBN:** *Delivery systems are needed to assist clients in achieving the goals of permanent abstinence from smoking and better personal and family health (Buchanan, 2002).* **EB:** *Acknowledgment of the attractive, pleasurable aspects of smoking may be seen as unacceptable and irresponsible, but doing so could well provide an opportunity to relate to the everyday and multiple practices of smoking and encourage cessation (McKie et al, 2003).*

evolve   See the EVOLVE website for World Wide Web resources for client education.

REFERENCES

Achille MA, Ouellette A, Fournier S et al: Impact of stress, distress and feelings of indebtedness on adherence to immunosuppressants following kidney transplantation, *Clin Transplant* 20(3):301-306, 2006.

Afonso C, Graca P, Kearney JM et al: Physical activity in European seniors: attitudes, beliefs and levels, *J Nutr Health Aging* 5(4):226-229, 2001.

Ahluwalia HK, Miller CE, Pickard SP et al: Prevalence and correlates of preventive care among adults with diabetes in Kansas, *Diabetes Care* 23(4):484-489, 2000.

Antai-Otong D: Antidepressant discontinuation syndrome, *Perspect Psychiatr Care* 39(3):127-128, 2003.

Battaglioli-Denero AM: Strategies for improving patient adherence to therapy and long-term patient outcomes, *J Assoc Nurses AIDS Care* 18(suppl 1):S17-S22, 2007.

Bowles KH, Foust JB, Naylor MD: Hospital discharge referral decision making: a multidisciplinary perspective, *Appl Nurs Res* 16(3):134-143, 2003.

Brown SA, Blozis S, Kouzekanani K et al: Dosage effects of diabetes self-management education for Mexican Americans, *Diabetes Care* 28(3):527-532, 2005.

Buchanan L: Implementing a smoking cessation program for pregnant women based on current clinical practice guidelines, *J Am Acad Nurse Pract* 14(6):243, 2002.

Carlson MC, Fried LP, Xue QL et al: Validation of the Hopkins Medication Schedule to identify difficulties in taking medications, *J Gerontol A Biol Sci Med Sci* 60(2):217-223, 2005.

Chen YC: Chinese values, health and nursing, *J Adv Nurs* 36(2):270, 2001.

Clark AM, Whelan HK, Barbour R et al: A realist study of the mechanisms of cardiac rehabilitation, *J Adv Nurs* 52(4):362-371, 2005.

Cox DJ, Kovatchev B, Koev D et al: Hypoglycemia anticipation, awareness and treatment training (HAATT) reduces occurrence of severe hypoglycemia among adults with type 1 diabetes mellitus, *Int J Behav Med* 11(4):212-218, 2004.

de Almeida MD, Graca P, Afonso C et al: Healthy eating in European elderly: attitudes, beliefs and levels, *J Nutr Health Aging* 5(4):217-219, 2001.

Florin J, Ehrenberg A, Ehnfor M: Patient participation in clinical decision-making in nursing: A comparative study of nurses' and patients' perceptions, *J Clin Nurs* 15(12):1498-1508, 2006.

Flynn KE, Smith MA, Freese J: When do older adults turn to the internet for health information? Findings from the Wisconsin Longitudinal Study, *J Gen Intern Med* 21(12):1295-1301, 2006.

French T, Weiss L, Waters M et al: Correlation of a brief perceived stress measure with nonadherence to antiretroviral therapy over time, *J Acquir Immune Defic Syndr* 38(5):590-597, 2005.

Frenn M, Malin S, Smith RL et al: Changing the tide: an Internet/video exercise and low-fat diet intervention with middle-school students, *Appl Nurs Res* 18(1):13-21, 2005.

Gillespie LD, Gillespie WJ, Robertson MC et al: Interventions for preventing falls in elderly people. *Cochrane Database Syst Rev* (4): CD000340, 2003.

Goldstein MG, Whitlock EP, DePue J et al: Multiple behavioral risk factor interventions in primary care: summary of research evidence, *Am J Prev Med* 27(2S):61-79, 2004.

Hernandez CA, Williamson KM: Evaluation of a self-awareness education session for youth education with type 1 diabetes, *Pediatr Nurs* 30(6):459-464, 502, 2004.

Hines SH, Seng JS, Messer KL: Adherence to a behavioral program to prevent incontinence, *West J Nurs Res* 29(1):36-56, 2007.

Holmes S: Nutrition and the prevention of cancer, *J Fam Health Care* 16(2):43-46, 2006.

Houts PS, Doak CC, Doak LG et al: The role of pictures in improving health communication: a review of research on attention, comprehension, recall, and adherence, *Patient Educ Couns* 61(2):173-190, 2006.

Johnson M, Griffiths R, Piper M et al: Risk factors for an untoward medication event among elders in community-based nursing caseloads in Australia, *Public Health Nurs* 22(1):36-44, 2005.

Kennedy AP, Nelson E, Reeves D et al: A randomized controlled trial to assess the effectiveness and cost of a patient orientated self management approach to chronic inflammatory bowel disease, *Gut* 53(11):1639-1645, 2004.

Kerkar N, Annunziato RA, Foley L et al: Prospective analysis of non-adherence in autoimmune hepatitis: a common problem, *J Pediatr Gastroenterol Nutr* 43(5):629-634, 2006.

Kroeze W, Werkman A, Brug J: A systematic review of randomized trials on the effectiveness of computer-tailored education on physical activity and dietary behaviors, *Ann Behav Med* 31(3):205-223, 2006.

Lancaster T, Stead LF: Self-help interventions for smoking cessation, *Cochrane Database Syst Rev* (3)CD001118, 2005.

Lefler LL, Bondy KN: Women's delay in seeking treatment with myocardial infarction: a meta-synthesis, *J Cardiovasc Nurs* 19(4):251-268, 2004.

Leininger MM, McFarland MR: *Transcultural nursing: concepts, theories, research, and practices,* ed 3, New York, 2002, McGraw-Hill.

Mann WC, Goodall S, Justiss MD et al: Dissatisfaction and nonuse of assistive devices among frail elders, *Assist Technol* 14(2):130-139, 2002.

McKie L, Laurier E, Taylor RJ et al: Eliciting the smoker's agenda: implications for policy and practice, *Soc Sci Med* 56(1):83-94, 2003.

Mudano AS, Casebeer L, Patino F et al: Racial disparities in osteoporosis prevention in a managed care population, *South Med J* 96(5):445-451, 2003.

Purk JK: Support groups: why do people attend? *Rehabil Nurs* 29(2):62-67, 2004.

Ravesloot CH, Seekins T, Cahill T et al: Health promotion for people with disabilities: development and evaluation of the Living Well with a Disability program, *Health Educ Res,* Oct 10, 2006 [Epub ahead of print].

Resnik B: Testing the effect of the WALC intervention on exercise adherence in older adults, *J Gerontol Nurs* 28(6):40-49, 2002.

Resnik DB: The patient's duty to adhere to prescribed treatment: an ethical analysis, *J Med Philos* 30(2):167-188, 2005.

Rich JS, Black WC: When should we stop screening? *Eff Clin Pract* 3(2):78, 2000.

Robinson-Whelen S, Hughes RB, Taylor HB et al: Improving the health and health behaviors of women aging with physical disabilities: a peer-led health promotion program, *Womens Health Issues* 16(6):334-345, 2006.

Rosenfeld AG: Treatment-seeking delay among women with acute myocardial infarction: decision trajectories and their predictors, *Nurs Res* 53(4):225-236, 2004.

Sagawa M, Oka M, Chaboyer W: The utility of cognitive behavioural therapy on chronic haemodialysis patients' fluid intake: a preliminary examination, *Int J Nurs Stud* 40(4):367-373, 2003.

Sarkisian CA, Liu H, Ensrud KE et al: Correlates of attributing new disability to old age. Study of Osteoporotic Fractures Research Group, *J Am Geriatr Soc* 49(2):134-141, 2001.

Saydah SH, Eberhardt MS: Use of complementary and alternative medicine among adults with chronic diseases: United States 2002, *J Altern Complement Med* 12(8):805-812, 2006.

Shemesh E, Yehuda R, Milo O et al: Posttraumatic stress, nonadherence, and adverse outcome in survivors of a myocardial infarction, *Psychosom Med* 66(4):521-526, 2004.

Sher I, McGinn L, Sirey JA, et al: Effects of caregivers' perceived stigma and causal beliefs on patients' adherence to antidepressant treatment, *Psychiatr Serv* 56(5):564-569, 2005.

Spindler H, Pedersen SS: Posttraumatic stress disorder in the wake of heart disease: prevalence, risk factors, and future research directions, *Psychosom Med* 67(5):715-723, 2005.

Stephenson PL: Before the teaching begins: managing patient anxiety prior to providing education, *Clin J Oncol Nurs* 10(2):241-245, 2006.

Uiters E, Deville WL, Foets M et al: Use of health care services by ethnic minorities in The Netherlands: do patterns differ? *Eur J Public Health* 16(4):388-393, 2006.

VonDras DD, Madey SF: The attainment of important health goals throughout adulthood: an integration of the theory of planned behavior and aspects of social support, *Int J Aging Hum Dev* 59(3):205-234, 2004.

Wade SL, Michaud L, Brown TM: Putting the pieces together: preliminary efficacy of a family problem-solving intervention for children with traumatic brain injury. *J Head Trauma Rehabil* 21(1):57-67, 2006.

Wang C, Chang S: Culturally tailored diabetes education program for Chinese Americans, *Nurs Res* 54(4):347-351, 2005.

Whitlock EP, Orleans CT, Pender N et al: Evaluating primary care behavioral counseling interventions: an evidence-based approach *Am J Prev Med* 22(4):267-284, 2002.

Wolf FM, Guevara JM, Grum CM et al: Educational interventions for asthma in children, *Cochrane Database Syst Rev* (1):CD000326, 2003.

H

Health-seeking behaviors (specify)

Kathaleen C. Bloom, PhD, CNM, and Barbara J. Olinzock, EdD, MSN, RN

NANDA   Definition

Active seeking (by a person in stable health) of ways to alter personal health habits and/or the environment in order to move toward a higher level of health

Defining Characteristics

Demonstrated lack of knowledge about health promotion behaviors; expressed concern about current environmental conditions on health status; expressed desire for increased control of health practice; expressed desire to seek a higher level of wellness; observed unfamiliarity with wellness community resources; stated unfamiliarity with wellness community resources

• = Independent;   ▲ = Collaborative;   EBN = Evidence-Based Nursing;   EB = Evidence-Based

NOC   Outcomes (Nursing Outcomes Classification)

Suggested NOC Outcomes

Adherence Behavior, Health Beliefs, Health Orientation, Health-Promoting Behavior, Health-Seeking Behavior

Example NOC Outcome with Indicators

Health-Seeking Behavior as evidenced by the following indicators: Completes health-related tasks/Performs self-screening when indicated/Seeks assistance from health professionals when indicated (Rate the outcome and indicators of **Health-Seeking Behavior:** 1 = never demonstrated, 2 = rarely demonstrated, 3 = sometimes demonstrated, 4 = often demonstrated, 5 = consistently demonstrated [see Section I].)

Client Outcomes

Client Will (Specify Time Frame):

- Maintain ideal weight and be knowledgeable about nutritious diet
- Demonstrate ways to fit newly prescribed change in health habits into lifestyle
- List community resources available for assistance with achieving wellness
- List ways to include wellness behaviors in current lifestyle

NIC   Interventions (Nursing Interventions Classification)

Suggested NIC Interventions

Health Education, Health System Guidance, Support System Enhancement

Example NIC Activities—Health Education

Prioritize identified learner needs based on client preference, skills of nurse, resources available, and likelihood of successful goal attainment; Emphasize immediate or short-term positive health benefits to be received by positive lifestyle behaviors rather than long-term benefits or negative effects of noncompliance

Nursing Interventions and *Rationales*

- Discuss the client's beliefs about health and his or her ability to maintain health. **EBN:** *Use of strategies responsive to the perceptions and concerns of the individual tends to be more successful because they target all aspect of people's lives (Telford, Kralik & Koch, 2006).*
- Identify barriers and benefits to being healthy. **EBN:** *Understanding perceived barriers to a healthy lifestyle is important in establishing effective health promotion interventions (Thanavaro et al, 2006).*
- Identify environmental and social factors that the client perceives as health promoting. **EBN:** *Health beliefs, attitudes, and behaviors are developed within and influenced by social systems (Drayton-Brooks & White, 2004; Shearer & Fleury, 2006).*

Nutritional

- Assess the role that stress plays in overeating and weight cycling. **EB:** *People who eat under stress tend to gain more weight and have elevated levels of nocturnal insulin, cortisol, and total/high density lipoprotein (HDL) cholesterol ratios under stress, indicating at least short-term consequences on metabolic health (Epel et al, 2004).*
- Encourage use of the nutritional guidelines developed by the U.S. Department of Agriculture (USDA). *Guidelines are available at http://www.health.gov/dietaryguidelines/dga2005/document/.*
- Refer to care plan **Readiness for enhanced Nutrition** for additional interventions.

Exercise

▲ Advise the client to consult with a healthcare provider to determine the ability to tolerate a specific regimen.

• = Independent;   ▲ = Collaborative;   EBN = Evidence-Based Nursing;   EB = Evidence-Based

- Engage in regular physical activity and reduce sedentary activities to promote health, psychological well-being, and a healthy body weight *(USDA, 2005; U.S. Department of Health and Human Services, 2001)*.
  - Engage in 30 or more minutes of moderate-intensity physical activity above usual activity level 4 or more days per week. **EB:** *For sedentary individuals, engagement in moderate physical activity for an accumulated 30 minutes daily is beneficial for many health outcomes (Bucksch & Schlicht, 2006).*
  - Engagement in more vigorous physical activity or for longer periods generally provides greater health benefits. **EB:** *Vigorous physical activity on a regular basis is cardioprotective (Swain & Franklin, 2006) and has a positive effect on blood pressure (Fagard, 2006) and sick leave (Proper et al, 2006).*
  - Engage in 60 minutes of moderate to vigorous activity on most days of the week to help manage body weight and prevent gradual, unhealthy body weight gain in adulthood.
  - Engage in 60 to 90 minutes of daily moderate physical activity to sustain weight loss in adulthood. **EB:** *High levels of physical activity and consumption of a low-calorie, moderate fat diet are the primary factors associated with long-term maintenance of weight loss (Phelan, Wyatt & Hill, 2006).*
  - Engage in stretching exercises for flexibility, and resistance exercises or calisthenics for muscle strength and endurance. NOTE: *The* USDA Dietary Guidelines for Americans 2005 *contains additional recommendations for specific populations. It is available at www.health.gov/dietary-guidelines/dga2005/ recommendations.htm.*
- Encourage appropriate exercise for individuals with chronic illnesses. **EBN:** *Exercise improves psychological and social well-being in some women survivors of cancer (Christopher & Morrow, 2004).* **EB:** *Progressive resistive exercise or a combination of progressive resistive exercise and aerobic exercise appears to be safe and may be beneficial for adults living with HIV/AIDS (O'Brien et al, 2004). Pulmonary rehabilitation, including exercise training, relieves symptoms, improves emotional function, and enhances sense of control over the condition (Lacasse et al, 2006).*
- Set up a support and reward system. **EBN:** *Use of multilevel supports (e.g., family, individual, and healthcare provider) is associated with meeting physical activity guidelines (Bull et al, 2006).* **EB:** *The use of incentives can increase participation in exercise programs (DeVahl, King & Williamson, 2005).*
- Consider using music to help the client focus on the enjoyment of exercise. **EB:** *Women in particular tend to exercise longer when listening to music (Macone et al, 2006).*
- Determine the exercises that the client prefers and encourage exercise at least three times per week (e.g., walking, jogging, aerobics, swimming, bicycling, yoga, tai chi). **EBN:** *Giving the individual choices increases feelings of control and thus motivation to participate (Wingham, Dalal & Sweeney, 2006).*

Stress Management

- Determine overall patterns of stress. **EB:** *Chronic stress has been found to be associated with increased blood pressure and impaired autonomic regulation of cardiovascular functions (Lucini et al, 2005) as well as a higher risk for depression (Shields, 2006) and chronic fatigue syndrome (Kato et al, 2006).*
- Determine the client's social support network. **EBN:** *Health beliefs, attitudes, and behaviors are developed within and are influenced by social systems (Drayton-Brooks & White, 2004; Shearer & Fleury, 2006).* **EB:** *Unpleasant symptoms and altered autonomic function associated with work stress can be altered through a work-site stress management program that includes cognitive restructuring and relaxation training (Lucini et al, 2007).*
- Teach stress-relieving techniques (e.g., deep and slow breathing, progressive muscle relaxation, meditation, imagery, problem solving). **EBN:** *Guided imagery significantly improves health-related quality of life in women with osteoarthritis (Baird & Sands, 2006).* **EB:** *A community based mind-body training program with individuals who self reported poor health-related quality of life at baseline showed moderate improvements after 3 months of practice (Lee, Mancuso & Charlson, 2004).*
- Implement nursing case management with chronic illness. **EBN:** *Nursing case management including self-management education and implementation of diabetes guidelines improved blood pressure and decreased diabetes-related emotional distress (Gabbay et al, 2006).*

Smoking, Drinking, Self-Medication

- Involve the client in mutual goal setting. **EB:** *Assessment of client needs with subsequent tailoring of behavioral interventions that include self monitoring, collaborative goal setting and active problem solving is associated with appropriate single and multiple risk factor reduction (Goldstein et al, 2004).*
- Refer a client who smokes to SmokEnders or a similar community-based program. Discuss ways in which the client can deal with a change in behavior. **EB:** *Individual and group counseling along with advice from a health professional are effective in inducing smoking cessation (Moher, Hey & Lancaster, 2005).*
- Alcoholic beverages should be avoided by individuals engaging in activities that require attention, skill, or coordination, such as driving or operating machinery. NOTE: *The* USDA Dietary Guidelines for Americans 2005 *contains additional recommendations for specific populations. It is available at www.health.gov/dietaryguidelines/ dga2005/recommendations.htm.*
- ▲ Refer a client who drinks alcohol excessively to Alcoholics Anonymous (AA). Identify a support person to help the client into the organization. **EB:** *There is an association between professional treatment for alcohol abuse and reduction in long-term alcohol-related outcomes that may be influenced by participation in AA (Moos & Moos, 2006).*
- ▲ Identify patterns of self medication with over-the-counter medications and herbal remedies, and excessive use of prescribed medications. *Medications and herbal preparations are most effective when taken as intended. Combining remedies predisposes the client to unwanted side effects.* **EBN:** *Older adults are especially at risk for drug and herbal interactions because they often have multiple health problems requiring treatment and are more susceptible to adverse drug effects (Yoon & Schaffer, 2006).*
- Refer to the care plans for **Dysfunctional Family processes: alcoholism, Ineffective Denial,** and **Defensive Coping.**

Health-Seeking Behaviors

- Recognize and allow the client to discuss the choice of complementary therapies available, such as spiritual practice, relaxation, imagery, exercise, lifestyle, diet (e.g., macrobiotic, vegetarian), and nutritional supplementation. **EBN:** *Individuals with cancer believe complementary therapies help improve quality of life by facilitating more effective coping, decreasing discomforts of treatment and illness, and providing a sense of control (Lengacher et al, 2006). Spirituality and religion are closely associated with health-promoting behaviors (Callaghan, 2006; Chester, Himburg & Weatherspoon, 2006).*

Health Screening, Appropriate Health Care

- Assess the frequency of illness-preventing practices, such as routine physical examinations, dental examinations, influenza immunization, breast self-examinations (BSEs), and mammograms, as recommended for women; testicular self-examinations (TSEs) and prostate examinations for men; and screening for familial diseases, such as glaucoma and elevated cholesterol level. **EBN:** *Frequency of BSE is related to perceived seriousness of breast cancer, benefits of BSE, and health motivation (Graham, Liggons & Hypolite, 2002).* **EB:** *Reducing uncertainty about how to perform breast self-examination is seen as a key to promoting self-examination (Babrow & Kline, 2000). Immunization against influenza is an effective intervention that reduces serologically confirmed cases (Hull et al, 2002).*
- Tailor health-related messages to stress the benefits of adherence (gain framed) and the costs of nonadherence (loss framed). **EB:** *Loss-framed relational messages and gain-framed health messages are the most persuasive in motivating behavior change (Kiene et al, 2005; Rivers et al, 2005).*
- Provide a phone call to remind the client of appointments. **EB:** *Use of telephone reminders (intention-to-treat analysis) significantly reduces nonattendance rate (Downer et al, 2006).*
- Refer to the care plan for **Ineffective Health maintenance.**

Pediatric

- Follow the recommended guidelines for childhood immunizations as laid out by the Centers for Disease Control and Prevention (CDC), available at http://www.cdc.gov/nip/recs/child-schedule.htm.

Geriatric

- Assess the client's awareness of deficits that may result from normal aging (e.g., changes in sleep patterns or frequency of urination, loss of visual acuity in night driving, loss of hearing, changes

---

• = Independent;   ▲ = Collaborative;   EBN = Evidence-Based Nursing;   EB = Evidence-Based

in diet, changes in memory, loss of significant others). **EB:** *Identifying unmet needs in five domains (senses, physical activity, incontinence, cognition, and emotional distress) in older people can lead to gains in their health status and functioning (Iliffe et al, 2004).*

▲ Find suitable housing that provides support, safety, protection, meals, and social events. Consider in-home care by adult children when possible. *Informal care by adult children reduces home health-care use and delays nursing home entry (Van Houtven & Norton, 2004).*

▲ Give the client information about community resources for older adults (e.g., services providing transportation to appointments, Meals on Wheels, home visitation services, pets, American Association of Retired Persons [AARP], Elder Hostel, informational websites). **EBN:** *Most older adult clients hope to be independent and useful for as long as possible without being a burden on others and prefer to receive care in the community when their health and/or other circumstances change (Cheek et al, 2007).*

▲ Assess for signs of elder abuse and report as appropriate. **EBN:** *Elder mistreatment includes acts of commission or omission, may be intentional or unintentional, and may occur in the community or in institutional settings (Baker & Heitkemper, 2005).* **EB:** *Elder abuse is any pattern of behavior that produces physical, psychological, financial, or social harm to an older person (Kurrle, 2004), and these types of abuse have indicators that may be both similar or dissimilar (Daly & Jogerst, 2005).*

▲ Teach health-protecting behaviors to older adult clients: monitoring cholesterol intake, exercising, having the stool checked for occult blood, or undergoing a mammogram, Pap test, or prostate or skin evaluation. **EBN:** *Age, chronic illnesses, degree of physical and mental health, and cognitive status influence older adults' participation in primary and secondary health behaviors (Resnick, 2003). Addition of individualized counseling regarding the pros and cons of health-promotion activities in established outpatient healthcare facilities significantly increases participation in health promotion behaviors, especially exercise (Resnick, 2001).*

▲ Consider the age of the client when suggesting screening for disease. **EB:** *The small benefit of screening in the older adults may be outweighed by the harms: anxiety, additional testing, and unnecessary treatment (Rich & Black, 2000).*

• Teach the importance of exercise. **EB:** *Educating older adults about the benefits of exercise increases the likelihood of their initiating and adhering to an exercise program (Boyette et al, 2002). Progressive resistance strength (PRT) appears to be an effective intervention to increase strength in older people and has a positive effect on some functional limitations (Latham et al, 2003).*

▲ Form collaborative, multidisciplinary partnerships with nurse-managed clinics for health promotion and chronic disease care management for community-residing older adults. **EBN:** *Senior citizens who participated in a community-based health promotion program reported better general health, performance of roles, and social functioning. (Nuñez et al, 2003).*

 ### Multicultural

• Assess for the influence of cultural beliefs, norms, and values on the client's beliefs about health behavior. **EBN:** *What the client considers normal and abnormal health behavior may be based on cultural perceptions (Leininger & McFarland, 2002). Religion and spirituality are associated with health-seeking behaviors of African-American women (Dessio et al, 2004). Factors underlying healthcare use among Hispanics included seriousness of symptoms, which had the most effect on visits to the doctor with more serious symptoms leading to more prompt visits (Larkey et al, 2001). Social, environmental, and cultural factors affect the willingness and ability of men of racial and ethnic minorities to participate in health screening and health promotion activities (Dallas & Burton, 2004).*

• Negotiate with the client the aspects of health behavior that will require further modification. **EBN:** *Give and take with the client will lead to culturally congruent care (Leininger & McFarland, 2002).*

• Use a community focus intervention. **EB:** *Korean-American women with access to a peer-group educational program and low-cost mammography had significantly improved attitudes and knowledge about breast cancer screening (Kim & Sarna, 2004).*

 ### Home Care

NOTE: All the previously listed nursing interventions are applicable to the home care setting. For more information, see Home Care interventions in the care plan for **Ineffective Health maintenance.**

• = Independent;   ▲ = Collaborative;   EBN = Evidence-Based Nursing;   EB = Evidence-Based

H

Client/Family Teaching

- Discuss the role of environmental and social factors in supporting a healthy family life. *The people are the community. Health beliefs, attitudes, and behaviors are developed within and influenced by social systems, including families and faith-based communities (Drayton-Brooks & White, 2004; Shearer & Fleury, 2006).*
- Use written, verbal, and video instruction to provide information about health-seeking opportunities and wellness, and provide the family with lists of addresses and where information can be found. Suggest use of the Internet. (Most libraries have Internet access with printing capabilities.) **EB:** *Online health information is accessed frequently and individuals make changes based on this information; only about half share this information with their healthcare provider (Liszka, Steyer & Hueston, 2006).* **EBN:** *The combination of verbal and written health information enables the provision of standardized care information to clients and/or significant others, which appears to improve knowledge and satisfaction (Johnson, Sandford & Tyndall, 2003).*
- ▲ Teach the importance of receiving a flu vaccine. Offer vaccinations in convenient locations free of charge, and discuss perceived barriers with clients. **EBN:** *Given the potential negative consequences of contracting influenza, prevention is the best strategy (Mayo & Cobbler, 2004).*
- Teach woman how to monitor ovarian health: monthly self-monitoring using a symptom checklist, including personal and family risks and early symptoms of gastrointestinal problems. *Critical review of general health-seeking models showed a need for expansion to include the early and atypical symptom period associated with ovarian cancer and the role of self and primary care in the diagnostic process (Koldjeski et al, 2004).*

 See the EVOLVE website for World Wide Web resources for client education.

REFERENCES

*See **ineffective Health maintenance** for additional references.*

Babrow AS, Kline KN: From "reducing" to "coping with" uncertainty: reconceptualizing the central challenge in breast self-exams, *Soc Sci Med* 51(12):1805, 2000.

Baird CL, Sands LP: Effect of guided imagery with relaxation on health-related quality of life in older women with osteoarthritis, *Res Nurs Health* 29(5):442-451, 2006.

Baker MW, Heitkemper MM: The roles of nurses on interprofessional teams to combat elder mistreatment, *Nurs Outlook* 53(5):253-259, 2005.

Boyette LW, Lloyd A, Boyette JE et al: Personal characteristics that influence exercise behavior of older adults, *J Rehabil Res Dev* 39(1):95, 2002.

Bucksch J, Schlicht W: Health-enhancing physical activity and the prevention of chronic diseases—an epidemiological review, *Soz Praventivmed* 51(5):281-301, 2006.

Bull S, Eakin E, Reeves M et al: Multi-level support for physical activity and healthy eating, *J Adv Nurs* 54(5):585-593, 2006.

Callaghan D: The influence of basic conditioning factors on healthy behaviors, self-efficacy, and self-care in adults, *J Holist Nurs* 24(3):178-185, 2006.

Cheek J, Ballantyne A, Byers L et al: From retirement village to residential aged care: what older people and their families say, *Health Soc Care Community* 15(1):8-17, 2007.

Chester DN, Himburg SP, Weatherspoon LJ: Spirituality of African-American women: correlations to health-promoting behaviors, *J Natl Black Nurses Assoc* 17(1):1-8, 2006.

Christopher KA, Morrow LL: Evaluating a community-based exercise program for women cancer survivors, *Appl Nurs Res* 17(2):100-108, 2004.

Dallas C, Burton L: Health disparities among men from racial and ethnic minority populations, *Annu Rev Nurs Res* 22:77-100, 2004.

Daly JM, Jogerst GJ: Definitions and indicators of elder abuse: a Delphi survey of APS caseworkers, *J Elder Abuse Negl* 17(1):1-19, 2005.

Dessio W, Wade C, Chao M et al: Religion, spirituality, and healthcare choices of African-American women: results of a national survey, *Ethn Dis* 14(2):189-197, 2004.

DeVahl J, King R, Williamson JW: Academic incentives for students can increase participation in and effectiveness of a physical activity program, *J Am Coll Health* 53(6):295-298, 2005.

Downer SR, Meara JG, Da Costa AC et al: SMS text messaging improves outpatient attendance, *Aust Health Rev* 30(3):389-396, 2006.

Drayton-Brooks S, White N. Health promoting behaviors among African American women with faith-based support, *ABNF J* 15(5):84-90, 2004.

Epel E, Jimenez S, Brownell K et al: Are stress eaters at risk for the metabolic syndrome? *Ann NY Acad Sci* 1032:208-210, 2004.

Fagard RH: Exercise is good for your blood pressure: effects of endurance training and resistance training, *Clin Exp Pharmacol Physiol* 33(9):853-856, 2006.

Gabbay RA, Lendel I, Saleem TM et al: Nurse case management improves blood pressure, emotional distress and diabetes complication screening, *Diabetes Res Clin Pract* 71(1):28-35, 2006.

Goldstein MG, Whitlock EP, DePue J et al: Multiple behavioral risk factor interventions in primary care: Summary of research evidence, *Am J Prev Med* 27(suppl 2):61-79, 2004.

Graham ME, Liggons Y, Hypolite M: Health beliefs and self breast examination in black women, *J Cult Divers* 9(2):49-54, 2002.

Hull S, Hagdrup N, Hart B et al: Boosting uptake of influenza immunisation: a randomised controlled trial of telephone appointing in general practice, *Br J Gen Pract* 52(482):712, 2002.

Iliffe S, Lenihan P, Orrell M et al: The development of a short instrument to identify common unmet needs in older people in general practice, *Br J Gen Pract* 54(509):914-918, 2004.

Johnson A, Sandford J, Tyndall J: Written and verbal information versus verbal information only for patients being discharged from acute hospital settings to home, *Cochrane Database Syst Rev* (4): CD003716, 2003.

Kato K, Sullivan PF, Evengard B et al: Premorbid predictors of chronic fatigue, *Arch Gen Psychiatry* 63(11):1267-1272, 2006.

Kiene SM, Barta WD, Zelenski JM et al: Why are you bringing up condoms now? The effect of message content on framing effects of condom use messages, *Health Psychol* 24(3):321-326, 2005.

Kim YH, Sarna L: An intervention to increase mammography use by Korean American women, *Oncol Nurs Forum* 31(1):105-110, 2004.

Koldjeski D, Kirkpatrick MK, Everett L et al: Health seeking related to ovarian cancer, *Cancer Nurs* 27(5):370-378, 2004.

Kurrle S: Elder abuse, *Aust Fam Physician* 33(10):807-812, 2004.

Lacasse Y, Goldstein R, Lasserson TJ et al: Pulmonary rehabilitation for chronic obstructive pulmonary disease, *Cochrane Database Syst Rev* (4):CD003793, 2006.

Larkey LK, Hecht ML, Miller K et al: Hispanic cultural norms for health-seeking behaviors in the face of symptoms, *Health Educ Behav* 28(1):65-80, 2001.

Latham N, Anderson C, Bennett D et al: Progressive resistance strength training for physical disability in older people, *Cochrane Database Syst Rev* (2):CD002759, 2003.

Lee SW, Mancuso CA, Charlson ME: Prospective study of new participants in a community-based mind-body training program, *J Gen Intern Med* 19(7):760-765, 2004.

Leininger MM, McFarland MR: *Transcultural nursing: concepts, theories, research, and practices*, ed 3, New York, 2002, McGraw-Hill.

Lengacher CA, Bennett MP, Kip KE et al: Relief of symptoms, side effects, and psychological distress through use of complementary and alternative medicine in women with breast cancer, *Oncol Nurs Forum* 33(1):97-104, 2006.

Liszka HA, Steyer TE, Hueston WJ: Virtual medical care: how are our patients using online health information? *J Community Health* 31(5):368-378, 2006.

Lucini D, Di Fede G, Parati G et al: Impact of chronic psychosocial stress on autonomic cardiovascular regulation in otherwise healthy subjects, *Hypertension* 46(5):1201-1206, 2005.

Lucini D, Riva S, Pizzinelli P et al: Stress management at the worksite: reversal of symptoms profile and cardiovascular dysregulation, *Hypertension* 49(2):291-297, 2007.

Macone D, Baldari C, Zelli A et al: Music and physical activity in psychological well-being, *Percept Mot Skills* 103(1):285-295, 2006.

Mayo AM, Cobbler S: Flu vaccines and patient decision making: what we need to know, *J Am Acad Nurse Pract* 16(9):402-410, 2004.

Moher M, Hey K, Lancaster T: Workplace interventions for smoking cessation. *Cochrane Database Syst Rev* (3), CD003440, 2005.

Moos RH, Moos BS: Participation in treatment and Alcoholics Anonymous: a 16-year follow-up of initially untreated individuals, *J Clin Psychol* 62(6):735-750, 2006.

Nuñez DE, Armbruster C, Phillips WT et al: Community-based senior health promotion program using a collaborative practice model: the Escalante Health Partnerships, *Public Health Nurs* 20(1):25, 2003.

O'Brien K, Nixon S, Glazier R et al: Progressive resistive exercise interventions for adults living with HIV/AIDS, *Cochrane Database Syst Rev* (4):CD004248, 2004.

Phelan S, Wyatt HR, Hill JO: Are the eating and exercise habits of successful weight losers changing? *Obesity* 14(4):710-716, 2006.

Proper KI, van den Heuvel SG, De Vroome EM et al: Dose-response relation between physical activity and sick leave, *Br J Sports Med* 40(2):173-178, 2006.

Resnick B: Promoting health in older adults: a four-year analysis, *J Am Acad Nurse Pract* 13(1):23-33, 2001.

Resnick B: Health promotion practices of older adults: model testing, *Public Health Nurs* 20(1):2-12, 2003.

Rich JS, Black WC: When should we stop screening? *Eff Clin Pract* 3(2):78, 2000.

Rivers SE, Salovey P, Pizarro DA et al: Message framing and pap test utilization among women attending a community health clinic, *J Health Psychol* 10(1):65-77, 2005.

Shearer N, Fleury J: Social support promoting health in older women, *J Women Aging* 18(4):3-17, 2006.

Shields M: Stress and depression in the employed population, *Health Rep* 17(4):11-29, 2006.

Swain DP, Franklin BA: Comparison of cardioprotective benefits of vigorous versus moderate intensity aerobic exercise, *Am J Cardiol* 97(1):141-147, 2006.

Telford K, Kralik D, Koch T: Acceptance and denial: implications for people adapting to chronic illness: literature review, *J Adv Nurs* 55(4):457-464, 2006.

Thanavaro JL, Moore SM, Anthony N et al: Predictors of health promotion behavior in women without prior history of coronary heart disease, *Appl Nurs Res* 19(3):149-155, 2006.

U.S. Department of Agriculture (USDA): *The dietary guidelines for Americans, 2005.* Available at http://www.health.gov/dietaryguidelines/dga2005/document/pdf/DGA2005.pdf, accessed on March 19, 2007.

U.S. Department of Health and Human Services: *Healthy people 2010*, ed 2, Washington, DC, 2001, U.S. Government Printing Office.

Van Houtven CH, Norton EC: Informal care and health use of older adults, *J Health Econ* 23(6):1159-1180, 2004.

Wingham J, Dalal HM, Sweeney KG: Listening to patients: choice in cardiac rehabilitation, *Eur J Cardiovasc Nurs* 5(4):289-294, 2006.

Yoon SL, Schaffer SD: Herbal, prescribed, and over-the-counter drug use in older women: prevalence of drug interactions, *Geriatr Nurs* 27(2):118-129, 2006.

H

Impaired Home maintenance   *Gail B. Ladwig, MSN, CHTP, RN*

NANDA   Definition

Inability to independently maintain a safe and growth-promoting immediate environment

Defining Characteristics

Objective

Disorderly surroundings; inappropriate household temperature; insufficient clothes; insufficient linen; lack of clothes; lack of linen; lack of necessary equipment; offensive odors; overtaxed family members; presence of vermin; repeated unhygienic disorders; repeated unhygienic infections; unavailable cooking equipment; unclean surroundings

Subjective

Household members describe financial crises; household members describe outstanding debts; household members express difficulty in maintaining their home in a comfortable fashion; household members request assistance with home maintenance.

Related Factors (r/t)

Deficient knowledge; disease; inadequate support systems; injury; impaired functioning; insufficient family organization; insufficient family planning; insufficient finances; lack of role modeling; unfamiliarity with neighborhood resources

NOC   Outcomes (Nursing Outcomes Classification)

Suggested NOC Outcomes

Family Functioning, Parenting: Psychosocial Safety, Parenting Performance, Role Performance, Self-Care: Instrumental Activities of Daily Living (IADLs)

Example NOC Outcome with Indicators
Family Functioning as evidenced by the following indicators: Regulates behavior of members/Obtains adequate resources to meet needs of members (Rate the outcome and indicators of **Family Functioning:** 1 = never demonstrated, 2 = rarely demonstrated, 3 = sometimes demonstrated, 4 = often demonstrated, 5 = consistently demonstrated [see Section I].)

Client Outcomes

Client Will (Specify Time Frame):

- Wear clean clothing, eat nutritious meals, and have a sanitary and safe home
- Have the resources to cope physically and emotionally with the chronic illness process
- Use community resources to assist with treatment needs

NIC   Interventions (Nursing Interventions Classification)

Suggested NIC Intervention

Home Maintenance Assistance

Example NIC Activities—Home Maintenance Assistance
Provide information on how to make home environment safe and clean; Help family use social support network

Nursing Interventions and *Rationales*

- Assess the concerns of family members, especially the primary caregiver, about long-term home care. **EB:** *Dementia severity was the key predictor of the decision to relinquish care (Bond & Clark, 2002).*
- Establish a plan of care with the client and family based on the client's needs and the caregiver's capabilities. **EBN:** *Health care workers need to provide support when the client and family are facing difficult decisions (Hurley and Volicer, 2002).*
- Set up a system of relief for the main caregiver in the home, and plan for sharing of household duties. **EB:** *The level of burden was affected directly by behavioral problems in the care receiver, frequency of getting a break, caregiver self-esteem, and caring for the client at odd hours (Chappell & Reid, 2002).*
- Consider the use of permethrin-impregnated mattress liners to control dust mites. **EB:** *A trial of*

• = Independent;   ▲ = Collaborative;   EBN = Evidence-Based Nursing;   EB = Evidence-Based

permethrin-impregnated bedding significantly reduced house dust mites and allergen concentrations. No adverse side effects were reported (Cameron & Hill, 2002).

▲ Initiate referral to community agencies as needed, including housekeeping services, Meals on Wheels (MOW), wheelchair-compatible transportation services, and oxygen therapy services. **EBN:** *Barriers to health promotion in people with chronic illness are fatigue, time, inadequate safety measures, and lack of accessible facilities (Stuifbergen, 1997). MOW programs improve dietary intake of recipients (Roy & Payette, 2006).*

▲ Obtain adaptive equipment and telemedical equipment, as appropriate, to help family members continue to maintain the home environment. **EBN:** *Telemedical equipment available for the home includes infusion pumps, pulse oximeters, 12-lead electrocardiogram (ECG) machines, and telestethoscopes (McNeal, 1998).*

▲ Ask the family to identify support people who can help with home maintenance. **EB:** *Supportive housing programs, which provide independent housing along with health and social services, hold great promise for mentally ill individuals who are homeless (Culhane, Metreaux & Hadley, 2002).*

Geriatric

▲ During the home visit, be alert for signs of elder abuse. Report any findings. **EBN:** *Activities categorized as mistreatment include force-feeding; overmedication/undermedication; withholding care or needed therapies; failure to provide safety precautions; and failure to provide health devices, such as dentures, glasses, or ambulatory devices (Rosenblatt, 1997).*

▲ Refer for telephone primary care management. **EB:** *Linking older adults in the community to telephone care-management decreased use of primary care physicians and hospital admissions (Shannon, Wilber & Allen, 2006).*

▲ Explore community resources to assist with home care (e.g., senior centers, Department of Aging, hospital case managers, the Internet, or church parish nurse). *Linkages between case managers, who build the service arrangements for older people, and community developers, who are responsible for building community capacity and social capital is essential for establishing the foundations of a caring community with the capacity to support older people (Austin, McClelland & Gursansky, 2006). An Internet resource is available at www.acsu.buffalo.edu/drstall.*

▲ Provide assistive technology devices: barrier-free environment (home modification), daily living aids, mobility aids, seating and positioning devices, and sensory aids. *Proper use of technology can help "aging in place" (Chu & Chen, 2006).*

• Encourage regular eye examinations. *Early detection of eye changes is imperative to prevent irreversible damage (AgeNet, 2003).*

• The following interventions should be considered for clients with diminished or failing sight:

  ▪ **Reduce glare:** use nonglare light bulbs; remove wax from floors (to reduce glare); encourage the client to wear sunglasses; use sheer curtains or blinds.

  ▪ **Use proper lighting:** use night lights in the bedroom, bathroom, and hallways; use dimmer switches and three-way bulbs to control light; put bright lights at the top and bottom of a staircase; use consistent lighting to minimize shadows.

  ▪ **Enhance color contrast:** use colored tape to define steps; paint walls and staircase to contrast with floor; put glow-in-the-dark tape on light switches and door knobs; use colored dishes.

  ▪ **Encourage the client to use low vision aids:** use magnifiers to improve near vision; hang magnifiers around the neck for convenience when sewing, doing crafts, or reading; request large-print medication labels, books, and phones; use handrails on stairs; keep flashlights in a convenient location.

    Vision loss can cause less hardship if adaptive strategies and aids are used. Use of aids increases safety and promotes a sense of independence (AgeNet, 2003).

• See the care plans for **Risk for Injury** and **Risk for Falls.**

Multicultural

• Acknowledge the stresses unique to racial/ethnic communities. **EBN:** *Targeted alcohol and tobacco marketing, high levels of unemployment, lack of health insurance, and racism are stresses unique to culturally diverse communities and often accompany poor housing (D'Avanzo et al, 2001). One in 10 Latino children lives in a "severely distressed neighborhood" (Annie E. Casey Foundation, 1994).*

• = Independent; ▲ = Collaborative; EBN = Evidence-Based Nursing; EB = Evidence-Based

H

Minority adults who moved to low-poverty neighborhoods were less likely to be exposed to violence and disorder, experience health problems, abuse alcohol, and receive cash assistance (Fauth, Leventhal & Brooks-Gunn, 2004).

Home Care

- The previously mentioned interventions incorporate these resources.
- ▲ Refer clients with mental illness and medical conditions to in-home behavioral health case management. *Clients in this program receive integrated medical and mental health services (Theis, Kozlowski & Behrens, 2006).*
- ▲ When the smart home becomes available, consider referral for use. *A groundbreaking home that uses the latest smart technology to give people with dementia and other serious long-term health conditions greater independence is being tested (Medical Devices & Surgical Technology Week, 2007).*
- See care plans **Contamination** and **Risk for Contamination.**

Client/Family Teaching

- Teach the caregiver the need to set aside some personal time every day to meet his or her own needs. **EBN:** *Family needs and need for relief are important (Hallström, Runesson & Elander, 2002).*
- ▲ Identify support groups within the community to assist families in the caregiver role. **EBN:** *A nurse-led support group may have a positive effect on the well-being of spouses of stroke clients (Larson, et al, 2005).*
- ▲ Provide counseling and support for caregivers of clients with Alzheimer's disease. **EBN:** *Clients whose spouses had counseling and support experienced a decrease in the rate of nursing home placement. Improvements in caregivers' satisfaction with social support, response to client behavior problems, and symptoms of depression were observed (Mittelman et al, 2006).*
- ▲ Provide written instructions for medication management and side effects, written instructions for equipment brought to the home, and resource phone numbers for emergency needs. **EBN:** *Verbal reinforcement of personalized written instructions appears to be the best intervention. In one study, the use of computer-generated, personalized instructions improved adherence (Hayes, 1998).*
- ▲ Promote food safety. Instruct client to avoid microbial food-borne illness by regularly washing hands, food contact surfaces, and fruits and vegetables. Meat and poultry should not be washed or rinsed. Separate raw, cooked, and ready-to-eat foods while shopping, preparing, or storing foods. Cook foods to a safe temperature to kill microorganisms. Chill (refrigerate) perishable food promptly and defrost foods properly. Avoid raw (unpasteurized) milk or any products made from unpasteurized milk, raw or partially cooked eggs, or foods containing raw eggs, raw or undercooked meat and poultry, unpasteurized juices, and raw sprouts. *The* Dietary Guidelines for Americans 2005 *contains additional recommendations for specific populations. It is available at www. health.gov/dietaryguidelines/dga2005/recommendations.htm.*
- ▲ Teach clients to prevent exposure that could result in adverse health effects from disturbed mold. Avoid areas where mold contamination is obvious; use environmental controls; use personal protective equipment; and keep hands, skin, and clothing clean and free from mold-contaminated dust. *Extensive water damage after major hurricanes and floods increases the likelihood of mold contamination in buildings. These measures help to limit exposure to mold and help to prevent mold-related health effects (Brandt, et al, 2006).*
- See care plans **Risk for Infection, Contamination,** and **Risk for Contamination.**

evolve See the EVOLVE website for World Wide Web resources for client education.

REFERENCES

AgeNet: Visual changes. Available at http://www.agenet.com/ ?Url=link.asp?DOC/36, accessed February 25, 2003.

Annie E. Casey Foundation: *Kids count data book: state profiles of child well-being,* ed 5, Baltimore, 1994, The Foundation.

Austin CD, McClelland RW, Gursansky D: Linking case management and community development, *Care Manag J* 7(4):162-168, 2006.

Bond MJ, Clark MS: Predictors of the decision to yield care of a person with dementia, *Aust J Ageing* 21(2):86, 2002.

Brandt M, Brown C, Burkhart J et al: Mold prevention strategies and possible health effects in the aftermath of hurricanes and major floods, *MMWR Recomm Rep* 55(RR-8):1-27, 2006.

Cameron MM, Hill N: Permethrin-impregnated mattress liners: a novel and effective intervention against house dust mites (Acari: Pyroglyphidae), *J Med Entomol* 39(5):755, 2002.

Chappell NL, Reid RC: Burden and well-being among caregivers: examining the distinction, *Gerontologist* 42(6):772, 2002.

• = Independent;   ▲ = Collaborative;   EBN = Evidence-Based Nursing;   EB = Evidence-Based

Chu HT, Chen MH: Assistive technology devices for the elderly at home [in Chinese], *Hu Li Za Zhi* 53(5):20-27, 2006.

Culhane DP, Metreaux S, Hadley T: Supportive housing for homeless people with severe mental illness, *LDI Issue Brief* 7(5):1, 2002.

D'Avanzo CE et al: Developing culturally informed strategies for substance-related interventions. In Naegle MA, D'Avanzo CE, editors: *Addictions and substance abuse: strategies for advanced practice nursing,* St Louis, 2001, Mosby.

Fauth RC, Leventhal T, Brooks-Gunn J: Short-term effects of moving from public housing in poor to middle-class neighborhoods on low-income, minority adults' outcomes, *Soc Sci Med* 59(11):2271-2284, 2004.

Hallström I, Runesson I, Elander G: International pediatric nursing. Observed parental needs during their child's hospitalization, *J Pediatr Nurs* 17(2):140, 2002.

Hayes K: Randomized trial of geragogy-based medication instruction in the emergency department, *Nurs Res* 47(4):211, 1998.

Hurley AC, Volicer L: Alzheimer disease: "It's okay, Mama, if you want to go, it's okay," *JAMA* 288(18):2324, 2002.

Larson J, Franzen-Dahlin A, Billing E et al: The impact of a nurse-led support and education programme for spouses of stroke patients: a randomized controlled trial, *J Clin Nurs* 14(8):995-1003, 2005.

McNeal G: Telecommunication techniques in high-tech home care, *Adv Pract Nurse* 10(3):279, 1998.

Medical Devices & Surgical Technology Week: Mental Health; Home uses technology to give people with dementia greater independence, *Medical Devices & Surgical Technology* Atlanta: p. 167, Feb 18, 2007.

Mittelman MS, Haley WE, Clay OJ et al: Improving caregiver well-being delays nursing home placement of patients with Alzheimer disease, *Neurology* 67(9):1592-1599, 2006.

Rosenblatt D: Elder mistreatment, *Crit Care Nurs Clin North Am* 9(2):183, 1997.

Roy MA, Payette H: Meals-on-wheels improves energy and nutrient intake in a frail free-living elderly population. *J Nutr Health Aging* 10(6):554-560, 2006.

Shannon GR, Wilber KH, Allen D: Reductions in costly healthcare service utilization: findings from the Care Advocate Program. *J Am Geriatr Soc.* 54(7):1102-1107, 2006.

Stuifbergen A: Health promotion: an essential component of rehabilitation for persons with chronic disabling conditions, *ANS Adv Nurs Sci* 19(4):1, 1997.

Theis GA, Kozlowski D, Behrens J: In-home behavioral health case management: an integrated model for high-risk populations. *Case Manager* 17(6):60-65, 68, 2006.

Readiness for enhanced Hope   *Margaret Lunney, RN, PhD, and Marie Giordano, MS, RN*

NANDA   Definition

A pattern of expectations and desires that is sufficient for mobilizing energy on one's own behalf and can be strengthened

Defining Characteristics

Expresses desire to enhance: ability to set achievable goals; belief in possibilities; congruency of expectations with desires; hope; interconnectedness with others; problem solving to meet goals; sense of meaning to life; spirituality

NOC   Outcomes (Nursing Outcomes Classification)

Suggested NOC Outcomes

Hope, Quality of Life

Example NOC Outcome with Indicators
Hope as evidenced by the following indicators: Expresses expectation of a positive future/Expresses faith/Expresses meaning in life/Exhibits a zest for life/Sets goals (Rate the outcome and indicators of **Hope**: 1 = never demonstrated, 2 = rarely demonstrated, 3 = sometimes demonstrated, 4 = often demonstrated, 5 = consistently demonstrated [see Section I].)

Client Outcomes

Client Will (Specify Time Frame):

- Describe values, expectations, and meanings
- Set achievable goals that are consistent with values
- Design strategies to achieve goals
- Express belief in possibilities

• = Independent;   ▲ = Collaborative;   EBN = Evidence-Based Nursing;   EB = Evidence-Based

NIC Interventions (Nursing Interventions Classification)

Suggested NIC Interventions

Cognitive Restructuring, Emotional Support, Hope Inspiration, Presence, Support System Enhancement

---

Example NIC Activities—Hope Inspiration

Assist patient/family to identify areas of hope in life; Demonstrate hope by recognizing the patient's intrinsic worth and viewing the patient's illness as only one facet of the individual; Encourage therapeutic relationships with significant others; Help the patient expand spiritual self

---

Nursing Interventions and *Rationales*

- Develop an open and caring relationship that enables the client to discuss hope. **EBN:** *Hope and well-being were strongly related in a study of 130 older adults. The authors concluded that nurses need to foster hope in a variety of ways, with development of an open and caring relationship being the first step (Davis, 2005).*
- Screen the client for hope using a valid and reliable instrument as indicated. **EBN:** *The Herth Hope Index was developed and tested for use in screening for hope in clinical settings (Herth 1992, 1993; Johnson, Cheffer & Roberts, 1996; Rustoen al, 2005). Use of the Herth Hope Index to compare the hope of 93 clients hospitalized with heart failure and 441 healthy control subjects showed that hope does not relate to disease; those with congestive heart failure (CHF) had higher levels of hope than the random group of healthy community dwelling persons (Rustoen et al, 2005).*
- Focus on the positive aspects of hope, rather than the prevention of hopelessness. **EBN:** *Numerous studies conducted during development of the health promotion model show that promotion differs from prevention and requires a positive rather than negative approach (Pender, Murdaugh & Parsons, 2006).*
- Provide emotional support. **EBN:** *A qualitative longitudinal study of the meaning of hope with 10 persons who had an acute spinal cord injury one year previous showed that emotional and motivational strategies were important to promote hope, and that hope is a powerful experience for health (Lohne & Severinsson, 2006).*
- Promote the client's awareness of the existential meanings in life events. **EB:** *In an undergraduate population (n = 191), research findings strongly supported that existential meanings, both explicit and implicit, were related to decreased depressive symptoms and increased levels of hope measured with two different instruments (Mascaro & Rosen, 2005).*
- Help the person to identify his or her desires and expectations. **EBN:** *In a concept analysis of hope, positive expectation and future orientation were two characteristics identified from previous literature sources (Benzein & Saveman, 1998). In a qualitative study with 14 adults aged 43 to 81 years with end stage renal disease, hope was identified as being able to see something in the future that keeps you going (Weil, 2000). Future orientation was one type of hope identified in a study of the nature of hope in chronically ill hospitalized clients (Kim et al, 2006).*
- Use a family-oriented approach when discussing hope. **EB:** *Including the family may facilitate the family's hope to be similar to the client's hope. In a study of 40 clients with cancer and 45 family members, the level of hope in family members was significantly lower than that in clients (p <.005) (Benzein & Berg, 2005).*
- Review internal and external resources to enhance hope. **EB:** *In a study of 1041 medical records over two years, higher levels of hope were associated with decreased likelihood of having or developing a disease (Richman et al, 2005).* **EBN:** *In a concept analysis of hope based on an extensive literature review, the consequences of hope were identified as ability to cope, renewal, development of new strategies, peace, and improved quality of life and physical health (Benzein & Saveman, 1998).*
- Identify spiritual beliefs and practices. **EBN:** *In a cross-sectional correlational study with 130 adults aged 60 to 89 years, spirituality was identified as a mediator of hope and well being (ß = .52, p <.001) (Davis, 2005). In the study by Weil (2000), hope was related to spiritual beliefs and other factors. Spiritual beliefs and practices are associated with higher levels of existential meaning, which is related to hope (Mascaro & Rosen 2005). Hope is a spiritual need, as identified in a study of 683 individuals (Flannelly, Galek & Flannelly, 2006).*

• = Independent;   ▲ = Collaborative;   EBN = Evidence-Based Nursing;   EB = Evidence-Based

- Assist the person to consider possible adaptations to changes. **EBN:** *A qualitative study of 14 men and women with end-stage renal disease showed that they maintained hope by attaching their hopes to reality and adapting to changes as needed (Weil, 2000).* **EB:** *The problem-solving strategies of college students who were classified as having high hope by scores on a hope scale (n = 119) were more positive and rational than the college students who were classified as having low hope (n = 92) (Chang, 1998). The findings suggest that fostering hope should include helping people to reconceptualize events as challenges rather than as threats (Chang, 1998).*

Home Care

- Previously mentioned interventions may be adapted for home care use.

Client/Family Teaching

- Assess client and family hope before teaching. **EBN:** *The degree and type of client and family hope may differ from each other, which may interfere with learning and use of knowledge for problem solving (Benzein & Berg, 2005; Chang, 1998).*
- Incorporate client and family goal setting with teaching content. **EBN:** *Realistic goal setting fosters and supports hope (Weil, 2000).*
- Provide information to the client and family regarding all aspects of the client's health condition. **EBN:** *Accurate and complete information is more likely to support hope than the perceptions that might occur without accurate and complete information (Johnson, Cheffer & Roberts 1996).*

evolve   See the EVOLVE website for World Wide Web resources for client education.

REFERENCES

Benzein EG, Berg AC: The level of and relation between hope, hopelessness and fatigue in patients and family members in palliative care, *Palliat Med* 19:234-240, 2005.

Benzein E, Saveman BL: One step towards the understanding of hope: a concept analysis, *Int J Nurs Stud* 35:322-329, 1998.

Chang EC: Hope, problem-solving ability, and coping in a college student population: some implications for theory and practice, *J Clin Psychol* 54(7):953-962, 1998.

Davis B: Mediators of the relationship between hope and well-being in older adults, *Clin Nurs Res* 14(3):253-272, 2005.

Flannelly KJ, Galek K, Flannelly LT: A test of the factor structure of the patient spiritual needs assessment scale, *Holist Nurs Pract* 20(4):187-190, 2006.

Herth K: Abbreviated instrument to measure hope: development and psychometric evaluation. *J Adv Nurs* 17:1251-1259, 1992.

Herth K: Hope in the family caregiver of terminally ill people, *J Adv Nurs* 18:538-548, 1993.

Johnson LH, Cheffer ND, Roberts SL: A hope and hopelessness model applied to the family of multitrauma injury patient, *J Trauma Nurs* 3(3):72-85, 1996.

Kim DS, Kim HS, Schwartz-Barcott D et al: The nature of hope in hospitalized chronically ill patients, *Int J Nurs Stud* 43(5):547-556, 2006.

Lohne V, Severinsson E: The power of hope: patient's experiences of hope a year after spinal cord injury, *J Clin Nurs* 15(3):315-323, 2006.

Mascaro N, Rosen DH: Existential meanings' role in the enhancement of hope and prevention of depressive symptoms, *J Pers* 73(4):985-1013, 2005.

Pender NJ, Murdaugh CL, Parsons MA: *Health promotion in nursing practice,* ed 5, Stamford, Conn, 2006, Appleton & Lange.

Richman LS, Kubzansky L, Maselko J et al: Positive emotion and health: going beyond the negative, *Health Psychol* 24(4):422-429, 2005.

Rustoen T, Howie J, Eidsmo I et al: Hope in patients hospitalized with heart failure, *Am J Crit Care* 14(5):417-425, 2005.

Weil CM: Exploring hope in patients with end stage renal disease on chronic hemodialysis, *Nephrol Nurs J* 27(2):219-224, 2000.

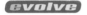

Hopelessness   *Gail Ladwig, RN, MSN, CHTP*

NANDA   ### Definition

Subjective state in which an individual sees limited or no alternatives or personal choices available and is unable to mobilize energy on own behalf

Defining Characteristics

Closing eyes; decreased affect; decreased appetite; decreased response to stimuli; decreased verbalization; lack of initiative; lack of involvement in care; passivity; shrugging in response to speaker;

• = Independent;   ▲ = Collaborative;   EBN = Evidence-Based Nursing;   EB = Evidence-Based

H

sleep pattern disturbance; turning away from speaker; verbal cues (e.g., despondent content, "I can't," sighing)

Related Factors (r/t)

Abandonment; deteriorating physiological condition; lost belief in spiritual power; lost belief in transcendent values; long-term stress; prolonged activity restriction creating isolation

NOC   Outcomes (Nursing Outcomes Classification)

Suggested NOC Outcomes

Decision Making, Hope, Mood Equilibrium, Nutritional Status: Food and Fluid Intake, Quality of Life, Sleep

Example NOC Outcome with Indicators
Has a presence of **Hope** as evidenced by the following indicators: Expresses expectation of a positive future/ Expresses faith/Expresses will to live (Rate the outcome and indicators of **Hope:** 1 = never demonstrated, 2 = rarely demonstrated, 3 = sometimes demonstrated, 4 = often demonstrated, 5 = consistently demonstrated [see Section I].)

Client Outcomes

Client Will (Specify Time Frame):

- Verbalize feelings, participate in care
- Make positive statements (e.g., "I can" or "I will try")
- Set goals
- Make eye contact, focus on speaker
- Maintain appropriate appetite for age and physical health
- Sleep appropriate length of time for age and physical health
- Express concern for another
- Initiate activity

NIC   Interventions (Nursing Interventions Classification)

Suggested NIC Intervention

Hope Inspiration

Example NIC Activities—Hope Inspiration
Assist patient/family to identify areas of hope in life; Demonstrate hope by recognizing client's intrinsic worth and viewing patient's illness as only one facet of the individual; Expand the patient's repertoire of coping mechanisms

Nursing Interventions and *Rationales*

- ▲ Monitor and document the potential for suicide. (Refer the client for appropriate treatment if a potential for suicide is identified.) Refer to the care plan **Risk for Suicide** for specific interventions. *Hopelessness associated with depression is an indicator of higher risk for suicidality (Szanto et al, 2002).*
- Be alert for symptoms of hopelessness in the general population. **EB:** *Hopelessness appears to be an important indicator of low subjective well-being in the general population (Haatainen et al, 2004).*
- Assist in identifying sources of hope and hopelessness. **EBN:** *Depending on the population being served, there may be specific interventions more helpful in promoting hope (Cutcliffe & Grant, 2001).* **EB:** *Hopelessness and depression were frequent and moderate to severe in a portion of clients in the early acute coronary syndrome (ACS) recovery period. An association between hopelessness and depression exists with clients after ACS (Dunn et al, 2006).*

• = Independent;   ▲ = Collaborative;   EBN = Evidence-Based Nursing;   EB = Evidence-Based

- Provide realistic feedback. **EBN:** *Accurate information allows the nurse-client relationship to redefine hope in the present (Kylma, Vehvilainen-Julkunen & Lahdevirta, 2001).*
- Assess for pain and respond with appropriate measures for pain relief. *Fear of pain and inability to cope with pain are significant risk factors for hopelessness (Duggleby, 2001).*
- Assist with problem solving and decision making. *Cognitive behavioral therapy (CBT) is a useful intervention when working on issues of hope (Collins & Cutliffe, 2003).*
- Determine appropriate approaches based on the underlying condition or situation that is contributing to feelings of hopelessness. *Understanding the source of the hopelessness, be it a victimizing relationship or a physical alteration, will indicate the approaches that may be most beneficial to the client (Schreiber, 2001).* **EB:** *Women with advanced breast cancer and their families benefit from specific strategies of intervention (Northouse et al, 2005).*
- Assist the client in looking at alternatives and setting goals that are important to him or her. *Use of the nurse's knowledge along with the client's experience within the context of a supportive relationship stimulates an unfolding of possibilities (Kylma, Vehvilainen-Julkunen & Lahdevirta, 2001).* **EB:** *When health professionals work with women with advanced beast cancer and their family caregivers, they should help them replace avoidant coping strategies (Northouse et al, 2005).*
- In dealing with possible long-term deficits, work with the client to set small, attainable goals. *Working on mutually agreed upon goals that are meaningful to the client will support hopefulness (Duggleby, 2001).* **EBN:** *Women with post–breast cancer lymphedema required individual attention to their specific needs and abilities (Radina et al, 2004).*
- Spend one-on-one time with the client. Use empathy; try to understand what the client is saying and communicate this understanding to the client and inspire hope. **EBN:** *Physical presence and active listening inspire hope in the client (Duggleby, 2001). The interview process itself can be therapeutic (Overcash, 2004). The inspiration of hope in psychiatric mental health nursing may be grounded in the relationship established between nurse and person in need of hope (Cutcliffe & Koehn, 2007).*
- Encourage decision making in the daily schedule. *Hopelessness may be an outgrowth of a perceived loss of control and/or self-efficacy. As changes occur, the nurse interacts with the client to evaluate their impact on life goals and assists in making adaptations that support hopefulness (Kylma, Vehvilainen-Julkunen & Lahdevirta, 2001).*
- Encourage expression of feelings and acknowledge acceptance of them. *Hope is ultimately dependent on external validation in the form of positive interpersonal relationships (Cutcliffe & Grant, 2001). The therapeutic relationship is an essential component of interventions to address hopelessness (Collins & Cutliffe, 2003).*
- Give the client time to initiate interactions. After an appropriate amount of time is allowed, approach the client in an accepting and nonjudgmental manner. *Establishing new relationships and control over events within them is constructive within the context of nurturing hopefulness (Kylma, Vehvilainen-Julkunen & Lahdevirta, 2001). The therapeutic relationship is an essential component of interventions to address hopelessness (Collins & Cutliffe, 2003).*
- Encourage the client to participate in group activities. *Group activities provide social support and help the client identify alternative ways to solve problems. They also allow the opportunity to care for others and to be cared for (Kylma, Vehvilainen-Julkunen & Lahdevirta, 2001).* **EBN:** *Women with cancer in church groups report a positive response (Ferrell et al, 2003).*
- Teach alternative coping strategies. **EB:** *Quality of life is enhanced in women with coronary syndrome X when they incorporate exercise and relaxation therapy into their coping behaviors (Tyni-Lenne et al, 2002).*
- Review the client's strengths with the client. *Have the client list his or her own strengths on a note card and carry this list for future reference. Working with the client to identify positive experiences and personal strengths facilitates the development of hopefulness (Kylma, Vehvilainen-Julkunen & Lahdevirta, 2001). CBT is a useful intervention when working on issues of hope and hopelessness (Collins & Cutliffe, 2003).*
- Communicate clearly what the illness trajectory and/or course of treatment will involve. *Efforts must be taken to eliminate as much uncertainty as possible (Kylma, Vehvilainen-Julkunen & Lahdevirta, 2001). People coping with nonhealing ulcers benefit from assistance with minimizing symptoms and normalizing their existence (Hopkins, 2004). Women who have had breast cancer surgery and their family and/or caregivers have specific needs for different types of information and interventions based on the stage of their cancer (Nikoletti et al, 2003).*

H

- = Independent; ▲ = Collaborative; EBN = Evidence-Based Nursing; EB = Evidence-Based

- Use humor as appropriate. *Humor is an effective intervention for hopelessness.* **EBN:** *There is a positive correlation between humor and psychosocial adjustment in children with cancer (Dowling, Hockenberry & Gregory, 2003).* **EB:** *Use of a specific humor intervention in hospital rehabilitation units produced a positive outcome in promoting psychosocial adjustment and healing (Scholl & Ragan, 2003).*
- Involve family and significant others in the plan of care. *Social support is a significant variable related to hope (Ehrenberger et al, 2002).* **EBN:** *Families of children who are technologically dependent benefit from an organized intervention for home care (Montagnino & Maurico, 2004).*
- Encourage the family and significant others to express care, hope, and love for the client. *Caring relationships have a positive influence on the presence of hope (Cutcliffe & Grant, 2001; Duggleby, 2001).* **EBN:** *Clients with non–small cell cancer feel a need for support from family (Kuo & Ma, 2002).*
- ▲ Consider use of integrative therapies, such as omega-3 fatty acids, *Hypericum perforatum* (St. John's wort), *S*-adenosylmethionine, folate, 5-hydroxytryptophan, acupuncture, exercise, and light therapy. **EB:** *Each of these are treatment interventions for depression. An evidence-based integrative medicine approach brings together treatment options with proven efficacy and the public's desire for complementary and alternative medicine treatments (Freeman, Helgason & Hill, 2004).*
- Use touch to demonstrate caring, if culturally appropriate and with the client's permission, and encourage the family to do the same. **EBN:** *Therapeutic touch (TT) produced positive, desired outcomes in women with breast cancer (Kelly et al, 2004). Women with fibromyalgia experienced a positive outcome with TT as an intervention (Denison, 2004).*
- Facilitate access to resources to support a positive spirituality. *Spiritual beliefs and practices that are practiced within a positive framework facilitate hope (Duggleby, 2001). Women with cancer who are involved in religious activities and groups report a more positive adaptation (Ferrell et al, 2003).*
- For additional interventions, see the care plans for **Readiness for enhanced Hope, Spiritual distress, Readiness for enhanced Spiritual well-being,** and **Disturbed Sleep pattern.**

Geriatric

- ▲ If depression is suspected, confer with the primary physician regarding referral for mental health services. *In older adults, hopelessness and suicidal wishes are present with high levels of depressive symptoms, suggesting a higher risk of suicidality (Szanto et al, 2002).*
- Take threats of self-harm or suicide seriously. *The elderly have the highest rate of completed suicide of all age groups (Szanto et al, 2002).*
- Identify significant losses that may be leading to feelings of hopelessness. *Helping clients to cope with grief and make more psychological energy available to them will support their hopefulness.* **EB:** *Specific intervention for individuals with HIV coping with bereavement issues produced improvement (Sikkema et al, 2004).*
- Discuss stages of emotional responses to multiple losses. **EB:** *Specific intervention for HIV individuals coping with bereavement issues produced improvement (Sikkema et al, 2004).*
- Use reminiscence and life-review therapies to identify past coping skills. *Older people in residential facilities benefit from this therapy (Wang, 2004). Life review produced a positive outcome when used with individuals with right hemisphere cerebral vascular accidents (Davis, 2004).*
- Express hope to the client and give positive feedback whenever appropriate. *The nurse's communication of caring for the client facilitates movement in the direction of hope. The therapeutic relationship has a positive effect on the alleviation of hopelessness (Collins & Cutliffe, 2003).*
- Identify the client's past and current sources of spirituality. Help the client explore life and identify those experiences that are noteworthy. The client may want to read the Bible or other religious text or have it read to him or her. **EBN:** *Spirituality is a significant factor in quality of life of women with ovarian cancer (Ferrell et al, 2003). Spirituality is positively related to self-transcendence in middle-aged adults. Self-transcendence is identified as a resource for well-being (Ellermann & Reed, 2001).*
- Encourage visits from children. *Social relationships foster hopefulness (Duggleby, 2001).*
- Position the client by a window, take the client outside, or encourage such activities as gardening (if ability allows). *Environmental changes can foster hope (Cutcliffe & Grant, 2001).*
- Provide esthetic forms of expression, such as dance, music, literature, and pictures. **EBN:**

Aesthetic experiences are related to feelings of timelessness and spacelessness, and serve as sources of gratification (Wikstrom, 2004).

Multicultural

- Assess for the influence of cultural beliefs, norms, and values on the client's feelings of hopelessness. **EBN:** *The client's expressions of hopelessness may be based on cultural perceptions (Leininger & McFarland, 2002).* **EB:** *Perceived racism is associated with higher levels of hopelessness for African-American boys (Nyborg & Curry, 2003). The interrelationship between contextual risk factors, rational choice theory, and opportunity cost provide a model to explain why African Americans die at a disproportionately higher rate from cardiovascular-related diseases (Appel, Giger & Davidhizar, 2005).*
- Assess the effect of fatalism on the client's expression of hopelessness. **EBN:** *Fatalistic perspectives, which involve the belief that one cannot control one's own fate, may influence health behaviors in some Asian, African-American, and Latino populations (Chen, 2001; Beutter & Davidhizar, 1999).*
- Assess for depression and refer to appropriate services. **EBN:** *Older Taiwanese-American adults with depressive symptoms report hopelessness as a symptom (Suen & Tusaie, 2004). The severity of depression in African Americans and Latinos may be predicted by feelings of hopelessness (Myers et al, 2002).*
- Encourage spirituality as a source of support for hopelessness. **EBN:** *African Americans and Latinos may identify spirituality, religiousness, prayer, and church-based approaches as coping resources (Samuel-Hodge et al, 2000).* **EBN:** *Spiritual beliefs, the role of prayer, and the role of family in caregiving were predominant aspects in the end of life experience in Mexican Americans. There is a need to focus on the role of religious institutions in Mexican American culture, where spirituality and religion are strong influences in the life experience (Gelfand et al, 2001).*

Home Care

- Previously mentioned interventions may be adapted for home care use.
- ▲ Assess for isolation within the family unit. Encourage the client to participate in family activities. If the client cannot participate, encourage him or her to be in the same area and watch family activities. Refer for telephone support. *Significant caring relationships foster hope (Duggleby, 2001). Participation in events increases energy and promotes a sense of belonging. Hope is facilitated by meaningful interpersonal relationships (Cutcliffe & Grant, 2001). Clients show significant improvements in depression and positive affect during the 16 weeks of telephone-administered treatment (Mohr et al, 2005).*
- Reminisce with the client about his or her life. *The process of remembering past pleasant activities and sharing them in a supportive environment inspires hope (Duggleby, 2001). Use of the self in the context of an interpersonal relationship with the client will facilitate hope (Cutcliffe & Grant, 2001). Older people in residential facilities benefit from this therapy (Wang, 2004). Life review produced a positive outcome when used with individuals with right hemisphere cerebral vascular accidents (Davis, 2004).*
- Identify areas in which the client can have control. Allow the client to set achievable goals in these areas. Assist the client when necessary to negotiate desirable outcomes. *Mobilization of resources to promote self-efficacy promotes hope (Kylma, Vehvilainen-Julkenen & Lahdevirta, 2001).*
- Clearly explain potential benefits and risks of a proposed intervention. *Clear, direct communication of the potential of an intervention to overcome a threat, along with honest discussion of negative aspects, empowers the client and promotes hope (Pinikahana & Happell, 2002).*
- If illness precipitated the hopelessness, discuss knowledge of and previous experience with the disease. Help the client to identify past coping strengths. *Uncertainty is a danger when it results in pessimism. Knowledge of the disease and previous positive coping experience with the illness provide hope for the future (Richer & Ezer, 2002).*
- ▲ Provide plant or pet therapy if possible. *Caring for pets or plants helps to redefine the client's identity and makes him or her feel needed and loved. Pet therapy has been reported to have a positive effect on a variety of client populations (Hooker, Freeman & Stewart, 2002).*

Client/Family Teaching

- Provide information regarding the client's condition, treatment plan, and progress. *Clear, direct communication of the potential of an intervention to overcome a threat along with honest discussion of negative aspects empowers the client and promotes hope (Pinikahana & Happell, 2002).*

• = Independent;   ▲ = Collaborative;   EBN = Evidence-Based Nursing;   EB = Evidence-Based

- Provide positive reinforcement, praise, and acknowledgment of the challenges of caregiving to family members. *Nurses provide much-needed support and encouragement to caregivers (Dibartolo, 2002).*
- Teach the use of stress-reduction techniques, relaxation, and imagery. Many cassette tapes on relaxation and meditation are available. Assist the client and caregivers with relaxation based on their preference from the initial assessment. *Stress management techniques are effective interventions for clients and their caregivers (Ducharme & Trudeau, 2002).* **EB:** *Women with coronary syndrome X benefited from physical training and relaxation therapy (Tyni-Lenne et al, 2002).*
- ▲ Refer the client to self-help groups, such as I Can Cope and Make Today Count. **EBN:** *Self-help and/or professionally led curriculum-based support programs for families are effective in reducing stress and facilitating coping and hope (Northouse et al, 2002).*
- ▲ Refer the family to community support groups targeted to the specific needs of the family caregivers. *Support groups provide validation of feelings, information, and an opportunity for sharing of creative strategies among participants (Fung & Chien, 2002).*

evolve See the EVOLVE website for World Wide Web resources for client education.

REFERENCES

Appel SJ, Giger JN, Davidhizar RE: Opportunity cost: the impact of contextual risk factors on the cardiovascular health of low-income rural southern African American women, *J Cardiovasc Nurs* 20:315-324, 2005.

Beutter M, Davidhizar R: A home care provider's challenge: caring for the Hispanic client in the home, *J Pract Nurs* 49(3):26-36, 1999.

Chen YC: Chinese values, health and nursing, *J Adv Nurs* 36(2):270, 2001.

Collins S, Cutcliffe JR: Addressing hopelessness in people with suicidal ideation: building upon the therapeutic relationship utilizing a cognitive behavioral approach, *J Psychiatr Ment Health Nurs* 10:175-185, 2003.

Cutcliffe JR, Grant G: What are the principles and processes of inspiring hope in cognitively impaired older adults within a continuing care environment? *J Psychiatr Ment Health Nurs* 8:427, 2001.

Cutcliffe JR, Koehn CV: Hope and interpersonal psychiatric/mental health nursing: a systematic review of the literature—part two, *J Psychiatr Ment Health Nurs* 14(2):141-147, 2007.

Davis MC: Life review therapy as an intervention to manage depression and enhance life satisfaction in individuals with right hemisphere cerebral vascular accidents, *Issues Ment Health Nurs* 25(5):503-515, 2004.

Denison B: Touch the pain away: new research on therapeutic touch and persons with fibromyalgia syndrome, *Holistic Nurs Pract* 18(3):142-151, 2004.

Dibartolo MC: Exploring self-efficacy and hardiness in spousal caregivers of individuals with dementia, *J Gerontol Nurs* 28(4):24, 2002.

Dowling JS, Hockenberry M, Gregory RL: Sense of humor, childhood cancer stressors, and outcomes of psychosocial adjustment, immune function, and infection, *J Pediatr Oncol Nurs* 20(6):271-292, 2003.

Ducharme F, Trudeau D: Qualitative evaluation of a stress management intervention for elderly caregivers at home: a constructivist approach, *Issues Ment Health Nurs* 23:691, 2002.

Duggleby W: Hope at the end of life, *J Hospice Palliat Nurs* 3(2):51, 2001.

Dunn SL, Corser W, Stommel M et al: Hopelessness and depression in the early recovery period after hospitalization for acute coronary syndrome, *J Cardiopulm Rehabil* 26(3):152-159, 2006.

Ehrenberger HE, Alligood MR, Thomas SP et al: Testing a theory of decision-making derived from King's systems framework in women eligible for a cancer clinical trial, *Nurs Sci Q* 15(2):156, 2002.

Ellermann CR, Reed PG: Self-transcendence and depression in middle-age adults, *West J Nurs Res* 23(7):689-713, 2001.

Ferrell, FR, Smith SL, Juarez G et al: Meaning of illness and spirituality in ovarian cancer survivors, *Oncol Nurs Forum* 30(2):249-257, 2003.

Freeman MP, Helgason C, Hill RA.: Selected integrative medicine treatments for depression: considerations for women, *J Am Med Womens Assoc* 59(3):216-224, 2004.

Fung W, Chien W: The effectiveness of a mutual support group for family caregivers of a relative with dementia, *Arch Psychiatr Nurs* 16(3):134, 2002.

Gelfand D, Balcazar H, Parzuchowski J et al: Mexicans and care for the terminally ill: family, hospice and the church, *Am J Hosp Palliat Care* 18(6):391-396, 2001.

Haatainen K, Tanskanen A, Kylma J et al: Factors associated with hopelessness: a population study, *Int J Soc Psychiatry* 50(2):142-152, 2004.

Hooker SD, Freeman LH, Stewart P: Pet therapy research: a historical review, *Holist Nurs Pract* 17(1):17-23, 2002.

Hopkins A: Disrupted lives: investigating coping strategies for non-healing leg ulcers, *Br J Nurs* 13(9):556-563, 2004.

Kelly AE, Sullivan P, Fawcett J et al: Therapeutic touch, quiet time, and dialogue: perceptions of women with breast cancer, *Oncol Nurs Forum* 31(3):625-631, 2004.

Kuo TT, Ma FC: Symptoms, distresses and coping strategies in patients with non-small-cell lung cancer, *Cancer Nurs* 25(4):309-317, 2002.

Kylma J, Vehvilainen-Julkunen K, Lahdevirta J: Hope, despair and hopelessness in living with HIV/AIDS: a grounded theory study, *J Adv Nurs* 33(6):764, 2001.

Leininger MM, McFarland MR: *Transcultural nursing: concepts, theories, research and practices,* ed 3, New York, 2002, McGraw-Hill.

Mohr DC, Hart SL, Julian L et al: Telephone-administered psychotherapy for depression, *Arch Gen Psychiatry*, 62(9):1007-1014, 2005.

Montagnino BA, Maurico RV: The child with a tracheostomy and gastrostomy: parental stress and coping in the home: a pilot study, *Pediatr Nurs* 30(5):373-401, 2004.

Myers HF, Lesser I, Rodriguez N et al: Ethnic differences in clinical presentation of depression in adult women, *Cultur Divers Ethnic Minor Psychol* 8(2):138-156, 2002.

Nikoletti S, Kristjanson LJ, Tataryn D et al: Information needs and coping styles of primary family caregivers of women following breast cancer surgery, *Oncol Nurs Forum* 30(6):987-996, 2003.

• = Independent; ▲ = Collaborative; EBN = Evidence-Based Nursing; EB = Evidence-Based

Northouse L, Kershaw T, Mood D et al: Effects of a family intervention on the quality of life of women with recurrent breast cancer and their family caregivers, *Psychooncology* 14(6):478-491, 2005.

Northouse LL, Walker J, Schafenacker A et al: A family-based program of care for women with recurrent breast cancer and their family members, *Oncol Nurs Forum* 29(10):1411, 2002.

Nyborg VM, Curry JF: The impact of perceived racism: psychological symptoms among African American boys, *J Clin Child Adolesc Psychol* 32(2):258-266, 2003.

Overcash JA: Using narrative research to understand the quality of life of older women with breast cancer, *Oncol Nurs Forum* 31(6):1153-1159, 2004.

Pinikahana J, Happell B: Exploring the complexity of compliance in schizophrenia, *Issues Ment Health Nurs* 23:513, 2002.

Radina ME, Armer JM, Culbertson S et al: Post-breast cancer lymphedema: understanding women's knowledge of their condition, *Oncol Nurs Forum* 31(1):97-104, 2004.

Richer MC, Ezer H: Living in it, living with it, and moving on: dimensions of meaning during chemotherapy, *Oncol Nurs Forum* 29(1):113, 2002.

Samuel-Hodge CD, Headen SW, Skelly AH et al: Influences on day-to-day self-management of type 2 diabetes among African American women: spirituality, the multi-caregiver role, and other social context factors, *Diabetes Care* 23(7):928, 2000.

Scholl JC, Ragan SL: The use of humor in promoting positive provider-patient interactions in a hospital rehabilitation unit, *Health Commun* 15(3):319-330, 2003.

Schreiber R: Wandering in the dark: women's experiences with depression, *Health Care Women Int* 22(1/2):85, 2001.

Sikkema KJ, Hansen NB, Kochman A et al: Outcomes from a randomized controlled trial of a group intervention for HIV positive men and women coping with AIDS-related loss and bereavement, *Death Stud* 28(3):187-209, 2004.

Suen LJ, Tusaie K: Is somatization a significant depressive symptom in older Taiwanese Americans, *Geriatr Nurs* 25(3):157-163, 2004.

Szanto K, Gildengers A, Mulsant B et al: Identification of suicidal ideation and prevention of suicidal behaviour in the elderly, *Drugs Aging* 19(1):11-24, 2002.

Tyni-Lenne R, Stryjan S, Eriksson B et al: Beneficial therapeutic effects of physical training and relaxation therapy in women with coronary syndrome X, *Physiother Res Int* 7(1):35-43, 2002.

Wang J: The comparative effectiveness among institutionalized and non-institutionalized elderly people in Taiwan of reminiscence therapy as a psychological measure, *J Nurs Res* 12(3):237-244, 2004.

Wikstrom B: Older adults and the arts: the importance of aesthetic forms of expression in later life, *J Gerontol Nurs* 30(9):30-36, 2004.

Hyperthermia   *Betty Ackley, MSN, EdS, RN*

NANDA   Definition

Body temperature elevated above normal range

Elevated body temperature can be either fever or hyperthermia.

Fever is a regulated rise in the core body temperature or variation in the temperature set point (Henker & Carlson, 2007). This elevation is in response to a chemical signal (endogenous pyrogen) released as part of an inflammatory response, with release of mediators such as interleukin-1B and interleukin-6. The immune system is enhanced by the fever, with lymphocyte proliferation and increased neutrophil activity. The client sleeps longer and deeper. The heart rate increases as well as the cardiac index. Also, the metabolic rate increases, and if the patient begins shivering, the rate may increase 200% or more.

Hyperthermia is an unregulated rise in body temperature, which is seen with heat illness, neurological disorders, or malignant hyperthermia, often with the temperature above 104° F (40° C). Hyperthermia is not adaptive (Holtzclaw, 2004) and should be treated as a medical emergency.

Defining Characteristics

Flushed skin; increase in body temperature above normal range; tachycardia; tachypnea; warm to touch; seizures (convulsions)

Related Factors (r/t)

Anesthesia; decreased perspiration; dehydration; exposure to hot environment; inappropriate clothing; increased metabolic rate; illness; medications; trauma; vigorous activity

NOC   Outcomes (Nursing Outcomes Classification)

Suggested NOC Outcomes

Thermoregulation, Thermoregulation: Newborn

• = Independent;   ▲ = Collaborative;   EBN = Evidence-Based Nursing;   EB = Evidence-Based

Client Outcomes

Client Will (Specify Time Frame):
- Maintain oral temperature within adaptive levels
- Remain free of complications of malignant hypertension (MH)
- Remain free of dehydration

NIC   Interventions (Nursing Interventions Classification)

Suggested NIC Interventions

Fever Treatment, Malignant Hyperthermia Precautions, Temperature Regulation

Nursing Interventions and *Rationales*

▲ Assess an afebrile hospitalized client's temperature per institutional policy, upon assessment of signs or symptoms of infection, if the client has chills, or at least once a day between 5 PM and 7 PM. *Body temperature has a daily circadian rhythm, in which the lowest temperature occurs in early morning hours, and the highest in late afternoon to evening (Bickley & Szilagyi, 2007).*

• Measure and record a febrile client's temperature using an oral or rectal thermometer at least every 4 to 6 hours or whenever a change in condition occurs (e.g., chills, change in mental status). **EBN:** *Oral temperature measurement provides a more accurate temperature than tympanic measurement (Fisk & Arcona, 2001; Giuliano et al, 2000). Axillary temperatures are often inaccurate. The oral temperature is usually accurate even in an intubated client (Fallis, 2002). The SolarTherm and DataTherm devices correlated strongly with core body temperatures obtained from a pulmonary artery catheter (Smith, 2004). Axillary and tympanic temperatures were less accurate than oral temperatures (Devrim et al, 2007).*

• Use the same site and method (device) for temperature measurement for a given client so that temperature trends are assessed accurately. **EBN and EB:** *A difference in the site (oral, rectal, axillary, or pulmonary) of temperature measurement results in a significant difference in temperature reading (Schmitz et al, 1995).*

▲ Notify the physician of temperature according to institutional standards or written orders, or when temperature reaches 100.5° F (38° C) and above. Also notify the physician of the presence of a change in mental status. *A change in mental status may indicate the onset of septic shock (Kasper et al, 2005).*

▲ Work with the physician to help determine the cause of the temperature increase, which will often help direct appropriate treatment. *It is generally more important to treat the underlying cause of the temperature increase than to treat the symptom of fever (Henker & Carlson, 2007).*

▲ Administer antipyretic medication per physician orders, when the cause of the temperature is not adaptive (neurological, heatstroke, or malignant hyperthermia), when infection-induced fever is greater than 39° C, and when the client cannot tolerate the increase in metabolic demand, such as when the client is the acutely ill or has cardiac or respiratory disease (Kasper et al, 2005). *Elimination of fever will interfere with its enhancement of the immune response, but temperature elevation is also accompanied by an increase in oxygen consumption and metabolic rate that may not be tolerated by the acutely ill client (Henker & Carlson, 2007).* **EB:** *A systematic review of three studies found little evidence to support the administration of antipyretics for fever (Hudgings et al, 2004).*

▲ Assess fluid loss and facilitate oral intake or administer intravenous fluids to replace fluids. *Increased metabolic rate and diaphoresis associated with fever cause loss of body fluids.*

• When diaphoresis is present, assist the client with bathing and changing into dry clothing. *Bathing and clothing changes increase comfort and decrease the possibility of continued shivering caused by water evaporation from the skin.*

• Do not use external cooling measures, such as ice packs, tepid water baths, or removal of blankets and clothing for fever management; these measures cause shivering and are ineffective. *If the client's temperature drops in response to rapid external cooling measures, shivering often results, which significantly increases oxygen consumption and cardiorespiratory effort (Holtzclaw, 2004).*

• Recognize that a hypothermia blanket is indicated for temperature reduction if the client's fever is above 104° F and cannot be controlled with antipyretics, or if a high body temperature is related to a disorder of temperature regulation (Kasper et al, 2005).

• When using a cooling blanket, choose a convective airflow system if possible, and set the temperature regulator to 1° to 2° F (0.6° to 1.1° C) below the client's current temperature. *Use higher cooling blanket temperatures because this will help prevent shivering and skin breakdown, and it is more comfortable (Henker & Carlson, 2007).* **EBN:** *Blankets that use convective airflow for cooling may be more effective than those that cool by conductive water flow (Creechan, Vollman & Kravutske, 2001). Airflow blankets were more effective than water-cooling blankets (Loke, Chan & Chan, 2005).*

• Use a nonsteroidal antipyretic (e.g., acetaminophen) as ordered instead of or in conjunction with a cooling blanket to improve fever reduction and decrease the duration of cooling blanket use. **EB:** *Although external cooling and use of antipyretics were equally effective in decreasing body temperature in critically ill clients, there was a 5% increase in energy expenditure with the use of the external cooling versus an 8% decrease of energy expenditure with the use of an antipyretic (Gozzoli et al, 2004).*

▲ Recognize that shivering can be harmful and prevent shivering when possible. Wrap extremities in towels to decrease shivering (Holtzclaw, 2004) before beginning use of the cooling blanket, or administer medications to prevent shivering as ordered. *Shivering results in aerobic muscle activity with increased metabolism, increased oxygen and glucose use, and increased heart rate, blood pressure and is poorly tolerated by clients who are weak, anemic or at risk for myocardial ischemia (Holtzclaw, 2004).*

Pediatric

• Assess risk factors of malignant hyperthermia, because this has an increased prevalence in the pediatric population. *The administration of inhalation anesthesia and succinylcholine is common in this age group. Risk assessment includes a personal or family history of anesthesia-related complications or death (Hommertzheim & Steinke, 2006).*

▲ Administer dantrolene and oxygen as ordered. *Dantrolene and oxygen should administered as treatment of malignant hyperthermia (Barone, Pablo & Barone, 2004).*

• Avoid routine sponging—especially cold sponging—to reduce body temperature in children. *There is a lack of evidence of the effectiveness of sponging for children to prevent febrile seizures. Washing the child with warm water may be comforting if the child is diaphoretic (Watts, 2001; Watts, Robertson & Thomas, 2003).*

Geriatric

• Recognize that an increase in oral temperature of 1° F above their baseline temperature or above 99° F should be considered a fever in older adults. *Febrile response to infection was found to be reduced with increasing age, and baseline temperatures were generally lower in older clients (Roghmann, Warner & Mackowiak, 2001; Woolery & Franco, 2004).*

• Rectal temperature may be more accurate to diagnose fever in older clients. However, nursing judgment must be used to determine if rectal temperature measurement is acceptable to the client, especially a client with mental changes or dementia. **EBN:** *Rectal thermometry identified fevers in elderly clients that were missed by the oral and tympanic routes (Varney et al, 2002).*

• Assess for other signs and symptoms of infection in addition to or in the absence of fever in older clients. Suspect infection when there has been a decline in function, including new or increased confusion, incontinence, falling, decreased mobility, or failure to cooperate. *The tempera-*

ture response is blunted in older adults because of changes in physiology resulting from aging (Woolery & Franco, 2004). The onset of pyrexia in older clients with infections can be delayed several hours; the delay was more than 12 hours for 12% of clients (McAlpine et al, 1986).

▲ Help the client seek medical attention immediately if fever is present. To diagnose the fever source, assess for possible precipitating factors, including medication changes, environmental changes, and recent medical interventions or infectious exposures. *Older adults are more susceptible to environmentally induced and medication induced hyperthermia because they have a greater incidence of underlying chronic medical conditions that impair thermal regulation or prevent removal from a hot environment (e.g., cardiovascular disease, neurological and psychiatric disorders, obesity, and use of anticholinergic and diuretic drugs [Woolery & Franco, 2004]).*

• In hot weather, encourage older adult clients to drink 8 glasses of fluid per day (within their cardiac and renal reserves) regardless of whether they are thirsty. Assess for the need for and presence of fans or air conditioning. *Older adults are more susceptible to a hot environment than are younger adults, because of a decreased sensitivity to heat, sweat gland function, and thirst. The number of deaths in geriatric populations rises as environmental temperatures increase in the hot summer months (Worfolk, 2000).*

• In hot weather, monitor older adult clients for signs of heatstroke, which include body temperature of 100° to 102° F (37.8°-38.9° C), orthostatic blood pressure drop, weakness, restlessness, mental status changes, faintness, thirst, nausea, and vomiting. If signs are present, move the client to a cool place, have the client lie down, give sips of water, check orthostatic blood pressure, spray with lukewarm water, cool with a fan, and seek medical assistance immediately. *Older adults are predisposed to heat exhaustion and should be watched carefully for its occurrence; if it is present, it should be treated promptly (Worfolk, 2000).*

 ### Home Care

• Some of the interventions described previously may be adapted for home care use.
• Assess whether the client or family has a thermometer and knows how to use it.
▲ Teach the client and family to use ordered antipyretic medication safely.
• Help the client and caregivers prevent and monitor for heatstroke/hyperthermia during times of high outdoor temperatures. *Preventive measures include minimizing time spent outdoors, using air conditioning or fans, increasing fluid intake, and resting frequently.*
• To prevent heat-related injury in athletes, laborers, and military personnel, instruct them to acclimate gradually to the higher temperatures, increase fluid intake, wear vapor-permeable clothing, and rest frequently.
• If body temperature increases above the adaptive range, institute measures to decrease temperature (e.g., get the client out of the sun and into a cool place, remove excess clothing, have the client drink fluids, spray the client with lukewarm water, and fan with cool air). *Hyperthermia is an acute and possibly life-threatening symptom. The client cannot stay at home safely.*
▲ If the client is in hospice or is terminally ill, follow the client's wishes and the physician's orders in determining the management of fever. *The goal of terminal care is to provide comfort and dignity during the dying process.*

 ### Client/Family Teaching

▲ Teach that infection-induced fever generally enhances the immune system, so the client can participate in the decision of whether to treat the fever. If treatment is elected or appropriate for comfort, instruct in the use of antipyretics as ordered.
• Teach the client that shivering with infection-induced fever has detrimental effects and that activities that can cause shivering (e.g., removing blankets, lowering the room temperature, taking tepid water baths, applying ice packs) should be avoided. *External cooling measures result in shivering and discomfort and are no longer recommended (Holtzclaw, 2004).*
• Instruct the client to increase fluids to prevent heat-induced hyperthermia and dehydration in the presence of fever. *Liberal fluid intake replaces fluid lost through perspiration and respiration.*
• Teach the client to stay in a cooler environment during periods of excessive outdoor heat or humidity. If the client does go out, instruct him or her to avoid vigorous physical activity, wear

lightweight, loose-fitting clothing, and wear a hat to minimize sun exposure. *Such methods reduce exposure to high environmental temperatures, which can cause heatstroke and hyperthermia.*

evolve See the EVOLVE website for World Wide Web resources for client education.

REFERENCES

Barone CP, Pablo CS, Barone GW: Postanesthetic care in the critical care unit, *Crit Care Nurs* 24(1):38-45, 2004.

Bickley LS, Szilagyi PG: *Bates' guide to physical examination and history taking,* ed 9, Philadelphia, 2007, Lippincott Williams & Wilkins.

Creechan T, Vollman K, Kravutske ME: Cooling by convection vs cooling by conduction for treatment of fever in critically ill adults, *Am J Crit Care* 10(1):52, 2001.

Devrim I, Kara A, Ceyhan M et al: Measurement accuracy of fever by tympanic and axillary thermometry, *Pediatr Emerg Care* 23(1):16-19, 2007.

Fallis WM: Monitoring urinary bladder temperature in the intensive care unit: state of the science, *Am J Crit Care* 11(1):38, 2002.

Fisk J, Arcona S: Comparing tympanic membrane and pulmonary artery catheter temperatures, *Dimens Crit Care Nurs* 20(2):44, 2001.

Giuliano KK, Giuliano AJ, Scott SS et al: Temperature measurement in critically ill adults: a comparison of tympanic and oral methods, *Am J Crit Care* 9(4):254, 2000.

Gozzoli V, Treggiari MM, Kleger GR et al: Randomized trial of the effect of antipyresis by metamizol, propacetamol or external cooling on metabolism, hemodynamics and inflammatory response, *Intens Care Med* 30(3):401, 2004.

Henker R, Carlson KK: Fever: applying research to bedside practice, *AACN Adv Crit Care* 18(1):76-87, 2007.

Holtzclaw BJ: Shivering in acutely ill vulnerable populations, *AACN Clin Issues* 15(2):267-269, 2004.

Hommertzheim R, Steinke E: Malignant hyperthermia: the perioperative nurses role, *AORN J* 83(1):149-168, 2006.

Hudgings L, Kelsberg G, Safranek SL et al: Do antipyretics prolong febrile illness? *J Fam Pract* 53(1):57-58, 61, 2004.

Kasper DL et al, editors: *Harrison's principles of internal medicine,* ed 16, New York, 2005, McGraw-Hill.

Loke AY, Chan HC, Chan TM: Comparing the effectiveness of two types of cooling blankets for febrile patients, *Nurs Crit Care* 10(5):247-254, 2005.

McAlpine CH, Martin BJ, Lennox IM et al: Pyrexia in infection in the elderly, *Age Ageing* 15:230, 1986.

Roghmann MC, Warner J, Mackowiak PA: The relationship between age and fever magnitude, *Am J Med Sci* 322:68, 2001.

Schmitz T, Bair N, Falk M et al: A comparison of five methods of temperature measurement in febrile intensive care patients, *Am J Crit Care* 4:286, 1995.

Smith LS: Temperature measurement in critical care adults: a comparison of thermometry and measurement routes, *Biol Res Nurs* 6(2):117, 2004.

Varney SM, Manthey DE, Culpepper VE et al: A comparison of oral, tympanic, and rectal temperature measurement in the elderly, *J Emerg Med* 22:153, 2002.

Watts R: Management of the child with fever, *Best Practice JBIEBNM* 5(5):1-6, Australia, 2001, Blackwell Science-Asia.

Watts R, Robertson J, Thomas G: Nursing management of fever in children: a systematic review, *Int J Nurs Pract* 9(1):S1-S8, 2003.

Woolery WM, Franco FR: Fever of unkown origin: keys to determining the etiology in older patients, *Geriatrics* 59(10):41-45, 2004.

Worfolk JB: Heat waves: their impact on the health of elders, *Geriatr Nurs* 21:70, 2000.

Hypothermia *Betty J. Ackley, MSN, EdS, RN*

NANDA Definition

Body temperature below normal range

Defining Characteristics

Body temperature below normal range; cool skin; cyanotic nail beds; hypertension; pallor; piloerection; shivering; slow capillary refill; tachycardia

Related Factors (r/t)

Aging; consumption of alcohol; damage to hypothalamus; decreased ability to shiver; decreased metabolic rate; evaporation from skin in cool environment; exposure to cool environment; illness; inactivity; inadequate clothing; malnutrition; medications; trauma

NOC Outcomes (Nursing Outcomes Classification)

Suggested NOC Outcomes

Thermoregulation, Thermoregulation: Newborn

• = Independent; ▲ = Collaborative; EBN = Evidence-Based Nursing; EB = Evidence-Based

Client Outcomes

Client Will (Specify Time Frame):
- Maintain body temperature within normal range
- Identify risk factors of hypothermia
- State measures to prevent hypothermia
- Identify symptoms of hypothermia and actions to take when hypothermia is present

H | NIC | Interventions (Nursing Interventions Classification)

Suggested NIC Interventions

Hypothermia Treatment, Temperature Regulation, Temperature Regulation: Intraoperative, Vital Signs Monitoring

Nursing Interventions and *Rationales*

- Remove the client from the cause of the hypothermic episode (e.g., cold environment, cold or wet clothing). Ensure that the client is in a warm environment. *The goal is to eliminate the causative or contributing factor and begin the warming process (Day, 2006).*
- Watch the client for signs of hypothermia: shivering, slurred speech, clumsy movements, fatigue, and confusion. As hypothermia progresses, the skin becomes pale, numb, and waxy. Muscles are tense, fatigue and weakness progress, and gradually there can be loss of consciousness with loss of a pulse and breathing (Elliott, 2004; Day, 2006).
- Cover the client with warm blankets and apply a covering to the head and neck to conserve body heat. *Layering of dry clothing including wearing a hat can be effective in warming a client with mild hypothermia (Elliott, 2004; Day, 2006).*
- Take the client's temperature at least hourly; if more than mild hypothermia is present (temperature lower than 95° F [35° C]), use a continuous temperature-monitoring device, preferably two of them, one in the rectum and the other in the esophagus (Kasper et al, 2005).
- If the client is awake, measure the oral temperature, instead of the tympanic or axillary temperature. **EBN:** *Oral temperature measurement provides a more accurate temperature than tympanic measurement (Fisk & Arcona, 2001; Giuliano et al, 2000). Axillary temperatures are often inaccurate. The oral temperature is usually accurate even in an intubated client (Fallis, 2002). The SolarTherm and DataTherm devices correlated strongly with core body temperatures obtained from a pulmonary artery catheter (Smith, 2004). A study performed in Turkey found that axillary and tympanic temperatures were less accurate than oral temperatures (Devrim et al, 2007).*
- ▲ Use a pulmonary artery catheter temperature-measuring device if available; if not, consider using a bladder catheter that measures temperature. **EBN:** *Measurement of the pulmonary artery temperature is considered the gold standard in assessing core body temperature. If a pulmonary artery catheter is not appropriate for the client, temperature measurement with a temperature-sensitive indwelling urinary catheter can be effective and provide a reliable indication of core temperature (Fallis, 2002).*
- Monitor the client's vital signs every hour and as appropriate. Note changes associated with hypothermia, such as initially increased pulse rate, respiratory rate, and blood pressure with mild

hypothermia, and then decreased pulse rate, respiratory rate, and blood pressure with moderate to severe hypothermia. *With mild hypothermia, there is activation of the sympathetic nervous system, which can increase the values of vital signs. As hypothermia progresses, decreased circulating volume develops, which results in decreased cardiac output and depressed oxygen delivery. Hypoxia, metabolic acidosis, and intrinsic irritability of a cold myocardium result in various dysrhythmias (Ruffolo, 2002; Day, 2006).*

▲ Attach electrodes and a cardiac monitor. Watch for dysrhythmias. *With hypothermia the client is prone to dysrhythmias because of the cold myocardium; dysrhythmias may include atrial fibrillation, ventricular fibrillation, or asystole (McCullough & Arora, 2004; Day, 2006).*

• Monitor for signs of coagulopathy (e.g., oozing of blood from open areas, intravascular catheter sites, or mucous membranes). Also note results of clotting studies as available. *Coagulopathy is a common occurrence during hypothermia in trauma clients (McCullough & Arora, 2004; Ruffolo, 2002).*

• For mild hypothermia (core temperature of 90°-95° F [32.2°-35° C]), rewarm client passively:
  ▪ Set room temperature to 70° to 75° F (21° to 24° C).
  ▪ Keep the client dry and remove damp or wet clothing.
  ▪ Layer clothing and blankets and cover the client's head; use insulated metallic blankets.
  ▪ Offer warm fluids, but no alcohol or caffeine.
  For mild hypothermia, allow the client to rewarm at his or her own pace. Heat is regained through the body's ability to generate heat. Passive rewarming is not encouraged for clients with temperatures lower than 82.4° F (28° C), because it is a slow process and may increase the risk of cardiac arrest in these circumstances (McCullough & Arora, 2004; Cochrane, 2001).

▲ For moderate hypothermia (core temperature 82.4° to 90° F [28° to 32.2° C]) use active external rewarming methods. The rewarming rate should not exceed 1.8° F (1° C) per hour. Methods include the following (Kasper et al, 2005):
  ▪ Forced-air warming blankets
  ▪ Carbon-fiber blanket
  ▪ Radiant heat lights
  EB: *A study of four forced-air warming systems demonstrated the Bair Hugger system was more effective in heat transfer from the peripheral body to the core (Giesbrecht, Ducharme & McGuire, 1994). Another study compared the effectiveness of the Bair Hugger to that of a thermostat electric undermattress, and found that the Bair Hugger raised the temperature faster (Janke, Pilkington & Smith, 1996). Resistive heating using a carbon-fiber blanket was shown to be much more effective at rewarming hypothermic subjects than metallic foil blankets (Greif et al, 2000). The carbon-fiber resistive heating blanket was shown to be more effective than regular blankets at maintaining the client's core body temperature during transport (Kober et al, 2001).*

▲ For severe hypothermia (core temperature below 82.4° F [28° C]) use active core-rewarming techniques as ordered (Kasper et al, 2005):
  ▪ Recognize that extracorporeal blood rewarming methods are most effective.
  ▪ Administer heated and humidified oxygen through the ventilator as ordered.
  ▪ Administer heated intravenous (IV) fluids at prescribed temperature.
  ▪ Perform peritoneal lavage and bladder irrigations as ordered.
  Severe hypothermia is associated with acidosis, coma, ventricular fibrillation, apnea, thrombocytopenia, platelet dysfunction, impaired clotting, and increased mortality in trauma clients and requires prompt core body rewarming (Eddy, Morris & Cullinane, 2000; McCullough & Arora, 2004).

• Check blood pressure frequently when rewarming; watch for hypotension. *As the body warms, formerly vasoconstricted vessels dilate, which results in hypotension (Day, 2006).*

▲ Administer IV fluids, using a rapid infuser IV fluid warmer as ordered. *Fluids are often needed to maintain adequate fluid volume. If the client develops untreated fluid depletion, hypotension with decreased cardiac output and acute renal failure can result. A rapid infuser warmer is needed to keep IV fluids warmed sufficiently to be effective in raising the body temperature (Ruffolo, 2002; Kasper et al, 2005).*

• Determine the factors leading to the hypothermic episode; see Related Factors. *It is important to assess risk factors and precipitating events to prevent another incident of hypothermia and to direct treatment (Day, 2006).*

H

• = Independent;   ▲ = Collaborative;   EBN = Evidence-Based Nursing;   EB = Evidence-Based

▲ Request a social service referral to help the client obtain the heat, shelter, and food needed to maintain body temperature. *A preventive approach that includes adequate food and fluid intake, shelter, heat, and clothing decreases the risk of hypothermia (Kasper et al, 2005).*

▲ Encourage proper nutrition and hydration. Request a referral to a dietitian to identify appropriate dietary needs. *Insufficient calorie and fluid intake predisposes the client to hypothermia.*

Pediatric

• Recognize that pediatric clients have a decreased ability to adapt to temperature extremes. Take the following actions to maintain body temperature in the infant/child:
  ▪ Keep the head covered.
  ▪ Use blankets to keep the client warm.
  ▪ Keep the client covered during procedures, transport, and diagnostic testing.
  ▪ Keep the room temperature at 72° F (22.2° C).

  The combination of a relatively larger body surface area, smaller body fluid volume, less well-developed temperature control mechanisms, and smaller amount of protective body fat limits the infant's and child's ability to maintain normal temperatures (Hockenberry, 2005).

• For the preterm or low birth weight newborn, use specially designed bags, skin-to-skin care, and transwarmer mattresses to keep preterm infants warm. **EB:** *These methods can help keep the vulnerable newborn warm in the delivery room, yet there is a need for more studies in this area (McCall et al, 2005).*

Geriatric

• Assess neurological signs frequently, watching for confusion and decreased level of consciousness. *Older adults are less likely to shiver or complain of feeling cold. Early signs of hypothermia are subtle (McCullough & Arora, 2004).*

• Recognize that older adults can develop indoor hypothermia from air conditioning or ice baths. *Clients present with vague complaints of mental and/or other skill deterioration (McCullough & Arora, 2004).*

• Recognize that older adults often wear socks and sweaters to protect themselves from feeling cold, even in warmer weather.

Home Care

NOTE: Hypothermia is not a symptom that appears in the normal course of home care. When it occurs, it is a clinical emergency and the client/family should access emergency medical services immediately.

• Some of the interventions described earlier may be adapted for home care use.

• Before a medical crisis occurs, confirm that the client or family has a thermometer and can read it. Instruct as needed. Verify that the thermometer registers accurately.

• Instruct the client or family to take the temperature when the client displays cyanosis, pallor, or shivering.

▲ Monitor temperature every hour, as noted previously. If the temperature of the client begins dropping below the normal range, apply layers of clothing or blankets, or adjust environmental heat to the comfort level. Do not overheat. Contact a physician. *Passive rewarming is the only method of rewarming that is appropriate for home care under normal circumstances.*

▲ If temperature continues to drop, activate the emergency system and notify a physician. *Hypothermia is a clinically acute condition that cannot be managed safely in the home.*

▲ If the client is in hospice care or is terminally ill, follow advance directives, client wishes, and the physician's orders. Keep the client free of pain. *The goal of terminal care is to provide dignity and comfort during the dying process.*

Client/Family Teaching

• Teach the client and family signs of hypothermia and the method of taking the temperature (age-appropriate).

• Teach the client methods to prevent hypothermia: wearing adequate clothing, including a hat and mittens; heating the environment to a minimum of 68° F (20° C); and ingesting adequate

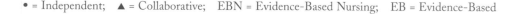

food and fluid. *Simple measures, such as layering clothes, wearing a hat, and avoiding extremes in temperature, prevent significant heat loss (Elliott, 2004; Laskowski-Jones, 2000).*

▲ Teach the client and family about medications, such as sedatives, opioids, and anxiolytics, that predispose the client to hypothermia (as appropriate). *If the client has had hypothermia in the past, using alternative medications is an option if there is no contra-indication (Elliott, 2004).*

evolve See the EVOLVE website for World Wide Web resources for client education.

REFERENCES

Cochrane DA: Hypothermia: a cold influence on trauma, *Int J Trauma Nurs* 7(1):8, 2001.

Day, MP: Hypothermia: a hazard for all seasons. *Nursing* 36(12):36-47, 2006.

Devrim I, Kara A, Ceyhan M et al: Measurement accuracy of fever by tympanic and axillary thermometry, *Pediatr Emerg Care* 23(1):16-19, 2007.

Eddy VA, Morris JA, Cullinane DC: Hypothermia, coagulopathy, and acidosis, *Surg Clin North Am* 80(3):845, 2000.

Elliott F: You'd better watch out, *Occup Health Saf* 73(11):76, 2004.

Fallis WM: Monitoring urinary bladder temperature in the intensive care unit: state of the science, *Am J Crit Care* 11(1):38, 2002.

Fisk J, Arcona S: Comparing tympanic membrane and pulmonary artery catheter temperatures, *Dimens Crit Care Nurs* 20(2):44, 2001.

Giesbrecht GG, Ducharme MB, McGuire JP: Comparison of forced-air patient warming systems for perioperative use, *Anesthesiology* 80(3):671, 1994.

Giuliano KK, Giuliano AJ, Scott SS et al: Temperature measurement in critically ill adults: a comparison of tympanic and oral methods, *Am J Crit Care* 9(4):254, 2000.

Greif R, Rajek A, Laciny S et al: Resistive heating is more effective than metallic-foil insulation in an experimental model of accidental hypothermia: a randomized controlled trial, *Ann Emerg Med* 35(4):337, 2000.

Hockenberry MJ: *Wong's essentials of pediatric nursing*, ed 7, St Louis, 2005, Mosby.

Janke EF, Pilkington SN, Smith DC: Evaluation of two warming systems after cardiopulmonary bypass, *Br J Anaesth* 77(2):268, 1996.

Kasper DL et al, editors: *Harrison's principles of internal medicine*, ed 16, New York, 2005, McGraw-Hill.

Kober A, Scheck T, Fulesdi B et al: Effectiveness of resistive heating compared with passive warming in treating hypothermia associated with minor trauma: a randomized trial, *Mayo Clin Proc* 76(4):369, 2001.

Laskowski-Jones L: Responding to winter emergencies, *Nursing* 30(1):34, 2000.

McCall E, Alderdice F, Halliday H et al: Interventions to prevent hypothermia at birth in preterm and/or low birth weight babies, *Cochrane Database Syst Rev* (1):CD004210, 2005.

McCullough L, Arora S: Diagnosis and treatment of hypothermia, *Am Fam Physician* 70(12):2325, 2004.

Ruffolo DC: Hypothermia in trauma: the cold, hard facts, *RN* 65(2):46, 2002.

Smith LS: Temperature measurement in critical care adults: a comparison of thermometry and measurement routes, *Biol Res Nurs* 6(2):117, 2004.

Disturbed personal Identity   Gail B. Ladwig, MSN, CHTP, RN

NANDA   Definition

Inability to distinguish between self and nonself

Defining Characteristics

To be developed

Related Factors (r/t)

To be developed

NOC   Outcomes (Nursing Outcomes Classification)

Suggested NOC Outcomes

Anxiety Self-Control, Identity

Example NOC Outcome with Indicators
Identity as evidenced by the following indicators: Verbalizes affirmations of personal identity/Exhibits congruent verbal and nonverbal behavior about self/Differentiates self from environment and other human beings (Rate the outcome and indicators of **Identity:** 1 = never demonstrated, 2 = rarely demonstrated, 3 = sometimes demonstrated, 4 = often demonstrated, 5 = consistently demonstrated [see Section I].)

• = Independent;   ▲ = Collaborative;   EBN = Evidence-Based Nursing;   EB = Evidence-Based

Client Outcomes

Client Will (Specify Time Frame):

- Show interest in surroundings
- Respond to stimuli with appropriate affect
- Perform self-care and self-control activities appropriate for age
- Acknowledge personal strengths
- Engage in interpersonal relationships
- Verbalize willingness to change lifestyle and use appropriate community resources

NIC   Interventions (Nursing Interventions Classification)

Suggested NIC Interventions

Decision-Making Support, Self-Esteem Enhancement

Example NIC Activities—Self-Esteem Enhancement
Monitor patient's statements of self-worth; Encourage patient to identify strengths

Nursing Interventions and _Rationales_

- Assess carefully for a history of abuse. **EB:** _Most of the clients with dissociative disorder report auditory hallucinations, symptoms associated with psychogenic amnesia, flashback experiences, and childhood abuse and/or neglect (Sar et al, 2007). Current levels of post-traumatic and dissociative symptomatology were significantly higher in the group reporting sexual abuse by a perpetrator in a relationship of trust, guardianship, or authority (Leahy, Pretty & Tenenbaum, 2004)._
- Assess for any history of seizure disorder; adhere to the diagnostic criteria for dissociative disorder in the Diagnostic and Statistical Manual of Mental Disorders, Fourth Edition (DSM-IV), and conduct a structured clinical interview. **EB:** _Misdiagnosis of persons with seizures and dissociative symptoms can be avoided by careful adherence to DSM-IV dissociative disorder criteria (Bowman & Coons, 2000)._
- Avoid labeling the client with terms such as multiple personality disorder (MPD). **EB:** _More clients attempted suicide after being diagnosed with MPD than before diagnosis (Fetkewicz, Sharma & Merskey, 2000)._
- Spend time communicating with the client. **EBN:** _Nursing presence is the foundation of a long-term nurse-client relationship that improves clinical decision making and ultimately client outcomes (Anderson, 2007)._
- Provide time for one-on-one interactions to establish a therapeutic relationship. **EBN:** _Nursing presence, one-on-one interaction, and connecting with the client helps the client grow in awareness of his or her own being (Doona, Chase & Haggerty, 1999)._
- Work with the client on setting personal goals. **EB:** _Clients develop for themselves, in conjunction with their therapists, a concept for treatment and setting goals that are as realistic and concrete as possible (Gierig & Hlsewiesche, 2002)._
- Provide communication, clear rules and aims, and safety procedures. **EBN:** _With these interventions, the use of seclusion for aggressive client behavior is substantially reduced (Mistral, Hall & McKee, 2002)._
- Work with the client to utilize their senses to deescalate problem behavior. **EBN:** _Sensory-based approaches and multisensory rooms are valuable resources (Champagne & Stromberg, 2004)._
- Give the client permission to share his or her experiences. **EB:** _An average of 6.8 years elapses between the time clients are first assessed and the time they receive an accurate diagnosis (Frye, 1990)._
- Use touch only after a thorough assessment and as appropriate. _Touch, which conveys caring, is an appropriate way of communicating, unless it makes the person touched feel uncomfortable (Wells-Federman et al, 1995)._
- Encourage the client to verbalize feelings about self and body image. Have the client make a list of strengths. **EB:** _These verbalizations help the client recognize the self; listing strengths promotes self-exploration (Sansone, Wiederman & Monteith, 2001)._

• = Independent;   ▲ = Collaborative;   EBN = Evidence-Based Nursing;   EB = Evidence-Based

▲ Support client's autonomy in a nurse-led shared care environment where the client is encouraged to participate in his or her care. **EBN:** *To achieve autonomy, clients prefer a mixed approach of negative freedom that emphasizes freedom of action and freedom from interference by others and positive freedom which stresses the idea that people should direct their lives according to their personal convictions and individual reasons and goals (Moser, Houtepen & Widdershoven, 2007).*

▲ Encourage participation in group therapy for building relationship skills and getting feedback from others with regard to behavior. **EB:** *Social skills training resulted in greater improvement in certain measures of social adjustment than did supportive group therapy (Marder et al, 1996).* **EBN:** *Group therapy could be a powerful tool for treating those who suffer profound wounds to self-esteem (Kurek-Ovshinsky, 1991).*

• Encourage the client to use a daily diary to set achievable and realistic goals and to monitor successes. *Journal writing has been found to improve physical and mental health measurably (Wells-Federman et al, 1995).*

▲ Refer for rational emotive therapy to help dispel underlying irrational thinking. **EBN:** *This therapy strives to produce sustained and profound cognitive, emotive, and behavioral change through active, vigorous disputation of underlying irrational philosophies (Sacks, 2004).*

Geriatric

• Address the client by his or her full name preceded by the proper title (i.e., Mr., Mrs., Ms., Miss); use a nickname or first name only if suggested by the client, and do not use terms of endearment (e.g., "honey"). **EBN:** *Research findings emphasize the importance of relationship-oriented experiences as part of assessment and intervention strategies for individuals with depression (Hagerty & Williams, 1999).*

• Practice reality orientation principles. **EB:** *Reality orientation therapy has benefits for both cognition and behavior of dementia sufferers (Spector et al, 2000).*

• Ask the client about important past experiences. **EBN:** *Factors that influence self-efficacy beliefs are personal expectations, personality, role models, verbal encouragement, progress, past experiences, spirituality, physical sensations, individualized care, social supports, and goals (Resnick, 2002).*

▲ If the client's symptoms are associated with a stroke, refer the client for longer rehabilitation that includes physical programs addressing psychological as well as neuromuscular issues. **EB:** *Clients who have had a stroke find the body unreliable, and the body appears separate from the self. These feelings may last a year or longer (Ellis-Hill, Payne & Ward, 2000).*

Multicultural

• Assess for the influence of cultural beliefs, norms, and values on the family's perceptions of infant/child behavior. **EBN:** *What the family considers normal infant/child behavior may be based on cultural perceptions (Leininger & McFarland, 2002).*

• Use a neutral, indirect style when addressing areas in which improvement is needed, such as a need for verbal or oral stimulation, when working with Native-American clients. **EBN:** *Using indirect statements such as "Other mothers have tried…" or "I had a client who tried 'X,' and it seemed to work very well" help avoid resentment on the part of the parent (Seideman et al, 1996).*

Home Care

• The interventions described previously may be adapted for home care use.

Client/Family Teaching

• Teach stress reduction and relaxation techniques. These techniques can be used when the client becomes anxious about the loss of self. *Muscle relaxation therapy (MRT) plays an important role in the modern treatment of anxiety disorders (Conrad & Roth, 2006).*

▲ Refer to community resources or other self-help groups appropriate for the client's underlying problem (e.g., Adult Children of Alcoholics, parent effectiveness group). **EBN:** *Group therapy provides an arena in which clients can experience the interdependent mode of adaptation without assaults to self-esteem (Kurek-Ovshinsky, 1991).*

▲ Refer to appropriate treatment as soon as signs of depression are noted. **EB:** *Between 15 and 19 treatment sessions of standard psychotherapy are required for a 50% recovery rate (Hansen & Lambert,*

2003). Most clients report residual symptoms despite successful treatment. Recovery should involve psychological well-being and therapeutic strategies for improving the level of remission, such as treatment of residual symptoms of depression (Fava, Ruini & Belaise, 2007).

evolve   See the EVOLVE website for World Wide Web resources for client education.

REFERENCES

Anderson JH: The impact of using nursing presence in a community heart failure program, *J Cardiovasc Nurs* 22(2):89-94, 2007.

Bowman ES, Coons PM: The differential diagnosis of epilepsy, pseudoseizures, dissociative identity disorder, and dissociative disorder not otherwise specified, *Bull Menninger Clin* 64(2):164-180, 2000.

Champagne T, Stromberg N: Sensory approaches in inpatient psychiatric settings: innovative alternatives to seclusion and restraint, *J Psychosoc Nurs Ment Health Serv* 42(9):34-44, 2004.

Conrad A, Roth WT: Muscle relaxation therapy for anxiety disorders: it works but how? *J Anxiety Disord,* Aug 30, 2006 [Epub ahead of print].

Doona M, Chase S, Haggerty L: Nursing presence: as real as a Milky Way bar, *J Holist Nurs* 17(1):54-70, 1999.

Ellis-Hill CS, Payne S, Ward C: Self-body split: issues of identity in physical recovery following a stroke, *Disabil Rehabil* 22(16):725-733, 2000.

Fava GA, Ruini C, Belaise C: The concept of recovery in major depression, *Psychol Med* 37(3):307-317, 2007.

Fetkewicz J, Sharma V, Merskey H: A note on suicidal deterioration with recovered memory treatment, *J Affect Disord* 58(2):155-159, 2000.

Frye B: Art and multiple personality disorder: an expressive framework for occupational therapy, *Am J Occup Ther* 44(11):1013-1022, 1990.

Gierig L, Hlsewiesche D: [Group of orientations: a systemic-draw-oriented beginning including the expression-centered method], *Ergother Rehabil* 41(7):15-18, 2002 [article in German].

Hagerty BM, Williams RA: The effects of sense of belonging, social support, conflict, and loneliness on depression, *Nurs Res* 48(4):215-219, 1999.

Hansen NB, Lambert MJ: An evaluation of the dose-response relationship in naturalistic treatment settings using survival analysis, *Ment Health Serv Res* 5(1):1-12, 2003.

Kurek-Ovshinsky C: Group psychotherapy in an acute inpatient setting: techniques that nourish self-esteem, *Issues Ment Health Nurs* 12(1):81-88, 1991.

Leahy T, Pretty G, Tenenbaum G: Perpetrator methodology as a predictor of traumatic symptomatology in adult survivors of childhood sexual abuse, *J Interpers Violence* 19(5):521-540, 2004.

Leininger MM, McFarland MR: *Transcultural nursing: concepts, theories, research and practices,* ed 3, New York, 2002, McGraw-Hill.

Marder SR, Wirshing WC, Mintz J et al: Two-year outcome of social skills training and group psychotherapy for outpatients with schizophrenia, *Am J Psychiatry* 153(12):1585-1592, 1996.

Mistral W, Hall A, McKee P: Using therapeutic community principles to improve the functioning of a high care psychiatric ward in the UK, *Int J Ment Health Nurs* 11(1):10-17, 2002.

Moser A, Houtepen R, Widdershoven G: Patient autonomy in nurse-led shared care: a review of theoretical and empirical literature, *J Adv Nurs* 57(4):357-365, 2007.

Resnick B: Geriatric rehabilitation: the influence of efficacy beliefs and motivation, *Rehabil Nurs* 27(4):152-159, 2002.

Sacks SB: Rational emotive behavior therapy: disputing irrational philosophies, *J Psychosoc Nurs Ment Health Serv* 42(5):22-31, 2004.

Sansone RA, Wiederman MW, Monteith D: Obesity, borderline personality symptomatology, and body image among women in a psychiatric outpatient setting, *Int J Eat Disord* 29(1):76, 2001.

Sar V, Koyuncu A, Ozturk E et al: Dissociative disorders in the psychiatric emergency ward. *Gen Hosp Psychiatry* 29(1):45-50, 2007.

Seideman RY, Jacobson S, Primeaux M et al: Assessing American Indian families, *MCN Am J Matern Child Nurs* 21(6):274-279, 1996.

Spector A, Orrell M, Davies S et al: Reality orientation for dementia, *Cochrane Database Syst Rev* (4):CD001119, 2000.

Wells-Federman CL, Stuart EM, Deckro JP et al: The mind-body connection: the psychophysiology of many traditional nursing interventions, *Clin Nurse Spec* 9(1):59-66, 1995.

Readiness for enhanced Immunization status   *Susan Mee Coleman, RN, PhD(c), CPNP*

NANDA   Definition

A pattern of conforming to local, national, and/or international standards of immunization to prevent infectious disease(s) that is sufficient to protect a person, family, or community and can be strengthened

Defining Characteristics

Expresses desire to enhance: behavior to prevent infectious disease; identification of possible problems associated with immunizations; identification of providers of immunizations; immunization status; knowledge of immunization standards; record-keeping of immunizations

• = Independent;   ▲ = Collaborative;   EBN = Evidence-Based Nursing;   EB = Evidence-Based

Outcomes (Nursing Outcomes Classification)

Suggested NOC Outcomes

Health Promoting Behavior, Immunization Behavior, Knowledge: Health Behavior, Knowledge: Health Promotion

Example NOC Outcomes with Indicators
Immunization Behavior as evidenced by the following indicators: Acknowledges disease risk without immunization/Brings updated immunization card to each visit/Obtains immunizations recommended for age by the AAP or USPHS/Describes relief measures for vaccine side effects/Reports any adverse reactions/Confirms date of next immunization/Identifies community resources for immunization (Rate the outcome and indicators of **Immunization Behavior**: 1 = never demonstrated, 2 = rarely demonstrated, 3 = sometimes demonstrated, 4 = often demonstrated, 5 = consistently demonstrated [see Section I].)

Client Outcomes

Client/Caregiver Will (Specify Time Frame):

- Review appropriate recommended immunization schedule with provider
- Ask questions about the benefits and risks of immunizations
- Ask questions regarding the risk of choosing not to be immunized
- Accurately respond to provider's questions related to pertinent information regarding individual health status as it relates to contraindications for individual vaccines.
- Inform provider of the health status of close contacts and household members
- Evidence understanding of the risks and benefits of individual immunization decisions
- Evidence understanding of the benefits of community immunization
- Communicate decisions about immunization decision to provider in relation to personal preferences, values, and goals
- Communicate to provider ongoing personal record of immunization
- Evidence understanding of the client's responsibility to maintain an accurate record of immunization

Interventions (Nursing Interventions Classification)

Suggested NIC interventions

Decision Making Support, Mutual Goal Setting

Example NIC Activities—Decision Making Support
Help patient identify the advantages and disadvantages of each alternative; Provide information requested by patient

Nursing Interventions and *Rationales*
Psychosocial

- Assess barriers to immunization:
  - Anxiety related to injection/parenteral pharmacologic therapy **EBN:** *Fear of needles is a reported barrier to immunization (Mayo & Cobler, 2004).*
  - Anxiety related to immunization side effects **EB:** *Parents who refuse to immunize their children may have personal cultural or experiential reasons for their refusal; parents experiencing omission bias benefit from reframing the decision from the viewpoint of the disease-vulnerable child (Ball, Evans & Bostram, 1998).*
  - Knowledge of risk associated with disease **EBN:** *Clients/caregivers who perceive the risk of a vaccine-preventable disease have lower vaccination status (Neiderhauser, Baruffi & Heck, 2001).*
  - Cost of health care **EB:** *Minorities report lesser self-rated general health and a higher cost barrier to health care, particularly in Hispanic communities. Removing barriers to health care is an impor-*

• = Independent;   ▲ = Collaborative;   EBN = Evidence-Based Nursing;   EB = Evidence-Based

tant aspect of health promotion and disease prevention (Liao et al, 2004). Programs to improve health insurance coverage and having a usual source of medical care positively impact age-appropriate immunization status (Dombroswki, Lantz & Freed, 2004).

- Assess client-provider relationship. **EBN:** *Shared decision making is embedded in the client-provider relationship (Wilkenson & Williams, 2002).* **EB:** *Clients who report trusting their healthcare provider have higher immunization rates (Norwalk et al, 2005). Faith-based, neighborhood health centers established to serve disadvantaged populations report high levels of provider trust (Zimmerman et al, 2003).*
- Assess client/caregiver level of participation in decision making process. **EB:** *Many parents elect not to vaccinate their children; clients and families should be involved in the decision making process.*
- Assess sources of information client has previously turned to. **EB:** *Lack of knowledge, fear of vaccine side effects, and misinformation perpetuated by antivaccine media contribute to low vaccination rates and vaccine refusal (Kimmel et al, 2007).*
- Assist client/caregiver to find appropriate educational resources. **EBN:** *Health information on vaccine efficacy should be accurate, consistent, and provided in a direct manner (Niederhauser, Baruffi & Heck, 2001).*
- Assess cultural or religious beliefs that may relate to either the decision making process or specific immunizations such as sexually transmitted disease. **EB:** *There is considerable dissension among parents in relation to attitude toward vaccination for sexually transmitted diseases (STDs). Public health policy makers, legislators, and school boards need to be sensitive to the concerns and rights of parents/caregivers regarding the potential mandate of immunization for STDs (Liddon et al, 2005).*

Physiological

- Perform comprehensive interview to elicit information regarding the client's susceptibility to adverse reactions to specific vaccines according to the manufacturer guidelines.
- Identify clients for whom a specific vaccine is contraindicated. **EBN:** *Client's perception of vaccine-related adverse effects and related allergy account for a proportion of vaccine refusal (Mayo & Cobler, 2004).*
- ▲ Report potential or actual adverse effects. **EB:** *Surveillance for adverse effects is important, and in some instances, mandated (Kretsinger et al, 2006).*
- Inform client/caregiver of the vaccine-specific risks to both women of childbearing age and the fetus. **EBN:** *Women's reproductive health overlaps with epidemiology of vaccine-preventable disease or physiological aspects of immunization (Schmidt, Kroger & Roy, 2004).*
- Discuss pregnancy planning with appropriate clients considering immunization. **EBN:** *Women's reproductive health overlaps with epidemiology of vaccine-preventable disease or physiological aspects of immunization. Prevention of vaccine-preventable disease is a critical element of women's health promotion (Schmidt, Kroger & Roy, 2004).*
- Identify high risk individuals for specific vaccine-preventable disease. **EBN:** *A meta-analysis of nursing sensitive interventions targeted to improve nursing sensitive client outcomes recommends clients with cancer and their household contact receive annual influenza immunization (Zitella et al, 2006).*
- Identify high risk groups for specific vaccine-preventable disease. **EB:** *Most deaths and serious illness resulting from vaccine-preventable influenza and pneumococcal disease occur in populations such as older adults at risk for complications of these diseases related to comorbidity (US Department of Health and Human Services, 2000).* **EB:** *In a study of female day care center educators, 10.2% presented as rubella seronegative. Women who are in contact with young children should be concerned due to the risk for infection and resultant congenital rubella syndrome (Gyorkos et al, 2005). Healthcare workers are a vulnerable population who benefit from influenza vaccination directly and indirectly by providing secondary benefit to healthcare facility consumers. In a study of 26,261 Mayo clinic employees, influenza vaccination compliance improved via the Peer Vaccination Program, which provided incentives and made raffles available only to vaccinated employees, offered vaccination during grand rounds, and provided e-mail encouragement (CDC, 2005).*
- Identify high risk populations for specific vaccine preventable disease. **EBN:** *Nurses engaged in both disaster planning and disaster interventions need to be proactive in emergency administration of vaccines such as tetanus (Walton, 2006). Vaccination rates for populations at high risk for hepatitis B virus (HBV) remain low (Willis et al, 2005).*

- Assess client's recent travel history and future travel plans. **EB:** *Communicable diseases that are currently not endemic in the United States persist among travelers, often resulting in delayed recognition and notification of public health authorities (CDC, 2007).*
- Identify vulnerable populations and marginalized populations. **EB:** *Residents of minority communities bear greater risk for disease; substantial variation in the use of preventive services among different minority populations provide opportunities for health interventions (Liao et al, 2004). High risk groups for HBV include men having sex with men, risk behaviors such as IV drug use, and multiple sex partners (Willis et al, 2005).*
- Tailor educational programs specific to these marginalized and vulnerable populations. **EB:** *In a study of 432 men having sex with men (MSM), researchers concluded that health education intervention that address perceived susceptibility and severity are likely to improve vaccination status. This study recommended interventions specific to influencing perceived susceptibility as a preferred intervention (deWit et al, 2005).*
- Adopt recommendations made by national and international professional groups advocating the use of Immunization Central Registries, Standing orders. **EBN:** *Adaptation of multimodal interventions targeted to improve immunization rates resulted in 97% compliance rate for 12-month-old children and 87% compliance rate for immunization standards for 24-month-old children. Recommendations include electronic medical record, phone calls, postcards and letters to clients, staff education, and client record surveillance (Parve, 2004).* **EB:** *Strategies to enhance immunization status include standing orders, computerized record reminder, chart reminder, performance feedback, home visits, mailed/telephone reminders, expanded access in clinical settings, client education, personal health records (Centers for Disease Control, 2007; Committee on Practice and Ambulatory Medicine, 2006; Ahmed et al, 2004).*
- Support access to health care that enables clients to access well preventive care on a walk-in basis during times that are consistent with client schedules. **EBN:** *Comprehensive efforts to identify population-specific barriers to access and targeted interventions to address barriers is effective in improving immunization rates (Parve, 2004).* **EB:** *More than 40 million Americans do not have a particular healthcare provider where they seek health care or health promoting advice. Financial, structural, and spiritual barriers limit access to health care (US Department of Health and Human Services, 2000).*

Multicultural

- Assess cultural beliefs and practices that may have an impact on the educational and decision making process specific to immunization as well as vaccine-specific illness. **EB:** *Variation exists both between and within cultural affiliations with respect to health beliefs and health seeking behaviors. In a study of Chinese Americans in New York City, Ma et al reports differences between attitudes and behavior of younger versus older members of the Chinese American community with respect to screening behavior, immunization acceptance, and willingness to discuss HPV with their healthcare provider (Ma et al, 2006).*
- Actively listen and be sensitive to how communication is shared culturally. **EB:** *Cultural sensitivity is the foundation of community outreach. In a study of Vietnamese-American children and their caregivers, attention to the information-sharing network of the subpopulation was integral to the study design. Media known to be respected and utilized by the community were considered in the study design (McPhee et al, 2003).*
- Employ culturally sensitive educational strategies to maximize the individual, family, or community response. **EB:** *In a study of patterns of immunization for HBV among Vietnamese-American children in the Houston, Texas, metropolitan area, awareness, knowledge, and immunization status improved significantly as a result of culturally sensitive interventions targeted to this vulnerable population (McPhee et al, 2003).*

Home Care

- Above interventions may be adapted for home care use.
- Develop clinical practice guidelines that include shared decision making. **EB:** *Both client-provider and system oriented interventions are effective in increasing vaccination status (Zimmerman et al, 2003).*

I

- Implement home care strategies that will enhance decision making and ability to maintain current immunization status. **EB:** *Provider-initiated phone calls to clients/caregivers, reminder postcards, and letters are effective strategies to improve immunization status (Norwalk et al, 2005).*
- Implement mechanisms to contact the client/caregiver at appropriate intervals with reminder literature or phone contact. **EB:** *The use of reminder postcards and/or employer-provided tool kits may enhance immunization status. The cost-benefit of these strategies should be regularly monitored to improve outcomes and make effective use of health resources (Ahmed et al, 2004).*

Client/Family Teaching

- Before teaching, evaluate the client preference for involvement with the decision making process.
- Use community-based and school-based interventions to teach school-age children and thereby provide vicarious education to the family. **EB:** *School-based curricula are effective in increasing immunization knowledge, enhancing positive attitude toward immunization, and improving health promotion behavior with respect to immunization (Glik et al, 2004). Community-based, culturally specific outreach programs improve immunization status (McPhee et al, 2003).*
- Develop curricula and media that enhance immunization education. **EB:** *Community-based, culturally specific educational programs result in an increase in client/caregiver knowledge and significantly improved vaccination rates (McPhee et al, 2003).*
- Employ media and curricula in office waiting rooms. **EB:** *Clients benefit when waiting room time is utilized as an educational opportunity (CDC, 2007; author, 2000).*
- Develop and distribute client log books that provide record keeping and foster ownership of the responsibility of current immunization status. **EB:** *Client/caregiver personal health records improve immunization rates (CDC, 2007; author, 2000).*

REFERENCES

Ahmed F, Friedman C, Franks A et al: Effect of the frequency of delivery of reminders and an influenza tool kit on increasing influenza vaccination rates among adults with high-risk conditions, *Am J Manag Care* 10(10):698-712, 2004.

Ball L, Evans G, Bostram A: A risky business: challenges in vaccine risk communication, *Pediatrics,* 101(3 Pt 1):453-458, 1998.

Centers for Disease Control and Prevention (CDC): Interventions to increase influenza vaccination of health-care workers—California and Minnesota, *MMWR Morb Mortal Wkly Rep* 54(8):196-199, 2005.

Centers for Disease Control and Prevention (CDC): Measles among adults associated with adoption of children in China—California, Missouri, and Washington, July-August 2006, *MMWR Morb Mortal Wkly Rep* 56(7):144-146, 2007.

Centers for Disease Control: Strategies for increasing adult vaccination rates, at http://www.cdc.gov/nip/registry/Default.htm. Accessed on April 20, 2007.

Committee on Practice and Ambulatory Medicine: Immunization information systems, *Pediatrics* 118(3):1293-1295, 2006.

deWit JBF, Vet R, Schitten M et al: Social-cognitive determinants of vaccination behavior against hepatitis B: an assessment among men who have sex with men, *Prev Med* 40(6):795-802, 2005.

Dombrowski KJ, Lantz PM, Freed GL: Role of health insurance and a usual source of medical care in age appropriate vaccination. *Am J Public Health,* 94(6):960-966, 2004.

Glik D, Macpherson F, Todd W et al: Impact of an immunization education program on middle school adolescents, *Am J Health Behav* 28(6):487-497, 2004.

Gyorkos TW, Beliveau C, Rahme E et al: High rubella seronegativity in daycare educators, *Clin Invest Med* 28(3):105-111, 2005.

Kimmel SR, Burns I, Wolfe RM et al: Addressing immunization barriers, benefits and risks, *J Fam Pract* 56(2):561-569, 2007.

Kretsinger K, Broder KR, Cortese MM et al: Preventing tetanus, diphtheria, and pertussis among adults: use of tetanus toxoid, reduced diphtheria toxoid and acellular pertussis vaccine recommendations of the Advisory Committee on Immunization Practices (ACIP) and recommendation of ACIP, supported by the Healthcare Infection Control Practices Advisory Committee (HICPAC), for use of Tdap among health-care personnel, *MMWR Recomm Rep* 55(RR-17):1-37, 2006.

Liao Y, Tucker P, Okoro CA et al: REACH 2010 Surveillance for Health Status in Minority Communities—United States, 2001-2002, *MMWR Surveill Summ* 53(6):1-36, 2004.

Liddon N, Pulley L, Cocherham WC et al: Parents'/guardians' willingness to vaccinate their children against genital herpes, *J Adolesc Health* 37(3):187-193, 2005.

Ma G, Shive S, Toubbeh J et al: Risk perceptions, barriers, benefits and self-efficacy of hepatitis B screening and vaccination among Chinese immigrants, *Int J Health Educ* 9:141-153, 2006.

Mayo AM, Cobler S: Flu vaccines and patient decision making: what we need to know, *J Am Acad Nurse Pract* 16(9):402-410, 2004.

McPhee SJ, Nguyen T, Euller GL et al: Successful promotion of hepatitis B vaccinations among Vietnamese-American children ages 3-18: results of a controlled trial, *Pediatrics* 111(6):1278-1288, 2003.

Neiderhauser VP, Baruffi G, Heck R: Parental decision making for the varicella vaccine, *J Pediatr Health Care* 15(5):236-243, 2001.

Norwalk MP, Lin CJ, Zimmerman RK et al: Tailored interventions to introduce influenza vaccine among 6-23 month old children at inner city health centers. *Am J Manag Care* 11:717-724, 2005.

Parve J: Remove vaccination barriers for children 12-24 months, *Nurse Pract* 29(4):35-38, 2004.

Schmidt JV, Kroger AT, Roy SL: Vaccines in women, *J Women's Health* 13(3):249-257, 2004.

US Department of Health and Human Services: *Healthy People 2010,* ed 2, (2 vols), Washington, DC, 2000, US Government Printing Office.

Walton F: One nurse can make a big difference, *Aust Nurs J* 14(2):15, 2006.

Wilkenson CR, Williams M: Strengthening patient-provider relationships, *Lippincotts Case Manag*, 7(3):86-100, 2002.

Willis BC, Ndiaye SM, Hopkins DP et al: Improving influenza, pneumococcal polysaccharide, and hepatitis B vaccination coverage among adults aged <65 years at high risk: a report on recommendations of the Task Force on Community Preventive Services, *MMWR Recomm Rep* 54(RR-5):1-11, 2005.

Zimmerman RK, Nowalk MP, Raymund M et al: Tailored interventions to increase influenza vaccination in neighborhood health centers serving the disadvantaged, *Am J Public Health* 93(10):1699-1705, 2003.

Zitella LJ, Friese CR, Hauser J et al: Putting evidence into practice: prevention of infection, *Clin J Oncol Nurs* 10:739-750, 2006.

Functional urinary Incontinence   *Mikel Gray, PhD, RN*   **evolve**

NANDA   Definition

Inability of usually continent person to reach toilet in time to avoid unintentional loss of urine (NANDA-I). Impairment or loss of continence due to functional deficits, including altered mobility, dexterity, or cognition, or environmental barriers (Gray, 2007).

Defining Characteristics

Although functional limitations (impaired mobility, dexterity, and cognition) are risk factors for urinary incontinence (UI) (Hunskaar et al, 2005; Jenkins & Fultz, 2005), the nature of their relationship is complex and only partly understood. For example, impaired cognition associated with Alzheimer's type dementia leads to detrusor overactivity (Rosenberg et al, 2005). Whether or not detrusor overactivity leads to UI (either urge UI or UI without sensory awareness) depends on multiple factors, including mobility, the severity of cognitive impairment, among other factors. Thus, while functional impairment exacerbates the severity of urinary incontinence, the underlying factors that contribute to these functional limitations themselves also contribute to abnormal lower urinary tract function and impaired continence.

Related Factors (r/t)

Cognitive disorders (delirium, dementia, severe or profound retardation); neuromuscular limitations impairing mobility or dexterity; environmental barriers to toileting

NOC   Outcomes (Nursing Outcomes Classification)

Suggested NOC Outcomes

Urinary Continence, Urinary Elimination

Example NOC Outcome with Indicators

Urinary Continence as evidenced by the following indicators: Recognizes urge to void/Responds to urge in timely manner/Voids in appropriate receptacle/Underclothing remains dry during day/Underclothing or bedding remains dry during night (Rate the outcome and indicators of **Urinary Continence:** 1 = never demonstrated, 2 = rarely demonstrated, 3 = sometimes demonstrated, 4 = often demonstrated, 5 = consistently demonstrated [see Section I].)

Client Outcomes

Client Will (Specify Time Frame):

- Eliminate or reduce incontinent episodes
- Eliminate or overcome environmental barriers to toileting
- Use adaptive equipment to reduce or eliminate incontinence related to impaired mobility or dexterity
- Use portable urinary collection devices or urine containment devices when access to the toilet is not feasible

• = Independent;   ▲ = Collaborative;   EBN = Evidence-Based Nursing;   EB = Evidence-Based

NIC   Interventions (Nursing Interventions Classification)

Suggested NIC Interventions

Urinary Habit Training, Urinary Incontinence Care

Example NIC Activities—Urinary Habit Training
Keep a continence specification record for 3 days to establish voiding pattern; Establish interval for toileting of preferably not less than 2 hours

Nursing Interventions and *Rationales*

▲ Perform a history taking and physical assessment focusing on bothersome lower urinary tract symptoms, cognitive status, functional status (particularly physical mobility and dexterity), frequency and severity of leakage episodes, and alleviating and aggravating factors. *The history provides clues to the causes, the severity of the condition, and its management (Reuben, 1999; Vickerman, 2002).* **EBN:** *Results of physical assessment, functional evaluation (mobility toileting skills, physical examination), and evaluation of cognitive status (Folstein Mini-Mental State Examination) and psychological status (Geriatric Depression Scale) for a group of 90 homebound revealed that functional impairments are associated with frequent and severe incontinence. Although these problems were perceived as particularly bothersome (despite multiple comorbid health issues), elders in this group remained optimistic about potential benefits of treatment (Folstein, Folstein & McHugh, 1975; McDowell et al, 1996).*

▲ Consult with the client and family, the client's physician, and other healthcare professionals concerning treatment of incontinence in the elderly client undergoing detailed geriatric evaluation. **EBN:** *Geriatric assessment units are designed to evaluate and assist clients and their families to deal with multiple problems experienced by geriatric clients, including urinary incontinence. Recommendations for no treatment of urinary incontinence may be based on a complex assessment of the client's physical health, comorbid conditions, and cognitive and psychological status (Silverman et al, 1997).*

• Teach the client, the client's care providers, or the family to complete a voiding diary (bladder log) by recording voiding frequency, the frequency of urinary incontinent episodes, and their association with urgency (a sudden and strong desire to urinate that is difficult to defer) over a 3- to 7-day period. An electronic voiding diary may be kept whenever feasible. In addition to these parameters, the client may be asked to record voided volume and fluid intake. *The voiding diary provides a more objective record of lower urinary tract function than the oral history, and it often provides a modest therapeutic effect by alerting the client to factors that promote urinary incontinence episodes (Sampselle, 2003). An electronic voiding diary provides an efficient and possibly more accurate method for documenting these parameters (Quinn, Goka & Richardson, 2003).*

• Assess the client for potentially reversible or modifiable causes of acute/transient urinary incontinence (e.g., urinary tract infection; atrophic urethritis; constipation or impaction; use of sedatives or narcotics, antidepressants or psychotropic medications interfering with efficient detrusor contractions, parasympatholytics, or alpha-adrenergic antagonists; polyuria caused by uncontrolled diabetes mellitus or insipidus). *Transient or acute incontinence may be relieved or eliminated by treating the underlying cause (Reilly, 2002).*

• Assess the client in an acute care or rehabilitation facility for risk factors for functional incontinence. **EBN:** *Risk factors include confusion, use of a wheelchair or assistive device for walking, and dependence on others for ambulation prior to admission (Palmer et al, 2002).*

• Assess the client for coexisting or premorbid urinary incontinence. *A history of premorbid urinary incontinence predicts a higher risk for persistent urinary leakage and poorer functional outcomes at 6 and 12 months (Jawad, Ward & Jones, 1999; Thommessen, Bautz-Holter & Laake, 1999).*

• Assess clients, regardless of frailty or age, residing in a long-term care facility for UI. **EB:** *UI significantly impairs quality of life, even among frail, and functionally or cognitively impaired elders residing in a nursing home (Dubeau, Simon & Morris, 2006).*

• = Independent;   ▲ = Collaborative;   EBN = Evidence-Based Nursing;   EB = Evidence-Based

- Assess the home, acute care, or long-term care environment for accessibility to toileting facilities, paying particular attention to the following:
  - Distance of the toilet from the bed, chair, and living quarters
  - Characteristics of the bed, including presence of side rails and distance of the bed from the floor
  - Characteristics of the pathway to the toilet, including barriers such as stairs, loose rugs on the floor, and inadequate lighting
  - Characteristics of the bathroom, including patterns of use, lighting, height of the toilet from the floor, presence of handrails to assist transfers to the toilet, and breadth of the door and its accessibility for a wheelchair, walker, or other assistive device

  Functional continence requires access to a toilet; environmental barriers blocking this access can produce functional incontinence (Chadwick, 2005; Wells, 1992).
- Assess the client for mobility, including the ability to rise from chair and bed, transfer to the toilet, and ambulate, and the need for physical assistive devices such as a cane, walker, or wheelchair. *Functional continence requires the ability to gain access to a toilet facility, either independently or with the assistance of devices to increase mobility (Jirovec & Wells, 1990; Wells, 1992).*
- ▲ Assess the client for dexterity, including the ability to manipulate buttons, hooks, snaps, loop and pile closure, and zippers as needed to remove clothing. Consult a physical or occupational therapist to promote optimal toilet access as indicated. *Functional continence requires the ability to remove clothing to urinate (Lekan-Rutledge, 2004; Maloney & Cafiero, 1999; Wells, 1992).*
- Evaluate cognitive status with a Neecham Confusion Scale (Neelan et al, 1992) in cases of acute cognitive change or with a Folstein Mini-Mental State Examination (Folstein et al, 1975) or other tool as indicated. *Functional continence requires sufficient mental acuity to respond to sensory input from a filling urinary bladder by locating the toilet, moving to it, and emptying the bladder (Maloney & Cafiero, 1999; McDowell et al, 1996).*
- Remove environmental barriers to toileting in the acute care, long-term care, or home setting. Assist the client in removing loose rugs from the floor and improving lighting in hallways and bathrooms. *Functional continence requires ready access to a urinal (Lekan-Rutledge, 2004; Wells, 1992).*
- Provide an appropriate, safe urinary receptacle such as a three-in-one commode, female or male hand-held urinal, no-spill urinal, or containment device when toileting access is limited by immobility or environmental barriers. *These receptacles provide access to a substitute toilet and enhance the potential for functional continence (Rabin, 1998; Wells, 1992).*
- ▲ Help the client with limited mobility to obtain evaluation by a physical therapist and to obtain assistive devices as indicated; assist the client in selecting shoes with a nonskid sole to maximize traction when arising from a chair and transferring to the toilet. *A physical therapist is an important member of the interdisciplinary team needed to manage urinary incontinence in the client with functional impairments (Maloney & Cafiero, 1999).*
- Assist the client in altering the wardrobe to maximize toileting access. Select loose-fitting clothing with stretch waistbands rather than buttoned or zippered waist; minimize buttons, snaps, and multilayered clothing; and substitute a loop and pile closure or other easily loosened systems for buttons, hooks, and zippers in existing clothing.
- Begin a prompted voiding program or patterned urge response toileting program for the elderly client in the home or a long-term care facility who has functional incontinence and dementia:
  - Determine the frequency of current urination using an alarm system or check-and-change device.
  - Record urinary elimination and incontinent patterns in a bladder log to use as a baseline for assessment and evaluation of treatment efficacy.
  - Begin a prompted toileting program based on the results of this program; toileting frequency may vary from every 1.5 to 2 hours to every 4 hours.
  - Praise the client when toileting occurs with prompting.
  - Refrain from any socialization when incontinent episodes occur; change the client and make her or him comfortable.

  EBN: *Prompted voiding or patterned urge response toileting executed during waking hours has been shown to markedly reduce or eliminate functional incontinence in selected clients in long-term care* *facilities and in the community setting (Colling et al, 1992; Engberg et al, 2002; Eustice, Roe & Paterson, 2000). It has not been shown to be effective for the reduction of nighttime voiding frequency or nocturnal enuresis in nursing home residents (Ouslander et al, 2001).*

Geriatric

- Institute aggressive continence management programs for the cognitively intact, community-dwelling client in consultation with the client and family. *Uncontrolled incontinence can lead to institutionalization of an elderly person who prefers to remain in a home care setting (O'Donnell et al, 1992).*
- Monitor the elderly client in a long-term care facility, acute care facility, or home for dehydration. *Dehydration can exacerbate urine loss, produce acute confusion, and increase the risk of morbidity and morality, particularly in the frail elderly client (Colling, Owen & McCreedy, 1994).*

Home Care

- The interventions described previously may be adapted for home care use.
- Assess current strategies used to reduce urinary incontinence, including limitation of fluid intake, restriction of bladder irritants, prompted or scheduled toileting, and use of containment devices. *Many elderly clients and care providers use a variety of self-management techniques to control urinary incontinence, such as fluid limitation, avoidance of social contacts, and use of absorptive materials, that may or may not be effective for reducing urinary leakage or beneficial to general health (Johnson, 2000).*
- Encourage a mind-set and program of self-care management. **EBN:** *Addressing self-care activities through exercise, diet, fluid intake, and use of protective devices helps the client to exercise control over incontinence (Leenerts, Teel & Pendleton, 2002).*
- Implement a bladder-training program, including self-monitoring activities (e.g., reducing caffeine intake, adjusting amount and timing of fluid intake, decreasing long voiding intervals while awake, instituting dietary changes to promote bowel regularity); bladder training; and pelvic muscle exercise. **EBN:** *In women age 55 years or older with involuntary urine loss associated with stress, urge, or mixed incontinence, clients responded to the aforementioned interventions with a 61% decrease in the severity of urinary incontinence at 2 years after intervention. Self-monitoring and bladder training accounted for most of the improvement (Dougherty et al, 2002).*
- For a memory-impaired elderly client, implement an individualized scheduled toileting program (on a schedule developed in consultation with the caregiver, approximately every 2 hours, with toileting reminders provided and existing patterns incorporated, such toileting before or after meals). **EBN:** *Functional incontinence in memory-impaired elderly clients decrease significantly with the described intervention. The client must be able to cooperate (Jirovec & Templin, 2001).*
- Teach the family the general principles of bladder health, including avoidance of bladder irritants, adequate fluid intake, and a routine schedule of toileting. (Refer to the care plan for **Impaired Urinary elimination.**)
- Teach prompted voiding to the family and client for the client with mild to moderate dementia (refer to previous description) (Colling, 1996; McDowell et al, 1999).
- Inspect the perineal and perianal skin for evidence of incontinence-associated dermatitis, including inflammation, vesicles in skin exposed to urinary leakage, and especially skin folds or denudation of the skin, particularly when incontinence is managed by absorptive pads or containment briefs. *Urinary incontinence, particularly when combined with fecal incontinence or use of absorptive pads or adult containment briefs, increases the risk of incontinence-associated dermatitis (Gray et al, 2007).* **EBN:** *In the acute care setting, 20% of clients with urinary and/or fecal incontinence were found to have perineal or perigenital skin damage, and 18% were found to have evidence of secondary cutaneous candidiasis (Junkin & Selekof, 2007, in press).*
- Begin a preventive skin care regimen for all clients with urinary and/or fecal incontinence and treat clients with incontinence-associated dermatitis or related skin damage (Refer to the care plan for **Total Incontinence.**)
- Advise the client about the advantages of using disposable or reusable insert pads, pad-pant systems, or replacement briefs specifically designed for urinary incontinence (or double urinary and fecal incontinence) as indicated. **EBN:** *Many absorptive products used by community-dwelling elders are not designed to absorb urine, prevent odor, and protect the perineal skin (McClish et al,*

1999). Disposable or reusable absorptive devices specifically designed to contain urine or double inconti-
nence are more effective than household products, particularly in cases of moderate to severe incontinence
(Gallo & Staskin, 1997; Shirran & Brazelli, 2000).

- Assist the family with arranging care in a way that allows the client to participate in family or favorite activities without embarrassment. Elicit discussion of the client's concerns about the social or emotional burden of incontinence. **EBN and EB:** *Careful planning can allow the dignity and integrity of family patterns to be retained. Urinary incontinence has a demonstrated influence on subjective well-being and quality of life, with depression, loneliness, or sadness possible (Fultz & Herzog, 2001). Discussing emotional concerns helps the client to develop a sense of control over inconti-nence (Leenerts, Teel & Pendleton, 2002).*

- ▲ Refer to occupational therapy for help in obtaining assistive devices and adapting the home for optimal toilet accessibility.

- ▲ Consider the use of an indwelling catheter for continuous drainage in the client who is both homebound and bed bound and is receiving palliative or end-of-life care (requires a physician's order). *An indwelling catheter may increase client comfort, ease care provider burden, and prevent urinary incontinence in bed-bound clients receiving end-of-life (palliative) care (Gray & Campbell, 2001).*

- ▲ When an indwelling urinary catheter is in place, follow prescribed maintenance protocols for managing the catheter, drainage bag, perineal skin, and urethral meatus. Teach infection control measures adapted to the home care setting. *Proper care reduces the risk of catheter-associated urinary tract infection.* **EBN:** *Frequent catheter changes increases the risk of a symptomatic urinary tract infec-tion by approximately 12-fold compared with catheter changes every 4 weeks or less often (White & Ragland, 1995).*

- Assist the client in adapting to the catheter. Encourage discussion of the client's response to the catheter. **EBN:** *Clients living with a catheter are often keenly aware of its presence; adaptation is served by normalizing the experience. Instruction could include the fact that the client will be more aware of some sensations and sounds (e.g., urine sloshing in the bag, the weight of the bag, pressure or pain when urine flow has been altered). Rehearsing emptying of the bag when away from home will support resumption of activities. Discussion of the client's response will assist him or her in dealing with embarrassment or frustration (Wilde, 2002).*

Client/Family Teaching

- Work with the client, family, and their extended support systems to assist with needed changes in the environment and wardrobe, and other alterations required to maximize toileting access.
- Work with the client and family to establish a reasonable and manageable prompted voiding program using environmental and verbal cues to remind caregivers of voiding intervals, such as television programs, meals, and bedtime.
- Teach the family to use an alarm system for toileting or to carry out a check-and-change program and to maintain an accurate log of voiding and incontinence episodes.

evolve See the EVOLVE website for World Wide Web resources for client education.

REFERENCES

Chadwick V: Assessment of functional incontinence in disabled living centers, *Nurs Times* 101(2):65-67, 2005.

Colling J: Noninvasive strategies to manage urinary incontinence among care-dependent persons, *J Wound Ostomy Continence Nurs* 23:302, 1996.

Colling J, Ouslander J, Hadley BJ et al: The effects of patterned urge response toileting (PURT) on urinary incontinence among nursing home residents, *J Am Geriatr Soc* 40:135, 1992.

Colling J, Owen TR, McCreedy MR: Urine volumes and voiding pat-terns among incontinent nursing home residents, *Geriatr Nurs* 15:188, 1994.

Dougherty MC, Dwyer JW, Pendergast JF et al: A randomized trial of

behavioral management for continence with older rural women, *Res Nurs Health* 25:3, 2002.

Dubeau CE, Simon SE, Morris JN: The effect of urinary incontinence on quality of life in older nursing home residents, *J Am Geriatr Soc* 54(9):1325-1333, 2006.

Engberg S, Sereika SM, McDowell BJ et al: Effectiveness of prompted voiding in treating urinary incontinence in cognitively impaired homebound older adults, *J Wound Ostomy Continence Nurs* 29(5):252-265, 2002.

Eustice S, Roe B, Paterson J: Prompted voiding for the management of urinary incontinence in adults, *Cochrane Database Syst Rev* (2): CD002113, 2000.

Folstein MF, Folstein SE, McHugh PR: Mini-mental state: a practical method of grading the cognitive state of patients for the clinician, *J Psychiatr Res* 12(3):189, 1975.

Fultz NH, Herzog AR: Self-reported social and emotional impact of urinary incontinence, *J Am Geriatr Soc* 49:892, 2001.

Gallo M, Staskin DR: Patient satisfaction with a reusable undergarment for urinary incontinence, *J Wound Ostomy Continence Nurs* 24:226, 1997.

Gray M, Bliss DZ, Doughty DB et al: Incontinence-associated dermatitis: a consensus, *J Wound Ostomy Continence Nurs* 24(1): 45-56, 2007.

Gray M, Campbell F: Urinary tract disorders. In Ferrell B, Coyle N, editors: *Textbook of palliative nursing,* Oxford, England, 2001, Oxford University Press.

Hunskaar S et al: Epidemiology of urinary (UI) and fecal (FI) incontinence and pelvic organ prolapse (POP) 3rd International Consultation on Incontinence, ed 3, Plymouth, England, 2005, Health Publication, Plymbridge Distributors.

Jawad SH, Ward AB, Jones P: Study of the relationship between premorbid urinary incontinence and stroke functional outcome, *Clin Rehabil* 13(5):447, 1999.

Jenkins KR, Fultz NH: Functional impairment as a risk factor for urinary incontinence among older Americans, *Neurourol Urodyn* 24(1):51-55, 2005.

Jirovec MM, Templin T: Predicting success using individualized scheduled toileting for memory-impaired elders at home, *Res Nurs Health* 24:1, 2001.

Jirovec MM, Wells TJ: Urinary incontinence in nursing home residents with dementia: the mobility-cognition paradigm, *Appl Nurs Res* 3:112, 1990.

Johnson ST: From incontinence to confidence, *Am J Nurs* 100(2):69, 2000.

Junkin J, Selekof J: Prevalence of incontinence and associated skin injury in an acute care population, *J Wound Ostomy Continence Nurs* 34(3), 2007 (in press).

Leenerts MH, Teel CS, Pendleton MK: Building a model of self-care for health promotion in aging, *J Nurs Sch* 34:355, 2002.

Lekan-Rutledge D: Urinary incontinence strategies for frail elderly women, *Urol Nurs* 24(4):281-302, 2004.

Maloney C, Cafiero M: Implementing an incontinence program in long-term care settings: a multidisciplinary approach, *J Gerontol Nurs* 25:47, 1999.

McClish DK, Wyman JF, Sale PG et al: Use and costs of incontinence pads in female study volunteers, *J Wound Ostomy Continence Nurs* 26(4):207, 1999.

McDowell BJ, Engberg SJ, Rodriguez E et al: Characteristics of urinary incontinence in homebound older adults, *J Am Geriatr Soc* 44(8):963, 1996.

McDowell BJ, Engberg S, Sereika S et al: Effectiveness of behavioral therapy to treat incontinence in homebound older adults, *J Am Geriatr Soc* 47(3):309, 1999.

Neelan VJ et al: Use of the NEECHAM confusion scale to assess acute confusional states of hospitalized older patients. In Funk SG et al, editors: *Key aspects of elder care: managing falls, incontinence and cognitive impairment,* New York, 1992, Springer.

O'Donnell BF, Drachman DA, Barnes HJ et al: Incontinence and troublesome behaviors predict institutionalization in dementia, *J Geriatr Psychiatry Neurol* 5:45, 1992.

Ouslander JG, Greendale GA, Uman G et al: Effects of oral estrogen and progestin on the lower urinary tract among female nursing home residents, *J Am Geriatr Soc* 49(6):803-807, 2001.

Palmer MH, Baumgarten M, Langenberg P et al: Risk factors for hospital acquired incontinence in elderly female hip fracture patients, *J Gerontol A Biol Sci Med Sci* 57(10):M672, 2002.

Quinn P, Goka J, Richardson H: Assessment of an electronic daily diary in patients with overactive bladder, *BJU Int* 91(7):647-652, 2003.

Rabin JM: Clinical use of the FemAssist device in female urinary incontinence, *J Med Syst* 22:257, 1998.

Reilly N: Assessment and management of acute or transient urinary incontinence. In Doughty D, editor: *Urinary and fecal incontinence: nursing management,* ed 2, St Louis, 2002, Mosby.

Reuben DB: A randomized clinical trial of outpatient comprehensive geriatric assessment coupled with an intervention to increase adherence to recommendations, *J Am Geriatr Soc* 47(3):269, 1999.

Rosenberg LJ, Griffiths DJ, Resnick NM: Factors that distinguish continent from incontinent older adults with detrusor overactivity, *J Urol* 174(5):1868-1872, 2005.

Sampselle CM: Bladder matters. Teaching women to use a voiding diary: what 'mind over bladder' can accomplish, *Am Nurs* 103(11):62-64, 2003.

Shirran E, Brazelli M: Absorbent products for the containment of urinary and/or fecal incontinence, *Cochrane Database Syst Rev* (2): CD0011406, 2000.

Silverman M, McDowell BJ, Musa D et al: To treat or not to treat: issues in decisions not to treat older persons with cognitive impairment, depression, and incontinence, *J Am Geriatr Soc* 45(9):1094, 1997.

Thommessen B, Bautz-Holter E, Laake K: Predictors of outcome of rehabilitation of elderly stroke patients in a geriatric ward, *Clin Rehabil* 13(2):123, 1999.

Vickerman J: Thorough assessment of functional incontinence, *Nurs Times* 98(28):58, 2002.

Wells TJ: Managing incontinence through managing the environment, *Urol Nurs* 12:48, 1992.

White MC, Ragland KE: Urinary catheter related infections among home care patients, *J Wound Ostomy Continence Nurs* 22:286, 1995.

Wilde MH: Urine flowing: a phenomenological study of living with a urinary catheter, *Res Nurs Health* 25:14, 2002.

Overflow urinary Incontinence   *Mikel Gray, PhD, RN*

NANDA   Definition

Involuntary loss of urine associated with overdistention of the bladder

Defining Characteristics

Bladder distention; high post-void residual volume; nocturia; observed involuntary leakage of small volumes of urine; reports involuntary leakage of small volumes of urine

Related Factors (r/t)

Bladder outlet obstruction; detrusor external sphincter dyssynergia; detrusor hypocontractility; fecal impaction; severe pelvic prolapse; side effects of anticholinergic medications; side effects of calcium channel blockers; side effects of decongestant medications; urethral obstruction

NOC   Outcomes (Nursing Outcomes Classification)

Urinary Continence, Urinary Elimination

Example NOC Outcome with Indicators
Urinary Continence as evidenced by the following indicators: Absence of urinary leakage between catheterizations or containment of micturition by condom catheter and drainage bag/Absence of UTI (negative leukocytes and bacterial growth negative or <100,000 CFU/mL)/Underclothing dry during day/Underclothing or bedding dry during night (Rate the outcome and indicators of **Urinary Continence:** 1 = never demonstrated, 2 = rarely demonstrated, 3 = sometimes demonstrated, 4 = often demonstrated, 5 = consistently demonstrated [see Section I].)

CFU, Colony-forming units; *UTI,* urinary tract infection.

Client Outcomes

Client Will (Specify Time Frame):

- Demonstrate consistent ability to urinate when desire to void is perceived or via timed schedule; measured urinary residual volume is <200-250 mL or 25% of total bladder capacity (voided volume plus urinary residual volume)
- Experience correction or relief from voiding and postvoid lower urinary tract symptoms (LUTS)
- Experience correction or alleviation of storage LUTS
- Be free of upper urinary tract distress (renal function remains sufficient; febrile urinary infections are absent)

NIC   Interventions (Nursing Interventions Classification)

Suggested NIC Intervention

Pelvic Muscle Exercises, Urinary Incontinence Care

Example NIC Activities—Urinary Incontinence Care
Explain etiology of problem and rationale for actions; Modify clothing and environment to provide easy access to toilet

Nursing Interventions and *Rationales*

- Please refer to the care plan for **Urinary retention**

• = Independent;   ▲ = Collaborative;   EBN = Evidence-Based Nursing;   EB = Evidence-Based

I

Reflex urinary Incontinence   *Mikel Gray, PhD, RN*

NANDA   Definition

Involuntary loss of urine at somewhat predictable intervals when a specific bladder volume is reached (North American Nursing Diagnosis Association International [NANDA-I], 2007). Involuntary loss of urine caused by a defect in the spinal cord between the nerve roots at or below the first cervical segment and those above the second sacral segment. Urine elimination occurs at unpredictable intervals; micturition may be elicited by tactile stimuli, including stroking of inner thigh or perineum (Gray, 2003).

Defining Characteristics

Urinary incontinence caused by neurogenic detrusor overactivity; disruption of spinal pathways leads to absent or diminished awareness of the desire to void or the occurrence of an overactive detrusor contraction; incomplete bladder emptying caused by dyssynergia of striated sphincter mechanism, which produces functional outlet obstruction of bladder; reflex urinary incontinence may be associated with sweating and acute elevation in blood pressure and pulse rate in clients with spinal cord injury. Refer to the care plan for **Autonomic dysreflexia.**

Related Factors (r/t)

Paralyzing spinal disorder affecting spinal segments C1 to S2

NOC   Outcomes (Nursing Outcomes Classification)

Suggested NOC Outcomes

Urinary Continence, Urinary Elimination

Example NOC Outcome with Indicators
Urinary Continence as evidenced by the following indicators: Absence of urinary leakage between catheterizations or containment of micturition by condom catheter and drainage bag/Absence of urinary tract infection (absence of leukocytes and absence of bacterial growth or <100,000 colony-forming units per milliliter)/ Underclothing dry during day/Underclothing or bedding dry during night (Rate the outcome and indicators of **Urinary Continence:** 1 = never demonstrated, 2 = rarely demonstrated, 3 = sometimes demonstrated, 4 = often demonstrated, 5 = consistently demonstrated [see Section I].)

Client Outcomes

Client Will (Specify Time Frame):

- Follow prescribed schedule for bladder evacuation
- Demonstrate successful use of triggering techniques to stimulate voiding
- Have intact perineal skin
- Remain clear of symptomatic urinary tract infection
- Demonstrate how to apply containment device or insert indwelling catheter or be able to provide caregiver with instructions for performing these procedures
- Demonstrate awareness of risk of autonomic dysreflexia, its prevention, and management

NIC   Interventions (Nursing Interventions Classification)

Suggested NIC Interventions

Urinary Catheterization: Intermittent, Urinary Elimination Management, Urinary Incontinence Care

• = Independent;   ▲ = Collaborative;   EBN = Evidence-Based Nursing;   EB = Evidence-Based

Example NIC Activities—Urinary Elimination Management
Monitor urinary elimination including frequency, consistency, odor, volume, and color as appropriate; Teach patient signs and symptoms of urinary tract infection

Nursing Interventions and *Rationales*

- Assess the client's neurological status, including the type of neurological disorder, the functional level of neurological impairment, its completeness (effect on motor and sensory function), and the ability to perform bladder management tasks, including intermittent catheterization, application of a condom catheter, and so on. *Knowledge of single, well-circumscribed neurological lesion level strongly correlates with bladder function. This correlation is weaker in clients with multilevel cord trauma due to secondary bleeding or swelling (Weld, Graney & Dmochowski, 2000).*

- Knowledge of functional impairments related to a spinal cord injury, including upper extremity function, is essential because it determines the client's ability to manage the bladder by self-catheterization (Gray, 2006).

- Inspect the perineal and perigenital skin. *Urinary and fecal incontinence associated with neurogenic bladder and bowel dysfunction in the client with a paralyzing disorder increases the risk of incontinence-associated dermatitis and pressure ulceration, particularly when a urine containment device such as an adult containment brief or condom catheter is used (Gray et al, 2007; Junkin & Selekof, 2007, in press).*

- Complete a bladder log to determine the pattern of urine elimination, incontinence episodes, and current bladder management program. *The bladder log provides an objective record of urine elimination that confirms the accuracy of the historical report, and a baseline for assessment and evaluation of treatment efficacy (Gray, 2006).*

- ▲ Consult with the physician concerning current bladder function and the potential of the bladder to produce upper urinary tract distress (hydronephrosis, vesicoureteral reflux, febrile urinary tract infection, or compromised renal function). **EBN:** *Reflex incontinence is typically accompanied by detrusor striated sphincter dyssynergia, which increases the risk of upper urinary tract distress (Gray et al, 1991; Killorin et al, 1992; Weld et al, 2000).*

- ▲ Determine a bladder management program in consultation with the client, family, and rehabilitation team. **EBN:** *The bladder management program profoundly affects the client and significant others; it is determined by holistic assessment that addresses the potential of the bladder to create upper urinary tract distress, the potential for incontinence and related complications, client and family preference, and the perceived impact of the bladder management program on the client's lifestyle (Anson & Gray, 1993; Gray, Rayome & Anson 1995).*

- ▲ In consultation with the rehabilitation team, counsel the client and family concerning the merits and potential risks associated with each possible bladder management program, including spontaneous voiding, intermittent self-catheterization, reflex voiding with condom catheter containment, and indwelling catheterization. *All bladder management programs carry some risk of urinary incontinence or serious urinary system complications (Wyndaele, Madersbacher & Kovindha, 2001).* **EBN:** *Spontaneous voiding and intermittent catheterization carry greater risk of urine loss than condom catheter containment or indwelling catheter, but these latter strategies carry higher risk for serious urinary system complications when evaluated over a period of years. Long-term indwelling catheterization carries the greatest risk for serious urologic complications (Anson & Gray, 1993; Gray, Rayome & Anson, 1995; Saint et al, 2006).*

- Teach the client with reflex incontinence to consume an adequate amount of fluids on a daily basis (approximately 30 mL/kg of body weight). *Dehydration exacerbates urine loss and increases the risk of related complications, including constipation and urinary tract infection. Increasing fluid intake has also been associated with a diminished risk for bladder cancer, which is particularly important for the client managed by long-term indwelling catheterization (Gray & Krissovich, 2003).*

- Advise clients that while consumption of cranberry products or cranberry tablets is in no way harmful or contraindicated, it does not reduce the risk for urinary tract infection. **EB:** *Consumption of 400 mg of cranberry tablets by clients with neurogenic bladder dysfunction and spinal*

---

cord injury does not reduce the risk for urinary tract infection as has been demonstrated in community-dwelling women without neurogenic bladder dysfunction (Linsenmeyer, House & Millis, 2004).

▲ Teach the client with reflex urinary incontinence that is managed by spontaneous voiding to self-administer an alpha-adrenergic blocking medication as directed and to recognize and manage potential side effects. *Clients who spontaneously urinate may take an alpha-adrenergic blocking drug to reduce urethral resistance during voiding (Linsenmeyer, Horton & Benevento, 2002).*

▲ Begin intermittent catheterization using a modified clean or sterile technique based on facility policies. *Modified clean intermittent catheterization may be used in an inpatient setting with appropriate staff and client education.*

▲ Teach intermittent catheterization as the client approaches discharge as directed. Instruct the client and at least one family member, spouse, or partner in the performance of catheterization using clean technique. Teach the client with quadriplegia how to instruct others to perform this procedure. **EBN:** *Intermittent catheterization is a safe and effective bladder management strategy for persons with reflex urinary incontinence. Inclusion of a family member, spouse, or significant other is particularly helpful for the client with limited upper extremity dexterity and reflex urinary incontinence (Anson & Gray, 1993; Chai et al, 1995; Gray, Rayome & Anson, 1995; Shekelle et al, 1999). Intermittent catheterization among children with spinal cord injuries and reflex urinary incontinence is safe and effective (Generao et al, 2004).*

▲ Teach the client managed by intermittent catheterization to self-administer antispasmodic (parasympatholytic) medications as directed, and to recognize and manage potential side effects. *Antimuscarinic medications enhance catheterized volumes and reduce the frequency of incontinence episodes in persons with reflex incontinence owing to spinal cord injury or multiple sclerosis (Ethans et al, 2004).*

▲ Consult with the physician and occupational therapist concerning the use of a neuroprosthesis or other device designed to improve hand use for the quadriplegic client with partial hand function. *Use of a neuroprosthetic device designed to improve hand function increases clients' independence when performing multiple functions, including bladder management (Creasey et al, 2000).*

▲ For a male client with reflex incontinence who cannot manage the condition effectively with spontaneous voiding, does not choose to perform intermittent catheterization, or cannot perform catheterization, teach the client and his family to obtain, select, and apply a condom catheter with drainage bag. Assist them in choosing a product that adheres to the penile shaft without allowing seepage of urine onto surrounding skin or clothing, contains a material and adhesive that does not produce hypersensitivity reactions on the skin, and includes a leg bag that is easily concealed under the clothing and does not cause irritation to the skin of the thigh. *Multiple components of the condom catheter affect the product's ability to contain urinary leakage, protect underlying skin, and preserve the client's dignity (Joseph, 1999; Watson, 1989; Watson & Kuhn, 1990).*

• Teach the client who uses a condom catheter to remove the condom device, inspect the skin, cleanse the penis thoroughly, and reapply a new catheter every day. *The risk of urinary tract infection increases if a condom catheter is worn for longer than 24 hours (Hirsh, Fainstein & Musher, 1979).*

• Teach the client whose incontinence is managed by a condom catheter to routinely inspect the skin with each catheter change for evidence of lesions caused by pressure from the containment device or by exposure to urine. *Skin breakdown is a common complication associated with routine use of the condom catheter (Anson & Gray, 1993).*

• Teach the client managed by intermittent or indwelling catheter to recognize signs of significant urinary tract infection and to seek care promptly when these signs occur. The signs of significant infection are the following:
  ▪ Discomfort over the bladder or during urination
  ▪ Acute onset of urinary incontinence
  ▪ Fever
  ▪ Markedly increased spasticity of muscles below the level of the spinal lesion
  ▪ Malaise, lethargy
  ▪ Hematuria
  ▪ Autonomic dysreflexia (hyperreflexia)

▲ Recognize that intermittent catheterization is typically associated with asymptomatic bacteriuria, and the indwelling catheter is routinely associated with asymptomatic colonization. *Antibiotic treatment of asymptomatic bacteriuria has not proven helpful (Morton et al, 2002; Murphy & Lampert, 2003), but prompt management of significant infection is necessary to prevent urosepsis or related complications (Siroky, 2002).*

Geriatric

▲ If difficulties are encountered in client teaching, refer the elderly client to a nurse who specializes in care of the aging client with urinary incontinence.

Home Care

• The interventions described previously may be adapted for home care use.
• Teach the client what the complications of reflex incontinence are and when to report changes to a physician or primary nurse. *Early detection allows for rapid diagnosis and treatment before irreversible damage to the renal parenchyma occurs (Burns, Rivas & Ditunno, 2001).*
▲ If the client is taught intermittent self-catheterization, arrange for contingency care in the event that the client is unable to perform self-catheterization. *Although self-catheterization has proved to be an effective and safe bladder management strategy, acute illness or surgery may render the client unable to perform self-catheterization and temporarily reliant on others to carry out this critical task (Joseph, 1999).*
• Assess and instruct the client and family in care of the catheter and supplies in the home. *Proper care of supplies reduces the risk of infection (Joseph, 1999).*
• Encourage a mind-set and program of self-care management. **EBN:** *Addressing self-care activities through exercise, diet, fluid intake, and protective devices helps the client to exercise control over incontinence (Leenerts, Teel & Pendleton, 2002).*
• Assist the family with arranging care in a way that allows the client to participate in family or favorite activities without embarrassment. Elicit discussion of the client's concerns about the social or emotional burden of incontinence. **EBN and EB:** *Careful planning can help the client retain dignity and maintain the integrity of family patterns. Urinary incontinence has a demonstrated influence on subjective well-being and quality of life, with depression, loneliness, or sadness possible (Fultz & Herzog, 2001). Discussing emotional concerns helps the client to develop a sense of control over incontinence (Leenerts, Teel & Pendleton, 2002).*
▲ If medications are ordered, instruct the family or caregivers and the client in medication administration, use, and side effects. *Adherence to a medication regimen increases its chances of success and decreases the risk of losing the regimen as an option for care when other alternatives are unacceptable.*

Client/Family Teaching

• Teach the client with a spinal injury the signs of autonomic dysreflexia, its relationship to bladder fullness, and management of the condition. Refer to the care plan for **Autonomic Dysreflexia.**
• Teach the client and several significant others the techniques of intermittent catheterization, indwelling catheter care and removal, or condom catheter management as appropriate.
• Teach the client and family techniques to clean catheters used for intermittent catheterization, including washing with soap and water and allowing to air dry, and using microwave cleaning techniques.

 See the EVOLVE website for World Wide Web resources for client education.

REFERENCES

Anson C, Gray ML: Secondary complications after spinal cord injury, *Urol Nurs* 13:107, 1993.
Burns AS, Rivas DA, Ditunno JF: The management of neurogenic bladder and sexual dysfunction after spinal cord injury, *Spine* 26(Suppl 24):S129, 2001.

Chai T, Chung AK, Belville WD et al: Compliance and complications of clean intermittent catheterization in the spinal cord injured patient, *Paraplegia* 33:161, 1995.
Creasey GH, Kilgore KL, Brown-Triolo DL et al: Reduction of costs of disability using neuroprostheses, *Assist Technol* 12(1):67, 2000.

• = Independent;   ▲ = Collaborative;   EBN = Evidence-Based Nursing;   EB = Evidence-Based

Ethans KD, Nance PW, Bard RJ et al: Efficacy and safety of toltero-dine in people with neurogenic detrusor overactivity, *J Spinal Cord Med* 27(3):214-218, 2004.

Fultz NH, Herzog AR: Self-reported social and emotional impact of urinary incontinence, *J Am Geriatr Soc* 49:892, 2001.

Generao SE, Dall'era JP, Stone AR et al: Spinal cord injury in children: long-term urodynamic and urological outcomes, *J Urol* 172(3):1092-1094, 2004.

Gray M: Reflex urinary incontinence. In Doughty DB, editor: *Urinary and fecal incontinence: nursing management*, ed 3, St Louis, 2006, Mosby.

Gray M, Bliss DZ, Doughty DB et al: Incontinence-associated dermati-tis: a consensus, *J Wound Ostomy Continence Nurs* 24(1):45-56, 2007.

Gray M, Krissovich M: Does fluid intake influence the risk for urinary incontinence, urinary tract infection and bladder cancer? *J Wound Ostomy Continence Nurs* 30(3):126-131, 2003.

Gray M, Rayome RG, Anson C: Incontinence and clean intermittent catheterization following spinal cord injury, *Clin Nurs Res* 4:6, 1995.

Gray ML et al: Urethral pressure gradient in the prediction of upper urinary tract distress following spinal cord injury, *J Am Paraplegia Soc* 14:105, 1991.

Hirsh DD, Fainstein V, Musher DM: Do condom catheter collecting systems cause urinary tract infection? *JAMA* 242:340, 1979.

Joseph AC: The challenge of developing the nursing clinical practice guideline: neurogenic bladder management, *Urol Nurs* 19(3):195-196, 1999.

Junkin J, Selekof J: Prevalence of incontinence and associated skin in-jury in an acute care population, *J Wound Ostomy Continence Nurs* 24(3), 2007 (in press).

Killorin W, Gray M, Bennett JK et al: Evaluative urodynamics and bladder management in the prediction of upper urinary infection in male spinal cord injury, *Paraplegia* 30:437, 1992.

Leenerts MH, Teel CS, Pendleton MK: Building a model of self-care for health promotion in aging, *J Nurs Scholarsh* 34:355, 2002.

Linsenmeyer TA, Horton J, Benevento J: Impact of alpha$_1$-blockers in men with spinal cord injury and upper tract stasis, *J Spinal Cord Med* 25(2):124, 2002.

Linsenmeyer TA, House JG, Millis SR: The role of abnormal congeni-tally displaced ureteral orifices in causing reflux following spinal cord injury, *J Spinal Cord Med* 27(2):116-119, 2004.

Morton SC, Shekelle PG, Adams JL et al: Antimicrobial prophylaxis for urinary tract infection in persons with spinal cord dysfunction, *Arch Phys Med Rehabil* 83(1):129, 2002.

Murphy DP, Lampert V: Current implications of drug resistance in spinal cord injury, *Am J Phys Med Rehabil* 82(1):72, 2003.

Saint S, Kaufman SR, Rogers MA et al: Condom versus indwelling urinary catheters: a randomized trial, *J Am Geriatr Soc* 54(7):1055-1061, 2006.

Shekelle PG, Morton SC, Clark KA et al: Systematic review of risk factors for urinary tract infection in adults with spinal cord dys-function, *J Spinal Cord Med* 22(4):258, 1999.

Siroky MB: Pathogenesis of bacteriuria and infection in the spinal cord injured patient, *Am J Med* 113(suppl 1A):67S, 2002.

Watson R: A nursing trial of urinary sheath systems on male hospital-ized patients, *J Adv Nurs* 14:467, 1989.

Watson R, Kuhn M: The influence of component parts on the perfor-mance of urinary sheath systems, *J Adv Nurs* 15:417, 1990.

Weld KJ, Graney MJ, Dmochowski RR: Clinical significance of detru-sor sphincter dyssynergia in patients with post traumatic spinal cord injury, *Urology* 56:565, 2000.

Weld KJ, Wall BM, Mangold TA et al: Influences on renal function in chronic spinal cord injured patients, *J Urol* 164(5):1490, 2000.

Wyndaele JJ, Madersbacher H, Kovindha A: Conservative treatment of the neuropathic bladder in spinal cord injured patients, *Spinal Cord* 39(6):294, 2001.

Stress urinary Incontinence   *Mikel Gray, PhD, RN*

NANDA   Definition

State in which the individual experiences urine loss of less than 50 mL accompanied by increased intraabdominal pressure

NOTE: The value of less than 50 mL for the volume of urine loss may be exceeded by women and men with severe stress incontinence caused by incompetence of the urethral sphincter mechanism. This is sometimes classified as *total incontinence*. In this book, however, *total incontinence* will be used to refer exclusively to incontinence due to extra-urethral causes, and all forms of stress inconti-nence are reviewed under this diagnosis, regardless of severity.

Defining Characteristics

Observed urine loss with physical exertion (sign of stress incontinence); reported loss of urine asso-ciated with physical exertion or activity (symptom of stress incontinence); urine loss associated with increased abdominal pressure (urodynamic stress urinary incontinence) (Abrams et al, 2002)

Related Factors (r/t)

Urethral hypermobility/pelvic organ prolapse (genetic factors/familial predisposition, multiple vaginal deliveries, delivery of infant large for gestational age, forceps-assisted or breech delivery, obesity, changes in estrogen levels at climacteric, extensive abdominopelvic, or pelvic surgery); ure-thral sphincter mechanism incompetence (multiple urethral suspensions in women, radical prosta-tectomy in men, uncommon complication of transurethral prostatectomy or cryosurgery of prostate, spinal lesion affecting sacral segments 2 to 4 or cauda equina, pelvic fracture)

NOC   Outcomes (Nursing Outcomes Classification)

Suggested NOC Outcomes

Urinary Continence, Urinary Elimination

Example NOC Outcome with Indicators
Urinary Continence as evidenced by the following indicators: Experiences no urine loss with physical activity or exertion, coughing, sneezing, or other maneuvers that precipitously raise abdominal pressure/Voids in appropriate receptacle/Able to move to toilet after strong desire to urinate is perceived/Underclothing remains dry during day/Underclothing or bedding remains dry during night (Rate the outcome and indicators of **Urinary Continence:** 1 = never demonstrated, 2 = rarely demonstrated, 3 = sometimes demonstrated, 4 = often demonstrated, 5 = consistently demonstrated [see Section I].)

Client Outcomes

Client Will (Specify Time Frame):

- Report fewer stress incontinence episodes and/or a decrease in the severity of urine loss
- Experience reduction in grams of urine loss measured objectively by a pad test
- Experience reduction in frequency of urinary incontinence episodes as recorded on voiding diary (bladder log)
- Identify containment devices that assist in management of stress incontinence

NIC   Interventions (Nursing Interventions Classification)

Suggested NIC Intervention

Pelvic Muscle Exercises, Urinary Incontinence Care

Example NIC Activities—Urinary Incontinence Care
Explain etiology of problem and rationale for actions; Modify clothing and environment to provide easy access to toilet

Nursing Interventions and *Rationales*

- Take a focused history addressing duration of urinary leakage and related lower urinary tract symptoms, including daytime voiding frequency, urgency, frequency of nocturia, frequency of urinary leakage, and factors provoking urine loss, focusing on the differential diagnosis of stress, urge or mixed stress and urge urinary symptoms. Consider using a symptom questionnaire that elicits relevant lower urinary tract symptoms and provides differentiation between stress and urge incontinence symptoms. *Some interventions used to treat stress and urge urinary incontinence are the same (such as pelvic floor muscle training), but some differ (such as pharmacotherapy). Over 23 validated symptom questionnaires have been developed for the evaluation of urinary and fecal incontinence (Avery et al, 2007).* **EBN:** *Several questionnaires have been developed that are specifically designed to enable the clinician to differentiate between stress and urge incontinence based on symptom report (Brown et al, 2006; Diokno et al, 1986).*
- ▲ Perform a focused physical assessment, including inspection of the perineal skin, vaginal examination to determine hypoestrogenic changes in the mucosa, pelvic examination to determine the presence of vaginal wall prolapse and uterine prolapse, and to reproduce the sign of stress urinary incontinence. **EBN:** *There is limited evidence supporting the diagnostic value of the physical examination in the diagnosis of urinary incontinence and differential diagnosis of stress versus urge incontinence in elderly women (van Gerwen & Lagro-Janssen, 2006).*
- Inspect the perineal and perianal skin for evidence of incontinence-associated dermatitis, including inflammation, vesicles in skin exposed to urinary leakage, and especially skin folds or denudation of the skin, particularly when incontinence is managed by absorptive pads or containment briefs. *Urinary incontinence, particularly when combined with fecal incontinence or use of absorptive*

• = Independent;   ▲ = Collaborative;   EBN = Evidence-Based Nursing;   EB = Evidence-Based

pads or adult containment briefs, increases the risk of incontinence-associated dermatitis (Gray et al, 2007). **EBN:** *20% of 608 clients with urinary and/or fecal incontinence in the acute care setting were found to have perineal or perigenital skin damage; 18% were found to have evidence of secondary cutaneous candidiasis (Junkin & Selekof, 2007, in press).*

- Attempt to reproduce the sign of stress urinary incontinence by asking the client to perform Valsalva maneuver or to cough while observing the urethral meatus for urine loss. **EBN:** *Urine loss, the sign of stress urinary incontinence, can be reproduced by asking the client to perform provocative maneuvers (cough or perform Valsalva maneuver) during physical examination. Mild to moderate stress urinary incontinence can be reproduced by asking the client to perform these maneuvers while standing and holding a paper towel in front of the urethral meatus (Miller et al, 1998). Urine loss volumes of less than 1 mL can be detected using this technique (Neumann et al, 2004). Among clients with moderately severe to severe cases associated with urethral sphincter mechanism incompetence, the sign of stress urinary incontinence can be elicited even when the client is lying in a supine position and has as little as 10 mL of urine in the bladder vesicle. Nevertheless, it is strongly recommended that the client be tested in both supine and upright positions and with a moderately filled bladder (Walter, Thornton & Steele, 2004).*

- ▲ Perform a focused pelvic examination, including visual inspection of the vaginal mucosa, observation of urethral hypermobility and related pelvic floor descent (prolapse), and digital assessment of pelvic floor muscle strength. **EBN:** *Digital assessment of pelvic muscle strength is completed by asking the female client to contract the pelvic floor muscles after placing one to two gloved fingers in the vaginal vault (Brink et al, 1989, 1992). Pelvic floor muscle strength can be similarly evaluated in men during the digital rectal examination. There is mixed evidence concerning the relationship of a digital assessment of pelvic floor muscle strength with dynamic manometric measurements, but it remains a well-accepted technique for determining the overall strength of the pelvic floor muscles and the client's ability to identify, contract, and relax this muscle group (Isherwood & Rane, 2000; Morin et al, 2004).*

- Determine the client's current use of containment devices; evaluate the devices for their ability to adequately contain urine loss, protect clothing, and control odor. Assist the client in identifying containment devices specifically designed to contain urinary leakage. **EBN:** *Clients, particularly women, tend to select feminine hygiene pads for urine containment. These devices, designed to contain menstrual flow, are not well-suited to address urine loss (McClish et al, 1999).*

- Teach the client to complete a voiding diary (bladder log) by recording voiding frequency, the frequency of urinary incontinent episodes, and their association with urgency (a sudden and strong desire to urinate that is difficult to defer) over a 3- to 7-day period. An electronic voiding diary may be kept whenever feasible. In addition to these parameters, the client may be asked to record voided volume and fluid intake. *The voiding diary provides a more objective record of lower urinary tract function than the oral history, and it often provides a modest therapeutic effect by alerting the client to factors that promote urinary incontinence episodes (Sampselle, 2003). An electronic voiding diary provides an efficient and possibly more accurate method for documenting these parameters (Quinn, Goka & Richardson, 2003).*

- ▲ With the client and in close consultation with the physician, review treatment options, including behavioral management; drug therapy; use of a pessary, vaginal device, or urethral insert; and surgery. Outline their potential benefits, efficacy, and side effects. *Multiple treatments have been used to manage stress incontinence; behavioral management options should be offered initially (Doughty & Burns, 2006).*

- ▲ Assess the client's pelvic muscle strength immediately prior to initiating a pelvic floor muscle rehabilitation using pressure manometry, a digital evaluation technique, or urine stop test. **EBN:** *A baseline of pelvic muscle strength is needed for initial assessment and for evaluation of treatment efficacy. Digital vaginal examination, a urine stream interruption test, or measurement of pelvic floor muscle contraction strength by a fluid-filled balloon are valid and reliable techniques for assessing pelvic floor muscle strength and contractile function (Brink et al, 1992; Sampselle & DeLancey, 1992).*

- ▲ Begin a pelvic floor muscle rehabilitation program. *Pelvic floor muscle rehabilitation is effective in the treatment of stress and mixed urinary incontinence (Bo, Talseth & Holme, 1999; Hay-Smith et al, 2006).*

- Teach the client undergoing pelvic muscle rehabilitation to identify, contract, and relax the pelvic floor muscles without contracting distant muscle groups (e.g., abdominal muscles) using tactile, audible, or visual biofeedback techniques. *Pelvic muscle rehabilitation is enhanced by the use of biofeedback (Berghmans et al, 1996; Bump et al, 1991).*

- Incorporate principles of exercise physiology into a pelvic muscle rehabilitation program using the following strategies:
  - Begin a graded exercise program, usually starting with 5 to 10 repetitions and advancing gradually to no more than 35 to 50 repetitions every day or every other day based on baseline and ongoing evaluation of maximal strength and endurance.
  - Continue exercise sessions over a period of 3 to 6 months.
  - Integrate muscle training into activities of daily living.
  - Assess progress every 2 weeks during the first month and every 4 to 6 weeks thereafter.

  EBN: *Pelvic muscle rehabilitation alleviates or cures stress incontinence using a combination of techniques, including biofeedback and strength training. Application of principles of physiotherapy maximizes the value of pelvic muscle rehabilitation (Brink et al, 1992; Dougherty et al, 1991, 1992; Johnson, 2001; Nygaard et al, 1996).*

- Alternatively, female clients may be taught pelvic muscle rehabilitation using weighted vaginal cones. **EBN:** *Weighted vaginal cones help women increase pelvic floor muscle tone and function and alleviate stress urinary incontinence (Laycock et al, 2001). The efficacy of weighted cones may be comparable to that achieved by pelvic muscle rehabilitation, but more comparative studies are needed before a definitive conclusion can be reached (Herbison, Plevnik & Mantle, 2002).*

▲ Begin transvaginal or transrectal electrical stimulation therapy in selected persons with stress incontinence in consultation with the client and physician. *Electrical stimulation alleviates stress incontinence in selected clients, probably by strengthening the pelvic muscles and possibly through a biofeedback effect (Sand et al, 1995).*

- Teach the principles of bladder training to women with stress urinary incontinence:
  - Assist the client in completing a voiding diary over a period of a minimum of 3 days or up to 7 days.
  - Review the results with the client, determining typical voiding frequency and establishing goals for voiding frequency.
  - Using baseline voiding frequency, as determined by the diary, teach the client to urinate by the clock when awake, typically every 30 to 120 minutes.
  - Encourage adherence to the program with timing devices, as well as verbal encouragement and support, and address individual reasons for schedule interruption.
  - Gradually increase the time between urinations to the negotiated goal. Time intervals between voiding are typically increased in increments of 15 to 30 minutes for clients with a baseline frequency of less than every 60 minutes and increments of 25 to 30 minutes for clients with a baseline frequency of more than every 60 minutes.

  EBN: *Bladder training reduces the frequency and severity of urinary leakage in women with stress incontinence, urge incontinence, and mixed incontinence. The results of bladder training in ambulatory, community-dwelling women is comparable to that achieved through pelvic floor muscle rehabilitation (Elser et al, 1999; Theofrastous et al, 2002; Wyman et al, 1998).*

▲ Teach the client to self-administer alpha-adrenergic agonist medications as ordered, imipramine, and topical estrogens as directed. *Pharmacotherapeutic agents alleviate stress incontinence symptoms in selected women (Andersson, 2000).*

▲ Refer the female client with stress urinary incontinence and pelvic organ prolapse who wishes to employ a pessary, vaginal device, or urethral insert to manage stress incontinence to a nurse specialist or gynecologist with expertise in the placement and maintenance of these devices. *Pessaries, vaginal devices, and urethral inserts alleviate or correct stress incontinence; however, they may cause serious complications unless inserted correctly and monitored closely (Shaikh et al, 2000). When fitted by an individual with adequate expertise, approximately 90% of bothersome symptoms associated with pelvic organ prolapse and 50% of lower urinary tract symptoms resolved, although occult stress urinary incontinence is uncovered in approximately 21% (Clemons et al, 2004).*

- Discuss potentially reversible or controllable risk factors with the client with stress incontinence and assist the client to formulate a strategy to alleviate or eliminate these conditions. *Although research supports a strong familial predisposition to stress incontinence among women, other risk factors associated with the condition, including obesity and chronic coughing from smoking, are reversible (Mushkat, Bukovsky & Langer, 1996; Skoner, Thompson & Caron, 1994).*

▲ Provide information about support resources such as the Simon Foundation for Continence or the National Foundation for Continence.

▲ Refer the client with persistent stress incontinence to a continence service, physician, or nurse who specializes in the management of this condition. **EBN:** *Complex stress incontinence can be successfully managed by a multidisciplinary approach (McDowell et al, 1996).*

Geriatric

• Evaluate the elderly client's functional and cognitive status to determine the effect of functional limitations on the frequency and severity of urine loss and on plans for management.

Home Care

• The interventions described previously may be adapted for home care use.

• Elicit discussion of the client's concerns about the social or emotional burden of stress incontinence. **EBN and EB:** *Urinary incontinence has a demonstrated influence on subjective well-being and quality of life, with depression, loneliness, or sadness possible (Fultz & Herzog, 2001). Discussing emotional concerns helps the client to develop a sense of control over incontinence (Leenerts, Teel & Pendleton, 2002).*

• Encourage a mind-set and program of self-care management. **EBN:** *Addressing self-care activities through exercise, diet, fluid intake, and protective devices helps the client to exercise control over incontinence (Leenerts, Teel & Pendleton, 2002).*

• Implement a bladder-training program, including self-monitoring activities (reducing caffeine intake, adjusting amount and timing of fluid intake, decreasing long voiding intervals while awake, making dietary changes to promote bowel regularity), bladder training, and pelvic muscle exercise. **EBN:** *Women age 55 years or older with involuntary urine loss associated with stress, urge, or mixed incontinence, responded to the aforementioned interventions with a 61% decrease in the severity of urinary incontinence at 2 years after intervention. Self-monitoring and bladder training accounted for most of the improvement (Dougherty et al, 2002).*

▲ Consider the use of an indwelling catheter for continuous drainage in the client with severe stress urinary incontinence who is homebound, bed bound, and receiving palliative or end-of-life care (requires a physician's order). *An indwelling catheter may increase client comfort, ease caregiver burden, and prevent urinary incontinence in bed-bound clients receiving end-of-life care.*

▲ When an indwelling catheter is in place, follow the prescribed maintenance protocols for managing the catheter, drainage bag, and perineal skin and urethral meatus. Teach infection control measures adapted to the home care setting. *Proper care reduces the risk of catheter-associated urinary tract infection.*

• Assist the client in adapting to the catheter. Encourage discussion of the client's response to the catheter. **EBN:** *Clients living with a catheter are keenly aware of its presence; adaptation is served by normalizing the experience. Rehearsing emptying of the bag when away from home will support resumption of activities. Discussion of the client's response will help him or her to deal with embarrassment or frustration (Wilde, 2002).*

• Begin a program of pelvic muscle rehabilitation in the homebound elderly client who is motivated to adhere to the program and has adequate cognitive function to understand and follow instructions. **EBN:** *Homebound elders are capable of completing a program of pelvic muscle rehabilitation and achieving clinically relevant relief from stress and urge urinary incontinence.*

Client/Family Teaching

• Teach the client to perform pelvic muscle exercise using an audiotape or videotape if indicated.

• Teach the client the importance of avoiding dehydration and instruct the client to consume fluid at the rate of 30 mL/kg of body weight daily (0.5 ounce/pound/day).

• Teach the client the importance of avoiding constipation by a combination of adequate fluid intake, adequate intake of dietary fiber, and exercise.

• = Independent; ▲ = Collaborative; EBN = Evidence-Based Nursing; EB = Evidence-Based

- Teach the client to apply and remove support devices such as a urethral insert.
- Teach the client to select and apply urine containment devices.

evolve See the EVOLVE website for World Wide Web resources for client education.

REFERENCES

Abrams P, Cardozo L, Fall M et al: The standardization of terminology of lower urinary tract function: report from the Standardisation Sub-committee of the International Continence Society, *Am J Obstet Gynecol* 187(1):116, 2002.

Andersson KE: Drug therapy for urinary incontinence, *Best Pract Res Clin Obstet Gynecol* 14(2):291, 2000.

Avery KN, Bosch JL, Gotoh M et al: Questionnaires to assess urinary and anal incontinence: review and recommendations, *J Urol* 177(1):39-49, 2007.

Berghmans LC, Frederiks CM, de Bie RA et al: Efficacy of biofeedback when included with pelvic muscle exercise treatment for stress incontinence, *Neurourol Urodyn* 15:37, 1996.

Bo K, Talseth T, Holme I: Single blind, randomized controlled trial of pelvic floor exercises, electrical stimulation, vaginal cones, and no treatment of genuine stress incontinence in women, *BMJ* 318:487, 1999.

Brink CA et al: Pelvic muscle exercise for elderly incontinence women. In Funk SG et al, editors: *Key aspects of elder care: managing falls, incontinence and cognitive impairment*, New York, 1992, Springer.

Brink CA, Sampselle CM, Wells TJ et al: A digital test for pelvic muscle strength in older women with urinary incontinence, *Nurs Res* 38(4):196-199, 1989.

Brown JS, Bradley CS, Subak LL et al: Diagnostic Aspects of Incontinence Study (DAISy) Research Group. The sensitivity and specificity of a simple test to distinguish between urge and stress urinary incontinence, *Ann Intern Med* 144(10):715-723, 2006.

Bump RC, Hurt WG, Fantl JA et al: Assessment of Kegel pelvic muscle exercise performance after brief verbal instruction, *Am J Obstet Gynecol* 165(2):322, 1991.

Clemons JL, Aguilar VC, Tillinghast TA et al: Patient satisfaction and changes in prolapse and urinary symptoms in women who were fitted successfully with a pessary for pelvic organ prolapse, *Am Obstet Gynecol* 190(4):1025-1029, 2004.

Diokno AC, Brock BM, Brown MB et al: Prevalence of urinary incontinence and other urological symptoms in the noninstitutionalized elderly, *J Urol* 136(5):1022-1025, 1986.

Doughty DB, Burns PA: Pathology and management of stress incontinence. In Doughty DB, editor: *Urinary and fecal incontinence: nursing management*, ed 3, St Louis, 2006, Elsevier/Mosby.

Dougherty MC et al: Graded exercise: effect of pressures developed by the pelvic muscles. In Funk SG et al, editors: *Key aspects of elder care: managing falls, incontinence and cognitive impairment*, New York, 1992, Springer.

Dougherty MC, Bishop KR, Mooney RA et al: Variation in intravaginal pressure measurements, *Nurs Res* 40:282, 1991.

Dougherty MC, Dwyer JW, Pendergast JF et al: A randomized trial of behavioral management for continence with older rural women, *Res Nurs Health* 25:3, 2002.

Elser DM, Wyman JF, McClish DK et al: The effect of bladder training, pelvic floor muscle training, or combination training on urodynamic parameters in women with urinary incontinence. Continence Program for Women Research Group, *Neurourol Urodyn* 18(5):427, 1999.

Fultz NH, Herzog AR: Self-reported social and emotional impact of urinary incontinence, *J Am Geriatr Soc* 49:892, 2001.

Gray M, Bliss DZ, Doughty DB et al: Incontinence-associated dermatitis: a consensus, *J Wound Ostomy Continence Nurs* 24(1):45-56, 2007.

Hay-Smith EJC, Dumoulin C: Pelvic floor muscle training versus no treatment, or inactive control treatments, for urinary incontinence in women, *Cochrane Database Syst Rev* (1):CD005654, 2006.

Herbison P, Plevnik S, Mantle J: Weighted vaginal cones for urinary incontinence, *Cochrane Database Syst Rev* (2):CD002114, 2002.

Isherwood PJ, Rane A: Comparative assessment of pelvic floor strength using a perineometer and digital examination, *BJOG* 107(8):1007-1011, 2000.

Johnson VY: How the principles of exercise physiology influence pelvic floor muscle training, *J Wound Ostomy Continence Nurs* 28(3):150, 2001.

Junkin J, Selekof J: Prevalence of incontinence and associated skin injury in an acute care population, *J Wound Ostomy Continence Nurs* 24(3), 2007 (in press).

Laycock J, Brown J, Cusack C et al: Pelvic floor reeducation for stress incontinence: comparing three methods, *Br J Community Nurs* 6(5):230, 2001.

Leenerts MH, Teel CS, Pendleton MK: Building a model of self-care for health promotion in aging, *J Nurs Scholarsh* 34:355, 2002.

McClish DK, Wyman JF, Sale PG et al: Use and costs of incontinence pads in female study volunteers, *J Wound Ostomy Continence Nurs* 26(4):207, 1999.

McDowell BJ, Burgio KL, Dombrowski M et al: An interdisciplinary approach to the assessment and behavioral treatment of urinary incontinence in geriatric outpatients, *Kango Kenkyu* 29(5):425, 1996.

Miller JM, Ashton-Miller JA, Delancey JO: Quantification of cough-related urine loss using the paper towel test, *Obstet Gynecol* 91 (5 pt 1):705, 1998.

Morin M, Dumoulin C, Bourbonnais D et al: Pelvic floor maximal strength using vaginal digital assessment compared to dynamometric measurements, *Neurourol Urodyn* 23(4):336-341, 2004.

Mushkat Y, Bukovsky I, Langer R: Female urinary stress incontinence—does it have familial prevalence? *Am J Obstet Gynecol* 174:617, 1996.

Neumann P, Blizzard L, Grimmer K et al: Expanded paper towel test: an objective test of urine loss for stress incontinence, *Neurourol Urodyn* 23(7):649-655, 2004.

Nygaard IE, Kreder KJ, Lepic MM et al: Efficacy of pelvic floor muscle exercise in women with stress, urge and mixed urinary incontinence, *Am J Obstet Gynecol* 174:120, 1996.

Quinn P, Goka J, Richardson H: Assessment of an electronic daily diary in patients with overactive bladder, *BJU Int* 91(7):647-652, 2003.

Sampselle CM: Bladder matters. Teaching women to use a voiding diary, *Am J Nurs* 103(11): 62-64, 2003.

Sampselle CM, DeLancey JOL: The urine stream interruption test and pelvic muscle function, *Nurs Res* 41:73, 1992.

Sand PK, Richardson DA, Staskin DR et al: Pelvic floor electrical stimulation in the treatment of genuine stress incontinence: a multicenter placebo controlled trial, *Am J Obstet Gynecol* 173:72, 1995.

Shaikh S, Ong EK, Glavind K et al: Mechanical devices for urinary incontinence in women, *Cochrane Database Syst Rev* (3):CD001756, 2006.

Skoner MM, Thompson WD, Caron VA: Factors associated with risk of stress urinary incontinence in women, *Nurs Res* 43:301, 1994.

Theofrastous JP, Wyman JF, Bump RC et al: Effects of pelvic floor muscle training on strength and predictors of response in the treatment of urinary incontinence, *Neurourol Urodyn* 21(5):486-490, 2002.

van Gerwen M, Lagro-Janssen AL: [Diagnostic value of patient history and physical examination in elderly patients with urinary in-

continence; a literature review], *Ned Tijdschr Geneesk* 150(32):1771-1775, 2006 [article in Dutch].

Walter AJ, Thornton JA, Steele AC: Further characterization of the supine empty stress test for predicting low Valsalva leak point pressures, *Int Urogynecol J* 15(5):298-301, 2004.

Wilde MH: Urine flowing: a phenomenological study of living with a urinary catheter, *Res Nurs Health* 25:14, 2002.

Wyman JF, Fantl JA, McClish DK et al: Comparative efficacy of behavioral interventions in the management of female urinary incontinence. Continence Program for Women Research Group, *Am J Obstet Gynecol* 179(4):999, 1998.

Total urinary Incontinence   *Mikel Gray, PhD, RN*

NANDA   Definition

State in which the individual experiences continuous and unpredictable loss of urine

NOTE: In this book, the diagnosis **Total urinary Incontinence** will be used to refer to continuous urine loss due to an extraurethral cause, and the diagnosis **Stress urinary Incontinence** will be used to refer to leakage caused by urethral sphincter incompetence, regardless of severity (Gray, 2007).

Defining Characteristics

Continuous urine flow varying from dribbling incontinence superimposed on an otherwise identifiable pattern of voiding to severe urine loss without identifiable micturition episodes

Related Factors (r/t)

Ectopia (ectopic ureter opens into vaginal vault or cutaneously; bladder ectopia with exstrophy/epispadias complex); fistula (opening from bladder or urethra to vagina or skin that bypasses urethral sphincter mechanism, allowing continuous urine loss)

NOC   Outcomes (Nursing Outcomes Classification)

Suggested NOC Outcomes

Tissue Integrity: Skin and Mucous Membranes, Urinary Continence, Urinary Elimination

Example NOC Outcome with Indicators
Tissue Integrity: Skin and Mucous Membranes as evidenced by the following indicators: Skin is lesion free/Skin intactness (Rate the outcome and indicators of **Tissue Integrity: Skin and Mucous Membranes:** 1 = severely compromised, 2 = substantially compromised, 3 = moderately compromised, 4 = mildly compromised, 5 = not compromised [see Section I].)

Client Outcomes

Client Will (Specify Time Frame):

* Experience urine loss that is adequately contained, with clothing remaining unsoiled and odor controlled
* Maintain intact perineal skin
* Maintain dignity, hide urine containment device in clothing, and minimize bulk and noise related to device

NIC   Interventions (Nursing Interventions Classification)

Suggested NIC Intervention

Urinary Incontinence Care

• = Independent;   ▲ = Collaborative;   EBN = Evidence-Based Nursing;   EB = Evidence-Based

Example NIC Activities—Urinary Incontinence Care
Provide protective garments, as needed; Cleanse genital skin area at regular intervals

Nursing Interventions and *Rationales*

- Obtain a history of the duration and severity of urine loss, prior management, and aggravating or alleviating features. *Urinary incontinence from an extraurethral source (fistula or ectopia) is often confused with other forms of incontinence. Total incontinence should be suspected whenever the client reports continuous urine loss irrespective of physical exertion or associated urgency (Flores-Carreras et al, 2001).*

- Query the client about risk factors for a fistula. *Women living in industrialized countries should be queried about recent pelvic surgery such as hysterectomy, radical hysterectomy, or pelvic exenteration, radiation therapy of the pelvis, or pelvic trauma (especially penetrating trauma). Women in third world countries, particularly those with limited access to advanced healthcare services, should be queried about traumatic labor and delivery. Fistulae are rare in developed countries and are usually associated with surgical misadventure, most commonly hysterectomy for benign indications (Kriplani et al, 2005). Fistulae among women in third world countries who lack rapid access to advanced health care are usually associated with obstructed or traumatic labor and delivery, complicated by the inability to rapidly gain access to surgical support before significant ischemia and tissue damage occurs (Ng'ang'a, 2006; Wall 2006).*

- ▲ Perform a focused physical assessment, including inspection of the perineal skin, examination of the vaginal vault, reproduction of the sign of stress incontinence (refer to the care plan for **Stress urinary Incontinence**), and testing of bulbocavernosus reflex and perineal sensations. *The physical examination will provide evidence supporting the diagnosis of extraurethral or another type of incontinence (stress, urge, or reflex) and provide the basis for further evaluation and/or treatment (Gray & Moore, 2006).*

- ▲ Consult a physician concerning the results of colposcopy, cystourethroscopy, intravenous urogram, cystogram, Pyridium pad test, methylene blue pad test, or pelvic examination. *Evaluation of the location and characteristics of a urinary fistula or ectopic ureter requires direct visualization or identification based on an imaging study of the urinary system (Flores-Carreras et al, 2001).*

- Assist the client in selecting and applying a urine containment device. Review types of containment products with the client, including advantages and potential complications associated with each type of product. *Urine containment products include a variety of absorptive pads, incontinence briefs, underpads for bedding, absorptive inserts that fit into specially designed undergarments, and condom catheters. Careful selection of an absorptive product and education concerning its use maximize its effectiveness in controlling urine loss in a particular individual (Dunn et al, 2002; Shirran & Brazelli, 2000).*

- Evaluate disposable versus reusable products for urine containment, considering the setting (home care versus acute care versus long-term care), preferences of the client and caregivers, and immediate versus long-term costs. *Economic factors as well as client and caregiver preferences affect the success and ultimate cost of a reusable versus disposable urine containment device (Dunn et al, 2002; Shirran & Brazelli, 2000).* **EBN:** *A study comparing a single reusable device with the "usual" containment device of a group of 175 community-dwelling subjects, which was most often a disposable pad, revealed that reusable garments provide comfort and perceived protection from visible urine loss equivalent to disposable pads (Gallo & Staskin, 1997).*

- Begin a structured skin care regimen that incorporates three essential steps: cleanse, moisturize, and protect. Select a cleanser with a pH range comparable to that of normal skin (usually labeled "pH balanced"), moisturize with an emollient to replace lipids removed with cleansing, and protect with a skin protectant containing a petrolatum, dimethicone, or zinc oxide base, or a no sting skin barrier. Skin that is exposed to urine and/or stool should be cleansed daily and following major incontinence episodes. Cleanse the skin gently with a soft cloth (either disposable or reusable). When feasible, select a product that combines two or all three of these processes into a single step. Ensure that products are available at the bedside when caring for a client with total incontinence in an inpatient facility. *Urinary incontinence, particularly when combined with fecal incontinence or use of absorptive pads or adult containment briefs, increases the risk of incontinence-associated dermatitis.* **EBN:** *Existing evidence demonstrates that a structured skin care regimen based on a three-step process (cleanse, moisturize, and protect) is effective for the prevention of incontinence-associated dermatitis (Gray et al, 2007).*

- Apply a thin layer of ointment as a skin protectant when using absorbent incontinence products such as adult containment briefs. **EBN:** *A randomized trial of petrolatum-based ointment skin protectant found transfer of the ointment from the skin to the absorbent product with resulting 54% to 90% loss of fluid uptake (Zehrer et al, 2005).*
- When cleansing a client with a moisture barrier containing zinc oxide, avoid vigorous scrubbing or use of a traditional washcloth to remove the paste. Instead, cleanse fecal materials away from the skin, leaving a clean layer of zinc oxide paste when cleansing after a single episode or gently removing the paste with mineral oil. *Pastes containing zinc oxide are difficult to remove, and it is not necessary to completely remove the product every time the perineal skin is cleansed. When deep cleansing and inspection of the underlying skin are indicated, mineral oil can be used to remove the paste without the need for brisk scrubbing.*
- ▲ Consult the physician or advanced practice nurse concerning use of a moisture barrier with active healing ingredients when incontinence-associated dermatitis exists. In addition, an antifungal powder may be applied underneath the ointment when perineal dermatitis is complicated by monilial infection. Teach the client to use the product sparingly when applying to affected areas. **EBN:** *An ointment made from Balsam Peru, trypsin, and castor oil (BCT ointment) has been shown to be more effective than placebo for the management of partial thickness wounds in clients with urinary or fecal incontinence (Gray & Jones, 2004). A thin layer of antifungal powder may be layered beneath the ointment, but application of excessive powder may paradoxically retain moisture and diminish its effectiveness (Evans & Gray, 2003; Gray, Ratliff & Donovan, 2002).*
- ▲ Consult the physician or advanced practice nurse concerning placement of an indwelling catheter when severe urine loss is complicated by urinary retention, when careful fluid monitoring or core body temperature monitoring is indicated in the critically ill client, or when urinary bypassing is required to promote healing of a stage III or IV pressure ulcer, or in the terminally ill client when use of absorbent products produces pain or distress. *Although not routinely indicated, the indwelling catheter provides an effective, transient management technique for carefully selected clients (Cravens & Zweig, 2000; Drinka, 2006; Gray & Campbell, 2006).*
- ▲ Refer the client with "intractable" or extraurethral incontinence to a continence service or specialist for further evaluation and management of urine loss. *The successful management of complex, severe urinary incontinence requires specialized evaluation and treatment from a health care provider with special expertise.*

Geriatric

- Provide privacy and support when changing incontinent devices in elderly clients. *Elderly, hospitalized clients frequently express feelings of shame, guilt, and dependency when undergoing urinary containment device changes (Biggerson et al, 1993).*
- Avoid brisk scrubbing and use of a washcloth when cleansing the skin of an aging client. *Brisk washing with a washcloth tends to strip superficial layers of skin, which potentially exacerbates erosion or damage to subcutaneous connective tissues (Gray, Ratliff & Donovan, 2002).*
- Employ meticulous infection control procedures when using an indwelling catheter.

Home Care

- The interventions described previously may be adapted for home care use.
- Encourage a mind-set and program of self-care management. **EBN:** *Addressing self-care activities through exercise, diet, fluid intake, and protective devices helps the client to exercise control over incontinence (Leenerts, Teel & Pendleton, 2002).*
- Assist the family with arranging care in a way that allows the client to participate in family or favorite activities without embarrassment. Elicit discussion of the client's concerns about the social or emotional burden of incontinence. **EBN and EB:** *Careful planning can help the client retain dignity and maintain the integrity of family patterns. Urinary incontinence has a demonstrated influence on subjective well-being and quality of life, with depression, loneliness, or sadness possible*

(Fultz & Herzog, 2001). Discussing emotional concerns helps the client to develop a sense of control over incontinence (Leenerts, Teel & Pendleton, 2002).

▲ Consider the use of an indwelling catheter for continuous drainage in the client with severe urinary incontinence who is homebound, bed bound, and receiving palliative or end-of-life care (requires a physician's order). *An indwelling catheter may increase client comfort, ease caregiver burden, and prevent urinary incontinence in bed-bound clients receiving end-of-life care.*

▲ When an indwelling catheter is in place, follow the prescribed maintenance protocols for managing the catheter, drainage bag, and perineal skin and urethral meatus. Teach infection control measures adapted to the home care setting. *Proper care reduces the risk of catheter-associated urinary tract infection.*

• Assist the client in adapting to the catheter. Encourage discussion of the client's response to the catheter. **EBN:** *Clients living with a catheter are keenly aware of its presence; adaptation is served by normalizing the experience. Rehearsing emptying of the bag when away from home will support resumption of activities. Discussion of the client's response will help him or her to deal with embarrassment or frustration (Wilde, 2002).*

Client/Family Teaching

• Teach the family to obtain, apply, and dispose of or clean and reuse urine containment devices.
• Teach the family a routine perineal skin care regimen, including daily or every other day hygiene and cleansing with containment product changes.
• Teach the client and family to recognize and manage perineal dermatitis, ammonia contact dermatitis, and monilial rash.
• Teach the client to maintain adequate fluid intake (30 mL/kg of body weight per day).
• Teach the client and family to recognize and manage urinary tract infection.

evolve   See the EVOLVE website for World Wide Web resources for client education.

REFERENCES

Biggerson AB et al: Elderly women's feelings about being incontinent, using napkins and being helped by nurses to change napkins, *J Clin Nurs* 2:165, 1993.

Cravens DD, Zweig S: Urinary catheter management, *Am Fam Physician* 61(2):369-376, 2000.

Drinka P: Complications of chronic indwelling urinary catheters, *J Am Med Dir Assoc* 7(6):388-392, 2006.

Dunn S, Kowanko I, Paterson J et al: Systematic review of the effectiveness of urinary continence products, *J Wound Ostomy Continence Nurs* 29(3):129-142, 2002.

Evans EC, Gray M: What interventions are effective for the prevention and treatment of cutaneous candidiasis? *J Wound Ostomy Continence Nurs* 30(1):11-16, 2003.

Flores-Carreras O, Cabrera JR, Galeano PA et al: Fistulas of the urinary tract in obstetric surgery, *Int Urogynecol J Pelvic Floor Dysfunct* 12(3):203-214, 2001.

Fultz NH, Herzog AR: Self-reported social and emotional impact of urinary incontinence, *J Am Geriatr Soc* 49(7):892-899, 2001.

Gallo M, Staskin DR: Patient satisfaction with a reusable undergarment for urinary incontinence, *J Wound Ostomy Continence Nurs* 24(4):226, 1997.

Gray M, Campbell F: Urinary tract disorders. In Ferrell B, Coyle N, editors: *Textbook of palliative nursing*, ed 2, Oxford, UK, 2006, Oxford University Press, pp 265-284.

Gray M, Jones D: The effect of different formulations of equivalent active ingredients on the performance of two topical wound treatment products, *Ostomy Wound Manage* 50(3):34-44, 2004.

Gray M, Moore KN: Assessment of patients with urinary incontinence. In Doughty DB, editor: *Urinary and fecal incontinence: management principles*, ed 3, St. Louis, 2006, Mosby, pp 341-412.

Gray M, Ratliff C, Donovan A: Perineal skin care for the incontinent patient, *Adv Skin Wound Care* 15(4):170-175, 2002.

Gray M, Bliss DZ, Doughty DB et al: Incontinence-associated dermatitis: a consensus, *J Wound Ostomy Continence Nurs* 34(1):45-54, 2007.

Kriplani A, Agarwal N, Parul GA et al: Observations on aetiology and management of genital fistulas, *Arch Gynecol Obstet* 271(1):14-18, 2005.

Leenerts MH, Teel CS, Pendleton MK: Building a model of self-care for health promotion in aging, *J Nurs Scholarsh* 34(4):355-361, 2002.

Ng'ang'a N: Women of the courtyard. A nurse's journey to treat obstetric fistulae in Niger, *AWHONN Lifelines*, 10(5):410-417, 2006.

Shirran E, Brazelli M: Absorbent products for the containment of urinary and/or fecal incontinence, *Cochrane Database System Rev* (2): CD0011406, 2000.

Wall LL: Obstetric vesicovaginal fistula as an international public-health problem, *Lancet* 368(9542):1201-1209, 2006.

Wilde MH: Urine flowing: a phenomenological study of living with a urinary catheter, *Res Nurs Health* 25(1):14-24, 2002.

Zehrer CL, Newman DK, Grove GL: Assessment of diaper-clogging potential of petrolatum moisture barriers, *Ostomy Wound Manag* 51(12):54-58, 2005.

Urge urinary Incontinence   *Mikel Gray, PhD, RN*

NANDA   Definition

State in which the individual experiences involuntary passage of urine occurring with precipitous desire to urinate. *Urge incontinence* is defined within the context of overactive bladder syndrome. The overactive bladder is characterized by bothersome urgency (a sudden and strong desire to urinate that is not easily deferred) (Abrams et al, 2002). Overactive bladder is typically associated with frequent daytime voiding and nocturia, and approximately 37% will experience urge urinary incontinence (Stewart et al, 2003).

Defining Characteristics

Diurnal urinary frequency (voiding more than once every 2 hours while awake); nocturia (awakening three or more times per night to urinate); voiding more than eight times within a 24-hour period as recorded on a voiding diary (bladder log); bothersome urgency (a sudden and strong desire to urinate that is not easily deferred); symptom of urge incontinence (urine loss associated with desire to urinate); enuresis (involuntary passage of urine while asleep)

Related Factors

Neurological disorders (brain disorders, including cerebrovascular accident, brain tumor, normal pressure hydrocephalus, traumatic brain injury); inflammation of bladder (calculi; tumor, including transitional cell carcinoma and carcinoma in situ; inflammatory lesions of the bladder; urinary tract infection); bladder outlet obstruction (see **Urinary retention**); stress urinary incontinence (mixed urinary incontinence; these conditions often coexist but relationship between them remains unclear); idiopathic causes (implicated factors include depression, sleep apnea/hypoxia)

NOC   Outcomes (Nursing Outcomes Classification)

Suggested NOC Outcomes

Tissue Integrity: Skin and Mucous Membranes, Urinary Continence, Urinary Elimination

Example **NOC** Outcome with Indicators
Urinary Continence as evidenced by the following indicators: Responds in timely manner to urge/Voids in appropriate receptacle/Has adequate time to reach toilet between urge and evacuation of urine/Underclothing remains dry during day/Underclothing or bedding remains dry during night (Rate the outcome and indicators of **Urinary Continence:** 1 = never demonstrated, 2 = rarely demonstrated, 3 = sometimes demonstrated, 4 = often demonstrated, 5 = consistently demonstrated [see Section I].)

Client Outcomes

Client Will (Specify Time Frame):

- Report relief from urge urinary incontinence or a decrease in the incidence or severity of incontinent episodes
- Identify containment devices that assist in the management of urge urinary incontinence

NIC   Interventions (Nursing Interventions Classification)

Suggested NIC Interventions

Urinary Habit Training, Urinary Incontinence Care

Example **NIC** Activities—Urinary Habit Training
Keep a continence specification record for 3 days to establish voiding pattern; Establish interval for toileting of preferably not less than 2 hours

• = Independent;   ▲ = Collaborative;   EBN = Evidence-Based Nursing;   EB = Evidence-Based

Nursing Interventions and *Rationales*

- Take a nursing history focusing on duration of urinary incontinence, diurnal frequency, nocturia, severity of symptoms, and alleviating and aggravating factors. *A focused history helps determine the cause of urinary incontinence and guides its subsequent management.* **EBN:** *Querying the client about the isolated symptom of urge incontinence shows a poor correlation with a diagnosis of detrusor overactivity incontinence. However, the agreement between urodynamic testing and the clinical diagnosis obtained by the history rises sharply when the client reports three symptoms: diurnal frequency, urge-related urine loss, and nocturia (Gray et al, 2001).*

- ▲ In close consultation with a physician of advanced practice nurse, consider administering a symptom questionnaire that elicits relevant lower urinary tract symptoms and differentiates stress and urge incontinence symptoms. *Some interventions used to treat stress and urge urinary incontinence are the same (such as pelvic floor muscle training) but some differ (such as pharmacotherapy). Over 23 validated symptom questionnaires have been developed for the evaluation of urinary and fecal incontinence (Avery et al, 2007).* **EBN:** *Several questionnaires have been developed that are specifically designed to enable the clinician differentiate between stress and urge incontinence based on symptom report (Brown et al, 2006; Diokno et al, 1986).*

- ▲ Perform a focused physical assessment, including inspection of the perineal skin, vaginal examination to determine hypoestrogenic changes in the mucosa, pelvic examination to determine the presence of vaginal wall prolapse and uterine prolapse, and to reproduce the sign of stress urinary incontinence. **EBN:** *There is limited evidence supporting the diagnostic value of the physical examination in the diagnosis of urinary incontinence and differential diagnosis of stress versus urge incontinence in elderly women (van Gerwen & Lagro-Janssen, 2006).*

- Inspect the perineal and perianal skin for evidence of incontinence-associated dermatitis, including inflammation, vesicles in skin exposed to urinary leakage, and especially skin folds or denudation of the skin, particularly when incontinence is managed by absorptive pads or containment briefs. *Urinary incontinence, particularly when combined with fecal incontinence or use of absorptive pads or adult containment briefs, increases the risk of incontinence-associated dermatitis (Gray et al, 2007).* **EBN:** *20% of clients with urinary and/or fecal incontinence in the acute care setting were found to have perineal or perigenital skin damage; 18% were found to have evidence of secondary cutaneous candidiasis (Junkin & Selekof, 2007, in press).*

- ▲ Perform a focused pelvic examination including visual inspection of the vaginal mucosa, observation of urethral hypermobility and related pelvic floor descent (prolapse), and digital assessment of pelvic floor muscle strength. Refer the woman with moderately severe to severe vaginal wall prolapse (descent to or beyond the introitus) to a female urologist or urogynecologist. *Severe pelvic organ prolapse complicates the management of urge urinary incontinence and predisposes the female client to urinary retention (Romanzi, 2002). Baseline of pelvic muscle strength is needed for initial assessment and for evaluation of treatment efficacy. It also provides an opportunity for the nurse to determine whether the client is able to identify, isolate, contract, and relax the pelvic floor muscles.*

- ▲ Complete a urinalysis, examining for the presence of nitrites, leukocytes, glucose, or hemoglobin (red blood cells). *The presence of nitrites and leukocytes raises a suspicion of urinary tract infection, the presence of glucosuria raises the risk of undiagnosed or poorly controlled diabetes mellitus, and the presence of red blood cells in the absence of signs of infection raises a suspicion of a bladder tumor. Each condition may produce acute urinary incontinence requiring treatment of the underlying cause (Fourcroy, 2001).*

- Teach the client to complete a voiding diary (bladder log) by recording voiding frequency, the frequency of urinary incontinent episodes and their association with urgency (a sudden and strong desire to urinate that is difficult o defer) over a 3- to 7-day period. An electronic voiding diary may be kept whenever feasible. In addition to these parameters, the client may be asked to record voided volume and fluid intake. *The voiding diary provides a more objective record of lower urinary tract function than the oral history, and it often provides a modest therapeutic effect by alerting the client to factors that promote urinary incontinence episodes (Sampselle, 2003). An electronic voiding diary provides an efficient and possibly more accurate method for documenting these parameters (Quinn, Goka & Richardson, 2003).*

- ▲ Review all medications the client is receiving, paying particular attention to sedatives, opioid analgesics, diuretics, antidepressants, psychotropic drugs, and cholinergics. Consult the physician or

I

• = Independent;   ▲ = Collaborative;   EBN = Evidence-Based Nursing;   EB = Evidence-Based

nurse practitioner about altering or eliminating these medications if they are suspected of affecting incontinence. *The side effects of multiple medications may produce or exacerbate urge incontinence (Fourcroy, 2001).*

- Assess the client for urinary retention (see the care plan for **Urinary retention**). *Urinary retention associated with bladder outlet obstruction may be a contributing cause of urge incontinence (Chai, Gray & Steers, 1998). Urinary retention associated with poor detrusor contraction strength has been described in frail elderly clients (Resnick & Yalla, 1987). Regardless of its cause, retention significantly affects the management of this condition (Gray, 2000).*

- Assess the client for functional limitations (environmental barriers, limited mobility or dexterity, impaired cognitive function; refer to the care plan for **Functional urinary Incontinence**). *Functional limitations affect the severity and management of urge urinary incontinence (Ouslander, 2002).*

▲ Consult the physician concerning diabetic management and pharmacotherapy for urinary tract infection when indicated. *In specific cases, urgency and an increased risk of urge incontinence may be related to urinary tract infection (Molander et al, 2000) or polyuria from undiagnosed or poorly managed diabetes mellitus (Samsioe et al, 1999).*

▲ Assess for signs and symptoms of atrophic vaginal changes in the perimenopausal or postmenopausal woman, including vaginal dryness, tenderness to touch, mucosal dryness, friability, and discomfort with gentle palpation. Specifically query the woman with atrophic vaginitis concerning associated lower urinary tract symptoms (usually voiding frequency, urgency, and dysuria). Refer the woman with atrophic vaginal changes and bothersome lower urinary tract symptoms to a gynecologist, urologist, or women's health nurse practitioner for further evaluation and management. *The relationship between atrophic vaginitis and urge incontinence risk remains unclear. However, several studies have observed that oral estrogen replacement may slightly increase the frequency of urinary incontinence episodes in postmenopausal women (Brown et al, 1999; Molander et al, 2000). Topical or intravaginal estrogen, particularly rings or tablets, may provide an alternative for relieving bothersome symptoms associated with atrophic vaginitis without the associated risks of oral preparations (Crandall, 2002). In addition, systematic reviews of existing evidence suggest that local hormone replacement therapy may reduce the risk of urinary tract infection in elderly women (Crandall, 2002; Rozenberg, 2004).*

- Teach the principles of bladder training to women with urge urinary incontinence.
  - Assist the client in completing a voiding diary over a period of a minimum of 3 days or up to 7 days.
  - Review the results with the client, determining typical voiding frequency and establishing goals for voiding frequency.
  - Using baseline voiding frequency, as determined by the diary, teach the client to urinate by the clock when awake, typically every 30 to 120 minutes.
  - Encourage adherence to the program with timing devices and verbal encouragement and support, and address individual reasons for schedule interruption.
  - Gradually increase the time between urinations to the negotiated goal. Time intervals between voiding are typically increased in increments of 15 to 30 minutes for clients with a baseline frequency of less than every 60 minutes and increments of 25 to 30 minutes for clients with a baseline frequency of more than every 60 minutes.

  EBN: *Bladder training reduces the frequency and severity of urinary leakage in women with urge, stress, or mixed urinary incontinence. Research suggests that the results of bladder training in ambulatory, community-dwelling women is comparable to that achieved through pelvic floor muscle rehabilitation (Elser et al, 1999; Theofrastous et al, 2002; Wyman et al, 1998). Bladder training has also been shown to augment the efficacy of pharmacotherapy for clients with urge urinary incontinence (Mattiasson et al, 2003; Song et al, 2006).*

- Review with the client the types of beverages consumed, focusing on the intake of caffeine, which is associated with a transient effect on lower urinary tract symptoms. Advise all clients to reduce or eliminate intake caffeinated beverages or over-the-counter medications of dietary aids containing caffeine. *Caffeine acts as a bladder irritant, increasing voiding frequency, urgency, and urge urinary incontinence episodes among those with this condition. Reducing the intake of caffeine alleviates these lower urinary tract symptoms (Gray, 2001).*

• = Independent;   ▲ = Collaborative;   EBN = Evidence-Based Nursing;   EB = Evidence-Based

- Review with the client the volume of fluids consumed and gradually adjust the fluid intake to meet the Adequate Intake recommendation of 3 L for the 19- to 30-year-old male and 2.2 L for the 19- to 30-year-old female. Water balance studies suggest that adult men require 2.5 L/day (Institute of Medicine, 2004). *Dehydration is postulated to exacerbate the symptoms of urgency (Pearson, 1992, 1993), and excessive fluid intake increases voided volume and urinary frequency (Fitzgerald & Brubaker, 2003). Increasing fluid intake in women with urinary incontinence may reduce the risk of urinary tract infection without increasing the frequency or severity of urine loss (Dougherty et al, 2002).*
- Instruct in techniques of urge suppression. Teach the client to identify, isolate, contract, and relax the pelvic floor muscles. When a strong or precipitous urge to urinate is perceived, teach the client to avoid running to the toilet. Instead, she or he should perform repeated, rapid pelvic muscle contractions until the urge is relieved. Relief is followed by micturition within 5 to 15 minutes, using non-hurried movements when locating a toilet and voiding. **EB:** *Randomized controlled trials comparing urge suppression techniques to pharmacotherapy or bladder training have shown it to be an effective method for reducing urge urinary incontinence episodes (Burgio, 2002).*
- ▲ Begin transvaginal or transrectal electrical stimulation using a low-frequency current (5 to 20 Hz) in consultation with the physician. *Electrical stimulation is an effective treatment for urge incontinence; in one randomized clinical trial it was found to completely eliminate symptoms of urge incontinence in 49% of a group of 121 subjects (Brubaker et al, 1997).*
- ▲ Teach the client to self-administer antimuscarinic (anticholinergic) drugs as directed. Teach dosage and administration of the medication and the importance of combining pharmacotherapy with scheduled voiding, adequate fluid intake, restriction of bladder irritants, and urge suppression techniques. *Antimuscarinic drugs increase bladder capacity, reduce the frequency of incontinence episodes, and diminish voiding frequency. However, they do not cure bladder dysfunction or reduce the time between perception of a strong urge and onset of an overactive detrusor contraction. The efficacy of pharmacotherapy for urge incontinence and overactive bladder dysfunction is enhanced when combined with behavioral interventions (Burgio, 2002; Burgio, Locher & Goode, 2000; Song et al, 2006).*
- ▲ Assist the client in selecting, obtaining, and applying a containment device for urine loss as indicated (refer to the care plan for **Total urinary Incontinence**).
- ▲ Provide the client with information about incontinence support groups such as the National Association for Continence and the Simon Foundation for Continence. *Self-help groups provide social support and a forum for sharing strategies for the management of all types of urinary incontinence (Irwin, 2000).*

Geriatric

- Assess the functional and cognitive status of the elderly client with urge incontinence. *Functional limitations affect the severity and management of urge urinary incontinence (Ouslander, 2002).*
- Plan care in long-term or acute care facilities based on knowledge of the elderly client's established voiding patterns, paying particular attention to patterns of nocturia.
- ▲ Carefully monitor the elderly client for potential adverse effects of antispasmodic medications, including a severely dry mouth interfering with the use of dentures, eating, or speaking, or confusion, nightmares, constipation, mydriasis, or heat intolerance. *Elderly persons are particularly susceptible to adverse effects associated with antispasmodic medications (Ghoneim & Hassouna, 1997).*

Home Care

- The interventions described previously may be adapted for home care use.
- Teach the importance of avoiding dehydration or excessive fluid consumption and the paradoxical relationship between dehydration and symptoms of urgency.
- Teach the family and client to identify and correct environmental barriers to toileting within the home.
- Encourage a mind-set and program of self-care management. **EBN:** *Addressing self-care activities through exercise, diet, fluid intake, and protective devices helps the client to exercise control over incontinence (Leenerts, Teel & Pendleton, 2002).*
- Implement a bladder-training program as appropriate, including self-monitoring activities (re-

ducing caffeine intake, adjusting amount and timing of fluid intake, decreasing long voiding intervals while awake, making dietary changes to promote bowel regularity), bladder training, and pelvic muscle exercise. **EBN:** *In one study of women age 55 years or older with involuntary urine loss associated with stress, urge, or mixed incontinence, clients responded to the aforementioned interventions with a 61% decrease in the severity of urinary incontinence at 2 years after intervention. Self-monitoring and bladder training accounted for most of the improvement (Dougherty et al, 2002).*

- Help the client and family to identify and correct environmental barriers to toileting within the home.

Client/Family Teaching

- Teach the client and family to recognize foods and beverages that are likely to irritate the bladder.
- Teach the family and client to recognize and manage side effects of antispasmodic medications used to treat urge incontinence.
- Help the client and family to recognize and manage side effect of anticholinergic medications used to manage irritative lower urinary tract symptoms.

evolve See the EVOLVE website for World Wide Web resources for client education.

REFERENCES

Abrams P, Cardozo L, Fall M et al: The standardisation of terminology of lower urinary tract function: report from the Standardization Sub-committee of the International Continence Society, *Am J Obstet Gynecol* 187(1):116-126, 2002.

Avery KN, Bosch JL, Gotoh M et al: Questionnaires to assess urinary and anal incontinence: review and recommendations, *J Urol* 177(1):39-49, 2007.

Brown JS, Bradley CS, Subak LL et al: The sensitivity and specificity of a simple test to distinguish between urge and stress urinary incontinence. Diagnostic Aspects of Incontinence Study (DAISy) Research Group, *Ann Intern Med* 144(10):715-723, 2006.

Brown JS, Grady D, Ouslander JG et al: Prevalence of urinary incontinence and associated risk factors in postmenopausal women. Heart & Estrogen/Progestin Replacement Study (HERS) Research Group, *Obstet Gynecol* 94:66, 1999.

Brubaker L, Benson JT, Bent A et al: Transvaginal electrical stimulation for female urinary incontinence, *Am J Obstet Gynecol* 177(3):536-540, 1997.

Burgio KL: Influence of behavior modification on overactive bladder, *Urology* 60(5 Suppl 1):72, 2002.

Burgio KL, Locher JL, Goode PS: Combined behavioral and drug therapy for urge incontinence in older women, *J Am Geriatr Soc* 48(4):370, 2000.

Chai TC, Gray ML, Steers WD: The incidence of a positive ice water test on bladder outlet obstructed patients: evidence for altered innervation, *J Urol* 160:34-38, 1998.

Crandall C: Vaginal estrogen preparations: a review of safety and efficacy for vaginal atrophy, *J Womens Health* 11(10):857-877, 2002.

Diokno AC, Brock BM, Brown MB et al: Prevalence of urinary incontinence and other urological symptoms in the noninstitutionalized elderly, *J Urol* 136(5):1022-1025, 1986.

Dougherty MC, Dwyer JW, Pendergast JF et al: A randomized trial of behavioral management for continence with older rural women, *Res Nurs Health* 25(1):3, 2002.

Elser DM, Wyman JF, McClish DK et al: The effect of bladder training, pelvic floor muscle training, or combination training on urodynamic parameters in women with urinary incontinence. Continence Program for Women Research Group, *Neurourol Urodyn* 18(5):427, 1999.

Fitzgerald MP, Brubaker L: Variability of 24-hour voiding diary variables among asymptomatic women, *J Urol* 169(1):207, 2003.

Fourcroy JL: Overactive bladder: a practical overview of diagnosis and treatment, *Adv Nurse Practit* 9(3):59, 2001.

Ghoneim GM, Hassouna M: Alternatives for the pharmacologic management of urge and stress urinary incontinence in the elderly, *J Wound Ostomy Continence Nurs* 24:311, 1997.

Gray M: Caffeine and urinary incontinence, *J Wound Ostomy Continence Nurs* 28:66, 2001.

Gray M: Urinary retention: management in the acute care setting, Part 2, *Am J Nurs* 100:36, 2000.

Gray M, Bliss DZ, Doughty DB et al: Incontinence-associated dermatitis: a consensus, *J Wound Ostomy Continence Nurs* 24(1):45-56, 2007.

Gray M, McClain R, Peruggia M et al: A model for predicting motor urge urinary incontinence, *Nurs Res* 50:116, 2001.

Institute of Medicine: Food and Nutrition Board: *Dietary reference intakes for water, potassium, sodium chloride and sulfate,* Washington, DC, 2004, The National Academies Press.

Irwin B: User support groups in continence care, *Nurs Times* 96(Suppl 31):24, 2000.

Junkin J, Selekof J: Prevalence of incontinence and associated skin injury in an acute care population, *J Wound Ostomy Continence Nurs* 24(3), 2007 (in press).

Leenerts MH, Teel CS, Pendleton MK: Building a model of self-care for health promotion in aging, *J Nurs Scholarsh* 34(4):355-361, 2002.

Mattiasson A, Blaakaer J, Hoye K et al: Simplified bladder training augments the effectiveness of tolterodine in patients with an overactive bladder. Tolterodine Scandinavian Study Group, *BJU Int* 91(1):54-60, 2003.

Molander U, Arvidsson L, Milsom I et al: A longitudinal cohort study of elderly women with urinary tract infection, *Maturitas* 34:127, 2000.

Ouslander JG: Geriatric considerations in the diagnosis and management of overactive bladder, *Urology* 60(5 suppl 1):50, 2002.

Pearson BD: Liquidate a myth: reducing liquids is not advisable for elderly with urine control problems, *Urol Nurs* 13:86, 1993.

Pearson BD: Urine control by elders: noninvasive strategies. In Funk SG et al editors: *Key aspects of elder care: managing falls, incontinence and cognitive impairment,* New York, 1992, Springer.

Quinn P, Goka J, Richardson H: Assessment of an electronic daily diary in patients with overactive bladder, *BJU Int* 91(7):647-652, 2003.

Resnick NM, Yalla SV: Detrusor hyperactivity with impaired contractile function. An unrecognized but common cause of incontinence in elderly patients, *JAMA* 257:3076, 1987.

Romanzi LJ: Management of the urethral outlet in patients with severe prolapse, *Curr Opin Urol* 12(4):339-344, 2002.

Rozenberg S et al: Estrogen therapy in older patients with recurrent urinary tract infections: a review, *Int J Fertil Womens Med* 49(2):71-74, 2004.

Sampselle CM: Teaching women to use a voiding diary, *Am J Nurs* 103(11):62-64, 2003.

Samsioe G, Heraib F, Lidfeldt J et al: Urogenital symptoms in women aged 50-59 years, *Gynecol Endocrinol* 13(2):113-117, 1999.

Song C, Park JT, Heo KO et al: Effects of bladder training and/or tolterodine in female patients with overactive bladder syndrome: a prospective, randomized study, *J Korean Med Sci* 21(6):1060-1063, 2006.

Stewart WF, Van Rooyen JB, Cundiff GW et al: Prevalence and burden of overactive bladder in the United States, *World J Urol* 20(6):327-336, 2003.

Theofrastous JP, Wyman JF, Bump RC et al: Effects of pelvic floor muscle training on strength and predictors of response in the treatment of urinary incontinence, *Neurourol Urodyn* 21(5):486-490, 2002.

van Gerwen M, Lagro-Janssen AL: [Diagnostic value of patient history and physical examination in elderly patients with urinary incontinence; a literature review], *Ned Tijdsch Geneesk* 150(32):1771-1775, 2006 [article in Dutch].

Wyman JF, Fantl JA, McClish DK et al: Continence Program for Women Research Group, Comparative efficacy of behavioral interventions in the management of female urinary incontinence. *Am J Obstet Gynecol* 179(4):999, 1998.

Risk for urge urinary Incontinence   *Mikel Gray, PhD, RN*

NANDA   Definition

At risk for involuntary loss of urine associated with a sudden, strong sensation or urinary urgency

Risk Factors

Overactive bladder dysfunction with associated detrusor overactivity; inflammation from urinary tract infection; inflammatory lesion; bladder or lower ureteral stone; bladder outlet obstruction; dietary risk factors; consumption of caffeine

Overactive bladder is a symptom syndrome characterized by bothersome urgency (a sudden and strong desire to urinate that is not easily deferred) typically associated with day and nighttime voiding frequency (more than eight urinations per day) (Abrams et al, 2002). Although urge urinary incontinence affects approximately 37% of patients with overactive bladder, 63% (Stewart, Van Rooyen & Cundiff, 2003) have an identifiable condition that is not adequately described by this diagnosis. It is hoped that **Risk for urge urinary Incontinence** will evolve in a manner that more clearly describes the underlying syndrome, overactive bladder.

NOC   Outcomes (Nursing Outcomes Classification)

Suggested NOC Outcomes

Tissue Integrity: Skin and Mucous Membranes, Urinary Continence, Urinary Elimination

---

Example NOC Outcome with Indicators

Urinary Continence as evidenced by the following indicators: Responds in timely manner to urge/Voids in appropriate receptacle/Has adequate time to reach toilet between urge and evacuation of urine/Underclothing remains dry during day/Underclothing or bedding remains dry during night (Rate the outcome and indicators of **Urinary Continence:** 1 = never demonstrated, 2 = rarely demonstrated, 3 = sometimes demonstrated, 4 = often demonstrated, 5 = consistently demonstrated [see Section I].)

Client Outcomes

Client Will (Specify Time Frame):

- Report relief from urge urinary incontinence or a decrease in the incidence or severity of incontinent episodes
- Identify containment devices that assist in the management of urge urinary incontinence

• = Independent;   ▲ = Collaborative;   EBN = Evidence-Based Nursing;   EB = Evidence-Based

NIC   Interventions (Nursing Interventions Classification)

Suggested NIC Interventions

Urinary Habit Training, Urinary Incontinence Care

Example NIC Activities—Urinary Habit Training
Keep a continence specification record for 3 days to establish voiding pattern; Establish interval for toileting of preferably not less than 2 hours

Nursing Interventions and *Rationales*

- Take a nursing history focusing on the following lower urinary tract symptoms: daytime voiding frequency, nocturia, presence of bothersome urgency (precipitous desire to urinate that interferes with activities of daily living [ADLs]), and presence of urine loss. *Bothersome lower urinary tract symptoms are strongly correlated with urge incontinence in adult women (Alling-Moller, Lose & Jorgensen, 2000).* **EBN:** *Diurnal voiding frequency (voiding every 2 hours or less often or more than 8 times within a 24-hour period), nocturia (arising to void more than once each night for younger clients and more than twice each night for adults age 65 years and older), and bothersome urgency are associated with urge incontinence (Gray et al, 2001).*

- ▲ In close consultation with a physician or advanced practice nurse, select and administer a validated questionnaire focusing on symptoms of overactive bladder. *A growing number of validated questionnaires have been developed to aid in diagnosis and management of overactive bladder syndrome (Coyne et al, 2003).* **EBN:** *The Overactive Bladder Questionnaire (OAB-q) is a valid, reliable, and responsive tool for the evaluation and management of overactive bladder syndrome, including clients with overactive bladder owing to neurological diseases such as Parkinsonism (Coyne, Matza & Thompson, 2005; Palleschi et al, 2006).*

- Query the client about specific risk factors for urge urinary incontinence, such as childhood enuresis, depression, prostate enlargement with bladder outlet obstruction, and neurological disorders, including stroke or Parkinsonism. *Bladder outlet obstruction and neurological disorders affecting modulatory areas in the brain are strongly associated with detrusor overactivity, bothersome lower urinary tract symptoms, and an increased risk for urge incontinence (Mostwin, 2002; Walter et al, 2006). Childhood enuresis may be a risk factor for overactive bladder symptoms in adults (Kuh, Cardozo & Hardy, 1999; Malmsten et al, 1997).*

- Assess the client's functional status, focusing on mobility, dexterity, and cognitive status. *The risk of urinary incontinence rises with increased impairment of mobility; clients who are bedridden are at greatest risk, followed by clients who are confined to a wheelchair, those relying on a walker, and those walking with minimal assistance (Aggazzotti et al, 2000). Cognitive impairment, particularly when accompanied by disoriented perception of time, is associated with an increased risk of urge urinary incontinence in the aging client (Griffiths et al, 2002).*

- ▲ Complete a urinalysis, focusing on the presence of nitrites, leukocytes, glucose, or hemoglobin (red blood cells). *The presence of nitrites and leukocytes raises a suspicion of urinary tract infection, the presence of glucosuria raises a risk of undiagnosed or poorly controlled diabetes mellitus, and the presence of red blood cells in the absence of signs of infection raises a suspicion of a bladder tumor. Each condition increases the risk of urgency symptoms and urge incontinence (Fourcroy, 2001).*

- Teach the client to complete a voiding diary (bladder log) by recording voiding frequency, the frequency of urgency episodes over a 3- to 7-day period. An electronic voiding diary may be kept whenever feasible. In addition to these parameters, the client may be asked to record voided volume and fluid intake. *The voiding diary provides a more objective record of lower urinary tract function than the oral history and it often provides a modest therapeutic effect by alerting the client to factors that promote urinary incontinence episodes (Sampselle, 2003). An electronic voiding diary provides an efficient and possibly more accurate method for documenting these parameters (Quinn, Goka & Richardson, 2003).*

- Advise all clients to reduce or eliminate intake caffeinated beverages or over-the-counter medications of dietary aids containing caffeine. *Caffeine acts as a bladder irritant, increasing voiding fre-*

• = Independent;   ▲ = Collaborative;   EBN = Evidence-Based Nursing;   EB = Evidence-Based

quency, urgency, and urge urinary incontinence episodes among those with this condition. Reducing the intake of caffeine alleviates these lower urinary tract symptoms (Gray, 2001).

- Advise community-dwelling men that moderate consumption of beer may reduce the risk of developing overactive bladder dysfunction and the associated risk for urge urinary incontinence. **EB:** *A longitudinal study of community-dwelling men found that moderate consumption of beer reduced the risk for developing overactive bladder (Dallosso et al, 2004a). Because this effect was not associated with intake of other alcoholic beverages, it seems likely that the protective effect is attributable to some other element of beer than its alcoholic content.*

- Advise community-dwelling women that intake of a balanced diet, and supplementation of vitamin D to ensure meeting daily recommended allowances may reduce the risk for of developing overactive bladder dysfunction and the associated risk for urge urinary incontinence. **EB:** *A longitudinal study of community-dwelling women found that deficits in a number of nutrients was modestly associated with the risk for developing overactive bladder dysfunction and the associated risk for urge urinary incontinence. Among these, vitamin D deficiency emerged as the strongest potential risk factor (Dallosso et al, 2004b).*

- Recognize that additional bladder irritants, including aspartame, carbonated drinks, decaffeinated coffee or tea, citrus juices, highly spiced foods, chocolates, and vinegar-containing foods, may be eliminated from the diet and added back singly to determine their impact on lower urinary tract symptoms and urgency. *Evidence is limited in support of the role of these substances as potential bladder irritants in clients at risk of urge urinary incontinence, but they do play a more significant role for those with interstitial cystitis (Bade, Peeters & Mensink, 1997; Interstitial Cystitis Association, 1999).*

- Review with the client the volume of fluids consumed and gradually adjust the fluid intake to meet the adequate intake recommendation of 3 L for the 19- to 30-year-old male and 2.2 L for the 19- to 30-year-old female. Water balance studies suggest that adult men require 2.5 L per day (Appel, 2004). *Dehydration is postulated to exacerbate symptoms of urgency (Pearson, 1992, 1993), and excessive fluid intake increases voided volume and urinary frequency. Consumption of fluids within the recommended daily allowance may reduce the risk of urinary tract infection without increasing the frequency or severity of urine loss (Dougherty, 1999).*

- ▲ Review all medications the client is receiving, paying particular attention to sedatives, opioid analgesics, diuretics, antidepressants, psychotropic drugs, and cholinergics. Consult the physician about altering or eliminating these medications if they are suspected of affecting incontinence. *The side effects of multiple medications may produce or exacerbate urge incontinence (Fourcroy, 2001).*

- ▲ Consult the physician concerning diabetic management and pharmacotherapy for urinary tract infection when indicated. *In specific cases, urgency and an increased risk of urge incontinence may be related to urinary tract infection (Molander et al, 2000) or polyuria from undiagnosed or poorly managed diabetes mellitus (Samsioe et al, 1999).*

- ▲ Assess for signs and symptoms of atrophic vaginal changes in the perimenopausal or postmenopausal woman, including vaginal dryness, tenderness to touch, dryness of mucosa on touch with friability, and discomfort with gentle palpation. Specifically query the client with atrophic vaginitis concerning storage lower urinary tract symptoms (voiding frequency, urgency, or dysuria). Refer the client with atrophic vaginal changes and bothersome lower urinary tract symptoms to a gynecologist, urologist, or women's health nurse practitioner for further evaluation and management. *The relationship between atrophic vaginitis and urge incontinence risk remains unclear. However, several studies have found that oral estrogen replacement slightly increases the frequency of urinary incontinence episodes (Brown et al, 1999; Molander et al, 2000).* **EB:** *A modest body of evidence suggests that intravaginal or topical estrogen replacement therapy reduces bothersome symptoms associated with atrophic urogenital changes, including urgency and dysuria. Local estrogen therapy also may reduce the risk for urinary tract infection in postmenopausal women (Rozenberg et al, 2004; Thacker, 2004).*

- Teach clients techniques of bladder training and pelvic muscle rehabilitation focusing on urge suppression. **EBN:** *An interdisciplinary research team, including a nurse researcher, has demonstrated that public education of community-dwelling middle-age and elderly women reduces the risk for incontinence and voiding frequency (Diokno et al, 2004; Sampselle et al, 2005).*

- Provide the client with information about incontinence support groups such as the National

Association for Continence and the Simon Foundation for Continence. *Self-help groups provide social support and a forum for sharing strategies for management of all types of urinary incontinence (Irwin, 2000).*

Geriatric

- Assess the functional and cognitive status of an elderly client with irritative lower urinary tract symptoms or urge incontinence.
- ▲ Advise a male client with bothersome lower urinary tract symptoms to see his physician or nurse practitioner, because these symptoms may be related to prostate enlargement.
- ▲ Carefully monitor the elderly client for potential adverse effects of anticholinergic medications, including severe dry mouth interfering with the use of dentures, eating, or speaking, or the occurrence of confusion, nightmares, constipation, mydriasis, or heat intolerance. *Elderly persons are particularly susceptible to adverse effects associated with anticholinergic medications.*

Home Care

- The interventions described previously may be adapted for home care use.
- Encourage a mind-set and program of self-care management. **EBN:** *Addressing self-care activities through exercise, diet, fluid intake, and protective devices helps the client take control of incontinence (Leenerts, Teel & Pendleton, 2002).*
- Implement a bladder-training program, including self-monitoring activities (reducing caffeine intake, adjusting amount and timing of fluid intake, decreasing long voiding intervals while awake, making dietary changes to promote bowel regularity), bladder training, and pelvic muscle exercise. **EBN:** *In one study of women age 55 years or older with involuntary urine loss associated with stress, urge, or mixed incontinence, clients responded to the aforementioned interventions with a 61% decrease in the severity of urinary incontinence at 2 years after intervention. Self-monitoring and bladder training accounted for most of the improvement (Dougherty et al, 2002).*
- Teach the client and family to recognize foods and beverages that are likely to irritate the bladder.
- Teach the importance of avoiding dehydration or excessive fluid consumption and the paradoxical relationship between dehydration and symptoms of urgency.
- Teach the family and client to recognize and manage side effects of anticholinergic medications used to treat irritative lower urinary tract symptoms.
- Teach the family and client to identify and correct environmental barriers to toileting within the home.
- Assist the family with arranging care in a way that allows the client to participate in family or favorite activities without embarrassment. Elicit discussion of the client's concerns about the social or emotional burden of incontinence. **EBN and EB:** *Careful planning can help the client retain dignity and maintain the integrity of family patterns. Urinary incontinence has a demonstrated influence on subjective well-being and quality of life, with depression, loneliness, or sadness possible (Fultz & Herzog, 2001). Discussing emotional concerns helps the client to develop a sense of control over incontinence (Leenerts, Teel & Pendleton, 2002).*

Client/Family Teaching

- Teach the client and family to recognize foods and beverages that are likely to irritate the bladder.
- Teach the importance of avoiding dehydration or excessive fluid consumption and the paradoxical relationship between dehydration and symptoms of urgency.

 See the EVOLVE website for World Wide Web resources for client education.

REFERENCES

Abrams P, Cardozo L, Fall M et al: The standardisation of terminology of lower urinary tract function: report from the Standardization Sub-committee of the International Continence Society, *Am J Obstet Gynecol* 187(1):116-126, 2002.

Aggazzotti G, Pesce F, Grassi D et al: Prevalence of urinary incontinence among institutionalized patients: a cross-sectional epidemiologic study in a midsized city in northern Italy, *Urology* 56(2):245, 2000.

Alling-Moller LA, Lose G, Jorgensen T: Risk factors for lower urinary tract symptoms in women 40 to 60 years of age, *Obstet Gynecol* 96:466, 2000.

Appel L et al: Dietary intake levels for water, salt, potassium, chloride and sulfate, Institute of Medicine, 2004.

Bade JJ, Peeters JM, Mensink HJ: Is the diet of patients with interstitial cystitis related to their disease? *Eur Urol* 32:179, 1997.

Brown JS, Grady D, Ouslander JG et al: Prevalence of urinary incontinence and associated risk factors in postmenopausal women, *Obstet Gynecol* 94:66, 1999.

Coyne KS, Matza LS, Thompson CL: The responsiveness of the Overactive Bladder Questionnaire (OAB-q), *Qual Life Res* 14(3):849-855, 2005.

Coyne KS, Zhou Z, Bhattacharyya SK et al: The prevalence of nocturia and its effect on health-related quality of life and sleep in a community sample in the USA, *BJU Int* 92(9):948-954, 2003.

Dallosso HM, Matthews RJ, McGrother CW et al: The association of diet and other lifestyle factors with the onset of overactive bladder: a longitudinal study in men, *Public Health Nutr* 7(7):885-891, 2004a.

Dallosso HM, McGrother CW, Matthews RJ et al: Nutrient composition of the diet and the development of overactive bladder: a longitudinal study in women, *Neurourol Urodyn* 23(3):204-210, 2004b.

Diokno AC, Sampselle CM, Herzog AR et al: Prevention of urinary incontinence by behavioral modification program: a randomized, controlled trial among older women in the community, *J Urol* 171(3):1165-1171, 2004.

Dougherty MC: *Establishing goals and lifestyle management*, WOCN Continence Conference, Austin, Tex, February 1999.

Dougherty MC, Dwyer JW, Pendergast JF et al: A randomized trial of behavioral management for continence with older rural women, *Res Nurs Health* 25(1):3, 2002.

Fourcroy JL: Overactive bladder: a practical overview of diagnosis and treatment, *Adv Nurse Practit* 9(3):59, 2001.

Fultz NH, Herzog AR: Self-reported social and emotional impact of urinary incontinence, *J Am Geriatr Soc* 49:892, 2001.

Gray M: Caffeine and urinary incontinence, *J Wound Ostomy Continence Nurs* 28:66, 2001.

Gray M, McClain R, Peruggia M et al: A model for predicting motor urge urinary incontinence, *Nurs Res* 50:116, 2001.

Griffiths DJ, McCracken PN, Harrison GM et al: Urge incontinence and impaired detrusor contractility in the elderly, *Neurourol Urodyn* 21(2):126, 2002.

Interstitial Cystitis Association: *Interstitial cystitis and diet*, Rockville, Md, 1999, The Association.

Irwin B: User support groups in continence care, *Nurs Times* 96(Suppl 31):24, 2000.

Kuh D, Cardozo L, Hardy R: Urinary incontinence in middle aged women: childhood enuresis and other lifetime risk factors in a British prospective cohort, *J Epidemiol Community Health* 53(8):453, 1999.

Leenerts MH, Teel CS, Pendleton MK: Building a model of self-care for health promotion in aging, *J Nurs Scholarsh* 34(4):355-361, 2002.

Malmsten UG, Milsom I, Molander U et al: Urinary incontinence and lower urinary tract symptoms: an epidemiological study of men aged 45 to 99 years, *J Urol* 158(5):1733, 1997.

Molander U, Arvidsson L, Milsom I et al: A longitudinal cohort study of elderly women with urinary tract infection, *Maturitas* 34:127, 2000.

Mostwin JL: Pathophysiology: the varieties of bladder overactivity, *Urology* 60(5 Suppl 1):22, 2002.

Palleschi G, Pastore AL, Stocchi F et al: Correlation between the Overactive Bladder questionnaire (OAB-q) and urodynamic data of Parkinson disease patients affected by neurogenic detrusor overactivity during antimuscarinic treatment, *Clin Neuropharmacol* 29(4):220-229, 2006.

Pearson BD: Liquidate a myth: reducing liquids is not advisable for elderly with urine control problems, *Urol Nurs* 13:86, 1993.

Pearson BD: Urine control by elders: noninvasive strategies. In Funk SG et al, editors: *Key aspects of elder care: managing falls, incontinence and cognitive impairment*, New York, 1992, Springer.

Quinn P, Goka J, Richardson H: Assessment of an electronic daily diary in patients with overactive bladder, *BJU Int* 91(7):647-652, 2003.

Rozenberg S, Pastijn A, Gevers R et al: Estrogen therapy in older patients with recurrent urinary tract infections: a review, *Int J Fertil Womens Med* 49(2):71-74, 2004.

Sampselle CM: Teaching women to use a voiding diary, *Am J Nurs* 103(11):62-64, 2003.

Sampselle CM, Messer KL, Seng JS et al: Learning outcomes of a group behavioral modification program to prevent urinary incontinence, *Int Urogynecol J* 16(6):441-446, 2005.

Samsioe G, Heraib F, Lidfeldt J et al: Urogenital symptoms in women aged 50-59 years. Women's Health in Lund Area (WHILSA) Study Group, *Gynecol Endocrinol* 13(2):113-117, 1999.

Stewart WF, Van Rooyen JB, Cundiff GW: Prevalence and burden of overactive bladder in the United States, *World J Urol* 20(6):327-336, 2003.

Thacker HL: Estrogen ring use for genitourinary atrophy and menopausal symptomatology, *Geriatrics* 59(5):34, 36-37, 2004.

Walter U, Dressler D, Wolters A et al: Overactive bladder in Parkinson's disease: alteration of brainstem raphe detected by transcranial sonography, *Eur J Neurol* 13(12):1291-1297, 2006.

I

Disorganized Infant behavior   Mary DeWys, RN, BS, and Peg Padnos, RN, BA, BSN

NANDA   Definition

Disintegrated physiological and neurobehavioral responses of infant to the environment

Defining Characteristics

Attention-Interaction System

Abnormal response to sensory stimuli (e.g., difficult to soothe, inability to sustain alert status)

Motor System

Altered primitive reflexes; changes to motor tone; finger splaying; fisting; hands to face; hyperextension of extremities; jittery; startles; tremors; twitches; uncoordinated movement

• = Independent;   ▲ = Collaborative;   EBN = Evidence-Based Nursing;   EB = Evidence-Based

Physiological

Arrhythmias; bradycardia; desaturation; feeding intolerances; skin color changes; tachycardia; time-out signals (e.g., gaze, grasp, hiccough, cough, sneeze, sigh, slack, jaw, open mouth, tongue thrust)

Regulatory Problems

Inability to inhibit startle; irritability

State-Organization System

Active-awake (fussy, worried gaze); diffuse sleep; irritable crying; state-oscillation; quiet-awake (staring, gaze aversion)

Related Factors (r/t)

Caregiver

Cue knowledge deficit; cue misreading; environmental stimulation contribution

Environmental

Lack of containment within environment; physical environment inappropriateness; sensory deprivation; sensory inappropriateness; sensory overstimulation

Individual

Gestational age; illness; immature neurological system; postconceptual age

Postnatal

Feeding intolerance; invasive procedures; malnutrition; motor problems; oral problems; pain; prematurity

Prenatal

Congenital disorders; genetic disorders; teratogenic exposure

NOC   Outcomes (Nursing Outcomes Classification)

Suggested NOC Outcomes

Child Development, Neurological Status, Preterm Infant Organization, Sleep, Thermoregulation: Newborn

---

Example NOC Outcome with Indicators

Preterm Infant Organization as evidenced by the following indicators: O_2 saturation >85%/ Thermoregulation/Feeding tolerance/Self-consolability/Quiet-alert/Attentiveness to stimuli/Responsive to stimuli (Rate the outcome and indicators of **Preterm Infant Organization:** 1 = severely compromised, 2 = substantially compromised, 3 = moderately compromised, 4 = mildly compromised, 5 = not compromised [see Section 1].)

Client Outcomes

Client Will (Specify Time Frame):

Infant/Child
- Display physiologic/autonomic stability: cardiorespiratory, visceral, neurofunctional
- Display organized motor system (Wyngarden, DeWys & Padnos, 1999)
- Display signs of state organization: ability to maintain organized sleep and awake states (Wyngarden, DeWys & Padnos, 1999)
- Demonstrate progress toward effective self-regulation (Wyngarden, DeWys & Padnos, 1999)
- Display clear behavior cues that communicate approach/engagement and stress/avoidance (Wyngarden, DeWys & Padnos, 1999)

• = Independent;   ▲ = Collaborative;   EBN = Evidence-Based Nursing;   EB = Evidence-Based

- Demonstrate ability to engage in positive interactive experiences with parent(s)
- Demonstrate ability to process, organize, and respond to sensory information in an adaptive way

Parent/Significant Other

- Recognize infant/child behaviors as a unique way of communicating needs
- Recognize infant behaviors used to communicate stress/avoidance and approach/engagement
- Recognize and support infant/child's coping behaviors used to self-regulate
- Read and respond to infant/child behavior cues in a way that facilitates autonomic/physiologic, motor, and state organization
- Recognize how the personal style of interactions can positively or negatively affect the infant/child's responses
- Recognize that following the infant's lead will help in fostering effective interactions
- Identify appropriate positioning and handling techniques that will enhance normal motor development and prevent positioning acquired abnormalities (Wyngarden, DeWys & Padnos, 1999)
- Promote infant/child's attention capabilities to orient to visual and auditory input (Wyngarden, DeWys & Padnos, 1999)
- Engage in pleasurable parent/infant/child interactions that encourage bonding and attachment (Wyngarden, DeWys & Padnos, 1999)
- Structure and modify the environment in response to infant/child's behavioral, personal, nurturing, medical, and sensory needs (Wyngarden, DeWys & Padnos, 1999)
- Identify available community resources that provide early intervention services, emotional support, community health nursing, and parenting classes (Wyngarden, DeWys & Padnos, 1999)

NIC   Interventions (Nursing Interventions Classification)

Suggested NIC Interventions

Developmental Care, Infant, Positioning, Sleep Enhancement

Example NIC Activities—Development Care
Teach parents to recognize infant states and cues and respond in sensitive way

Nursing Interventions and *Rationales*

- Identify infant/child's behavioral organization as unique way of communicating in five subsystems of functioning (i.e., physiologic/autonomic, motor, state, self-regulatory, attention-interactional). The Assessment of Preterm Infants' Behavior (APIB) is a newborn neurobehavioral assessment appropriate for preterm, at risk, and full-term newborns, from birth to 1 month after expected due date. *The APIB is based in ethological-evolutionary thought and focuses on the assessment of mutually interacting behavioral subsystems in simultaneous interaction with the environment (Als et al, 2005).*
- Provide individualized developmental care for low-birth-weight, preterm infants that positively influences neurodevelopmental functioning and reduces the severity of medical illness. **EB:** *Positive outcomes include earlier transition to full oral feedings; younger discharge age; reduced hospital charges; improved weight, length, and head circumference; and lower family stress (Als et al, 2003).*
- Identify appropriate positioning and handling techniques that enhance normal development and motor organization and prevent position-acquired abnormalities. *Developmentally correct positioning (e.g., positioning in flexion, frequent positioning changes, using comforting physical containment as appropriate, giving opportunities for sucking and finger grasping) has been shown to be effective in providing comfort, decreasing stress, conserving energy, enhancing sleep, and facilitating normal development of the preterm infant (Aita & Snider, 2003; Sweeney & Gutierrez, 2002). EB: Prone positioning may improve quality of sleep and respiratory function and decrease stress for ventilated preterm infants (Chang, Anderson & Lin, 2002; see also Monterosso, Kristjanson & Cole, 2002).*

• = Independent;   ▲ = Collaborative;   EBN = Evidence-Based Nursing;   EB = Evidence-Based

- Demonstrate ways to facilitate state organization and control. *Pacing type, intensity, and timing of stimulation according to infant state and behavior cues is critical to facilitating state organization (Fajardo et al, 1990).* **EBN:** *Effective developmental handling during caregiving has been shown to promote behavioral state organization (Becker, Brazy & Grunwald, 1997).*
- Support the infant's need for uninterrupted sleep periods. Consider swaddling in supine position for sleep. *Physical containment decreases startles in quiet sleep (QS) and increases duration of rapid eye movement (REM) sleep that helps infants return to sleep without intervening. Handle infant slowly and gently, observing for cues of stress/stability (VandenBerg, 1999).*
- Cluster care whenever possible, allowing for longer periods of uninterrupted sleep. *Introduce one intervention at a time and observe infant cues, taking care not to overstimulate (Als et al, 1994).*
- Structure and organize the environment. *A developmental care approach designed to reduce environmental stress and facilitate motor and sleep-wake organization may result in improved behavioral organization during the preterm period (Als, 1998; Als et al, 1994; Buehler et al, 1995).*
- Identify and support the infant/child's use of self-regulatory/consoling behaviors needed for mastering the environment. **EBN:** *When providing infant stimulation, it can be helpful to modify developmental interventions based on physiologic and behavioral cues (Burns et al, 1994).*
- Recognize behavior used to communicate stress/avoidance and approach/engagement. *The ability to read and interpret infant/child behavior provides a framework for responding contingently, that is, in a way that communicates the infant/child's importance and ability to affect the environment (Als et al, 2005). When mothers evaluated their caregiving from birth through their infant's first year of life, they said that their most frequent source of confidence and competence came from their infant's contentedness of mood and soothability (Pridham, Chin-Yu & Brown, 2001).*
- Correlate stress/disorganized behaviors to internal factors (e.g., pain, hunger, discomfort) and/or external factors (e.g., lights, noise, handling). *Noise is one of the common stressors in hospital intensive care units (ICUs), resulting in sensory overload that has the potential to alter development adversely (DePaul & Chambers, 1995; Elander & Hellstrom, 1995). Intrauterine cocaine exposure can result in disorganized behavior patterns of infants (DeWys & McComish-Fry, 1992). Provide ongoing support during and after procedures (e.g., heel stick); stay with infant throughout recovery period (VandenBerg, 1999).*
- Provide opportunities for physical closeness, loving touch, massage, cuddling, skin-to-skin (Kangaroo Care), and rocking. *Infant massage has been found to be a therapeutic tool that improves developmental outcomes, decreases stress, increases weight gain, improves motor function, aids sleep, increases alert/awake periods, improves pain tolerance, leads to improved feeding tolerance, improves attachment, helps parents understand infant's cues, and enhances feelings of parental confidence (Beachy, 2003; Manious, 2002).* **EBN and EB:** *Parents have been found to be more sensitive and to show more positive affect when participating in skin-to-skin "Kangaroo" care (Feldman et al, 2002). Kangaroo Care provides an environment that supports autonomic stability and fosters improvement in basic physiological functions (Ludington-Hoe & Swinth, 1996). Infants who have had Kangaroo Care have been found to benefit with cardiorespiratory stabilization, improved oxygenation, improved thermoregulation, increased weight gain, earlier breastfeeding, less crying, increased quiet sleep, and decreased length of stay (Chwo et al, 2002; Ludington-Hoe et al, 1999; see also Ludington, 1990; Tessier et al, 1998).*
- Provide opportunities for parent/caregiver to engage in positive parent-infant interactions. *Engagement and disengagement are infant cues signaling responses to internal and external stimuli (Blackburn, 1978). The parent/caregiver becomes the mediator between infant and environment (Blackburn, 1983).*
- Encourage parents' competence by affirming their strengths and capabilities when caring for their infants. **EBN:** *New neonatal intensive care unit (NICU) mothers who participated in one parent-to-parent support program had less anxiety during the first four months post-discharge than the comparison group; at twelve months postdischarge, self-esteem was found to have increased, and mothers also had better maternal–infant relationships and more nurturing home environments (Roman et al, 1995). Parents must be supported and welcomed as active collaborators in their infant's care (Lawhon, 2002).*
- Identify and support infant/child's attention capabilities. *In organized quiet-alert states, infants are able to focus their attention and interact with their environment in a purposeful way. It is important to*

• = Independent;   ▲ = Collaborative;   EBN = Evidence-Based Nursing;   EB = Evidence-Based

give the baby opportunities to attend to sensory input, but not at the cost of behavioral disorganization (Burns et al, 1994). **EBN:** *A study of state organization of very low birth weight infants demonstrated the positive effects of developmental handling and recognized that alertness may be promoted without physiological and behavioral disorganization (Becker, Brazy & Grunwald, 1997).*

- Provide pleasurable experiences (i.e., visual, auditory, tactile, vestibular, proprioceptive) that enhance development of sensory pathways. *Healthy 33-34-week postconceptual age infants who received 15 minutes of auditory, visual, tactile, and vestibular stimulation each day were found to have improved state modulation and better ability to maintain quiet-alert state, resulting in enhanced parent-infant interactions and feedings (White-Traut et al, 1993). Observe how the infant responds to different sensations and modify as appropriate. Promote behavioral organization, positive patterns of maternal-infant interactions, and conserve energy for growth (Burns et al, 1994).*

▲ Provide information or refer to community based follow-up programs for preterm/at-risk infants and their families. *Seamless communication between NICU staff and community agencies enhances parent's feelings of confidence during the difficult transition from NICU discharge to home (Sherman et al, 2002).*

Multicultural

- Assess for the influence of cultural beliefs, norms, and values on the family's perceptions of infant/child behavior. **EBN:** *What the family considers normal infant/child behavior may be based on cultural perceptions (Guarnaccia, 1998; Leininger & McFarland, 2002).* **EBN:** *The theory of hot and cold espoused by many Mexican Americans have symbolic significance for the nature and process of reproduction and for the relationship between mother and child (Giger & Davidhizar, 2000). Beliefs related to the phenomena of communication, time, space, social organization, environmental control, and biological variations can all influence the family's perceptions of infant/child behavior (Giger & Davidhizar, 2000).*

- Use a neutral, indirect style when addressing areas where improvement is needed (such as a need for verbal or oral stimulation) when working with Native American clients. **EBN:** *Using indirect statements such as "Other mothers have tried…" or "I had a client who tried 'X' and it seemed to work very well" will assist in avoiding resentment from the parent (Seideman et al, 1996).*

- Use therapeutic communication techniques that emphasize acceptance, offer the self, validate the client's concerns, and convey respect when discussing the infant/child behavior. **EBN:** *Validation is a therapeutic communication technique that lets the client know that the nurse has heard and understands what was said, and it promotes the nurse-client relationship (Heineken, 1998).*

Family Teaching

- Assist family's support systems in recognizing and responding to infant's unique behavioral cues. *Demonstrating and modeling appropriate interactional skills is an integral component of family education and will improve family-infant interactions (McGrath & Conliffe-Torres, 1996).*

- Demonstrate calming interventions to provide parents with tools for positive interactions with their infant/child (Karl, 1999).

- Nurture parents so that they in turn can nurture their infant/child. *The psychological trauma to parents when their infant is hospitalized in the NICU cannot be underestimated (Doering, Dracup & Moser, 1999). The most difficult and overlooked aspects of care of the high risk neonate is effective, timely, and compassionate information delivery to parents and family by the medical staff (Sherman et al, 2002).*

- Establish a nurturing environment in which parents can interact with their infant/child (Goulet et al, 1998).

- Have knowledge of community early intervention services and follow-up programs for preterm and at-risk infants and families (Akers et al, 2007).

Home Care

- Above interventions may be adapted for home care use.

- Educate families in preparing home environment. *Patterns of sound, light, and caregiving tasks should minimize stress, conserve energy, and protect the developing neonate from inappropriate environmental stimuli (Akers et al, 2007; VandenBerg, 1999).*

• = Independent;   ▲ = Collaborative;   EBN = Evidence-Based Nursing;   EB = Evidence-Based

- Prepare families for realistic challenges of caring for preterm and at-risk infants prior to discharge. Areas include corrected versus chronological age, feeding skills, poor endurance/easy fatiguability, shorter sleep-wake cycles, decreased alertness and increased fussiness, overstimulation, and so forth. *Help parents identify their infant's characteristics, developmental capabilities and limitations, along with interventions that will support optimal growth and development. Facilitate creation of a support network that will help parents ease the transition from NICU to home (VandenBerg, 1999).*
- Encourage families to teach friends/visitors to recognize and respond to infant's unique behavioral cues. *It is important for families to feel comfortable obtaining support from their regular support systems; therefore, supportive persons need to be taught how to interact in the environment in a way that supports both the family and the infant (Als et al, 2005).*
- Provide information about community resources, developmental follow-up services, and parent-to-parent support programs. *Parents benefit from knowledge of their infant's autonomic sensitivity, lower sensory threshold, potential difficulties with self-calming, and more tentative ability to orient and attend to environmental and social stimuli. Additional anticipatory guidance should include knowledge about prevention of overstimulation and exhaustion of these more sensitive infants (Mouradian, Als & Coster, 2000).*

REFERENCES

Aita M, Snider L: The art of developmental care in the NICU: a concept analysis, *J Adv Nurs* 41(3):223, 2003.

Akers AL et al: InReach: connecting NICU infants and their parents with community early intervention services, *Zero to Three* 27(3), 2007.

Als H: Developmental care in the newborn intensive care unit, *Curr Opin Pediatr* 10:138, 1998.

Als H, Butler S, Kosta S et al: The Assessment of Preterm Infants' Behavior (APIB): furthering the understanding and measurement of neurodevelopmental competence in preterm and full-term infants, *Ment Retard Dev Disabil Res Rev* 11(1):94-102, 2005.

Als H, Gilkerson L, Duffy FH et al: A three-center, randomized, controlled trial of individualized developmental care for very low birth weight preterm infants: medical, neurodevelopmental, parenting, and caregiving effects, *J Dev & Behav Pediatr* 24(6):399-408, 2003.

Als H, Lawhon G, Duffy FH et al: Individualized developmental care for the very-low-birth-weight preterm infant: medical and neurofunctional effects, *JAMA* 272(11):853-858, 1994.

Beachy JM: Premature infant massage in the NICU, *Neonatal Netw* 22(3):39-45, 2003.

Becker PT, Brazy JE, Grunwald PC: Behavioral state organization of very low birth weight infants: effects of developmental handling during caregiving, *Infant Behav Dev* 20(4):503, 1997.

Blackburn S: Fostering behavior development of high-risk infants, *J Obst Gynecol Neonatal Nurs* 12:76-86, 1983.

Blackburn S: State related behaviors and individual differences. In Barnard KE, editor: *Nursing child assessment satellite training: learning resource manual,* Seattle, 1978, University of Washington, pp 29-39.

Buehler D, Als H, Duffy FH et al: Effectiveness of individualized developmental care for low-risk preterm infants: behavioral and electrophysiologic evidence, *Pediatrics* 96(5):923-932, 1995.

Burns K, Cunningham M, White-Traut R et al: Infant stimulation: modification of an intervention based on physiologic and behavioral cues, *J Obstet Gynecol Neonatal Nurs* 23(7):581-589, 1994.

Chang Y, Anderson G, Lin C: Effects of prone and supine positions on sleep state and stress responses in mechanically ventilated preterm infants during the first postnatal week, *J Adv Nurs* 40(2):161, 2002.

Chwo M, Anderson GC, Good M et al: A randomized controlled trial of early kangaroo care for preterm infants: effects on temperature, weight, behavior, and acuity, *J Nurs Res* 10(2):129-142, 2002.

DePaul D, Chambers SE: Environmental noise in the neonatal intensive care unit: implications for nursing practice, *J Perinatal Neonatal Nurs* 8:71, 1995.

DeWys M, McComish-Fry J: *Infants states and cues: facilitating effective parent-infant interactions.* In *Caring for infants: a resource manual for caring for infant trainers,* East Lansing, MI, 1992, Michigan State University Board of Trustees.

Doering LV, Dracup K, Moser D: Comparison of psychosocial adjustment of mothers and fathers of high-risk infants in the neonatal intensive care unit, *J Perinatol* 19(3):132-137, 1999.

Elander G, Hellstrom G: Reduction of noise levels in intensive care units for infants: evaluation of an intervention program, *Heart Lung* 24:376, 1995.

Fajardo B, Browning M, Fisher D et al: Effect of nursery environment on state regulation in very-low-birth-weight premature infants, *Infant Behav Dev* 13:287-303, 1990.

Feldman R, Eidelman AI, Sirota L et al: Comparison of skin-to-skin (kangaroo) and traditional care: parenting outcomes and preterm infant development, *Pediatrics* 110(1 Pt 1):16-26, 2002.

Giger J, Davidhizar R: *Transcultural nursing: assessment and intervention,* St. Louis, 2000, Mosby.

Goulet C, Bell L, St-Cyr D et al: A concept analysis of parent-infant attachment, *J Adv Nurs* 28(5):1071, 1998.

Guarnaccia PJ: Multicultural experiences of family caregiving: a study of African American, European American, and Hispanic American families, *New Direct Ment Health Serv* (77):45-61, Spring 1998.

Heineken J: Patient silence is not necessarily client satisfaction: communication in home care nursing, *Home Healthc Nurse* 16(2):115, 1998.

Karl D: The interactive newborn bath: using infant neurobehavior to connect parents and newborns, *MCN Am J Matern Child Nurse* 24(6):280, 1999.

Lawhon G: Facilitation of parenting the premature infant within the newborn intensive care unit, *J Perinatal Neonatal Nurs* 16(1):71, 2002.

Leininger MM, McFarland MR: *Transcultural nursing: concepts, theories, research and practices,* ed 3, New York, 2002, McGraw-Hill.

Ludington SM: Energy conservation during skin-to-skin contact between preterm infants and their mothers, *Heart Lung* 19(5 pt 1):445, 1990.

Ludington-Hoe SM, Anderson GC, Simpson S et al: Birth-related fatigue in 34-36–week preterm neonates: rapid recovery with very early kangaroo (skin-to-skin) care, *J Obstet Gynecol Neonatal Nurs* 28(1):94-103, 1999.

Ludington-Hoe SM, Swinth JY: Developmental aspects of kangaroo care, *J Obstet Gynecol Neonatal Nurs* 25(8):691, 1996.

Manious R: Infant massage as a component of developmental care: past, present, and future, *Holist Nurs Pract* 16(5):1, 2002.

McGrath J, Conliffe-Torres S: Integrating family-centered developmental assessment and intervention into routine care in the neonatal intensive care unit, *Nurs Clin North Am* 31(2):367, 1996.

Monterosso L, Kristjanson L, Cole J: Neuromotor development and the physiologic effects of positioning in very low birth weight infants, *J Obstet Gynecol Neonatal Nurs* 31(2):128, 2002.

Mouradian LE, Als H, Coster WJ: Neurobehavioral functioning of healthy preterm infants of varying gestational ages, *J Dev Behav Pediatr*, 21(6):408-427, 2000.

Pridham K, Chin-Yu CY, Brown R: Mothers' evaluation of their caregiving for premature and full-term infants through the first: contributing factors, *Res Nurs Health* 24(3):157-169, 2001.

Roman LA, Lindsey JK, Boger RP et al: Parent-to-parent support initiated in the neonatal intensive care unit, *Res Nurs Health* 18(5):385-394, 1995.

Seideman RY, Jacobson S, Primeaux M et al: Assessing American Indian families, *MCN Am J Matern Child Nurs* 21(6):274, 1996.

Sherman MP et al: *Follow-up of the NICU patient,* www.emedicine Medicine: Instant Access to the Minds of Medicine, 2002.

Sweeney J, Gutierrez T: Musculoskeletal implications of preterm infant positioning in the NICU, *J Perinatal Neonatal Nurs* 16(1):58, 2002.

Tessier R, Cristo M, Velez S et al: Kangaroo mother care and the bonding hypothesis, *Pediatrics* 102(2):e17, 1998.

VandenBerg KA: What to tell parents about the developmental needs of their baby at discharge, *Neonatal Netw* 18(1):57, 1999.

White-Traut R, Nelson MN, Silvestri JM et al: Patterns of physiological and behavioral response of intermediate care preterm infants to intervention, *Pediatr Nurs* 19(6):625-629, 1993.

Wyngarden K, DeWys M, Padnos P: *Learnings from the field: the impact of using two new nursing diagnoses, organized infant behavior and disorganized infant behavior* (abstract), Classification of Nursing Diagnoses: Proceedings of the Thirteenth Conference, NANDA, 1999.

I

Risk for disorganized Infant behavior
Mary DeWys, RN, BS, Kathy Wyngarden, MSN, FNP, RN, and Peg Padnos, RN, BA, BSN

NANDA   Definition

Risk for alteration in integrating and modulation of the physiological and behavioral systems of functioning (i.e., autonomic, motor, state, organizational, self-regulatory, and attentional-interactional systems)

Risk Factors

Environmental overstimulation; invasive procedures; lack of containment within environment; motor problems; oral problems; pain; painful procedures; prematurity

NOC   Outcomes (Nursing Outcomes Classification)

Suggested NOC Outcomes

Child Development, Neurological Status, Preterm Infant Organization, Sleep, Thermoregulation: Newborn

Example NOC Outcome with Indicators
Preterm Infant Organization as evidenced by the following indicators: O_2 saturation >85%/Thermoregulation/Feeding tolerance/Self-consolability/Quiet-alert/Attentiveness to stimuli/Response to stimuli (Rate the outcome and indicators of **Preterm Infant Organization:** 1 = severely compromised, 2 = substantially compromised, 3 = moderately compromised, 4 = mildly compromised, 5 = not compromised [see Section 1].)

Client Outcomes

Client Will (Specify Time Frame):
Infant/Child
- Display physiologic/autonomic stability: cardiorespiratory, visceral, neurofunctional
- Display organized motor system (Wyngarden, DeWys & Padnos, 1999)
- Display signs of state organization (Wyngarden, DeWys & Padnos, 1999)

• = Independent;   ▲ = Collaborative;   EBN = Evidence-Based Nursing;   EB = Evidence-Based

- Demonstrate progress toward effective self-regulation: display range of effective self-regulatory behaviors (Wyngarden, DeWys & Padnos, 1999)
- Display clear behavior cues that communicate approach/engagement and stress/avoidance (Wyngarden, DeWys & Padnos, 1999)
- Demonstrate ability to engage in positive interactive experiences with parent(s)
- Demonstrate ability to process, organize, and respond to sensory information in an adaptive way

Parent/Significant Other

- Recognize infant/child behaviors as a unique way of communicating needs
- Recognize infant behaviors used to communicate stress/avoidance and approach/engagement
- Recognize and support infant/child's coping behaviors used to self-regulate
- Read and respond to infant/child behavior cues in a way that facilitates autonomic/physiologic, motor, and state organization
- Recognize how the personal style of interactions can positively or negatively affect the infant/child's responses
- Recognize that following the infant's lead will help in fostering effective interactions
- Identify appropriate positioning and handling techniques that will enhance normal motor development and prevent positioning acquired abnormalities (Wyngarden, DeWys & Padnos, 1999)
- Promote infant/child's attention capabilities to orient to visual and auditory input (Wyngarden, DeWys & Padnos, 1999)
- Engage in pleasurable parent/infant/child interactions that encourage bonding and attachment (Wyngarden, DeWys & Padnos, 1999)
- Structure and modify the environment in response to infant/child's behavioral, personal, nurturing, medical, and sensory needs (Wyngarden, DeWys & Padnos, 1999)
- Identify available community resources that provide early intervention services, emotional support, community health nursing, and parenting classes (Wyngarden, DeWys & Padnos, 1999)

NIC   Interventions (Nursing Interventions Classification)

Suggested NIC Interventions

Developmental Care, Infant Care, Positioning, Sleep Enhancement

Example NIC Activities—Developmental Care
Teach parents to recognize infant cues and states; Assist parents in planning care responsiveness to infant cues and states

Nursing Interventions and *Rationales*

Refer to **Disorganized Infant behavior**

REFERENCE

Wyngarden K, DeWys M, Padnos M: Learnings from the field: the impact of using two new nursing diagnoses, organized infant behavior and disorganized infant behavior (abstract), *Classification of nursing diagnoses: proceedings of the thirteenth conference,* NANDA, 1999.

Readiness for enhanced organized Infant behavior

Mary DeWys, RN, BS, and Peg Padnos, RN, BA, BSN

NANDA   Definition

A pattern of modulation of the physiological and behavioral systems of functioning (i.e., autonomic, motor, state-organizational, self-regulatory, and attentional-interactional systems) in an infant that is satisfactory but that can be improved

Defining Characteristics

Definite sleep-wake states; response to stimuli (e.g., visual, auditory); stable physiologic measures; use of some self-regulatory behaviors

Related Factors (r/t)

Pain, prematurity

NOC   Outcomes (Nursing Outcomes Classification)

Suggested NOC Outcomes

Child Development, Neurological Status, Preterm Infant Organization, Sleep, Thermoregulation: Newborn

Example NOC Outcome with Indicators
Preterm Infant Organization as evidenced by the following indicators: O_2 saturation >85%/ Thermoregulation/Feeding tolerance/Self-consolability/Quiet-alert/Attentiveness to stimuli/Response to stimuli (Rate the outcome and indicators of **Preterm Infant Organization:** 1 = severely compromised, 2 = substantially compromised, 3 = moderately compromised, 4 = mildly compromised, 5 = not compromised [see Section I].)

Client Outcomes

Client Will (Specify Time Frame):

Infant/Child

- Display stable vital signs and skin color
- Display smooth, synchronous, and purposeful body movements
- Display range of clear sleep and awake states
- Display smooth transitions between sleep and wake states
- Demonstrate range of effective self-consoling behaviors
- Demonstrate smooth visceral/digestive functioning without feeding intolerances
- Ability to effectively attend and interact with the environment with minimal stress
- Enjoy engaging in reciprocal social play experiences
- Display pleasure with sensory-motor experiences
- Is not "over-" or "under reactive" to sensory-motor experiences (visual, auditory, tactile, movement, body awareness)
- Continue to demonstrate progressive growth and development

Parents/Significant Other

- Demonstrate ways to structure and modify the environment that enhances the infant/child's own adaptive capacity for achieving optimal physiologic and neurobehavioral functioning
- Identify their infant/child's behaviors that signal "stress/avoidance" or "approach"
- Demonstrate ways to facilitate motor organization and development by appropriate handling and positioning techniques
- Demonstrate care that is contingent with the state of the infant/child
- Demonstrate additional ways to facilitate state organization/development

● = Independent;   ▲ = Collaborative;   EBN = Evidence-Based Nursing;   EB = Evidence-Based

- Support and expand infant's/child's self-regulatory skills
- Demonstrate ways to help infant/child achieve an attentive state that allows him/her to orient to visual and auditory sensory stimuli
- Support and expand infant/child's calm alert periods, the ideal state for learning and interacting
- Demonstrate ways to engage the infant/child in social interactions and allow the infant/child to lead the interaction
- Demonstrate contingent responses to the infant/child's approach/engagement and avoidance/disengagement cues
- Demonstrate ways to provide pleasurable and developmentally appropriate sensory-motor experiences (visual, auditory, tactile, movement, body awareness)

NIC Interventions (Nursing Interventions Classification)

Suggested NIC Interventions

Developmental Care, Environmental Management, Kangaroo Care, Newborn Monitoring, Nonnutritive Sucking, Positioning, Sleep Enhancement

Example NIC Activities—Developmental Care
Provide water mattress and sheepskin, as appropriate; Use smallest diaper to prevent hip abduction

Nursing Interventions and *Rationales*

Refer to care plans for **Disorganized Infant behavior** and **Risk for disorganized Infant behavior.**
NOTE: Interventions should be based on individual response of the infant/child to each intervention. Interventions appropriate for one infant/child may not be appropriate for another. In addition, a particular intervention that seems appropriate for one infant/child at a particular time may not be as effective with the same infant/child at another time. Carefully observe for the desired adaptive response or expected outcomes and continually reevaluate. Nursing care that is responsive and contingent with the state of the infant is ideal; however, if stressful events occur, provide appropriate interventions to minimize stress and facilitate self-regulation.

Ineffective Infant feeding pattern *Mary DeWys, RN, BS, and Peg Padnos, RN, BSN*

NANDA Definition

Impaired ability of an infant to suck or coordinate the suck/swallow response resulting in inadequate oral nutrition for metabolic needs

Defining Characteristics

Inability to coordinate sucking, swallowing, and breathing; inability to initiate an effective suck; inability to sustain an effective suck

Related Factors (r/t)

Anatomic abnormality; neurological delay; neurological impairment; oral hypersensitivity; prematurity; prolonged NPO status

NOC Outcomes (Nursing Outcomes Classification)

Suggested NOC Outcomes

Breastfeeding Establishment: Infant, Maternal, Breastfeeding: Maintenance, Hydration, Nutritional Status: Food and Fluid Intake

Example NOC Outcome with Indicators
Breastfeeding Establishment: Infant as evidenced by the following indicators: Proper alignment and latch on/Correct suck and tongue placement/Urinations per day appropriate for age/Weight gain appropriate for age (Rate the outcome and indicators of **Breastfeeding Establishment: Infant**: 1 = not adequate, 2 = slightly adequate, 3 = moderately adequate, 4 = substantially adequate, 5 = totally adequate [see Section I].)

Client Outcomes

Infant Will (Specify Time Frame):

- Consume adequate calories that will result in appropriate weight gain and optimal growth and development
- Have opportunities for skin-to-skin (kangaroo care) experiences
- Have opportunities for "trophic" (i.e., small volume of breastmilk/formula) enteral feedings prior to full oral feedings
- Progress to stable, neurobehavioral organization (i.e., motor, state, self-regulation, attention-interaction)
- Demonstrate presence of mature oral reflexes that are necessary for safe feeding
- Progress to safe, self-regulated oral feedings
- Coordinate the suck-swallow-breathe sequence while nippling
- Display clear behavioral cues related to hunger and satiety
- Display approach/engagement cues, with minimal avoidance/disengagement cues
- Have opportunities to pace own feeding, taking breaks as needed
- Display evidence of being in the "quiet-alert" state while nippling
- Progress to and engage in mutually positive parent/caregiver-infant/child interactions during feedings

Parent/Family Will (Specify Time Frame):

- Recognize necessity of adequate calories for appropriate weight gain and optimal growth and development
- Learn to read and respond contingently to infant's behavioral cues (e.g., hunger, satiety, approach/engagement, stress/avoidance/disengagement)
- Learn strategies that promote organized infant behavior
- Learn appropriate positioning and handling techniques
- Learn effective ways to relieve stress behaviors during nippling
- Learn ways to help infant coordinate suck-swallow-breathe sequence (i.e., external pacing techniques)
- Engage in mutually positive interactions with infant during feeding
- Recognize ways to facilitate effective feedings: feed in quiet-alert state; keep length of feeding appropriate; burp; prepare/structure environment; recognize signs of sensory overload; encourage self-regulation; respect need for breaks and breathing pauses; avoid pulling and twisting nipple during pauses; allow infant to resume sucking when ready; provide oral support (cheek and/or jaw) as needed; use appropriate nipple hole size and flow rate

NIC   Interventions (Nursing Interventions Classification)

Suggested NIC Interventions

Bottle Feeding, Breastfeeding Assistance, Fluid Monitoring, Kangaroo Care, Lactation Counseling, Teaching: Infant Safety

Example NIC Activities—Lactation Counseling
Provide information about advantages and disadvantages of breastfeeding; Discuss alternative methods of feeding

Nursing Interventions and *Rationales*

- Refer to care plans for **Disorganized Infant behavior and Risk for disorganized Infant behavior, Effective, Ineffective,** and **Interrupted Breastfeeding** and assess as needed.
- Interventions follow a sequential pattern of implementation that can be adapted as appropriate.
- Assess infant's functional oral reflexes (i.e., root, gag, suck, swallow, cough). *Postnatal development of oral functional reflexes is necessary for effective oral feedings: gag at 34 weeks, suck/swallow at 28-30 weeks; nonnutritive sucking (NNS) at 33 weeks; coordinated ability to suck-swallow-breathe at 36-38 weeks (Lau et al, 2000).*
- Assess infant's suck, swallow, and breathing coordination in a 1:1:1 ratio. *As infants mature they become more able to coordinate breathing with sucking and swallowing (Medoff-Cooper, McGrath & Bilker, 2000).* **EB:** *The inability to maintain a 2-minute pattern is attributed to fatigue, habituation, and respiratory compromise (Palmer, Crawley & Blanco, 1993).*
- Assess infant's baseline cardiopulmonary parameters prior to, during, and 10 minutes after feeding. *Determine oxygen requirements for infants with bronchopulmonary dysplasia (BPD), respiratory distress syndrome (RDS), and chronic lung disease (CLD) because these clients work hard at breathing, gulp their feedings and become exhausted, all of which increase risk of aspiration (VandenBerg, 1990).*
- Assess for attachment behaviors that can affect a feeding, negatively or positively. *Mothers who are warm, emotionally available, and sensitive in reading and responding to cues and communicated needs for comfort and nurturance are more likely to have infants who are securely attached to them (Boris, Aoki & Zeanah, 1999). Insecure attachment may intensify feeding problems and may lead to severe malnutrition (Chatoor et al, 1998).*
- ▲ Provide developmentally supportive neonatal intensive care for preterm infants. *Developmentally supportive care refers to the provision of social interactions and necessary nursing interventions in a fashion that supports the neurodevelopmental and physiological stability of the neonate (Taquino & Lockridge, 1999).*
- Provide opportunities for kangaroo (i.e., skin-to-skin) care. *Very early skin-to-skin contact enhanced breastfeeding success during the early postpartum period. No significant differences were found at 1 month (Moore & Anderson, 2007).*
- ▲ Before the infant is ready for oral feedings, implement gavage feedings (or other alternative) as ordered, using breast milk whenever possible. *Gavage feedings may be necessary because serious illness can interfere with a neonate's ability to suck; calories and nutrient needs are increased by the stress of illness (Medoff-Cooper, McGrath & Bilker, 2000).*
- ▲ Provide a naturalistic environment for tube feedings (naso-oro-gastric, gavage, or other) that approximates a pleasurable oral feeding experience: hold in semi-upright/flexed position; offer NNS; pace feedings; allow for semi-demand feedings contingent with infant cues; offer rest breaks; burp, as appropriate. **EBN:** *Sucking helps calm infants, thus raising oxygen level, aiding digestion, increasing average daily weight gain, and preparing them for earlier nipple feedings and discharge (McCain et al, 2001; Shiao, 1997).*
- Provide 10 minutes of NNS prior to oral feeding. **EBN:** *Ten minutes of NNS has been found to promote the awake state and lower heart rate before feeding (McCain, 1995).*
- ▲ Consider trophic (i.e., small volume) feedings for high-risk hospitalized infants if appropriate. **EB:** *Trophic feedings provide minimum enteral nutrition, help infants attain earlier full oral, and contribute to earlier hospital discharge (Anderson & Loughead, 2002).*
- Structure the environment and modify sensory stimuli according to infant's physiologic and behavioral organization. *Full-term infants are able to show appropriate and organized physiological and state behavior in response to internal and external stimuli, whereas preterm infants' state behavior is less well-organized and less well-communicated to caregivers. Cardiorespiratory stability is necessary for nipple feedings (Shiao, 1997).*
- Position preterm infant in semi-upright position, with head in neutral alignment, chin slightly tucked, back straight, shoulders/arms forward, hands in midline, hips flexed 90 degrees. **EBN:** *"Total sucking pattern" of the full-term newborn combines strong physiological flexion and high rib cage position to provide support for the tongue and jaw, which is essential for effective nippling (Brandon, Holditch-Davis & Beylea, 1999; Brown & Heermann, 1997). The modified, upright, side-*

lying position used in breastfeeding may be effective for some premature infants (Fraker & Walbert, 2003).

- Feed infant in the quiet-alert state. *The quiet-alert state was found to be optimal for feeding preterm infants (Brandt, Andrews & Kvale, 1998; McCain, 1997; Medoff-Cooper, McGrath & Bilker, 2000).*
- Determine the appropriate shape, size, and hole of nipple to provide flow rate for preterm infants that facilitates 1:1:1 ratio of suck-swallow-breathe sequence. *High-flow and soft nipples, which are often incorrectly used to feed preterm infants, may exacerbate difficulties in coordinated sucking, swallowing, and breathing (Matthews, 1994).*
- Implement external pacing for infants having difficulty coordinating breathing with sucking and swallowing. *Tip infant and bottle forward so no liquid collects in the nipple. Once infant takes a breath, gently tip him or her and bottle back to semi-upright position so that liquid returns to nipple. Repeat until infant is able to maintain a coordinated pattern (Matthews, 1994).*
- Provide infants with jaw and/or cheek support, as needed. **EBN:** *Oral support provided stability for the preterm infant's jaw and cheeks and resulted in decreased frequency and length of pauses between bursts without interfering with cardiopulmonary functioning (Hill, Kurkowski & Garcia, 2000).*
- Allow appropriate time for nipple feeding to ensure infant's safety. **EBN:** *Nipple feeding can lead to nutritional deficits because of increased metabolic demands. (Hill, Kurkowski & Garcia, 2000; Shiao, 1997).*
- Monitor length of feeding so that it does not exceed 30 minutes. *Efficient feeders will consume half of the amount within the first five minutes (Case-Smith, Cooper & Scala, 1989).* **EBN:** *Feeding length correlates with presence of stress indicators that interfere with feeding effectiveness (Glass & Wolf, 1994; McCain, 2003).*
- Encourage transitioning from scheduled to semi-demand feedings, contingent with infant behavior cues. **EBN:** *Healthy preterm infants 32 to 33 weeks postconceptual age, who followed a semi-demand protocol that included NNS to promote awake behavior, were found to be more often in a quiet-alert state for feedings, more efficient feeders, and more often in a sleep state after feedings than their control counterparts (McCain, 2003).*
- Progress to self-regulatory feedings based on the infant's hunger and satiety cues. **EBN:** *"Hunger signs include movement of the hand to the mouth, pacifier sucking, sucking on the fingers or fist, restlessness, and fussy crying" (McCain, 2003).*
- Encourage the parents to engage other family members in the feeding process. *Nurses can promote the psychosocial development of the at-risk infant and family by encouraging the parents' caregiving ability (Moran et al, 1999).*
- ▲ Refer to a multidisciplinary team (e.g., neonatal/pediatric nutritionist, physical or occupational therapist, speech pathologist, lactation specialist, as needed. *Collaborative practice with others who are specially trained to meet the needs of this vulnerable population will help ensure feeding and parenting success (Caretto et al, 2000).*

Home Care

- The above appropriate interventions may be adapted for home care use.
- ▲ Infants with risk factors and clinical indicators of feeding problems present prior to hospital discharge should be referred to appropriate community early-intervention service providers (e.g., community health nurses, Early-On, occupational therapy, speech pathologists, feeding specialists) to facilitate adequate weight gain for optimal growth and development. *Home visitation by maternal-child nurses and/or certified lactation consultants, working collaboratively with the attending physician, midwife, or nurse practitioner, is recommended for breastfeeding mothers whose infants are at risk for dehydration, weight loss, and hyperbilirubinemia (Locklin & Jansson, 1999). Feeding difficulties and jaundice top the list of non-life-threatening reasons for rehospitalization of infants discharged from NICU during the first two weeks postdischarge (Escobar et al, 1999).*

Family Teaching

- Provide anticipatory guidance for infant's expected feeding course. *Knowing what to anticipate helps the family feel involved and enhances attachment (Caretto et al, 2000; Huckabay, 1999).*
- Teach various effective feeding methods and strategies to parent(s). *Parents should be involved in*

---

the feeding process as soon as possible to enhance attachment and increase their confidence in their ability to nurture a child (Bruschweiler, 1998; Huckabay, 1999).

- Teach parents how to read, interpret, and respond contingently to infant cues. *Parents' understanding of infant cues may increase their involvement in caring for the infant by improving their perception of the infant's abilities (Medoff-Cooper, McGrath & Bilker, 2000).*
- Provide a family-focused caring environment that supports parents in their primary caregiving role. **EB:** *It is important to build nurturing relationships within the NICU environment among infants, parents, nurses, and staff where "strengths are emphasized while vulnerabilities are partnered" (Gilkerson & Als, 1995).*
- Help parents identify support systems prior to hospital discharge. *This should include immediate and extended family members and friends; if necessary, include these persons in family teaching sessions (Griffin & Abraham, 2006).*
- Provide anticipatory guidance for the infant's discharge. *Parents need assistance in assuming responsibility for infant care as the day of discharge approaches (Davis, Lodgson & Birkmer, 1996; Elliot & Reimer, 1998).*

evolve See the EVOLVE website for World Wide Web resources for client education.

REFERENCES

Anderson DM, Loughead JL: Feeding the ill or preterm infant, *Neonatal Netw* 21(7):7, 2002.

Boris NW, Aoki Y, Zeanah CH: The development of infant-parent attachment: considerations for assessment, *Infants Young Child* 11(4):1, 1999.

Brandon DH, Holditch-Davis D, Beylea M: Nursing care and the development of sleeping and waking behaviors in preterm infants, *Res Nurs Health* 22(3):217, 1999.

Brandt KA, Andrews CM, Kvale J: Mother-infant interaction and breast-feeding outcome six weeks after birth, *J Obstet Gynecol Neonatal Nurs* 27:169, 1998.

Brown LD, Heerman JA: The effect of developmental care on preterm infant outcome, *Appl Nurs Res* 10(4):190, 1997.

Bruschweiler SN: Early emotional care for mothers and infants, *Pediatrics* 102(5 suppl E):1278, 1998.

Caretto V, Topolski KF, Linkous CM et al: Current parent education on infant feeding in the neonatal intensive care unit: the role of the occupational therapist, *Am J Occup Ther* 54(1):59, 2000.

Case-Smith J, Cooper P, Scala V: Feeding efficiency of premature neonates, *Am J Occup Ther* 43(4):245, 1989.

Chatoor I, Ganiban J, Colin V et al: Attachment and feeding problems: a reexamination of nonorganic failure to thrive and attachment insecurity, *J Am Acad Child Adolesc Psychiatry* 37(11):1217, 1998.

Davis DW, Logsdon MC, Birkmer JC: Types of support expected and received by mothers after their infants' discharge from the NICU, *Issues Compr Pediatr Nurs* 19(4):263, 1996.

Elliott S, Reimer C: Postdischarge telephone follow-up program for breastfeeding preterm infants discharged from a special care nursery, *Neonatal Netw* 17(6):41, 1998.

Escobar GJ, Joffe S, Gardner MN et al: Rehospitalization in the first two weeks after discharge from the neonatal intensive care unit, *Pediatrics* 104(1):e2, 1999.

Fraker C, Walbert L, editors: *Evaluation and treatment of pediatric feeding disorders from NICU to childhood,* Austin, Tex, 2003, Pro-ed.

Gilkerson L, Als H: Role of reflective process in the implementation of developmentally supportive care in the newborn intensive care nursery, *Inf Young Child* 7(4):20, 1995.

Glass RP, Wolf LS: A global perspective on feeding assessment in the neonatal intensive care unit, *Am J Occup Ther* 48(6):514, 1994.

Griffin T, Abraham M: Transition to home from the newborn intensive care unit: applying the principles of family-centered care in the discharge process, *J Perinatal Neonatal Nurs* 20(3):243-249, 2006.

Hill AS, Kurkowski TB, Garcia J: Oral support measures used in feeding the preterm infant, *Nurs Res* 49(1):2, 2000.

Huckabay LM: The effect on bonding behavior of giving a mother her premature baby's picture, *Sch Inq Nurs Pract* 13(4):349, 1999.

Lau C, Alagugurusamy R, Schanler RJ et al: Characterization of the developmental stages of sucking in preterm infants during bottle feeding, *Acta Paediatr* 89(7):846, 2000.

Locklin MP, Jansson MJ: Home visits: strategies to protect the breast-feeding newborn at risk, *J Obstet Gynecol Neonatal Nurs* 28(1):34, 1999.

Matthews GL: Supporting suck-swallow-breathe coordination during nipple feeding, *Am J Occup Ther* 48(6):561, 1994.

McCain GC: An evidence-based guideline for introducing oral feeding to healthy preterm infants, *Neonatal Netw* 22(5):45, 2003.

McCain GC: Behavioral state activity during nipple feedings for preterm infants, *Neonatal Netw* 16(5):43, 1997.

McCain GC: Promotion of preterm infant nipple feeding with nonnutritive sucking, *J Pediatr Nurs* 10(1):3, 1995.

McCain GC, Gartside PS, Greenberg JM et al: A feeding protocol for healthy preterm infants that shortens time to oral feeding, *J Pediatr* 139(3):374, 2001.

Medoff-Cooper B, McGrath JM, Bilker W: Nutritive sucking and neurobehavioral development in preterm infants from 34 weeks PCA to term, *MCN Am J Matern Child Nurs* 25(2):64, 2000.

Moore ER, Anderson GC: Randomized controlled trial of very early mother-infant skin-to-skin contact and breastfeeding status, *J Midwifery Womens Health* 52(2):116-125, Apr 2007.

Moran M, Radzyminski SG, Higgins KR et al: Maternal kangaroo (skin-to-skin) care in the NICU beginning 4 hours postbirth, *MCN Am J Matern Child Nurs* 24(2):74, 1999.

Palmer MM, Crawley K, Blanco IA: Neonatal Oral-Motor Assessment Scale: a reliability study, *J Perinatol* 13(1):28, 1993.

Shiao SY: Comparison of continuous versus intermittent sucking in very-low-birth-weight infants, *J Obstet Gynecol Neonatal Nurs* 26:313, 1997.

Taquino LT, Lockridge T: Caring for critically ill infants: strategies to promote physiological stability and improve developmental outcomes, *Crit Care Nurse* 19(6):64, 1999.

VandenBerg KA: Nippling management of the sick neonate in the NICU: the disorganized feeder, *Neonatal Netw* 9(1):9, 1990.

• = Independent; ▲ = Collaborative; EBN = Evidence-Based Nursing; EB = Evidence-Based

Risk for Infection   *Gail B. Ladwig, MSN, CHTP, RN*   *evolve*

NANDA   **Definition**

At increased risk for being invaded by pathogenic organisms

Risk Factors

Chronic disease; inadequate acquired immunity; inadequate primary defenses (broken skin, traumatized tissue, decrease in ciliary action, stasis of body fluids, change in pH secretions, altered peristalsis); inadequate secondary defenses (decreased hemoglobin, leucopenia, suppressed inflammatory response); increased environmental exposure to pathogens; immunosuppression; invasive procedures; insufficient knowledge to avoid exposure to pathogens; malnutrition; pharmaceutical agents (e.g., immunosuppressants); rupture of amniotic membranes; trauma; tissue destruction

NOC   **Outcomes (Nursing Outcomes Classification)**

Suggested NOC Outcomes

Immune Status, Knowledge: Infection Control, Risk Control, Risk Detection

Example NOC Outcome with Indicators
Immune Status as evidenced by the following indicators: Recurrent infections not present/Skin and mucosa integrity/Gastrointestinal (GI), Respiratory, Genitourinary (GU) function/Weight and body temperature in expected range (Rate the outcome and indicators of **Immune Status:** 1 = severely compromised, 2 = substantially compromised, 3 = moderately compromised, 4 = mildly compromised, 5 = not compromised [see Section I].)

Client Outcomes

Client Will (Specify Time Frame):

- Remain free from symptoms of infection
- State symptoms of infection of which to be aware
- Demonstrate appropriate care of infection-prone site
- Maintain white blood cell count and differential within normal limits
- Demonstrate appropriate hygienic measures such as hand washing, oral care, and perineal care

NIC   **Interventions (Nursing Interventions Classification)**

Suggested NIC Interventions

Immunization/Vaccination Administration, Infection Control, Infection Protection

Example NIC Activities—Infection Control
Wash hands before and after each patient care activity; Ensure aseptic handling of all intravenous lines; Ensure appropriate wound care technique; Teach patient and family members how to avoid infections

Nursing Interventions and *Rationales*

- ▲ Consider targeted surveillance for methicillin-resistant Staphylococcus aureus (MRSA) (screen clients at risk for MRSA on admission). *Targeted surveillance for MRSA colonization was cost-effective and provided substantial benefits by reducing the rate of nosocomial MRSA infections in a community hospital system (West et al, 2006).*
- ▲ Observe and report signs of infection such as redness, warmth, discharge, and increased body temperature. **EB:** *Prospective surveillance study for nosocomial infection on hematology-oncology units should include fever of unknown origin as the single most common and clinically important entity (Engelhart et al, 2002).*

• = Independent;   ▲ = Collaborative;   EBN = Evidence-Based Nursing;   EB = Evidence-Based

- ▲ Assess temperature of neutropenic clients; report a single temperature of greater than (100.5° F) *Fever is often the first sign of an infection (NCCN, 2006).*
- Oral or tympanic thermometers may be used to assess temperature in adults and infants. **EBN:** *The use of tympanic thermometers in addition to oral thermometers in obtaining temperatures is supported (Gilbert, Barton & Counsell, 2002). Tympanic membrane temperature recordings in healthy preterm neonates are safe, accurate, easy, and comfortable for the baby (Bailey & Rose, 2001).*
- The chemical (Tempa.DOT) thermometer may be used with intensive care unit (ICU) clients. *This study demonstrated the accuracy of the chemical thermometer but the pulmonary artery catheter remains the "gold standard" (Farnell et al, 2005).*
- ▲ Note and report laboratory values (e.g., white blood cell count and differential, serum protein, serum albumin, and cultures). **EB:** *The white blood cell count and the automated absolute neutrophil count are better diagnostic tests for adults and most children (Cornbleet, 2002).*
- Assess skin for color, moisture, texture, and turgor (elasticity). Keep accurate, ongoing documentation of changes. *The skin is the body's first line of defense in protecting the body from infection (NCCN, 2006).*
- Carefully wash and pat dry skin, including skinfold areas. Use hydration and moisturization on all at-risk surfaces. **EBN:** *Atopic dermatitis is a common, chronic skin condition that can be managed in most clients by prescribing avoidance measures, good skin care, antihistamines, and conservative topical medications (Mack, 2004).* Refer to care plan for **Risk for impaired Skin integrity.**
- Monitor weight loss, leaving 25% or more of food uneaten at most meals. **EBN:** *This study demonstrated the above criteria as significant predictors of protein calorie malnutrition (Crogan, Corbett & Short, 2002).* Refer to care plan **Readiness for enhanced Nutrition** for additional interventions.
- Use strategies to prevent nosocomial pneumonia (NP): assess lung sounds, sputum; use sterile water rather than tap water for mouth care of immunosuppressed clients; provide a clean manual resuscitation bag for each client; use sterile technique when suctioning; suction secretions above tracheal tube before suctioning; drain accumulated condensation in ventilator tubing into a fluid trap or other collection device before repositioning the client; assess patency and placement of nasogastric tubes; elevate the client's head to 30 degrees or higher to prevent gastric reflux of organisms in the lung. **EB:** *Ventilator-associated pneumonia is the most common nosocomial infection seen in the intensive care unit (Hunter, 2006).*
- Encourage fluid intake. *Fluid intake helps thin secretions and replace fluid lost during fever (Calianno, 1999).*
- Use appropriate "hand hygiene" (i.e., hand washing or use of alcohol-based hand rubs). **EBN:** *Meticulous infection control precautions are required to prevent health care–associated infection, with particular attention to hand hygiene and universal precautions (Gould, 2004).*
- When using an alcohol-based hand rub, apply product to palm of one hand and rub hands together, covering all surfaces of hands and fingers, until hands are dry. Note that the volume needed to reduce the number of bacteria on hands varies by product. **EB:** *By introducing the use of hand rubbing with an alcoholic solution, there was significant improved hand-cleansing compliance (Girou & Oppein, 2001).*
- Follow Standard Precautions and wear gloves during any contact with blood, mucous membranes, nonintact skin, or any body substance except sweat. Use goggles, powder-free gloves, and gowns when appropriate. Standard Precautions apply to all clients. You must assume all clients are carrying blood-borne pathogens. Standard Precautions exceed Universal Precautions (CDC, 2002). **EBN:** *Research has shown that several postsurgical complications can occur when powder particles from surgical and exam gloves fall into an open incision or are accidentally placed in the body with an instrument on which the particles have attached themselves (Same-Day Surgery, 2004).*
- Follow Transmission-Based Precautions for airborne-, droplet-, and contact-transmitted microorganisms:
  - **Airborne:** Isolate the client in a room with monitored negative air pressure, with the room door closed and the client remaining in the room. Always wear appropriate respiratory protection when you enter the room. For tuberculosis, you should wear an approved particulate respirator mask. Limit the movement and transport of the client from the room to essential purposes only. If at all possible, have the client wear a surgical mask during transport.

- ■ **Droplet:** Keep the client in a private room, if possible. If not possible, maintain a spatial separation of 3 feet from other beds or visitors. The door may remain open. You should wear a mask when you must come within 3 feet of the client. Some hospitals may choose to implement a mask requirement for droplet precautions for anyone entering the room. Limit transport to essential purposes and have the client wear a mask if possible.
- ■ **Transmission:** Place the client in a private room if possible or with someone who has an active infection from the same microorganism. Wear clean, nonsterile gloves when entering the room. When providing care, change gloves after contact with any infective material such as wound drainage. Remove the gloves and wash your hands before leaving the room and take care not to touch any potentially infectious items or surfaces on the way out. Wear a gown if you anticipate your clothing may have substantial contact with the client or other potentially infectious items. Remove the gown before leaving the room. Limit transport of the client to essential purposes and take care that the client does not contact other environmental surfaces along the way. Dedicate the use of noncritical client care equipment to a single client. If use of common equipment is unavoidable, adequately clean and disinfect equipment before use with other clients. *Standard Precautions are based on the likely routes of transmission of pathogens. The second tier of the new CDC guidelines is Transmission-Based Precautions. This replaces many old categories of isolation precautions and disease-specific precautions with three simpler sets of precautions. These three sets of precautions are designed to prevent airborne transmission, droplet transmission, and contact transmission (CDC, 2002).*
- • Use alternatives to indwelling catheters whenever possible (external catheters, incontinence pads, bladder control techniques). Sterile technique must be used when inserting urinary catheters. **EB:** *Urinary tract infections (UTIs) account for almost half of all healthcare–associated infection (HAI), and a significant number of these infections are related to the insertion of urinary catheters (Bissett, 2005).*
- • If a urinary catheter is necessary, follow catheter management practices: All indwelling catheters should be connected to a sterile closed drainage system (i.e., not broken), except for good clinical reasons. Cleanse the perineum and meatus twice daily using soap and water. *Nosocomial UTIs account for up to 40% of all hospital-acquired infections with 80% of these associated with the use of urinary catheters (Hampton, 2004).*
- • Use evidence-based practices and education personal in care of peripheral catheters: use aseptic technique for insertion and care, label insertion sites and all tubing with date and time of insertion, inspect every 8 hours for signs of infection, record, and report. **EB:** *This study demonstrated that an education-based intervention that uses evidence-based practices can be successfully implemented in a diverse group of medical and surgical units and reduce catheter-associated bloodstream infection rates (Warren et al, 2006).* **EBN:** *Care in selection of site and catheter is important. The shortest catheter and smallest size should be used when possible. Accommodate the need to replace catheters before they occlude (Schmid, 2000).*
- • Use careful sterile technique wherever there is a loss of skin integrity. **EB:** *Extensive literature search revealed that sterile gloves should be used for postoperative wound dressing changes (St. Clair & Larrabee, 2002).*
- • Use clean gloves for all high-risk hospitalized clients. **EB:** *This study demonstrated the effectiveness of using clean gloves to prevent cross-contamination of all multiresistant nosocomial pathogens (Safdar et al, 2006).*
- • Ensure the client's appropriate hygienic care with hand washing; bathing; and hair, nail, and perineal care performed by either the nurse or the client. *Hygienic care is important to prevent infection in at-risk clients (Wujcik, 1993).*
- ▲ Recommend responsible use of antibiotics; use antibiotics sparingly. *Widespread use of certain antibiotics, particularly third-generation cephalosporins, has been shown to foster development of generalized beta-lactam resistance in previously susceptible bacterial populations (Yates, 1999).* **EB:** *The reduction of endometritis by two thirds to three quarters and a decrease in wound infections justify a policy of recommending prophylactic antibiotics to women undergoing elective or nonelective cesarean section (Smaill & Hofmeyr, 2002).*

I

▲ Carefully screen and treat women with infertility who may have female genital tuberculosis. **EB:** *Female genital tuberculosis is a symptomless disease inadvertently uncovered during investigation for infertility (Aliyu, Aliyu & Salihu, 2004).*

Pediatric

NOTE: Many of the above interventions are appropriate for the pediatric client.

• Follow meticulous hand hygiene when working with premature infants. **EB:** *In this study of Serratia marcescens in a neonatal intensive care unit (NICU) transmission was likely to occur through the hands of staff (Sarvikivi et al, 2004). Cross-transmission through transient hand carriage of a healthcare worker appeared to be the probable route of transmission in NICU (Milisavljevic et al, 2004).*

• Cluster nursing procedures to decrease number of contacts with infants allowing time for appropriate hand hygiene. **EBN:** *Enhancement of minimal handling and clustering of nursing procedures reduced the total client contact episodes, which could help to overcome the major barrier of time constraints (Lam, Lee & Lau, 2004).*

• Avoid the prophylactic use of topical cream in premature infants. **EB:** *Prophylactic application of topical ointment increases the risk of coagulase negative staphylococcal infection and any nosocomial infection. A trend toward increased risk of any bacterial infection was noted in infants prophylactically treated (Conner, Soll & Edwards, 2004).*

Geriatric

• Suspect pneumonia when the client has symptoms of lethargy or confusion. **EB:** *Many elderly persons do not have the classic symptoms of community acquired pneumonia; instead, they may present with confusion, lethargy, tachypnea, anorexia, or abdominal pain (Patel & Criner, 2003).*

• Most clients develop NP by either aspirating contaminated substances or inhaling airborne particles. Refer to care plan for **Risk for Aspiration.**

▲ Carefully screen elderly women for salmonella with symptoms of urinary tract infections. **EB:** *Salmonellosis is a major cause of gastroenteritis in the United States and can lead to septicaemia and other extraintestinal illness, including urinary tract infections (Sivapalasingam et al, 2004).*

▲ Observe and report if the client has a low-grade temperature or new onset of confusion. **EB:** *Residents of long-term care facilities who are suspected of having an infection and have one temperature reading of greater than 100° F (37.8° C), more than two readings of greater than 99° F (37.2° C), or an increase of 2° F (1.1° C) over baseline should be reported immediately to the on-site nurse, and appropriate testing should be done to determine site of infection (Bentley et al, 2001).* **EBN:** *Those caring for elderly clients must be alerted to the potential presence of infection when even low-grade temperature elevations appear for short periods (Holtzclaw, 2003). In the majority of acute confusion in the elderly, the etiology was multifactorial infections and dehydration as the most common causes (Cacchione et al, 2003).*

▲ Recommend that the geriatric client receive an annual influenza immunization and one-time pneumococcal vaccine. **EB:** *Immunization against influenza is an effective intervention that reduces serologically confirmed cases by between 60% and 70% (Hull et al, 2002). Oseltamivir prophylaxis was very effective in protecting nursing home residents from influenza-like illnesses and in halting an outbreak of influenza B (Parker, Loewen & Skowronski, 2001).*

• Recognize that chronically ill geriatric clients, particularly those with depression, have an increased susceptibility to infection; practice meticulous care of all invasive sites. *Depression has been noted as a risk factor for lethal infectious disease in disabled older adults, with reduced reactivity in humoral and cellular immunity (Shinkawa et al, 2002). A successful infection control program can provide the foundation for expanding performance improvement throughout the long-term care facility (Stevenson & Loeb, 2004).*

• Recognize that older adults are at risk for human immunodeficiency virus (HIV)/acquired immune deficiency syndrome (AIDS); institute Universal Precautions and appropriate instruction for all age groups. *Older adults are less likely to use a condom or to participate in routine HIV testing. Survival rates of elders with HIV are lower compared with younger clients (Chiao, Ries & Sande, 1999).*

Home Care

- Some of the above interventions may be adapted for home care use.
- Assess and treat wounds in the home. **EBN:** *Wound treatment in the community, when combined with comprehensive nursing assessment, can be effective while reducing costs (Carville, 2004).*
- Review standards for surveillance of infections in home care. *Home care has expanded in the United States, but infection surveillance, prevention, and control have lagged behind. In this article, it is recommended that infectious disease control principles form the basis of training for home care providers to assess infection risk and develop prevention strategies (Rhinehart, 2001).*
- Maintain strong infection control policies. *Strong guidelines are important to avoid infection in the home setting, especially addressing such issues as storage and use of irrigation solutions and supplies (Friedman, 2003).*
- ▲ Monitor recurrent antibiotic use in infants. Instruct parents on appropriate indicators for medical visits and on the influence of breastfeeding and day care at home for avoiding increased need for antibiotics. **EB:** *Families who sought frequent antibiotic therapy for infants with fever or cold had a low threshold for seeking medical help. Breastfeeding and care at home was found to decrease medical visits for antibiotics (Louhi-Pirkanniemi, 2004).*
- ▲ Monitor for the occurrence of infectious exacerbation of chronic obstructive pulmonary disease (COPD); refer to physician for treatment. *Nontypable* Haemophilus influenzae, Streptococcus pneumoniae, *and* Moraxella *can cause exacerbation of COPD (Sheikh & Sethi, 2001).*
- ▲ Refer for nutritional evaluation; implement dietary changes to support recovery and address antibiotic side effects. *Overgrowth of* Clostridium difficile *can cause abdominal pain, fever, and diarrhea. Inclusion of probiotics in the diet can counteract antibiotic-associated diarrhea (Vogelzang, 2001).*

 Client/Family Teaching

- Teach the client risk factors contributing to surgical wound infection, smoking, and higher body mass index. **EB:** *These are some of the factors associated with risk of surgical wound infection (Reilly, 2002).*
- ▲ Teach the client and family the symptoms of infection that should be promptly reported to a primary medical caregiver (e.g., redness, warmth, swelling, tenderness or pain, new onset of drainage or change in drainage from wound, increase in body temperature). **EB:** *Two thirds of wound infections occur after discharge (Reid et al, 2002).*
- ▲ Teach signs of HBV and AIDS symptoms: malaise, abdominal pain, vomiting or diarrhea, enlarged glands, rash; tuberculosis symptoms: cough, night sweats, dyspnea, changes in sputum, changes in breath sounds; insulin-dependent diabetes mellitus (IDDM) symptoms: sores or wounds that do not heal. *A high prevalence of HBV/AIDS, an increasing incidence of tuberculosis, and the general risk of diabetes are related to increased rate of infection.*
- ▲ Encourage high-risk persons, including healthcare workers, to have influenza vaccinations. *Vaccinations help to prevent viral NP (Calianno, 1999).*
- Influenza: Teach frequent hand washing, limited contact with sick person, use of masks by caregiver and sick person, and keeping sick person in the "sick room." *Respiratory droplets from sneezing or coughing spread the influenza virus, and the virus can live on items for days (Allen, 2006).*
- Assess whether the client and family know how to read a thermometer; provide instructions if necessary. Chemical dot thermometers are easy to use and decrease risk of infection. Clients need to know that the instructions should be followed carefully and that electronic thermometers may be the best choice for accuracy. *Single-use clinical thermometers provide a safe alternative to the traditional mercury in glass thermometers for routine temperature taking (MacQueen, 2001).*

 See the EVOLVE website for World Wide Web resources for client education.

REFERENCES

Aliyu MH, Aliyu SH, Salihu HM: Female genital tuberculosis: a global review, *Int J Fertil Womens Med* 49(3):123-136, 2004.

Allen P: Home Care Fact Sheet: Influenza, *Pediatric Nurs* 32(6):573-576, 2006.

Bailey J, Rose P: Axillary and tympanic membrane temperature recording in the preterm neonate: a comparative study, *J Adv Nurs* 34(4):465-471, 2001.

Bentley DW, Bradley S, High K et al: Practice guidelines for evalua-

• = Independent;   ▲ = Collaborative;   EBN = Evidence-Based Nursing;   EB = Evidence-Based

tion of fever and infection in long-term care facilities, *Clin Infect Dis* 31(3):640-653, 2000.

Bissett L: Reducing the risk of catheter-related urinary tract infection. *Nurs Times* 101(12):64-65, 2005.

Cacchione PZ, Culp K, Laing J et al: Clinical profile of acute confusion in the long-term care setting, *Clin Nurs Res* 12(2):145-158, 2003.

Calianno C: *Nosocomial pneumonia,* Springnet, Springhouse. Available at www.springnet.com/ce/ce965a.htm, accessed on March 29, 1999.

Carville K: A report on the effectiveness of comprehensive wound assessment and documentation in the community, *Prim Intent* 12(1):41, 2004.

CDC, Centers for Disease Control and Prevention, Hospital Infection Control Practices Advisory Committee: recommendations for isolation precautions in hospitals, revised November 9, 2002. Available at www.cdc.gov/ncidod/hip/isolat/isopart2.htm, accessed on March 16, 2003.

Chiao EY, Ries KM, Sande MA: AIDS and the elderly, *Clin Infect Disease* 28:740, 1999.

Conner JM, Soll RF, Edwards WH: Topical ointment for preventing infection in preterm infants, *Cochrane Database Syst Rev* (1): CD001150, 2004.

Cornbleet PJ: Clinical utility of the band count, *Clin Lab Med* 22(1):101, 2002.

Crogan NL, Corbett CF, Short RA: The minimum data set: predicting malnutrition in newly admitted nursing home residents, *Clin Nurs Res* 11(3):341, 2002.

Engelhart S, Glasmacher A, Exner M et al: Surveillance for nosocomial infections and fever of unknown origin among adult hematology-oncology patients, *Infect Control Hosp Epidemiol* 23(5):244, 2002.

Farnell S, Maxwell L, Tan S, Rhodes A, Philips B: Temperature measurement: comparison of non-invasive methods used in adult critical care, *J Clin Nurs* 14(5):632-639, May 2005.

Friedman MM: Infection control update for home care and hospice organizations, *Home Healthc Nurse* 21(11):753, 2003.

Gilbert M, Barton AJ, Counsell CM: Comparison of oral and tympanic temperatures in adult surgical patients, *Appl Nurs Res* 15(1):42, 2002.

Girou E, Oppein F: Handwashing compliance in a French university hospital: new perspective with the introduction of hand-rubbing with a waterless alcohol-based solution, *J Hosp Infect* 48(Suppl A): S55, 2001.

Gould D: Systematic observation of hand decontamination, *Nurs Stand* 18(47):39-44, 2004.

Hampton S: Nursing management of urinary tract infections for catheterized patients, *Br J Nurs* 13(20):1180-1184, 2004.

Holtzclaw BJ: Use of thermoregulatory principles in patient care: fever management, *Online J Clin Innovat* 5(5):1-23, 2003.

Hull S, Hagdrup N, Hart B et al: Boosting uptake of influenza immunization: a randomized controlled trial of telephone appointing in general practice, *Br J Gen Pract* 52(482):710, 2002.

Hunter JD: Ventilator associated pneumonia, *Postgrad Med J,* 82(965):172-178, 2006.

Lam BC, Lee J, Lau YL: Hand hygiene practices in a neonatal intensive care unit: a multimodal intervention and impact on nosocomial infection, *Pediatrics* 114(5):e565-e571, 2004.

Louhi-Pirkanniemi K: Recurrent antibiotic use in a small child and the effects on the family, *Scand J Prim Health Care* 22(1):16, 2004.

Mack S: Atopic dermatitis: an overview for the nurse practitioner, *J Am Acad Nurse Pract* 16(10):451-454, 2004.

Macqueen S: Clinical benefits of 3M Tempa Dot thermometer in paediatric setting, *Br J Nurs* 10(1):55-58, 2001.

Milisavljevic V, Wu F, Larson E et al: Molecular epidemiology of *Serratia marcescens* outbreaks in two neonatal intensive care units, *Infect Control Hosp Epidemiol* 25(9):719-721, 2004.

NCCN (National Comprehensive Cancer Network): Fever and Neutropenia Treatment Guidelines for Patients with Cancer — Version II/March 2006, *NCCN (National Cancer Comprehensive Network),* www.nccn.org/patients/patient_gls/_english/_fever_and_neutropenia/1_introduction.asp retrieved Feb 26, 2007.

Parker R, Loewen N, Skowronski D: Experience with oseltamivir in the control of a nursing home influenza B outbreak, *Can Commun Dis Rep* 27(5):37, 2001.

Patel N, Criner G: Community-acquired pneumonia in the elderly: update on treatment strategies, *Consultant* 43(6):689-690, 692, 695-697, 2003.

Reid R, Simcock JW, Chisholm L et al: Postdischarge clean wound infections: incidence underestimated and risk factors overemphasized, *ANZ J Surg* 72(5):339, 2002.

Reilly J: Evidence-based surgical wound care on surgical wound infection, *Br J Nurs* 11(Suppl 16):S4, 2002.

Rhinehart E: Infection control in home care, *Emerg Infect Dis* 7(2): 208-211, 2001.

Safdar N, Marx J, Meyer N, et al: Effectiveness of preemptive barrier precautions in controlling nosocomial colonization and infection by methicillin-resistant Staphylococcus aureus in a burn unit, *Am J Infect Control* 34(8):476-483, 2006.

Same-Day Surgery: Powdered gloves increase surgical complication risk: adhesions, granulomas, decreased resistance linked, 28(5):54-55, 2004.

Sarvikivi E, Lyytikinen O, Salmenlinna S et al: Clustering of *Serratia marcescens* infections in a neonatal intensive care unit, *Infect Control Hosp Epidemiol* 25(9):723-729, 2004.

Schmid MW: Risks and complications of peripherally and centrally inserted intravenous catheters, *Crit Care Nurs Clin North Am* 12(2):165, 2000.

Sheikh S, Sethi S: Management of infectious exacerbation of COPD, *Home Health Care Consult* 8(5):21, 2001.

Shinkawa M, Nakayama K, Hirai H et al: Depression and immunoreactivity in disabled older adults, *J Am Geriatr Soc* 50:198, 2002.

Sivapalasingam S, Hoekstra RM, McQuiston JR et al: Salmonella bacteriuria: an increasing entity in elderly women in the United States, *Epidemiol Infect* 132(5):897-902, 2004.

St Clair K, Larrabee JH: Clean versus sterile gloves: which to use for postoperative dressing changes? *Outcomes Manag* 6(1):17, 2002.

Stevenson KB, Loeb M: Topics in long-term care. Performance improvement in the long-term-care setting: building on the foundation of infection control, *Infect Control Hosp Epidemiol* 25(1):72-79, 2004.

Vogelzang JL: Nutrition in home care. Nonfunctional gut? Try a probiotic food, *Home Healthc Nurse* 19:467, 2001.

Warren D, Cosgrove S, Diekema D et al: A multicenter intervention to prevent catheter-associated bloodstream infections, *Infect Control Hosp Epidemiol* 27(7):662-669, 2006.

West TE, Guerry C, Hiott M et al: Effect of targeted surveillance for control of methicillin-resistant Staphylococcus aureus in a community hospital system, *Infect Control Hosp Epidemiol* 27(3):233-238, 2006.

Wujcik D: Infection control in oncology patients, *Nurs Clin North Am* 28:639, 1993.

Yates RR: New intervention strategies for reducing antibiotic resistance, *Chest* 115(Suppl):24S, 1999.

Risk for Injury   *Betty J. Ackley, MSN, EdS, RN*   `evolve`

NANDA   Definition

At risk of injury as a result of the interaction of environmental conditions interacting with the individual's adaptive and defensive resources

NOTE: This nursing diagnosis overlaps with other diagnoses such as **Risk for Falls, Risk for Trauma, Risk for Poisoning, Risk for Suffocation, Risk for Aspiration,** and if the client is at risk of bleeding, **Ineffective Protection.** Refer to care plans for these diagnoses if appropriate.

Risk Factors

External

Biological (e.g., immunization level of community, microorganism); chemical (e.g., poisons, pollutants, drugs, pharmaceutical agents, alcohol, nicotine, preservatives, cosmetics, dyes); human (e.g., nosocomial agents; staffing patterns; cognitive, affective, psychomotor factors); mode of transport; nutritional (e.g., vitamins, food types); physical (e.g., design, structure, and arrangement of community, building, and/or equipment)

Internal

Abnormal blood profile (leukocytosis/leucopenia, altered clotting factors, thrombocytopenia, sickle cell, thalassemia, decreased hemoglobin); biochemical dysfunction; developmental age (physiological, psychosocial); effector dysfunction; immune-autoimmune dysfunction; integrative dysfunction; malnutrition; physical (e.g., broken skin, altered mobility); psychological (affective orientation); sensory dysfunction; tissue hypoxia

NOC   Outcomes (Nursing Outcomes Classification)

Suggested NOC Outcomes

Personal Safety Behavior, Psychosocial Safety, Risk Control, Safe Home Environment

> #### Example NOC Outcome with Indicators
>
> **Risk Control** as evidenced by the following indicators: Monitors environmental risk factors/Develops effective risk control strategies/Follows selected risk control strategies (Rate the outcome and indicators of **Risk Control:** 1 = never demonstrated, 2 = rarely demonstrated, 3 = sometimes demonstrated, 4 = often demonstrated, 5 = consistently demonstrated [see Section I].)

Client Outcomes

Client Will (Specify Time Frame):

- Remain free of injuries
- Explain methods to prevent injury

NIC   Interventions (Nursing Interventions Classification)

Suggested NIC Interventions

Behavior Modification, Health Education, Patient Contracting, Self-Modification Assistance

> #### Example NIC Activities—Health Education
>
> Identify internal or external factors that may enhance or reduce motivation for healthy behavior; Determine current health knowledge and lifestyle behaviors of individual, family, or target group

• = Independent;   ▲ = Collaborative;   EBN = Evidence-Based Nursing;   EB = Evidence-Based

I

Nursing Interventions and *Rationales*

- Prevent iatrogenic harm to the hospitalized client by following the 2007 National Patient Safety goals:
    - Accuracy of Patient Identification
        - Use at least two methods (e.g., client's name and medical record number or birth date) to identify the client before administering medications, blood products, treatments, or procedures.
        - Prior to beginning any invasive or surgical procedure, have a final verification to confirm the correct client, the correct procedure, and the correct site for the procedure using active communication techniques.
    - Effectiveness of Communication among Care Staff
        - When taking verbal or telephone orders, the orders should be written down and then read back for verification to the individual giving the order.
        - Standardize use of abbreviations, acronyms, symbols, and dose designations that are used in the institution.
        - Make sure of timeliness of reporting and taking action of critical test results and values.
        - Utilize a standardized approach of "handing off" communications, including opportunities to ask and answer questions.
    - Medication Safety
        - Standardize and limit the number of drug concentrations utilized by the institution (e.g., concentrations of medications such as morphine in patient controlled analgesia [PCA] pumps).
        - Label all medications and medication containers (e.g., syringes, medication cups, or other solutions on or off the surgical field).
        - Identify all of the client's current medications upon admission to a healthcare facility, and ensure that all healthcare staff have access to the information.
        - Reconcile all medication at discharge, and provide list to the client.
        - Improve the effectiveness of alarm systems in the clinical area.
    - Reduce the risk of infections by following Centers for Disease Control (CDC) hand hygiene guidelines.
    - Evaluate all clients for fall risk and take appropriate actions to prevent falls.
    - Prevent pressure ulcer formation.

These actions have been shown to increase client safety and are required actions for accreditation by the Joint Commission (2007).

- See care plan for **Risk for Falls.**
- ▲ Avoid use of restraints if at all possible. Restraint free is now the standard of care for hospitals and long-term care facilities. Obtain a physician's order if restraints are necessary. *The use of restraints has been associated with serious injuries, including rhabdomyolysis, brachial plexus injury, neuropathy, dysrhythmias, as well as strangulation, traumatic brain injuries, and all the consequences of immobility (Capezuti, 2004; Park & Tang, 2007). Restraint-free extended care facilities were shown to have fewer residents with activities of daily living (ADL) deficiencies and fewer residents with bowel or bladder incontinence than facilities that use restraints (Castle & Fogel, 1998).* **EBN and EB:** *There was no increase in falls or injuries in a group of clients that were not restrained compared with a similar group that was restrained in a nursing home (Capezuti et al, 1999). Substantial evidence shows restraints pose a safety risk of their own (Capezuti & Braun, 2001; Capezuti & Wexler, 2003; Dunn, 2001; Talerico & Capezuti, 2001).*
- In place of restraints, use the following:
    - Well-staffed and educated nursing personnel with frequent client contact
    - Continuity of care with familiar staff
    - Nursing units designed to care for clients with cognitive or functional impairments
    - Avoiding use of IVs or tubes that are susceptible to being removed
    - Alarm systems with ankle, above the knee, or wrist sensors
    - Bed or wheelchair alarms
    - Increased observation of the client
    - Providing exercise to diffuse and deflect client behavior

---

- Low or very low height beds
- Border-defining pillow/mattress to remind the client to stay in bed

These alternatives to restraints can be helpful to prevent falls (Capezuti, 2004; McCarter-Bayer, Bayer & Hall, 2005; Park & Tang, 2007).

- For an agitated client, consider providing individualized music of the client's choice. **EBN:** *Clients who previously were in restraints demonstrated more positive behaviors when listening to individualized music than did clients who were out of restraints but were not exposed to music (Janelli, Kanski & Wu, 2002). Calming music was shown to be effective in decreasing agitation in persons with dementia (Remington, 2002).*

- Review drug profile for potential side effects that may increase risk of injury. **EB:** *Benzodiazepines have a fivefold increase injury risk for drivers (Movig et al, 2004).*

- Use one quarter– to one half–length side rails only, and maintain bed in a low position. Ensure that wheels are locked on bed and commode. Keep dim light in room at night. *Use of full side rails can result in the client climbing over the rails, leading with the head, and sustaining a head injury. Side rails with widely spaced vertical bars and side rails not situated flush with the mattress have been associated with asphyxiation deaths because of rail and in bed entrapment and should not be used (Capezuti, 2004; Hanger, Ball & Wood, 1999).*

- If the client has a new onset of confusion (delirium), refer to the care plan for **Acute Confusion.** If the client has chronic confusion, see the care plan for **Chronic Confusion.**

- Ask family to stay with the client to prevent the client from accidentally falling or pulling out tubes.

- Remove all possible hazards in environment such as razors, medications, and matches.

- Place an injury-prone client in a room that is near the nurses station. *Such placement allows more frequent observation of the client.*

- Help clients sit in a stable chair with armrests. Avoid use of wheelchairs and geri-chairs except for transportation as needed. *Clients are likely to fall when left in a wheelchair or geri-chair because they may stand up without locking the wheels or removing the footrests.*

▲ Refer to physical therapy for strengthening exercises and gait training to increase mobility.

▲ For the agitated psychotic client, use nonphysical forms of behavior management, such as verbal intervention or show of force. If medication is required, use oral medications if at all possible. *Nonphysical behavior management is first-line strategy when dealing with the psychotic client; oral medications can be just as effective as intramuscular injections when used for agitation if the client will swallow them and avoid possible injury from intramuscular injections (Murphy, 2002).*

 Pediatric

- Teach parents the need for close supervision of all young children playing near water, including washing machines. **EB:** *Children can be harmed by washing machines by the wringer mechanism, also by hot water, and by drowning (Warner, Kenney & Rice, 2003).*

- If child has epilepsy, recommend showers instead of tub baths, and no unsupervised swimming is ever allowed. *Most drowning accidents involving children are preventable if basic safety measures are taken (Bolte, 2000).*

- Assess the client's social economic status. **EB:** *Pediatric clients living in poverty are at higher risk for injury (Shenassa, Stubbendick & Brown, 2004).*

- Never leave young children unsupervised around cooking areas. **EB:** *Some identified hazards to young children include burns and scalds, water temperatures set at greater than 54 degrees Celsius, kettles or appliances with dangling wires, or no stove guards to prevent a child from grabbing pots (Leblanc et al, 2006).*

- Teach parents and children the need to maintain safety for the exercising child, including wearing helmets when biking and using breakaway bases for baseball. *A parents' use of helmets appears to affect a child's use (Martin, 2002).* **EB:** *Use of breakaway bases was shown to reduce the number of injuries in baseball and softball by 96% (Janda, Bir & Kedroske, 2001).*

- Teach both parents and children the need for gun safety. There are a number of programs available to teach gun safety, including Eddie the Eagle Gun Safe Program, Straight Talk about Risks (STAR), Steps to Prevent Firearm Injury in the Home, and the Emergency Nurses Association Gun Safety Program (Howard, 2001).

Geriatric

- Encourage the client to wear glasses and hearing aids and to use walking aids when ambulating.
- If the client experiences dizziness because of orthostatic hypotension when getting up, teach methods to decrease dizziness, such as rising slowly, remaining seated several minutes before standing, flexing feet upward several times while sitting, sitting down immediately if feeling dizzy, and trying to have someone present when standing. *If orthostatic hypotension is present and there is minimal change in the heart rate, most likely the baroreceptors are not working to maintain blood pressure on arising. This is common in the elderly and can be from cardiovascular disease, neurological disease, or a medication effect (Sclater & Alagiakrishnan, 2004).*
- Discourage driving at night. *A decline in depth perception, slower recovery from glare, and night blindness are common in the elderly and make night driving a difficult and unsafe task.*

Multicultural

- Acknowledge racial/ethnic differences at the onset of care. **EBN:** *Acknowledgment of race/ethnicity issues will enhance communication, establish rapport, and promote treatment outcomes (D'Avanzo et al, 2001). A recent study found that burns, guns, drowning, and being pierced/cut appeared to be particularly important mechanisms of injury for Hispanic children (Karr, Rivara & Cummings, 2005). Death by violence has increased significantly among Alaska Natives, who have a suicide rate, frequently related to alcohol and self-inflicted gunshot wounds, three times that of the general U.S. population (National Center for Health Statistics, 2002).*
- Assess for the influence of cultural beliefs, norms, and values on the client's perceptions of risk for injury. **EBN:** *What the client considers risky behavior may be based on cultural perceptions (Giger & Davidhizar, 2004). Young, African-American, and Hispanic pregnant women are at higher risk for trauma in pregnancy and are most likely to benefit from primary trauma prevention efforts (Ikossi et al, 2005). African Americans, American Indians, and Alaska Natives were identified as high-risk groups who engaged in the following risky traffic-related behavior: not wearing seat belts, not using child safety seats, not wearing bicycle or motorcycle helmets, driving after drinking, driving while fatigued or distracted, speeding, running red lights, and aggressive driving (Schlundt, Warren & Miller, 2004).*
- Assess whether exposure to community violence is contributing to risk for injury. **EBN:** *Exposure to community violence has been associated with increases in aggressive behavior and depression (Gorman-Smith & Tolan, 1998). Minority students, especially African-American and Hispanic students in lower grades, may participate in and may more often be victims of school violence (Hill & Drolet, 1999).*
- Use culturally relevant injury prevention programs whenever possible.
- Validate the client's feelings and concerns related to environmental risks. **EBN:** *Ethnic minority families were less likely to engage in some safety practices and have less access to information regarding the availability and fitting of safety equipment (Mulvaney & Kendrick, 2004). Injuries were identified as the third leading cause of death among Hispanics and the leading cause for those Hispanic individuals 1 to 44 years of age (Mallonee, 2003).*

Home Care/Client/Family Teaching

- For interventions and rationales see **Risk for Trauma.**

evolve See the EVOLVE website for World Wide Web resources for client education.

REFERENCES

Bolte R: Drowning: a preventable cause of death, *Patient Care* 34(7):129, 2000.

Capezuti E: Minimizing the use of restrictive devices in dementia patients at risk for falling, *Nurs Clin North Am* 39:625, 2004.

Capezuti EA, Braun JA: Medico-legal aspects of hospital siderail use. In Kapp MD, editor: *Ethics, law, and aging review: liability issues and risk management in caring for older person,* New York, 2001, Springer.

Capezuti E, Strumpf N, Evans L et al: Outcomes of nighttime physical restraint removal for severely impaired nursing home residents, *Am J Alzheimer's Dis Other Demen* 14(3):157, 1999.

Capezuti E, Wexler SS: Choosing alternatives to restraints. In Siegler EL, Mirafzail S, Foust JB, editors: *An introduction to hospitals and inpatient care,* New York, 2003, Springer.

Castle NG, Fogel B: Characteristics of nursing homes that are restraint free, *Gerontologist* 38(2):181, 1998.

• = Independent;   ▲ = Collaborative;   EBN = Evidence-Based Nursing;   EB = Evidence-Based

D'Avanzo CE et al: Developing culturally informed strategies for substance-related interventions. In Naegle MA, D'Avanzo CE, editors: *Addictions and substance abuse: strategies for advanced practice nursing*, St Louis, 2001, Mosby.

Dunn KS: The effect of physical restraints on fall rates in older adults who are institutionalized, *J Gerontol Nurs* 27(10):40-48, 2001.

Giger J, Davidhizar R: *Transcultural nursing: assessment and intervention*, St. Louis, 2004, Mosby.

Gorman-Smith D, Tolan P: The role of exposure to community violence and developmental problems among inner city youth, *Dev Psychopathol* 10(1):101, 1998.

Hanger HC, Ball MC, Wood LA: An analysis of falls in the hospital: can we do without bedrails? *J Am Geriatr Soc* 47(5):529-531, 1999.

Hill SC, Drolet JC: School related violence among high school students in the United States 1993-1995, *J Sch Health* 69(7):264, 1999.

Howard PK: An overview of a few well-known national children's gun safety programs and ENA's newly developed program, *J Emerg Nurs* 27(5):485, 2001.

Ikossi DG, Lazar AA, Morabito D et al: Profile of mothers at risk: an analysis of injury and pregnancy loss in 1,195 trauma patients, *J Am Col Surg* 200(1):49-56, 2005.

Janda DH, Bir C, Kedroske B: A comparison of standard versus breakaway bases: an analysis of a preventative intervention for softball and baseball foot and ankle injuries, *Foot Ankle Int* 22:810, 2001.

Janelli LM, Kanski GW, Wu YB: Individualized music—a different approach to the restraint issue, *Rehabil Nurs* 27(6):221, 2002.

Joint Commission 2007 National Patient Safety Goals: Available at http://www.jointcommission.org/PatientSafety/NationalPatient-SafetyGoals/07_npsg_facts.htm. Accessed March 20, 2007.

Karr CJ, Rivara FP, Cummings P: Severe injury among Hispanic and non-Hispanic white children in Washington state, *Public Health Rep* 120(1):19-24, 2005.

Leblanc J, Pless I, King W et al: Home safety measures and the risk of unintentional injury among young children: a multi-centre case control study, *Can Med Assoc J* 175(8):883-887, 2006.

Mallonee S: Injuries among Hispanics in the United States: implications for research, *J Transcult Nurs* 14(3):217-226, 2003.

Martin S: Everyone should wear a helmet, *Can Med Assoc J* 167(11):1282, 2002.

McCarter-Bayer A, Bayer F, Hall K: Preventing falls in acute care: an innovative approach, *J Gerontol Nurs* 31(3):25-33, 2005.

Movig KL, Mathijssen MP, Nagel PH et al: Psychoactive substance use and the risk of motor vehicle accidents, *Accid Anal Prev* 36(4):631, 2004.

Mulvaney C, Kendrick D: Engagement in safety practices to prevent home injuries in preschool children among white and non-white ethnic minority families, *Inj Prev* 10(6):375, 2004.

Murphy MC: The agitated psychotic patient: guidelines to ensure staff and patient safety, *J Am Psychiatr Nurses Assoc* 8(Suppl 4):S2, 2002.

National Center for Health Statistics: *Health: United States, 2002 with urban and rural chartbook*, Washington, DC, 2002, US Government Printing Office.

Park M, Tang JH: Changing the practice of physical restraint use in acute care, *J Gerontol Nurs* 33(2):9-16, 2007.

Remington R: Calming music and hand massage with agitated elderly, *Nurs Res* 51(5):317, 2002.

Schlundt D, Warren R, Miller S: Reducing unintentional injuries on the nation's highways: a literature review, *J Health Care Poor Underserved* 15(1):76-98, 2004.

Sclater A, Alagiakrishnan K: Orthostatic hypotension. A primary care primer for assessment and treatment, *Geriatrics* 59(8):22, 2004.

Shenassa ED, Stubbendick A, Brown MJ: Social disparities in housing and related pediatric injury: a multilevel study, *Am J Public Health* 94(4):633, 2004.

Talerico KA, Capezuti E: Myths and facts about side rails, *Am J Nurs* 101(7):43-48, 2001.

Warner BL, Kenney BD, Rice M: Washing machine related injuries in children: a continuing threat, *Injury Prev* 9(4):357, 2003.

Risk for perioperative positioning Injury   Terri Foster, BSN, CNOR, RN

NANDA   Definition

At risk for inadvertent anatomical and physical changes as a result of posture or equipment used during an invasive/surgical procedure

Risk Factors

Disorientation; edema; emaciation; immobilization; muscle weakness; obesity; sensory/perceptual disturbances due to anesthesia

NOTE: The following systems are most frequently affected by surgical positioning: neurological, musculoskeletal, integumentary, respiratory, and cardiovascular. Risk factors contributing to the incidence of injury related to surgical positioning include, but are not limited to, the client's age; height; weight; nutritional status; skin condition; the presence of preexisting conditions such as diabetes, vascular, and/or respiratory disease; anemia; hypovolemia; immuno-compromise; impaired nerve function; physical mobility limitations such as arthritis, limited range of motion (ROM), presence of implants/prosthesis or malignancy; effects of anesthesia; staff's knowledge of the equipment; required position for the procedure; use of a heating blanket; extracorporeal circulation; and the duration of the procedure—3 hours or more (AORN, 2006; Steris, 2004). Studies have shown statistical significance between pressure ulcer development and length of surgical procedure (Schultz, 2005). As a result of

I

these factors, there is the potential for impaired tissue perfusion, impaired skin integrity, or neuromuscular or joint injury related to surgical positioning. The anesthetized client is at increased risk of injury due to positioning because anesthesia prevents the body's defense mechanism from warning the client of exaggerated stretching, twisting, or compression of his or her body (Power, 2002).

Complications of Surgical Positioning

Complications of positioning include, but are not limited to, mechanical restriction of the rib cage, vasodilatation, hyper/hypotension, decreased cardiac output, inhibition of normal compensatory mechanisms, redistribution and congestion of the blood supply, and nerve and muscle trauma due to stretching and compression (AORN, 2006). Studies have shown that procedures lasting more than 2.5 to 3 hours significantly increase the risk for pressure ulcer formation (AORN, 2006). Studies have also shown that a normal capillary interface pressure of 32 mm Hg or less should be maintained due to higher pressures causing occlusion and subsequent restriction/blockage of blood flow and ultimately tissue breakdown/ischemia (AORN, 2006). Research has shown that pressure ulcers will develop in 8.5% of all surgical patients whose procedure lasted more than 3 hours (Rothrock, 2003).

Transient physiological reactions to surgical positioning include skin redness and/or bruising, lumbar backache, stiffness in the limbs and neck, numbness, and generalized muscle aches that usually resolve within 24 to 48 hours without treatment. Lumbar back pain, previously considered a transient physiological reaction to positioning, may be an indication of rhabdomyolysis (Alterman et al, 2007).

More serious complications of surgical positioning include pressure ulcers, peripheral nerve injury, deep venous thrombosis, joint dislocation, compartment syndrome (impairment of microcirculation in soft tissue), rhabdomyolysis, and joint injury.

NOC   Outcomes (Nursing Outcomes Classification)

Suggested NOC Outcomes

Circulation Status, Neurological Status, Risk Control, Tissue Integrity: Skin and Mucous Membranes, Tissue Perfusion: Peripheral

Example NOC Outcome with Indicators
Tissue Perfusion: Peripheral as evidenced by the following indicators: Peripheral edema/Localized extremity pain/Skin integrity/Muscle function/Sensation/Peripheral pulses (Rate the outcome and indicators of **Tissue Perfusion: Peripheral:** 1 = severely compromised, 2 = substantially compromised, 3 = moderately compromised, 4 = mildly compromised, 5 = not compromised [see Section I].)

Client Outcomes

Client Will (Specify Time Frame):

- Demonstrate unchanged skin condition, with exception of the incision, between admission and discharge from the operating room
- Demonstrate redness of the skin for less than 30 minutes at points of pressure
- Be free of injury related to positioning during the surgical procedure, including intact skin and free from pain or numbness associated with surgical positioning
- Demonstrate unchanged or improved physical mobility from preoperative status
- Demonstrate unchanged or improved cardiovascular and respiratory status from preoperative status
- Demonstrate unchanged or improved peripheral sensory integrity from preoperative status
- Maintain sense of privacy and dignity

NIC   Interventions (Nursing Interventions Classification)

Suggested NIC Interventions

Positioning: Intraoperative, Pressure Ulcer Prevention, Risk Identification, Skin Surveillance

• = Independent;   ▲ = Collaborative;   EBN = Evidence-Based Nursing;   EB = Evidence-Based

Example NIC Activities—Positioning: Intraoperative
Use an adequate number of personnel to transfer patient; Maintain patient's proper body alignment

Nursing Interventions and *Rationales*

General Interventions for Any Surgical Client

Prevention of Pressure Ulcers

- Identify clients at risk for pressure ulcer development so that cost-effective, evidence-based preventive measures can be instituted. *Pressure ulcers, regardless of whether they originate in surgery or elsewhere, represent a negative client outcome (Schultz, 2005). Pressure ulcers are associated with an increased risk of death one year posthospital discharge. The cost of treating pressure ulcers depends on the severity, but averages anywhere from $5000 to $40,000 (Sewchuk, Padula & Osborne, 2006).* **EB:** *Research has shown that in addition to using appropriate positioning devices, completing a preoperative, intraoperative, and postoperative assessment (for several days postop) decreases the risk of pressure ulcer development.* **EB:** *In a study group containing 50 clients where a fluid pressure-reducing mattress and continuous assessment were both utilized, only 2 clients developed a pressure ulcer (Sewchuk, Padula & Osborne, 2006). Repeated assessment during hospitalization can predict risk for pressure ulcer development (Pokorny, Koldjeski & Swanson, 2003).*
- Recognize that clients undergoing cardiac surgical procedures are at increased risk of developing a pressure ulcer, especially below the waist or in the occiput area. **EB:** *In one study, 52.9% of all pressure ulcers occurred on the heels, and most of these clients underwent cardiac surgery (26 out of 37) (Sewchuk, Padula & Osborne, 2006).*
- Use of pressure-reducing devices is necessary to prevent ulcer formation. **EB:** *Pressure greater than 32 mm Hg has been determined to be the force necessary to occlude arteriolar capillary blood flow (Schultz, 2005).*
- Pad the operating room table well. Avoid use of gel overlays. **EB:** *Research, along with comparative pressure maps shows that gel overlays actually increase rather than decrease pressure on bony prominences (Steris, 2005). Research shows that pressure ulcer occurrence decreases with the use of a fluid pressure-reducing mattress along with comprehensive staff education (Sewchuk, Padula & Osborne, 2006). Studies have shown that the standard 2-inch thick operating room (OR) table mattress significantly contributes to the development of pressure ulcer (Scott-Williams, 2006).*
- Avoid using rolled towels and bolsters made using towels, sheets, and so on, as they tend to produce high and inconsistent pressures (Goodman, 2006).
- Avoid covering positioning devices as the material used to cover the device reduces the effectiveness of the positioning device (Goodman, 2006).
- Appropriate numbers of personnel should be present to assist in positioning the client. *Use of transfer devices and adequate staff, when moving/positioning clients, decreases frictional forces, tissue bruising, and pressure injury (Scott-Williams, 2006).* **EBN:** *Two people should assist an awake client to transfer from a cart/bed to the OR table: one person on the stretcher side to assist the client onto the OR table and a second person on the far side of the OR table to prevent the client from falling off the table (Phillips, 2007). A minimum of four persons are necessary when transferring/positioning an anesthetized, unconscious, obese, or weak client (Evans, 2005; Phillips, 2007).*
- Monitor pressure being applied to the client intraoperatively by staff, equipment, and/or instruments. *Staff leaning on the client or equipment and/or instruments resting on the client can cause redness and bruising and lead to pressure ulcers (Rothrock, 2003). An adequate clearance of 2 to 3 inches should be maintained in order to protect feet and protuberant parts from over bed tables, mayo stands, and frames (Phillips, 2007).* **EB:** *Injury due to retraction and manipulation of tissue has been observed during pelvic procedures (femoral nerve injuries) as well as during hip surgery (sciatic nerve injuries) (Phillips, 2007). Head straps that are too tight can cause facial nerve injury (Phillips, 2007).*
- Pad all bony prominences. **EB:** *Pressure over bony prominences causes blood vessel compression, which in turn diminishes the flow of oxygen and nutrients to the area, which eventually results in cell death (Goodman, 2006).*
- Reddened areas or areas injured by pressure should not be massaged. **EB:** *One research study showed that pressure ulcer incidence was reduced 38% in non-massaged versus massaged areas*

I

(Goodman, 2006). The added stress of massaging tissue can cause additional damage (Steris, 2005). **EB:** *Clients undergoing epidural anesthesia should wear heel pads and be placed on a large celled ripple type mattress to prevent pressure ulcer formation (Roeder et al, 2005).*

- Keep linens on the OR table free of wrinkles. *Folds and creases in linen can cause pressure on the skin (Phillips, 2007).*
- Lift rather than pull or slide the client when positioning. *Sliding and pulling increase the incidence of skin injury (dermal abrasion or soft tissue injury) from shearing and friction (Phillips, 2007).* **EBN:** *The use of technical aids and techniques when correctly positioning the client has been shown to decrease the intensity of pressure and shearing forces (Defloor et al, 2000).*
- Recognize that the longer the surgery, the greater the chance of the client developing pressure ulcers. **EBN:** *The risk of developing an intraoperative pressure ulcer increases as the length of the surgical procedure increases, especially in procedures lasting longer than 3 hours (Rothrock, 2003).*

Positioning the Perioperative Client

- Equipment should be checked to verify it is in good working order and it should be used according to manufacturer's instructions. **EB:** *Equipment that is working properly leads to client safety and aids in improved exposure of the surgical site (AORN, 2006). Many beds have a weight limit for safe use; therefore, it is necessary to check the equipment to ensure that it will tolerate the client's weight (Phillips, 2007).* **EBN:** *Preplanning ensures that the correct positioning devices are available and in good working condition, and that appropriate numbers of personnel are available to position the client safely and appropriately (AORN, 2006).*
- Recognize that the nurse must demonstrate knowledge of not only the equipment, but also anatomy and the application of physiological principles in order to properly position the client (AORN, 2006). **EBN:** *Preplanning ensures that the correct positioning devices are available and in good working condition, and that appropriate numbers of personnel are available to position the client safely and appropriately (AORN, 2006).*
- A preoperative assessment should be completed prior to the surgical procedure to "identify physical alterations that may require additional precautions for procedure-specific positioning" (AORN, 2006). *The client's overall condition, procedure length, equipment to be used during surgery (i.e., x-ray), amount of exposure needed at the operative site, and the expected anatomic and physiologic changes associated with the type of anesthesia should be considered during the preoperative assessment (Steris, 2004).*
- Lock the OR table, cart, or bed and stabilize the mattress before transfer/positioning of the client (Phillips, 2007). *An unlocked OR table, cart, or bed could lead to the client's sustaining a fall injury.*
- Clients, especially those with limited range of motion/mobility, should be asked to position themselves under the nurse's guidance before induction of anesthesia so that he or she can verify that a position of comfort has been obtained. **EB:** *Having the awake client assist in positioning is helpful for assessing range of comfort when the skeleton is distorted and for evaluating alternate positioning that will allow for maximum surgical site exposure (Martin, 2000).*
- Ensure nerves are protected by positioning extremities carefully. *Improperly positioned arms, hands, shoulders, legs, or feet can lead to serious injury or paralysis.*
- Avoid hyperextension of joints. **EB:** *Hyperextension of joints can cause postoperative pain and permanent injury to extremities (Phillips, 2007).*
- Movements during positioning should be slow and smooth. **EB:** *Quick, jerky movements can cause musculo-skeletal injury (Rothrock, 2003). Slow movements allow the body time to adjust to circulatory and respiratory changes, and also allow the staff to have better control of the client's body (Phillips, 2007; Steris, 2004).*
- Reassess the client after positioning and periodically during the procedure for maintenance of proper alignment and skin integrity. *Changes in position can expose or injure body parts (e.g., shearing, friction, compression) that were originally protected (AORN, 2006). Once the client has been positioned, lifting him or her slightly for a moment may allow skin to realign with the skeleton and decrease potential for shearing, and so on (Rothrock, 2003).*
- Do not allow extremities to extend beyond/off the OR table. *Many beds have an extension that can be added to accommodate tall clients (Phillips, 2007).*

- Monitor intraocular pressure when client is in prone position. **EB:** *The prone position significantly increases intraocular pressure, which places the client at increased risk for vision loss (Greenberg & Tymms, 2003).*
- Extended pressure on the scalp can cause localized alopecia in that area postoperatively. **EB:** *Research shows that the likelihood of alopecia developing can be reduced if the head is repositioned every 30 minutes (Steris, 2004).*
- Avoid contact with metal when positioning the client. *Prior to draping, observe the client to ensure that pressure isn't being exerted on tissue (Steris, 2005).*
- Position hips in proper alignment with knees flexed. *Unaligned hips can cause pressure to the low back and hip joints. When strained, hips are prone to lumbar plexus damage (Millsap, 2006).*
- Monitor vulnerable areas such as ulnar nerves, brachial plexus, occiput, and so on.
- To decrease the potential for a brachial plexus injury, position arms so that they don't extend beyond a 90-degree angle.
- When positioning arms at sides, place the arm on the sheet; pass the sheet over the top of the arm, and then have another person roll the client up so that the arm can be tucked under the client. **EB:** *When the arm is placed beneath the sheet and the sheet brought over the top of the arm and then tucked beneath the mattress, the arm can fall off the mattress and hang over the metal edge of the table, where it is exposed to being leaned against by the surgical team (GASNet, 2001; Millsap, 2006).*
- Prevent pooling of preparative solutions, blood, irrigation, urine, and feces. Prior to initiating the skin prep, absorbent pads should be placed to collect any preoperative solutions that run off the area being prepped. Clean up as necessary. *Pooling in areas of high pressure can increase the chances for the development of a more severe pressure sore, and prolonged exposure to skin prep chemicals in pressure areas can lead to chemically induced contact dermatitis (Rothrock, 2003).*
- Ensure that the airway and chest are free from obstruction, that is, arms not pressing on chest, gown not causing neck or chest constriction.
- Keep the client appropriately covered during the procedure. Reducing unnecessary exposure provides privacy and dignity for the client during positioning and also helps in the prevention of hypothermia (AORN, 2006; Phillips, 2007).
- Implement measures to prevent inadvertent hypothermia (Beyea, 2002). **EBN:** *One study demonstrated that the use of warming blankets under clients was statistically significant in the increased development of pressure ulcers (Armstrong & Bortz, 2001). Other research has shown that forced air warming over non-pressure areas can decrease the risk of pressure ulcers developing, by slowing the detrimental effects of hypothermia (Rothrock, 2003). Another study with results of clinical significance showed the incidence of pressure ulcers was reduced by almost half when intraoperative warming occurred (Rothrock, 2003).*
- If the client is positioned in Trendelenburg/reverse Trendelenburg or with the head of the bed raised/lowered, every attempt should be made to lift the client for several seconds, prior to prepping and draping, to allow the skin to realign itself. *When raising/lowering the head of the bed or placing the client in Trendelenburg/reverse Trendelenburg position, gravity can cause the skeleton to be pulled, which in turn can lead to tearing, folding, and/or stretching of tissue (Rothrock, 2003).*
- Position the client's legs parallel and uncrossed. *Crossing of the client's ankles and legs creates occlusive pressure on blood vessels and nerves that can lead to pressure necrosis and also place the client at risk for development of a deep vein thrombosis (Phillips, 2007).*
- Maintain alignment of head with cervical, thoracic, and lumbar spine. *Misalignment, flexion, and twisting may cause muscle and nerve damage, as well as airway interference. Proper alignment of the head and spine prevents neuromuscular strain. The head should be in a neutral position and turned as little as possible so that airway and cerebral circulation are maintained (Phillips, 2007).*
- Body supports and restraint straps (safety belt) should be loose and secured over waist or mid-thigh at least 2 inches above knees, avoiding bony prominences by placing a blanket between the strap and the client. *Adequate arterial circulation must be maintained to avoid changes in blood pressure, tissue perfusion (oxygenation), venous return, and thrombus formation. Occlusion and pressure on peripheral blood vessels should be avoided (Phillips, 2007).*
- Clients positioned in lithotomy should be kept in this position for as short a time as possible.

• = Independent;   ▲ = Collaborative;   EBN = Evidence-Based Nursing;   EB = Evidence-Based

EB: *One study showed that for every hour past the first hour in lithotomy, there is a 100-fold increase in risk for neuropathy (Warner, 2003).*

- Recognize that complete, concise, accurate documentation of client assessment and use of positioning devices is imperative. For information on specific positioning—Supine, Prone, Lateral, Lithotomy, Trendelenburg, Reverse Trendelenburg—please refer to Phillips NF: *Berry & Kohn's Operating Room Technique*, ed 11, Philadelphia, 2007, Mosby.

evolve See the EVOLVE website for World Wide Web resources for client education.

REFERENCES

Alterman I, Sidi A, Azamfirei L et al: Rhabdomyolysis: another complication after prolonged surgery, *J Clin Anesth* 19(1):64-66, 2007.

AORN: Recommended practices for positioning the patient in the perioperative practice setting, *AORN Standards and Recommended Practices for Perioperative Nursing,* Denver, 587-592, 2006, The Association of Perioperative Registered Nurses.

Armstrong D, Bortz P: An integrative review of pressure relief in surgical patients, *AORN J* 73(3):645-674, 2001.

Beyea S: *Perioperative nursing data set: the perioperative nursing vocabulary,* ed 2, Denver, 2002, AORN, Inc.

DeFloor T, De Schuijmer JD: Preventing pressure ulcers: an evaluation of four operating table mattresses, *Appl Nurs Res* 13(3):134-141, 2000.

Evans G: Time out: patient positioning a safety essential, *OR Today* 36-37, 2005.

GASNet Anesthesiology: Positioning: "tucking" the arms. http://gasnet.org/tips/armtuck_br.php.

Goodman T: *Positioning: a patient safety initiative,* Infection Control Education Institute, 2006.

Greenberg R, Tymms A: Alert for perioperative visual loss: an unusual presentation of an orbital haemangioma during spinal surgery, *Anaesth Intensive Care* 31(6):679-682, 2003.

Martin JT: Positioning aged patients, *Geriatr Anesth* 18:1, 2000.

Millsap CC: Pay attention to patient positioning! *RN* 69(1):59-63, 2006.

Phillips NF: *Berry and Kohn's operating room technique, positioning the patient,* ed 11, St Louis, 2007, Mosby.

Pokorny ME, Koldjeski D, Swanson M: Skin care intervention for patients having cardiac surgery, *Am J Crit Care* 12(6):535-544, 2003.

Power H: Patient positioning outcomes for women undergoing gynaecological surgeries, *Can Oper Room Nurs J* 20(3):7-10, 27-30, 2002.

Roeder BA, Geddes LA, Corson N et al: Heel and calf capillary–support: pressure in lithotomy positions, *AORN J* 81(4):821-830, 2005.

Rothrock J: *Alexander's care of the patient in surgery,* ed 12, St. Louis, 2003, Mosby.

Schultz A: Predicting and preventing pressure ulcers in surgical patients, *AORN J* 81(5):986-1006, 2005.

Scott-Williams S: Prevent patient positioning problems, *Outpatient Surgery Magazine,* December 2006.

Sewchuk D, Padula C, Osborne E: Prevention and early diction of pressure ulcers in patients undergoing cardiac surgery, *AORN J* 84(1):75-96, 2006.

Steris: Intraoperative patient positioning: It's more than just comfort [study guide], No. M1721EN, 2004, available at www.steris.com. Accessed April 23, 2007.

Steris: Perioperative pressure management: It's a "sore" subject [study guide], No. M2832EN, 2005, available at www.steris.com. Accessed April 23, 2007.

Warner M: 7 patient positioning strategies, *Outpatient Surgery Magazine,* August 2003.

Insomnia   Judith A. Floyd, PhD, RN, and Jean D. Humphries, MSN, RN   **evolve**

NANDA   Definition

A disruption in amount and quality of sleep that impairs functioning

Defining Characteristics

Observed changes in affect; observed lack of energy; increased work/school absenteeism; patient reports changes in mood; patient reports decreased health status; patient reports decreased quality of life; patient reports difficulty concentrating; patient reports difficulty falling asleep; patient reports difficulty staying asleep; patient reports dissatisfaction with sleep (current); patient reports increased accidents; patient reports lack of energy; patient reports nonrestorative sleep; patient reports sleep disturbances that produce next-day consequences; patient reports waking up too early

Related Factors (r/t)

Activity pattern (e.g., timing, amount); anxiety; depression; environmental factors (e.g., ambient noise, daylight/darkness exposure, ambient temperature/humidity, unfamiliar setting, fear, gender-

---

• = Independent;   ▲ = Collaborative;   EBN = Evidence-Based Nursing;   EB = Evidence-Based

related hormonal shifts, grief, inadequate sleep hygiene [current], intake of stimulants, intake of alcohol, impairment of normal sleep pattern (e.g., travel, shift work, parental responsibilities, interruptions for interventions); medications; physical discomfort (e.g., body temperature, pain, shortness of breath, cough, gastroesophageal reflux, nausea, incontinence/urgency); stress (e.g., ruminative presleep pattern)

NOC   Outcomes (Nursing Outcomes Classification)

Suggested NOC Outcomes

Comfort Level, Pain Level, Personal Well-Being, Psychosocial Adjustment: Life Change, Quality of Life, Rest, Sleep

Example NOC Outcome with Indicators
Sleep as evidenced by the following indicators: Hours of sleep/Sleep pattern/Sleep quality/Sleep efficiency/Feels rejuvenated after sleep/Napping appropriate for age (Rate the outcome and indicators of **Sleep:** 1 = severely compromised, 2 = substantially compromised, 3 = moderately compromised, 4 = mildly compromised, 5 = not compromised [see Section I].)

I

Client Outcomes

Client Will (Specify Time Frame):

- Wake up less frequently during night
- Awaken refreshed and not be fatigued during day
- Fall asleep without difficulty
- Verbalize plan to implement sleep promoting routines

NIC   Interventions (Nursing Interventions Classification)

Suggested NIC Intervention

Sleep Enhancement

Example NIC Activities—Sleep Enhancement
Monitor/record patient's sleep pattern and number of sleep hours; Encourage patient to establish a bedtime routine to facilitate transition from wakefulness to sleep

Nursing Interventions and *Rationales*

- Obtain a sleep history including bedtime routines, history of sleep problems, changes in sleep with present illness, and use of medications and stimulants. *Assessment of sleep behavior and patterns are an important part of any health status examination (Landis, 2002).*
- ▲ Assess level of pain and use available pharmacological and non-pharmacological approaches to pain management. *Pain leads to sleep disruption and sleep disruption increases the perception of pain (Roehrs & Roth, 2005; Stiefel & Stagno, 2004).*
- Provide pain relief shortly before bedtime and position the client comfortably for sleep. *Clients have reported that uncomfortable positions and pain are common factors of sleep disturbance (Sateia et al, 2000).*
- Determine level of anxiety. If the client is anxious, use relaxation techniques. See Nursing Interventions and Rationales for **Anxiety. EBN and EB:** *The use of relaxation techniques to promote sleep in people with chronic insomnia has been shown to be effective (Floyd et al, 2000; Johnson, 1991b; Morin et al, 1994).*
- Teach methods for calming the mind. **EBN:** *Guided imagery and meditation decreased sleep disturbance and improved sleep quality (Carlson & Garland, 2005; Richardson, 2003).*

• = Independent;   ▲ = Collaborative;   EBN = Evidence-Based Nursing;   EB = Evidence-Based

▲ Assess for signs of new onset of depression: depressed mood state, statements of hopelessness, poor appetite. Refer for counseling as appropriate. *Many symptoms associated with sleep disruption probably arise from central nervous system hyperarousal in the depressed client (Sateia et al, 2000).*

▲ If the client is waking frequently during the night, consider the presence of sleep apnea problems and refer to a sleep clinic for evaluation. **EB:** *Survey study identified that 36% of adults had high probability for sleep apnea (Netzer et al, 2003).*

▲ Monitor for presence of sleep disordered breathing as evidenced by loud snoring with periods of apnea, or other sleep disorders such as restless leg syndrome or periodic limb movement disorder. Refer to an accredited sleep disorder center. *Polysomnography evaluation is recommended if a sleep disorder exists (Epstein & Bootzin, 2002).* **EB:** *Up to 15% of all chronic poor sleep is associated with breathing disturbances (Sateia, Doghramji & Hauri, 2000).*

• Observe the client's medication, diet, and caffeine intake. Look for hidden sources of caffeine, such as over-the-counter medications. *Difficulty sleeping can be a side effect of medications such as bronchodilators; caffeine can also interfere with sleep (Benca, 2005).* **EB:** *Caffeine use after 2 PM is associated with poor sleep (Ellis et al, 2002).*

• Provide measures to take before bedtime to assist with sleep (e.g., quiet time to allow the mind to slow down, carbohydrates such as crackers). *Simple measures can increase quality of sleep. Carbohydrates cause release of the neurotransmitter serotonin, which helps induce and maintain sleep (Somer, 1999).*

• Provide a back massage before bedtime. *Use of a back massage has been shown effective for promoting relaxation, which likely leads to improved sleep (Richards et al, 2003).*

• Provide pain relief shortly before bedtime and position the client comfortably for sleep. *Clients have reported that uncomfortable positions and pain are common factors of sleep disturbance (Sateia, Doghramji & Hauri, 2000).*

• Keep environment quiet for sleeping (e.g., avoid use of intercoms, lower the volume on radio and television, keep beepers on nonaudio mode, anticipate alarms on intravenous [IV] pumps, talk quietly on unit). *Attention to environmental sources of noise can eliminate or reduce them (Barr, 1993).* **EBN:** *Healthy volunteers exposed to recorded critical care noise levels experienced poor quality sleep (Topf et al, 1996). Excessive noise disrupts sleep (Floyd, 1999). Quiet time increased sleep duration in hospitalized adults (Olson et al, 2001).*

• Use soothing sound generators with sounds of the ocean, rainfall, or waterfall to induce sleep, or use "white noise" such as a fan to block out other sounds. Also consider the use of earplugs. **EBN:** *Ocean sounds promoted sleep for a group of postoperative open-heart surgery clients (Williamson, 1992). Earplugs have been found to decrease the effects of simulated intensive care unit noise on sleep (Wallace et al, 1999).*

• Encourage the client to use soothing music to facilitate sleep. **EBN:** *Music results in better sleep quality, longer sleep duration, greater sleep efficiency, shorter sleep latency, less sleep disturbance, and less daytime dysfunction (Lai & Good, 2005).*

• For hospitalized stable clients, consider instituting the following sleep protocol to foster sleep:
  - Night shift: Give the client the opportunity for uninterrupted sleep from 1 AM–5 AM. Keep environmental noise to a minimum.
  - Evening shift: Limit napping between 4 PM and 9 PM. At 10 PM, lower intensity of room and unit lights, provide sleep medication according to individual assessment, and keep noise and conversation on the unit to a minimum.
  - Day shift: Encourage short naps before 11 AM. Enforce a physical activity regimen as appropriate. Schedule newly ordered medications to avoid waking the client between 1 AM and 5 AM.

  EBN: *The high frequency of nocturnal care interactions has been found to leave clients with few uninterrupted periods for sleep (Edwards & Schuring, 1993a; Tamburri et al, 2004). Critical care nurses can take effective actions to promote sleep (Edwards & Schuring, 1993b).*

Geriatric

• Determine if the client has new onset of a physiological problem that could result in insomnia, such as pain, cardiovascular disease, pulmonary disease, neurological problems such as dementia,

---

or urinary problems. *Sleep disturbances in the elderly may represent a complex interaction of age-related changes and pathological causes (Sateia, Doghramji & Hauri, 2000).*

- Assess urinary elimination patterns. Instruct the client to decrease fluid intake in the evening and take diuretics early in the morning unless contraindicated. *Many elderly people awaken to void during the night. Increasing water intake at night or taking diuretics late in the day increases nocturia, which results in disrupted sleep (Avidan, 2005).*

- Obtain a list of all medications including over-the-counter medications and alcohol intake. *Alcohol intake and medication effects are common causes of insomnia in the elderly. Rebound insomnia associated with the use of shorter-acting hypnotics may perpetuate a cycle of sleep disturbance and chronic hypnotic use (Sateia, Doghramji & Hauri, 2000).*

▲ If the client is waking frequently during the night, consider the presence of sleep apnea problems and refer to a sleep clinic for evaluation. *Sleep apnea in the elderly may be caused by changes in the respiratory drive of the central nervous system or may be obstructive and associated with obesity (Foyt, 1992).*

▲ Evaluate the client for presence of depression or anxiety, which can result in insomnia. Refer for treatment as appropriate. *Anxiety and depression are common in the elderly and can result in insomnia (Sateia, Doghramji & Hauri, 2000).*

- Suggest light reading or TV viewing that does not excite as an evening activity. *Soothing activities decrease stimulation of the reticular activating system and help sleep come naturally (Labyak, 2002).*

- Recommend avoidance of hypnotics and alcohol to induce sleep. *Avoid alcohol ingestion 4 to 6 hours before bedtime. Long-term use of hypnotics can induce a drug-related insomnia. Sleep induced by alcohol is often disrupted later in the night (Epstein & Bootzin, 2002).* **EB:** *In nonalcoholic sleepers, bedtime alcohol use decreased sleep latency but increased wakefulness during the latter part of the sleep period (Roehrs & Roth, 1997).*

- Reduce daytime napping in the late afternoon; limit naps to short intervals as early in the day as possible. *The majority of elderly nap during the day (Evans & Rogers, 1994). Avoiding naps in the late afternoon makes it easier to fall asleep at night.* **EBN:** *Naps longer than 50 minutes were associated with increased nighttime awakening (Floyd, 1995).* **EB:** *Napping short intervals early in the day enhanced cognitive and psychomotor performance (Campbell, Murphy & Stauble, 2005).*

- Help the client recognize that changes in length of sleep occur with aging, as well as nature of sleep experience. *Client may not be able to sleep for 8 hours as when younger, and more frequent awakening is part of the aging process (Floyd, 2002).* **EB:** *Only two studies report that older adults with insomnia reveal a greater problem with sleep maintenance. The prevalence of apnea increases significantly with age, risk factors include being male, snoring, and obesity. Community-based studies have indicated this is common among older adults, affecting approximately 24% of those over age 65 (Espie, 2001).*

 Home Care

- Previously discussed interventions may be adapted for home care use.

- Provide support to the family of the client with chronic sleep pattern disturbance. *Ongoing sleep pattern disturbances can disrupt family patterns and cause sleep deprivation in client or family members, which creates increased stress on the family.*

- Instruct the client/family in expectations for normal sleep. Elicit expectations for sleep, previous sleep patterns; correct misconceptions that influence emotional responses to deviation from expectations. **EBN:** *Client/family may be unduly disturbed by normal changes in sleep patterns. As persons age, increased time is needed to fall asleep; frequency of waking after sleep onset increases; length of waking after sleep onset increases (which may be related to unrecognized sleep apnea); and nighttime sleep amount tends to decrease (Floyd, Falahee & Fhobir, 2000).* **EBN:** *A study found that older adults often have insomnia, frequent nocturnal awakenings, snoring, restlessness, and periodic limb movements during sleep; daytime sleepiness often is a symptom (Piani et al, 2004).*

- Assess the client for sleep apnea, particularly poststroke (e.g., interview partner regarding the client's sleep pattern and behaviors, have the client maintain sleep log). *Perceived sleep disturbance may be an indication of sleep apnea, which tends to increase with age. In one study poststroke, 59% of*

• = Independent;   ▲ = Collaborative;   EBN = Evidence-Based Nursing;   EB = Evidence-Based

I

participants met criteria for sleep apnea. More clients with sleep apnea than without were delirious, depressed, or activities of daily living (ADL) dependent; and had a higher frequency of ischemic heart disease and latency in reaction and in response to verbal stimuli. Clients may benefit from continuous positive airway pressure (CPAP) treatment (Sandberg et al, 2001).

▲ Assess the client for depression or other psychiatric disorder. Refer for mental health services as indicated. *Sleep disturbance is part of the syndrome of depression and other psychiatric disorders. Improvement in sleep pattern is unlikely unless the underlying disorder is treated.*

• Have the client maintain a sleep diary, describing daily activity levels, use of stimulants, activities, or physical sensations around bedtime. Assess diary for potential areas of intervention. *Details about daily activities may yield clues to change sleep pattern (e.g., exercise timing or excessive coffee use, meals before bedtime, acid indigestion while lying flat).*

• Assess environment for possible hazards to the client during periods of disturbance (e.g., appliances, stairs). Ensure that, if client awakens during the night, there will be sufficient light (consider a night light), with passageways clear of obstruction between bed and bathroom. *Client safety is a primary goal of care in the home setting.* **EB:** *Older adults frequently wake during the night with an urge to void (Piani et al, 2004).*

• Initiate nonpharmacological interventions for insomnia: control of environmental stimuli, sleep restriction, relaxation techniques, increasing sunlight exposure, acupuncture, cognitive and educational interventions to address dysfunctional attitudes about sleep. **EBN and EB:** *Nonpharmacological interventions can improve sleep efficiency and continuity and increase satisfaction with sleep pattern while reducing hypnotic use (Morin, Mimeault & Gagne, 1999; Woodward, 1999). Nursing interventions are directed at making environments conducive to sleep, relaxing the client, or entraining the circadian sleep-wake cycle (Floyd, 1999).*

• Use the scent of lavender. **EB:** *The scent of lavender has improved the sleep quality in adults and elderly (Cannard, 1995; Lewith, Godfrey & Prescott, 2005).*

• In the presence of a cognitive disorder, reassure family regarding sleep expectations for the client and address potential problems (e.g., enuresis will require frequent cleansing of client and changes of bed linens); procurement of a hospital bed with side rails may be necessary to prevent falling out of bed. **EB:** *A study showed that older adults with cognitive disorders had fewer nighttime awakenings than those without a cognitive disorder but were the only participants to be enuretic or to fall out of bed. Individuals with cognitive dysfunctions had more daytime sleepiness and more difficulty maintaining attention and concentration; sleep attacks were much more common in participants with cognitive disorders (Piani et al, 2004).*

▲ In the presence of a psychiatric disorder, refer for psychiatric home healthcare services for client reassurance and implementation of therapeutic regimen. *Psychiatric home care nurses can address issues relating to client's sleep disturbance. Behavioral interventions in the home can assist client to participate more effectively in treatment plan (Patusky et al, 1996).*

• Provide support to the family of the client with chronic sleep pattern disturbance. *Ongoing sleep pattern disturbances can disrupt family patterns and cause sleep deprivation in the client or family members, which creates increased stress on the family.*

Client/Family Teaching

• Encourage the client to avoid coffee and other caffeinated foods and liquids and also to avoid eating large high-protein or high-fat meals close to bedtime. *Caffeine intake increases the time it takes to fall asleep and increases awake time during the night (Evans & Rogers, 1994).*

• Advise the client to avoid use of alcohol or hypnotics to induce sleep. Avoid alcohol ingestion 4 to 6 hours before bedtime. *Sleep induced by alcohol is often disrupted later in the night (Epstein & Bootzin, 2002). Clients can easily become dependent on hypnotics for sleep and develop rebound insomnia if they are discontinued. Nonpharmacological interventions to maintain sleep are more effective than pharmacological treatments in the long term (Epstein & Bootzin, 2002).*

• Ask the client to keep a sleep diary for several weeks. *Often the client can find the cause of the sleep deprivation when the pattern of sleeping is examined (Pagel et al, 1997).*

• Teach somatic and cognitive relaxation techniques to induce the relaxation response and facilitate sleep. **EBN and EB:** *The use of relaxation techniques to promote sleep in people with chronic insomnia has been shown to be effective (Floyd et al, 2000; Johnson, 1991a; Morin, Culbert & Schwartz, 1994).*

• = Independent; ▲ = Collaborative; EBN = Evidence-Based Nursing; EB = Evidence-Based

- Teach the client need for increased exercise. Encourage to take a daily walk 5 to 6 hours before retiring. *Moderate activity such as walking can increase the quality of sleep (King et al, 1997).*
- Encourage the client to develop a bedtime ritual that includes quiet activities such as reading, television, or crafts. **EBN:** *The use of a bedtime routine has been shown to be effective in inducing and maintaining sleep in a population of older women (Johnson, 1991a).*
- Teach the following guidelines for good sleep hygiene to improve sleep habits:
  - Go to bed only when sleepy.
  - When awake in the middle of the night, go to another room, do quiet activities, and go back to bed only when sleepy.
  - Use the bed only for sleeping.
  - Avoid afternoon and evening naps.
  - Get out of bed at the same time every morning.
  - Recognize that not everyone needs 8 hours of sleep.
  - Move the alarm clock away from the bed so that it cannot be seen.
  - Do not associate lulls in performance with sleeplessness; sleeplessness should not be blamed for everything that goes wrong during the day.

  EB: *These guidelines on sleep hygiene have been shown to effectively improve quality of sleep (Morin et al, 1994; Morin et al, 2005).*

evolve See the EVOLVE website for World Wide Web resources for client education.

REFERENCES

Avidan AY: Sleep in the geriatric patient population, *Semin Neurol* 25(1):52, 2005.

Barr WJ: Noise notes: working smart, *Am J Nurs* 93:16, 1993.

Benca RM: Diagnosis and treatment of chronic insomnia: review, *Psychiatr Serv* 56(3):334, 2005.

Campbell SS, Murphy PJ, Stauble TN: Effects of a nap on nighttime sleep and waking function in older subjects, *J Am Geriatr Soc* 53(1):48, 2005.

Cannard G: Complementary therapies: on the scent of a good night's sleep, *Nurs Stand* 9(34):17, 1995.

Carlson LE, Garland SN: Impact of mindfulness-based stress reduction (MBSR) on sleep, mood, stress and fatigue symptoms in cancer outpatients, *Int J Behav Med* 12(4):278, 2005.

Edwards GB, Schuring LM: Pilot study: validating staff nurses' observations of sleep and wake states among critically ill patients using polysomnography, *Am J Crit Care* 2(2):125, 1993a.

Edwards GB, Schuring LM: Sleep protocol: a research-based practice change, *Crit Care Nurse* 13:84, 1993b.

Ellis J, Hampson SE, Cropley M et al: Sleep hygiene or compensatory sleep practices: an examination of behaviours affecting sleep in older adults, *Psychol Health Med* 7(2):157, 2002.

Epstein DR, Bootzin RR: Insomnia, *Nurs Clin North Am* 37(4):611, 2002.

Espie CA: The clinical effectiveness of cognitive behavior therapy for chronic insomnia: implementation and evaluation of a sleep clinic in general medical practice, *Behav Resp Ther* 39:45-60, 2001.

Evans BD, Rogers AE: 24-hour sleep/wake patterns in healthy elderly persons, *Appl Nurs Res* 7:75, 1994.

Floyd JA: Another look at napping in the older adult, *Geriatr Nurs* 16(3):136, 1995.

Floyd JA: Sleep and aging, *Nurs Clin North Am* 37(4):719, 2002.

Floyd JA: Sleep promotion in adults, *Annu Rev Nurs Res* 17:27, 1999.

Floyd JA, Falahee ML, Fhobir RH: Creation and analysis of a computerized database of interventions to facilitate adult sleep, *Nurs Res* 49(4):236, 2000.

Floyd JA, Medler SM, Ager JW et al: Age-related changes in initiation and maintenance of sleep: a meta-analysis, *Res Nurs Health* 23(2):106, 2000.

Foyt MM: Impaired gas exchange in the elderly, *Geriatr Nurs* 13:262, 1992.

Johnson JE: A comparative study of the bedtime routines and sleep of older adults, *J Commun Nurs* 8(3):129, 1991a.

Johnson JE: Progressive relaxation and the sleep of older noninstitutionalized women, *Appl Nurs Res* 4(4):165, 1991b.

King AC, Oman RF, Brassington GS et al: Moderate-intensity exercise and self-rated quality of sleep in older adults, *JAMA* 277(1):32, 1997.

Labyak S: Sleep and circadian schedule disorders, *Nurs Clin North Am* 37:599, 2002.

Lai HL, Good M: Music improves sleep quality in older adults, *J Adv Nurs* 49(3):234, 2005.

Landis CA: Sleep and methods of assessment, *Nurs Clin North Am* 37:583, 2002.

Lewith GT, Godfrey AD, Prescott P: A single-blinded, randomized pilot study evaluating the aroma of Lavandula augustifolia as a treatment for mild insomnia, *J Alt Complementary Med* 11(4):631, 2005.

Morin C, Beaulieu-Bonneau S, LeBlanc M et al: Self-help treatment for insomnia: a randomized controlled trial, *Sleep* 28(1):1319-1327, 2005.

Morin CM, Culbert JP, Schwartz SM: Nonpharmacological interventions for insomnia, *Am J Psychiatry* 151(8):1172, 1994.

Morin CM, Mimeault V, Gagne A: Nonpharmacologic treatment of chronic insomnia, *J Psychosom Res* 46(2):103, 1999.

Netzer NC, Hoegel JJ, Loube D et al: Prevalence of symptoms and risk of sleep apnea in primary care, *Chest* 124:1406, 2003.

Olson DM, Borel CO, Laskowitz DT et al: Quiet time: a nursing intervention to promote sleep in neurocritical care units, *Am J Crit Care* 10(2):74, 2001.

Pagel JF et al: How to prescribe a good night's sleep, *Patient Care* 31(4):87, 1997.

Patusky KL et al: Clinical lessons in psychiatric home health care: a case study approach, *Home Healthc Manag Pract* 9(1):18, 1996.

Piani A, Brotini S, Dolso P et al: Sleep disturbances in elderly: a subjective evaluation over 65, *Arch Gerontol Geriatr* 9(Suppl):325, 2004.

Richards K, Nagel C, Markie M et al: Use of complementary and alternative therapies to promote sleep in critical ill patients, *Crit Care Nurs Clin North Am* 15(3):329-340, 2003.

Richardson S: Effects of relaxation and imagery on the sleep of critically ill adults, *Dimen Crit Care Nurs* 22(4):182, 2003.

Roehrs T, Roth T: Hypnotics, alcohol, and caffeine: relation to insomnia. In Pressman MR, Orr WC, editors: *Understanding sleep: the evaluation and treatment of sleep disorders,* Washington, DC, 1997, American Psychological Association.

Roehrs T, Roth T: Sleep and pain: interaction of two vital functions, *Semin Neurol* 25(1):106, 2005.

Sandberg O, Franklin K, Bucht G et al: Sleep apnea, delirium, depressed mood, cognition, and ADL ability after stroke, *J Am Geriatr Soc* 49:391, 2001.

Sateia MJ, Doghramji K, Hauri PJ et al: Evaluation of chronic insomnia. An American Academy of Sleep Medicine review, *Sleep* 23(2):243-308, 2000.

Somer E: *Food and mood: the complete guide to eating well and feeling your best,* ed 2, New York, 1999, Henry Holt.

Stiefel F, Stagno D: Management of insomnia in patients with chronic pain conditions, *CNS Drugs* 18(5):285, 2004.

Tamburri LM, DiBrienza R, Zozula R et al: Nocturnal care interactions with patients in critical care units, *Am J Crit Care* 13(2):102, 2004.

Topf M, Bookman M: Effects of critical care unit noise on the subjective quality of sleep, *J Adv Nurs* 24(3):545-551, 1996.

Wallace CJ, Robins J, Alvord LS et al: The effect of earplugs on sleep measures during exposure to simulated intensive care unit noise, *Am J Crit Care* 8:210-219, 1999.

Williamson J: The effect of ocean sounds on sleep after coronary artery bypass graft surgery, *Am J Crit Care* 1(1):91, 1992.

Woodward M: Insomnia in the elderly, *Aust Fam Phys* 28:653, 1999.

Decreased Intracranial Adaptive Capacity   Laura Mcilvoy, PhD, RN, CCRN, CNRN

NANDA   Definition

Intracranial fluid dynamic mechanisms that normally compensate for increases in intracranial volumes are compromised, resulting in repeated disproportionate increases in intracranial pressure (ICP) in response to a variety of noxious and non-noxious stimuli

Defining Characteristics

Baseline ICP greater than 10 mm Hg; disproportionate increases in ICP following a single environmental or nursing maneuver stimulus; elevated P2 component of ICP waveform; repeated increases in ICP of greater than 10 mm Hg for more than = minutes following any of a variety of external stimuli; volume-pressure response test variation (volume-pressure ratio of 2, pressure-volume index of less than 10); wide-amplitude ICP waveform (Kirkness, Burr & Cain, 2006; Rauch, Mitchell & Tyler, 1990)

Related Factors (r/t)

Brain injuries: decreased cerebral perfusion less than or equal to 50 to 60 mm Hg; sustained increase in ICP greater than 10 to 15 mm Hg; systemic hypotension with intracranial hypertension

NOC   Outcomes (Nursing Outcomes Classification)

Suggested NOC Outcomes

Neurological Status, Neurological Status: Consciousness

Example NOC Outcome with Indicators
Neurological Status as evidenced by the following indicators: Consciousness/Intracranial pressure/Vital signs/Central motor control/Cranial sensory-motor function/Spinal sensory-motor function (Rate the outcome and indicators of **Neurological Status:** 1 = severely compromised, 2 = substantially compromised, 3 = moderately compromised, 4 = mildly compromised, 5 = not compromised [see Section I].)

Client Outcomes

Client Will (Specify Time Frame):

• Experience fewer than five episodes of disproportionate increases in intracranial pressure (DIICP) in 24 hours

• = Independent;   ▲ = Collaborative;   EBN = Evidence-Based Nursing;   EB = Evidence-Based

- Have neurological status changes that are not triggered by episodes of DIICP
- Have cerebral perfusion pressure (CPP) remaining greater than 60 to 70 mm Hg in adults

NIC   Interventions (Nursing Interventions Classification)

Suggested NIC Interventions

Cerebral Edema Management, Cerebral Perfusion Promotion, Intracranial Pressure (ICP) Monitoring, Neurological Monitoring

Example NIC Activities—Cerebral Edema Management
Monitor for confusion, changes in mentation, complaints of dizziness, syncope; Allow ICP to return to baseline between nursing activities

Nursing Interventions and *Rationales*

- To assess ICP and CPP effectively:
  - Maintain and display ICP and CPP continuously. ICP data guide therapy and predict outcome. *The only way to determine CPP is to continuously monitor ICP and blood pressure (CPP = MAP – ICP). Continuous monitoring of CPP improves odds of survival at hospital discharge in clients with traumatic brain injury (TBI) (Brain Trauma Foundation & American Association of Neurological Surgeons, 2000; Kirkness, Burr & Cain, 2006).*
  - Maintain ICP <20 mm Hg and CPP >60 mm Hg. *The Guidelines for the Management of Severe Brain Injury established the treatment threshold for ICP as >20 mm Hg. These guidelines also state CPP should be maintained at a minimum of 60 mm Hg.*
  - Monitor neurological status frequently using the Glasgow Coma Scale (GCS), noting changes in eye opening, motor response to painful stimuli, and awareness of self, time, and place. *The GCS is the most widely used tool to assess level of consciousness in neurologically injured clients. A decrease of 2 points in a GCS score without identifiable cause (administration of sedation, narcotics, or anesthetic agents) should be reported to the physician.*
- ▲ To prevent harmful increases in ICP:
  - Administer sedation per collaborative protocol. **EB:** *Propofol infusions, compared with morphine sulfate infusions, lower ICP; decrease need for paralytic agents, benzodiazepines, pentobarbital, and cerebrospinal fluid (CSF) drainage; and improve outcomes in terms of disability and mortality at 6 months (Kelly et al, 1999).*
  - Administer pain medication per collaborative protocol. *Propofol in combination with narcotics prevents elevations of ICP in TBI clients. Narcotics do not adversely affect ICP in post-craniotomy clients (Englehard et al, 2004; Ferber et al, 2000).*
  - Maintain normothermia. *Elevation in brain temperature is associated with a rise in ICP. However, antipyretics and external cooling methods are only 40% effective in reducing fever in neurologically injured clients. Research into effective fever management continues (Mcilvoy, in press; O'Donnell & Lorber, 1997; Ogden, Mayer & Connolly, 2005; Rossi et al, 2001).*
  - Maintain optimal oxygenation and ventilation, applying positive end expiratory pressure (PEEP) as needed and avoiding hyperventilation. *Hypoxia causes increased mortality and morbidity in neurologically injured clients. It must be scrupulously avoided or corrected immediately. PEEP markedly improves gas exchange by increasing pulmonary volumes and is an effective treatment for refractory hypoxemia. PEEP levels of 10 cm H_2O have been found to produce no significant changes in ICP, especially when combined with head of bed elevation of 30°. PEEP levels of 15 cm H_2O produced a significant increase in ICP in one study but did not approach intracranial hypertension. Hyperventilation, especially in the absence of intracranial hypertension, has been found to worsen outcomes in TBI clients and should be avoided, especially in the first 24 hours postinjury (Brain Trauma Foundation & American Association of Neurological Surgeons, 2000; Huynh et al, 2002; Schulz-Stubner & Thiex, 2006; Schwarz et al, 2002b; Videtta et al, 2002).*
  - Limit endotracheal suction passes to two in order to limit ICP increases. Premedicate clients with adequate sedation, opiates, and/or neuromuscular blocking agents to prevent coughing

• = Independent;   ▲ = Collaborative;   EBN = Evidence-Based Nursing;   EB = Evidence-Based

and associated increases in ICP. **EBN and EB:** *Suctioning is known to increase ICP and CPP. In well-sedated or paralyzed clients, these elevations in ICP are attenuated. Particular care must be taken in suctioning clients with spiking ICP patterns, as increases in ICP may be cumulative with each suction pass (Gemma et al, 2002; Joanna Briggs Institute for Evidence Based Nursing and Midwifery, 2000; Kerr et al, 2001).*

- Allow auditory stimuli (family voices and music). **EBN:** *Taped messages by family, ear plugs, music tapes, or tapes of environmental noise have not been shown to increase ICP (Schinner et al, 1995; Walker, Eakes & Siebelink, 1998).*

- To prevent harmful decreases in CPP:
  - Maintain euvolemia. *Infusing intravenous fluids to sustain normal circulating volume helps maintain normal cerebral blood flow. A fluid balance lower than 594 ml is associated with poor outcomes in traumatic brain injury (Bullock, Chestnut & Clifton, 2001).*
  - Maintain head of bed flat or less than 30° in acute stroke clients. *Both mean blood flow velocity in the middle cerebral artery and CPP are increased with lowering head position from 30° to 0° in both ischemic and hemorrhagic stroke clients (Moraine, Berre & Melot, 2000; Schwarz et al, 2002b; Wojner-Alexandrov et al, 2005).*

- To treat sustained intracranial hypertension (ICP >20 mm Hg):
  - Elevate head of bed at least 30° with head in midline position. **EB:** *Elevating the head of the bed to 30° or greater allows for increased venous drainage that decreases ICP. However, if client is suffering acute stroke, CPP may be compromised with head elevation (Fan, 2004; Hung, Hare & Brien, 2000; Moraine, Berre & Melot, 2000; Murphy et al, 2004; Schwarz et al, 2002b; Winkleman, 2000; Wojner-Alexandrov et al, 2005).*
  - Remove or loosen rigid cervical collars. **EB:** *Most TBI clients are maintained in a rigid cervical collar until cervical spines are clear or as a treatment for cervical injury. Loosening or removing these collars allows for unrestricted venous drainage that lowers ICP (Hunt, Hallworth & Smith, 2001; Mobbs, Stoodley & Fuller, 2002).*
  - ▲ Administer a bolus dose of mannitol and/or hypertonic saline per collaborative protocol. **EB:** *Mannitol is recommended for control of raised ICP after a severe brain injury with a dose range of 0.25 g/kg to 1.0 g/kg body weight. Mannitol provides an immediate plasma expanding effect that reduces blood viscosity and increases cerebral blood flow. Fifteen to thirty minutes later, the osmotic diuretic effect occurs with eventual decrease of cerebral edema. Infusion of hypertonic saline also produces immediate volume expansion and provides an osmotic effect. Initial studies demonstrate that hypertonic saline may decrease ICP more effectively than mannitol with the effect lasting longer. However, the optimal concentration and dosage is unknown (Battison et al, 2005; Brain Trauma Foundation & American Association of Neurological Surgeons, 2000; Murphy et al, 2004; Schwarz et al, 2002b; Vialet et al, 2003).*
  - ▲ Drain CSF from an intraventricular catheter system per collaborative protocol. **EB:** *A withdrawal of 3 ml of CSF decreases ICP by 10.1% sustained for 10 minutes (Kerr et al, 2001).*
  - ▲ Administer barbiturates per collaborative protocol. **EB:** *Barbiturates decrease ICP but are associated with clinically significant hypotension that produces detrimental decreases in MAP and CPP. They should only be used in clients that are hemodynamically stable and monitored closely for decreases in blood pressure (Brain Trauma Foundation & American Association of Neurological Surgeons, 2000; Roberts, 2000).*
  - ▲ Induce moderate hypothermia (32°-35° C) per collaborative protocol. **EB:** *Reducing body/brain temperatures has been effective in reducing ICP in both traumatic and ischemic brain injuries. However, the odds of clients developing pneumonia with hypothermia are nearly double those of normothermia. The optimal degree of hypothermia and the timing of induction are under investigation, though it is known that rapid rewarming can increase ICP (Clifton et al, 2001; Jiang, Yu & Zhu, 2000; Polderman et al, 2002; Tokutomi et al, 2003).*
- ▲ To treat decreased CPP (sustained CPP <60 mm Hg):
  - Administer norepinephrine to raise MAP per collaborative protocol. **EB:** *Vasopressors are frequently used to maintain adequate MAP in support of cerebral perfusion. Norepinephrine is effective in raising MAP and CPP, and may be more effective than dopamine (Biestro et al, 1998; Schwarz et al, 2002b; Steiner et al, 2004).*

• = Independent;   ▲ = Collaborative;   EBN = Evidence-Based Nursing;   EB = Evidence-Based

■ Administer hypertonic saline per collaborative protocol. **EB:** *Infusions of hypertonic saline have been found to raise CPP while decreasing ICP (Al-Rawl et al, 2005; Bentsen et al, 2004; Schwarz et al, 2002a).*

REFERENCES

Al-Rawl P, Zygun D, Tseng M et al: Cerebral blood flow augmentation in patients with severe subarachnoid haemorrhage, *Acta Neurchir Suppl* 95:123-127, 2005.

Battison C, Andrews P, Graham C et al: Randomized, controlled trial on the effect of a 20% mannitol solution and a 7.5% saline/6% dextran solution on increased intracranial pressure after brain injury, *Crit Care Med* 33(11):196-202, 2005.

Bentsen G, Breivik H, Lundar T et al: Predictable reduction of intracranial hypertension with hypertonic saline hydroxyethyl starch: a prospective clinical trial in critically ill patients with subarachnoid haemorrhage, *Acta Anaesthesiol Scand* 48(9):1089-1095, 2004.

Biestro A, Barrios E, Baraibar J et al: Use of vasopressors to raise cerebral perfusion pressure in head injured patients, *Acta Neurochir Suppl* 71:5-9, 1998.

Brain Trauma Foundation & American Association of Neurological Surgeons: Management and Prognosis of Severe Traumatic Brain Injury: Part 1 Guidelines for the Management of Severe Traumatic Brain Injury, 2000. Retrieved June 1, 2006, from www.braintrauma.org

Bullock R, Chestnut R, Clifton G: Management and prognosis of severe traumatic brain injury, *J Neurotrauma* 17(6 & 7):451-627, 2001.

Clifton G, Miller E, Choi S et al: Lack of effect of induction of hypothermia after acute brain injury, *New Engl J Med* 344(8):556-563, 2001.

Englehard K, Reeker W, Kochs E et al: Effect of remifentanil on intracranial pressure and cerebral blood flow velocity in patients with head trauma, *Acta Anaesthesiol Scand* 48(4):396-399, 2004.

Fan J: Effect of backrest position on intracranial pressure and cerebral perfusion pressure in individuals with brain injury: a systematic review, *J Neurosci Nurs* 36(5):278-288, 2004.

Ferber J, Juniewicz H, Glogowska E et al: Tramadol for postoperative analgesia in intracranial surgery. Its effect on ICP and CPP, *Neurol Neurochir Polska* 34(6 Suppl):70-79, 2000.

Gemma M, Tommasino C, Cerri M et al: Intracranial effects of endotracheal suctioning in the acute phase of head injury, *J Neurosurg Anesthesiol* 14(1):50-54, 2002.

Hung O, Hare G, Brien S: Head elevation reduces head-rotation associated with increased ICP in patients with intracranial tumors, *Can J Anesth* 47(5):415-420, 2000.

Hunt K, Hallworth S, Smith M: The effects of rigid collar placement on intracranial and cerebral perfusion pressures, *Anaesthesia* 56(6):511-513, 2001.

Huynh T, Messer M, Sing R et al: Positive end-expiratory pressure alters intracranial and cerebral perfusion pressure in severe traumatic brain injury, *J Trauma* 53(3):488-493, 2002.

Jiang J, Yu M, Zhu C: Effect of long-term mild hypothermia therapy in patients with severe traumatic brain injury: 1-year follow-up review of 87 cases, *J Neurosurg* 93(4):546-549, 2000.

Joanna Briggs Institute for Evidence Based Nursing and Midwifery: Tracheal suctioning of adults with an artificial airway. *Best Practice: Evidence Based Practice Information Sheets for Health Professionals*, 4(4):1-5, 2000.

Kelly D, Goodale D, Williams J et al: Propofol in the treatment of moderate and severe head injury: a randomized prospective double-blinded pilot trial, *J Neurosurgery* 90(6):1042-1052, 1999.

Kerr M, Weber B, Sereika S et al: Dose response to cerebrospinal fluid drainage on cerebral perfusion in traumatic brain-injured adults, *Neurosurg Focus* 11(4):E1, 2001.

Kirkness C, Burr R, Cain K: Effect of continuous display of cerebral perfusion pressure on outcomes in patients with traumatic brain injury, *Am J Crit Care* 15(6):600-610, 2006.

Mcilvoy LH: Impact of brain temperature and core temperature on ICP and CPP, *J Neurosci Nurs* (in press).

Mobbs R, Stoodley M, Fuller J: Effect of cervical hard collar on intracranial pressure after head injury, *ANZ J Surg* 72(6):389-391, 2002.

Moraine J, Berre J, Melot C: Is cerebral perfusion pressure a major determinant of cerebral blood flow during head elevation in comatose patients with severe intracranial lesions? *J Neurosurg* 92(4):606-614, 2000.

Murphy N, Auzinger G, Bernel W et al: The effect of hypertonic sodium chloride on intracranial pressure in patients with acute liver failure, *Hepatology* 39(2):464-470, 2004.

O'Donnell J, Lorber B: Use and effectiveness of hypothermia blankets for febrile patients in the intensive care unit, *Clin Infect Dis* 24:1208-1213, 1997.

Ogden A, Mayer S, Connolly E: Hyperosmolar agents in neurosurgical practice: the evolving role of hypertonic saline, *Neurosurgery* 57(2):207-215, 2005.

Polderman KH, Tjong Tjin Joe R, Peerdeman S et al: Effects of therapeutic hypothermia on intracranial pressure and outcome in patients with severe head injury, *Intensive Care Med* 28(11):1563-1573, 2002.

Rauch ME et al: Validation of risk factors for the nursing diagnosis decreased intracranial adaptive capacity, *J Neurosci Nurs* 22(3):173-178, 1990.

Roberts I: Barbiturates for acute traumatic brain injury, *Cochrane Database Syst Rev* (2):CD000033, 2000.

Rossi S, Zanier E, Mauri I et al: Brain temperature, core temperature, and intracranial pressure in acute cerebral damage, *J Neurol Neurosurg Psychiatr* 71(4):448-454, 2001.

Schinner K, Chisholm A, Grap M et al: Effects of auditory stimuli on intracranial pressure and cerebral perfusion pressure in traumatic brain injury, *J Neurosci Nurs* 27(6):348-354, 1995.

Schulz-Stubner S, Thiex R: Raising the head-of-bed by 30 degrees reduces ICP and improves CPP without compromising cardiac output in euvolemic patients with traumatic brain injury and subarachnoid hemorrhage: a practice audit, *Eur J Anaesthesiol* 23:177-180, 2006.

Schwarz S, Georgiadis D, Aschoff A et al: Effects of hypertonic (10%) saline in patients with raised intracranial pressure after stroke, *Stroke* 33(1):136-140, 2002a.

Schwarz S, Georgiadis D, Aschoff A et al: Effects of induced hypertension on intracranial pressure and flow velocities of the middle cerebral arteries in patients with large hemispheric stroke, *Stroke* 33(4):998-1004, 2002b.

I

Steiner L, Johnson A, Czosnyka M et al: Direct comparison of cerebrovascular effects of norepinephrine and dopamine in head-injured patients, *Crit Care Med* 32(4):1049-1054, 2004.

Tokutomi T, Morimoto K, Miyagi T et al: Optimal temperature for the management of severe traumatic brain injury: Effect of hypothermia on intracranial pressure, systemic and intracranial hemodynamics, and metabolism, *Neurosurgery* 52(1):102-111, 2003.

Vialet R, Albanese J, Thomachot L et al: Isovolume hypertonic solutes (sodium chloride and mannitol) in the treatment of refractory post-traumatic intracranial hypertension: 2ml/kg 7.5% saline is more effective than 2 ml/kg 20% mannitol, *Crit Care Med* 31(6):1683-1687, 2003.

Videtta W, Villarejo F, Cohen M et al: Effects of positive end-expiratory pressure on intracranial pressure and cerebral perfusion pressure, *Acta Neurochir Suppl* 81:93-97, 2002.

Walker J, Eakes G, Siebelink E: The effects of familial voice interventions on comatose head-injured patients, *J Trauma Nurs* 5(2):41-45, 1998.

Winkleman C: Effect of backrest position on intracranial and cerebral perfusion pressure in traumatically brain-injured adults, *Am J Crit Care* 9(6):373-380, 2000.

Wojner-Alexandrov A, Gerami Z, Chernyshev O et al: Heads down: Flat positioning improves blood flow velocity in acute ischemic stroke, *Neurology* 64:1354-2357, 2005.

Deficient Knowledge (specify)

Barbara J. Olinzock, EdD, MSN, RN, and Kathaleen C. Bloom, PhD, CNM

NANDA   Definition

Absence or deficiency of cognitive information related to a specific topic

Defining Characteristics

Exaggerated behaviors; inaccurate follow through of instruction; inaccurate performance of test; inappropriate behaviors (e.g., hysterical, hostile, agitated, apathetic); verbalization of the problem

Related Factors (r/t)

Cognitive limitation; information misinterpretation; lack of exposure; lack of interest in learning; lack of recall; unfamiliarity with information resources

NOC   Outcomes (Nursing Outcomes Classification)

Suggested NOC Outcomes

Knowledge: Diet, Disease Process, Energy Conservation, Health Behavior, Health Resources, Infection Control, Medication, Personal Safety, Prescribed Activity, Substance Use Control, Treatment Procedure(s), Treatment Regimen

Example NOC Outcome with Indicators
Knowledge: Health Behavior as evidenced by the following indicators: Description of: Healthy nutritional practices/Benefits of activity and exercise/Safe use of prescription and nonprescription drugs (Rate the outcome and indicators of **Knowledge: Health Behavior:** 1 = none, 2 = limited, 3 = moderate, 4 = substantial, 5 = extensive [see Section I].)

Client Outcomes

Client Will (Specify Time Frame):

- Explain disease state, recognize need for medications, and understand treatments
- Explain how to incorporate new health regimen into lifestyle
- State an ability to deal with health situation and remain in control of life
- Demonstrate how to perform health-related procedure(s) satisfactorily
- List resources that can be used for more information or support after discharge

NIC   Interventions (Nursing Interventions Classification)

Suggested NIC Interventions

Teaching: Disease Process, Individual, all categories Learning Facilitation

• = Independent;   ▲ = Collaborative;   EBN = Evidence-Based Nursing;   EB = Evidence-Based

Example NIC Activities—Teaching: Disease Process
Discuss therapy/treatment options; Describe rationale behind management/therapy/treatment recommendations

Nursing Interventions and *Rationales*

- Observe the client's ability and readiness to learn (e.g., mental acuity, ability to see or hear, no existing pain, emotional readiness, absence of language or cultural barriers) and previous knowledge. **EBN:** *Learning best occurs when learners are motivated and attend to the important aspects of what is to be learned (Forrest, 2004).* **EBN:** *Learning readiness changes over time based upon situational, physical, and emotional challenges (Olinzock, 2004).*

- Assess personal context and meaning of illness (e.g., perceived change in lifestyle, financial concerns, cultural patterns, and lack of acceptance by peers or coworkers). **EBN:** *Improved symptom management and client satisfaction were noted as a result of interventions that focused on the client's meaning and perspective of their illness (Forrest, 2004; Hornsten et al, 2005).*

- Monitor the information needs of clients over time. **EBN:** *Clients are unique in how they process information. Some clients will be more uncertain than others and may need more educational intervention over time (Suhonen & Leino-Kilpi, 2006).*

- Use approaches that support client priorities, preferences, and choice. **EBN:** *Clients will express preferences about information needs and the when, how, and under what circumstances they want to learn if given the opportunity to do so (Rutten et al, 2005; Suhonen & Leino-Kilpi, 2006).* **EBN:** *A mismatch can occur between what information the client wants to know at a given time and providers' expectations (Suhonen et al, 2005).*

- Provide information to support self-efficacy, self-regulation, and self-management. **EB:** *When focusing on information about problem solving and decision making, significant improvement in symptom limitations were noted (Doorenbos et al, 2005).* **EB:** *Educational programs based upon empowerment and client participation have demonstrated effectiveness (Deakin et al, 2005).*

- Focus teaching on wellness versus "disease state." *Illness representation appears to be an important psychosocial factor in learning (Cherrington et al, 2004).*

- Consider the client's literacy skill when using written information. **EB:** *Computerized methods have been used to individualize and tailor written materials to the needs of the client and caregivers (Hoffmann & McKenna, 2006). Materials that are written simply, on a fifth grade reading level are recommended (Thrall, 2004).*

- Tailor the delivery of instruction to the client's cognitive abilities. **EB:** *Clients with both higher and lower literacy benefited with the use of well-tailored materials including audio, visual, computerized, and written (Bosworth et al, 2005; DeWalt et al, 2004).*

- Provide visual aids to enhance learning. **EB:** *Visual aids such as pictures and simple word captions have proven to be effectively used to highlight important information, especially when working with clients with low literacy (Houts et al, 2006).*

- Consider multifaceted methods of disbursing information. **EB:** *The use of written educational materials as the sole source of information may be ineffective (Urek et al, 2005). A combination of written and verbal information was beneficial for knowledge comprehension and client satisfaction (Johnson, Sandford & Tyndall, 2003; Sheard & Garrud, 2006).*

- Consider using phone calls to monitor and reinforce learning. **EBN:** *Telephone follow-up by expert nurses has been proven effective in improving symptom management and increased client satisfaction (Kim, Yoo & Shim, 2005).*

- ▲ Help the client identify community resources for continuing information and support. **EBN:** *Advocating for clients through participation in a community-based case management program has demonstrated improved clinical and financial outcomes for clients with complex chronic conditions (Schiefalacqua, Ulch & Schmidt, 2004).*

- ▲ Consider using a group educational program. **EB:** *Group care that tailors learning to individual information needs has proven more effective than standard one-to-one teaching. The group care was the major factor associated with improved knowledge, problem-solving ability, and quality of life (Deakin et al, 2005). More intensive one-to-one attention may be needed for socially disadvantaged populations (Glazier et al, 2006).*

- Use computer- and web-based methods as appropriate. **EB:** *Information disbursed as a web-based method contributed to greater behavioral changes and increased knowledge, participation, and social*

K

• = Independent;   ▲ = Collaborative;   EBN = Evidence-Based Nursing;   EB = Evidence-Based

support (Wantland et al, 2004). However, possible disparities between advantaged and disadvantaged populations and computer use have been noted (Murray et al, 2005).

- Provide adequate time for mastery of content. *Long-term multiple follow-up contact points have proven effective in improving symptom management with chronic conditions and improved quality of life (Tankova, Dakovska & Koev, 2004).*
- Evaluate learning outcomes. Using evaluation strategies such as return demonstrations, verbalizations, or the application of skills to new situations is recommended (Thrall, 2004).

Pediatric

- Use family-centered approaches when teaching children and adolescents. *Parents expressed a need to negotiate and participate with healthcare providers about decisions regarding the care of their children (Corlett & Twylcross, 2006; Hopia et al, 2005).*
- Use educational strategies that are interactive and engaging for younger children and toddlers. *Information transfer that is highly individualized and interactive is recommended (Bradlyn et al, 2004; McPherson et al, 2006).*
- Provide a developmentally appropriate environment when addressing the health education needs of adolescents. **EBN:** *The unique developmental needs of the pregnant adolescent, for example, require attention when designing prenatal care services (Grady & Bloom, 2004). Simulated experiences such as Baby Think can be a powerful strategy for effective learning about complex decisions regarding the risks of sexual activity and the realities of parenting (Didion & Gatzke, 2004).*

Geriatric

- Adapt the teaching process for the physical constraints of the aging process (e.g., speak clearly, use a variety of audio-visual-psychomotor methods, provide examples, and allow time for the client to repeat and review. **EBN:** *Adults are capable of learning at any age. Age modifies but does not inhibit learning (Zurakowski, Taylor & Bradway, 2006).*
- Ensure that the client uses necessary reading aids (e.g., eyeglasses, magnifying lenses, large-print text) or hearing aids. **EBN:** *Visual and hearing deficits require amplification or clarification of sensory input (Zurakowski, Taylor & Bradway, 2006).*
- Use printed material, videotapes, lists, diagrams, and Internet. *Methods that clients can refer to at another time are recommended (Zurakowski, Taylor & Bradway, 2006).*
- Repeat and reinforce information during several brief sessions. **EBN:** *Brief sessions focus attention on essential information. Older clients benefit from repeated follow-up sessions (Zurakowski, Taylor & Bradway, 2006).* **EBN:** *Information that is simple, targeted, and reinforced has been identified as most beneficial for older adults (Sahyoun, Pratt & Anderson, 2004).*
- Discuss healthy lifestyle changes that promote wellness for the older adult. **EBN:** *Greater efforts must be made both to improve preventive health care and enhance quality-of-life interventions of older people (Nakasato & Carnes, 2006).*
- Offer opportunities for practice of psychomotor skills. **EBN:** *Older adults indicate a preference for hands-on learning. They learn with hands on and rehearsal when teaching psychomotor skills (Zurakowski, Taylor & Bradway, 2006).*
- Deliver education within a social context and appropriate physical environment. *Interpersonal and social relationships are an important part of learning for older adults (Sahyoun, Pratt & Anderson, 2004).*
- Consider health education programs using television and newspapers. *There was a significant increase in stroke knowledge following this health education program as demonstrated through a telephone pretest and posttest (Becker et al, 2001).*
- Consider using technology including interactive computer programs to disperse health education to older adults. **EB:** *Older adults will use technology based upon a decision-making process of costs versus benefits regardless of previous positive or negative experiences (Melenhorst, Rogers & Bouwhuis, 2006).*

Multicultural

- Acknowledge racial/ethnic differences at the onset of care. **EBN:** *Show respect, acknowledge racial ethnic/differences, show sensitivity and self-awareness to enhance communication and rapport, and promote treatment outcomes (Rust et al, 2006).*
- Assess for the influence of cultural beliefs, norms, and values on the client's knowledge base.

• = Independent; ▲ = Collaborative; EBN = Evidence-Based Nursing; EB = Evidence-Based

EBN: *The client's knowledge base may be influenced by cultural perceptions (Leininger & McFarland, 2002).* **EBN:** *Illness beliefs guide health behavior (Russell, 2006).*

- Provide written healthcare information to clients with limited English proficiency in their native language. **EB:** *Clients with limited English proficiency were unable to understand routinely dispensed medication instructions written in English (Leyva, Sharif & Ozuah, 2005).*
- Assess for cultural/ethnic self-care practices. **EBN:** *Folk and home remedies may interact with medications and treatment (Russell, 2006).*
- Use teaching methods that are culturally sensitive and support client customs, values, and lifestyle. **EBN:** *Teaching focused on preferred language, cultural dietary preferences, family and social involvement, and discussion of cultural health beliefs resulted in significant improvement knowledge and self-care behavior (Brown et al, 2007; Wang & Chan, 2005).*

 Home Care

- All of the previously mentioned interventions are applicable to the home setting.
- Assess the client/family learning needs, information needs, and current level of knowledge. **EB:** *Caregivers express a need for having their informational needs met (Van Heugten et al, 2006).*
- Monitor the appropriateness of using telehome health care as a teaching method for clients and family caregivers. *Interactive teleconferencing and on-site training for family caregivers positively influenced knowledge, self-perceived competence, and resourcefulness (Hartford, 2005). While clients report satisfaction with telehome health methods, they also express that they do not want to lose the personal contact (Bowles & Baugh, 2007).*
- Consider using an outreach home-based educational intervention. **EB:** *A home-based educational intervention targeted at symptom identification for inner-city families found the program was effective in improving symptom identification and overall medication management (Butz et al, 2005).* **EBN:** *The use of post-hospitalization outreach from a nurse for clients with chronic conditions and their family/caregivers found significant improvement in psychosocial outcomes, less social isolation, reduced physical dependence, and reduced caregiver strain (Burton & Gibbons, 2005).*
- Encourage family and peer support. **EB:** *A partner-guided protocol that included integrated education and training of clients and partners improved symptom management. There was also significant improvement in self-efficacy and caregiver strain (Keefe et al, 2005; Dunbar et al, 2005).*
- Assess for specific areas of learning that have the potential for strong emotional responses by the client or family/caregiver. **EBN:** *Attending to physical care and failing to assess for distress in clients and family caregivers can impact health outcomes and quality of life (Madden, 2006).*
- Encourage self-care management of illness. **EB:** *Reducing self-management education reduces positive outcomes (Powell & Gibson, 2003).*

evolve See the EVOLVE website for World Wide Web resources for client education.

REFERENCES

Becker K, Fruin M, Gooding T et al: Community-based education improves stroke knowledge, *Cerebrovasc Dis* 11(1):34-43, 2001.

Bosworth HB, Olsen MK, Gentry P et al: Nurse administered telephone intervention for blood pressure control: a patient-tailored intervention, *Patient Educ Couns* 57(1):5-14, 2005.

Bowles KH, Baugh AC: Applying research to optimize telehomecare, *J Cardiovasc Nurs* 22(1):5-15, 2007.

Bradlyn AS, Beale IL, Kato PM et al: Pediatric oncology professionals' perceptions of information needs of adolescent patients with cancer, *J Pediatr Oncol Nurs* 21(6):335-342, 2004.

Brown A, Blozis S, Kouzekanani K et al: Health beliefs of Mexican Americans with type 2 diabetes: the Starr County border health initiative, *Diabetes Educ* 33(2):300-308, 2007.

Burton C, Gibbons R: Expanding the role of the stroke nurse: a pragmatic clinical trial, *J Adv Nurs* 52(6):640-650, 2005.

Butz AM, Syron L, Johnson B et al: Home-based asthma self-management education for inner city children, *Public Health Nurs* 22(3):189-199, 2005.

Cherrington CC, Moser DK, Lennie TA et al: Illness representation after acute myocardial infarction: impact on in-hospital recovery, *Am J Crit Care* 13(2):136-145, 2004.

Corlett J, Twylcross A: Negotiation of parental roles within family-centered care: a review of the research, *J Clin Nurs* 15(10):1308-1316, 2006.

Deakin T, McShane CE, Cade JE et al: Group based training for self-management strategies in people with type 2 diabetes mellitus, *Cochrane Database Syst Rev* (2):CD003417, 2005.

DeWalt DA, Pignone M, Malone R et al: Development and pilot testing of a disease management program for low literacy patients with heart failure, *Patient Educ Couns* 55(1):78-86, 2004.

Didion J, Gatzke H: The Baby Think It Over experience to prevent teen pregnancy: a postintervention evaluation, *Public Health Nurs* 21(4):331-337, 2004.

Doorenbos A, Given B, Given C et al: Reducing symptom limitations: a cognitive behavioral intervention randomized trial, *Psycho-Oncolog* 14(7):574-584, 2005.

• = Independent;   ▲ = Collaborative;   EBN = Evidence-Based Nursing;   EB = Evidence-Based

Dunbar SB, Clark PC, Deaton C et al: Family education and support interventions in heart failure: a pilot study. *Nurs Res* 54(3):158-166, 2005.

Forrest S: Learning and teaching: the reciprocal link, *Contin Educ Nurs* 35(2):74-79, 2004.

Glazier RH, Bajcar J, Kennie R et al: A systematic review of interventions to improve diabetes care in socially disadvantaged populations, *Diabetes Care* 29(7):1675-1688, 2006.

Grady MA, Bloom KC: Pregnancy outcomes of adolescents enrolled in a Centering Pregnancy program, *J Midwifery Womens Health* 49(5):412-420, 2004.

Hartford K: Telenursing and patients' recovery from bypass surgery, *J Adv Nurs* 50(5):459-468, 2005.

Hoffmann T, McKenna K: Analysis of stroke patients' and carers' reading ability and the content and design of written materials: recommendations for improving stroke information, *Patient Educ Couns* 60(3):286-293, 2006.

Hopia H, Tomlinson PS, Paavilainen E et al: Child in hospital: family experiences and expectations of how nurses can promote family health, *J Clin Nurs* 14(2):212-222, 2005.

Hornsten A, Lundman B, Stenlund H et al: Metabolic improvement after intervention focusing on personal understanding in type 2 diabetes, *Diabetes Res Clin Pract* 68(1):65-74, 2005.

Houts PS, Doak CC, Doak LG et al: The role of pictures in improving health communication: a review of research on attention, comprehension, recall, and adherence, *Patient Educ Couns* 61(2):173-190, 2006.

Johnson A, Sandford J, Tyndall J: Written and verbal information versus verbal information only for patients being discharged from acute hospital settings to home, *Cochrane Database Syst Rev* (4):CD003716, 2003.

Keefe FJ, Ahles TA, Sutton L et al: Partner-guided cancer pain management at the end of life: a preliminary study, *Pain Symptom Manage* 29(3):263-272, 2005.

Kim H, Yoo Y, Shim H: Effects of an internet-based intervention on plasma glucose levels in patients with type 2 diabetes, *J Nurs Care Qual* 20(4):335-340, 2005.

Leininger MM, McFarland MR: *Transcultural nursing: concepts, theories, research and practices*, ed 3, New York, 2002, McGraw-Hill.

Leyva M, Sharif I, Ozuah PO: Health literacy among Spanish-speaking Latino parents with limited English proficiency, *Ambul Pediatr* 5(1):56-59, 2005.

Madden J: The problem of distress in patients with cancer: more effective assessment, *Clin J Oncol Nurs* 10(5):615-619, 2006.

McPherson AC, Glazebrook C, Forster D et al: A randomized, controlled trial of an interactive educational computer package for children with asthma, *Pediatrics* 117(4):1046-1054, 2006.

Melenhorst AS, Rogers WA, Bouwhuis DG: Older adults' motivated choice for technological innovation: evidence for benefit-driven selectivity, *Psycho Aging* 21(1):190-195, 2006.

Murray E, Burns J, See TS et al: Interactive health communication applications for people with chronic disease, *Cochrane Database Syst Rev* (4):CD004274, 2005.

Nakasato YR, Carnes BA: Health promotion in older adults: promoting successful aging in primary care settings, *Geriatrics* 61(4):27-31, 2006.

Olinzock BJ: A model for assessing learning readiness for self-direction of care in individuals with spinal cord injuries: a qualitative study, *SCI Nurs* 21(2):69-74, 2004.

Powell H, Gibson PG: Options for self-management for adults with asthma, *Cochrane Database Syst Rev* (2):CD004107, 2003.

Russell S: An overview of adult learning processes, *Urol Nurs* 26(5):349-352, 2006.

Rust G, Kondwani K, Martinez R et al: A crash-course in cultural competence, *Ethn Dis* 16(2 Suppl 3):S3-S29-S36, 2006.

Rutten LJ, Arora NK, Bakos AD et al: Information needs and sources of information among cancer patients: a systematic review of research (1980–2003), *Patient Educ Couns* 57:250–261, 2005.

Sahyoun NR, Pratt CA, Anderson A: Evaluation of nutrition education interventions for older adults: a proposed framework, *J Am Diet Assoc* 104(1):58-69, 2004.

Schiefalacqua NM, Ulch PO, Schmidt M: How to make a difference in the health care of a population. One person at a time, *Nurs Adm Q* 28(1):29-35, 2004.

Sheard C, Garrud P: Evaluation of generic patient information: effects on health outcomes, knowledge and satisfaction, *Patient Educ Couns*, 61(1):43-47, 2006.

Suhonen R, Leino-Kilpi H: Adult surgical patients and the information provided to them by nurses: a literature review, *Patient Educ Couns* 61(1):5-15, 2006.

Suhonen R, Nenonen H, Laukka A et al: Patients' informational needs and information do not correspond in hospital, *J Clin Nurs* 14(10):1167-1176, 2005.

Tankova T, Dakovska G, Koev D: Education and quality of life in diabetic patients, *Patient Educ Couns* 53(3):285-290, 2004.

Thrall TH: Dump the mumbo jumbo, *Hosp Health Netw* 78(10):70-72, 74, 2004.

Urek MC, Tudoric N, Plavec D et al: Effect of educational programs on asthma control and quality of life in adult asthma patients, *Patient Educ Coun* 58:47-54, 2005.

Van Heugten C, Visser-Meily A, Post M et al: Care for carers of stroke patients: evidence-based clinical practice guidelines, *J Rehabil Med* 38(3):153-158, 2006.

Wang C, Chan S: Culturally tailored diabetes education program for Chinese Americans, *Nurs Res* 54(5):347-353, 2005.

Wantland DJ, Portillo CJ, Holzemer WL et al: The effectiveness of Web-based vs. non-Web-based interventions: a meta-analysis of behavioral change outcomes, *J Med Internet Res* 6(4):e40, 2004.

Zurakowski T, Taylor M, Bradway C: Effective teaching strategies for the older adult with urologic concerns, *Urol Nurs* 6(5):355-360, 2006.

Readiness for enhanced Knowledge (specify)   *evolve*

Barbara J. Olinzock, EdD, MSN, RN, and Kathaleen C. Bloom, PhD, CNM

NANDA Definition

The presence or acquisition of cognitive information related to a specific topic is sufficient for meeting health-related goals and can be strengthened

Defining Characteristics

Behaviors congruent with expressed knowledge; explains knowledge of the topic; expresses an interest in learning; describes previous experiences pertaining to the topic

• = Independent;   ▲ = Collaborative;   EBN = Evidence-Based Nursing;   EB = Evidence-Based

NOC   Outcomes (Nursing Outcomes Classification)

Suggested NOC Outcome

Knowledge: Health Promotion

Example NOC Outcome with Indicators
Knowledge: Health Promotion as evidenced by the following indicator: Description of health behaviors that promote health/Description of relevant health resources (Rate the outcome and indicators of **Knowledge: Health Promotion:** 1 = none, 2 = limited, 3 = moderate, 4 = substantial, 5 = extensive [see Section I].)

Client Outcomes

Client Will (Specify Time Frame):

- Demonstrate knowledge of new information
- Meet personal health-related goals
- Explain how to incorporate new health regimen into lifestyle
- List sources to obtain information

NIC   Interventions (Nursing Interventions Classification)

Suggested NIC Interventions

Health Education, Learning Readiness Enhancement

Example NIC Activities—Health Education
Prioritize identified learner needs based on client preference, skills of nurse, resources available, and likelihood of successful goal attainment

Nursing Interventions and *Rationales*

- ▲ Include clients as members of the healthcare team in mutual goal setting when providing education. **EBN:** *Clients should be considered as co-team members who should be consulted about the information they need (Edwards, 2002).* **EB:** *Approaches that included collaborative goal setting and shared decision making associated with increased sense of personal control were more effective for behavioral change and were less likely to cause resistance (Kennedy et al, 2003).*
- Use open-ended questions and encourage two-way communication. **EBN:** *Intervention strategies that use interpersonal communication, including an open-ended interview process versus a structured didactic approach, are recommended (Timmins, 2006).*
- Support client priorities, preferences, and choice. **EBN:** *Clients will express preferences about information needs and the when, how, and from whom they want to learn (Rutten et al, 2005; Russell, 2006).*
- Use strategies to promote client motivation and sustain learning. **EBN:** *The use of motivational and disease management interventions has demonstrated promise for improved adherence and lifestyle change (Beswick et al, 2005).*
- Provide information to support self-efficacy, self-regulation, and self-management. **EB:** *Educational programs based upon empowerment, client participation, and adult learning principles have demonstrated effectiveness (Deakin et al, 2005; Kennedy et al, 2003).*
- Seek teachable moments to encourage health promotion. **EBN:** *The provision of information should not be restricted just to treatment information but also to any information that prepares clients to manage health-related issues (Timmins, 2006). Hospitalized clients were shown to be in a "window of opportunity" for focusing on health-related issues (Narsavage & Idemoto, 2003).*
- Consider the client's literacy skill when using written information. **EBN:** *Well-designed education materials will facilitate client learning and the transfer of education from inpatient to community settings (Pryor & Jannings, 2004).*

● = Independent;   ▲ = Collaborative;   EBN = Evidence-Based Nursing;   EB = Evidence-Based

- Ensure that the client's literacy levels, including English as a second language, are considered when developing and selecting written health information for clients. **EB:** *The use of simplified educational materials generally had a positive effect on knowledge and comprehension (Berkman et al, 2004; Pignone et al, 2005).*
- Use computer and web-based methods as appropriate. **EB:** *Web-based interventions contributed to greater behavioral changes and increased knowledge, participation, and social support (Wantland et al, 2004).* **EB:** *Providers should consider that there may be possible disparities between advantaged and disadvantaged populations and computer use (Murray et al, 2005).*
- Individualize health education interventions. **EB:** *Interventions such as individualized computer use, brochures, and teaching sessions tailored to the learning needs of clients have demonstrated positive effects on risk reduction and lifestyle changes (Lancaster & Stead, 2005; Fernander et al, 2006; Jones et al, 2006).*
- Assist clients to access the Internet, libraries, and schools to locate appropriate health resources and information. **EB:** *Using effective technology has been demonstrated to enhance learning (Mead et al, 2003).*
- Facilitate individualized proactive planning with clients before visits to their healthcare provider. **EBN:** *A pre-visit questionnaire facilitates individualized proactive planning before a healthcare visit (Glynne-Jones et al, 2006).*
- Provide appropriate healthcare information and screening for clients with physical disabilities. **EB:** *Health promotion activities for clients with disabilities have been proven to contribute significantly to quality of life (Ennis et al, 2006).*
- Encourage group and peer support as appropriate to enhance learning. **EBN:** *Individual and group counseling in conjunction with advice from a health professional has proven effective in supporting self-care management (Moher, Hey & Lancaster, 2005).* **EB:** *Specific forms of social support such as Internet and telephone peer support has proven effective in lifestyle and self-care changes (van Dam et al, 2004).*
- Use a combination of teaching methods. **EB:** *The use of intensive, multiple modalities in lifestyle modification programs such as structured sessions in conjunction with "hands on" and creative activities is associated with a positive effect on health knowledge and on lifestyle changes (Aldana et al, 2005; Gallegos, Ovalle-Berumen & Gomez-Meza, 2006).*
- Reinforce learning through educational follow-up. **EBN:** *Longer periods of participation over time and consistent structured education programs have resulted in symptom management and risk reduction (Snethen, Broome & Cashin, 2006; Chouinard & Robichaud-Eckstrand, 2005).*
- Refer to care plan for **Deficient Knowledge.**

Pediatric

- Consider the delivery of alternative settings for teaching parents of children with chronic conditions. **EBN:** *Teaching children about chronic conditions can be structured to fit busy schedules. Educational interventions can be provided through newsletters, parent-teacher conferences in schools, churches, or community centers (Homer, 2004).*
- Use educational strategies that are interactive and engaging for younger children and toddlers. *Information transfer that is highly individualized and interactive is recommended (McPherson et al, 2006).*
- Provide a developmentally appropriate environment when addressing the health education needs of adolescents. **EBN:** *The unique developmental needs of the pregnant adolescent, for example, require attention when designing prenatal care services (Grady & Bloom, 2004). Simulated experiences such as Baby Think can be a powerful strategy for effective learning about complex decisions regarding the risks of sexual activity and the realities of parenting (Didion & Gatzke, 2004).*
- Refer to **Deficient Knowledge** care plan.

Geriatric and Multicultural

- Refer to **Deficient Knowledge** care plan.

Home Care

- Consider high-tech options for delivery of home-based instruction. **EBN:** *Interactive teleconferencing and on-site training for family caregivers positively influenced knowledge, self-perceived compe-*

tence, and resourcefulness, with no significant difference between the types of program delivery (Rosswurm, Larrabee & Zhang, 2002). Positive outcomes are reported in the use of telehome care, but clients prefer to continue with some amount of personal contact (Bowles & Baugh, 2007).

evolve   See the EVOLVE website for World Wide Web resources for client education.

REFERENCES

Aldana SG, Greenlaw RL, Diehl HA et al: Effects of an intensive diet and physical activity modification program on the health risks of adults, *J Am Diet Assoc* 105(3):371-381, 2005.

Berkman ND, Dewalt DA, Pignone MP et al: Literacy and health outcomes, *Evidence Report/Technology Assessment (Summary)*, 87:1-8, 2004, available online at http://www.ahrq.gov/downloads/pub/evidence/pdf/literacy/literacy.pdf. Accessed June 1, 2006.

Beswick AD, Ree K, West RR et al: Improving uptake and adherence in cardiac rehabilitation: literature review, *J Adv Nurs* 49(5):538-555, 2005.

Bowles KH, Baugh AC: Applying research to optimize telehomecare, *J Cardiovasc Nurs* 22(1):5-15, 2007.

Chouinard MC, Robichaud-Eckstrand S: The effectiveness of a nursing inpatient smoking cessation program in individuals with cardiovascular disease, *Nurs Res* 54(4):243-254, 2005.

Deakin T, McShane CE, Cade JE et al: Group based training for self-management strategies in people with type 2 diabetes mellitus, *Cochrane Database Syst Rev* (2):CD003417, 2005.

Didion J, Gatzke H: The Baby Think It Over experience to prevent teen pregnancy: a postintervention evaluation, *Public Health Nurs* 21(4):331-337, 2004.

Edwards C: A proposal that patients be considered honorary members of the healthcare team, *J Clin Nurs* 11(3):340-348, 2002.

Ennis M, Thain J, Boggild M et al: A randomized controlled trial of a health promotion education programme for people with multiple sclerosis, *Clin Rehabil* 20(9):783-792, 2006.

Fernander AF, Patten CA, Schroeder DR et al: Characteristics of six-month tobacco use outcomes of Black patients seeking smoking cessation intervention, *J Health Care Poor Underserved* 17(2):413-424, 2006.

Gallegos EC, Ovalle-Berumen F, Gomez-Meza MV: Metabolic control of adults with type 2 diabetes mellitus through education and counseling. *J Nurs Scholarsh* 38(4):344-351, 2006.

Glynne-Jones R, Ostler P, Lumley-Graybow S et al: Can I look at my list? An evaluation of a 'prompt sheet' within an oncology outpatient clinic, *Clin Oncol (R Coll Radiol)* 18(5):395-400, 2006.

Grady MA, Bloom KC: Pregnancy outcomes of adolescents enrolled in a Centering Pregnancy program, *J Midwifery Womens Health* 49(5):412-420, 2004.

Homer SD: Effect of education on school-age children's and parents' asthma management. *Speci Pediatr Nurs* 9(3):95-102, 2004.

Jones RB, Pearson J, Cawsey AJ et al: Effect of different forms of information produced for cancer patients on their use of the information, social support, and anxiety: randomized trial, *BMJ* 332(7547):942-948, 2006.

Kennedy A, Nelson E, Reeves D et al: A randomised controlled trial to assess the impact of a package comprising a patient-orientated, evidence-based self-help guidebook and patient-centered consultations on disease management and satisfaction in inflammatory bowel disease, *Health Technol Assess* 7(28):3, 1-113, 2003.

Lancaster T, Stead LF: Self-help interventions for smoking cessation, *Cochrane Database Syst Rev* (3):CD001118, 2005.

McPherson AC, Glazebrook C, Forster D et al: A randomized, controlled trail of an interactive educational computer package for children with asthma, *Pediatrics* 117(4):1046-1054, 2006.

Mead N, Varnam R, Rogers A et al: What predicts patients' interest in the Internet as a health resource in primary care in England, *J Health Serv Res Policy* 8(1):33-39, 2003.

Moher M, Hey K, Lancaster T: Workplace interventions for smoking cessation, *Cochrane Database Syst Rev* (2):CD003440, 2005.

Murray E, Burns J, See TS et al: Interactive health communication applications for people with chronic disease, *Cochrane Database Syst Rev* (4):CD004274, 2005.

Narsavage G, Idemoto BK: Smoking cessation interventions for hospitalized patients with cardio-pulmonary disorders, *Online J Issues Nurs* 8(2):8, 2003.

Pignone MP, Dewalt DA, Sheridan S et al: Interventions to improve health outcomes for patients with low literacy: a systematic review, *J Gen Intern Med* 20(2):185-192, 2005.

Pryor J, Jannings W: Preparing patients to self-manage faecal continence following spinal cord injury, *J Aust Rehabil Nurses Assoc* 7(2):20-23, 2004.

Rosswurm MA, Larrabee JH, Zhang J: Training family caregivers of dependent elderly adults through on-site and telecommunications programs, *J Gerontol Nurs* 28(7):27-38, 2002.

Russell S: An overview of adult learning processes, *Urol Nurs* 26(5):349-352, 370, 2006.

Rutten LJ, Arora NK, Bakos AD et al: Information needs and sources of information among cancer patients: a systematic review of research (1980-2003), *Patient Educ Couns* 57(3):250-261, 2005.

Snethen JA, Broome ME, Cashin SE: Effective weight loss for overweight children: a meta-analysis of intervention studies, *Pediatr Nurs* 21(1):45-56, 2006.

Timmins F: Exploring the concept of 'information need,' *Int J Nurs Pract* 12(6):375-381, 2006

van Dam HA, van der Horst FG, Knoops L et al: Social support in diabetes: a systematic review of controlled intervention studies, *Patient Educ Couns* 59(1):1-12, 2004.

Wantland DJ, Portillo CJ, Holzemer WL et al: The effectiveness of Web-based vs. non-Web-based interventions: a meta-analysis of behavioral change outcomes, *J Med Internet Res* 6(4):e40, 2004.

K

Sedentary Lifestyle   *Betty J. Ackley, MSN, EdS, RN*

NANDA   **Definition**

Reports a habit of life that is characterized by a low physical activity level

Defining Characteristics

Chooses a daily routine lacking physical exercise; demonstrates physical deconditioning; verbalizes preference for activities low in physical activity

Related Factors

Deficient knowledge of health benefits of physical exercise; lack of training for accomplishment of physical exercise; lack of resources (time, money, companionship, facilities); lack of motivation; lack of interest

NOC   **Outcomes (Nursing Outcomes Classification)**

Suggested NOC Outcome

Ambulation

Example NOC Outcome with Indicators
Ambulation as evidenced by the following indicators: Walks with effective gait/Walks at moderate pace/Walks up and down steps/Walks moderate distance (Rate the outcome and indicators of **Ambulation:** I = severely compromised, 2 = substantially compromised, 3 = moderately compromised, 4 = mildly compromised, 5 = not compromised [see Section I].)

Client Outcomes

Client Will (Specify Time Frame):

- Increase physical activity to minimum of 10,000 steps per day
- Meet mutually defined goals of increased exercise
- Verbalize feeling of increased strength and ability to move

NIC   **Interventions (Nursing Interventions Classification)**

Suggested NIC Interventions

Exercise Therapy: Ambulation, Joint Mobility, Positioning

Example NIC Activities—Exercise Therapy: Ambulation
Assist patient to use footwear that facilitates walking and prevents injury; Instruct in availability of assistive devices, if appropriate

Nursing Interventions and *Rationales*

- Observe the client for cause of sedentary lifestyle. Determine whether cause is physical or psychological. *Some clients choose not to move because of psychological factors such as an inability to cope or depression.* See care plan for **Ineffective Coping** or **Hopelessness.**
- ▲ Assess for reasons why the client would be unable to participate in an exercise program; refer for evaluation by a primary care practitioner as needed.
- Use the Outcome Expectation for Exercise Scale to determine client's self-efficacy expectations and outcomes expectations toward exercise. **EBN:** *The client's self-efficacy expectations and outcome expectations for exercise will greatly influence his or her willingness to exercise. Interventions can be implemented to strengthen the expectations and hopefully improve exercise behavior (Resnick, Zimmerman & Orwig, 2001).*

• = Independent;   ▲ = Collaborative;   EBN = Evidence-Based Nursing;   EB = Evidence-Based

- Recommend the client enter an exercise program with a friend. **EBN:** *Findings from a study of exercise behavior found that friends have the strongest influence to keep on an exercise program, more than family members or experts (Resnick, Orwig & Magaziner, 2002).*
- Recommend the client begin a walking program using the following criteria:
  - Purchase a pedometer
  - Determine common times when walking can be incorporated into usual lifestyle
  - Set goal of walking 10,000 steps per day, which equals = miles per day
  - If, after coming home from work, does not have required number of steps, go for a walk until reach designated goal of 10,000 steps per day

EB: *Use of a pedometer resulted in two times the usual amount of activity and weight loss in overweight adults (VanWormer, 2004). Middle-aged women who walked more frequently and for longer periods of time had lower body mass index (BMI), and if walked 10,000 plus steps per day were in the normal range for BMI (Thompson, Rakow & Perdue, 2004).*

Pediatric

- Encourage child to increase the amount of walking done per day; if child is willing, ask him or her to wear a pedometer to measure number of steps. **EB:** *A study demonstrated that the recommended number of steps per day to have a healthy body composition for the 6- to 12-year-old is 12,000 for a girl and 15,000 for a boy (Tudor-Locke et al, 2004).*
- Encourage the adolescent to increase exercise to help feel better. **EBN:** *Adolescents had positive feeling states once they began to exercise (Robbins et al, 2004).*

Geriatric

- Assess ability to move using the Get Up and Go test. Ask the client to rise from a sitting position, walk 10 feet, turn, and return to the chair to sit. *Performance on this screening examination demonstrates the client's mobility and ability to leave the house safely (Robertson & Montagnini, 2004).*
- Recommend the client begin a regular exercise program, even if generally active. **EB:** *A research program demonstrated that people who exercise with a defined program had greater functional capacity or reserve than clients who had an active lifestyle but no defined exercise program (Wellbery, 2005).*
- ▲ Refer the client to physical therapy for resistance exercise training as able including abdominal crunch, leg press, leg extension, leg curl, calf press, and more. **EB:** *Six months of resistance exercise for the elderly greatly increased their aerobic capacity, possibly from increased skeletal muscle strength (Vincent et al, 2002). Clients in an extended care facility were put on a strength-, balance-, and endurance-training program; the client's balance and mobility improved significantly (Rydwik, Kerstin & Akner, 2005). Progressive resistance strength training for physical disability in older clients may result in increased strength and positive improvements in some limitations (Latham et al, 2003).*
- Use the WALC Intervention (Walk; Address pain, fear, fatigue during exercise; Learn about exercise; Cue by self-modeling) to improve exercise adherence in the older adult. **EBN:** *The WALC Intervention resulted in more exercise and had greater self-efficacy expectations regarding exercise (Resnick, 2002).*
- Recommend the client begin a Tai Chi practice. **EB and EBN:** *Studies have demonstrated that Tai Chi improves balance in the elderly and may help prevent falls (Wolf et al, 2003; Taggart, 2002).*
- If client is frail, ensure good nutrition, appropriate medications, attention to vision and hearing deficits, and increase social support along with exercise. *Frailty in the elderly can be multifactorial and often can be ameliorated or reversed (Storey & Thomas, 2004).*
- If client is scheduled for an elective surgery that will result in admission into the intensive care unit (ICU) and immobility, or recovery from a knee replacement, initiate a prehabilitation program that includes a warm-up, aerobic strength, flexibility, and functional task work. **EBN and EB:** *By increasing the functional capacity of the individual prior to the stressor of inactivity, the predictable declines in physical activity can be prevented or alleviated (Topp et al, 2002). Clients who performed strength activities preoperatively walked significantly greater distances postoperatively after total hip replacement (Whitney & Parkman, 2002). Aerobic training along with strength and interval training was effective in fewer postoperative complications, shorter postoperative stays, and reduced functional disabilities (Carli & Zavorsky, 2005).*
- ▲ Evaluate the client for signs of depression (flat affect, insomnia, anorexia, frequent somatic com-

plaints) or cognitive impairment (use Mini-Mental State Exam [MMSE]). Refer for treatment or counseling as needed. **EBN:** *Cognitive impairment is frequently found in association with depression in older subjects. Several depression screening instruments have been developed for use in older people. Community and primary studies suggest that only a small minority of older clients with depression receive treatment (Tallis, 2003).*

Home Care

- Above interventions may be adapted for home care use.
- ▲ Assess home environment for factors that create barriers to mobility. Refer to occupational therapy services if needed to assist the client in restructuring home and daily living patterns.

Client/Family Teaching

- Work with the client using the Transtheoretical Model of behavior change and determine if the client is in the precontemplation, contemplation, preparation, action, or maintenance state of behavior change about exercise. Provide appropriate strategies to support change to exercising based on determined state of change. **EBN:** *The Transtheoretical Model of behavior change can be very useful for nurses to utilize to increase exercise behavior with stage-appropriate interventions (Burbank, Reibe & Padula, 2002). Use of the Transtheoretical Model of behavior change plus theory of self-efficacy suggests that both of these theories are helpful to increase exercise in the older adult (Resnick & Nigg, 2003).*
- Develop a series of contracts with mutually agreed on goals of increased activity. Include measurable landmarks of progress, consequences for meeting or not meeting goals, and evaluation dates. Sign the contracts with the client. **EBN:** *Using a series of evolving contracts to modify behavior toward increasing activity helps the client learn skills to change behavior (Boehm, 1989; Steckel, 1974).*

evolve   See the EVOLVE website for World Wide Web resources for client education.

REFERENCES

Boehm S: Patient contracting, *Annu Rev Nurs Res* 7:143-153, 1989.

Burbank PM, Reibe D, Padula CA: Exercise and older adults: changing behavior with the transtheoretical model, *Orthop Nurs* 21(4):51-61, 2002.

Carli F, Zavorsky GS: Optimizing functional exercise capacity in the elderly surgical population, *Curr Opin Clin Nutr Metab Care* 8(1):23-32, 2005.

Latham N, Anderson C, Bennett D et al: Progressive resistance strength training for physical disability in older people, *Cochrane Database Syst Rev* (2):CD002759, 2003.

Resnick B: Testing the effect of the WALC intervention on exercise adherence in older adults, *J Gerontol Nurs*, 28(6):40-49, 2002.

Resnick B, Nigg C: Testing a theoretical model of exercise behavior for older adults, *Nurs Res* 52(2):80-88, 2003.

Resnick B, Orwig D, Magaziner J: The effect of social support on exercise behavior in older adults, *Clin Nurs Res* 11(1):52-70, 2002.

Resnick B, Zimmerman S, Orwig D: Model testing for reliability and validity of the outcome expectations for exercise scale, *Nurs Res* 50(5):293-299, 2001.

Robbins LB, Pis MB, Pender NJ et al: Exercise self-efficacy, enjoyment, and feeling states among adolescents, *West J Nurs Res* 26(7):716-721, 2004.

Robertson RG, Montagnini M: Geriatric failure to thrive, *Am Fam Physician* 70(2):343-350, 2004.

Rydwik E, Kerstin F, Akner G: Physical training in institutionalized elderly people with multiple diagnoses—a controlled pilot study, *Arch Gerontol Geriatr* 40(1):29-44, 2005.

Steckel SB: The use of positive reinforcement in order to increase patient compliance, *AANNT J* 1:1, 1974.

Storey E, Thomas RL: Understanding and ameliorating frailty in the elderly, *Top Geriatr Rehabil* 20(1):4-13, 2004.

Taggart HM: Effects of tai chi exercise on balance, functional mobility, and fear of falling among older women, *Appl Nurs Res* 15(4):235-242, 2002.

Tallis R: *Geriatric medicine and gerontology*, ed 6, London, 2003, Churchill Livingstone, pp 838-843.

Thompson DL, Rakow J, Perdue SM: Relationship between accumulated walking and body composition in middle-aged women, *Med Sci Sports Exerc* 36(5):911-914, 2004.

Topp R, Ditmyer M, King K et al: The effect of bed rest and potential of prehabilitation on patients in the intensive care unit, *AACN Clin Issues* 13(2):263-276, 2002.

Tudor-Locke C, Pangrazi RP, Corbin CB et al: BMI-referenced standards for recommended pedometer-determined steps/day in children, *Prev Med* 38(6):857-864, 2004.

VanWormer JJ: Pedometers and brief e-counseling: increasing physical activity for overweight adults, *J Appl Behav Anal* 37(3):421-425, 2004.

Vincent KR, Braith RW, Feldman RA et al: Improved cardiorespiratory endurance following 6 months of resistance exercise in elderly men and women, *Arch Intern Med* 162:673-678, 2002.

Wellbery C: Physical function and levels of activity in the elderly, *Am Fam Physician* 71(3):557, 2005.

Whitney JA, Parkman S: Preoperative physical activity, anesthesia, and analgesia: effects on early postoperative walking after total hip replacement, *Appl Nurs Res* 15(1):19-27, 2002.

Wolf SL, Sattin RW, Kutner M et al: Intense Tai Chi exercise training and fall occurrences in older, transitionally frail adults: a randomized, controlled trial, *J Am Geriatr Soc* 51(12):1693-1701, 2003.

● = Independent;   ▲ = Collaborative;   EBN = Evidence-Based Nursing;   EB = Evidence-Based

Risk for impaired Liver function   *Nancy Beyer, MS, CEN, RN, and Betty Ackley, MSN, EdS, RN*

NANDA   **Definition**

At risk for liver dysfunction

Risk Factors

Hepatotoxic medications (e.g., acetaminophen, statins); HIV co-infection; substance abuse (e.g., alcohol, cocaine); viral infection (e.g., hepatitis A, B, C, D, E, Epstein-Barr); chronic biliary obstruction and infection; right heart failure; acute fatty liver of pregnancy; Reye's syndrome, nutritional deficiencies

NOC   **Outcomes (Nursing Outcomes Classification)**

Suggested NOC Outcomes

Knowledge: Health Behavior

Example NOC Outcome with Indicators—Knowledge: Health Behavior
Knowledge: Health Behavior as evidenced by the following indicators: Description of safe use of prescription drugs/Description of adverse health effects of alcohol misuse/Description of adverse health effects of recreational drug use/Description of healthy nutritional practices/Description of appropriate use of self-screening (Rate the outcome and indicators of **Knowledge: Health Behavior:** 1 = none, 2 = limited, 3 = moderate, 4 = substantial, 5 = extensive [see Section I].)

Client Outcomes

Client Will (Specify Time Frame):

- State the upper limit of the amount of acetaminophen can safely take per day
- Have normal liver enzymes, serum and urinary bilirubin levels, white blood cell count (WBC), red blood cell count (RBC)
- Be free of jaundice, pruritus, bruising, petechiae, gastrointestinal bleeding, hemorrhage
- Have coagulation studies within normal limits
- Report abdominal girth of normal dimensions
- Be oriented to time, place, and person
- Be able to eat frequent small meals per day without nausea and/or vomiting
- State rationale for seeking medical attention for gallbladder/biliary disease
- If alcohol abuse is factor, state relationship between abuse and worsening gastrointestinal and liver disease
- Be free of cardiovascular and/or renal compromise: fluid retention, peripheral edema, ascites, decreased urinary output, changes in serum blood urea nitrogen (BUN) and creatinine levels
- Be free of abdominal tenderness/pain and have normal colored stool

NIC   **Interventions (Nursing Interventions Classification)**

Suggested NIC Intervention

Teaching: Disease Process, Substance Use Treatment

Example NIC Activities—Teaching Disease Process
Discuss lifestyle changes that may be required to prevent future complications and/or control the disease process

Nursing Interventions and *Rationales*

- Watch for signs of liver dysfunction including: jaundice of the eyes or skin, pruritus, gastrointestinal bleeding, coagulopathy, infections, increasing abdominal girth, fluid overload, shortness of breath, and mental status changes, changes in the color of the stool, changes in urinary function concurrent with increased serum and urinary bilirubin levels (Whiteman & McCormick, 2005).

- Evaluate liver function tests. *Standard liver panels include the serum enzymes aspartate transaminase (AST), alanine transaminase (ALT), alkaline phosphatase, and g-glutamyltransferase; total, direct, and indirect serum bilirubin; and serum albumin. The ALT is thought to be the most cost-effective screening test for identifying metabolic or drug-induced hepatic injury, but like other liver function tests, it is of limited use in predicting degree of inflammation and of no use in estimating severity of fibrosis.* **EB:** *A platelet count of less than 160 K per mm³ has a sensitivity of 80% for detecting cirrhosis in clients with chronic hepatitis C (Heidelbaugh & Bruderly, 2006).*

- Evaluate coagulation studies such as international normalized ratio (INR), prothrombin time (PT), and partial thromboplastin time (PTT), especially with concurrent bleeding of mouth/gums. *Prolonged prothrombin time and decreased production of clotting factors can result in bleeding (Whiteman & McCormick, 2005).*

- Monitor for signs and symptoms of electrolyte and acid-base imbalances, especially hyperkalemia, hypoglycemia, and metabolic acidosis. *The cause of these imbalances are nutritional deficits, nausea and vomiting, fluid losses/shifts, and renal complications.*

- Instruct client about possibility of a liver biopsy if he or she has other symptoms of possible liver problems, such as abnormal liver function tests, bleeding, jaundice, and nutritional deficits. *Liver biopsy is not necessary for diagnosis but is helpful for grading the severity of disease and staging the degree of fibrosis and permanent architectural damage (Wolfe, 2005; Luxon, 2006).*

- ▲ Determine the total amount of acetaminophen the client is taking per day and administer medications for an overdose as ordered. The amount of acetaminophen ingested should not exceed 4 g per day as a limit. *It is common for clients to take multiple pain medications, all containing acetaminophen (Cohen, 2006). Acetaminophen overdose is the leading cause of liver failure in the United States (US Health Facts, 2006; Perkins, 2006).* **EB:** *Charcoal and N-acetylcysteine are the usual treatments of acetaminophen overdose. At times liver transplantation is needed (Brok, Buckley & Gluud, 2006).*

- Evaluate the serum acetaminophen-protein adducts in the client with possible liver failure from excessive intake of acetaminophen. **EB:** *This diagnostic test was helpful in determining if liver failure is associated with acetaminophen toxicity (Davern, James & Hinson, 2006).*

- ▲ If the client is an alcoholic, refer to a cessation program. *It is essential the client stop drinking as soon as possible to allow the liver to heal. Alcoholism is associated with malnutrition, which is harmful to the liver (DiCecco & Francisco-Ziller, 2006). Alcoholism is also associated with formation of proteins called cytokines, which cause inflammation and resultant damage to the liver (Neuman, 2003).* See care plan for **Ineffective Denial** and **Dysfunctional Family processes: alcoholism.**

- Recognize that severe malnutrition may result in acute liver failure, which is reversible with improved nutrition. *Severe malnutrition from anorexia nervosa resulted in liver disease in two young females (De Caprio et al, 2006).*

- Encourage vaccinations for hepatitis A and B for all ages. *Hepatitis A can affect anyone in the United States. Vaccination can prevent hepatitis A and B, which at times can cause liver failure (CDC, 2006; Rein, 2007).*

- Measure abdominal girth if individual presents with abdominal distention and pain. *Increasing abdominal distention and pain are signs of impending portal hypertension with presence of fluid shifts resulting in ascites (Whiteman & McCormick, 2005).*

- Assess for tenderness and/or pain level in the right upper quadrant. *Tenderness in this area is a symptom of biliary, liver, and/or pancreatic problems.*

- Recognize that new onset of symptoms of liver dysfunction such as jaundice, fatigue, and nausea may be caused by infection with hepatitis C (Wolfe, 2005).

- Provide frequent smaller meals for easier digestion. Provide diet with optimal carbohydrates, proteins, and fats. Proteins can be increased as client can tolerate, and serum protein, albumin levels, and bilirubin levels indicate improved liver function. Provide essential vitamins and minerals (Kimber, 1998).

- Observe for signs and symptoms of mental status changes such as confusion from encephalopathy. Assess ammonia level if mental changes occur.

Pediatric

- Encourage vaccinations for hepatitis A and B for all ages. *Hepatitis A can affect anyone in the United States. Vaccination can prevent hepatitis A and B, which at times can cause liver failure. Children should be vaccinated between ages 12 months to 23 months for hepatitis A (CDC, 2006; Rein, 2007).*
- Recognize that children can develop fatty liver disease, which can result in liver failure. Most children are asymptomatic, but others complain of malaise, fatigue, or vague recurrent abdominal pain. *Risk factors for fatty liver disease include obesity, insulin resistance, and hypertriglyceridemia. The diagnosis is made by liver biopsy, and the mainstay of treatment is weight loss (Marion, Baker & Dhawan, 2004).*

 Geriatric

- The interventions above are appropriate for the elderly. *Liver disease in the elderly varies little from liver disease in younger people (Zaw & Joglekar, 2005).*

 Home Care

- Encourage rest, optimal nutrition (high carbohydrates, low protein, essential vitamins and minerals) during initial inflammatory processes of the liver.
- Watch for liver dysfunction in the client receiving long-term parenteral nutrition. *There can be multiple causes of liver disease in this client population including hepatoxic medications, infections, other chronic conditions, pre-existing liver disease, and sometimes the parenteral formula (Hamilton & Austin, 2006).*

 Client/Family Teaching

- Teach the client and family to examine all medications the client is taking, looking for acetaminophen as an ingredient, and reinforce the 4 GM upper limit of intake of acetaminophen to protect liver function.
- For the caregiver and client with hepatitis A, B, and C, teach the need for careful handwashing, use of gloves, and other precautions to prevent spread of any of these diseases.
- Teach avoidance of high-risk behaviors that cause hepatitis and ways to avoid those behaviors.
- Educate clients and their caregivers about treatment options and interventions for hepatitis.
- Teach client and family to report signs and symptoms that may indicate further complications including increased abdominal girth, bleeding, bruising, petechiae, jaundice, pruritus, confusion, rapid weight gain, or weight loss (fluid overload versus anorexia and nausea/vomiting), shortness of breath.

REFERENCES

Brok J, Buckley N, Gluud C: Interventions for paracetamol (acetaminophen) overdose, *Cochrane Database Syst Rev* (2):CD003328, 2006.

CDC: *Viral hepatitis A,* 2006, available at http://www.cdc.gov/ncidod/diseases/hepatitis/b/index.htm. Accessed on March 30, 2007.

CDC: *Viral hepatitis B,* 2006, available at http://www.cdc.gov/ncidod/diseases/hepatitis/a/index.htm. Accessed on March 30, 2007.

Cohen MR: Medication errors. Acetaminophen toxicity: undercover agent, *Nursing* 36(7):15, 2006.

Davern TJ II, James LP, Hinson JA: Measurement of serum acetaminophen-protein adducts in patients with acute liver failure, *Gastroenterol* 130(3):687-694, 2006.

De Caprio C, Alfano A, Senatore I et al: Severe acute liver damage in anorexia nervosa: two case reports, *Nutrition* 22(5):572-575, 2006.

DiCecco SR, Francisco-Ziller N: Nutrition in alcoholic liver disease, *Nutr Clin Pract* 21(3):245-254, 2006.

Hamilton C, Austin T: Liver disease in long-term parenteral nutrition, *Supp Line* 28(1):16-18, 2006.

Heidelbaugh JJ, Bruderly M: Cirrhosis and chronic liver failure: part I. diagnosis and evaluation, *Am Fam Physician* 74(5):756-763, 2006.

Kimber H: Nutritional approaches to liver detoxification, *Posit Health* 33:37-39, 1998.

Luxon BA: Symposium on liver disease. Noninvasive tests for liver fibrosis, *Postgrad Med* 119(3):8-13, 2006.

Marion AW, Baker AJ, Dhawan A: Fatty liver disease in children, *Arch Dis Child* 89(7):648-652, 2004.

Neuman MG: Cytokines—central factors in alcoholic liver disease, *Alcohol Res Health* 27(4):307-316, 2003.

Perkins JD: Acetaminophen sets records in the United States: number 1 analgesic and number 1 cause of acute liver failure, *Liver Transpl* 12(4):682-683, 2006.

Rein DB, Hicks KA, Wirth KE et al: Cost-effectiveness of routine childhood vaccination for hepatitis A in the United States, *Pediatrics* 119(1):e12-e21, 2007.

US HEALTHFACTS: Overdose of acetaminophen, aka Tylenol, the leading cause of liver failure in the U.S. 31(4):6, 2006.

Whiteman K, McCormick C: When your patient is in liver failure, *Nursing* 35(4):58-63, 2005.

Wolfe G: Hepatitis C: Laboratory tests to be done before the diagnosis can be made, *Lippincott's Case Manag* 10(2):115-117, 2005.

Zaw K, Joglekar M: Liver disease and the elderly, *Geriatr Med* 35(5):33-39, 2005.

Risk for Loneliness   *Gail B. Ladwig, MSN, CHTP, RN*

NANDA   **Definition**

At risk for experiencing discomfort associated with a desire or need for more contact with others

Risk Factors

Affectional deprivation; cathectic deprivation; physical isolation; social isolation

NOC   **Outcomes (Nursing Outcomes Classification)**

Suggested NOC Outcomes

Loneliness Severity, Social Interaction Skills, Social Involvement, Social Support

Example NOC Outcome with Indicators
Loneliness Severity as evidenced by the following indicator: Sense of social isolation/Difficulty in establishing contact with other people (Rate the outcome and indicators of **Loneliness Severity:** 1 = severe, 2 = substantial, 3 = moderate, 4 = mild, 5 = none [see Section I].)

Client Outcomes

Client Will (Specify Time Frame):

- Maintain one or more meaningful relationships (growth enhancing versus codependent or abusive in nature)—relationships allowing self-disclosure—and demonstrate a balance between emotional dependence and independence
- Participate in ongoing positive and relevant social activities and interactions that are personally meaningful
- Demonstrate positive use of time alone when socialization is not possible

NIC   **Interventions (Nursing Interventions Classification)**

Suggested NIC Interventions

Family Integrity Promotion, Socialization Enhancement, Visitation Facilitation

Example NIC Activities—Socialization Enhancement
Encourage enhanced involvement in already established relationships; Use role playing to practice improved communication skills and techniques

Nursing Interventions and *Rationales*

- Assess the client's perception of loneliness. (Is the person alone by choice, or do others impose the aloneness?) **EBN:** *Among persons with severe mental illness, more than half identify problems with loneliness and social isolation (Perese, Getty & Wooldridge, 2003; Perese & Wolf, 2005).* Refer to care plan for **Social isolation.**
- Assess the client's ability and/or inability to meet physical, psychosocial, spiritual, and financial needs and how unmet needs further challenge the ability to be socially integrated. NOTE: See care plan for **Disturbed Body image** if loneliness is associated with impaired skin integument. **EB:** *Existential loneliness is an issue that arises for women with human immunodeficiency virus (HIV) (Mayers & Svartberg, 2001).* **EBN:** *Clients' perception of general health, symptoms, and social support influences health status outcome (Lindsay et al, 2001).*
- ▲ Assess the bereaved client who is alone for suicide and make appropriate referrals. *Bereaved persons are at excess risk of suicidal ideation compared to nonbereaved people. Heightened suicidal ideation in bereavement is associated with loneliness and severe depressive symptoms (Stroebe, Stroebe & Abakoumkin, 2005).* Refer to care plan Risk for **Suicide.**

• = Independent;   ▲ = Collaborative;   EBN = Evidence-Based Nursing;   EB = Evidence-Based

▲ Assess the client who is alone for substance abuse and make appropriate referrals. *Women who abused substances in this study reported negative feelings of boredom and loneliness (Harris, Fallot & Berley, 2005).*

• Evaluate the client's desire for social interaction in relation to actual social interaction. **EB:** *The lonelier the student, the more dishonest, the more negative, and the less revealing was the quality of the self-disclosure in their ICQ ("I seek you") chat interaction (Leung, 2002).*

• Use active listening skills. Establish therapeutic relationship and spend time with the client. **EBN:** *Being truly present was listed as one behavior that demonstrated caring (Yonge & Molzahn, 2002). Presence and caring communication is important (Sundin, Jansson & Norberg, 2002).*

▲ Assist the client with identifying loneliness as a feeling and the causes related to loneliness; make appropriate referrals. **EBN:** *Loneliness was the number one fear identified by the homeless who did not stay in shelters (Reichenbach, McNamee & Seibel, 1998). This study demonstrated that providing care for chronic conditions of the homeless at a nurse-managed clinic has the potential to improve health and reduce use of the Emergency Department (Savage et al, 2006).*

• Explore ways to increase the client's support system and participation in groups and organizations. **EB:** *Satisfaction with support networks was a potent predictor of self-esteem, emotional health, and loneliness in female survivors of violence and abuse (Fry & Barker, 2002).* **EBN:** *Encouragement by nurses is important in helping clients with mental illness to become part of support groups (Perese, Getty & Wooldridge, 2003). Psychosocial group intervention on loneliness and social support in Japanese women with breast cancer demonstrated significantly lower scores for loneliness (Fukui et al, 2003).*

• Encourage the client to be involved in meaningful social relationships and support personal attributes. **EBN:** *Personal attributes and social support mediated the effects of emotional distress by decreasing its impact on activities of daily living (ADL) functioning. (Gulick, 2001).*

• Encourage the client to develop closeness in at least one relationship. **EBN:** *Dependence and independence should be balanced in healthy relationships. The development of a balanced level of emotional dependence and the ability to self-disclose are important factors in reducing the risk for loneliness (Mahon & Yarcheski, 1992).*

Adolescents

• Assess the client's social support system. **EBN:** *Use a social support tool or validated assessment tool if possible (e.g., Personal Lifestyle Questionnaire [PLQ]) (Mahon, Yarcheski & Yarcheski, 2003).*

• Evaluate the family stability of younger and middle adolescent clients and advocate and encourage healthy, growth-producing relationships with family and support systems. **EB:** *This study showed a fear of intimacy and loneliness among adolescents who were taught during childhood not to trust strangers (Terrell, Terrell & Von Drashek, 2000). Younger adolescents are at a higher risk for loneliness if they are shy or have low self-esteem. Younger adolescents rely more on parental relationships (Mahon & Yarcheski, 1992).*

• Evaluate peer relationships. **EB:** *Peer relations appear to be the best predictors of adolescent loneliness (Uruk & Demir 2003).*

• Encourage social support for clients with visual impairments. **EB:** *Personal networks and social support for Dutch adolescents with visual impairments indicate that social support, especially the support of peers, is important to adolescents with visual impairments (Kef, 2002).*

• For older adolescents, encourage close relationships with peers and involvement with groups and organizations. **EBN:** *A positive relationship with friends and parents promotes psychological well-being in adolescents and reduces malaise. Loneliness can be a risk for the adolescent's well-being (Corsano, Majorano & Champretavy, 2006).*

• Consider use of pets to cope with loneliness. **EBN:** *Homeless youths identified pets as companions that provide unconditional love and decrease feelings of loneliness (Rew, 2000).* **EBN:** *Equine-facilitated psychotherapy is a little-known experiential intervention that offers the opportunity to achieve healing (Vidrine, Owen-Smith & Faulkner, 2002).*

Geriatric

• Refer to care plan **Social isolation** for additional interventions.

• Assess the client's adaptive sensory functions or any other health deviations that may limit or decrease his or her ability to interact with others. **EB:** *Greater loneliness was found to be associated*

• = Independent;   ▲ = Collaborative;   EBN = Evidence-Based Nursing;   EB = Evidence-Based

with an increased probability of having a coronary condition, as were low levels of both emotional support and companionship (Sorkin, Rook & Lu, 2002).

- Assess caregivers for Alzheimer's disease clients for depression related to loneliness. **EBN:** *Loneliness was significantly related to depression of husbands, wives, and daughters providing care for Alzheimer's disease family members (Beeson et al, 2000).*

- ▲ Identify community support systems specific to elderly populations. **EB:** *Aging is often accompanied by significant losses of family members and other social support. Residents of a nursing facility show that social relationships with other residents were a strong predictor of decreased depression and loneliness (Fessman & Lester, 2000).*

- To keep older people independent, interventions to prevent loneliness should be explored. Consider using art as an intervention. **EBN:** *Integrating masterworks of art with care of the chronically ill elderly demonstrates that masterworks of art can generate energy exchange between the elderly and caregivers (Hodges, Keeley & Grier, 2001).*

- Consider a retirement village. **EB:** *Participants reported that isolation and loneliness decreased when clients relocated to a retirement village (Buys, 2001).*

- Encourage support by friends and family when the decision to stop driving must be made. **EBN:** *Increased loneliness and isolation affected the older driver, although an enhanced sense of responsibility was evident among friends and family. Findings suggest that the support offered by friends and family played a significant role in the decision to stop driving (Johnson, 1998).*

- Provide opportunities for indoor gardening. **EBN:** *Indoor gardening enhances socialization, activities of daily living (ADLs), and perceptions of loneliness in elderly nursing home residents (Brown et al, 2004).*

- Provide reading materials for clients who are able to read. *Older people who enjoyed reading for pleasure were rarely lonely (Rane-Szotak & Herth, 1994).*

L

Multicultural and Home Care

- Refer to care plan **Social isolation.**

Home Care

- Refer to care plan **Social isolation** for additional interventions.
- ▲ Above interventions may be adapted for home care use. Assess for depression with lonely elderly client and make appropriate referrals. **EBN:** *Findings have related loneliness in older adults to mental health problems, especially depression (McInnis & White, 2001).*
- ▲ If the client is experiencing somatic complaints, evaluate client complaints to ensure physical needs are being met, and then identify relationship between somatic complaints and loneliness. **EBN:** *Three factors have been found to increase levels of loneliness among elderly individuals residing in a nursing home: lack of intimate relationships, increased dependency, and loss (Hicks, 2000).*
- Identify alternatives to being alone (e.g., telephone contact). **EBN:** *Social support can be provided to low-income pregnant women who may have little or no social support and feel alienated in a clinical setting by telephone (Bullock, Browning & Geden, 2002).*
- Consider using computers and the Internet to alleviate or reduce loneliness and social isolation. **EBN:** *Residents age 65 years and older who were living alone used the computer to combat loneliness (Clark, 2002). Internet use was found to decrease loneliness and depression significantly, while perceived social support and self-esteem increased significantly (Shaw & Gant, 2002). Among Internet users there were trends toward less loneliness and less depression (White et al, 2002).*

Client/Family Teaching

- Refer to care plan **Social isolation** for additional interventions.
- Encourage positive use of solitude to prevent loneliness (e.g., reading, listening to music, enjoying nature and art). *A positive use of solitude plays a strong role in preventing or alleviating loneliness. The mentioned activities are activities that enhance well-being and decrease feelings of loneliness (Rane-Szotak & Herth, 1994).*
- Include the family in all client-teaching activities, and give them accurate information regarding the illness severity. **EBN:** *By listening to residents and family members, nurses can improve life for residents and dignify them as individuals (Iwasiw et al, 2003).*

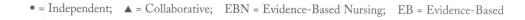

• = Independent;   ▲ = Collaborative;   EBN = Evidence-Based Nursing;   EB = Evidence-Based

- Give family members something to do such as holding a hand, applying lotion, or assisting with feeding. **EB:** *Perceived family support was predictive of reduced loneliness in this study of women with HIV (Serovich et al, 2001).*
- Encourage family members to express caring by telling the client where they will be and sending messages when they cannot be present. **EBN:** *If people could spare a smile or a word for others who might be perceived as lonely, such a small gesture might just make the day of a lonely person a little less of an ordeal (Killeen, 1998). Loneliness can only be alleviated and made less painful. This can only be achieved by increasing humankind's awareness of this distressing condition that all people endure sometime during their lives (Killeen, 1998).*
- ▲ Provide appropriate education for clients and their support persons about hepatitis C: transmission and treatment. *Clients with hepatitis C often face significant social problems, ranging from social isolation, living alone, and familial stress. Data from this study suggest that educational interventions targeting support persons of clients and their relatives and friends about the disease, the risk factors for its spread, and about potential consequence and the stressors may lessen or alleviate the social strains clients with hepatitis C experience (Blasiole et al, 2006).*

evolve See the EVOLVE website for World Wide Web resources for client education.

REFERENCES

Beeson R, Horton-Deutsch S, Farran C et al: Loneliness and depression in caregivers of persons with Alzheimer's disease or related disorders, *Issues Ment Health Nurs* 21(8):779-806, 2000.

Blasiole JA, Shinkunas L, Labrecque DR et al: Mental and physical symptoms associated with lower social support for patients with hepatitis C, *World J Gastroenterol* 12(29):4665-4672, 2006.

Brown VM, Allen AC, Dwozan M et al: Indoor gardening and older adults: effects on socialization, activities of daily living, and loneliness, *J Gerontol Nurs* 30(10):34-42, 2004.

Bullock LF, Browning C, Geden E: Telephone social support for low-income pregnant women, *J Obstet Gynecol Neonatal Nurs* 31(6):658-664, 2002.

Buys LR: Life in a retirement village: implications for contact with community and village friends, *Gerontology* 47(1):55-59, 2001.

Clark DJ: Older adults living through and with their computers, *Comput Inform Nurs* 20(3):117-124, 2002.

Corsano P, Majorano M, Champretavy L: Psychological well-being in adolescence: the contribution of interpersonal relations and experience of being alone, *Adolescence* 41(162):341-353, 2006.

Fessman N, Lester D: Loneliness and depression among elderly nursing home patients, *Int J Aging Hum Dev* 51(2):137-141, 2000.

Fry PS, Barker LA: Quality of relationships and structural properties of social support networks of female survivors of abuse, *Genet Soc Gen Psychol Monogr* 128(2):139-163, 2002.

Fukui S, Koike M, Ooba A et al: The effect of a psychosocial group intervention on loneliness and social support for Japanese women with primary breast cancer, *Oncol Nurs Forum* 30(5):823-830, 2003.

Gulick E: Emotional distress and activities of daily living functioning in persons with multiple sclerosis, *Nurs Res* 50(3):147-154, 2001.

Harris M, Fallot RD, Berley RW: Qualitative interviews on substance abuse relapse and prevention among female trauma survivors, *Psychiatr Serv* 56(10):1292-1296, 2005.

Hicks TJ Jr: What is your life like now? Loneliness and elderly individuals residing in nursing homes, *J Gerontol Nurs* 26(8):15-19, 2000.

Hodges HF, Keeley AC, Grier EC: Masterworks of art and chronic illness experiences in the elderly, *J Adv Nurs* 36(3):389-398, 2001.

Iwasiw C, Goldenberg D, Bol N et al: Resident and family perspectives. The first year in a long-term care facility, *J Gerontol Nurs* 29(1):45-54, 2003.

Johnson J: Older rural adults and the decision to stop driving: the influence of family and friends, *J Community Health Nurs* 15(4):205-216, 1998.

Kef S: Psychosocial adjustment and the meaning of social support for visually impaired adolescents, *J Vis Impair Blind* 96(1):22, 2002.

Killeen C: Loneliness: an epidemic in modern society, *J Adv Nurs* 28(4):762-770, 1998.

Leung L: Loneliness, self-disclosure, and ICQ ("I seek you") use, *Cyberpsychol Behav* 5(3):241-251, 2002.

Lindsay GM, Smith LN, Hanlon P et al: The influence of general health status and social support on symptomatic outcome following coronary artery bypass grafting, *Heart* 85(1):80-86, 2001.

Mahon NE, Yarcheski A: Alternate explanations of loneliness in adolescents: a replication and extension study, *Nurs Res* 41:151-156, 1992.

Mahon NE, Yarcheski T, Yarcheski A: The revised Personal Lifestyle Questionnaire for early adolescents, *West J Nurs Res* 25(5):533-547, 2003.

Mayers AM, Svartberg M: Existential loneliness: a review of the concept, its psychosocial precipitants and psychotherapeutic implications for HIV-infected women, *Br J Med Psychol* 74(Pt 4):539-553, 2001.

McInnis GJ, White JH: A phenomenological exploration of loneliness in the older adult, *Arch Psychiatr Nurs* 15(3):128-139, 2001.

Perese EF, Getty C, Wooldridge P: Psychosocial club members' characteristics and their readiness to participate in a support group, *Issues Ment Health Nurs* 24(2):153-174, 2003.

Perese EF, Wolf M: Combating loneliness among persons with severe mental illness: social network interventions' characteristics, effectiveness, and applicability, *Issues Ment Health Nurs* 26(6):591-609, 2005.

Rane-Szotak D, Herth K: A new perspective on loneliness in later life, *Issues Ment Health Nurs* 16:583-592, 1994.

Reichenbach E, McNamee M, Seibel L: The community health nursing implications of the self-reported health status of a local homeless population, *Public Health Nurs* 15(6):398-405, 1998.

Rew L: Friends and pets as companions: strategies for coping with loneliness among homeless youth, *J Child Adolesc Psychiatr Nurs* 13(3):125-132, 2000.

Savage CL, Lindsell CJ, Gillespie GL et al: Health care needs of homeless adults at a nurse-managed clinic, *J Community Health Nurs* 23(4):225-234, 2006.

Serovich JM, Kimberly JA, Mosack KE et al: The role of family and friend social support in reducing emotional distress among HIV-positive women, *AIDS Care* 13(3):335-341, 2001.

Shaw LH, Gant LM: In defense of the Internet: the relationship between Internet communication and depression, loneliness, self-esteem, and perceived social support, *Cyberpsychol Behav* 5(2):157-171, 2002.

Sorkin D, Rook KS, Lu JL: Loneliness, lack of emotional support, lack of companionship, and the likelihood of having a heart condition in an elderly sample, *Ann Behav Med* 24(4):290-298, 2002.

Stroebe M, Stroebe W, Abakoumkin G: The broken heart: suicidal ideation in bereavement, *Am J Psychiatry* 162(11):2178-2180, 2005.

Sundin K, Jansson L, Norberg A: Understanding between care providers and patients with stroke and aphasia: a phenomenological hermeneutic inquiry, *Nurs Inq* 9(2):93-103, 2002.

Terrell F, Terrell IS, Von Drashek SR: Loneliness and fear of intimacy among adolescents who were taught not to trust strangers during childhood, *Adolescence* 35(140):611-617, 2000.

Uruk AC, Demir A: The role of peers and families in predicting the loneliness level of adolescents, *J Psychol* 137(2):179-193, 2003.

Vidrine M, Owen-Smith P, Faulkner P: Equine-facilitated group psychotherapy: applications for therapeutic vaulting, *Issues Ment Health Nurs* 23(6):587-603, 2002.

White H, McConnell E, Clipp E et al: A randomized controlled trial of the psychosocial impact of providing Internet training and access to older adults, *Aging Ment Health* 6(3):213-221, 2002.

Yonge O, Molzahn A: Exceptional nontraditional caring practices of nurses, *Scand J Caring Sci* 16(4):399-405, 2002.

Impaired Memory *Graham J. McDougall Jr., PhD, RN, APRN, BC, FAAN*

NANDA Definition

Inability to remember or recall bits of information or behavioral skills; impaired memory may be attributed to pathophysiological or situational causes that are either temporary or permanent

Defining Characteristics

Experience of forgetting; forgets to perform a behavior at a scheduled time; inability to determine if a behavior was performed; inability to learn new information; inability to learn new skills; inability to perform a previously learned skill; inability to recall events; inability to recall factual information; inability to retain new information; inability to retain new skills

Related Factors (r/t)

Anemia; decreased cardiac output; excessive environmental disturbances; fluid and electrolyte imbalance; hypoxia; neurological disturbances

NOC Outcomes (Nursing Outcomes Classification)

Suggested NOC Outcomes

Cognitive Orientation, Memory, Neurological Status: Consciousness

Example NOC Outcome with Indicators
Memory as evidenced by the following indicators: Recalls immediate information accurately/Recalls recent information accurately/Recalls remote information accurately (Rate the outcome and indicators of **Memory:** 1 = severely compromised, 2 = substantially compromised, 3 = moderately compromised, 4 = mildly compromised, 5 = not compromised [see Section I].)

Client Outcomes

Client Will (Specify Time Frame):

• Demonstrate use of techniques to help with memory loss
• State has improved memory for everyday concerns

NIC   **Interventions (Nursing Interventions Classification)**

Suggested NIC Intervention
Memory Training

Example NIC Activities—Memory Training
Stimulate memory by repeating patient's last expressed thought, as appropriate; Provide opportunity to use memory for recent events, such as questioning patient about a recent outing; Assist in associate-learning tasks, such as practice learning and recalling verbal and pictoral information presented, as appropriate

Nursing Interventions and *Rationales*

- Assess overall cognitive function and memory. The emphasis of the assessment is everyday memory, the day-to-day operations of memory in real-world ordinary situations (Cohen, 1989). Use an assessment tool such as the Mini-Mental State Examination (MMSE) and/or the Metamemory in Adulthood (MIA) questionnaire. *The MMSE can help determine whether the client has cognitive impairment and/or memory loss or delirium and needs to be referred for further evaluation and treatment (Agostinelli et al, 1994; Breitner and Welsh, 1995; McDougall, 1990). The MIA is a reliable and nonthreatening assessment for nonimpaired individuals and has been validated to be effective (McDougall, 1990).*

- Assess for memory complaints since memory loss may be the earliest manifestation of mild cognitive impairment (MCI). *An MCI diagnosis includes the five criteria of cognitive complaints not normal for the age of the individual, no dementia, cognitive decline, memory impairment, and essentially normal functional activities (Winblad et al, 2004).*

- ▲ Determine whether onset of memory loss is gradual or sudden. If memory loss is sudden, refer the client to a physician or neuropsychologist for evaluation. *Acute onset of memory loss may be associated with neurological disease, medication effect, electrolyte disturbances, hypoxia, hypothyroidism, mental illness, or many other physiological factors (Elliott, 2000; Foreman et al, 2001).*

- Determine amount and pattern of alcohol intake. *Alcohol intake has been associated with blackouts; clients may function but not remember their actions. Long-term alcohol use causes Korsakoff's syndrome with associated memory loss; however, moderate consumption of alcohol may be health promoting (Britton, Singh-Manoux & Marmot, 2004; Perreira & Sloan, 2002; Zimmerman, McDougall & Becker, 2004). Dementia and cognitive decline are positively associated with silent brain infarcts (Vermeer et al, 2003).*

- Note the client's current medications and intake of any mind-altering substances such as benzodiazepines, ecstasy, marijuana, cocaine, or glucocorticoids. *Benzodiazepines can produce memory loss for events that occur after taking the medication; information is not stored in long-term memory (Fluck et al, 1998). They can also decrease retrieval of memory (Beracochea, 2006). Cocaine abuse has been shown to decrease memory (Butler & Frank, 2000). The ingestion of ecstasy has been associated with impaired memory, both learning and recall (Gowing et al, 2002; Quednow et al, 2006).* **EB:** *Glucocorticoid therapy may cause a decrease in memory function that is usually reversible once a person is off the medications (Wolkowitz et al, 1997). Clients receiving long-term prednisone performed significantly worse on memory tasks than matched control subjects (Keenan, 1996). Both infrequent and long-term use of marijuana is associated with impaired memory function (Curran et al, 2002; Solowij et al, 2002) and may become more of a concern to evaluate with the aging of the baby boomers.*

- Note the client's current level of stress. Ask if there has been a recent traumatic event. *Post-traumatic stress and anxiety-inducing general life factors may induce memory problems (Diamond, Park & Woodson, 2004; Jelicic & Merckelbach, 2004). Elevated cortisol levels associated with stress have been shown to impair memory (Greendale et al, 2000; Lupien et al, 1997).*

- ▲ If stress is associated with memory loss, refer to a stress reduction clinic. If not available, suggest that the client meditate, receive massages, and participate in moderate physical activity, all of which may promote stress reduction and reduce anxiety and depression (Rees et al, 2004). Encourage the client to develop an aerobic exercise program. **EB:** *Aerobic exercise may improve*

memory and executive function in depressed middle-aged and older adults (Khatri et al, 2001). An increase in memory function has been shown in the elderly after a strength training program (Lachman, 2006).

• Determine the client's sleep patterns. If insufficient, refer to care plan for **Insomnia. EB:** *Memory consolidation is enhanced by sleep (Gais et al, 2002; Peigneux et al, 2001).*

▲ Determine the client's blood sugar levels. If they are elevated, refer to physician for treatment and encourage healthy diet and exercise to improve memory. *Elevated blood sugar levels were associated with impaired memory (Convit, 2003).*

▲ If signs of depression such as weight loss, insomnia, or sad affect are evident, refer the client for psychotherapy. *Depression can result in source memory errors, in which case the client is not sure if he or she did something or just thought about doing it (Elias, 2001).*

▲ Perform a nutritional assessment. If nutritional status is marginal, confer with a dietitian and primary care practitioner to evaluate whether the client needs supplementation with foods or vitamins. Teach the client the need to eat a healthy diet with adequate intake of whole grains, fruits, and vegetables to decrease cerebrovascular infarcts. *Moderate, long-term deficiencies of nutrients may lead to loss of memory. This condition may be preventable or diminished through diet (Cataldo, DeBruyne & Whitney, 2003). Adequate levels of vitamin E may help protect memory (Miller, 2000).* **EB:** *People who eat mostly fruits and vegetables (9 or 10 servings per day) have decreased incidence of ischemic strokes (Joshipura et al, 1999).*

▲ Question the client about cholesterol level. If it is high, refer to physician or dietitian for help in lowering. Encourage the client to eat a healthy diet, avoiding saturated fats and *trans*-fatty acids. **EB:** *Individuals who are prescribed statin medications that lowered cholesterol have a substantially lower risk of developing dementia (Jick et al, 2000). High intake of saturated or* trans-*fatty acids may increase the risk of Alzheimer's disease (Morris et al, 2006).*

• Suggest clients use cues, including alarm watches, electronic organizers, calendars, lists, or pocket computers, to trigger certain actions at designated times. *Cues and external cognitive strategies can help remind clients of certain actions (McDougall, 1999).*

• Encourage the client to use external memory devices, such as a calendar for appointments, keep reminder lists, place a string around finger or rubber band around wrist as reminders, or enlist someone else to remind him or her of important events. *Using reminders can serve as cues for memory-impaired clients.*

• Help the client set up a medication box that reminds the client to take medication at needed times; assist the client with refilling the box at intervals if necessary. *Medication boxes are effective because clients will know whether medication has been taken when corresponding compartments are empty.*

• If safety is an issue with certain activities (e.g., the client forgets to turn off stove after use or forgets emergency telephone numbers), suggest alternatives such as using a microwave or whistling teakettle for heating water and programming emergency numbers in telephone so that they are readily available.

▲ Refer the client to a memory clinic (if available), a neuropsychologist, or an occupational therapist. Memory clinics can help the client learn ways to improve memory. *Clinics may be more effective if work is done in groups because of increased support, reinforcement, and motivation (McDougall, 1999).*

• For clients with memory impairments associated with dementia, see care plan for **Chronic Confusion.**

Geriatric

• Assess for signs of depression. *Depression is the most important affective variable for memory loss in the older adult (McDougall, 1999).* **EB:** *Cognitive impairment is not an inevitable consequence of aging, even in very old age (Snowdon, 1997).*

• Evaluate all medications that the client is taking to determine whether they are causing the memory loss. *Many medications, both prescription and over the counter, may cause memory loss in the elderly, including anticholinergics, H2-receptor antagonists, beta-blockers, digitalis, benzodiazepines, barbiturates, and even mild opiates (Dergal et al, 2002; Sjogren, Thomsen & Olsen, 2000).*

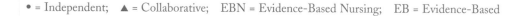

• = Independent;   ▲ = Collaborative;   EBN = Evidence-Based Nursing;   EB = Evidence-Based

- Evaluate all herbal and/or nutraceutical products that the individual might be using to improve their memory function. *Products that claim to enhance some aspect of cognitive function may not be known outside of the homeopathic field, and their stated benefits may not have been clearly researched (McDougall, Austin-Wells & Zimmerman, 2005).*
- Recommend that elderly clients maintain a positive attitude and active involvement with the world around them and that they maintain good nutrition. **EB:** *It is possible to maintain good cognitive function until extreme old age if elderly persons maintain active involvement with their environment and are able to avoid having vascular disease with infarction of brain tissue (Snowdon, 1997).* **EB:** *Activities such as chess and crossword puzzles have been found useful in assisting memory and cognitive function (Dowd & Davidhizar, 2003).*
- Encourage the elderly to believe in themselves and to work to improve their memory. *Negative attitudes and belief may decrease motivation and impair everyday memory function (McDougall, 1999).* **EB:** *Elderly clients may be able to improve their memory function up to 50% if they use appropriate strategies and invest the energy and time (Ball et al, 2002). Stimulation of the brain is necessary for neurogenesis (the formation of new neurons in the brain) to occur throughout the lifespan (Eriksson et al, 1998).*
- ▲ Refer the client to a memory class that focuses on helping older adults learn memory strategies. **EBN and EB:** *Classes that focus on memory strategies could improve memory (McDougall, 2002). In memory impairment associated with strokes, there is insufficient evidence to determine if memory training is effective (Majid, Lincoln & Weyman, 2000).*
- Help family develop a memory aid booklet or wallet that contains pictures and labels from the client's life, or develop a video movie that includes familiar pictures with narration (Cohen, 2002). *Using memory aids helps clients with dementia make more factual statements and stay on topic and decreases the number of confused, erroneous, and repetitive statements made (Bourgeois, 1992).* **EB:** *Use of the memory book may also help decrease the number of depressive statements by the client (Bourgeois et al, 2001).*
- Help family label items such as the bathroom or sock drawer to increase recall. *A supportive environment that includes orientation can help increase the client's awareness (Green & Gildemeister, 1994).*

Multicultural

- Assess for the influence of cultural beliefs, norms, and values on the family or caregiver's understanding of impaired memory. *There is more age-specific prevalence of dementia among African Americans than Caucasians. A greater familial risk of Alzheimer's exists among African-American families. The cumulative risk of dementia among first-degree relatives of African Americans who suffer from Alzheimer's is 43.7%. (McDougall & Holston, 2003). Older Hispanic Americans are twice as likely as Caucasians to have impairments that prevent them from shopping or attending social functions, with 28% of older Hispanic Americans rating their health as poor or very poor.*
- Use bias-free instruments when assessing memory in the culturally diverse client. **EBN:** *Use of the MMSE without modification for ethnic bias resulted in younger Hispanics being categorized as more severely impaired than others (Mulgrew et al, 1999).*
- Inform the client's family or caregiver of meaning of and reasons for common behavior observed in the client with impaired memory. *An understanding of impaired memory behavior will enable the client family/caregiver to provide the client with a safe environment.*
- Validate family members' feelings regarding the impact of the client's behavior on family lifestyle. **EBN:** *Even though validation therapy for dementia is a communication technique that lets the client know that the nurse has heard and understands what was said, and it promotes the nurse-client relationship, there is insufficient evidence from randomized trials to make any conclusion about its efficacy for people with dementia or cognitive impairment (Neal & Briggs, 2003; Heineken, 1998).*

Home Care

- Above interventions may be adapted for home care use.
- Arrange cues for medication taking that are focused around daily events (e.g., meals and bed-

M

times). **EBN:** *Older adults report the use of internal memory strategies to compensate for age-related memory loss; specifically they prefer event-based prescription medication instructions (Branin, 2001).*

- Assess the client's need for outside assistance with recall of treatment, medications, and willingness/ability of family to provide needed support. *During initial phase of home care, increased frequency of visits may be necessary to compensate for the client's inability to recall treatment and medications. Counting of medications may be needed to determine if the client is following medication regimen. Telephone calls from family/friends may help to remind the client of treatment schedule.*

- Identify a checking-in support system (e.g., Lifeline or significant others). *Checking in ensures the client's safety.*

- Keep furniture placement and household patterns consistent. *Change increases risk of impaired memory and decreased functioning.*

- ▲ In the presence of a medical disorder, institute case management of frail elderly to support continued independent living. *Memory difficulties often represent and can lead to increasing needs for assistance in using the healthcare system effectively. Case management can help coordinate services to help the memory-impaired person.*

Client/Family Teaching

- When teaching the client, determine what the client knows about memory techniques and then build on that knowledge. *New material is organized in terms of what knowledge already exists, and efficient teaching should attempt to take advantage of what is already known in order to graft on new material (McDougall, 1999).*

- When teaching a skill to the client, set up a series of practice attempts. Begin with simple tasks so that the client can be positively reinforced and progress to more difficult concepts. *Distributed practice with correct recall attempts can be a very effective teaching strategy. Widely distribute practice over time if possible (Camp, Cohen-Mansfield & Capezuti, 2002).*

- Teach clients to use memory techniques such as repeating information they want to remember, making mental associations to remember information, and placing items in strategic places so that they will not be forgotten. *These methods increase recall of information the client thinks is important. The internal methods of increasing memory can be effective, especially if used along with external methods such as calendars, lists, and other methods (McDougall, 1999).*

evolve   See the EVOLVE website for World Wide Web resources for client education.

REFERENCES

Agostinelli B, Demers K, Garrigan D et al: Targeted interventions. Use of the Mini-Mental State Exam, *J Gerontol Nurs* 20(8):15-23, 1994.

Ball K, Berch DB, Helmers KF et al: Advanced Cognitive Training for Independent and Vital Elderly Study Group, *JAMA* 288(18):2271-2281, 2002.

Beracochea D: Antegrade and retrograde effects of benzodiazepines on memory. *Sci World J* 6:1460-1465, 2006.

Bourgeois MS: *Conversing with memory impaired individuals using memory aids: a memory aid workbook,* Gaylord, Mich, 1992, Northern Speech Services.

Bourgeois MS, Dijkstra K, Burgio L et al: Memory aids as an augmentative and alternative communication strategy for nursing home residents with dementia, *Augment Altern Commun* 17(3):196-210, 2001.

Branin JJ: The role of memory strategies in medication adherence among the elderly, *Home Health Care Serv Q* 20(2):1-16, 2001.

Breitner JC, Welsh KA: Diagnosis and management of memory loss and cognitive disorders among elderly persons, *Psychiatr Serv* 46:29-35, 1995.

Britton A, Singh-Manoux A, Marmot M: Alcohol consumption and cognitive function in the Whitehall II Study, *Am J Epidemiol* 160(3):240-247, 2004.

Butler LF, Frank EM: Neurolinguistic function and cocaine abuse, *J Med Speech Lang Pathol* 8(3):199, 2000.

Camp CJ, Cohen-Mansfield J, Capezuti EA: Use of nonpharmacologic interventions among nursing home residents with dementia, *Psychiatr Serv* 53(11):1397-1401, 2002.

Cataldo CB, DeBruyne LK, Whitney EN: *Nutrition and diet therapy: principles and practice,* ed 6, Belmont, Calif, Wadsworth, 2003.

Cohen G: Everyday memory. In Cohen G, editor: *Memory in the real world,* Hillsdale, 1989, Lawrence Erlbaum, pp. 1-15.

Cohen GD: Creative interventions for Alzheimer's disease: familiar activities, videos can help patients copy with memory loss, *Geriatrics* 57(3):62, 65, 2002.

Convit A, Wolf OT, Tarshish C et al: Reduced glucose tolerance is associated with poor memory performance and hippocampal atrophy among normal elderly, *Proc Natl Acad Sci U S A* 100(4):2019-2022, 2003.

Curran HV, Brignell C, Fletcher S et al: Cognitive and subjective dose-response effects of acute oral Delta 9-tetrahydrocannabinol (THC) in infrequent cannabis users, *Psychopharmacology (Berl)* 164(1):61-70, 2002.

Dergal JM, Gold JL, Laxer DA et al: Potential interactions between herbal medicines and conventional drug therapies used by older adults attending a memory clinic, *Drugs Aging* 19(11):879-886, 2002.

Diamond DM, Park CR, Woodson JC: Stress generates emotional memories and retrograde amnesia by inducing an endogenous form of hippocampal LTP, *Hippocam* 14(3):281-291, 2004.

Dowd SB, Davidhizar R: Can mental and physical activities such as chess and gardening help in the prevention and treatment of Alzheimers? *J Pract Nurs* 53(3):11-13, 2003.

Elias J: Why caregiver depression and self-care abilities should be part of the PPS case mix methodology, *Home Healthc Nurse* 19(1):23-30, 2001.

Elliott B: Case report. Diagnosing and treating hypothyroidism, *Nurs Pract* 25(3):92-94, 99-105, 2000.

Eriksson PS, Perfilieva E, Bjork-Eriksson T et al: Neurogenesis in the adult human hippocampus, *Nat Med* 4(11):1313-1317, 1998.

Fluck E, File SE, Springett J et al: Does the sedation resulting from sleep deprivation and lorazepam cause similar cognitive deficits? *Pharmacol Biochem Behav* 59(4):909-915, 1998.

Foreman MD, Wakefield B, Culp K et al: Delirium in elderly patients: an overview of the state of the science, *J Gerontol Nurs* 27(4):12-20, 2001.

Gais S et al: Learning-dependent increases in sleep spindle density, *J Neurosci* 22(15):6830-6834, 2002.

Gowing LR, Henry-Edwards SM, Irvine RJ et al: The health effects of ecstasy: a literature review, *Drug Alcohol Rev* 21(1):53-63, 2002.

Green PM, Gildemeister JE: Memory aging research and memory support in the elderly, *J Neurosci Nurs* 26:241-244, 1994.

Greendale GA, Kritz-Silverstein D, Seeman T et al: Higher basal cortisol predicts verbal memory loss in postmenopausal women: Rancho Bernardo Study, *J Am Geriatr Soc* 48(12):1655-1658, 2000.

Heineken J: Patient silence is not necessarily client satisfaction: communication in home care nursing, *Home Healthc Nurse* 16(2):115-120, 1998.

Jelicic M, Merckelbach H: Traumatic stress, brain changes, and memory deficits: a critical note, *J Nerv Ment Dis* 192(8):548-553, 2004.

Jick H, Zornberg GL, Jick SS et al: Statins and risk of dementia, *Lancet* 356(9242):1627-1631, 2000.

Joshipura KJ, Ascherio A, Manson JE et al: Fruit and vegetable intake in relation to ischemic stroke, *JAMA* 6(282):1233-1239, 1999.

Keenan PA: Chronic prednisone use causes memory loss, *Neurology* 47:1396, 1996.

Khatri P, Blumenthal JA, Babyak MA et al: Effects of exercise training on cognitive functioning among depressed older men and women, *J Aging Phys Act* 9(1):43-57, 2001.

Lachman ME, Neupert SD, Bertrand R et al: The effects of strength training on memory in older adults, *J Aging Phys Act* 14(1):59-73, 2006.

Lupien SJ, Gaudreau S, Tchiteya BM et al: Stress-induced declarative memory impairment in healthy elderly subjects: relationship to cortisol reactivity, *J Clin Endocrinol Metab* 82(7):2070-2075, 1997.

Majid MJ, Lincoln NB, Weyman N: Cognitive rehabilitation for memory deficits following stroke, *Cochrane Database Syst Rev* (3): CD002293, 2000.

McDougall GJ: Cognitive interventions among older adults, *Annu Rev Nurs Res* 17:219-240, 1999.

McDougall GJ: Memory improvement in octogenarians, *Appl Nurs Res* 15(1):2-10, 2002.

McDougall GJ: A review of screening instruments for assessing cognition and mental status in older adults, *Nurs Pract* 15(11):18-28, 1990.

McDougall GJ, Austin-Wells V, Zimmerman T: Utility of nutraceutical products marketed for cognitive and memory enhancement, *J Holist Nur* 23:415-433, 2005.

McDougall GJ, Holston EC: Black and white men at risk for memory impairment, *Nurs Res* 52(1):42-46, 2003.

Miller JW: Vitamin E and memory: is it vascular protection? *Nutr Rev* 58(4):109-111, 2000.

Morris MC et al: Dietary copper and high saturated and trans fat intakes associated with cognitive decline, *Arch Neurol* 63(8):1085-1088, 2006.

Mulgrew CL, Morganstern N, Shetterly SM et al: Cognitive functioning and impairment among rural elderly Hispanics and non-Hispanic whites as assessed by the Mini-Mental State Exam, *J Gerontol B Psychol Sci Soc Sci* 54B(4):223-230, 1999.

Neal M, Briggs M: Validation therapy for dementia, *Cochrane Database Syst Rev* (3):CD001394, 2003.

Peigneux P et al: Sleeping brain, learning brain. The role of sleep for memory systems, *Neuroreport* 12(18):A111-A124, 2001.

Perreira KM, Sloan FA: Excess alcohol consumption and health outcomes: a 6-year follow-up of men over age 50 from the health and retirement study, *Addiction* 97(3):301-310, 2002.

Quednow BB, Jessen F, Kuhn KU et al: Memory deficits in abstinent-MDMA (ectasy) users: neuropsychological evidence of frontal dysfunction, *J Psychopharmacol* 20(3):373-384, 2006.

Rees K, Bennett P, West R et al: Psychological interventions for coronary heart disease, *Cochrane Database Syst Rev* 2:CD002902, 2004.

Sjogren P, Thomsen AB, Olsen AK: Impaired neuropsychological performance in chronic nonmalignant pain patients receiving long-term oral opioid therapy, *J Pain Symptom Manage* 19(2):100-108, 2000.

Snowdon DA: Aging and Alzheimer's disease: lessons from the Nun Study, *Gerontologist* 37(2):150-156, 1997.

Solowij N, Stephens RS, Roffman RA et al: Cognitive functioning of long-term heavy cannabis users seeking treatment, *JAMA* 287(9):1123-1131, 2002.

Vermeer SE, Prins ND, den Heijer T et al: Silent brain infarcts and the risk of dementia and cognitive decline, *N Engl J Med* 348(13):1215-1222, 2003.

Winblad B, Palmer K, Kivipelto M et al: Mild cognitive impairment—beyond controversies, towards a consensus: report of the International Working Group on Mild Cognitive Impairment, *J Intern Med* 256(3):240-246, 2004.

Wolkowitz OM, Reus VI, Canick J et al: Glucocorticoid medication, memory and steroid psychosis in medical illness, *Ann N Y Acad Sci* 823:81-96, 1997.

Zimmerman T, McDougall GJ Jr, Becker H: Older women's cognitive and affective response to moderate drinking, *Int J Geriatr Psychiatry*, 19(11):1095-1102, 2004.

Impaired bed Mobility *Brenda Emick-Herring, RN, MSN, CRRN*

NANDA **Definition**

Limitation of independent movement from one bed position to another

Defining Characteristics

Impaired ability to: move from supine to sitting; to move from sitting to supine; to move from supine to prone; to move from prone to supine; to move from supine to long sitting; to move from long sitting to supine; to "scoot" or reposition self in bed; to turn from side to side

Related Factors (r/t)

Cognitive impairment; deconditioning; deficient knowledge; environmental constraints (i.e., bed size, bed type, treatment equipment, restraints); insufficient muscle strength; musculoskeletal impairment; neuromuscular impairment; obesity; pain; sedating medications. NOTE: specify level of independence using a standardized functional scale

NOC Outcomes (Nursing Outcomes Classification)

Suggested NOC Outcomes

Mobility, Self-Care: Activities of Daily Living (ADLs)

Example NOC Outcome with Indicators
Mobility as evidenced by the following indicators: Body positioning performance/Gait/Joint movement (Rate the outcome and indicators of **Mobility:** 1 = severely compromised, 2 = substantially compromised, 3 = moderately compromised, 4 = mildly compromised, 5 = not compromised [see Section I].)

Client Outcomes

Client Will (Specify Time Frame):

- Demonstrate optimal independence in positioning, exercising, and performing functional activities in bed
- Demonstrate ability to direct others on how to do bed positioning, exercising, and functional activities

NIC Interventions (Nursing Interventions Classification)

Suggested NIC Intervention

Bed Rest Care

Example NIC Activities—Bed Rest Care
Position in proper body alignment; Teach bed exercises, as appropriate

Nursing Interventions and *Rationales*

- Assess/determine client's risk for intracranial pressure (ICP)/aspiration/pressure ulcer/pain and for respiratory/cardiovascular/muscle tone abnormalities. *These conditions warrant certain bed positions to prevent complications (Sullivan, 2000; WOCN Society, 2003).* **EBN:** *Authors recommend a semirecumbent position to reduce risk of aspiration with enteral feedings even with little quality research to prove it (Williams & Leslie, 2004). Head of bed elevation (HOB) at 30° reduced ICP (Fan, 2004).*
- Critically think/set priorities to use most therapeutic bed positions/frequency of turns based on client's history, risk profile, preventative needs; realize positioning for one condition may negatively affect another. **EBN:** *Therapeutic bed positions are recommended from author's assimilation of results of multisystem research (Sullivan, 2000).*
- Raise HOB 30° for clients with acute increased ICP (Fan, 2004; Sullivan, 2000) and 0° to 15° for those with acute cerebral ischemia. Refer to care plan for **Decreased Intracranial adaptive capacity. EB:** *Head elevation of 30° in acute closed head injured clients reduced ICP significantly (Ng, Lim & Wong, 2004). Flat to 15° HOB elevation may increase blood flow to ischemic tissue in acute stroke survivors (Wojner, El-Mitwalli & Alexandrov, 2002).*
- Turn clients at high risk for pressure/shear/friction frequently (Salcido, 2006). *Turn clients **at least** every 2 to 4 hours on pressure-reducing mattress/every 2 hours on standard foam mattress (WOCN Society, 2003).* **EBN:** *Staff improved identifying clients at high risk for pressure ulcers/need for repositioning bed-bound clients using a prevention model (Lyder et al, 2004).*

• = Independent; ▲ = Collaborative; EBN = Evidence-Based Nursing; EB = Evidence-Based

- Tilt clients 30° or less while lying on side. *Full (versus tilt) side-lying position places high pressure on trochanter (Defloor, 2000; Hoeman, 2002).*
- Assist client to sit as upright as possible during meals/ingestion of pills if dysphagic. Refer to care plan for **Impaired Swallowing.** *Helps prevent aspiration of food, liquids, and pills (Flannery & Pugh, 2004; Gavin-Dreschnack, 2004).*
- Periodically sit client as upright as tolerated in bed, if vital signs/oxygen saturation levels remain stable. Dangle client at the bedside if possible. *Being vertical reduces work of heart and abnormal posturing, changes intravascular pressure, improves lung ventilation and aeration, and stimulates neural reflexes/awareness of surroundings (Metzler & Harr, 1996).* **EB:** *Bed rest may delay recovery/cause harm (Allen, Glasziou & Del Mar, 1999). Sitting inpatients with community-acquired pneumonia 20 minutes the first day with progressive mobilization thereafter shortened the length of stay by one day (Mundy et al, 2003).*
- Maintain HOB at lowest elevation that is medically possible to prevent pressure ulcers; check sacrum often. *Sacral shearing risk is high when HOB is above 30°; skin may stick to linen if clients slide down, causing skin to pull away from underlying muscle tissue/bone (WOCN Society, 2003).*
- Position bed flat at intervals unless medically contraindicated. *Helps maintain body alignment/normalize tone; is the start position for bed mobility tasks; and is position of most beds at home (Kumagai, 1998).*
- Place pillows under legs of immobile supine-lying clients unless contraindicated, for example, after total knee replacement. *Lengthwise pillows under calves lowers heel pressure (WOCN Society, 2003).*
- Therapeutically (re)position joints/limbs in neutral alignment; safely pad pressure points/body parts needing support preoperatively/intraoperatively. *This prevents pressure ulcers, trauma, nerve injury, and restricted blood flow to immobile and strapped body parts during surgery (Murphy, 2004).*
- Use static/dynamic bed surfaces and assess for "bottoming out" under susceptible bony areas (body sinks onto mattress, thus the recommended 1 inch between mattress/bones is absent). Refer to care plan for **Risk for impaired Skin integrity.** *Devices help prevent/treat pressure ulcers (WOCN Society, 2003; Gutierrez, 2002; Johnson & Nolde-Lopez, 2002).*
- Place clients with stage III or IV pressure ulcers on low-air-loss surface or air-fluidized bed or consult enterostomal therapy nurse to determine appropriate surfaces (WOCN Society, 2003).
- Recognize and actively prevent complications associated with immobility. *The inability to be upright disturbs many body systems (Metzler & Harr, 1996; Olson, 1967).*
- Use a formalized screening tool to identify persons at high risk for deep vein thrombosis (DVT). *Early detection of high risk prompts early initiation of prophylaxis (Hums & Blostein, 2006).*
- Assess clients for venous thromboembolism and implement prophylaxis as ordered, for example, anticoagulants, antiembolic stockings, elastic wraps, sequential compression devices, feet/ankle exercises, and hydration. Refer to care plan for **Ineffective Tissue perfusion.** *Anticoagulants prevent blood clot formation; mechanical devices/exercises prevent venous stasis (Anderson & Spencer, 2003; Grande & Caparro, 2005; Kehl-Pruett, 2006).*
- Start oxygen/manage airway/follow protocols for clients with unexplained acute cardiopulmonary problems. *Pulmonary emboli may quickly arise in immobilized persons (Koschel, 2004).*
- Implement the following interventions during bed mobility activities:
  - Place positioning devices such as pillows/foam wedges between bony prominences (knees, etc.).
  - Use transferring devices such as trapeze, draw sheet, mechanical lateral transfer aid, ceiling-mounted lifts to move (rather than drag) dependent/obese persons (Jenkins & Egersett, 2004; APTA, ARN, VHA Task Force, 2005). *Devices prevent musculoskeletal injuries in staff and protect clients' skin against pressure, friction, and shear (WOCN Society, 2003).* **NOTE:** *Trapeze has isotonic effect and may be contraindicated with cardiac disease/stroke and with hemiplegics; gripping with sound hand elicits tonicity in affected side (Bobath, 1978; Hoeman, 2002).* **EBN:** *Manual lifting often causes overexertion back stress injuries to staff; may be uncomfortable to clients (Owen, Welden & Kane 1999). Ergonomic equipment likely improves nurses' back pain outcomes; cognitive behavioral training may improve back pain/self-care outcomes (Menzel, Lilley & Robinson, 2006).*
- Use special beds/equipment to move bariatric (very obese) clients, such as mattress overlay, sliding/roller board, trapeze, stirrup, and pulley attached to overhead traction system (holds one

leg up during pericare). *This reduces skin shear and frictional burn plus decreases resistance for staff to overcome when repositioning obese clients (Dionne 2000, 2002; Daus 2001, 2003).*

- Place bariatric beds along a corner wall. *Helps keep bed from moving as staff reposition clients.*
- Logroll and tilt dependent bariatric clients (avoid full side-lying position) until familiar with his or her ability to help turn in bed. *If client starts to slide out of bed in full side-lying position, it is difficult for staff to stop the motion (Dionne, 2002).*
- Apply elbow pads to comatose/restrained clients and to those who use elbows to prop/scoot up in bed; apply nocturnal elbow splint if ulnar nerve palsy exists or if painful elbow with paresthesia in ulnar side of fourth/fifth fingers develops. *Prolonged compression or flexion puts pressure on ulnar nerve, causing neuropathy/damage; pads prevent this. Elbow splints provide joint extension (Congress of Neurological Surgeons, 2002). NOTE: An enclosure bed for agitated clients may alleviate restraints, thus preventing arm abrasions/nerve damage/pain.*
- Range/exercise joints and apply padded foot splints/boots on a rotating schedule. *Immobility, chronic spasticity, and muscle weakness/atrophy from connective tissue changes contribute to joint contractures (Fried & Fried, 2001).*
- Explain importance of exhaling (versus holding one's breath/straining) during bed activities. *Exhaling prevents increased intraabdominal/intrathoracic pressure, which elevates blood pressure and impairs myocardial/cerebral perfusion, and the Valsalva maneuver (Rodriguez, 1998).*
- If bed movement intensifies pain, administer analgesics and accept clients' rating of pain (McCaffery & Pasero, 1999). *Certain drugs help neuropathic pain associated with peripheral nerve injury/disuse (Robinson & Shannon, 2002).* **EBN:** *A phenomenological study demonstrated nurses intervened for postoperative pain, thus affecting quality of care (Soderhamn & Idvall, 2003).*
- Assess for effects of antispasmodic medications. *A therapeutic level is one that prevents spasms but does not produce muscle weakness (Finocchiaro & Herzfeld, 1998).*
- ▲ Assess for increased joint resistance, spasms, and related pain/sensations. **EB:** *A multicenter trial where intramuscular botulinum toxin A was injected into flexed wrists/fingers of stroke survivors resulted in less spasticity and disability (Brashear et al, 2002). Researchers concluded professionals' clinical "muscle tone" spasticity rating should be in conjunction with spinal cord injury clients' rating, plus sensations experienced along with the tonicity (Lechner, Frotzler & Eser, 2006).*
- ▲ Recognize benefits of continuous intrathecal baclofen infusion (CITB) via an implanted pump in the spinal canal as ordered. *Intractable chronic spasticity/pain interrupts function, positioning, hygiene, and quality of life.* **EBN:** *The majority of clients receiving CITB had a significant decrease in tone/nursing care and increased function (Rawicki, 1999).* **EB:** *Spasticity decreased per Ashworth scores, and answers to questions relating to quality of life were positive (Gianino et al, 1998).*
- Assist clients to splint incisions/wounds/painful abdominal areas with a pillow as they change positions, cough, or perform functional activities in bed.
- ▲ Refer clients to dietitian or provide dietary information to promote normal weight. *Extra weight causes work/stress on body parts during bed mobility activities and intolerance to prone position.*
- Identify/modify hospital beds with large gaps within the side rail/mattress system that potentially create an entrapment hazard. Act to ensure mattresses fit the bed, and instill gap fillers, rail inserts/pads/covers, and bumper wedges; monitor their effectiveness. *Entrapment can be life threatening (Powell-Cope, Baptiste & Nelson, 2005).*

Exercising

- Perform passive range of motion (ROM) at least twice a day to immobile joints; support limb above/below joint being ranged. *This maintains joint/muscle movement and prevents contractures; muscles gain strength by working. Joint support allows staff to detect ease/resistance to movement (Hoeman, 2002).*
- Perform ROM slowly/rhythmically. Do not range beyond point of pain. Range only to point of resistance in those with loss of sensation/mentation. *Fast, jerky ROM creates pain and increases tone. Slow, rhythmical movements relax/lengthen spastic muscles so they can be ranged further. NOTE: This is not the case with rigidity, as in Parkinson's disease (Palmer & Wyness, 1988).*
- Range a hemiplegic arm with the shoulder slightly externally rotated. *Spasticity prevents normal gliding movements of shoulder; thus soft tissue gets pinched between bones, causing pain. External rotation prevents this (Borgman & Passarella, 1991).*

M

▲ Reinforce self-initiated practice of exercises taught by therapists (muscle setting, strengthening, and contraction against resistance, and weight lifting). *This promotes self-responsibility. Active exercises/weight lifting help maintain muscle tone/strength; muscle setting shortens fibers without moving limb/joints; resistive exercises cause muscles to work against gentle force/gravity, thus stimulating muscle lengthening (Hoeman, 2002).*

• Intervene for misalignment, flaccidity, spasticity, reduced sensation, and excessive effort while moving. *Therapeutic bed positioning/moving restores more normal tone/postures (Bobath, 1978; Gee & Passarella, 1985; Kumagai, 1998; Palmer & Wyness, 1988).*

• Allow clients to do as many bed activities as they can; help with light manual guidance and verbal cues if needed. *Clients need the opportunity to feel more normal tone and postures so they do not relearn abnormal patterns (Ossman & Campbell, 1990; Passarella & Lewis, 1987).*

Bed Positioning

• Incorporate the following measures to promote normal tone and prevent complications. Refer to Ossman & Campbell (1990), Kumagai (1998), and Gee & Passarella (1985) for detailed instructions.

  ▪ Position head and neck in midline. *Head, neck, and trunk alignment normalizes muscle tone in the extremities, thus decreasing spasticity (Bobath, 1978).*

  ▪ Use a flat head pillow when clients are supine if their neck tends to flex forward; use a small pillow behind the head and/or between shoulder blades if extension occurs. *Prevents flexor or extensor tone/contractures of the head and neck (Bobath, 1978; Palmer & Wyness, 1988).*

  ▪ Lay a sandbag under the pillow along one or both sides of the head when clients with lateral neck rotation are supine, and one thick/two thin pillows under the head, when they are side-lying. *Lateral head flexion and rotation, if allowed, may occlude the internal jugular vein, thus preventing cerebral ventricular outflow, which can increase ICP (Palmer & Wyness, 1988).*

  ▪ Change the position of clients' shoulders/arms frequently. Abduct the shoulders of persons with high paraplegia or quadriplegia horizontally to 90° briefly twice a day. *Positioning their arms in the horizontal plane provides full range of motion (Pires, 1984).*

  ▪ Position a hemiplegic shoulder fairly close to the client's body. *Too much abduction increases spasticity around the scapula, inhibits normal gliding movements, and pinches soft tissue, causing pain (Borgman & Passarella, 1991).*

  ▪ Apply resting forearm, wrist, and hand splints. Strictly adhere to on/off orders. Routinely check underlying skin for signs of pressure/poor circulation. *Devices maintain hands/wrists in neutral alignment and/or immobilize inflamed joints as a means of controlling pain.*

  ▪ Use hard hand cone or splint as ordered. This helps prevent hand contractures. **EBN:** *A hard cone likely inhibits the long flexors of the hand versus a soft roll, which may elicit flexor patterns (Jamieson & Dayhoff, 1980).*

  ▪ Periodically elevate paralyzed arms on pillows and apply isotoner gloves. *Lymph fluid collects in dependent hands, causing venous insufficiency and limited motion; elevation/gravity prevents fluid accumulation (Borgman & Passarella, 1991).*

  ▪ Place a thin pillow under the weak pelvis/hip/upper thigh of persons with hemiplegia and a trochanter roll along the outside of a hemiplegic leg or paralyzed legs. *Maintains hip and leg alignment (Bobath, 1978).*

  ▪ Strictly maintain leg abduction in persons with a surgical hip pinning or replacement by placing an abductor splint/pillow between legs. *Abduction stabilizes new prosthesis in the joint (Hoeman, 2002).*

  ▪ Apply foot splints, boots, or high-top tennis shoes as recommended by the physical therapist; routinely assess underlying skin for signs of pressure. *This helps prevent foot drop and spasticity (Hoeman, 2002; Palmer & Wyness, 1988).*

  ▪ Assist clients to lie prone/semiprone periodically unless contraindicated (cardiopulmonary disturbances or increased intracranial pressure). *This promotes drainage and mobilizes secretions from dependent lobes of lung and enhances hip/trunk extension, so it is therapeutic for persons with leg amputation and/paralysis (Kumagai, 1998; Palmer & Wyness, 1988).*

  ▪ Tilt hemiplegics onto both unaffected/affected sides with the affected shoulder slightly forward (move/lift the affected shoulder, <u>not</u> the forearm/hand. *Weight bearing on and place-*

M

ment of the affected shoulder slightly forward reduces tone. Moving the affected shoulder versus the wrist or hand prevents shoulder pain (Bobath, 1978; Borgman & Passarella, 1991).

- Components of normal bed mobility include rolling, bridging, scooting, long sitting, and sitting upright. Most movements start with the client supine, flat in bed. Normal movements are bilateral, segmental, well-timed, and effortless. They involve set positions, weight bearing and shifting, trunk centering, and stabilization against gravity. **For information on how to therapeutically perform and teach Bed Mobility—rolling, bridging, scooting laterally, long sitting, and moving from side-lying to sitting upright—please refer to Borgman & Passarella, 1991; Gee & Passarella, 1985; Kumagai, 1998.**

Geriatric

- Discriminately raise bed side rails; instead try body pillows, low beds, bed alarms, and antislip floor mats next to beds. *Falls/entrapment related to bed rails can cause injury/death (Todd, Rhul & Gross, 1997).* **EBN:** *A project demonstrated careful assessment of residents, education, and trials/ evaluation of alternative measures decreased use of bedrails/falls (Hoffman et al, 2003).*
- Assess caregivers' strength, health history, and cognitive status to predict ability/risk for assisting bed-bound clients at home. Explore alternatives if risk is too high. *Caregivers are often frail elders with chronic health problems who cannot physically help loved ones (McAnaw, 2001).*
- Assess the client's stamina and energy level during bed mobility/activities; if limited, spread out activities and allow rest breaks. *Elders may have fatigue and poor energy reserves due to cardiopulmonary impairments (McAnaw, 2001).*

Home Care

- ▲ Utilize nurse case managers, care coordinators, or social workers to assess support systems and identify need for durable medical equipment, assistive technology, and home health services. *Professional advocates can help clients understand coverage issues and locate resources (Berry & Ignash, 2003).*
- Encourage use of the client's bed unless contraindicated. Raise HOB with commercial blocks or grooved-out pieces of wood under legs; set bed against walls in a corner. *Emotionally, persons may benefit from sleeping in their own bed with their partner. Blocks/walls help secure the bed.*
- Suggest rearranging furniture for accessibility and to meet sleeping/toileting/living needs on one level. *Converting to a suite area for both living/sleeping purposes and decorating it cozily yet functionally may be emotionally soothing and less taxing for client and caregiver (Yearns, 1995).*
- Stress psychological/physical benefits of clients being as self-sufficient as possible with bed mobility/cares even though it may be time-consuming. *Allowing independence and autonomy may help prevent disuse syndromes and feelings of helplessness and low self-esteem.*
- Prepare family for potential regression in clients' self-care during the transition from hospital to home. *Relocation may produce anxiety; client may cope by withdrawing (Theuerkauf, 1996).*
- Offer emotional support and suggest community support systems to help with adjustment and coping issues. *The home environment may trigger the reality of lost function and disability.*
- Discuss support systems available for caregivers to help them cope. **EBN:** *Caregivers used and reported benefiting from an Internet site that offered stroke education, support, and group discussion (Pierce et al, 2004).*
- ▲ In the presence of medical disorders, institute case management for the frail elderly to support continued independent living.
- Refer to the Home Care interventions of the care plan for **Impaired physical Mobility.**

Client/Family Teaching

- Use various sensory modalities to teach client/caregivers correct techniques for ROM, exercises, repositioning, self-care activities, and using devices. *Readiness and learning styles vary but may be enhanced with visual/auditory/tactile/cognitive stimulus as described below (Allen, 2002).*
  - Provide visual information such as demonstrations, sketches, instructional videos, written directions, stickems, or other notes.
  - Encourage/offer auditory information such as verbal instructions/cueing, audio recorded tapes, timers, audiovisual tapes, reading aloud written directions, and self-talk during activities.

• = Independent;   ▲ = Collaborative;   EBN = Evidence-Based Nursing;   EB = Evidence-Based

- ■ Use tactile stimulation such as motor task practice/repetition, return demonstrations, note taking, manual guidance, or hand-on-hand technique as needed.
- • Schedule time with family/caregivers for education and practice. Suggest they come prepared with questions and wear comfortable, safe clothing/shoes. *Motor practice provides opportunity for hands-on learning; repetition helps learning/memory retention (Allen, 2002).*
- • Implement ergonomic approaches and reinforce sound body mechanics during bed mobility/exercises/hygiene. *Risk of injury is high because home care staff and caregivers often work alone, without mechanical aids and in crowded spaces (Galinsky, Waters & Malit, 2001).*
- • Use memory aids/strategies such as written schedules, directions, sketches, and timers for bed mobility and exercises with clients with cognitive decline. *This helps them function as independently as possible*

evolve See the EVOLVE website for World Wide Web resources for client education.

REFERENCES

Allen C, Glasziou P, Del Mar C: Bed rest: a potentially harmful treatment needing more careful evaluation, *Lancet* 354(9186):1229-1233, 1999.

Allen JC: Outcome-directed client and family education. In Hoeman SP, editor: *Rehabilitation nursing: process, application, and outcomes,* ed 3, St. Louis, 2002, Mosby.

American Physical Therapy Association, Association of Rehabilitation Nurses, Veterans Health Administration Task Force: Strategies to improve patient and healthcare provider safety in patient handling and movement tasks, *Rehab Nurs* 30(3):80-83, 2005.

Anderson FA, Spencer FA: Risk factors for venous thromboembolism, *Circulation* 107(23 Suppl 1):I9-I16, 2003.

Berry BE, Ignash S: Assistive technology: providing independence for individuals with disabilities, *Rehabil Nurs* 28(1):6-14, 2003.

Bobath B: *Adult hemiplegia: evaluation and treatment,* London, 1978, William Heinemann Medical Books.

Borgman MF, Passarella PM: Nursing care of the stroke patient using Bobath principles: an approach to altered movement, *Nurs Clin North Am* 26(4):1019-1035, 1991.

Brashear A, Gordon MF, Elovic E et al: Intramuscular injection of botulinum toxin for the treatment of wrist and finger spasticity after a stroke, *N Engl J Med* 347(6):395-400, 2002.

Congress of Neurological Surgeons: Medical student curriculum in neurosurgery. Available at www.neurosurgery.org/cns/ meetings/curriculum/d1.html, 2002.

Daus C: Rehab and the bariatric patient, *Rehab Manag* 14(9):42, 44-45, 2001.

Daus C: The right fit, *Rehab Manag* 16(7):32-35, 2003.

Defloor T: The effect of position and mattress on interface pressure, *Appl Nurs Res* 13(1):2-11, 2000.

Dionne M: Maximizing efficiency with minimum effort: transferring the bariatric patient, *Rehab Manag* 13(6):64, 2000.

Dionne M: 10 tips for safe mobility in the bariatric population, *Rehab Manag* 15(8):28, 2002.

Fan JY: Effect of backrest position on intracranial pressure and cerebral perfusion pressure in individuals with brain injury: a systematic review, *J Neurosci Nurs* 36(5):278-288, 2004.

Finocchiaro D, Herzfeld S: Neurological deficits associated with spinal cord injury. In Chin PA, Finocchiaro D, Rosebrough A, editors: *Rehabilitation nursing practice,* New York, 1998, McGraw-Hill.

Flannery J, Pugh SB: Stroke rehabilitation. In Flannery J: *Rehabilitation nursing secrets,* St Louis, 2004, Mosby.

Fried KM, Fried GW: Immobility. In Derstine J, Hargrave SD, editors: *Comprehensive rehabilitation nursing,* Philadelphia, 2001, WB Saunders.

Galinsky T, Waters T, Malit B: Overexertion injuries in home health

care workers and the need for ergonomics, *Home Health Care Serv Q* 20(3):57-73, 2001.

Gavin-Dreschnack D: Effects of wheelchair posture on patient safety, *Rehabil Nurs* 29(6):221-226, 2004.

Gee ZL, Passarella PM: *Nursing care of the stroke patient: therapeutic approach,* Pittsburgh, 1985, AREN.

Gianino JM, York MM, Paice JA et al: Quality of life: effect of reduced spasticity from intrathecal baclofen, *J Neurosci Nurs* 30(1):47-54, 1998.

Gracies JM, Elovic E, McGuire J et al: Traditional pharmacological treatments for spasticity. Part I: local treatments, *Muscle Nerve Suppl* 6:S61-S91, 1997.

Grande C, Caparro M: Use of low-molecular-weight heparins in the treatment and secondary prevention of cancer-associated thrombosis, *Semin Oncol Nurs* 21(4):41-49, 2005.

Gutierrez A: Pressure lessons, *Rehabil Manag* 15(9):44, 2002.

Hoeman SP: Movement, functional mobility, and activities of daily living. In Hoeman SP, editor: *Rehabilitation nursing: process, application, and outcomes,* ed 3, St. Louis, 2002, Mosby.

Hoffman SB, Powell-Cope G, MacClellan L et al: BedSAFE. A bed safety project for frail older adults, *J Gerontol Nurs* 29(11):34-42, 2003.

Hums W, Blostein P: A comparative approach to deep vein thrombosis risk assessment, *J Trauma Nurs* 13(1):28-30, 2006.

Jamieson S, Dayhoff NE: A hard bed-positioning device to decrease wrist and finger hypertonicity: a sensorimotor approach for the patient with nonprogressive brain damage, *Nurs Res* 29:285-289, 1980.

Jenkins L, Egersett M: Better lifts and transfers, *Rehabil Manag* 17(9):24-27, 2004.

Johnson KMM, Nolde-Lopez G: Skin integrity. In Hoeman SP, editor: *Rehabilitation nursing: process, application, and outcomes,* ed 3, St Louis, 2002, Mosby.

Kehl-Pruett W: Deep vein thrombosis in hospitalized patients: a review of evidence based guidelines for prevention, *Dimens Crit Care Nurs* 25(2):53-59, 2006.

Koschel MJ: Pulmonary embolism: quick diagnosis can save a patient's life, *Am J Nurs* 104(6):46-50, 2004.

Kumagai KAS: Physical management of the neurologically involved client: techniques for bed mobility and transfers. In Chin PA, Finocchiaro D, Rosebrough A, editors: *Rehabilitation nursing practice,* New York, 1998, McGraw-Hill.

Lechner HE, Frotzler A, Eser P: Relationship between self- and clinically rated spasticity in spinal cord injury, *Arch Phys Med Rehabil* 87(1):15-19, 2006.

Lyder CH, Grady J, Mathur D et al: Preventing pressure ulcers in

M

Connecticut hospitals by using the plan—study-act model of quality improvement, *Jt Comm J Qual Saf* 30(4):205-214, 2004.

McAnaw MB: Normal changes with aging. In Maas ML et al, editors: *Nursing care of older adults: diagnoses, outcomes and interventions,* St Louis, 2001, Mosby.

McCaffery M, Pasero C: *Pain: clinical manual,* ed 2, St Louis, 1999, Mosby.

Menzel NN, Lilley S, Robinson ME: Interventions to reduce back pain in rehabilitation hospital nursing staff, *Rehabil Nurs* 31(4):138-147, 2006.

Metzler DJ, Harr J: Positioning your patient properly, *Am J Nurs* 96(3):33-37, 1996.

Mundy LM, Leet TL, Darst K et al: Early mobilization of patients hospitalized with community-acquired pneumonia, *Chest* 124(3):883-889, 2003.

Murphy EK: Negligence cases concerning positioning injuries, *AORN J* 80(2):311-314, 2004.

Ng I, Lim J, Wong HB: Effects of head posture on cerebral hemodynamics: its influence on intracranial pressure, cerebral perfusion pressure, and cerebral oxygenation, *Neurosurg* 54(3):593-597, 2004.

Olson EV: The hazards of immobility, *Am J Nurs* 67:781-783, 1967.

Ossman NJ, Campbell M: *Therapist guide: adult positions, transitions, and transfers—reproducible instruction cards for caregivers,* Tucson, 1990, Communication Skill Builders.

Owen BD, Welden N, Kane J: What are we teaching about lifting and transferring patients? *Res Nurs Health* 22(1):3-13, 1999.

Palmer M, Wyness MA: Positioning and handling: important considerations in the care of the severely head-injured patient, *J Neurosurg Nurs* 20(1):42-49, 1988.

Passarella PM, Lewis N: Nursing application of Bobath principles in stroke care, *J Neurosurg Nurs* 19(2):106-109, 1987.

Pierce LL, Steiner V, Govoni AL et al: Internet-based support for rural caregivers of persons with stroke shows promise, *Rehab Nurs* 29(3):95-99, 2004.

Pires M: Spinal cord injuries: coping with devastating damage. In Ursevich PR, editor: *Coping with neurologic problems proficiently,* ed 2, Springhouse, Penn, 1984, Springhouse.

Powell-Cope G, Baptiste AS, Nelson A: Modification of bed systems and use of accessories to reduce the risk of hospital-bed entrapment, *Rehabil Nurs* 30(1):9-17, 2005.

Rawicki B: Treatment of cerebral origin spasticity with continuous intrathecal baclofen delivered via an implantable pump: long-term follow-up review of 18 patients, *J Neurosurg* 91(5):733-736, 1999.

Robinson MD, Shannon S: Rehabilitation of peripheral nerve injuries, *Phys Med Rehabil Clin North Am* 13(1):109-135, 2002.

Rodriguez L: Medical-surgical complications in the rehabilitation client. In Chin PA, Finocchiaro D, Rosebrough A, editors: *Rehabilitation nursing practice,* New York, 1998, McGraw-Hill.

Salcido R: Patient turning schedules: why and how often? *Adv Skin Wound Care* 17 (4 pt 1):156, 2006.

Soderhamn O, Idvall E: Nurses' influence on quality of care in postoperative pain management: a phenomenological study, *Int J Nurs Pract* 9:26-32, 2003.

Sullivan J: Positioning of patients with severe traumatic brain injury: research-based practice, *J Neurosci Nurs* 32(4):204-209, 2000.

Theuerkauf A: Self-care and activities of daily living. In Hoeman SP, editor: *Rehabilitation nursing: process and application,* ed 2, St Louis, 1996, Mosby.

Todd JF, Ruhl CE, Gross TP: Injury and death associated with hospital bed side-rails: reports to the US Food and Drug Administration from 1985-1995, *Pub Health Briefs* 87(10):1675-1677, 1997.

Williams TA, Leslie GD: A review of the nursing care of enteral feeding tubes in critically ill adults: Part I, *Intens Crit Care Nurs* 20(6):330-343, 2004.

Wojner AW, El-Mitwalli A, Alexandrov AV: Effect of head positioning on intracranial blood flow velocities in acute ischemic stroke: a pilot study, *Crit Care Nurs Q* 24(4):57-66, 2002.

Wound, Ostomy, and Continence Nurses Society (WOCN): *Guideline for prevention and management of pressure ulcers* (WOCN clinical practice guideline, no 2), Glenview, Ill, 2003, The Society.

Yearns MH: Modest home makeovers to improve farmhouse accessibility: how our AgrAgbility team used this fast, affordable alternative to remodeling with the Miller family, *Technol Disabil* 4:49, 1995.

Impaired physical Mobility Betty J. Ackley, MSN, EdS, RN

NANDA Definition

A limitation in independent, purposeful physical movement of the body or of one or more extremities

Defining Characteristics

Decreased reaction time; difficulty turning; engages in substitutions for movement (e.g., increased attention to other's activity, controlling behavior, focus on pre-illness disability/activity); exertional dyspnea; gait changes; jerky movements; limited ability to perform gross motor skills; limited ability to perform fine motor skills; limited range of motion; movement-induced tremor; postural instability; slowed movement; uncoordinated movements

Related Factors

Activity intolerance; altered cellular metabolism; anxiety; body mass index above 75th age-appropriate percentile; cognitive impairment; contractures; cultural beliefs regarding age-appropriate activity; deconditioning; decreased endurance; depressive mood state; decreased muscle control; decreased

---

• = Independent; ▲ = Collaborative; EBN = Evidence-Based Nursing; EB = Evidence-Based

muscle mass; decreased muscle strength; deficient knowledge regarding value of physical activity; developmental delay; discomfort; disuse; joint stiffness; lack of environmental supports (e.g., physical or social); limited cardiovascular endurance; loss of integrity of bone structures; malnutrition; medications; musculoskeletal impairment; neuromuscular impairment; pain; prescribed movement restrictions; reluctance to initiate movement; sedentary lifestyle; sensoriperceptual impairments
Suggested functional level classifications include the following:
0—Completely independent
1—Requires use of equipment or device
2—Requires help from another person for assistance, supervision, or teaching
3—Requires help from another person and equipment device
4—Dependent (does not participate in activity)

NOC Outcomes (Nursing Outcomes Classification)

Suggested NOC Outcomes

Ambulation, Ambulation: Wheelchair, Mobility, Self-Care: Activities of Daily Living (ADLs), Transfer Performance

Example NOC Outcome with Indicators
Ambulation as evidenced by the following indicators: Walks with effective gait/Walks at moderate pace/Walks up and down steps/Walks moderate distance (Rate the outcome and indicators of **Ambulation:** 1 = severely compromised, 2 = substantially compromised, 3 = moderately compromised, 4 = mildly compromised, 5 = not compromised [see Section I].)

Client Outcomes

M

Client Will (Specify Time Frame):

- Increase physical activity
- Meet mutually defined goals of ambulation
- Verbalize feeling of increased strength and ability to move
- Demonstrate use of adaptive equipment (e.g., wheelchairs, walkers) to increase mobility

NIC Interventions (Nursing Interventions Classification)

Suggested NIC Interventions

Exercise Therapy: Ambulation, Joint Mobility, Positioning

Example NIC Activities—Exercise Therapy: Ambulation
Assist patient to use footwear that facilitates walking and prevents injury; Instruct in availability of assistive devices, if appropriate

Nursing Interventions and *Rationales*

- Screen for mobility skills in the following order: (1) bed mobility; (2) supported and unsupported sitting; (3) transition movements such as sit to stand, sitting down, and transfers; and (4) standing and walking activities. Use a tool such as the **Assessment Tool for Safe Patient Handling and Movement.** Additional measures of physical function include: unassisted leg stand, use of a balance platform, elbow flexion and knee extension strength, grip strength, timed chair stands, and the 6-minute walk. *The abilities of the client should be assessed to determine how best to facilitate movement and protect the nurse from harm (Nelson et al, 2003; Curb et al, 2006).*
- Observe the client for cause of impaired mobility. Determine whether cause is physical or psychological. *Some clients choose not to move because of psychological factors such as an inability to cope or depression.* Refer to care plan for **Ineffective Coping** or **Hopelessness.**

- Monitor and record the client's ability to tolerate activity and use all four extremities; note pulse rate, blood pressure, dyspnea, and skin color before and after activity. Refer to the care plan for **Activity intolerance.**
▲ Before activity, observe for and, if possible, treat pain. Ensure that the client is not oversedated. *Pain limits mobility and is often exacerbated by movement.*
▲ Consult with physical therapist for further evaluation, strength training, gait training, and development of a mobility plan. *Techniques such as gait training, strength training, and exercise to improve balance and coordination can be very helpful for rehabilitating clients (Tempkin, Tempkin & Goodman, 1997).*
▲ Obtain any assistive devices needed for activity, such as gait belt, walker, cane, crutches, or wheelchair, before the activity begins. *Assistive devices can help increase mobility (Nelson et al, 2004).*
- If the client is immobile, perform passive range of motion (ROM) exercises at least twice a day unless contraindicated; repeat each maneuver three times. *Inactivity rapidly contributes to muscle shortening and changes in periarticular and cartilaginous joint structure. The formation of contractures starts after 8 hours of immobility (Fletcher, 2005).*
▲ If the client is immobile, consult with physician for a safety evaluation before beginning an exercise program; if program is approved, begin with the following exercises:
  ■ Active ROM exercises using both upper and lower extremities (e.g., flexing and extending at ankles, knees, hips)
  ■ Chin-ups and pull-ups using a trapeze in bed (may be contraindicated in clients with cardiac conditions)
  ■ Strengthening exercises such as gluteal or quadriceps sitting exercises
  These exercises help reverse weakening and atrophy of muscles (Kasper et al, 2005).
- If client is immobile, consider use of a transfer chair, a chair that becomes a stretcher. *Utilizing a transfer chair where the client is pulled onto a flat surface and then seated upright in the chair can help previously immobile clients get out of bed (Nelson et al, 2003).*
- Help the client achieve mobility and start walking as soon as possible if not contraindicated. **EB:** *Bed rest for primary treatment of medical conditions or after healthcare procedures is associated with worse outcomes than early mobilization (Allen, Glasziou & Del Mar, 1999). Early mobilization for acute limb injuries generally resulted in improved function, less pain, and earlier return to work and sports (Ebell, 2005).*
- Use a gait-walking belt when ambulating the client. *Gait belts help improve the caregiver's grasp, reducing the incidence of injuries (Nelson et al, 2003).*
- Apply any ordered brace before mobilizing the client. *Braces support and stabilize a body part, allowing increased mobility.*
- Initiate a "No Lift" policy where appropriate assistive devices are utilized for manual lifting. **EBN:** *Workman's comp costs decreased significantly after initiation of a "No Lift" program, and it was predicted that $5 million would be saved within 9 years (Nelson et al, 2003). A "No Lift" policy along with other measures such as the "Back Injury Resource Nurses" and an algorithm on safe client handling resulted in decreased workers' compensation expenses with reduced lost and modified word days, along with nurse and client satisfaction (Nelson et al, 2006).*
- Increase independence in activities of daily living (ADLs), encouraging self-efficacy and discouraging helplessness as the client gets stronger. *Providing unnecessary assistance with transfers and bathing activities may promote dependence and a loss of mobility.*
▲ If the client has osteoarthritis or rheumatoid arthritis, ask for a referral to a physical therapist to begin an exercise program that includes aerobic exercise, resistance exercise, and gentle stretching. **EB:** *Exercise has been shown to be beneficial in both kinds of arthritis (Westby & Li, 2006).*
- If client has had a cerebrovascular accident (CVA) with hemiparesis, consider use of constraint-induced movement therapy (CIMT), where the functional extremity is purposely constrained and the client is forced to use the involved extremity. *Constraint therapy is estimated to benefit about half of the total CVA population (Barker, 2005).* **EB:** *The plasticity of the brain allows the brain to rewire and reroute neural connections to take up the work of the injured area of the brain (National Institute of Neurological Disorders and Stroke, 2004). Constraint therapy improved motor function and health-related quality of life (Wu et al, 2007).*

- If the client has had a CVA, recognize that balance is likely impaired and protect from falling. **EB:** *Clients did not have normal balance after therapy, even if only a mild CVA (Garland, 2007).*
- If the client does not feed or groom self, sit side-by-side with the client, put your hand over the client's hand, support the client's elbow with your other hand, and help the client feed self; use the same technique to help the client comb hair. *This feeding technique increases client mobility, range of motion, and independence, and clients often eat more food (Pedretti, 1996).*

Geriatric

- Assess ability to move using the "Get Up and Go" test. Ask the client to rise from a sitting position, walk 10 feet, turn, and return to the chair to sit. *Performance on this screening exam demonstrates the client's mobility and ability to leave the house safely (Robertson & Montagnini, 2004).*
- Help the mostly immobile client achieve mobility as soon as possible, depending on physical condition. *In the elderly, mobility impairment can predict increased mortality and dependence; however, this can be prevented by physical exercise (Fletcher, 2005; Hirvensalo, Rantanen & Heikkinen, 2000).*
- If client is frail, ensure good nutrition, appropriate medications, attention to vision and hearing deficits, and increase social support along with exercise. *Frailty in the elderly can be multifactorial and often can be ameliorated or reversed (Storey & Thomas, 2004).*
- Use the Outcome Expectation for Exercise Scale to determine client's self-efficacy expectations and outcomes expectations toward exercise. **EBN:** *The client's self-efficacy expectations and outcome expectations for exercise will greatly influence his or her willingness to exercise. If the individual has a low outcome, interventions can be implemented to strengthen the expectations and hopefully improve exercise behavior (Resnick et al, 2001).*
- For a client who is mostly immobile, minimize cardiovascular deconditioning by positioning the client in the upright position several times daily. *The hazards of bed rest in the elderly are multiple, serious, quick to develop, and slow to reverse. Deconditioning of the cardiovascular system occurs within days and involves fluid shifts, fluid loss, decreased cardiac output, decreased peak oxygen uptake, and increased resting heart rate (Fletcher, 2005; Kasper et al, 2005; Resnick & Daly, 1998).* **EB:** *Studies indicate that to prevent the functional decline of older clients that often results from restricted activity during hospitalization, an exercise program designed to educate clients about remaining mobile during their stay and to provide assistance in walking is beneficial. Screening procedures often identify clients who can benefit from physical therapy (Tucker, Molsberger & Clark, 2004).*
- ▲ Refer the client to physical therapy for resistance exercise training as able, including abdominal crunch, leg press, leg extension, leg curl, calf press, and more. **EB:** *Six months of resistance exercise for the elderly greatly increased their aerobic capacity, possibly from increased skeletal muscle strength (Vincent et al, 2002). When clients in an extended care facility were put on a strength, balance, and endurance training program, the clients' balance and mobility improved significantly (Rydwik, Kerstin & Akner, 2005).*
- Use the WALC Intervention (Walk; Address pain, fear, fatigue during exercise; Learn about exercise; Cue by self-modeling) to improve exercise adherence in the older adult. **EBN:** *The WALC Intervention resulted in more exercise and had greater self-efficacy expectations regarding exercise (Resnick, 2002).*
- ▲ If client is scheduled for an elective surgery that will result in admission into an intensive care unit (ICU) and immobility, or recovery from a knee replacement, initiate a prehabilitation program that includes a warm-up, aerobic strength, flexibility, and functional task work. **EBN and EB:** *By increasing the functional capacity of the individual prior to the stressor of inactivity, the predictable declines in physical activity can be prevented or alleviated (Topp et al, 2002). Clients who performed strength activities preoperatively walked significantly greater distances postoperatively after total hip replacement (Whitney & Parkman, 2002). Aerobic training along with strength and interval training was effective in fewer postoperative complications, shorter postoperative stays, and reduced functional disabilities (Carli & Zavorsky, 2005).*
- ▲ Evaluate the client for signs of depression (flat affect, insomnia, anorexia, frequent somatic complaints) or cognitive impairment (use Mini-Mental State Exam [MMSE]). Refer for treatment or counseling as needed. **EBN:** *Depression and decreased cognition in the elderly correlate with decreased levels of functional ability (Fletcher, 2005).*

• = Independent;   ▲ = Collaborative;   EBN = Evidence-Based Nursing;   EB = Evidence-Based

- Watch for orthostatic hypotension when mobilizing elderly clients. Have the client dangle at the side of the bed with legs hanging over the edge of the bed, flex and extend feet several times after sitting up, then stand up slowly with someone holding the client. If client becomes light-headed or dizzy, return them to bed immediately. *Orthostatic hypotension as a result of cardiovascular system changes, chronic diseases, and medication effects is common in the elderly (Dingle, 2003).*
- Be very careful when getting a mostly immobile client up. Be sure to lock the bed and wheelchair and have sufficient personnel to protect the client from falls. **EB:** *The most important preventative measure to reduce the risk of injurious falls for nonambulatory residents involves increasing safety measures while transferring, including careful locking of equipment such as wheelchairs and beds before moves (Thapa et al, 1996).*
- Do not routinely assist with transfers or bathing activities unless necessary. *The nursing staff may contribute to impaired mobility by helping too much. Encourage client independence (Kasper et al, 2005).*
- Use gestures and nonverbal cues when helping clients move if they are anxious or have difficulty understanding and following verbal instructions. *Nonverbal gestures are part of a universal language that can be understood when the client is having difficulty with communication.*
- Recognize that wheelchairs are not a good mobility device and often serve as a mobility restraint. **EB:** *Wheelchairs can be very effective restraints (Simmons et al, 1995).*
- Ensure that chairs fit clients. Chair seat should be 3 inches above the height of the knee. Provide a raised toilet seat if needed. *Raising the height of a chair can dramatically improve the ability of many older clients to stand up. Low, deep, soft seats with armrests that are far apart reduce a person's ability to get up and down without help.*
- If the client is mainly immobile, provide opportunities for socialization and sensory stimulation (e.g., television and visits). Refer to the care plan for **Deficient Diversional activity.**
- Recognize that immobility and a lack of social support and sensory input may result in confusion or depression in the elderly (Fletcher, 2005). Refer to nursing interventions for **Acute Confusion** or **Hopelessness** as appropriate.

 ### Home Care

- Above interventions may be adapted for home care use.
- ▲ Begin discharge planning as soon as possible with case manager or social worker to assess need for home support systems, assistive devices, and community or home health services.
- ▲ Assess home environment for factors that create barriers to physical mobility. Refer to occupational therapy services if needed to assist the client in restructuring home and daily living patterns.
- ▲ Refer to home health aide services to support the client and family through changing levels of mobility. Reinforce need to promote independence in mobility as tolerated. *Providing unnecessary assistance with transfers and bathing activities may promote dependence and a loss of mobility (Fletcher, 2005).*
- ▲ Refer to physical therapy for gait training, strengthening, and balance training. *Physical therapists can provide direct interventions as well as assess need for assistive devices (e.g., cane, walker).*
- Discuss with client and caregiver the possibility of a service dog to support the more immobile client. **EB:** *Service dogs can pull wheelchairs, find keys, open the door, bring the telephone, and more. Use of service dogs was found to increase socialization, increase self-esteem, and give peace of mind to caregivers (Rintala et al, 2005).*
- Assess skin condition at every visit. Establish a skin care program that enhances circulation and maximizes position changes. *Impaired mobility decreases circulation to dependent areas. Decreased circulation and shearing place the client at risk for skin breakdown.*
- Once the client is able to walk independently, suggest the client enter an exercise program, or walk with a friend. **EBN:** *Findings from a study of exercise behavior found that friends have the strongest influence to keep on an exercise program, more than family members or experts (Resnick, Orwig & Magaziner, 2002).*
- Provide support to the client and family/caregivers during long-term impaired mobility. *Long-term impaired mobility may necessitate role changes within the family and precipitate caregiver stress.* Refer to the care plan for **Caregiver role strain.**
- ▲ Institute case management of frail elderly to support continued independent living.

Client/Family Teaching

- Teach the client to get out of bed slowly when transferring from the bed to the chair.
- Teach the client relaxation techniques to use during activity.
- Teach the client to use assistive devices such as a cane, a walker, or crutches to increase mobility.
- Teach family members and caregivers to work with clients during self-care activities such as eating, bathing, grooming, dressing, and transferring rather than having the client be a passive recipient of care.
- Work with the client using self-efficacy interventions using single or multiple methods **EBN:** *Use of self-efficacy-based interventions resulted in increased exercise (Resnick, 2007 in press).*
- Work with the client using the Transtheoretical Model of behavior change and determine if the client is in the precontemplation, contemplation, preparation, action, or maintenance state of behavior change about exercise. Provide appropriate strategies to support change to exercising based on determined state of change. **EBN:** *The Trans-theoretical Model of behavior change can be very useful for nurses to increase exercise behavior utilizing stage-appropriate interventions (Burbank, Reibe & Padula, 2002). Use of the Transtheoretical Model of behavior change plus theory of self-efficacy suggests that both of these theories are helpful in increasing exercise in the older adult (Resnick & Nigg, 2003).*

evolve See the EVOLVE website for World Wide Web resources for client education.

REFERENCES

Allen C, Glasziou P, Del Mar C: Bed rest: a potentially harmful treatment needing more careful evaluation, *Lancet* 354(9186):1229-1233, 1999.

Barker E: New hope for stroke patients, *RN* 68(2):38-42, 2005.

Burbank PM, Reibe D, Padula CA: Exercise and older adults: changing behavior with the transtheoretical model, *Orthop Nurs* 21(4):51-61, 2002.

Carli F, Zavorsky GS: Optimizing functional exercise capacity in the elderly surgical population, *Curr Opin Clin Nutr Metab Care* 8(1):23-32, 2005.

Curb JD, Ceria-Ulep CD, Rodriguez BL et al: Performance-based measures of physical function for high-function populations, *J Am Geriatr Soc* 54(5):737-742, 2006.

Dingle M: Role of dangling when moving from supine to standing position, *Br J Nurs* 12(6):346-350, 2003.

Ebell M: Early mobilization better for acute limb injuries, *Am Fam Physician* 71(4), 2005. Accessed online March 30, 2007, at: http://www.InfoPOEMs.com.

Fletcher K: Immobility: geriatric self-learning module, *Medsurg Nurs* 14(1):35-37, 2005.

Garland SJ: Recovery of standing balance and health-related quality of life after mild or moderately severe stroke, *Arch Phys Med Rehabil* 88(2):218-227, 2007.

Hirvensalo M, Rantanen T, Heikkinen E: Mobility difficulties and physical activity as predictors of mortality and loss of independence in the community-living older population, *J Am Geriatr Soc* 48(5):493-498, 2000.

Kasper DL et al, editors: *Harrison's principles of internal medicine,* ed 16, New York, 2005, McGraw-Hill.

National Institute of Neurological Disorders and Stroke: Stroke: hope through research. Available at www.ninds.nih.gov/ disorders/ stgroke/detail_stroke.htm, accessed March 5, 2005.

Nelson A, Matz M, Chen F et al: Development and evaluation of a multifaceted ergonomics program to prevent injuries associated with patient handling tasks, *Int J Nurs Stud* 43(6):717-733, 2006.

Nelson A, Owen B, Lloyd JD et al: Safe patient handling movement, *AJN* 103(3):32-43, 2003.

Nelson A, Powell-Cope G, Gavin-Dreschnack D et al: Technology to promote safe mobility in the elderly, *Nurs Clin North Am* 39:649-671, 2004.

Pedretti LW: *Occupational therapy: practice skills for physical dysfunction*, ed 4, St Louis, 1996, Mosby.

Resnick B: Exercise Promotion: Motivational Techniques. In Ackley B, et al: *Evidence-based Nursing Care: Guidelines: Medical Surgical Interventions*, Philadelphia, 2007 in press, Mosby.

Resnick B: Testing the effect of the WALC intervention on exercise adherence in older adults, *J Gerontol Nurs,* 28(6):40-49, 2002.

Resnick B, Daly MP: Predictors of functional ability in geriatric rehabilitation patients, *Rehabil Nurs* 23(1):21-29, 1998.

Resnick B, Nigg C: Testing a theoretical model of exercise behavior for older adults, *Nurs Res* 52(2):80-88, 2003.

Resnick B, Orwig D, Magaziner J: The effect of social support on exercise behavior in older adults, *Clin Nurs Res* 11(1):52-70, 2002.

Resnick B, Zimmerman S, Orwig D et al: Model testing for reliability and validity of the outcome expectations for exercise scale, *Nurs Res* 50(5):293-299, 2001.

Rintala DH et al: The effects of service dogs on the lives of persons with mobility impairments: a pre-post study design, *Sci Psychosoc Process* 18(4):236-249, 2005.

Robertson RG, Montagnini M: Geriatric failure to thrive, *Am Fam Physician* 70(2):343-350, 2004.

Rydwik E, Kerstin F, Akner G: Physical training in institutionalized elderly people with multiple diagnoses—a controlled pilot study, *Arch Gerontol Geriatr* 40(1):29-44, 2005.

Simmons SF, Schnelle JF, MacRae PG et al: Wheelchairs as mobility restraints: predictors of wheelchair activity in nonambulatory nursing home residents, *J Am Geriatr Soc* 43:384-388, 1995.

Storey E, Thomas RL: Understanding and ameliorating frailty in the elderly, *Top Geriatr Rehabil* 20(1):4, 2004.

Tempkin T, Tempkin A, Goodman H: Geriatric rehabilitation, *Nurs Pract Forum* 8(2):59-63, 1997.

Thapa PB, Brockman KG, Gideon P et al: Injurious falls in nonambulatory nursing home residents: a comparative study of circumstances, incidence, and risk factors, *J Am Geriatr Soc* 44(3):273-278, 1996.

Topp R, Ditmyer M, King K et al: The effect of bed rest and potential

M

of prehabilitation on patients in the intensive care unit. *AACN Clin Issues* 13(2):263-276, 2002.

Tucker D, Molsberger SC, Clark A: Walking for wellness: a collaborative program to maintain mobility in hospitalized older adults, *Geriatr Nurs* 25(4):242-245, 2004.

Vincent KR, Braith RW, Feldman RA et al: Improved cardiorespiratory endurance following 6 months of resistance exercise in elderly men and women, *Arch Intern Med* 162:673-678, 2002.

Westby MD, Li L: Physical therapy and exercise for arthritis: do they work? *Geriatr Aging* 9(9):624-630, 2006.

Whitney JA, Parkman S: Preoperative physical activity, anesthesia, and analgesia: effects on early postoperative walking after total hip replacement, *Appl Nurs Res* 15(1):19-27, 2002.

Wu CY, Chen CL, Tsai WC et al: A randomized controlled trial of modified constraint-induced movement therapy for elderly stroke survivors: changes in motor impairment, daily functioning, and quality of life, *Arch Phys Med Rehabil* 88(3):273-278, 2007.

Impaired wheelchair Mobility   *Brenda Emick-Herring, RN, MSN, CRRN*

NANDA   Definition

Limitation of independent operation of wheelchair within environment

Defining Characteristics

Impaired ability to operate: manual or power wheelchair on curbs; manual or power wheelchair on even surface; manual or power wheelchair on an uneven surface; manual or powered wheelchair on an incline; manual or powered wheelchair on a decline

Related Factors (r/t)

Intolerance to activity; decreased strength and endurance; pain or discomfort; perceptual or cognitive impairment; neuromuscular impairment; musculoskeletal impairment; depression; severe anxiety. Suggested functional level classifications include the following:

0—Completely independent
1—Requires use of equipment or device
2—Requires help from another person for assistance, supervision, or teaching
3—Requires help from another person and equipment or device
4—Dependent—does not participate in activity

NOC   Outcomes (Nursing Outcomes Classification)

Suggested NOC Outcome

Ambulation: Wheelchair

Example NOC Outcome with Indicators
Ambulation: Wheelchair as evidenced by the following indicators: Propels wheelchair safely/Transfers to and from wheelchair/Maneuvers curbs, doorways, ramps (Rate the outcome and indicators of **Ambulation: Wheelchair:** 1 = severely compromised, 2 = substantially compromised, 3 = moderately compromised, 4 = mildly compromised, 5 = not compromised [see Section I].)

Client Outcomes

Client Will (Specify Time Frame):

- Demonstrate independence in operating and moving a wheelchair or other device with wheels
- Demonstrate the ability to direct others in operating and moving a wheelchair or other device
- Demonstrate therapeutic positioning, pressure relief, and safety principles while operating and moving wheelchair or other device equipped with wheels

NIC   Interventions (Nursing Interventions Classification)

Suggested NIC Interventions

Exercise Therapy: Muscle Control, Positioning: Wheelchair

Example NIC Activities—Positioning: Wheelchair
Select the appropriate wheelchair for the patient: standard adult, semi-reclining, fully reclining, amputees; Monitor for patient's inability to maintain correct posture in wheelchair

Nursing Interventions and *Rationales*

- Assist client to put on and take off equipment (e.g., braces, orthoses, abdominal binders) in bed. *Provide stabilization and alignment; abdominal binder prevents postural hypotension and increases vital capacity (for hemodynamic stability, binder must be put on and taken off in bed).*
- Inspect skin where orthoses, braces, and so on rested, once they are removed. *Early detection of pressure allows for early pressure relief strategy implementation (WOCN Society, 2003).*
- ▲ Obtain referrals for physical and occupational therapy, or wheelchair seating clinic. *Individualized wheelchair seating system fits client abilities and provides postural alignment, comfort, and reduced pressure (Gavin-Dreschnack, 2004). The correct seating system allows client to propel chair safely and use the hands. Correct seating also allows function and prevents slouching/leaning/sliding down, which all can cause deformity, discomfort, and overuse of physical restraints (Cox, 2004; Cooper et al, 2000; Minkel, 2001).*
- Keep the right cushion and wheelchair with the right client (Gavin-Dreschnack, 2004). *Cushions lessen shock, pressure, vibration, pain, and fatigue (Cooper et al, 2000; Paleg, 2002).*
- Use of properly contoured surfaces/cushions/supports, and continence management, nutrition, hydration, and repositioning help prevent sitting-acquired pressure ulcers (Cooper et al 2000; Paleg, 2002; WOCN Society, 2003). *This allows immobile clients to remain seated longer and distributes body mass, thus lowering peak pressure over bones.* **EBN:** *Four cushions tested had varying pressure-reducing abilities at buttock-seat interface when clients slid down or slouched (Defloor & Grypdonck, 1999).*
- ▲ Obtain physical therapist (PT), occupational therapist (OT), or wheelchair clinic referral for cushion reevaluation if signs of pressure exist. *Professionals do pressure mapping to evaluate cushion properties and assess pressure distribution (Swaine, 2003).* **EB:** *A pilot study indicated high buttock-cushion interface pressure was associated with pressure ulcers (Brienza et al, 2001). Pressure mapping is a reliable means of evaluating interface pressures (Stinson, Porter-Armstrong & Eakin, 2003).*

- Emphasize importance of weight shifts every 15 minutes with safety belts in place (leaning and pushups). *This prevents capillary occlusion/force on skin over small bony areas (Minkel, 2000).* **EB:** *A controlled trial without randomization (N=10 with spinal cord injury) found no effective reduction in pressure on ischial tuberosities with clients in a reclined position at 35° (Henderson et al, 1994).*
- Activate passive standing position of wheelchair (if available) or, if applicable, stand client briefly (WOCN Society, 2003). *This removes tissue pressure over bony prominences.*
- Place both feet on floor when clients are passively sitting in a wheelchair. *Less pressure exists on sacral/buttock tissue sitting upright with feet on the floor than on foot rests (Rader, Jones & Miller, 1999).*
- Routinely assess client's sitting posture and frequently reposition him/her into sound alignment as needed. **EBN:** *Nurses spent only 6% of their time deliberately repositioning stroke clients with poor posture and asymmetry (Dowswell, Dowswell & Young, 2000).*
- Place client's feet securely on foot rests and fasten seat belts across the top of the thighs before propelling the wheelchair. *This prevents foot injuries and helps stabilize and hold the pelvis in place (Rader, Jones & Miller, 1999).* **EB:** *Use of seat belts and appropriately adjusted leg rests likely improves control and safety of occupants of electric wheelchairs going up various inclines (Corfman et al, 2003).*
- Implement use of friction-coated projection hand rims and leather gloves as clients propel manual wheelchairs. *Friction-coated projection rims are less invasive and slippery than aluminum rims; gloves absorb forces of propulsion and help prevent nerve damage/carpel tunnel.*
- Manually guide or explain to push forward on both wheel rims to move ahead, push the right rim to turn left and vice versa, and pull backward on both wheel rims to back up.

- Recommend that clients back wheelchairs into an elevator. If entering face first, instruct them to turn chair around to face the elevator doors. *Clients can see the control panel, floor monitor display, and doors opening and can exit wheeling forward (Minor & Minor, 1999).*
- Reinforce principle of descending a curb backward ("popping a wheelie") if balance, trunk control, strength, and timing are adequate. *Backward descent carries less risk of clients losing control and falling forward out of wheelchair (Minor & Minor, 1999).*
- Ascend curbs in a forward position by popping a wheelie or having aid tilt chair back, place front wheels over curb, and roll chair up. If surface is muddy or sandy, ascend backwards. *Front casters will not roll on soft surfaces; a backward approach requires less energy and prevents getting stuck or falling forward.*
- During assisted wheelies, helper must hold wheelchair until all four wheels are back on the ground and client has control of wheelchair. *Releasing one's grip too soon may alter client's balance and cause injury.*
- Reinforce compensatory strategies for unilateral neglect and agnosia (visual scanning, self-talk, self-questioning as to what could be wrong) as clients propel wheelchair through doorways and around obstacles. *Too often nurses physically move wheelchair or obstacle instead of cueing client to detect and solve problems.*
- Sit dysphagic clients as upright as possible in individualized wheelchair versus geri-chair when eating. *When fed in this position, there is less risk of aspiration (Gavin-Dreschnack, 2004).*
- ▲ Follow therapist recommendations as to how clients should propel manual wheelchairs to prevent upper extremity pain and joint degeneration *Overuse and repetitive strain is common (Cooper, Cooper & Boninger, 2004; Nylund et al, 2000).*
  - Stress that clients maintain normal versus extra body weight.
  - Reinforce use of long/smooth strokes to limit high force on the pushrim, and let the hand "naturally drift down" when letting go of the pushrim (Koontz & Boninger, 2003). **EB:** *Individualized forward adjustment of axle position on ultra lightweight wheelchair and personal wheelchair fitting lessened upper extremity nerve injury (Boninger et al, 2000). Tetraplegics had more frequent/intense shoulder pain than paraplegics; pushing up an incline and wheeling longer than 10 minutes created pain in both groups (Curtis et al, 1999).*
  - Remind clients to press with length of arm (not elbows) during repositioning and weight shifts. Nocturnal splints, elbow pads, and use of ultra lightweight, pushrim-activated, power-assisted, or electric wheelchair may relieve tendonitis. *Arms are overworked during propulsion, transfers, and upper dressing and thus are at risk for painful syndromes (Congress of Neurological Surgeons, 2002; Minkel, 2000).*
- Recognize value systems of clients/nurses regarding use of a wheelchair may differ and create tension. *A wheelchair may symbolize weakness and loss of autonomy to clients, whereas it may symbolize independence to professionals (Minkel, 2000).* **EBN:** *Wheelchair users had frustration with barriers, accessibility, independence issues, and societal attitudes toward people with disabilities (Pierce, 1998).*
- ▲ Offer support/referrals to help clients cope with issues related to physical disability and loss. *Clients may experience depression and anxiety with physical loss and disability.* **EB:** *Support group members to attend meetings to meet others with the same diagnosis/issues and to obtain information; married couples also attend for socialization (Purk, 2004).*
- Suggest and help clients transition from a manual to a powered wheelchair or device if progressive physical disability occurs. **EB:** *Powered mobility devices positively affected subject's roles, occupational performance, interests, independence, and self-esteem (Buning, Angelo & Schmeler, 2001).*
- ▲ Reduce floor clutter and establish safety rules for drivers of power mobility devices; make referrals to PT or OT for driver reevaluations if accidents occur or client's health deteriorates. *This promotes safe driving and helps prevent injury to client, pedestrians, and property.* **EB:** *A study identified risks related to power mobility devices and solutions to reduce risks to improve safety (Mortenson et al, 2005).*
- Request and receive clients' permission before moving unoccupied wheelchair in room or out to hallway (Cox, 2004; Gavin-Dreschnack, 2004). *Chronic wheelchair users may view chair as part of their identity and independence and may become stressed if it's not readily available.*

M

Geriatric

- Alternate wheelchair mobility with rest periods. *Increased resting heart rate and blood pressure and decreased maximal oxygen uptake, vital capacity, and strength indicate activity intolerance (Radwanski, 2002).*
- Avoid using restraints on fidgeting clients who slide down in a wheelchair; rather, assess for deformities, spinal curvatures, abnormal tone, discomfort, and limited joint range. *Elders may move to get comfortable or do a task that inadvertently results in poor posture and sliding (Rader, Jones & Miller, 1999); special seating system aids posture/comfort (Minkel, 2001; Taylor, 2003).*
- Ensure proper seat depth leg positioning when elders are sitting up and use custom foot rests (not elevated leg rests) to prevent sliding down in wheelchairs. *Tight hamstrings and a posterior pelvic tilt are common in elders and may pull pelvis toward front of chair; special leg/foot rests are needed (Gavin-Dreschnack, 2004).* **EB:** *Trained research staff conducted studies on wheelchair use and exercise. Time-measured studies indicate increase in independence with locomotion and toileting when activity is conducted on a regular basis. Repetition of exercise with a maximum weight also indicate improvement with endurance, strength, and urinary continence (Ouslander et al, 2005).*
- ▲ Assess for side effects of medications and potential need for dosage readjustments to increase wheelchair tolerance. *Medications can cause orthostatic hypotension, dizziness, and altered cardiac output (Halm, 2001).* **EB:** *Study review/meta analysis showed a "weak association" between Digoxin, type IA antiarrhythmics, and diuretics and falling elders; taking three to four or more meds increased recurrent fall rates (Leipzig, Cumming & Tinetti, 1999).*
- Allow client to propel wheelchair independently at his or her own speed. *Elders may move slowly due to diminished ROM/strength, stiff/sore joints, and cardiopulmonary compromise.*

Home Care

- Assess home environment for barriers and for a support system for emergency and contingency care (e.g., Lifeline). *Immobility and wheelchair use may pose a threat during health crises.* **EB:** *In two connected studies, 37% of respondents at home had fallen from wheelchairs and 46% of fallers had injuries; 36% had not made home modifications (Berg, Hines & Allen, 2002).*

- Arrange traffic patterns so they are wide enough to maneuver a wheelchair. *This prevents damage to skin/walls/woodwork/furniture and increases independence (Yearns & Huntoon, 1997).*
- Explain a 5-foot turning space is necessary to maneuver wheelchairs, doorways need to be 32 to 36 inches wide, and entrance ramps/paths should slope 1 inch per foot (Yearns & Huntoon, 1997).
- Suggest simple changes such as replacing door hardware with fold-back hinges, removing doorway encasements (if too narrow), and removing or replacing thresholds (if too high). *Universal design literature recommends ways to modify and build homes and appliances to make them more accessible.*
- Suggest rearranging room functions, furniture, and storage so that toileting, sleeping, bathing, and preparing and eating meals can safely take place on one level of the home. *The ability to perform these activities is critical for staying in one's own home (Yearns & Huntoon, 1997).*
- ▲ Request PT/OT referrals to evaluate wheelchair skills and safety, to suggest home modifications and ways to propel wheelchairs on irregular surfaces and get back into a chair after a fall (Berg et al, 2002). **EB:** *A study concluded the Wheelchair Skills Test (WST) is a short, reliable test for professionals to assess clients' manual wheelchair skills (Kirby et al, 2004). Pilot testing indicates this tool effectively evaluates driver ability of powered mobility devices in the community (Letts, Dawson & Kaiserman-Goldenstein, 1998).*
- ▲ Provide support to clients and teach about pertinent local support groups and internet resources (Purk, 2004). *Loss, chronic illness, and injury often trigger serious emotional responses.* **EBN:** *Caregivers used and benefited from an Internet site that offered stroke education, support, and group discussion (Pierce, Steiner & Govoni, 2004).*
- ▲ Provide client with information about advocacy, resources, accessibility, assistive technology, potential funding, and issues under the Americans with Disabilities Act. *This creates the potential for greater accessibility to such services and to independence (Berry & Ignash, 2003).*
- ▲ Suggest community resources for servicing and tuning up wheelchairs and/or locating parts so clients can service their own chairs, since an annual tune-up is recommended.

• = Independent;   ▲ = Collaborative;   EBN = Evidence-Based Nursing;   EB = Evidence-Based

Client/Family Teaching

- Suggest that the client test-drive wheelchairs and try out cushions and postural supports before purchasing them. *Equipment is very expensive, and different makes and models have different advantages and disadvantages (Minkel, 2000).*
- Assess pain levels of long-term wheelchair users and make referrals to therapists or wheelchair clinics for modifications. **EB:** *Most subjects experienced pain relief with ergonomic, individualized seating interventions (Samuelsson et al, 2001). Seating prototype testing found seat adjustability and low-back support improved comfort (Crane & Hobson, 2003).*
- Instruct and have client return demonstrate re-inflation of pneumatic tires; encourage client to monitor tire pressure every 2 to 3 weeks. **EB:** *Tire pressure that is at or below 50% of what the manufacturer recommends increases wheeling/rolling resistance and energy expenditure (Sawatzky, Denison & Kim, 2002).*
- Instruct clients to remove large wheelchair parts when lifting wheelchair into car for transport; when reassembling it, check that all parts are fastened securely and temperature is tepid. *This reduces weight that needs to be lifted; locked parts and a safe temperature prevents injury/burns.*
- ▲ Make social service referral to educate clients on financial coverage/regulations of third-party payors and Health Care Financing Association for equipment. *It is important to recognize the advantages, cost, and durability of different wheelchair models before purchasing one (Cooper et al, 2000).*
- Teach the importance of using seatbelts or chair tie-downs when riding in motor vehicles; if unavailable, clients in wheelchairs should be transported in large heavy vehicles only. *Clients need restraint protection in case of abrupt vehicle maneuvers (Shaw, 2000).*
- For further information, refer care plans for **Impaired Transfer ability** and **Impaired bed Mobility.**

evolve See the EVOLVE website for World Wide Web resources for client education.

REFERENCES

Berg K, Hines M, Allen S: Wheelchair users at home: few modifications and many injurious falls, *Am J Pub Health* 92(1):48, 2002.

Berry BE, Ignash S: Assistive technology: providing independence for individuals with disabilities, *Rehabil Nurs* 28(1):6-14, 2003.

Boninger ML, Baldwin M, Cooper RA et al: Manual wheelchair pushrim biomechanics and axle position, *Arch Phys Med Rehabil* 81:608-613, 2000.

Brienza DM, Karg PE, Geyer MJ et al: The relationship between pressure ulcer incidence and buttock-seat cushion interface pressure in at-risk elderly wheelchair users, *Arch Phys Med Rehabil* 82(4):529-533, 2001.

Buning ME, Angelo JA, Schmeler MR: Occupational performance and the transition to powered mobility: a pilot study, *Am J Occup Ther* 55(3):339-344, 2001.

Congress of Neurological Surgeons: Medical student curriculum in neurosurgery: diagnosis and management of peripheral nerve injury and entrapment 2002, available at www.neurosurgery.org/cns/meetings/curriculum/dl.html.

Cooper RA, Cooper R, Boninger ML: Push for power, *Rehabil Manag* 17(2):32-36, 2004.

Cooper RA, Schmeler MR, Cooper R et al: Long-term rehab: advanced seating systems, parts I and II, *Rehabil Manag* 13(2-3):58, 2000.

Corfman TA, Cooper RA, Fitzgerald SG et al: Tips and falls during electric-powered wheelchair driving: effects of seatbelt use, legrests, and driving speed, *Arch Phys Med Rehabil* 84(12):1797-1802, 2003.

Cox DI: Not your parent's wheelchair, *Rehabil Manag* 17(7):26-27, 2004.

Crane B, Hobson D: No room for discomfort, *Rehabil Manag* 16(1):30, 2003.

Curtis KA, Drysdale GA, Lanza RD et al: Shoulder pain in wheelchair users with tetraplegia and paraplegia, *Arch Phys Med Rehabil* 80(4):453-457, 1999.

Defloor T, Grypdonck MH: Sitting posture and prevention of pressure ulcers, *Appl Nurs Res* 12(3):136-142, 1999.

Dowswell G, Dowswell T, Young J: Adjusting stroke patients' poor position: an observational study, *J Adv Nurs* 32(2):286-291, 2000.

Gavin-Dreschnack D: Effects of wheelchair posture on patient safety, *Rehabil Nurs* 29(6):221-226, 2004.

Halm M: Altered tissue perfusion. In Maas ML et al, editors: *Nursing care of older adults: diagnoses, outcomes, and interventions,* St Louis, 2001, Mosby.

Henderson JL, Price SH, Brandstater ME et al: Efficacy of three measures to relieve pressure in seated persons with spinal cord injury, *Arch Phys Med Rehabil* 75(5):535-539, 1994.

Kirby RL, Dupuis DJ, Macphee AH et al: The wheelchair skills test (version 2.4): measurement properties, *Arch Phys Med Rehabil* 85(5):794-804, 2004.

Koontz AM, Boninger M: Proper propulsion, *Rehabil Manag* 16(6):18-22, 2003.

Leipzig RM, Cumming RG, Tinetti ME: Drugs and falls in older people: a systematic review and meta-analysis: II. Cardiac and analgesic drugs, *J Am Geriatr Soc* 47(1):40-50, 1999.

Letts L, Dawson D, Kaiserman-Goldenstein E: Development of the power-mobility community driving assessment, *Can J Rehabil* 11(3):123, 1998.

Minkel JL: Seating and mobility considerations for people with spinal cord injury, *Phys Ther* 80(7):701-709, 2000.

Minkel JL: Sitting outside of the box, *Rehabil Manag* 14(8):50, 2001.

Minor MAD, Minor SD: *Patient care skills,* ed 4, Stamford, Conn, 1999, Appleton and Lange.

Mortenson WB, Miller WC, Boily J et al: Perceptions of power mobility use and safety within residential facilities, *Can J Occup Ther* 72(3):142-152, 2005.

Nyland J, Quigley P, Huang C et al: Preserving transfer independence among individuals with spinal cord injury, *Spinal Cord* 38:649-657, 2000.

Ouslander JG, Griffiths PC, McConnell E et al; Functional incidental training: a randomized, controlled, crossover trial in Veterans Affairs nursing homes, *J Am Geriatr Soc* 53(7):1091-1100, 2005.

Paleg G: The prevention struggle, *Rehabil Manag* 15(8):40-42, 2002.

Pierce LL: Barriers to access: frustrations of people who use a wheelchair for full-time mobility, *Rehabil Nurs* 23(3):120-125, 1998.

Pierce LL, Steiner V, Govoni AL: Internet-based support for rural caregivers of persons with stroke shows promise, *Rehabil Nurs* 29(3):95-99, 2004.

Purk JK: Support groups: why do people attend? *Rehabil Nurs* 29(2):62-67, 2004.

Rader J, Jones D, Miller LL: Individualized wheelchair seating: reducing restraints and improving comfort and function, *Top Geriatr Rehabil* 15(2):34, 1999.

Radwanski MB: Gerontological rehabilitation nursing. In Hoeman SP, editor: *Rehabilitation nursing: process, application, and outcomes,* ed 3, St Louis, 2002, Mosby.

Samuelsson K, Larsson H, Thyberg M et al: Wheelchair seating intervention. Results from a client-centered approach, *Disabil Rehabil* 23(15):677-682, 2001.

Sawatzky BJ, Denison I, Kim W: Rolling, rolling, rolling, *Rehabil Manag* 15(6):36-39, 2002.

Shaw G: Wheelchair rider risk in motor vehicles: a technical note, *J Rehabil Res Dev* 37(1):89-100, 2000.

Stinson MD, Porter-Armstrong AP, Eakin PA: Pressure mapping systems: reliability of pressure map interpretation. *Clin Rehabil,* 17(5):504-511, 2003.

Swaine JM: Seeing the difference, *Rehabil Manag* 16(9):26-28, 30-31, 2003.

Taylor SJ: An overview of evaluation for wheelchair seating for people who have had strokes, *Top Stroke Rehabil* 10(1):95, 2003.

Wound, Ostomy, and Continence Nurses Society (WOCN): *Guideline for prevention and management of pressure ulcers,* Glenview, Ill, 2003, The Society.

Yearns MH, Huntoon R: *A home for all ages: convenient, comfortable, and attractive,* handout for 47th Annual Conference of the National Council on the Aging, HDFS-H-294, March 1997.

Nausea   *Betty J. Ackley, EdS, MSN, RN*

NANDA   Definition

A subjective, unpleasant, wavelike sensation in the back of the throat, epigastrium, or the abdomen that may lead to the urge or need to vomit

Defining Characteristics

Aversion to food; gagging sensation; increased salivation; increased swallowing; report of nausea; sour taste in mouth

Related Factors (r/t)

Biophysical

Biochemical disorders (e.g., uremia, diabetic ketoacidosis, pregnancy); esophageal disease; gastric distention; gastric irritation; increased intracranial pressure; intraabdominal tumors; labyrinthitis; liver capsule stretch; localized tumors (e.g., acoustic neuroma, primary or secondary brain tumors, bone metastases at base of skull); meningitis; Meniere's disease; motion sickness; pain; pancreatic disease; splenetic capsule stretch; toxins (e.g., tumor-produced peptides, abnormal metabolites due to cancer)

Situational

Anxiety; fear; noxious odors; noxious taste; pain; psychological factors; unpleasant visual stimulation

Treatment Related

Gastric distention; gastric irritation: pharmaceuticals

NOC   Outcomes (Nursing Outcomes Classification)

Suggested NOC Outcomes

Comfort Level, Hydration, Nausea & Vomiting Severity, Nutritional Status: Food and Fluid Intake, Nutrient Intake

• = Independent;   ▲ = Collaborative;   EBN = Evidence-Based Nursing;   EB = Evidence-Based

Example NOC Outcome with Indicators
Nausea & Vomiting Severity as evidenced by the following indicators: Frequency of nausea/Intensity of nausea/Distress of nausea (Rate the outcome and indicators of **Nausea & Vomiting Severity:** I = severe, 2 = substantial, 3 = moderate, 4 = mild, 5 = none [see Section I].)

Client Outcomes

Client Will (Specify Time Frame):

* State relief of nausea
* Explain methods they can use to decrease nausea and vomiting (N&V)

NIC   Interventions (Nursing Interventions Classification)

Suggested NIC Interventions

Distraction, Medication Administration, Progressive Muscle Relaxation, Simple Guided Imagery, Therapeutic Touch

Example NIC Activities—Distraction
Encourage the individual to choose the distraction technique(s) desired, such as music, engaging in conversation or telling a detailed account of event or story, guided imagery, or humor; Advise patient to practice the distraction technique before the time needed, if possible

Nursing Interventions and *Rationales*

N

* Determine cause of N&V (e.g., medication effects, viral illness, food poisoning, extreme anxiety, anesthetic agents, pregnancy). *Since most episodes of N&V are now preventable, it is important for the cause to be determined (Garrett et al, 2003).*
* Provide distraction from the sensation of nausea, using soft music, television, and videos per the client preference. *Distraction can help direct attention away from the sensation of nausea (Garrett et al, 2003).* **EBN:** *Music therapy has been shown to decrease N&V in chemotherapy clients (Ezzone et al, 1998).*
* Apply a cold washcloth to the forehead of a nauseated client. *This is a distraction technique to help the client deal with nausea.*
* Maintain a quiet, well-ventilated environment free of strong odors from food, perfume or cleaning solutions. *Odors can cause or exacerbate N&V (Garrett et al, 2003).*
* Avoid sudden movement of the client; allow the client to lie still. *Movement can trigger further N&V (Garrett et al, 2003).*
* If nausea is associated with frequent vomiting, assess client for fluid and electrolyte imbalances. *Protracted vomiting can cause hyponatremia, hypokalemia, or dehydration (Garrett et al, 2003).*
* Keep a clean emesis basin and tissues within the client's reach.
* Provide oral care after the client vomits. *Oral care helps remove the taste and smell of vomitus, thus reducing the stimulus for further vomiting.*
* Stay with the client to give support, place hand on shoulder, and hold the emesis basin. **EBN:** *A study demonstrated that clients with nausea that received purposeful touch as an intervention, had decreased nausea (Dune, 2002).*
* After vomiting is controlled and nausea abates, begin offering the client small amounts of clear fluids, such as water, clear soda, or preferably ginger ale, and then bland foods, such as crackers or dry toast; progress to a soft diet. *Ginger root (found in some ginger ales) has been shown to be more effective than a placebo for treatment of postoperative N&V (Chaiyakunapruk et al, 2006).*
* Remove cover of food tray before bringing it into the client's room. *The sudden, concentrated food odors that come when the cover is removed in front of the client can trigger nausea.*
* ▲ Refer clients with HIV for management of antiretroviral-related nausea. **EBN:** *A nursing study*

• = Independent;   ▲ = Collaborative;   EBN = Evidence-Based Nursing;   EB = Evidence-Based

demonstrated that nausea associated with combination antiretroviral therapy was quite common and may adversely affect medication adherence (Reynolds & Neidig, 2002).

Nausea in Pregnancy

- Recommend that the woman eat dry crackers or dry toast in bed before arising and then get up slowly. Also advise to chew gum or suck hard candies, eat small frequent meals, avoid foods with offensive odors, and avoid preparing food or shopping when nauseated. *These are traditional strategies for alleviating nausea (Grodner, Long & DeYoung, 2004).*
- ▲ Discuss with the primary care practitioner the possibility of using transcutaneous electrical stimulation in the form of Relief Band Device (Woodside Biomedical) to help relieve nausea. **EB:** *The results of a systematic review of the studies showed that the results of using P6 acupressure during pregnancy are equivocal (Jewell & Young, 2005).*
- ▲ Consider the use of continuous acupressure applied by Sea-Bands with acupressure buttons or by hand to P6 on both wrists. **EBN:** *Sea-Bands with acupressure buttons were demonstrated to be a noninvasive, inexpensive, safe, and effective treatment for the N&V of pregnancy (Steele et al, 2001).*
- ▲ Refer client for acupuncture. **EB:** *Acupuncture is an effective treatment for women who experience nausea and dry retching in early pregnancy (Smith, Crowther & Beilby, 2002).*

Nausea Following Surgery

- ▲ Medicate the client for nausea as ordered. **EB:** *Antiemetic medications can reduce the incidence of postoperative nausea and vomiting (PONV), and use of more than one medication may be needed (Apfel et al, 2004).*
- ▲ Alleviate postoperative pain using ordered analgesic agents (refer to care plan for **Acute Pain**). *Pain is known to be a factor in the development of PONV.*
- Ensure that the nauseated client is not hypotensive. Check blood pressure and note signs of postural hypotension. *Postural hypotension can be caused by deficient fluid volume following surgery and can result in nausea (Garrett et al, 2003).*
- Consider use of a recliner chair postoperatively for clients who have had laparoscopy if not contraindicated. **EBN:** *A study demonstrated that clients who used a recliner chair postoperatively after laparoscopy had fewer adverse symptoms, such as nausea, severe pain, and delayed voiding (Agodoa, Holder & Fowler, 2002).*
- Recommend that the client sit down when experiencing nausea. **EB:** *Women undergoing gynecological surgery presenting with orthostatic dysregulation and arterial hypotension in their history exhibit an increased risk of PONV (Pusch et al, 2002).*
- ▲ Consider use of isopropyl alcohol (IPA) inhalation for treatment of PONV for clients who have general anesthesia for a surgical procedure. *Positive results may be due to controlled breathing during inhalation rather than IPA.* **EBN:** *Study results show IPA to be somewhat effective for PONV (Merritt, Okyere & Jasinski, 2002; Anderson & Gross 2004; Winston et al, 2003).*
- ▲ Consult with primary care practitioner for use of nonpharmacological techniques, such as acupuncture, electroacupuncture, or transcutaneous electrical nerve stimulation as an adjunct for controlling PONV. **EB:** *A study of the use of acupuncture for PONV demonstrated a significant reduction in vomiting in clients after gynecological surgery (Streitberger et al, 2004). P6 acupoint stimulation seems to reduce the risk of nausea in postoperative surgical clients (Lee & Done, 2005).*
- Teach the use of acupressure on two points on the wrist, or use of bands providing pressure to prevent or relieve nausea in some kinds of surgery. **EBN:** *Studies confirmed the effectiveness of acupressure in preventing PONV (Ming et al, 2002; Alkaissi et al, 2002; Streitberger et al, 2004).*
- Use relaxation, imagery, and distraction techniques for nausea; encourage the client to take slow, deep breaths. *Deep breaths can serve as a distraction technique and can help rid the body of the anesthetic agent.*

Nausea Following Chemotherapy

- ▲ Consult with physician regarding need for antiemetic medications, either prophylactic or when N&V occurs. *Preventing N&V is important; one serious bout can result in anticipatory nausea for the remainder of the client's treatments (Garrett et al, 2003).*
- ▲ Use antiemetics and a nursing intervention program of increased access to support and increased

N

information. **EBN:** *In comparative antiemetic trials of 162 women with ovarian cancer receiving cisplatin-based chemotherapy, the group receiving antiemetics and the nursing intervention above reported less nausea (Borjeson et al, 2002).*

▲ If nausea is associated with the use of opioids, consult with the primary care practitioner for possible use of alternative pain medication. *Opioids can stimulate the vomiting center (Garrett et al, 2003).*

• Help the client learn how to use acupressure for nausea, applying pressure bilaterally at P6 points using fingers or bands to decrease the amount and severity of nausea. **EBN and EB:** *Finger acupressure can be effective to relieve chemotherapy-induced nausea (Dibble et al, 2000, 2006; Shin et al, 2004; Ezzone, Streitberger & Schneider, 2006). Use of pressure bands can be effective (Roscoe et al, 2006). Research supports the use of acupressure along with antiemetic drugs; this is supported by a National Institutes of Health (NIH) consensus statement (Collins & Thomas, 2004).*

▲ For clients who continue to experience nausea after antiemetic drugs or other treatments, consult with the primary care practitioner regarding the possibility of using acupuncture to help control nausea. Such devices as the Relief Band are not effective. *Acupuncture has been shown to effectively control chemotherapy-induced N&V in adults (Collins & Thomas, 2004; Acupuncture, 2000).* **EB:** *A systematic review pooled the results of 11 clinical trials (N = 1247) and determined that there was no benefit to using the Relief Band (Ezzone, Streitberger & Schneider, 2006).*

• Recognize that the use of ginger root *(Zingiber officinale)* may relieve nausea. **EBN:** *In a study of use of ginger after compazine treatment, the group that received ginger had better relief of nausea (Pace, 1987).* **EB:** *Another study demonstrated that ginger was helpful for delayed nausea (Manusirivithaya et al, 2004).*

• Work with the client, using guided imagery and progressive muscle relaxation to reduce nausea. **EB:** *Studies have shown that guided imagery and progressive muscle relaxation can decrease nausea (Luebbert, Dahme & Hasenbring 2001; Yoo et al, 2005; Molassiotis et al, 2002).*

• Offer the nauseated client a 10-minute foot massage. **EBN:** *Foot massage was shown to be an effective way to decrease nausea, pain, and anxiety in a group of oncology clients (Grealish, Lomasney & Whiteman, 2000).*

• If client has anticipatory nausea, use such interventions as education, relaxation therapy, and imagery to help client decrease nausea associated with the event. **EBN:** *Nurses can identify clients at highest risk for developing anticipatory nausea and implement strategies to prevent/minimize it (Eckert, 2001).*

Geriatrics

▲ Administer antiemetic drugs carefully; watch for side effects. *Management hinges on correction of the reversible cause, employing nondrug measures as appropriate and prescribing the correct antiemetic. Nondrug measures may include avoiding the smell or even the sight of food, avoiding exposure to foods that precipitate nausea, and presenting food in smaller quantities (Tallis, 2003).*

▲ Evaluate nonsteroidal antiinflammatory drugs (NSAIDs) as a possible cause of nausea. *NSAIDs are commonly taken for arthritis pain in older adult clients and can cause nausea as well as abdominal pain and ulcers (Peura, 2003).*

Home Care

• Previously mentioned interventions may be adapted for home care use.

▲ In hospice care clients, assess for causes of nausea, such as constipation, bowel obstruction, adverse effects of medications, and onset of increased intracranial pressure. Refer the client to a primary care practitioner if needed. *There can be multiple causes of nausea in clients with advanced cancer (Haughney, 2004).*

• Assist the client and family with identifying and avoiding irritants in the home that exacerbate nausea (e.g., strong odors from food, plants, perfume, and room deodorizers).

Client/Family Teaching

• Teach the client techniques to use when uncomfortable, including relaxation techniques, guided imagery, hypnosis, and music therapy (Garrett et al, 2003).

evolve   See the EVOLVE website for World Wide Web resources for client education.

• = Independent;   ▲ = Collaborative;   EBN = Evidence-Based Nursing;   EB = Evidence-Based

REFERENCES

Acupuncture: National Institutes of Health consensus development conference statement, *Dermatol Nurs* 12(2):126-133, 2000.

Agodoa SE, Holder MA, Fowler SM: Effects of recliner-chair versus traditional hospital bed on postsurgical diagnostic laparoscopic recovery time, *J Perianesth Nurs* 17(5):318, 2002.

Alkaissi A, Everttson K, Johnsson V et al: P6 acupressure may relieve nausea and vomiting after gynecological surgery: an effectiveness study in 410 women, *Can J Anaesth* 49(10):1034-1039, 2002.

Anderson LA, Gross J: Aromatherapy with peppermint, isopropyl alcohol, or placebo is equally effective in relieving postoperative nausea, *J Perianesth Nurs* 19(1):29-35, 2004.

Apfel CC, Korttila K, Abdalla M et al: A factorial trial of six interventions for the prevention of postoperative nausea and vomiting, *N Eng J Med* 350(24):2441, 2004.

Borjeson S, Hursti TJ, Tishelman C et al: Treatment of nausea and emesis during cancer chemotherapy. Discrepancies between antiemetic effect and well-being, *J Pain Sympt Manag* 24(3):345, 2002.

Chaiyakunapruk N, Kitikannakorn N, Nathisuwan S et al: The efficacy of ginger for the prevention of postoperative nausea and vomiting: a meta-analysis, *Am J Obstet Gynecol* 194(1):95-99, 2006.

Collins KB, Thomas DJ: Acupuncture and acupressure for the management of chemotherapy-induced nausea and vomiting, *J Am Acad Nurse Pract* 16(2):76, 2004.

Dibble SL, Chapman J, Mack KA et al: Acupressure for nausea: results of a pilot study, *Oncol Nurs Forum* 27(1):41-47, 2000.

Dibble SL, Luce J, Cooper BA et al: Acupressure for delayed chemotherapy induced nausea & vomiting: a RCT. *Oncol Nurs Forum*, 2007 (in press).

Dune LS: Nausea relief and purposeful touch: decreasing distress by altering the perceptual field, Texas Woman's University PhD, Order No AA13046305, 2002.

Eckert RM: Understanding anticipatory nausea, *Oncol Nurs Forum* 28(10):1553, 2001.

Ezzone S, Baker C, Rosselet R et al: Music as an adjunct to antiemetic therapy, *Oncol Nurs Forum* 25(9):1551, 1998.

Ezzone J, Streitberger, K, Schneider A: Cochrane systematic reviews examine P6 acupuncture-point stimulation for nausea and vomiting, *J Altern Complement Med* 12(5):489-495, 2006.

Garrett K, Tsuruta K, Walker S et al: Managing nausea and vomiting. Current strategies, *Crit Care Nurse* 23(1):31-50, 2003.

Grealish L, Lomasney A, Whiteman B: Foot massage: a nursing intervention to modify the distressing symptoms of pain and nausea in patients hospitalized with cancer, *Cancer Nurs* 23(3):237, 2000.

Grodner M, Long S, DeYoung S: *Foundations and clinical applications of nutrition: a nursing approach*, ed 3, St Louis, 2004, Mosby.

Haughney A: Nausea and vomiting in end-stage cancer, *Am J Nurs* 104(11):40-48, 2004.

Jewell D, Young G: Interventions for nausea and vomiting in early pregnancy, *Cochrane Database Syst Rev* (4):CD000145, 2005.

Lee A, Done ML: Stimulation of the wrist acupuncture point P6 for preventing postoperative nausea and vomiting, *Cochrane Database Syst Rev* (3):CD003281, 2005.

Luebbert K, Dahme B, Hasenbring M: The effectiveness of relaxation training in reducing treatment-related symptoms and improving emotional adjustment in acute non-surgical cancer treatment: a meta-analytical review, *Psychooncology* 10(6):490-502, 2001.

Manusirivithaya S, Sripramote M, Tangjitgamol S et al: Antiemetic effect of ginger in gynecologic oncology patients receiving cisplatin, *Int J Gynecol Cancer* 14(6):1063-1069, 2004.

Merritt BA, Okyere CP, Jasinski DM: Isopropyl alcohol inhalation: alternative treatment of postoperative nausea and vomiting, *Nurs Res* 51(2):125, 2002.

Ming JL, Kuo BI, Lin JG et al: The efficacy of acupressure to prevent nausea and vomiting in post-operative patients, *J Adv Nurs* 39(4):343, 2002.

Molassiotis A, Yung HP, Yam BM et al: The effectiveness of progressive muscle relaxation training in managing chemotherapy-induced nausea and vomiting in Chinese breast cancer patients: a randomised controlled trial, *Support Care Cancer* 10(3):237-246, 2002.

Pace JC: Oral ingestion of encapsulated ginger and reported self-care actions for the relief of chemotherapy associated nausea and vomiting, *Diss Abstr Int* 47:3297-B, 1987.

Peura DA: Evaluating the approaches to safe and effective analgesia for older patients with arthritis, *Adv Stud Med* 3(3):128, 2003.

Pusch F, Berger A, Wildling E et al: Preoperative orthostatic dysfunction is associated with an increased incidence of postoperative nausea and vomiting, *Anesthesiology* 96(6):1381, 2002.

Reynolds NR, Neidig JL: Characteristics of nausea reported by HIV-infected patients initiating combination antiretroviral regimens, *Clin Nurs Res* 11(1):71, 2002.

Roscoe JA, Jean-Pierre P, Morrow GR et al: Exploratory analysis of the usefulness of acupressure bands when severe chemotherapy-related nausea is expected, *J Soc Integr Oncol* 4(1):16-20, 2006.

Shin YH et al: Effect of acupuncture on nausea and vomiting during chemotherapy cycle for Korean postoperative stomach cancer patients, *Cancer Nurs* 27(4):267-274, 2004.

Smith C, Crowther C, Beilby J: Acupuncture to treat nausea and vomiting in early pregnancy: a randomized controlled trial, *Birth* 29(1):1, 2002.

Steele NM, French J, Gatherer-Boyles J et al: Effect of acupressure by Sea-Bands on nausea and vomiting of pregnancy, *J Obstet Gynecol Neonatal Nurs* 30(1):61, 2001.

Streitberger K, Diefenbacher M, Bauer A et al: Acupuncture compared to placebo-acupuncture for postoperative nausea and vomiting prophylaxis: a randomized placebo-controlled patient and observer blind trial, *Anaesthesia* 59(2):142, 2004.

Tallis R: *Geriatric medicine and gerontology*, ed 6, 2003, Churchill Livingstone, pp 262-264.

Winston AW, Rinehart RS, Riley GP et al: Comparison of inhaled isopropyl alcohol and intravenous ondansetron for treatment of postoperative nausea, *AANA J* 71(2):127-132, 2003.

Yoo HJ, Ahn SH, Kim SB et al: Efficacy of progressive muscle relaxation training and guided imagery in reducing chemotherapy side effects in patients with breast cancer and in improving their quality of life, *Support Care Cancer* 13:826-833, 2005.

N

Unilateral Neglect   *Lori M. Rhudy, PhDc, RN*

NANDA   Definition

Impairment in sensory and motor response, mental representation, and spatial attention of the body and the corresponding environment characterized by inattention to one side and overattention to the opposite side. Left side neglect is more severe and persistent than right side neglect.

Defining Characteristics

Appears unaware of positioning of neglected limb; difficulty remembering details of internally represented familiar scenes that are on the neglected side; displacement of sounds to the nonneglected side; distortion of drawing on the half of the page on the neglected side; failure to cancel lines on the half of the page on the neglected side; failure to eat food from portion of the plate on the neglected side; failure to dress neglected side; failure to groom neglected side; failure to move eyes, head, limbs, trunk in the neglected hemispace, despite being aware of a stimulus in that space; failure to notice people approaching from the neglected side; lack of safety precautions with regard to the neglected side; marked deviation of the eyes to the nonneglected side to stimuli and activities on that side; marked deviation of the head to the nonneglected side to stimuli and activities on that side; marked deviation of the trunk to the nonneglected side to stimuli and activities on that side; omission of drawing on the half of the page on the neglected side; perseveration of visual motor tasks on nonneglected side; substitution of letters to form alternative words that are similar to the original in length when reading; transfer of pain sensation to the nonneglected side; use of only vertical half of page when writing

Related Factors (r/t)

Brain injury from cerebrovascular problems; brain injury from neurological illness; brain injury from trauma; brain injury from tumor; left hemiplegia from CVA of the right hemisphere; hemianopsia NOTE: Because the right hemisphere is dominant in directing attention, unilateral neglect is more common if neurological pathology occurs in the right hemisphere of the brain, which results in left-sided neglect (Ringman et al, 2004). Also, unilateral neglect often occurs with damage to the right parietal lobe, the right frontal lobe, the thalamus, and basal ganglia (Ringman et al, 2004)

NOC   Outcomes (Nursing Outcomes Classification)

Suggested NOC Outcomes

Body Image, Body Positioning: Self-Initiated, Mobility, Self-Care: Activities of Daily Living (ADLs)

Example NOC Outcome with Indicators
Mobility as evidenced by the following indicators: Balance/Coordination/Gait/Muscle movement (Rate the outcome and indicators of **Mobility:** 1 = severely compromised, 2 = substantially compromised, 3 = moderately compromised, 4 = mildly compromised, 5 = not compromised [see Section I].)

Client Outcomes

Client Will (Specify Time Frame):

- Use techniques that can be used to minimize unilateral neglect
- Care for both sides of the body appropriately and keep affected side free from harm
- Return to the highest functioning level possible based on personal goals and abilities
- Remain free from injury

NIC   Interventions (Nursing Interventions Classification)

Suggested NIC Intervention

Unilateral Neglect Management

• = Independent;   ▲ = Collaborative;   EBN = Evidence-Based Nursing;   EB = Evidence-Based

| **Example NIC Activities—Unilateral Neglect Management** |
| Provide realistic feedback about patient's perceptual deficit; Touch unaffected shoulder when initiating conversation |

Nursing Interventions and *Rationales*

- Assess the client for signs of unilateral neglect (e.g., not washing, shaving, or dressing one side of the body; sitting or lying inappropriately on affected arm or leg; failing to respond to environmental stimuli contralateral to the side of lesion; eating food on only one side of plate; or failing to look to one side of the body). *Looking, listening, touching, and searching deficits occur on the affected side of the body and may or may not be associated with a loss of vision, sensation, or motion on the affected side (Plummer, Morris & Dunai, 2003).*

- It is strongly recommended that stroke recovery is assessed using the National Institutes of Health Stroke Scale (NIHSS) at the time of admission or within the first 24 hours. *The Neglect subscale of the NIHSS includes extinction and inattention (Ringman et al, 2004). Of the 62 assessment tools for evaluation of the presence of unilateral neglect, 28 of them are standardized (Menon & Korner-Bitensky, 2004).*

- It is practical to postpone evaluation for unilateral neglect until a couple of weeks after a stroke. **EB:** *Many of the clients who have unilateral neglect at that point are likely to retain it, although many will improve (Appelros et al, 2004).*

- Provide a safe, well-lighted, and clutter-free environment. Place call light and other personal items (such as a urinal) on the unaffected side. Cue the client to environmental hazards when mobile. *Cognitive impairment may accompany neglect; safety is of paramount importance.*

- ▲ Refer to a rehabilitation team (including, but not limited to, rehabilitation clinical nurse specialist, physical medicine and rehabilitation physician, neuropsychologist, occupational therapist, physical therapist, and speech and language pathologist) for continued help in dealing with unilateral neglect. **EB:** *Research has shown there is some evidence that cognitive rehabilitation for unilateral spatial neglect improves performance, but its effect on disability is not clear. Further studies are needed (Bowen, Lincoln & Dewey, 2002; Cicerone et al, 2005; Jutai et al, 2003; Teasell et al, 2005).*

- Use the principles of rehabilitation to progressively increase the client's ability to compensate for unilateral neglect by using assistive devices, feedback, and support, depending on phase of recovery:
  - ■ **Stage I** (Stabilization) Focus attention mainly on nonneglected side.
    - ❑ Set up environment so that most activity is on unaffected side.
    - ❑ Place the client's personal items within view and on unaffected side.
    - ❑ Position the bed so that client is approached from the unaffected side.
    - ❑ Monitor and assist the client to achieve adequate food and fluid intake.

    The initial priorities are client safety and identification of rehabilitation needs.
  - ■ **Stage II** (Early recovery): Help the client develop an awareness of neglected side.
    - ❑ Gradually focus the client's attention on affected side.
    - ❑ Gradually move personal items and activity to affected side.
    - ❑ Stand on the client's affected side when assisting with ambulation or ADLs.

    The goal now is for the client to develop an awareness of the neglected side.
  - ■ **Stage III** (Rehabilitation): Help the client compensate for neglect.
    - ❑ Use cues and anchors to promote attention to the neglected side and help the client develop compensatory mechanisms to deal with the neglect syndrome (Kalbach, 1991). Use reminders to keep the client scanning the entire environment.
    - ❑ Use bright yellow or red stickers on outer margins in reading or writing exercises. Have the client look for the sticker while reading or writing. Similar markers can be applied to a meal tray or plate to encourage scanning of the entire meal.
    - ❑ Encourage the client to bathe and groom the affected side first.
    - ❑ Focus touch and talking on affected side; use a positive approach (e.g., "Mary, turn your head to the left and you'll see your daughter").

    The goal now is for the client to compensate for neglect by attending to the affected side.
    EB: *A study demonstrated that clients discovered and gradually compensated for their unilateral neglect during stroke recovery (Tham & Kielhofner, 2003).*

• = Independent;   ▲ = Collaborative;   EBN = Evidence-Based Nursing;   EB = Evidence-Based

- Recognize that unilateral neglect can improve following a stroke. **EB:** *A study demonstrated that some degree of neglect was common at baseline, but rapid recovery occurred during the first 7 days, and by 3 months only 8.6% of the 31.1 % of clients exhibiting neglect continued to demonstrate neglect (Ringman et al, 2004).*

Home Care

- Many of the previously listed interventions may be adapted for use in the home care setting.
- Position bed at home so that client gets out of bed on unaffected side. *Positioning the bed so that the client gets out on the unaffected side can increase safety.*

Client/Family Teaching

- Explain pathology and symptoms of unilateral neglect to both the client and family.
- Teach the client how to scan regularly to check the position of body parts and to regularly turn head from side to side for safety when ambulating, using a wheelchair, or doing self-care tasks. Recommend the client think of self like a horizon-illuminating lighthouse. **EB:** *The use of the visual image of being a lighthouse was shown to improve function in a neglect client when walking, using a wheelchair, or engaging in problem-solving activities (Niemeier, 1998).*
- Teach caregivers to cue the client to the environment.

evolve   See the EVOLVE website for World Wide Web resources for client education.

REFERENCES

Appelros P, Nydevik I, Karlsson GM et al: Recovery from unilateral neglect after right-hemisphere stroke, *Disabil Rehabil* 26(8):471-477, 2004.

Bowen A, Lincoln NB, Dewey M: Cognitive rehabilitation for spatial neglect following stroke, *Cochrane Database Syst Rev* (2): D003586, 2002.

Cicerone KD, Dahlberg C, Malec JF et al: Evidence-based cognitive rehabilitation: updated review of the literature from 1998 through 2002, *Arch Phys Med Rehabil* 86(8):1681-1692, 2005.

Jutai JW, Bhogal SK, Foley NC et al: Treatment of visual perceptual disorders post stroke, *Top Stroke Rehabil* 10(2):77-107, 2003.

Kalbach LR: Unilateral neglect: mechanisms and nursing care, *J Neurosci Nurs* 23(2):125-129, 1991.

Menon A, Korner-Bitensky N: Evaluating unilateral spatial neglect post stroke: working your way through the maze of assessment choices, *Top Stroke Rehabil* 11(3):41-66, 2004.

Niemeier JP: The lighthouse strategy: use of a visual imagery technique to treat visual inattention in stroke patients, *Brain Inj* 12(5):399-406, 1998.

Plummer P, Morris ME, Dunai J: Assessment of unilateral neglect, *Phys Ther* 83(8):732-740, 2003.

Ringman JM, Saver JL, Woolson RF et al: Frequency, risk factors, anatomy, and course of unilateral neglect in an acute stroke cohort, *Neurology* 63(3):468-474, 2004.

Teasell R, Salter K, Bitensky J et al: *Evidence-based review of stroke rehabilitation: perceptual disorders,* Module 13, 2005, available at http://www.ebrsr.com/modules.html. Accessed June 20, 2006.

Tham K, Kielhofner G: Impact of the social environment on occupational experience and performance among persons with unilateral neglect, *Am J Occup Ther* 57(4):403-412, 2003.

N

Noncompliance   *Betty J. Ackley, MSN, EdS, RN*

NANDA   Definition

Behavior of person and/or caregiver that fails to coincide with a health-promoting or therapeutic plan agreed on by the person (and/or family and/or community) and healthcare professional; in the presence of an agreed-on, health-promoting, or therapeutic plan, person's or caregiver's behavior is fully or partially nonadherent and may lead to clinically ineffective or partially ineffective outcomes

Defining Characteristics

Behavior indicative of failure to adhere (directly observed or verbalized by patient or significant others) (critical); objective tests (e.g., physiological measures, detection of physiological markers); evidence of development of complications; evidence of exacerbation of symptoms; failure to keep appointments; failure to progress

Related Factors (r/t)

Healthcare plan

Duration; significant others; cost; intensity; complexity; financial flexibility of plan

---

• = Independent;   ▲ = Collaborative;   EBN = Evidence-Based Nursing;   EB = Evidence-Based

Individual Factors

Cultural influences; developmental abilities; health beliefs; individual's value system; knowledge relevant to the regimen behavior; motivational forces; personal abilities; significant others; skill relevant to the regimen behavior; spiritual values

Health System

Access to care; client/provider relationships; communication skills of the provider; convenience of care; credibility of provider; individual health coverage; provider continuity; provider regular follow-up; provider reimbursement; satisfaction with care; teaching skills of the provider

Network

Involvement of members in health plan; social value regarding plan; perceived beliefs of significant others

NOTE: The nursing diagnosis **Noncompliance** is judgmental and places blame on the client (Ward-Collins, 1998). The authors recommend use of the diagnosis **Ineffective Therapeutic regimen management** in place of the diagnosis **Noncompliance.** The diagnosis **Ineffective Therapeutic regimen management** has interventions that are developed by both the healthcare providers and the client. It is a more respectful and efficacious nursing diagnosis than **Noncompliance.**

NOC   Outcomes (Nursing Outcomes Classification)

Suggested NOC Outcomes

Adherence Behavior, Compliance Behavior, Treatment Behavior: Illness or Injury

> #### Example NOC Outcome with Indicators
>
> **Adherence Behavior** as evidenced by the following indicators: Uses strategies to maximize health/Uses strategies to eliminate unhealthy behavior/Provides rationale for adopting a health regimen/Uses health services congruent with need (Rate the outcome and indicators of **Adherence Behavior:** 1 = never demonstrated, 2 = rarely demonstrated, 3 = sometimes demonstrated, 4 = often demonstrated, 5 = consistently demonstrated [see Section I].)

Client Outcomes

Client Will (Specify Time Frame):

- Describe consequence of continued noncompliance with treatment regimen
- State goals for health and the means by which to obtain them
- Communicate an understanding of disease and treatment
- List treatment regimens and expectations and agree to follow through
- List alternative ways to meet goals
- Describe the importance of family participation to help achieve goals

NIC   Interventions (Nursing Interventions Classification)

Suggested NIC Interventions

Health System Guidance, Self-Modification Assistance

> #### Example NIC Activities—Health System Guidance
>
> Inform patient of appropriate community resources and contact persons; Inform patient how to access emergency services by telephone and vehicle, as appropriate

Nursing Interventions and *Rationales*

- Ask the client why he or she has not complied with the prescribed treatment. Have the client "tell his or her story." Listen nonjudgmentally. *Compliance assessment should begin with a nonthreatening discussion with the client.*

• = Independent;   ▲ = Collaborative;   EBN = Evidence-Based Nursing;   EB = Evidence-Based

- Make the client an active partner in his or her own healthcare management. Recognize that the client has absolute control over whether he or she follows the healthcare regimen. Always treat the client with respect, and develop mutual outcomes for treatment. *If the client feels respected and is involved in decision making, compliance will increase. Many clients report that how they are treated by health professionals has a great impact on whether they will follow advice. The traditional paternalistic approach to healthcare results in many clients failing to follow the prescribed treatment (Tsoneva & Shaw, 2004).*

- Instruct the client about the purpose, action, side effects, and administration of medications. **EB:** *A Cochrane systematic review found that telling people about their medications was an effective strategy to improve medication compliance both in the short term (<6 months) and long term (at least 6 months). Telling clients about side effects of medications did not make noncompliance more likely (Haynes et al, 2005).* **EBN:** *Teaching clients with cancer about analgesics and their appropriate use resulted in a decrease in pain levels (Devine, 2003).*

- Assess the likelihood of medication-related problems and noncompliance with medication regimen. **EB:** *Using a 5-item questionnaire with the usual teaching regarding medications enabled providers to identify 14% more individuals at risk for medication-related problems than the usual care practice (Langford et al, 2006). Examining client's beliefs about anticoagulation therapy and satisfaction, researchers were able to correctly predict compliance with warfarin therapy 85% of the time (Orensky & Holdford, 2005).*

- Determine the client's ability to obtain required medications. **EB:** *A client's inability to acquire or pay for medications was a significant barrier to adherence (Krueger, Berger & Felkey, 2005). Adherence is enhanced when the underlying reasons for nonadherence are assessed and dealt with (Krueger, Felkey & Berger, 2003).* **EBN:** *Clients often are forced to choose between paying bills and buying medication. They often skip doses to make their medications last longer, buy only a few doses at a time, or go out of the country to obtain their medications more cheaply (Ostwald et al, 2006).*

- Instruct the client on self-monitoring and self-regulation of medications as appropriate. **EB:** *Comprehensive programs that include self-monitoring and self-regulation were effective in improving medication adherence (Haynes et al, 2005). Inclusion of self-monitoring and reinforcement within complex interventions were effective for long-term medication adherence (McDonald, Garg & Haynes, 2002). Self-monitoring and self-adjustment of oral anticoagulation therapy resulted in fewer thrombolic events and lower mortality than those who self-monitor only, making self-management preferable for those clients who are capable of it (Heneghan et al, 2006).*

- Provide structured education tailored to the individual. **EB:** *Educational interventions that were personalized and that involved frequent contact with the nurse or pharmacist to learn about antihypertensive and lipid-lowering medications were the most effective (Petrilla et al, 2005). Clients who received structured education involving both verbal and written instruction followed by discussion had greater knowledge and compliance with psychotropic medication therapy (Fernandez et al, 2006).* **EBN:** *The use of an intervention specifically tailored to perceived benefits and barriers to self-care for heart failure was found to change the perceived benefits and barriers of these clients (Sethares & Elliott, 2004).*

- Provide written educational materials at an appropriate reading level. **EB:** *A review of studies investigating the use and impact of written drug information revealed that the readability and presentation of the written information influence knowledge, compliance, and satisfaction (Koo, Krass & Aslani, 2003).*

- Work with the client to determine how he or she will handle the illness and need for medications or prescribed care. **EBN:** *Self-efficacy was enhanced when people solved problems that they themselves identified (Bodenheimer et al, 2002).*

- Arrange for follow-up via telephone. **EB:** *Telephone follow-up is significant both in the short term (<6 months) and the long term (at least 6 months) (Haynes et al, 2005). In one study, 46% of clients who were nonadherent with their medications at baseline were adherent 6 months into the study when they received bimonthly telephone counseling by a nurse. Only 34% of clients who received usual care were adherent at 6 months (Bosworth et al, 2005). Telephone follow-up was found to improve compliance with antibiotic therapy in clients with tonsillitis or pharyngitis. Educational intervention that included a telephone call 4 days into the therapy was superior to education alone for ensuring completion of the full course of antibiotic (Urién et al, 2004).*

• = Independent; ▲ = Collaborative; EBN = Evidence-Based Nursing; EB = Evidence-Based

- If the client is in denial, provide information, communicate unconditional positive regard, avoid distancing yourself, and look for opportunities for authentic contact with your client, being present psychologically and physically. *The most important thing you can do for someone who appears to be in denial is to take the time to genuinely connect (Robinson, 1999).* **EBN:** *The relationship between the client and provider is very important in increasing adherence (Russell, Krantz & Neville, 2004).* See care plan for **Ineffective Denial.**
- Observe for cause of noncompliance (see Related Factors). Recognize that noncompliance is very common. **EBN:** *Lack of adherence to treatment among persons with chronic disorders constitutes a significant problem; half of clients have difficulty following their regimen (Dunbar-Jacob et al, 2000).*
- Recognize that behavioral change comes slowly and often in stages (Prochaska, Norcross & DiClemente, 1995):
  - Precontemplation: change is not contemplated; unaware of problem or risk
  - Contemplation: aware that problem exists; no specific plans or commitment to change
  - Preparation: plan to take action within the next 30 days
  - Action: now taking action to improve health; often behavior not consistently carried out
  - Maintenance: consistently engages in healthful behavior for more than 6 months
  Individuals tend to cycle through the stages of change, often not in a linear progression, and may go through the cycle several times. The most important thing is unconditional acceptance of the person, understanding of the behavior, and subtle encouragement when asked. Make information available, but do not preach or force information on clients (Samuelson, 1998).
- Determine the client's and family's knowledge of illness and treatment. Teach them about the illness and purpose of the treatment regimen if necessary. *Knowledge is power, and with it comes increased control; the more control clients have, the more likely they are to comply with the prescribed regimen.*
- ▲ Monitor the client for signs of depression that may cause noncompliance. Refer for treatment if appropriate. **EBN:** *Depression can cause increased incidence of "source memory errors," resulting in the client being unable to remember if he or she did something or just thought about doing it, which can be very serious when it involves taking needed medications (Elias, 2001). Depression was a factor resulting in noncompliance in taking glaucoma medications (Pappa et al, 2006).*
- Monitor the client's ability to follow directions, solve problems, concentrate, and read. **EB:** *Half of the adult population has deficiencies in reading or computation skills. Up to 48% of English-speaking clients do not have adequate functional health literacy (Andrus & Roth, 2002). More than 90 million Americans have limited literacy skills. Almost 2 million U.S. residents cannot speak English, and millions more speak it poorly (Dreger & Tremback, 2002).*
- Avoid using threats, pressure, and inappropriate fear arousal to increase compliance. *These measures are unethical and generally ineffective. If clients are "browbeaten" and attempts are made to shame, induce guilt, or embarrass the client, the noncompliant client will only dig deeper in his or her resolve not to change (Samuelson, 1998).*
- Determine whether the client's support system helps or hinders therapy. Bring family members and significant others into the educational process as desired by the client. **EB:** *Schizophrenic clients who have little family support are more likely to be noncompliant than are those with family support, especially if there is a history of substance abuse and difficulty recognizing own symptoms (Olfson et al, 2000).*
- Listen to the client's descriptions of abilities; encourage the client to use these abilities in self-care. When dealing with complex healthcare regimens, start the client with small behavioral changes (e.g., have a client receiving chemotherapy rinse mouth with a saliva substitute twice daily). When one step has been accomplished, add another step. *The client is often overwhelmed by what is expected and needs help with managing behavioral changes (Boehm, 1992).*
- Work with the client to develop cues that trigger needed healthcare behaviors (e.g., checking blood sugar level before putting on makeup each morning), including weekends, holidays, and vacations. *Associating cues with desired behaviors increases the frequency of these behaviors. Compliance often decreases when the client no longer has a usual routine.*
- Work with the client to develop an instruction and reminder sheet that fits medications and treatments into the client's lifestyle. *Visual reminders help increase compliance (Schlenk, Dunbar-Jacob & Engberg, 2004).*

N

- Observe the noncompliant client for possibility of secondary gain, such as increased attention, if the client continues to be ill and noncompliant. *Adolescent clients may use noncompliance as a passive form of manipulation to control their relationships with others to avoid school, work, or the legal system. Also, sometimes the illness has become part of the client's self-concept and identity and therefore meets needs (Muscari, 1998).*
- ▲ Consult with the primary care practitioner about simplifying the healthcare regimen so that it more easily fits into the client's lifestyle (e.g., taking medications once daily versus four times daily). *Complex regimens and inconvenient dose scheduling decrease compliance.*
- ▲ Refer the client for compliance therapy (motivational interviewing and cognitive behavioral therapy) for medication management for clients with schizophrenia. **EBN:** *Failure to keep up their antipsychotic medication is a major cause of relapse in people with psychosis. Compliance therapy is effective in enhancing concordance and reducing the risk of relapse (Gray, Robson & Bressington, 2002).* **EBN:** *Compliance therapy, based on cognitive-behavioral techniques, appears to be effective in enhancing compliance and preventing relapse in people with schizophrenia who are taking antipsychotic medication (Gray, Wykes & Gournay, 2002; White, 2004).*

Geriatric

- Make the client an explicit medication instruction using bulleted lists and simple icons. **EB:** *Several studies have demonstrated that use of a medication schedule increased compliance (Esposito, 1995; Raynor, Booth & Blenkinsopp, 1993).*
- ▲ If the client has sensory and coordination deficits, use a medication organizer and have the home health nurse or family place the client's medications in daily compartments. *Careful labeling, self-administration of medicine programs, simplification of drug regimens, and the use of medication compliance devices can help promote adherence in older clients (McGraw & Drennan, 2001).*
- Assess for cognitive ability to understand medication use. *Many older adult clients stop medication because of high cost and because they do not understand the importance of taking medication. Often these clients will state that they feel fine and no longer need the medication to avoid cost.*
- ▲ Ask clients if they can afford medications. Refer clients for financial help from social worker or case manager if needed. **EB:** *A small but growing proportion of Americans are unable to afford prescribed medications (Kennedy, Coyne & Sclar, 2004).*
- ▲ Monitor the client for signs of depression associated with noncompliance (e.g., refusing to eat or take medications). Refer the client for treatment of depression as needed. *Noncompliance in older adults may be a form of indirect self-destructive behavior that is associated with depression and leads to suicide (Meisekothen, 1993).* **EBN:** *One study demonstrated that depressed clients were three times more likely than nondepressed clients to be noncompliant (DiMatteo, Lepper & Croghan, 2000).*
- Use repetition, verbal cues, and memory aids, such as pictures, schedules, or reminder sheets, when teaching the healthcare regimen. Use events, such as meals, bedtime, and so on, as reminders when to take medications. **EBN:** *There may be age-related memory deficits that necessitate an increased use of measures that cue the client to perform needed healthcare behaviors (Dunbar-Jacob et al, 2000). This research demonstrated that older adults reported greater use of internal memory strategies and a preference for event-based over time-based prescription medication instructions (Branin, 2001).*
- Consider assistive medication technology, such as talking reminders and pill dispensers. *Older adult clients are relying on technology to help them adhere to increasingly complex medication regimens (Logue, 2002; Schlenk, Dunbar-Jacob & Engberg, 2004).*

Multicultural

- Assess for the influence of cultural beliefs, norms, and values on the client's ability to modify health behavior. *What the client considers normal and abnormal health behavior may be based on cultural perceptions (Leininger & McFarland, 2002). Adherence to medical treatment is influenced by the person's health beliefs, health practices, specific disease, treatment time frame, medication regimen, cognitive-affective status, worldview, and language (Barron et al, 2004). Minority clients expressed concerns and barriers to adherence that included cost, difficulty of obtaining medication, daily life hassles, and a general distrust of the medical establishment (Bender & Bender, 2005).*
- Discuss with the client those aspects of their health behavior/lifestyle that will remain unchanged by their health status. **EBN:** *Aspects of the client's life that are meaningful and valuable to him or her should be understood and preserved without change (Leininger & McFarland, 2002).*

• = Independent;   ▲ = Collaborative;   EBN = Evidence-Based Nursing;   EB = Evidence-Based

- Negotiate with the client regarding the aspects of health behavior that will need to be modified. **EBN:** *Give and take with the client will lead to culturally congruent care (Leininger & McFarland, 2002).*
- Assess the role of fatalism on the client's ability to modify health behavior. **EBN:** *Fatalistic perspectives, which involve the belief that you cannot control your own fate, may influence health behaviors in some African-American and Latino populations (Chen, 2001; Gonzalez & Kuipers, 2004).*
- Validate the client's feelings regarding the impact of health status on current lifestyle. **EBN:** *Validation is a therapeutic communication technique that lets the client know that the nurse has heard and understands what was said, and it promotes the nurse-client relationship (Heineken, 1998). Latinas' cognitions about medications were directly related to inadequate adherence (Arcia, Fernandez & Jaquez, 2004).*
- Use mechanical reminders to cue clients and improve adherence. **EBN:** *African-American and Hispanic women who used an electronic monitoring bottle for 6 months showed significant increases in adherence (Robbins et al, 2004).*

 ## Home Care

NOTE: Because the home care nurse enters the client's home as a guest, the ability of the nurse to establish a supportive, therapeutic relationship is especially important. A paradigm shift in nurses' view of noncompliance has been proposed, to include the recognition of clients as experts on their own lives, and the assessment of client social context to determine possible rationales for not following professional advice (Russell et al, 2003).

- Previously mentioned interventions may be adapted for home care use.
- Before providing any care, review the Home Health Care Bill of Rights with the client, including the right to refuse treatment. *Identifying the rights of the client demonstrates respect of the healthcare system and its representatives for client wishes.*
- If included in agency policies and procedures, also review client responsibilities with the client, which is often part of a printed Bill of Rights. *Reviewing responsibilities helps the client define roles of mutual respect and partnership with the healthcare provider.*
- When the client is noncompliant, redefine personal and health priorities (contract for services) with the client to determine alternative motivational strategies or health actions to meet health goals. *For clients to carry out desired health actions, they must perceive actions as beneficial to self and the cost of the health action as not being greater than the benefit (Rosenstock, 1974).*
- ▲ Institute self-care management to maximize client responsibility for own care. Refer to the care plan for **Powerlessness. EB:** *Client participation in care has been increased by using multiple components of self-regulation in interventions for asthma, anxiety, and smoking (Clark, Gong & Kaciroti, 2001; Clark & Nothwehr, 1997).*
- Elicit and answer questions respectfully regarding illness and treatment, correcting any misconceptions and highlighting the importance of assisting the client to incorporate treatment plan into daily lifestyle. Do not use medical jargon in explanations.
- Explore barriers to medical regimen adherence. Review medications and treatment regularly for needed modifications. Take complaints of side effects seriously and serve as the client advocate to address changes as indicated.
- ▲ If noncompliance compromises the client's health status, refer for psychiatric home healthcare services to assess the client's motivation and implement therapeutic regimen. **EBN:** *Psychiatric home care nurses can address issues relating to the client's nonadherence to treatment and inability to adjust to changes in health status. Behavioral interventions in the home can assist the client to participate more effectively in treatment plan (Patusky, Rodning & Martinez-Kratz, 1996).*
- ▲ If noncompliant behavior continues and the client chooses not to cooperate with medical regimen, the home healthcare agency cannot continue to provide services. *Reimbursement guidelines and agency policies do not support the continued use of healthcare resources when the client makes an informed decision to not follow the prescribed regimen.*
- If care is to be terminated, identify all possible alternatives for the client, and assist with making an informed choice about future health actions. *Some regulatory guidelines require healthcare providers to give written notice of discontinuance of care using established time frames. Noncompliance and a plan for termination of care notwithstanding, it remains the goal and ethical responsibility of home healthcare providers to promote optimal wellness, independence, and safety.*

• = Independent;   ▲ = Collaborative;   EBN = Evidence-Based Nursing;   EB = Evidence-Based

- Respect the wishes of terminally ill clients to refuse selected aspects of medical regimen. With terminally ill clients, do not terminate care. Provide those aspects of care that the client and family or caregivers will accept. *The goal of hospice care is to provide comfort and dignity in the dying process.*

Client/Family Teaching

▲ Teach clients about medication side effects (e.g., mental changes, sexual dysfunction) so that they understand them and feel comfortable discussing them.

- Teach clients to control their "self-talk" by giving themselves positive messages to promote desired behaviors, such as taking medications and controlling food intake. **EBN:** *Self-talk has been shown to be a common motivating method for behavior changes (McSweeney, 1993).*

evolve See the EVOLVE website for World Wide Web resources for client education.

REFERENCES

Andrus MR, Roth MT: Health literacy: a review, *Pharmacotherapy* 22(3):282, 2002.

Arcia E, Fernandez MC, Jaquez M: Latina mothers' stances on stimulant medication: complexity, conflict, and compromise, *J Dev Behav Pediatr* 25(5):311-317, 2004.

Barron F, Hunter A, Mayo R et al: Acculturation and adherence: issues for health care providers working with clients of Mexican origin, *J Transcult Nurs* 15(4):331-337, 2004.

Bender BG, Bender SE: Patient-identified barriers to asthma treatment adherence: responses to interviews, focus groups, and questionnaires, *Immunol Allergy Clin North Am* 25(1):7-30, 2005.

Bodenheimer T, Lorig K, Holman H et al: Patient self-management of chronic disease in primary care, *JAMA* 288(19):2469, 2002.

Boehm S: Patient contracting. In Bulechek GM, McCloskey JC, editors: *Nursing interventions: essential nursing treatments,* Philadelphia, 1992, WB Saunders.

Bosworth HB, Olsen MK, Gentry P et al: Nurse administered telephone intervention for blood pressure control: a patient-tailored multifactorial intervention, *Patient Educ Couns* 57:5-14, 2005.

Branin JJ: The role of memory strategies in medication adherence among the elderly, *Home Health Care Serv Q* 20(2):1, 2001.

Chen YC: Chinese values, health and nursing, *J Adv Nurs* 36(2):270, 2001.

Clark NM, Gong M, Kaciroti N: A model of self-regulation for control of chronic diseases, *Health Educ Behav* 28:769, 2001.

Clark NM, Nothwehr F: Self-management of asthma by adult patients, *Patient Educ Couns* 32:S5, 1997.

Devine EC: Meta-analysis of the effect of psychoeducational interventions on pain in adults with cancer, *Oncol Nurs Forum* 30:75-89, 2003.

DiMatteo MR, Lepper HS, Croghan TW: Depression is a risk factor for noncompliance with medical treatment: meta-analysis of the effects of anxiety and depression on patient adherence, *J Psychosoc Nurs Ment Health Serv* 38(5):37, 2000.

Dreger V, Tremback T: Optimize patient health by treating literacy and language barriers, *AORN J* 75(2):280, 2002.

Dunbar-Jacob J, Erlen JA, Schlenk EA et al: Adherence in chronic disease, *Annu Rev Nurs Res* 18:48, 2000.

Elias JW: Why caregiver depression and self-care abilities should be part of the PPS case mix methodology, *Home Healthc Nurse* 19(1):23, 2001.

Esposito L: The effects of medication education on adherence to medication regimens in an elderly population, *J Adv Nurs* 21:935, 1995.

Fernandez RS, Evans V, Griffiths RD et al: Educational interventions for mental health consumers receiving psychotropic medication: a review of the evidence, *Int J Ment Health Nurs* 15:70-80, 2006.

Gonzalez T, Kuipers J: Mexican Americans. In Giger JN, Davidhizar RE, editors: *Transcultural nursing: assessment and intervention,* St Louis, 2004, Mosby.

Gray R, Robson D, Bressington D: Medication management for people with a diagnosis of schizophrenia, *Nurs Times* 98(47):38, 2002.

Gray R, Wykes T, Gournay K: From compliance to concordance: a review of the literature on interventions to enhance compliance with antipsychotic medication, *J Psychiatr Ment Health Nurs* 9(3):277, 2002.

Haynes RB, Yao X, Degani A et al: Interventions to enhance medication adherence, *Cochrane Database Syst Rev* (4):CD000011, 2005.

Heineken J: Patient silence is not necessarily client satisfaction: communication in home care nursing, *Home Healthc Nurs* 16(2):115, 1998.

Heneghan C, Alonso-Coello P, Garcia-Alamino JM et al: Self-monitoring of oral anticoagulation: a systematic review and meta-analysis, *Lancet* 367(9508):404-411, 2006.

Kennedy J, Coyne J, Sclar D: Drug affordability and prescription non-compliance in the United States: 1997-2002, *Clin Ther* 26(4):607, 2004.

Koo M, Krass I, Aslani P: Factors influencing consumer use of written drug information, *Ann Pharmacother* 37:259-267, 2003.

Krueger KP, Berger BA, Felkey BG: Medication adherence and persistence: a comprehensive review, *Adv Ther* 22(4):313-356, 2005.

Krueger KP, Felkey BG, Berger BA: Improving adherence and persistence: a review and assessment of interventions and description of steps toward a national adherence initiative, *J Am Pharm Assoc (Wash DC)* 43(6):668-678, 2003.

Langford BJ, Jorgenson D, Kwan D et al: Implementation of a self-administered questionnaire to identify patients at risk for medication-related problems in a family health center, *Pharmacotherapy* 26:260-268, 2006.

Leininger MM, McFarland MR: *Transcultural nursing: concepts, theories, research and practices,* ed 3, New York, 2002, McGraw-Hill.

Logue RM: Self-medication and the elderly: how technology can help, *Am J Nurs* 102(7):51, 2002.

McDonald HP, Garg AX, Haynes RB: Interventions to enhance patient adherence to medication prescriptions: scientific review, *JAMA* 288(22):2868-2879, 2002.

McGraw C, Drennan V: Self-administration of medicine and older people, *Nurs Stand* 15(18):33, 2001.

McSweeney JC: Making behavior changes after a myocardial infarction, *West J Nurs Res* 15(4):441, 1993.

Meisekothen LM: Noncompliance in the elderly: a pathway to suicide, *J Am Acad Nurse Pract* 5(2):67, 1993.

Muscari ME: Rebels with a cause, *Am J Nurs* 98(12):26, 1998.

Olfson M, Mechanic D, Hansell S et al: Predicting medication noncompliance after hospital discharge among patients with schizophrenia, *Psychiatr Serv* 51(2):216, 2000.

Orensky IA, Holdford DA: Predictors of noncompliance with warfarin therapy in an outpatient anticoagulation clinic, *Pharmacotherapy* 25:1801-1808, 2005.

Ostwald SK, Wasserman J, Davis S: Medications, comorbidities, and medical complications in stroke survivors: the CAReS study, *Rehabil Nurs* 31:10-14, 2006.

Pappa C, Hyphantis T, Pappa S et al: Psychiatric manifestations and personality traits associated with compliance with glaucoma treatment, *J Psychosom Res* 61(5):609-617, 2006.

Patusky KL, Rodning C, Martinez-Kratz M: Clinical lessons in psychiatric home care: a case study approach, *J Home Healthc Manag* 9:18, 1996.

Petrilla AA, Benner JS, Battelman DS et al: Evidence-based interventions to improve patient compliance with antihypertensive and lipid-lowering medications, *Int J Clin Pract* 59:1441-1451, 2005.

Prochaska JO, Norcross J, DiClemete C: *Changing for good: a revolutionary six stage program for overcoming bad habits and moving your life positively forward,* New York, 1995, Collins.

Raynor OK, Booth TG, Blenkinsopp A: Effects of computer generated reminder charts on patients' compliance with drug regimens, *BMJ* 306:1158, 1993.

Robbins B, Rausch KJ, Garcia RI et al: Multicultural medication adherence: a comparative study, *J Gerontol Nurs* 30(7):25-32, 2004.

Robinson AW: Getting to the heart of denial, *Am J Nurs* 99(5):38, 1999.

Rosenstock I: Health belief model and preventive behavior. In Becker M, editor: *The health belief model and personal health behavior,* Thorofare, NJ, 1974, CB Slack.

Russell J, Krantz S, Neville S: The patient-provider relationship and adherence to highly active antiretroviral therapy, *J Assoc Nurses AIDS Care* 15(5):40, 2004.

Russell S, Daly J, Hughes E et al: Nurses and 'difficult' patients: negotiating noncompliance, *J Adv Nurs* 43(3):281, 2003.

Samuelson M: Stages of change: from theory to practice, *Art Health Promot* 2(5):1, 1998.

Schlenk EA, Dunbar-Jacob J, Engberg S: Medication non-adherence among older adults: a review of strategies and interventions for improvement, *J Gerontol Nursing* 30(7):33, 2004.

Sethares KA, Elliott K: The effect of a tailored message intervention on heart failure readmission rates, quality of life, and benefit and barrier beliefs in persons with heart failure, *Heart Lung* 33:249-260, 2004.

Tsoneva J, Shaw J: Understanding patients' beliefs and goals in medicine-taking, *Prof Nurse* 19(8):466-468, 2004.

Urién AM, Guillén VF, Beltran DO et al: Telephonic back-up improves antibiotic compliance in acute tonsillitis/pharyngitis, *Int J Antimicrob Agents* 23:138-143, 2004.

Ward-Collins D: "Noncompliant": isn't there a better way to say it? *Am J Nurs* 98(5):27-31, 1998.

White RB: Adherence to the dialysis prescription: partnering with patients for improved outcomes, *Nephrol Nurs J* 31(4):432, 2004.

N

Imbalanced Nutrition: less than body requirements   Betty J. Ackley, MSN, EdS, RN

NANDA   Definition

Intake of nutrients insufficient to meet metabolic needs

Defining Characteristics

Abdominal cramping; abdominal pain; aversion to eating; body weight 20% or more under ideal; capillary fragility; diarrhea; excessive loss of hair; hyperactive bowel sounds; lack of food; lack of information; lack of interest in food; loss of weight with adequate food intake; misconceptions; misinformation; pale mucous membranes; perceived inability to ingest food; poor muscle tone; reported altered taste sensation; reported food intake less than RDA (recommended daily allowance); satiety immediately after ingesting food; sore buccal cavity; steatorrhea; weakness of muscles required for swallowing or mastication

Related Factors (r/t)

Biological factors; economic factors; inability to absorb nutrients; inability to digest food; inability to ingest food; psychological factors

NOC   Outcomes (Nursing Outcomes Classification)

Suggested NOC Outcomes

Nutritional Status, Nutritional Status: Food and Fluid Intake, Nutrient Intake, Weight Control

• = Independent;   ▲ = Collaborative;   EBN = Evidence-Based Nursing;   EB = Evidence-Based

Example NOC Outcome with Indicators
Nutritional Status as evidenced by the following indicators: Food and fluid intake/Weight/height ratio/ Hematocrit (Rate the outcome and indicators of **Nutritional Status:** 1 = severe deviation from normal range, 2 = substantial deviation from normal range, 3 = moderate deviation from normal range, 4 = mild deviation from normal range, 5 = no deviation from normal range [see Section I].)

Client Outcomes

Client Will (Specify Time Frame):
- Progressively gain weight toward desired goal
- Weigh within normal range for height and age
- Recognize factors contributing to underweight
- Identify nutritional requirements
- Consume adequate nourishment
- Be free of signs of malnutrition

NIC   Interventions (Nursing Interventions Classification)

Suggested NIC Interventions

Feeding, Nutrition Management, Nutrition Therapy, Weight Gain Assistance

Example NIC Activities—Nutrition Management
Ascertain patient's food preferences; Provide patient with high-protein, high-calorie, nutritious finger foods and drinks that can be readily consumed, as appropriate

N

Nursing Interventions and _Rationales_

- ▲ Utilize a nutritional screening tool to determine possibility of malnutrition on admission into any healthcare facility. Watch for recent weight loss of over 10 pounds; 10% under healthy weight; not eating for more than three days; half of normal eating for more than five days; Body Mass Index (BMI) of less than 20; presence of large wound or surgical area; multiple trauma; or other reasons why the client may be malnourished, and refer client to a dietitian for a complete nutritional assessment (Lutz & Przytulski, 2005; Thomas et al, 2005). **EB:** _Research has shown that up to 50% of all clients are malnourished on admission, and the presence of malnutrition influences the length of stay (De Luis et al, 2006)._
- • Monitor for signs of malnutrition, including brittle hair that is easily plucked, bruises, dry skin, pale skin and conjunctiva, muscle wasting, smooth red tongue, cheilosis, "flaky paint" rash over lower extremities, and disorientation (Kasper, 2005).
- • Recognize that severe protein calorie malnutrition can result in septicemia from impairment of the immune system, organ failure including heart failure, liver failure, respiratory dysfunction, especially in the critically ill client. _Untreated malnutrition can result in death (Kasper, 2005)._
- ▲ Note laboratory test results as available: serum albumin, prealbumin, serum total protein, serum ferritin, transferrin, hemoglobin, hematocrit, and electrolytes. _A serum albumin level of less than 3.5 g/100 milliliters is considered an indicator of risk of poor nutritional status (DiMaria-Ghalili & Amella, 2005). Prealbumin level was reliable in evaluating the existence of malnutrition (Devoto et al, 2006)._
- • Weigh the client daily in acute care, weekly in extended care, at the same time of day (usually before breakfast) and with same amount of clothing.
- ▲ Monitor food intake; record percentages of served food that is eaten (25%, 50%); consult with dietitian for actual calorie count if needed.
- • Observe the client's relationship to food. Attempt to separate physical from psychological causes for eating difficulty. _Refusing to eat may be the only way the client can express some control, and it may also be a symptom of depression._

• = Independent;   ▲ = Collaborative;   EBN = Evidence-Based Nursing;   EB = Evidence-Based

- Compare usual food intake with the Food Guide Pyramid, noting slighted or omitted food groups. *Omission of entire food groups increases risk of deficiencies.*
- If the client is a vegetarian, evaluate vitamin B_{12} and iron intake. Strict vegetarians may be at particular risk for vitamin B_{12} and iron deficiencies. *Special care should be taken when implementing vegetarian diets for pregnant women, infants, children, and older adults. A dietitian can furnish a balanced vegetarian diet (with adequate substitutes for omitted foods) for inpatients and can provide instruction for outpatients (Lutz & Przytulski, 2005).*
- Observe the client's ability to eat (time involved, motor skills, visual acuity, and ability to swallow various textures). If the client needs to be fed, allocate *at least 35 minutes* to feeding. *Clients in institutions are susceptible to protein-calorie malnutrition (PCM) or protein-energy malnutrition when they are unable to feed themselves.* **EB:** *Research demonstrates it takes at least 35 minutes to feed the client who is willing to eat (Simmons, Osterweil & Schnelle, 2001; Simmons & Schnelle, 2004).*

NOTE: If the client is unable to feed self, refer to Nursing Interventions and Rationales for **Feeding Self-care deficit.** If the client has difficulty swallowing, refer to Nursing Interventions and Rationales for **Impaired Swallowing.** If the client is receiving tube feedings, refer to the Nursing Interventions and Rationales for **Risk for Aspiration.**

- ▲ If the client has a minimally functioning gastrointestinal tract and is on a diet of clear fluids, consult with a dietitian regarding use of a clear liquid product that contains increased amounts of protein and calories, such as Citrotein, Boost Breeze, or Resource Fruit Beverage.
- For the client with anorexia who will not eat foods, consider offering 30 mL of a nutritional supplement in a medication cup every hour. **EB:** *A Cochrane review found that use of oral nutritional supplements was more effective than dietary advice from a dietitian, but further studies are needed (Baldwin, Parsons & Logan, 2001). Another Cochrane review demonstrated that there was a small but consistent weight gain along with a positive effect on mortality and a shorter length of hospital stay in older adult clients who received a nutritional supplement (Milne, Potter & Avenell, 2005).*
- For the client who is malnourished and can eat, offer small quantities of energy-dense and protein-enriched food, served in an appetizing fashion, at frequent intervals. **EB:** *Small, frequent feedings of **usual food** were not effective in increasing energy intake in older adult clients (Taylor & Barr, 2006). Fortified foods were acceptable to clients if they tasted the same as regular foods, and intake resulted in increased blood levels of vitamins (Chin et al, 2001; de Jong, Chin & Paw, 2001; Dunne & Dahl, 2007).*
- If the client lacks endurance, schedule rest periods before meals, open packages, and cut up food for the client. *Nursing assistance will conserve the client's energy for eating.*
- When the client is malnourished, watch carefully for signs of infection and maintain every action possible to protect the client from infection. *Protein-energy malnutrition is associated with a significant decrease in immunity (Ritz & Gardner, 2006). Infection may result in confusion, anorexia, and negative nitrogen balance, all of which contribute to protein-energy malnutrition (Kamel, Thomas & Morley, 1998).*
- If the client is pregnant, ensure that she is receiving adequate folic acid by eating a balanced diet and taking prenatal vitamins as ordered. *All women of child-bearing potential are urged to consume 400 mcg of synthetic folic acid from fortified foods or supplements in addition to food folate from a varied diet (Lutz & Przytulski, 2005).*
- Provide companionship at mealtime to encourage nutritional intake. *Mealtime usually is a time for social interaction; often clients will eat more food if other people are present at mealtimes.* **EB:** *Compared with married subjects, mean weight loss and the prevalence of weight loss were significantly higher among widowed subjects who ate more solitary meals, more commercial meals per week, and fewer snacks and homemade meals (Shahar et al, 2001).*
- Monitor state of oral cavity (gums, tongue, mucosa, teeth). Provide good oral hygiene before and after meals. *Good oral hygiene enhances appetite; the condition of the oral mucosa is critical to the ability to eat. The oral mucosa must be moist, with adequate saliva production to facilitate the digestion of food.*
- If a client has anorexia and dry mouth from medication side effects, offer sips of fluids throughout the day, along with sugarless hard candy and chewing gum to stimulate saliva formation (DiMaria-Ghalili & Amella, 2005).

N

• = Independent;   ▲ = Collaborative;   EBN = Evidence-Based Nursing;   EB = Evidence-Based

- Determine relationship of eating and other events to onset of nausea, vomiting, diarrhea, or abdominal pain.
- Determine time of day when the client's appetite is the greatest. Offer highest calorie meal at that time. *Clients with liver disease often have their greatest appetite at breakfast time.*
- ▲ Administer antiemetics and pain medications as ordered and needed before meals. *The presence of nausea or pain decreases the appetite.*
- Prepare the client for meals. Clear unsightly supplies and excretions. Avoid invasive procedures before meals. *A pleasant environment helps promote intake.*
- If client is nauseated, remove cover of food tray before bringing it into the client's room. *The sudden, concentrated food odors that come when the cover is removed in front of the client can trigger nausea (Quinton, 1998).*
- Work with the client to develop a plan for increased activity. *Immobility leads to negative nitrogen balance that fosters anorexia.*
- If the client is anemic, offer foods rich in iron and vitamins B_{12}, C, and folic acid. *Iron in meat, fish, and poultry is absorbed more readily than iron in plants. Vitamin C increases the solubility of iron. Vitamin B_{12} and folic acid are necessary for erythropoiesis (Lutz & Przytulski, 2005).*
- For the agitated pacing client, offer finger foods (sandwiches, fresh fruit) and fluids. *If a client cannot be still, food can be consumed while pacing.*
- ▲ If a client has been malnourished for a significant length of time, consult with a dietitian and refeed carefully after correcting electrolyte balance. Watch for heart and respiratory failure. *Refeeding syndrome, a potentially fatal condition, occurs in some malnourished clients when nutrients are given (orally, by tube feeding, or parenterally) in excess of the client's ability to metabolize them. Clients at risk of refeeding syndrome must be monitored carefully for electrolyte imbalances, congestive heart failure, and respiratory failure (Lutz & Przytulski, 2005).*

Pediatric

- Watch for symptoms of malnutrition, including short stature, thin arms and legs, poor condition of skin and hair, visible vertebrae and rib cage, wasted buttocks, wasted facial appearance, lethargy, and in extreme cases, edema (Recognizing Malnutrition, 2006).
- Weigh and measure the length (height) of the child and use a growth chart to help determine growth pattern, which reflects nutrition. *Age-related growth charts are available from the Child Growth Foundation, www.childgrowthfoundation.org.*
- Determine the child's BMI after the age of 3 years (Fowler-Brown & Kahwati, 2004).
- ▲ Refer to a physician and a dietician a child who is underweight for any reason. **EB:** *Good nutrition is extremely important for children to ensure sufficient growth and development of all body systems (Morgan, Ward & Murdoch, 2004).*
- ▲ Work with parents of the underweight child to improve the child's nutritional status as needed by:
  - Referring to a breast feeding specialist if needed
  - Teaching how to select, prepare, and handle appropriate food for the age of the child
  - Teaching when to introduce solid foods and progress weaning
  - Advising on the appropriate range of food and portion sizes for children
  - Advising the parent to accept the child's natural size and shape, because the child needs the parents' unconditional love
  - Make family meals a priority (Neumark-Sztainer et al, 2003)
  - Involving the child in menu planning, cooking, and preparing food, as appropriate for the child's age
  - Encouraging children to love their bodies

  Areas of concern that may be causing malnutrition should be discussed with the parents, and referrals made as necessary, including to physician, dietitian, or specialist, such as a speech therapist, to help with swallowing (Recognizing Malnutrition, 2006).
- Work with the child and parent to develop an appropriate weight gain plan. *The goal with a child is sometimes to maintain existing weight as the body grows taller (Fowler-Brown & Kahwati, 2004).*
- Recognize that a large percentage of girls and teenagers are dieting, which can result in nutritional problems.

Geriatric

- Assess for protein-energy malnutrition in older adult clients regardless of setting. Use a screening tool, such as the Nutritional Risk Screening (NRS) if in acute care, or the Mini Nutritional Assessment (MNA) if in long term care or living in the community (Sieber, 2006). *It is imperative to assess older adult clients for malnutrition, because it is so common in this population (DiMaria-Ghalili & Amella, 2005).* **EB:** *Underweight older adults with a BMI less than 20 who have difficulty feeding themselves or bathing were found to be at greatest risk of dying in the hospital (Thomas et al, 2005).* **EBN:** *Malnutrition is a frequent and serious problem in older adults; there is no doubt that malnutrition contributes significantly to morbidity and mortality in older clients (Chen, Schilling & Lyder, 2001).*
- Assess for factors contributing to a current acute illness, such as dehydration and the presence of diarrhea. **EBN:** *Dehydration is the most common fluid and electrolyte imbalance in older adults. Offering fluids and maintaining intake of 1600 mL/day ensures adequate hydration (Hodgkinson, Evans & Wood, 2003).* **EB:** *Diarrhea and malabsorption can cause unexplained weight loss. Clients may not admit to having chronic diarrhea, particularly if they also are incontinent (Holt, 2001).*
- ▲ Interpret laboratory findings cautiously. *Compromised kidney function makes reliance on blood and urine samples for nutrient analyses less reliable in older adults than in younger persons.* **EBN:** *Because it is correlated to urine specific gravity and urine osmolality, observing urine color is a low-cost method of monitoring dehydration (Wakefield et al, 2002).*
- Offer high-protein supplements based on individual needs and capabilities. *Clients with decreased kidney function may not be able to excrete the waste products from protein metabolism.*
- Recognize that constipation is a common problem with older clients, therefore they avoid many types of food for fear of problems with their bowel regimen. **EBN:** *A fiber supplement in the form of raw bran is not always tolerated by older adults. Studies indicate that daily consumption of fruit and fiber-rich porridge has a positive effect on stool frequency and consistency when compared to laxative use (Wisten, 2005).*
- Give the client a choice of supplements, including a taste test, to increase personal control. If the client is unwilling to drink a glass of liquid supplement, offer 30 mL/hr in a medication cup. **EB:** *Alternatively, offer 3 oz supplement with each medication pass (Lewis & Boyle, 1998). Older adults will often take medications when they will not take food. The supplement is then served as a medicine.*
- Offer liquid energy supplements. **EB:** *Older nursing home residents gained an average of 3.3 lb in 60 days when consuming an average of 400 kilocalories (kcal) per day of oral supplements (Lauque et al, 2000). A Cochrane Review demonstrated that there was a small but consistent weight gain along with a positive effect on mortality and a shorter length of hospital stay in older clients who received a nutritional supplement (Milne, Potter & Avenell, 2005).*
- Unless medically contraindicated, permit self-selected seasonings and foods.
- Serve food in a restaurant style manner if possible. **EB:** *Older adults generally eat more when they go out to eat (Castro, 2002). Food served family style increased food ingestion and decreased the number of older clients with malnutrition in a nursing home (Nijs et al, 2006).*
- Encourage physical activity and toileting assistance before meals. **EB:** *Exercise and scheduling toileting intervention may improve oral food and fluid consumption during meals and bowel movement frequency in nursing home residents (Simmons, 2004).*
- Assess components of bone health: older adults need 1200 mg calcium daily and adequate vitamin D.
- Recognize that older women may continue their younger preoccupation with weight and recurrent dieting, despite being at normal weight.
- Assess for psychological and mental factors that impact nutrition. Watch for signs of depression. *Malnutrition is commonly found with depression in the elderly (Stewart, 2004).* **EB:** *Nutritional risk independently increased the likelihood of death in cognitively impaired older adults (Keller & Ostbye, 2000). Emotions affect food intake. The presence of anxiety and anger decreased food intake in older adults (Paquet et al, 2003).*
- Provide soothing music during meals. **EBN:** *Findings from this study suggest that soothing music selections have beneficial effects on relaxation in community-residing older adults (Lai, 2004).*

N

● = Independent;   ▲ = Collaborative;   EBN = Evidence-Based Nursing;   EB = Evidence-Based

▲ Provide appropriate diet for ability to chew food. Insert dentures (if needed) before meals. Assess the fit of dentures. Refer the client for dental consultation if needed.

NOTE: If the client is unable to feed self, refer to Nursing Interventions and Rationales for **Feeding Self-care deficit.** If the client has impaired physical function, malnutrition, depression and cognitive impairment, please refer to care plan on **Adult Failure to thrive.**

Multicultural

- Assess for dietary intake of essential nutrients. **EB:** *African-American women have calcium intakes of less than 75% of the RDA (Zablah et al, 1999). Hispanics with type 2 diabetes also often have inadequate protein nutritional status (Castaneda, Bermudez & Tucker, 2000). Mexican-American women have a higher prevalence of iron-deficiency anemia than non-Hispanic white females (Frith-Terhune et al, 2000). Rural African-American men had low caloric intakes coupled with high fat intakes and nutrient deficiencies (Vitolins et al, 2000). African-American adolescents have some of the highest levels of vitamin D deficiency (Gordon et al, 2004).*
- Assess for the influence of cultural beliefs, norms, and values on the client's nutritional knowledge. *What the client considers normal dietary practices may be based on cultural perceptions (Leininger & McFarland, 2002). Among African Americans, there was a general perception that "eating healthfully" meant giving up part of their cultural heritage, trying to conform to the dominant culture, and feeling that friends and relatives usually were not supportive of dietary changes (James, 2004).*
- Discuss with the client those aspects of their diet that will remain unchanged. Negotiate with the client regarding the aspects of his or her diet that will need to be modified. *Aspects of the client's life that are meaningful and valuable to them should be understood and preserved without change (Leininger & McFarland, 2002).*
- Encourage family meals. **EB:** *Frequency of family meals was positively associated with intake of fruits, vegetables, grains, and calcium-rich foods, and negatively associated with soft drink consumption (Neumark-Sztainer et al, 2003).*

Home Care

- Previously mentioned interventions may be adapted for home care use.
- Monitor food intake. Instruct the client in intake of small frequent meals of foods with increased calories and protein.
- Assess a client's willingness to eat; fashion interventions accordingly. **EBN:** *Older adults reported that factors influencing appetite included mood, personal value, wholesomeness, food (preparation, consistency, and freshness), pleasantness of eating environment, and meal companionship (Wikby & Fagerskiold, 2004).*
- ▲ Assess the client for depression. Refer for mental health services as indicated. *Decreased appetite with weight loss is part of the syndrome of depression. Return of appetite is unlikely unless the underlying depression is treated.*
- Consider social factors that may interfere with nutrition (e.g., lack of transportation, inadequate income, lack of social support). **EB:** *Increasing the number of people present at meals was effective in increasing food intake in free-living elderly (DeCastro, 2002).*
- ▲ Monitor the effect of total parenteral nutrition (TPN) as ordered by physician, and use appropriate interventions including weight, blood glucose levels, electrolytes, symptoms of fluid overload or deficit, and symptoms of infection at entry site of catheter. Please refer to the guideline entitled "Total Parenteral Nutrition Administration" in *Evidence-Based Nursing Care Guidelines: Medical Surgical Interventions* for more information on care (Gorski, in press).
- ▲ In the presence of a diagnosis of depression, refer the client for psychiatric home healthcare services for client reassurance and implementation of therapeutic regimen. *Poor appetite and weight loss are symptoms of depression.*

Client/Family Teaching

- Help the client/family identify the area to change that will make the greatest contribution to improved nutrition.
- Build on the strengths in the client's/family's food habits. Adapt changes to their current practices.

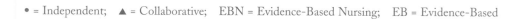

- Select appropriate teaching aids for the client's/family's background.
- Implement instructional follow-up to answer the client's/family's questions.
- Suggest community resources as suitable (food sources, counseling, Meals on Wheels, senior centers).
- Teach the client and family how to manage tube feedings or parenteral therapy at home.

 See the EVOLVE website for World Wide Web resources for client education.

REFERENCES

Baldwin C, Parsons T, Logan S: Dietary advice for illness-related malnutrition in adults, *Cochrane Database Syst Rev* (2):CD002008, 2001.

Castaneda C, Bermudez OI, Tucker KL: Protein nutritional status and functions are associated with type II diabetes in Hispanic elders, *Am J Clin Nutr* 72(1):89, 2000.

Chen CC, Schilling LS, Lyder CH: A concept analysis of malnutrition in the elderly, *J Adv Nurs* 36(1):131-142, 2001.

Chin A, Paw MJ, de Jong N et al: Physical exercise and /or enriched foods for functional improvement in frail, independently living elderly: a randomized controlled trial, *Arch Phys Med Rehabil* 82(6):811-817, 2001.

DeCastro JM: Age-related changes in the social, psychological, and temporal influences on food intake in free-living, healthy, adult humans, *J Gerontol* 57A(6):M368-M377, 2002.

de Jong N, Chin A, Paw MJ et al: Appraisal of 4 months consumption of nutrient-dense foods within the daily feeding pattern of frail elderly, *J Aging Health* 13(2):200-216, 2001.

De Luis DA, Izaola O, Cuellar L et al: Nutritional assessment: predictive variables at hospital admission related with length of stay, *Ann Nutr Metab* 50(4):394-398, 2006.

Devoto G, Gallo F, Marchello C et al: Prealbumin serum concentrations as a useful tool in the assessment of malnutrition in hospitalized patients, *Clin Chem* 52(12):2281-2285, 2006.

DiMaria-Ghalili RA, Amella E: Nutrition in older adults, *Am J Nurs* 105(3):40, 2005.

Dunne JL, Dahl WJ: A novel solution is needed to correct low nutrient intakes in elderly long-term care residents, *Nutr Rev* 65(3):135-139, 2007.

Fowler-Brown A, Kahwati LC: Prevention and treatment of overweight in children and adolescents, *Am Fam Physician* 69(11):2591-2598, 2004.

Frith-Terhune AL, Cogswell ME, Khan LK et al: Iron deficiency anemia: higher prevalence in Mexican American than in non-Hispanic white females in the third National Health and Nutrition Examination Survey, 1988-1994, *Am J Clin Nutr* 72(4):963-968, 2000.

Gordon CM, DePeter KC, Feldman HA et al: Prevalence of vitamin D deficiency among healthy adolescents, *Arch Pediatr Adolesc Med* 158(6):531-537, 2004.

Gorski LA: Total parenteral nutrition administration. In Ackley B et al, editors. *Evidence-based nursing care guidelines: medical surgical interventions*, Philadelphia, Mosby (in press).

Hodgkinson B, Evans D, Wood J: Maintaining oral hydration in older adults: a systematic review, *Int J Nurs Pract* 9(3):S19-S28, 2003.

Holt PR: Diarrhea and malabsorption in the elderly, *Gastroenterol Clin North Am* 30(2):427, 2001.

James DC: Factors influencing food choices, dietary intake, and nutrition-related attitudes among African Americans: application of a culturally sensitive model, *Ethn Health* 9(4):349-367, 2004.

Kamel HK, Thomas DR, Morley JE: National deficiencies in long-term care: part II. Management of protein-energy malnutrition and dehydration, *Ann Long Term Care* 6:250, 1998.

Kasper DL: *Harrison's principles of internal medicine*, ed 16, New York, 2005, McGraw-Hill.

Keller HH, Ostbye T: Do nutrition indicators predict death in elderly Canadians with cognitive impairment? *Can J Public Health* 91:220, 2000.

Lai H: Music preference and relaxation in Taiwanese elderly people, *Geriatr Nurs* 25(5):286-291, 2004.

Lauque S, Arnaud-Battandier F, Mansourian R et al: Protein-energy oral supplementation in malnourished nursing-home residents. A controlled trial, *Age Ageing* 29(1):51-56, 2000.

Leininger MM, McFarland MR: *Transcultural nursing: concepts, theories, research and practices*, ed 3, New York, 2002, McGraw-Hill.

Lewis DA, Boyle KD: Nutritional supplement use during medication administration: selected case studies, *J Nutr Elderly* 17:53, 1998.

Lutz CA, Przytulski KR: *Nutrition and diet therapy*, ed 4, Philadelphia, 2005, FA Davis.

Milne AC, Potter J, Avenell A: Protein and energy supplementation in elderly people at risk from malnutrition, *Cochrane Database Syst Rev* (2):CD003288, 2005.

Morgan A, Ward E, Murdoch B: Clinical characteristics of acute dysphagia in pediatric patients following traumatic brain injury, *J Head Trauma Rehabil* 19(3):226-240, 2004.

Neumark-Sztainer D, Hannan PJ, Story M et al: Family meal patterns: associations with sociodemographic characteristics and improved dietary intake among adolescents, *J Am Diet Assoc* 103(3):317-322, 2003.

Nijs KA, deGraaf C, Siebelink E et al: Effect of family-style meals on energy intake and risk of malnutrition in Dutch nursing home residents: a randomized controlled trial, *J Gerontol A Biol Sci Med Sci* 61(9):935-942, 2006.

Paquet C, St-Arnaud-McKenzie D, Kergoat MJ et al: Direct and indirect effects of everyday emotions on food intake of elderly patients in institutions, *J Gerontol A Biol Sci Med Sci* 58(2):153-158, 2003.

Quinton D: Anticipatory nausea and vomiting in chemotherapy, *Prof Nurse* 13(10): 663, 1998.

Recognizing malnutrition, *Paediatr Nurs* 18(5):30, 2006.

Ritz, BS, Gardner EM: Recent advances in nutritional sciences, *J Nutr* 136(5):1141-1145, 2006.

Shahar DR, Schultz R, Shahar A et al: The effect of widowhood on weight change, dietary intake, and eating behavior in the elderly population, *J Aging Health* 13(2):189-199, 2001.

Sieber CC: Nutritional screening tools—How does the MNA compare? Proceedings of the session held in Chicago May 2-3, 2006, *J Nutr Health Aging* 10(6):488-492, 2006.

Simmons S: Effects of an exercise and scheduled toileting intervention on appetite and constipation in nursing home residents, *J Nutr Health Aging* 8(2):116-121, 2004.

N

Simmons SF, Osterweil D, Schnelle JF: Improving food intake in nursing home residents with feeding assistance: a staffing analysis, *J Gerontol A Biol Sci Med Sci* 56(12):M790-M794, 2001.

Simmons SF, Schnelle JF: Individualized feeding assistance care for nursing home residents: staffing requirements to implement two interventions, *J Gerontol A Biol Sci Med Sci* 59(9):M966-M973, 2004.

Stewart JT: Why don't physicians consider depression in the elderly? *Postgrad Med* 115(6):57, 2004.

Taylor KA, Barr S: Provision of small, frequent meals does not improve energy intake of elderly residents with dysphagia who live in an extended-care facility. *J Am Diet Assoc* 106(7):115, 2006.

Thomas DR, Kamel H, Azharrudin M et al: The relationship of functional status, nutritional assessment, and severity of illness to in-hospital mortality, *J Health Nutr Aging* 9(3):169-175, 2005.

Vitolins MZ, Quandt SA, Case LD et al: Ethnic and gender variation in the dietary intake of rural elders, *J Nutr Elderly* 19(3):15-30, 2000.

Wakefield B, Mentes J, Diggleman L et al: Monitoring hydration status in elderly veterans, *West J Nurs Res* 24(2):132-142, 2002.

Wikby K, Fagerskiold A: The willingness to eat: an investigation of appetite among elderly people, *Scand J Caring Sci* 18:120, 2004.

Wisten A: Fruit and fiber (Pajala porridge) in the prevention of constipation, *Scand J Caring Sci,* 19(1):71-76, 2005.

Zablah EM, Reed DB, Hegsted M et al: Barriers to calcium intake in African American women, *J Hum Nutr Diet* 12(2):123-132, 1999.

Imbalanced Nutrition: more than body requirements

Betty J. Ackley, MSN, EdS, RN

NANDA   Definition

Intake of nutrients that exceeds metabolic needs

Defining Characteristics

Concentrating food intake at the end of the day; dysfunctional eating pattern (e.g., pairing food with other activities); eating in response to external cues (e.g., time of day, social situation); eating in response to internal cues other than hunger (e.g., anxiety); sedentary activity level; triceps skin fold >25 mm in women, >15 mm in men; weight 20% over ideal for height and frame

Related Factors (r/t)

Excessive intake in relation to metabolic need

NOC   Outcomes (Nursing Outcomes Classification)

Suggested NOC Outcomes

Nutritional Status: Food and Fluid Intake, Nutrient Intake, Weight Control

Example NOC Outcome with Indicators
Weight Control as evidenced by the following indicators: Demonstrates progress toward target weight/Balances exercise with caloric intake/Maintains recommended eating pattern/Controls preoccupation with food (Rate the outcome and indicators of **Weight Control:** 1 = never demonstrated, 2 = rarely demonstrated, 3 = sometimes demonstrated, 4 = often demonstrated, 5 = consistently demonstrated [see Section I].)

Client Outcomes

Client Will (Specify Time Frame):

- State pertinent factors contributing to weight gain
- Identify behaviors that remain under client's control
- Design dietary modifications to meet individual long-term goal of weight control
- Lose weight in a reasonable period (1 to 2 lb per week)
- Incorporate appropriate activities requiring energy expenditure into daily life

• = Independent;   ▲ = Collaborative;   EBN = Evidence-Based Nursing;   EB = Evidence-Based

| NIC | Interventions (Nursing Interventions Classification) |

Suggested NIC Interventions

Eating Disorders Management, Nutrition Management, Nutritional Counseling, Weight Management, Weight Reduction Assistance

Example NIC Activities—Weight Management
Determine individual's motivation for changing eating habits; Develop with the individual a method to keep daily record of intake, exercise sessions, and by changes in body weight

Nursing Interventions and *Rationales*

- Ask the client to keep a food diary for 1-3 days, where everything ingested (food and drink) is recorded. **EB:** *Use of self-monitoring tools that meet the needs of clients increases dietary reporting and promotes self-efficacy (Mossavar-Rahmani et al, 2004).*
- Advise the client to measure food periodically. Help the client learn usual portion sizes. *Measuring food alerts the client to normal portion sizes. Estimating amounts can be extremely inaccurate.* **EB:** *Women who were served either larger portions or more calorie-dense foods in the same portion size ate the extra calories instead of decreasing their calorie intake (Kral, Roe & Rolls, 2004). Young adults who self-selected portion sizes for breakfast and dinner chose larger portions (Schwartz & Byrd-Bredbenner, 2006). Group training effectively teaches how to accurately estimate and measure food portion sizes (Ayala, 2006).*
- Help the client determine their body mass index (BMI). *Use a chart or a website, such as http://www.bcm.edu/cnrc/caloriesneed.htm. A normal BMI is 20 to 25, 26 to 29 is overweight, and a BMI of greater than 30 is obese (Nix, 2005).*
- Recommend the client follow the U.S. Dietary Guidelines, which can be found at www.healthierus.gov/dietaryguidelines. *Dietary guidelines are written by national experts and based on research in nutrition.*
- Recommend the client use the interactive Food Guide Pyramid site at www.MyPyramid.gov to determine the number of calories to eat, and gain more information on how to eat in a healthy fashion. *To lose weight, the client must eat fewer calories.* **EB**: *Safe choices for weight loss include low calorie diets, such as the DASH diet or a Weight Watchers type of diet (Strychar, 2006). Eating a low calorie, low fat diet is one of many factors associated with maintenance of the weight loss (Wing & Phelan, 2005).*
- Recommend that the client lose weight slowly, no more than 1-2 pounds per week, based on a healthy eating pattern and increased exercise. The number of calories consumed should be at least 1600 for men, and 1300 for women. *Slower weight loss is generally more likely to be lasting weight loss. It is important that increased activity is included to help burn more calories (Ruser, Federman & Kashaf, 2005).*
- Demonstrate the use of food labels to make healthful choices. Alert the client/family to focus on serving size, total fat, and simple carbohydrates. *The standardized food label in bold type simplifies the search for information. Fats and sugars contribute the least to a healthful diet and the most to excessive calorie intake. Generally, clients should eat foods that are no more than 30% fat (Nix, 2005).*
- Weigh the client twice a week under the same conditions. *It is important to most clients and contributes to their progress to have the tangible reward that the scale shows. Monitoring twice a week allows for frequent feedback to encourage the client to continue with the program.*
- Watch the client for signs of depression, such as flat affect, poor sleeping habits, or lack of interest in life. *Depression is found in at least one third of all obese persons (Ruser, Federman & Kashaf, 2005).*

Pattern of Dietary Intake

- Recommend the client eat a healthy breakfast every morning. **EB:** *People who skip breakfast are more likely to overeat in the evening and are 450 times more likely to be obese (deCastro, 2004; Ma et al, 2003). Less than half of the people who binge on food eat breakfast; those people who eat breakfast weigh less than those who do not (Masheb & Grillo, 2006). Eating breakfast regularly is one of many factors associated with maintenance of weight loss (Wing & Phelan, 2005).*

N

• = Independent;   ▲ = Collaborative;   EBN = Evidence-Based Nursing;   EB = Evidence-Based

- Recommend the client avoid eating in fast food restaurants. **EB:** *People who often eat fast foods gain an average of 10 lb more than those who eat fast food less often, and are two times more likely to develop insulin resistance, which can lead to diabetes (Pereira, Kartashov & Ebbeling, 2005).*
- ▲ Obtain a thorough history. Refer to a dietitian if the client has a medical condition. *The most appropriate clients for the nursing intervention of weight management are adults with no other major health problems requiring medical nutritional therapy.*

Recommended Foods/Fluids

- Encourage the client to increase intake of vegetables and fruits to at least five servings per day, preferably 9 servings per day. **EB:** *Women who increase their fruit and vegetable intake to 4 servings per day have a 24% lower risk of obesity than those who eat only 2 servings per day (He et al, 2004).*
- Encourage the client to eat at least 3 servings of whole grains per day, preferably more. **EB:** *Men who eat more whole grains have decreased weight gain (Koh-Banerjee et al, 2004).*
- Evaluate the client's usual intake of fiber. *In general, high-fiber foods take longer to eat and contain fewer calories than most other foods.*
- Discuss the possibility of using a primarily plant-based or vegetarian diet to lose weight. **EB:** *The weight and BMI of vegetarians is on average 3% to 20% lower than that of nonvegetarians (Berkow & Barnard, 2006). People who voluntarily choose a lacto-ovo-vegetarian diet as part of a weight loss treatment are able to continue with the diet for 18 months (Burke et al, 2006).*
- Encourage the client to **decrease** intake of sugars, including soft drinks, desserts, and candy. *Sugar predisposes to dental caries, and also is a source of calories that is empty of other nutrients (Nix, 2005). Consuming excessive amounts of fructose, which is used to sweeten soft drinks, other foods with a high glycemic index, and insufficient high-fiber grains may result in development of type 2 diabetes (Wu et al, 2004).*
- Recommend client increases intake of water to at least 2000 mL, or 2 quarts per day. A guideline is 1-1.5 mL of fluid per each calorie needed, so an average intake would be between 2000 and 3000 mL/day, or at least 8 cups of fluid (Grodner, Long & DeYoung, 2004). *The adequate intake recommendation is 3 L for the 19- to 30-year-old male and 2.2 L for the 19- to 30-year-old female. Water balance studies suggest that adult men require 2.5 liters per day (Institute of Medicine, 2004).*
- For more information on healthy eating, refer to nursing interventions for **Readiness for enhanced Nutrition.**

Behavioral Methods for Weight Loss

- Familiarize the client with the following behavior modification techniques:
  - Self-monitoring of food intake, including keeping a food and exercise diary
  - Graphing weight weekly
  - Controlling stimuli that causes overeating, such as watching television with frequent food-related commercials
  - Limiting food intake to one site in the home
  - Sitting down at the table to eat
  - Planning food intake for each day
  - Rearranging the schedule to avoid inappropriate eating
  - Avoiding boredom that results in eating; keeping a list of activities on the refrigerator
  - For a party, eating before arriving, sitting away from the snack foods, and substituting lower-calorie beverages for alcoholic ones
  - Deciding beforehand what to order in a restaurant
  - Bringing only healthy foods into the house to decrease temptation
  - Slowing mealtime by swallowing food before putting more food on the utensil, pausing for a minute during the meal and attempting to increase the number of pauses, and trying to be the last one to finish eating
  - Drinking a glass of water before each meal; taking sips of water between bites of food
  - Charting one's progress
  - Making an agreement with oneself or a significant other for a meaningful reward and not rewarding oneself with food
  - Changing one's mindset, as in control of eating behavior

• = Independent;   ▲ = Collaborative;   EBN = Evidence-Based Nursing;   EB = Evidence-Based

- Viewing exercise as a means of controlling hunger
- Practicing relaxation techniques
- Visualizing oneself enjoying a fresh apple in preference to apple pie

EB: *Cognitive-behavior therapy, when combined with a diet and exercise intervention, results in more weight loss than diet and exercise alone. Behavioral therapy used independently as a stand-alone therapy also results in significant weight loss (Shaw et al, 2006). Weight loss methods including dietary, exercise, or behavioral interventions result in significant weight loss among people with prediabetes. These methods also decrease development of diabetes (Norris et al, 2005).*

Physical Activity

▲ Assess for reasons why the client would be unable to participate in an exercise program; refer the client for evaluation by a primary care practitioner as needed. *Encourage activity to help with weight loss.*

- Use the Outcome Expectation for Exercise Scale to determine the client's self-efficacy expectations and outcomes expectations toward exercise. **EBN:** *The client's self-efficacy expectations and outcome expectations for exercise will greatly influence his or her willingness to exercise. If the individual has a low outcome, interventions can be implemented to strengthen the expectations and hopefully improve exercise behavior (Resnick, Zimmerman & Orwig, 2001).*
- Recommend the client enter an exercise program with a friend. **EBN:** *Findings from a study of exercise behavior found that friends have the strongest influence to keep on an exercise program, more than family members or experts (Resnick, Orwig & Magaziner, 2002).*
- Recommend the client begin a walking program using the following guidelines:
  - Buy a pedometer
  - Determine times when walking can be incorporated into usual lifestyle
  - Set a goal of walking 10,000 steps per day, or 5 miles per day.
  - If the client does not have required number of steps when he or she comes home from work, go for another walk until the designated goal of 10,000 steps per day is reached.

EB: *Use of a pedometer results in two times the usual amount of activity and weight loss in overweight adults (VanWormer, 2004). Middle-aged women who walk more have lower BMIs; women who walk 10,000 or more steps per day are in the normal range for BMI (Thompson, Rakow & Perdue, 2004).*

 Pediatric

- Work with parents of the overweight child by encouraging the following behaviors:
  - Emphasize providing good food, not depriving children of food. *Trying to get children to eat less or move more for weight control generally backfires and makes the child preoccupied with food and unwilling to move unless forced.*
  - Accept the child's natural size and shape, because the child needs the parents' unconditional love
  - Make family meals a priority
  - Involve the child in planning menus, cooking, and preparing foods as appropriate for the child's age
  - Educate parents to participate in activities with children
  - Encourage children to love their bodies

  These methods can help children who are overweight without causing harm to the child (Satter, 2005).
- Determine the child's BMI after the child is 3 years old (Fowler-Brown & Kahwati, 2004). *The Centers for Disease Control and Prevention (CDC) BMI chart for children and teens is available at www.cdc.gov/nccdphp/dnpa/bmi/bmi-for-age.htm.* **EB:** *Children who are overweight or obese have a higher risk for being overweight or obese as adults; children in the high normal weight range also have an elevated risk of becoming overweight or obese (Field, Cook & Gillman, 2005).*
- Work with the child and parent to develop an appropriate weight maintenance plan, including behavioral methods of weight loss as well as increased activity. *The goal with a child is often to maintain existing weight as the body grows taller (Fowler-Brown & Kahwati, 2004).* **EB:** *There is insufficient data to determine the effectiveness of obesity prevention programs, although reduction in sedentary behaviors and increased activity are probably appropriate (Campbell et al, 2002).*

• = Independent;   ▲ = Collaborative;   EBN = Evidence-Based Nursing;   EB = Evidence-Based

- Encourage children to increase the amount of walking done per day, if they are willing, and ask them to wear a pedometer to measure number of steps. **EB:** *The recommended number of steps per day to have a healthy body composition is 12,000 for a 6- to 12-year-old girl and 15,000 for a boy (Tudor-Locke et al, 2004).*
- Do not use food as a reward for good behavior, especially foods that are concentrated sources of sugar or fat. *This practice may make "bad" food more desirable (www.obesity.org).*
- Recommend the child decrease television viewing, watching movies, and playing video games. Ask parents to limit television to 1 to 2 hours per day maximum (Calamaro & Faith, 2004). **EB:** *Girls who watch more TV have a higher BMI and percentage of body fat (Davison, Downs & Birch, 2006).*

Geriatric

- Assess changes in lifestyle and eating patterns. *Energy needs decrease an estimated 5% per decade after the age of 40 years, but eating patterns often remain unchanged from youth.*
- Assess fluid intake. Recommend routine drinks of water regardless of thirst. *Thirst sensation becomes dulled in older adults.*
- Observe for socioeconomic factors that influence food choices (e.g., inadequate funds or cooking facilities). *Even those on restricted budgets and with limited facilities can be helped to choose food sources for a balanced diet.*
- Suggest a variety of seasonings. *The ability to taste sweet, bitter, sour, and salty declines in most but not all older persons (Miller, 2004).*

Multicultural

- Assess for the influence of cultural beliefs, norms, acculturation, and values on the client's nutritional knowledge and practices. *What the client considers normal dietary practices may be based on cultural perceptions (Leininger & McFarland, 2002). Among African Americans, there was a general perception that "eating healthfully" meant giving up part of their cultural heritage (James, 2004). A higher risk for obesity among Latino immigrants was associated with length of residence in the United States and may be due to acculturation processes, such as the adoption of a diet high in fat and low in fruits and vegetables and sedentary lifestyles of the host country (Kaplan et al, 2004). Another study suggests that acculturation to the United States is a risk factor for obesity-related behaviors among Asian-American and Hispanic adolescents (Unger et al, 2004).*

- Encourage parental efforts at increasing physical activity and decreasing dietary fat for their children. **EB:** *Physical activity and dietary fat consumption were inversely related among African-American girls (Thompson et al, 2004). Interventions to increase physical activity among preadolescent African-American girls may benefit from a parental component to encourage support and self-efficacy for daughters' physical activity (Adkins et al, 2004).*
- Assess for the influence of cultural beliefs, norms, and values on the client's idea of acceptable body weight and body size. *Ideal body weight and size may be based on cultural perceptions (Leininger & McFarland, 2002).* **EB:** *African-American women report more satisfaction with body size than other women (Miller et al, 2000). Overweight Hispanic women with high levels of binge eating and depression preferred a slim body ideal (Fitzgibbon et al, 1998).*
- Discuss with the client those aspects of his or her diet that will remain unchanged, and work with the client to adapt cultural core foods. *Aspects of the client's life that are meaningful and valuable to the client should be understood and preserved without change (Leininger & McFarland, 2002).* **EB:** *Dramatic weight loss was achieved in Hawaii using a culturally appropriate methodology (Shintani et al, 1991).*
- Negotiate with the client regarding the aspects of his or her diet that will need to be modified. *Give and take with the client will lead to culturally congruent care (Leininger & McFarland, 2002).*
- Validate the client's feelings regarding the impact of current lifestyle, finances, and transportation on the ability to obtain and prepare nutritious food.
- Limit television viewing and consumption of soft drinks.
- Encourage family meals. **EB:** *Frequency of family meals was positively associated with intake of fruits, vegetables, grains, and calcium-rich foods, and negatively associated with soft drink consumption (Neumark-Sztainer et al, 2003).*

• = Independent;   ▲ = Collaborative;   EBN = Evidence-Based Nursing;   EB = Evidence-Based

Client/Family Teaching

- Provide the client and family with information regarding the treatment plan options. *If the client and family select the treatment plan, they are more likely to comply with it, particularly if the client does not do the marketing and cooking.*
- Inform the client about the health risks associated with obesity, which include cancer, diabetes, heart disease, strokes, hypertension, gastroesophageal reflux, gallstones, osteoarthritis, and venous thrombosis (Nutrition Action, 2004).
- Inform the client and family of the disadvantages of trying to lose weight by dieting alone. *Resting metabolic rate is decreased as much as 45% with extreme calorie restriction. The decrease persists after the diet period has ended, which leads to the "yo-yo effect." With a reduced-calorie diet alone, as much as 25% of the weight lost can be lean body mass rather than fat. Resting energy expenditure is positively related to lean body mass (Lutz & Przytulski, 2005).*
- Teach the importance of exercise in a weight control program.
- Recommend the client receive adequate amounts of sleep. **EB:** *Sleep deprivation, less than 7 hours per night, is associated with an increased risk of obesity (Tufts University, 2005). Another study demonstrated an association between short sleep duration and obesity in young adults (Hasler et al, 2004). Sleep curtailment in young healthy men resulted in increased hunger and appetite (Spiegel et al, 2004).*
- Teach stress reduction techniques as alternatives to eating. *The client should have available a variety of healthy behaviors to substitute for unhealthy ones.*

evolve   See the EVOLVE website for World Wide Web resources for client education.

REFERENCES

Adkins S, Sherwood NE, Story M et al: Physical activity among African-American girls: the role of parents and the home environment, *Obes Res* 12(suppl):S38-S45, 2004.

Ayala GX: An experimental evaluation of a group- versus computer-based intervention to improve food portion size estimation skills, *Health Educ Res* 21(1):133-145, 2006.

Berkow SE, Barnard N: Vegetarian diets and weight status, *Nutr Rev* 64(4):175-188, 2006.

Burke LE, Choo J, Music E et al: PREFER study: a randomized clinical trial testing treatment preference and two dietary options in behavioral weight management-rationale, design and baseline characteristics, *Contemp Clin Trials* 27(1):34-48, 2006.

Calamaro CJ, Faith MS: Preventing childhood overweight, *Nutr Today* 39(5):194, 2004.

Campbell K, Waters E, O'Meara S et al: Interventions for preventing obesity in children, *Cochrane Database Syst Rev* (2):CD001871, 2002.

Davison KK, Downs DS, Birch LL: Pathways linking perceived athletic competence and parental support at age 9 years to girls' physical activity at age 11 years, *Res Q Exerc Sport* 77(1):23-31, 2006.

deCastro JM: The time of day of food intake influences overall intake in humans, *J Nutr* 134(1):104-111, 2004.

Field AE, Cook NR, Gillman MW: Weight status in childhood as a predictor of becoming overweight or hypertensive in early adulthood, *Obes Res* 13(1):163, 2005.

Fitzgibbon ML, Spring B, Avellone ME et al: Correlates of binge eating in Hispanic, black and white women, *Int J Eat Disord* 24(1):43, 1998.

Fowler-Brown A, Kahwati LC: Prevention and treatment of overweight in children and adolescents, *Am Family Physician* 69(11):2591, 2004.

Grodner M, Long S, DeYoung S: *Foundations and clinical applications of nutrition,* St Louis, 2004, Mosby.

Hasler G, Buysse DJ, Klaghofer R et al: The association between short sleep duration and obesity in young adults: a 13-year prospective study, *Sleep* 27(4):661, 2004.

He K, Hu FB, Colditz GA et al: Changes in intake of fruits and vegetables in relation to risk of obesity and weight gain among middle-aged women, *Int J Obes Relat Metab Disord* 28(12):1569, 2004.

Institute of Medicine: Applications of dietary reference intakes for electrolytes and water, Washington, DC, 2004, National Academies Press.

James DC: Factors influencing food choices, dietary intake, and nutrition-related attitudes among African Americans: application of a culturally sensitive model, *Ethn Health* 9(4):349-367, 2004.

Kaplan MS, Huguet N, Newsom JT et al: The association between length of residence and obesity among Hispanic immigrants, *Am J Prev Med* 27(4):323-326, 2004.

Koh-Banerjee P, Franz M, Sampson L et al: Changes in whole-grain, bran, and cereal fiber consumption in relation to 3 year weight gain among men, *Am J Clin Nutr* 80(5):1237, 2004.

Kral TV, Roe LS, Rolls BJ: Combined effects of energy density and portion size on energy intake in women, *Am J Clin Nutr* 79(6):962, 2004.

Leininger MM, McFarland MR: *Transcultural nursing: concepts, theories, research and practices,* ed 3, New York, 2002, McGraw-Hill.

Lutz CA, Przytulski KR: *Nutrition and diet therapy,* ed 4, Philadelphia, 2005, FA Davis.

Ma Y, Bertone ER, Stanek III EJ et al: Association between eating patterns and obesity in a free-living US adult population, *Am J Epidemiol* 158(1):85, 2003.

Masheb RM, Grillo CM: Eating patterns and breakfast consumption in obese patients with binge eating disorder, *Behav Res Ther* 44(11):1545-1553, 2006.

Miller CA: *Nursing for wellness in older adults,* ed 4, Philadelphia, 2004, JB Lippincott.

Miller KJ, Gleaves DH, Hirsch TG et al: Comparisons of body image dimensions by race/ethnicity and gender in a university population, *Int J Eat Disord* 27(3):310-316, 2000.

Mossavar-Rahmani Y, Henry H, Rodabough R et al: Additional self-monitoring tools in the dietary modification component of the women's health initiative, *J Am Diet Assoc* 104(1):76, 2004.

N

• = Independent;   ▲ = Collaborative;   EBN = Evidence-Based Nursing;   EB = Evidence-Based

Neumark-Sztainer D, Hannan PJ, Story M et al: Family meal patterns: associations with sociodemographic characteristics and improved dietary intake among adolescents, *J Am Diet Assoc* 103(3):317-322, 2003.

Nix S: *Williams' basic nutrition and diet therapy*, St Louis, 2005, Mosby.

Norris SL, Zhang X, Avenell A et al: Long-term non-pharmacological weight loss interventions for adults with prediabetes, *Cochrane Database Syst Rev* (2):CD005270, 2005.

Nutrition Action: Ten myths that won't quit, *Nutrition Action Health Letter* 32(10):3-4, 2004.

Pereira MA, Kartashov AI, Ebbeling CB: Fast-food habits, weight gain, and insulin resistance (the CARDIA study): 15-year prospective analysis, *Lancet* 365(9453):36, 2005.

Resnick B, Orwig D, Magaziner J: The effect of social support on exercise behavior in older adults, *Clin Nurs Res* 11(1):52, 2002.

Resnick B, Zimmerman S, Orwig D: Model testing for reliability and validity of the outcome expectations for exercise scale, *Nurs Res* 50:5, 2001.

Ruser CB, Federman DG, Kashaf SS: Whittling away at obesity and overweight, *Postgrad Med* 117(1):31, 2005.

Satter E: *Your child's weight, helping without harming*, Madison, Wisc, 2005, Kelcy Press.

Schwartz J, Byrd-Bredbenner C: Portion distortion: typical portion sizes selected by young adults, *J Am Diet Assoc* 106(9):1412-1418, 2006.

Shaw K, Gennat H, O'Rourke P et al: Exercise for overweight or obesity, *Cochrane Database Syst Rev* (4):CD003817, 2006.

Shintani TT, Hughes CK, Beckham S et al: Obesity and cardiovascular risk intervention through the ad libitum feeding of traditional Hawaiian diet, *Am J Clin Nutr* 53(suppl 6):1647S-1651S, 1991.

Spiegel K, Tasali E, Penev P et al: Brief communication: sleep curtailment in healthy young men is associated with decreased leptin levels, elevated ghrelin levels, and increased hunger and appetite, *Ann Intern Med* 141(11):846, 2004.

Strychar I: Diet in the management of weight loss, *CMAJ* 174(1):56-63, 2006.

Thompson D, Jago R, Baranowski T et al: Covariability in diet and physical activity in African-American girls, *Obes Res* 12(suppl):S46-S54, 2004.

Thompson DL, Rakow J, Perdue SM: Relationship between accumulated walking and body composition in middle-aged women, *Med Sci Sports Exerc* 36(5):911, 2004.

Tudor-Locke C, Pangrazi RP, Corbin CB et al: BMI-referenced standards for recommended pedometer-determined steps/day in children, *Prev Med* 38(6):857, 2004.

Tufts University: Getting enough sleep helps you stay slim, *Health Nutr Let* 22(11):2, 2005.

Unger JB, Reynolds K, Shakib S et al: A. Acculturation, physical activity, and fast-food consumption among Asian-American and Hispanic adolescents, *J Community Health* 29(6):467-481, 2004.

VanWormer JJ: Pedometers and brief e-counseling: increasing physical activity for overweight adults, *J Appl Behav Anal* 37(3):421, 2004.

Wing RR, Phelan S: Long-term weight loss maintenance, *Am J Clin Nutr* 82(suppl 1):222S-225S, 2005.

Wu T, Giovannucci E, Pischon T et al: Fructose, glycemic load, and quantity and quality of carbohydrate in relation to plasma C-peptide concentrations in U.S. women, *Am J Clin Nutr* 80(4):1043, 2004.

N

Readiness for enhanced Nutrition   *Betty J. Ackley, MSN, EdS, RN*

NANDA   Definition

A pattern of nutrient intake that is sufficient for meeting metabolic needs and can be strengthened

Defining Characteristics

Attitude toward drinking is congruent with health goals; attitude toward eating is congruent with health goals; consumes adequate fluid; consumes adequate food; eats regularly; expresses knowledge of health fluid choices; expresses knowledge of health food choices; expresses willingness to enhance nutrition; follows an appropriate standard for intake (e.g., the food pyramid or American Diabetic Association guidelines); safe preparation for fluids; safe preparation for food; safe storage for food and fluids

NOC   Outcomes (Nursing Outcomes Classification)

Suggested NOC Outcomes

Nutritional Status, Nutritional Status: Food and Fluid Intake, Nutrient Intake, Weight Control

Example NOC Outcome with Indicators
Nutritional Status as evidenced by the following indicators: Food and fluid intake/Weight/height ratio/Hematocrit (Rate the outcome and indicators of **Nutritional Status:** 1 = severe deviation from normal range, 2 = substantial deviation from normal range, 3 = moderate deviation from normal range, 4 = mild deviation from normal range, 5 = no deviation from normal range [see Section I].)

• = Independent;   ▲ = Collaborative;   EBN = Evidence-Based Nursing;   EB = Evidence-Based

Client Outcomes

Client Will (Specify Time Frame):

- Explain how to eat according to the *Dietary Guidelines for Americans 2005*
- Design dietary modifications to meet individual long-term goal of health, using principles of variety, balance, and moderation
- Weigh within normal range for height and age

NIC   Interventions (Nursing Interventions Classification)

Suggested NIC Interventions

Nutrition Management, Nutritional Counseling, Weight Management

Example NIC Activities—Nutrition Management
Determine individual's motivation for changing eating habits; Develop with the individual a method to keep a daily record of intake, exercise sessions, and/or changes in body weight

Nursing Interventions and *Rationales*

- See the Nursing Interventions for **Imbalanced Nutrition: more than body requirements.**
- Ask the client to keep a food diary for 1-3 days, where everything consumed (food or drink) is recorded. Analyze the quality, quantity, and pattern of food intake. *Using a food diary will help both the client and the nurse examine usual foods eaten and patterns of eating.* **EB:** *Development of self-monitoring tools that meet the needs of clients increase dietary reporting and promote self-efficacy (Mossavar-Rahmani et al, 2004).*
- ▲ Review the client's current exercise level. With the client and primary healthcare provider, design a long-term exercise program. Encourage the client to adopt an exercise program that involves walking 3-5 hours per week at an average pace. *This is the amount of exercise recommended by the* Dietary Guidelines for Americans 2005 *and results in lowering the risk for cardiovascular disease, diabetes, osteoporosis, and other chronic illnesses (Wright, 2007).*
- Determine the client's knowledge of the need for supplements. Discourage the client from taking excessive amounts of vitamins unless prescribed by a physician. *If the client eats a healthy diet, there is generally no need for supplementation. If the client is over age 50 years, one multivitamin per day is generally recommended.* **EB:** *A review of clinical trials concluded that antioxidant supplements are unlikely to reduce the risk of heart disease, and high doses of individual supplements can have adverse effects (Kris-Etherton et al, 2004). Another review of 14 randomized trials demonstrated that intake of antioxidant supplementation did not prevent gastrointestinal (GI) cancers, and intake seemed to increase mortality (Bjelakovic et al, 2004).*

Carbohydrates

- Encourage the client to **decrease** intake of sugars, including soft drinks, desserts, and candy. Limit sugar intake to 12 teaspoons of added sugar daily. *Sugar predisposes to dental caries, and also is a source of calories that is empty of other nutrients (Nix, 2005). A 20-ounce cola drink contains 17 teaspoons of sugar (Tufts University, 2004).* **EB:** *Consuming excessive amounts of fructose, which is used to sweeten soft drinks, and insufficient high-fiber grains is associated with development of type 2 diabetes (Wu et al, 2004).*
- Recommend the client eat whole grains whenever possible, and explain how to find whole grains using the food label. **EB:** *Intake of whole grains (3 servings per day) has been shown to decrease the incidence of type 2 diabetes in men and women (McKeown, Meigs & Liu, 2002; Meyer et al, 2000). It has also been shown to decrease heart disease (Liu et al, 1999; Jensen et al, 2004). Intake of refined grains in women was associated with an increased risk of hemorrhagic strokes (Oh et al, 2005).*
- Evaluate the client's usual intake of fiber. Recommended intake is 25 grams per day. *In general, high-fiber foods take longer to eat and contain fewer calories than most other foods.* **EB:** *Increased dietary fiber was associated with lower body weight and waist-to-hip ratios, and it predicted weight gain more strongly than fat consumption did (Slavin, 2005).*

N

• = Independent;   ▲ = Collaborative;   EBN = Evidence-Based Nursing;   EB = Evidence-Based

- Recommend the client eat five to nine fruits and vegetables per day, with a minimum of two servings of fruit and three servings of vegetables. Encourage client to eat a rainbow of fruits and vegetables, because bright colors are associated with increased nutrients. *Both fruits and vegetables are excellent sources of vitamins and also phytochemicals that help protect against disease.* **EB:** *An epidemiological study demonstrated a decreased incidence of cardiovascular disease deaths and overall mortality with an increased intake of fruits and vegetables (Bazzano et al, 2002). Intake of fruits and vegetables can help prevent heart disease, stroke, hypertension, high cholesterol, some types of cancer, and diverticulitis, and guard against cataracts and macular degeneration (Hung, Joshipura & Jiang, 2004).*

Fats

- Recommend the client limit intake of saturated fats and *trans*-fatty acids; instead increase intake of vegetable oils, such as canola oil and olive oil. Limit fat intake to around 30% of total calories per day. *Intake of both saturated fat and* trans-*fatty acids raise the low-density lipoprotein (LDL) level, which predisposes to atherosclerosis (Welland, 2007). Eating even small amounts of trans fats have been associated with an increase in risk of heart disease, strokes, and diabetes (EN Comments, 2007).*
- Recommend client use low-fat choices when selecting and cooking meat, and also when selecting dairy products.
- Recommend that the client eat cold-water fish, such as salmon, tuna, or mackerel, at least two times per week to ensure adequate intake of omega-3 fatty acids. If the client is unwilling to eat fish, suggest other sources, such as flaxseed, soy, or walnuts. NOTE: Fish oil capsules should be taken cautiously; some brands can be contaminated with mercury or pesticides. *Intake of excessive omega-3 fatty acids can result in bleeding.* **EB:** *The intake of omega-3 fatty acids by eating fish or taking fish oil capsules results in decreased incidence of sudden cardiac death (Jones, 2002; Marchioli et al, 2002; von Schacky, 2007). Consumption of fish was associated with a significantly reduced progression of coronary artery atherosclerosis in postmenopausal women with coronary artery disease (Erkkila et al, 2004).Omega-3 fatty acids were found to be effective in helping psychiatric clients with both unipolar and bipolar depression (Freeman et al, 2006).*

Protein

- Recommend the client decrease intake of red meat and processed meats, instead eat more poultry, fish, and dairy sources of protein. *Women who eat more red and processed meats, along with processed grains and sweets, have higher rates of cerebrovascular accidents (CVAs) (Fung et al, 2004).*
- Recommend the client eat meatless meals at intervals and try alternative sources of protein, including nuts, especially almonds (one handful), and nut butters. **EB:** *Consumption of nuts was associated with a reduced risk of coronary heart disease in a study of registered nurses (Hu et al, 1998). Consumption of nuts and peanut butter was shown to probably decrease the incidence of type 2 diabetes in women (Jiang et al, 2002). In a study conducted on physicians, nut consumption demonstrated that those whose diet included the most nuts had the lowest risk of dying from heart disease (Albert et al, 2002). An additional study demonstrated that regular consumption of almonds decreased risk factors for cardiovascular disease and other chronic diseases (Jaceldo-Siegl et al, 2004).*
- Recommend the client eat beans and especially soybeans as an alternative to animal proteins at intervals. Introduce the client to soy products, such as flavored soy milk. *Eating soy protein as a substitute for animal products reduces the incidence of coronary artery disease by reducing blood lipids, oxidized LDL, homocysteine, and blood pressure (Jenkins et al, 2002).* NOTE: *Women with diagnosed estrogen-dependent cancer of the breast should generally avoid eating soy foods.*

Fluid and Electrolytes

- Recommend the client choose and prepare foods with less salt, aiming for a maximum of 2300 mg per day, which is approximately 1 teaspoon (*Dietary Guidelines for Americans 2005;* Welland, 2007).
- If the client drinks alcohol, encourage him or her to drink in moderation—no more than one drink per day for women and two drinks per day for men. *Consuming more than a moderate amount of alcohol is one of the main causes of hypertension in both men and women (Krousel-Wood et al, 2004).*
- Recommend that the client increase intake of water to at least 2000 mL or 2 quarts per day. A guideline is 1 to 1.5 mL of fluid per each calorie needed, so an average intake would be between

2000 and 3000 mL/day, or at least 8 cups of fluid (Grodner, Long & DeYoung, 2004). *The adequate intake recommendation is 3 L for the 19- to 30-year-old male and 2.2 L for the 19- to 30-year-old female. Water balance studies suggest that adult men require 2.5 L per day (Institute of Medicine, 2004).*

Pediatric

- Provide appropriate nutrition for children (see Box III-3). *Although the health status of American children has improved, the number of children who are overweight has more than doubled among 2- to 5-year-olds and more than tripled among 6- to 11-year-olds, which has major health consequences (Nicklas & Johnson, 2004).*

Geriatric

- Use a nutritional screening tool designed for older adults, such as the Mini Nutrition Assessment (MNA), the Malnutrition Universal Screening Tool (MUST), or the Nutrition Risk Screening (NRS). *The MNA is helpful for older clients living in the community or in an extended care facility, and the NRS is more helpful for clients in the acute care setting (Sieber, 2006).*
- Assess changes in lifestyle and eating patterns. *Energy needs decrease an estimated 5% per decade after age 40 years, but eating patterns often remain unchanged from youth (Lutz & Przytulski, 2005).*
- ▲ Recommend the client discuss the need for a low-dose balanced multiple vitamin and mineral supplement with physician. *It is generally recommended that anyone over age 50 years should take a multivitamin every day to ensure that adequate vitamins and minerals are obtained.* **EB:** *Some studies have demonstrated increased immunity and decreased rate of infections in older people who take vitamin supplements (Dossey, 2005).*

BOX III-3 PEDIATRIC NUTRITION GUIDELINES

- Aim for five servings of fruits and vegetables each day. You can gradually build up to this amount. Eat fruit with each meal for a week.
- Reduce fat. Opt for low-fat substitutes, such as the following:
  - Low-fat dairy skim or 1% milk (after age 2 years), cheese with 2 to 6 g fat per oz
  - Lean meats and poultry (95% lean ground beef or turkey); remove visible fat from meat and skin from poultry
  - Low-fat or fat-free salad dressings, mayonnaise, and margarine
  - Desserts, such as angel food cake, low-fat ice cream or frozen yogurt, animal crackers, vanilla wafers, gingersnaps, or graham crackers
- Eat sugary foods in moderation. If your child eats a healthy diet, one sweet a day is fine.
- Drink water or skim or 1% milk (after age 2 years) instead of high-calorie, sugary drinks.
- Check ingredients on nutrition labels. Foods with sugar listed as one of the first three or four ingredients may be high in sugar and should be eaten in moderation.
- Eat healthy snacks. Keep healthy foods on hand for snacks. Good snack ideas include the following:
  - Fresh fruit
  - Cereal with low-fat milk
  - Low-fat cheese with low-fat crackers
  - Graham crackers with low-fat hot chocolate
  - Raw vegetables with low-fat dip
  - Applesauce

From Kosharek SM: *If your child is overweight: a guide for parents,* ed 3, Chicago, 2006, American Dietetic Association.

N

- Assess fluid intake. Recommend routine drinks of water regardless of thirst. *Older adults are predisposed to deficient fluid volume because of decreased fluid in body, decreased thirst sensation, and decreased ability to concentrate urine (Bennett, 2000; Suhayda & Walton, 2002).*
- Observe for socioeconomic factors that influence food choices (e.g., finances, cooking facilities). *Even those on restricted budgets and with limited facilities can be assisted to choose food sources of a balanced diet.*
- Suggest a variety of seasonings. *The ability to taste sweet, bitter, sour, and salty declines in most but not all older persons (Morley, 1997).*

 ### Multicultural

- Assess for dietary intake of essential nutrients. **EBN:** *Hispanics with type 2 diabetes also often have inadequate protein nutritional status (Castenada, Bermudez & Tucker, 2000). Rural African-American men had low caloric intakes coupled with high fat intakes but also had nutrient deficiencies (Vitolins et al, 2000). African-American adolescents have some of the greatest vitamin D deficiencies (Gordon et al, 2004). Approximately 50% to 75% of the Mexican population suffer from malnutrition, making it one of the leading causes of death among children. The problem is primarily economic, although lack of education is a contributing faction (Giger & Davidhizar, in press).*
- Assess for the influence of cultural beliefs, norms, and values on the client's nutritional knowledge. *What the client considers normal dietary practices may be based on cultural perceptions (Leininger & McFarland, 2002; Giger & Davidhizar, in press). Among African-Americans, there was a general perception that "eating healthfully" meant giving up part of their cultural heritage (James, 2004).*
- Discuss with the client those aspects of their diet that will remain unchanged. *Aspects of the client's life that are meaningful and valuable to them should be understood and preserved without change (Leininger & McFarland, 2002).*
- Determine the motivational factors operating within the client at the present time. **EBN:** *African-American women were motivated to increase their physical activity by personal and familial histories of heart disease and related risk factors (Banks-Wallace, 2000).*
- Negotiate with the client regarding the aspects of his or her diet that will need to be modified. *Give and take with the client will lead to culturally congruent care (Leininger & McFarland, 2002).*
- Explore strategies that appeal to the client. **EBN:** *Group interventions that include spiritual and community building may be especially effective for promoting physical activity among African-American women (Banks-Wallace, 2000). A recent study using the Parents as Teachers site to deliver a dietary change program via personal visits, newsletters, and group meetings was successful in reducing the percentage of calories from fat and increasing fruit and vegetable consumption among participating parents (Haire-Joshu et al, 2003).*
- Validate the client's feelings regarding the impact of current lifestyle, finances, and transportation on ability to obtain nutritious food.
- Encourage family meals. **EB:** *Frequency of family meals was positively associated with intake of fruits, vegetables, grains, and calcium-rich foods and was negatively associated with soft drink consumption (Neumark-Sztainer et al, 2003).*

 ### Client/Family Teaching

- The majority of interventions previously described involve teaching.
- Work with the family members regarding information on how to improve nutritional status.
- Teach the importance of exercise in a weight control program.

evolve See the EVOLVE website for World Wide Web resources for client education.

REFERENCES

Albert CM, Gaziano JM, Willett WC et al: Nut consumption and decreased risk of sudden cardiac death in the Physician's Health Study, *Arch Intern Med* 162(2):1382-1387, 2002.

Banks-Wallace J: Staggering under the weight of responsibility: the impact of culture on physical activity among African American women, *Multicult Nurs Health* 6:24, 2000.

Bazzano LA, He J, Ogden LG et al: Fruit and vegetable intake and risk of cardiovascular disease in U.S. adults: the first National Health and Nutrition Examination Survey epidemiologic follow-up study, *Am J Clin Nutr* 76(1):93-99, 2002.

Bennett JA: Dehydration: hazards and benefits, *Geriatr Nurs* 21(2):84, 2000.

• = Independent;   ▲ = Collaborative;   EBN = Evidence-Based Nursing;   EB = Evidence-Based

Bjelakovic G, Nikolova D, Simonetti RG et al: Antioxidant supplements for prevention of gastrointestinal cancers: a systematic review and meta-analysis, *Lancet* 364(9441):1219-1228, 2004.

Castenada C, Bermudez OI, Tucker KL: Protein nutritional status and functions are associated with type II diabetes in Hispanic elders, *Am J Clin Nutr* 72(1):89, 2000.

Dietary Guidelines for Americans 2005, available at http://www.healthierus.gov/dietaryguidelines.

Dossey B: *Holistic nursing: a handbook for practice*, ed 4, Boston, 2005, American Holistic Nurses Association.

EN Comments: Trans fats get the boot thanks to you; how to spur more change, *Environ Nutr* 30(3):3, 2007.

Erkkila AT, Lichtenstein AH, Mozaffarian D et al: Fish intake is associated with a reduced progression of coronary artery atherosclerosis in postmenopausal women with coronary artery disease, *Am J Clin Nutr* 80(3):626-632, 2004.

Freeman MP, Hibbeln JR, Wisner KL et al: Omega-3 fatty acids: evidence bases for treatment and future research in psychiatry. *J Clin Psychiatry* 67(12):1954-1964, 2006.

Fung TT, Stampfer MJ, Manson JE et al: Prospective study of major dietary patterns and stroke risk in women, *Stroke* 35(9):2014-2019, 2004.

Giger J, Davidhizar, R: *Transcultural nursing: assessment and intervention*, ed 5, St Louis, Mosby Year Book (in press).

Gordon CM, DePeter KC, Feldman HA et al: Prevalence of vitamin D deficiency among healthy adolescents, *Arch Pediatr Adolesc Med* 158(6):531-537, 2004.

Grodner M, Long SL, DeYoung SL: *Foundations and clinical applications of nutrition, a nursing approach*, ed 3, St. Louis, 2004, Mosby.

Haire-Joshu D, Brownson RC, Nanney MS et al: Improving dietary behavior in African Americans: the Parents As Teachers High 5, Low Fat Program, *Prev Med* 36(6):684-691, 2003.

Hu FB, Stampfer MJ, Manson JE et al: Frequent nut consumption and risk of coronary heart disease in women: prospective cohort study, *BMJ* 317(7169):1341-1345, 1998.

Hung HC, Joshipura KJ, Jiang R: Fruit and vegetable intake and risk of major chronic disease, *J Natl Cancer Inst* 96:1577, 2004.

Institute of Medicine: Applications of dietary reference intakes for electrolytes and water, Washington, DC, 2004, National Academies Press.

Jaceldo-Siegl K, Sabate J, Rajaram S et al: Almond supplementation without advice on food replacement induces favourable nutrient modifications to the habitual diets of free-living individuals, *Br J Nutr* 92(3):533-540, 2004.

James DC: Factors influencing food choices, dietary intake, and nutrition-related attitudes among African Americans: application of a culturally sensitive model, *Ethn Health* 9(4):349-367, 2004.

Jenkins DJ, Kendall CW, Jackson CJ et al: Effects of high- and low-isoflavone soyfoods on blood lipids, oxidized LDL, homocysteine, and blood pressure in hyperlipidemic men and women, *Am J Clin Nutr* 76(2):365, 2002.

Jensen, MK, Koh-Banerjee, P, Hu FB et al: Intakes of whole grains, bran and germ and the risk of coronary heart disease in men, *Am J Clin Nutr* 80(6):1492-1499, 2004.

Jiang R, Manson JE, Stampfer MJ et al: Nut and peanut butter consumption and risk of type 2 diabetes in women, *JAMA* 288(20):2554-2560, 2002.

Jones PJ: Effect of n-3 polyunsaturated fatty acids on risk reduction of sudden death, *Nutr Rev* 60:12, 2002.

Kris-Etherton PM, Lichtenstein AH, Howard BV et al: Antioxidant

vitamin supplements and cardiovascular disease, *Circulation* 110(5):637-641, 2004.

Krousel-Wood MA, Muntner P, He J et al: Primary prevention of essential hypertension, *Med Clin North Am* 88(1):223-238, 2004.

Leininger MM, McFarland MR: *Transcultural nursing: concepts, theories, research and practices,* ed 3, New York, 2002, McGraw-Hill.

Liu S, Stampfer MJ, Hu FB et al: Whole grain consumption and risk of coronary heart disease: results from the Nurses' Health Study, *Am J Clin Nutr* 70(3):412-419, 1999.

Lutz CA, Przytulski KR: *Nutrition and diet therapy*, ed 4, Philadelphia, 2005, FA Davis.

Marchioli R, Barzi F, Bomba E et al: Early protection against sudden death by n-3 polyunsaturated fatty acids after myocardial infarction: time-course analysis of the results of the Gruppo Italiano per lo Studio della Sopravvivenza nell'Infarto Miocardico (GISSI)-Prevenzione, *Circulation* 105(16):1987-1993, 2002.

McKeown NM, Meigs JB, Liu S: Whole-grain intake is favorably associated with metabolic risk factors for type 2 diabetes and cardiovascular disease in the Framingham Offspring Study, *Am J Clin Nutr* 76:2, 2002.

Meyer KA, Kushi LH, Jacobs Jr DR et al: Carbohydrates, dietary fiber, and incident type 2 diabetes in older women, *Am J Clin Nutr* 71(4):921-930, 2000.

Morley JE: Anorexia of aging: physiologic and pathologic, *Am J Clin Nutr* 66:760, 1997.

Mossavar-Rahmani Y, Henry H, Rodabough R et al: Additional self-monitoring tools in the dietary modification component of the Women's Health Initiative, *J Am Diet Assoc* 104(1):76-85, 2004.

Nicklas T, Johnson R: Position of the American Dietetic Association: dietary guidance for healthy children ages 2 to 11 years, *J Am Diet Assoc* 104(4):660-677, 2004.

Nix S: *Williams' basic nutrition and diet therapy*, St Louis, 2005, Mosby.

Neumark-Sztainer D, Hannan PJ, Story M et al: Family meal patterns: associations with sociodemographic characteristics and improved dietary intake among adolescents, *J Am Diet Assoc,* 103(3):317-322, 2003.

Oh K, Hu FB, Cho E et al: Carbohydrate intake, glycemic index, glycemic load, and dietary fiber in relation to risk of stroke in women, *Am J Epidemiol* 161(2):161-169, 2005.

Sieiber CC: Nutritional screening tools—How does the MNA compare? Proceedings of the session held in Chicago May 2-3, 2006 (15 Years of Mini Nutritional Assessment), *J Nutr Health Aging* 10(6):488-492, 2006.

Slavin JL: Dietary fiber and body weight, *Nutrition* 21(3):411, 2005.

Suhayda R, Walton JC: Preventing and managing dehydration, *Medsurg Nurs* 11(6):267, 2002.

Tufts University: How much sugar is right? *Health Nutr Let* 22(4), 2004.

Vitolins MZ, Quandt SA, Case LD et al: Ethnic and gender variation in the dietary intake of rural elders, *J Nutr Elder* 19(3):15-30, 2000.

von Schacky C: Omega 3 fatty acids and cardiovascular disease, *Curr Opin Clin Nutr Metab Care* 10(2):129-135, 2007.

Welland D: Red-flagging food labels: 8 tips to sift fact from fiction, *Environ Nutr* 30(3):2, 2007.

Wright H: Get active to increase your chances of surviving cancer, *Environ Nutr* 30(3):1-4, 2007.

Wu T, Giovannucci E, Pischon T et al: Fructose, glycemic load, and quantity and quality of carbohydrate in relation to plasma C-peptide concentrations in US women, *Am J Clin Nutr* 80(4):1043-1049, 2004.

N

• = Independent; ▲ = Collaborative; EBN = Evidence-Based Nursing; EB = Evidence-Based

Risk for imbalanced Nutrition: more than body requirements

Betty J. Ackley, MSN, EdS, RN

NANDA   Definition

At risk for intake of nutrients that exceeds metabolic needs

Risk Factors

Concentrating food at the end of day; dysfunctional eating patterns; eating in response to external cues (e.g., time of day, social situation); eating in response to internal cues other than hunger (e.g., anxiety); higher baseline weight at beginning of each pregnancy; observed use of food as comfort measure; observed use of food as reward; pairing food with other activities; parental obesity; rapid transition across growth percentiles in children; reported use of solid food as major food source before 5 months of age

NOC   Outcomes (Nursing Outcomes Classification)

Suggested NOC Outcomes

Nutritional Status: Food and Fluid Intake, Nutrient Intake, Weight Control

Example NOC Outcome with Indicators
Weight Control as evidenced by the following indicators: Demonstrates progress toward target weight/Balances exercise with caloric intake/Maintains recommended eating pattern/Controls preoccupation with food (Rate the outcome and indicators of **Weight Control**: 1 = never demonstrated, 2 = rarely demonstrated, 3 = sometimes demonstrated, 4 = often demonstrated, 5 = consistently demonstrated [see Section I].)

Client Outcomes

Client Will (Specify Time Frame):

- Explain concept of a balanced diet
- Compare current eating pattern with recommended healthy one
- Design dietary modifications to meet individual long-term goal of weight control, using principles of variety, balance, and moderation
- Identify role of exercise in weight control

NIC   Interventions (Nursing Interventions Classification)

Suggested NIC Interventions

Nutrition Management, Nutritional Counseling, Weight Management

Example NIC Activities—Weight Management
Determine individual's motivation for changing eating habits; Develop with the individual a method to keep daily record of intake, exercise sessions, and/or changes in body weight

Nursing Interventions and *Rationales*

- Refer to care plan for **Imbalanced Nutrition: more than body requirements.**

Impaired Oral mucous membrane   *Betty J. Ackley, MSN, EdS, RN*   evolve

NANDA Definition

Disruptions of lips and soft tissues of oral cavity

Defining Characteristics

Bleeding; cheilitis; coated tongue; desquamation; difficult speech; difficulty eating; difficulty swallowing; diminished taste; edema; enlarged tonsils; fissures; geographic tongue; gingival hyperplasia; gingival pallor; gingival recession; halitosis; hyperemia; macroplasia; mucosal denudation; mucosal pallor; nodules; oral discomfort; oral lesions; oral pain; oral ulcers; papules; pocketing deeper than 4 mm; presence of pathogens; purulent drainage; purulent exudates; red or bluish masses (e.g., hemangiomas); reports bad taste in mouth; smooth atrophic tongue; spongy patches; stomatitis; vesicles; white curdlike exudates; white patches/plaques; xerostomia

Related Factors (r/t)

Barriers to oral self-care; barriers to professional care; chemotherapy; chemical irritants (e.g., alcohol, tobacco, acidic foods, drugs, regular use of inhalers or other noxious agents); cleft lip; cleft palate; decreased platelets; decreased salivation; deficient knowledge of appropriate oral hygiene; dehydration; depression; diminished hormone levels (women); ineffective oral hygiene; infection; immunocompromised; immunosuppression; loss of supportive structures; malnutrition; mechanical factors (e.g., illfitting dentures); braces; tubes (endotracheal/nasogastric); surgery in oral cavity; medication side effects; mouth breathing; NPO for more than 24 hours; radiation therapy; stress; trauma

NOC Outcomes (Nursing Outcomes Classification)

Suggested NOC Outcomes

Oral Hygiene, Tissue Integrity: Skin and Mucous Membranes

Example NOC Outcome with Indicators
Oral Hygiene as evidenced by the following indicators: Cleanliness of mouth/Moisture of oral mucosa and tongue/Color of mucosa membranes/Oral mucosa integrity (Rate the outcome and indicators of **Oral Hygiene:** 1 = severely compromised, 2 = substantially compromised, 3 = moderately compromised, 4 = mildly compromised, 5 = not compromised [see Section I].)

Client Outcomes

Client Will (Specify Time Frame):

- Maintain intact, moist oral mucous membranes that are free of ulceration and debris
- Demonstrate measures to regain or maintain intact oral mucous membranes

NIC Interventions (Nursing Interventions Classification)

Suggested NIC Intervention

Oral Health Restoration

Example NIC Activities—Oral Health Restoration
Use a soft toothbrush for removal of dental debris; Instruct patient to avoid commercial mouthwashes

Nursing Interventions and *Rationales*

▲ Inspect the oral cavity at least once daily and note any discoloration, lesions, edema, bleeding, exudate, or dryness. Refer to a physician or dental specialist as appropriate. *Oral inspection can*

• = Independent;   ▲ = Collaborative;   EBN = Evidence-Based Nursing;   EB = Evidence-Based

reveal signs of oral disease, symptoms of systemic disease, drug side effects, or trauma of the oral cavity (Gonsalves, Chi & Neville, 2007).

- Assess for mechanical agents such as ill-fitting dentures and chemical agents such as frequent exposure to tobacco that could cause or increase trauma to oral mucous membranes. **EB:** *Denture wearing and being edentulous can be related to a decreased quality of life and risk for undiagnosed oral disease (Weyant et al, 2004).*
- Monitor the client's nutritional and fluid status to determine if it is adequate. Refer to the care plan for **Deficient Fluid volume** or **Imbalanced Nutrition: less than body requirements** if applicable. *Dehydration and malnutrition predispose clients to impaired oral mucous membranes.*
- Encourage fluid intake of up to 3000 mL/day if not contraindicated by the client's medical condition. *Fluids help increase moisture in the mouth, which protects the mucous membranes from damage and helps the healing process (Roberts, 2000).*
- Determine the client's mental status. If the client is unable to care for himself or herself, oral hygiene must be provided by nursing personnel. The nursing diagnosis **Bathing/hygiene Self-care deficit** is then applicable.
- Determine the client's usual method of oral care and address any concerns regarding oral hygiene. *Whenever possible, build on the client's existing knowledge base and current practices to develop an individualized plan of care.*
- If the client does not have a bleeding disorder and is able to swallow, encourage the client to brush the teeth with a soft toothbrush using fluoride-containing toothpaste at least twice per day. **EBN and EB:** *The toothbrush is the most important tool for oral care. Brushing the teeth is the most effective method for reducing plaque and controlling periodontal disease (American Dental Association [ADA], 2007; Pearson & Hutton, 2002).*
- Encourage the client to brush the tongue with the toothbrush or use a tongue scraper twice a day. **EB:** *The tongue scraper was shown to be more effective than brushing in removing volatile sulfur compounds, which are associated with halitosis (Pedrazzi et al, 2004). Tongue brushing or scraping resulted in improved taste sensation and reduced the coating on the tongue (Quirynen et al, 2004).*
- If the client does not have a bleeding disorder, encourage the client to floss once per day or use an interdental cleaner. **EB:** *Floss is useful to remove plaque buildup between the teeth (Brown & Yoder, 2002; ADA, 2007).*

Client Receiving Chemotherapy/Radiation

- Ensure that the client receives a comprehensive oral examination before initiation of chemotherapy or radiation, with aggressive preventative dental care given as needed (National Institutes of Health [NIH], 1990; Sonis & Kunz, 1988).
- Provide instructions about the need for and method of providing frequent oral care to the client 1 week before radiation therapy. **EBN:** *Instructions on oral care given 1 week before radiation resulted in reduced mucositis as opposed to instructions given 1 day before or no instructions (Shieh et al, 1997).*
- For measurement of presence or severity of mucositis, use the Oral Mucositis Assessment Scale (OMAS). **EB:** *This is an instrument that has two components: the clinician's assessment of presence and severity of mucositis, and client report about pain, difficulty swallowing, and ability to eat (Sonis et al, 1999). For more information about measurement of oral mucositis, refer to Eilers & Epstein (2004).*
- Use cryotherapy with ice chips dissolved in the client's mouth before, during, and after bolus administration of fluorouracil to reduce the severity of mucositis (Cascinu et al, 1994; Rocke et al, 1993). Also use cryotherapy for clients receiving bolus edatrexate (Edelman et al, 1998) and melphalan (Asia et al, 2005; Tartarone et al, 2005).
- Give the client frequent sips of water, and ask client to rinse the mouth with water regularly. **EBN:** *The use of water to moisten the mouth has been shown to be as effective as many other agents (Joanna Briggs Institute, 2004).*
- If client has a dry mouth (xerostomia):
  - Provide saliva substitutes as ordered. *Saliva substitutes are helpful to decrease the discomfort of dry mouth and may help prevent stomatitis (National Institute of Dental and Craniofacial Research, 2000).*

• = Independent;   ▲ = Collaborative;   EBN = Evidence-Based Nursing;   EB = Evidence-Based

■ Suggest the client chew sugarless gum or sugarless sour candy to promote salivary flow. *The ADA and NIDCR support the use of sugarless gum or candy to promote salivary flow (ADA, 2007; NIDCR, 2000).*

■ Provide ice chips frequently to keep the mouth moist. **EB:** *There is some evidence that ice chips help prevent mucositis (Clarkson, Worthington & Eden, 2003).*

• Help client use a mouth rinse of salt and soda every 1 to 2 hours for prevention and treatment of stomatitis. **EBN:** *A study demonstrated that there was no difference in the rate of cessation of symptoms of stomatitis when four different mouthwashes were used: chlorhexidine, lidocaine, Benadryl and Maalox, and salt and soda (Dodd et al, 2000).*

▲ If the mouth is severely inflamed and it is painful to swallow, contact the physician for a topical anesthetic or analgesic order. Modification of oral intake (e.g., soft or liquid diet) may also be necessary to prevent friction trauma. The nursing diagnosis **Imbalanced Nutrition: less than body requirements** may apply.

• If the client's platelet count is lower than 50,000/mm^3 or the client has a bleeding disorder, use a specially made toothbrush designed for sensitive or diseased tissue, or a toothette that is not soaked in glycerin or flavorings; if the client cannot tolerate a toothbrush or a toothette, a piece of gauze wrapped around a finger can be used to remove plaque and debris (Brown & Yoder, 2002).

• Use tap water or normal saline to provide oral care; do not use commercial mouthwashes containing alcohol or hydrogen peroxide. Also do not use lemon-glycerin swabs. *Alcohol dries the oral mucous membranes (Rogers, 2001).* **EBN:** *Hydrogen peroxide can cause mucosal damage and is extremely foul tasting to clients (Tombes & Gallucci, 1993). Use of lemon-glycerin swabs can result in decreased salivary amylase and oral moisture as well as erosion of tooth enamel (Foss-Durant & McAffee, 1997; Poland, 1987).*

• Use foam sticks to moisten the oral mucous membranes, clean out debris, and swab out the mouth of the edentulous client. Do not use foam sticks to clean the teeth unless the platelet count is very low and the client is prone to bleeding gums. *Foam sticks are useful for cleansing the oral cavity of a client who is edentulous (Curzio & McCowan, 2000).* **EBN:** *Foam sticks are not effective for removing plaque; the toothbrush is much more effective (Pearson & Hutton, 2002).*

• Keep the lips well lubricated by using a lip balm that is water or aloe based. *This is a comfort measure (Joanna Briggs Institute, 2004; Sadler et al, 2003).*

Client on a Ventilator

• Use a child-sized toothbrush to brush teeth; use suction to remove secretions. **EBN:** *Brushing the teeth is effective in removing dental plaque (Stiefel et al, 2000). Increased plaque on the teeth is associated with increased contamination of the mouth and incidence of ventilator-associated pneumonia (Munro et al, 2006).*

• Use water as a rinsing agent and mouthwash. **EBN:** *The use of water to moisten the mouth has been shown to be as effective as many other agents (Joanna Briggs Institute, 2004).*

▲ Apply chlorhexidine gluconate in the oral cavity by swab or spray early after intubation and at intervals if ordered. **EBN:** *The use of chlorhexidine gluconate administered early after intubation and at intervals decreased positive cultures of bacteria and may decrease ventilator-associated pneumonia (Grap et al, 2004; Koeman et al, 2006).*

• Refer to the care plan for **Impaired Dentition** if the client has problems with the teeth.

Geriatric

• Determine the functional ability of the client to provide his or her own oral care. Refer to **Bathing/hygiene Self-care deficit.** *Interventions must be directed toward both treatment of the functional loss and care of oral health (Avlund, Holm-Pedersen & Schroll, 2001).*

• Provide appropriate oral care to the elderly with a self-care deficit by brushing the teeth after every meal. *Oral care is often poor for clients with dementia in long-term facilities (Sigal, 2006).* **EB:** *Several studies have shown that the rate of pneumonia was decreased by providing oral care after every meal (Watando et al, 2004; Yoneyama et al, 2002).*

• Carefully observe the oral cavity and lips for abnormal lesions such as white or red patches, masses, ulcerations with an indurated margin, or a raised granular lesion. *Malignant lesions are*

• = Independent;   ▲ = Collaborative;   EBN = Evidence-Based Nursing;   EB = Evidence-Based

more common in elderly persons than in younger persons, especially if there is a history of smoking or alcohol use, and many elderly persons rarely visit a dentist (Aubertin, 1997).

- Ensure that dentures are removed and scrubbed at least once daily, removed and rinsed thoroughly after every meal, and removed and kept in an appropriate solution at night. *This is an evidence-based protocol for denture care (Curzio & McCowan, 2000). Denture plaque containing* Candida *organisms can cause denture-induced stomatitis, which is more common in clients with unhealthy lifestyles and poor oral hygiene than in others (Lyon et al, 2006).*
- If the client has xerostomia, evaluate medications to see if they could be the cause, provide synthetic saliva products to moisten the oral cavity as ordered, and offer frequent sips of water and sugarless gum or candy to provide lubrication. *Xerostomia is common in the elderly for many reasons, including medication use and aging. The goal is to keep the mouth moist to prevent stomatitis (Walton, Miller & Tordecilla, 2001).*

Home Care

- The interventions previously described may be adapted for home care use.
- ▲ If dryness is a side effect of the client's medication(s), instruct the client in the use of artificial saliva.
- Instruct the client to avoid alcohol-based or hydrogen peroxide–based commercial products for mouth care and to avoid other irritants to the oral cavity (e.g., tobacco, spicy foods). *Oral irritants can further damage the oral mucosa and increase the client's discomfort.*
- Instruct the client in ways to soothe the oral cavity (e.g., cool beverages, ice pops, viscous lidocaine).
- If the client often breathes by mouth, add humidity to the room unless contraindicated.
- ▲ If necessary, refer for home health aide services to support the family in oral care and observation of the oral cavity.

Client/Family Teaching

- Teach the client how to inspect the oral cavity and monitor for signs and symptoms of infection or complications as well as when to call the healthcare practitioner (Rogers, 2001).
- Teach the client and family how to perform appropriate mouth care if necessary.
- Recommend the client use a powered toothbrush for removal of dental plaque and prevention of gingivitis. **EB:** *A Cochrane systematic review and other studies found that use of powered toothbrushes reduced plaque and incidence of gingivitis more than use of a manual toothbrush (Robinson et al, 2005; Zimmer et al, 2005; Sjogren et al, 2004).*

 See the EVOLVE website for World Wide Web resources for client education.

REFERENCES

American Dental Association (ADA): *Cleaning your teeth and gums,* www.ada.org/public/topics/cleaning_faq.asp, accessed March 23, 2007.

Asia Y, Mori T, Kudo M et al: Oral cryotherapy for the prevention of high-dose melphalan-induced stomatitis in allogeneic hematopoietic stem cell transplant recipients, *Support Care Cancer,* 13(4):266-269, 2005.

Aubertin MA: Oral cancer screening in the elderly: the home healthcare nurse's role, *Home Healthc Nurse* 15(9):594, 1997.

Avlund K, Holm-Pedersen P, Schroll M: Functional ability and oral health among older people: a longitudinal study from age 75 to 80, *J Am Geriatr Soc* 49:7, 2001.

Brown CG, Yoder LH: Stomatitis: an overview, *Am J Nurs* 102(suppl 4):20, 2002.

Cascinu S, Fedeli A, Fedeli SL et al: Oral cooling (cryotherapy), an effective treatment for the prevention of 5-fluorouracil-induced stomatitis, *Eur J Cancer B Oral Oncol* 30B(4):234-236, 1994.

Clarkson JE, Worthington HV, Eden OB: Interventions for preventing oral mucositis or oral candidiasis for patients with cancer receiving chemotherapy, *Cochrane Database Syst Rev* (3):CD000978, 2003.

Curzio J, McCowan M: Getting research into practice: developing oral hygiene standards, *Br J Nurs* 9(7):434, 2000.

Dodd MJ, Dibble SL, Miaskowski C et al: Randomized clinical trial of the effectiveness of three commonly used mouthwashes to treat chemotherapy-induced mucositis, *Oral Surg Oral Med Oral Pathol Oral Radiol Endod* 90(1):39, 2000.

Edelman MJ, Gandara DR, Perez EA et al: 1998 Phase I trial of edatrexate plus carboplatin in advanced solid tumors: amelioration of dose-limiting mucositis by ice chip cryotherapy, *Invest New Drugs* 16(1):69-75, 1998.

Eilers J, Epstein JB: Assessment and measurement of oral mucositis, *Semin Oncol Nurs* 20(1):22, 2004.

Foss-Durant AM, McAffee A: A comparison of three oral care products commonly used in practice, *Clin Nurs Res* 6:1, 1997.

Gonsalves WC, Chi, AC, Neville BW: Common oral lesions: part I. Superficial mucosal lesions, *Am Fam Physician* 75(4):501-506, 2007.

Grap MJ, Munro CL, Elswick RK Jr et al: Duration of action of a single, early oral application of chlorhexidine on oral microbial flora in mechanically ventilated patients: a pilot study, *Heart Lung* 33(2):83, 2004.

Joanna Briggs Institute: *Prevention and treatment of oral mucositis in cancer patients: best practice information sheet*, www.joannabriggs.edu.au/best_practice/bp5.php, accessed March 23, 2007.

Koeman M, van der Ven AJ, Hak E et al: Oral decontamination with chlorhexidine reduces the incidence of ventilator-associated pneumonia, *Am J Respir Crit Care Med* 173(12):1348-1356, 2006.

Lyon JP, da Costa SC, Totti VM et al: Predisposing conditions for *Candida* spp. carriage in the oral cavity of denture wearers and individuals with natural teeth, *Can J Microbiol* 52(5):462-467, 2006.

Munro CL, Grap MJ, Elswick RK Jr et al: Oral health status and development of ventilator-associated pneumonia: a descriptive study, *Am J Crit Care* 15(5):453-461, 2006.

National Institute of Dental and Craniofacial Research: *Cancer treatment and oral health*, www.nidcr.nih.gov/HealthInformation/DiseasesAndConditions/CancerTreatmentAndOralHealth/default.htm, accessed January 10, 2007.

National Institutes of Health Consensus Development Panel: NIH consensus statement: oral complications of cancer therapies, *NCI Monogr* 3, 1990.

Pearson LS, Hutton JL: A controlled trial to compare the ability of foam swabs and toothbrushes to remove dental plaque, *J Adv Nurs* 39:5, 2002.

Pedrazzi V, Sato S, de Mattos MG et al: Tongue-cleaning methods: a comparative clinical trial employing a toothbrush and a tongue scraper, *J Periodontol* 75(7):1009, 2004.

Poland JM: Comparing Moi-Stir to lemon-glycerin swabs, *Am J Nurs* 87(4):422, 1987.

Quirynen M, Avontroodt P, Soers C et al: Impact of tongue cleaners on microbial load and taste, *J Clin Periodontol* 31(7):5-6, 2004.

Roberts J: Developing an oral assessment and intervention tool for older people: 2, *Br J Nurs* 9(18):2033, 2000.

Robinson PG, Deacon SA, Deery C et al: Manual versus powered toothbrushing for oral health, *Cochrane Database Syst Rev* (2): CD002281, 2005.

Rocke LK, Loprinzi CL, Lee JK et al: A randomized clinical trial of two different durations of oral cryotherapy for prevention of 5-fluorouracil-related stomatitis, *Cancer* 72:2234, 1993.

Rogers BB: Mucositis in the oncology patient, *Nurs Clin North Am* 36:4, 2001.

Sadler GR, Stoudt A, Fullerton JT et al: Managing the oral sequelae of cancer therapy, *Medsurg Nurs* 12(1):28, 2003.

Shieh SH, Wang ST, Tsai ST et al: Mouth care for nasopharyngeal cancer patients undergoing radiotherapy, *Oral Oncol* 33(1):36-41, 1997.

Sigal MJ: Dental considerations for persons with dementia, *Oral Health* 96(9):53-55, 2006.

Sjogren K, Lundberg AB, Birkhed D et al: Interproximal plaque mass and fluoride retention after brushing and flossing—a comparative study of powered toothbrushing, manual toothbrushing and flossing, *Oral Health Prev Dent* 2(2):119-124, 2004.

Sonis S, Kunz A: Impact of improved dental services on the frequency of oral complications of cancer therapy for patients with non-head-and-neck malignancies, *Oral Surg Oral Med Oral Pathol* 65, 1988.

Sonis ST, Eilers JP, Epstein JB et al: Validation of a new scoring system for the assessment of clinical trial research of oral mucositis induced by radiation or chemotherapy, Mucositis Study Group, *Cancer* 85(10):2103-2113, 1999.

Stiefel KA, Damron S, Sowers NJ et al: Improving oral hygiene for the seriously ill patient: implementing research-based practice, *Medsurg Nurs* 9(1):40, 2000.

Tartarone A, Matera R, Romano G et al: Prevention of high-dose melphalan-induced mucositis by cryotherapy, *Leuk Lymphoma* 46(4):633-634, 2005.

Tombes MB, Gallucci B: The effects of hydrogen peroxide rinses on the normal oral mucosa, *Nurs Res* 42(6):332, 1993.

Walton JC, Miller J, Tordecilla L: Elder oral assessment and care, *Medsurg Nurs* 10:1, 2001.

Watando A, Ebihara S, Ebihara T et al: Daily oral care and cough reflex sensitivity in elderly nursing home patients, *Chest* 126(4):1066, 2004.

Weyant RJ, Pandav RS, Plowman JL et al: Medical and cognitive correlates of denture wearing in older community-dwelling adults, *J Am Geriatr Soc* 52(4):596, 2004.

Yoneyama T, Yoshida M, Ohrui T et al: Oral care reduces pneumonia in older patients in nursing homes, *J Am Geriatr Soc* 50(3):340, 2002.

Zimmer S, Strauss J, Bizhang M et al: Efficacy of the Cybersonic in comparison with the Braun 3D Excel and a manual toothbrush, *J Clin Periodontol* 32(4):360-363, 2005.

Pain: Assessment Guide   *Chris Pasero, MS, RN-BC, FAAN, and Margo McCaffery, MS, RN-BC, FAAN*

ASSESSMENT: USE OF PAIN RATING SCALES

Nursing Assessment/Diagnosis of Pain Sensation

Ask the client about the current level of pain, if possible. The client's self-report of pain is the single most reliable indicator of how much pain the client is experiencing. The pain intensity rating given by the client is always what is recorded in the client's record.

Basic Measures of Pain

The hierarchy of importance of basic measures of pain is as follows:
1. Obtain the client's self-report of pain. **EBN:** *The patient's self report is the single most reliable indicator of pain (American Pain Society, 2003).*
2. Consider underlying painful or potentially painful pathology or condition:
   a. Search for causes of pain, such as endotracheal intubation and suctioning.
   b. If there is a reason to suspect pain, assume pain is present (document "APP") (Pasero & McCaffery 2002; Pasero 2003).
   c. Formulate an appropriate pain treatment plan if pain is assumed to be present.
3. Observe behaviors (e.g., facial expressions, body movements, crying) in patients who are unable to report pain (Herr et al, 2004). **EBN:** *In the absence of self report, observation of behavior is a valid approach to pain assessment (Herr et al, 2006).*
   a. Surrogate's report of possible pain behaviors. **EBN:** *Credible information can be obtained from a parent or another person who knows the client well (Herr et al, 2006).*
   b. Physiological measures may be considered but are not sensitive or specific indicators of pain and should not be emphasized (American Pain Society, 2004; Herr et al, 2006).
   c. The absence of behavioral or physiological indicators does not mean the absence of pain (Pasero & McCaffery 2002; Pasero 2003).
4. Attempt an analgesic trial with low-dose nonopioid or opioid analgesic in patients who are unable to report pain.
   a. Administer nonopioid for mild pain; add opioid for more severe pain.
   b. Observe for reduction or other positive change in behavior after analgesic administration. If behaviors continue and the previous dose was safe (e.g., opioid dose), increase dose and observe behavior. Continue to titrate upward until a therapeutic effect is seen, bothersome side effects occur, or no benefit is determined.
   c. Formulate a pain treatment plan based on response.
   d. Explore other causes for behavior if no benefit is derived from analgesic trial.

Client/Family Teaching: Use of Pain Rating Scale

NOTE: When it is obvious that pain is severe (e.g., after trauma or major surgery), a pain rating scale need not be used initially. Give an analgesic and wait until the client is better able to understand and use the pain rating scale.
- Explain the primary purposes of a pain rating scale. Show the client and family the scale. This step allows quick, consistent communication between client and caregiver, nurse, or physician. Emphasize that the client must volunteer information because the caregivers may not know when the client feels pain. *This step also helps establish a pain relief goal that is satisfactory to the client.*
- Explain the specific pain rating scale (e.g., 0 to 10; 0 = no pain and 10 = worst possible pain). When a numerical scale is used, verify that the client can count to the number used. If the client does not understand what scale is standard in that clinical setting, use another scale.
- Discuss the word *pain*. Explain that pain is discomfort that may occur anywhere in the body; may have various characteristics such as aching, hurting, pulling, tightness, burning, or pricking; and may be mild to severe. If the client prefers some other term such as hurt, use that word. To verify that the client understands how the word pain (or other word preferred by client) is used, ask client to give two examples of pain he or she has now or has experienced.

• = Independent;   ▲ = Collaborative;   EBN = Evidence-Based Nursing;   EB = Evidence-Based

- Ask client to practice using the pain rating scale by rating the current pain or past painful experiences.
- Establish a comfort-function goal. Ask the client what pain rating would be acceptable or satisfactory while at rest and active. *This helps set a realistic initial goal. Zero pain is not always possible.*
- Once the initial goal is achieved, the possibility of better pain relief can be considered. Emphasize to the client that satisfactory pain relief is a level of pain that is noticeable but not distressing and enables the client to sleep, eat, and perform other required or desired physical activities. Pain rated at higher than 3 on a 0 to 10 pain rating scale interferes significantly with daily function. *Perceived quality of life appears to be comparable across cultures, with pain ratings of higher than 5 markedly interfering with a person's ability to enjoy life (Pasero & McCaffery, 2004b).* (See **Acute Pain.**)

0–10 Numerical Descriptive Pain Intensity Scale

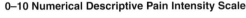
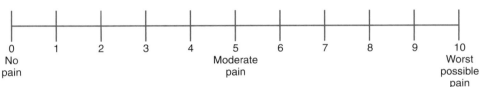

0	1	2	3	4	5	6	7	8	9	10
No pain					Moderate pain					Worst possible pain

HOW TO USE THE WONG-BAKER FACES PAIN SCALE

Wong–Baker FACES Pain Rating Scale

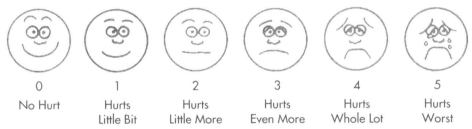

0	1	2	3	4	5
No Hurt	Hurts Little Bit	Hurts Little More	Hurts Even More	Hurts Whole Lot	Hurts Worst

From Wong DL, Hockenberry-Eaton M, Wilson D, Winkelstein ML: *Wong's Essentials of Pediatric Nursing,* ed 6, St Louis, 2001, Mosby. Reprinted with permission.

Original instructions: Explain to the person that each face is for a person who feels happy because he has no pain (hurt) or sad because he has some or a lot of pain. "**Face 0** is very happy because he does not hurt at all. **Face 1** hurts just a little bit. **Face 2** hurts a little more. **Face 3** hurts even more. **Face 4** hurts a whole lot. **Face 5** hurts as much as you can imagine, although you do not have to be crying to feel this bad." Ask the person to choose the face that best describes how he is feeling. A rating scale is recommended for persons age 3 years and older.

Brief word instructions: Point to each face using the words to describe the pain intensity. Ask the child to choose the face that best describes his or her own pain and record the number.

• = Independent;   ▲ = Collaborative;   EBN = Evidence-Based Nursing;   EB = Evidence-Based

HOW TO USE THE FACES PAIN SCALE—REVISED

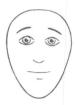 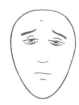 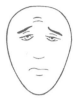 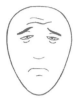 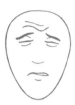 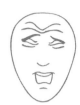

From the *Pediatric Pain Sourcebook*. Original copyright © 2001. Used with permission of the International Association for the Study of Pain and the Pain Research Unit, Sydney Children's Hospital, Randwick NSW 2031, Australia, www.painsourcebook.ca.

"These faces show how much something can hurt. This face [point to the left-most face] shows no pain (or hurt). The faces show more and more pain [point to each face from left to right] up to this one [point to the right-most face]; it shows very much pain. Point to the face that shows how much you hurt (right now)." NOTE: Numbers are not shown to children. **EB:** *The Faces Pain Scale was shown to be valid in 4- to 12-year-olds postoperatively. It was further validated with 600 children ages 4 to 5 years receiving immunizations (Wood et al, 2003; Hicks et al, 2001).*

REFERENCES

American Pain Society: *Principles of analgesic use in the treatment of acute pain and cancer,* ed 5, Glenview, Ill, 2003, APS.

American Pain Society: *Pain: current understanding, emerging therapies, and novel approaches to drug discovery,* 2007, available at http://www.ampainsoc.org/pub/bulletin/sum05/res01.htm. Accessed April 26, 2007.

American Pain Society: *The assessment and management of acute pain in infants, children, and adolescents: a position statement from the American Academy of Pediatrics Committee on psychosocial aspects of child and family health and American Pain Society Task Force on pain in infants, children and adolescents,* 2007, available at http://www.ampainsoc.org/advocacy/pediatric2.htm. Accessed April 26, 2007.

Ardery G, Herr UA, Titler MG et al: Assessing and managing acute pain in older adults: a research base to guide practice, *Med Surg Nurs* 12(1):7, 2003.

Giuffre M et al: Postoperative joint replacement pain: description and opioid requirement, *J Post Anesth Nurs* 6(4):239-245, 1991.

Herr K, Coyne P, McCaffery M et al: Pain assessment in the nonverbal patient: position statement with clinical recommendations, *Pain Manage Nurs* 7(2):44-52, 2006.

Hicks CL et al: The Faces Pain Scale-Revised: toward a common metric in pediatric pain measurement, *Pain* 93:2, 2001.

Passero C: Pain in the critically ill, *J Perianesth Nurs* 18(6):422-425, 2003.

Passero C, McCaffery M: Pain in the critically ill, *Am J Nurs* 102(1):59-60, 2002.

Passero C, McCaffery M: Comfort-function goals, *Am J Nurs* 104(9):77, 2004.

Wood C et al: *Self-assessment by the Faces Pain Scale: revised of immediate post-vaccination pain following administration of Priorix versus MMRII as a second dose in 4 to 6 year old children.* Presented at the Sixth International Symposium on Pediatric Pain, Sydney, Australia, 2003.

Acute Pain   *Chris Pasero, MS, RN-BC, FAAN, and Margo McCaffery, MS, RN-BC, FAAN*   *evolve*

NANDA   Definition

Pain is whatever the experiencing person says it is, existing whenever the person says it does (McCaffery, 1968). Unpleasant sensory and emotional experience arising from actual or potential tissue damage or described in terms of such damage (Mersky & Bogduk, 1994); sudden or slow onset of pain of any intensity from mild to severe with anticipated or predictable end and a duration of less than 6 months.

Defining Characteristics

Subjective

Pain is always subjective and cannot be proved or disproved. A client's report of pain is the most reliable indicator of pain (American Pain Society [APS], 2004). A client with cognitive ability who can speak or point should use a pain rating scale (e.g., 0 to 10) to identify the current level of pain intensity (self-report) and determine a comfort-function goal (Pasero & McCaffery, 2004). Establishment of a comfort-function goal involves helping the client to select a pain rating level that will allow the client to easily perform identified functional goals (e.g., a pain rating of 3 on a scale of 0 to 10 to cough, deep breathe, and ambulate).

Objective

Expressions of pain are extremely variable and cannot be used in lieu of self-report. Neither behavior nor vital signs can substitute for the client's self-report (McCaffery & Pasero, 1999; 2003). However, observable responses to pain may be helpful in assessing clients who cannot or will not use a self-report pain rating scale (Pasero & McCaffery, 2005; Herr et al, 2006). Observable responses may be loss of appetite and inability to deep breathe, ambulate, sleep, or perform ADLs. Clients may show guarding, self-protective behavior, self-focusing or narrowed focus, distraction behavior ranging from crying to laughing, and muscle tension or rigidity. In sudden and severe pain, autonomic responses such as diaphoresis, blood pressure and pulse changes, pupillary dilation, or increases or decreases in respiratory rate and depth may be present, but physiologic indicators are considered the least sensitive for pain as they may be a sign of other pathology, such as hypovolemia and anxiety. Physiological indicators may be used to confirm other findings; however, the absence of any physiological or behavioral indicator does not mean the absence of pain. A hierarchy of pain measures is recommended for the assessment of pain in patients who cannot report pain: (1) attempt to obtain self-report; (2) consider the presence of underlying painful pathology or condition and assume pain is present if appropriate; (3) observe behaviors that may indicate the presence of pain in patients who cannot report pain; (4) obtain a proxy (parent, caregiver, or significant other who knows patient very well) report of behaviors that might indicate pain; (5) attempt an analgesic trial whereby a dose of analgesia is administered and any reduction in pain behaviors is noted. From this analgesic trial a pain treatment plan can be developed (Pasero & McCaffery, 2005; Herr et al, 2006). (See Pain: Assessment Guide and Appendix D for specific guidelines.)

Related Factors (r/t)

Injury agents (biological, chemical, physical, psychological)

NOC   Outcomes (Nursing Outcomes Classification)

Suggested Outcomes

Comfort Level, Pain Control, Pain Level

Example Outcome
Pain Level as evidenced by the following indicators: Reported pain/Length of pain episodes/Facial expressions of pain/Muscle tension (Rate the outcome and indicators of **Pain Level:** 1 = severe, 2 = substantial, 3 = moderate, 4 = mild, 5 = none [see Section I].)

• = Independent;   ▲ = Collaborative;   EBN = Evidence-Based Nursing;   EB = Evidence-Based

Client Outcomes

Client Will (Specify Time Frame):

- Use pain rating scale to identify current pain intensity and determine comfort/function goal (if client has cognitive abilities)
- Describe how unrelieved pain will be managed
- Report that pain management regimen relieves pain to satisfactory level with acceptable and manageable side effects
- Perform activities of recovery with reported acceptable level of pain (if pain is above comfort-function goal, take action that decreases pain or notify a member of the health care team)
- If cognitively impaired, demonstrate a reduction in pain behaviors, have manageable and tolerable side effects, and perform recovery activities satisfactorily
- State ability to obtain sufficient amounts of rest and sleep
- Describe nonpharmacological method that can be used to help control pain

NIC   Interventions (Nursing Interventions Classification)

Suggested NIC Interventions

Analgesic Administration, Pain Management, Patient-Controlled Analgesia (PCA) Assistance

Example NIC Activities—Pain Management
Assure patient attentive analgesic care; Perform a comprehensive assessment of pain, to include location, characteristics, onset/duration, frequency, quality, intensity or severity of pain, and precipitating factors

Nursing Interventions and *Rationales*

- ▲ Determine whether the client is experiencing pain at the time of the initial interview. If so, intervene at that time to provide pain relief. Assess and document the intensity, character, onset, duration, and aggravating and relieving factors of pain during the initial evaluation of the client. *The initial assessment and documentation provide direction for the pain treatment plan. A comprehensive pain assessment includes all characteristics of the pain that the client can provide. The client's report of the pain is considered the single most reliable indicator of pain (APS, 2004; JCAHO, 2000).*
- Assess pain in a client by using a self-report such as the 0 to 10 numerical pain rating scale, Wong-Baker FACES Scale, or the Faces Pain Scale (see Pain: Assessment Guide and Appendix D). *Systematic ongoing assessment and documentation provide direction for the pain treatment plan; adjustments are based on the client's response (Berry et al, 2006).* **EB:** *Single-item ratings of pain intensity are valid and reliable as measures of pain intensity (Jensen, 2003).* **EBN:** *An investigation of nursing attitudes and beliefs about pain assessment revealed that effective use of pain rating scales is often determined by the nurse's personal attitude about its effectiveness (Layman Young, Horton & Davidhizar, 2006).*
- Question the client regarding pain at frequent intervals, often at the same time as taking vital signs. *Pain assessment is as important as taking vital signs, and the APS suggests applying the concept of pain assessment as the "fifth vital sign" (APS, 2004).*
- Ask the client to describe past experiences with pain and the effectiveness of methods used to manage pain, including experiences with side effects, typical coping responses, and the way the client expresses pain. **EBN:** *Surveyed clients with cancer pain revealed that they had a number of concerns (barriers) that affected their willingness to report pain and use analgesics (Vallerand et al, 2007). Many harbored fears and misconceptions regarding the use of analgesics, management of side effects, and risk of addiction.*
- Establish a comfort-function goal with the client. Question the client regarding the level of pain that he or she believes is appropriate to achieve a state of comfort and appropriate function. Attempt to keep pain at a level that will allow the client to achieve functional and quality-of-life goals with relative ease (Pasero & McCaffery, 2004). *The pain rating that allows the client to have comfort and appropriate function should be determined because this allows a tangible way to measure outcomes of pain management (Griffie, 2003).*

● = Independent;   ▲ = Collaborative;   EBN = Evidence-Based Nursing;   EB = Evidence-Based

- Describe the adverse effects of unrelieved pain. **EBN:** *Numerous pathophysiological and psychological morbidity factors may be associated with pain (Noble, 2006).*
- Assess and document the intensity of the pain and discomfort after any known pain-producing procedure, with each new report of pain, and at regular intervals. *Systematic ongoing assessment and documentation provide direction for the pain treatment plan; adjustments are based on the client's responses. The client's report of pain is the single most reliable indicator of pain (APS, 2004; TJC, 2000).*
- If the client is cognitively impaired and unable to report pain or use a pain rating scale, assess and document behaviors that may indicate pain (e.g., change in activity, loss of appetite, guarding, grimacing, moaning) (Herr, 2002). A hierarchy of pain assessment is recommended in these clients: (1) attempt to obtain self-report because it is the single most reliable indicator of pain; (2) consider the presence of underlying painful pathology or condition and assume pain is present; (3) observe behaviors that may indicate the presence of pain; (4) obtain a proxy (parent, caregiver, or significant other who knows client very well) report of behaviors that might indicate pain; (5) attempt an analgesic trial in which a dose of analgesia is administered and any reduction in pain behaviors is noted. *From this analgesic trial a pain treatment plan can be developed (Pasero & McCaffery, 2005; Herr et al, 2006). (See Pain: Assessment Guide and Appendix D for specific guidelines.) The absence of behaviors thought to be indicative of pain does not necessarily mean that pain is absent (Pasero, 2003b; Pasero & McCaffery, 2002, 2005).* **EBN:** *Certain behaviors have been shown to be indicative of pain and can be used to assess pain in clients who cannot use a self-report pain rating tool (e.g., in the cognitively impaired client). The clinician should be aware that pain expression is highly individual and what may be a pain behavior in one client may not be in another. Pain assessment must be individualized (Herr, 2002).*
- Assume that pain is present and treat accordingly in a client who has a pathological condition or who is undergoing a procedure thought to be painful. *Pain is associated with certain pathological conditions (e.g., fractures) and procedures (e.g., surgery). In the absence of the client's report of pain (e.g., anesthetized, critically ill, or cognitively impaired client), the clinician should assume pain is present and treat accordingly (Pasero, 2003b; Pasero & McCaffery, 2002, 2005; Herr, 2002; Herr et al, 2006).*
- Attempt an analgesic trial in clients who are unable to report pain but have an underlying pathology or condition that is thought to be painful or have behaviors that may indicate the presence of pain. Administer a nonopioid if pain is thought to be mild and an opioid if pain is thought to be moderate to severe. Observe for any change in behavior. *Understand that there may be no change in unresponsive clients or when a trial is attempted with a low dose. The trial is used as a basis for establishment of an ongoing pain treatment plan (Herr et al, 2006; Pasero & McCaffery, 2005).*
- Prevent pain when possible during procedures such as venipuncture, nasogastric tube insertion, and male Foley catheter insertion. Use a topical local anesthetic such as EMLA cream. **EBN:** *EMLA cream can significantly decrease venipuncture and IV insertion pain (Fetzer, 2002).*
- Determine the client's current medication use. *Obtain a complete history of medications the client is taking or has taken to help prevent drug-drug interactions and toxicity problems that can occur when incompatible drugs are combined or when allergies are present. The history also provides the clinician an understanding of what medications have been tried and were or were not effective in treating the client's pain (APS, 2004).*
- ▲ Explore the need for both opioid (narcotic) and nonopioid analgesics. *Pharmacological interventions are the cornerstone of management of moderate to severe pain (APS, 2004; Pasero 2003a). Unless contraindicated, all clients with acute pain should receive a nonopioid agent around the clock.*
- Use a multimodal analgesic approach (Pasero, 2003a) *The analgesic regimen should include a nonopioid even if pain is severe enough to require the addition of an opioid (Pasero, 2003a). Combining analgesics can result in acceptable pain relief with lower dosages of each analgesic than would be possible with one analgesic alone. Lower dosages can result in fewer or less-severe side effects (APS, 2004; Pasero, 2003a).*
- ▲ Obtain a prescription to administer an opioid analgesic if indicated, especially for severe pain. *Opioid analgesics are indicated for the treatment of moderate to severe pain (APS, 2004; Pasero, 2003a).*
- ▲ Administer opioids orally or IV. Provide client-controlled analgesia (PCA), perineural infusions, and intraspinal analgesia as ordered and when appropriate and available. *The least invasive route of administration capable of providing adequate pain control is recommended. The IV route is preferred*

P

for rapid control of severe pain. For ongoing pain, give analgesia around the clock. For intermittent pain, as-needed dosing is appropriate (APS, 2004; Pasero, 2003a; Pasero & McCaffery, in press). **EBN:** *PCA was more effective in controlling pain than on-demand intramuscular injections (Chang, Ip & Cheung, 2004; Bainbridge, Martin & Cheng, 2006).*

- Avoid giving pain medication intramuscularly (IM). *The IM route is avoided because of unreliable absorption, pain, and inconvenience (Pasero, 2003; APS, 2004). Repeated IM injections can cause sterile abscesses and fibrosis of muscle and soft tissue. In addition, IM injection may lead to nerve injury with persistent neuropathic pain (APS, 2004).* **EBN:** *PCA was more effective in controlling pain than on-demand IM injections (Chang, Ip & Cheung, 2004).*

- Explain to the client the pain management approach that has been ordered, including therapies, medication administration, side effects, and complications. *One of the most important steps toward improved control of pain is a better client understanding of the nature of pain, its treatment, and the role the client needs to play in pain control (APS, 2004).*

- Plan nursing care when the client is comfortable based on the reality that oral opioid medications begin to work in approximately 1 hour and IV medications work in 5 to 30 minutes depending on the medication. Most transdermal medications become effective in 12 to 16 hours, with steady blood levels within 48 hours (APS, 2004). *Pain diminishes the client's activity. Knowing when the medication becomes effective helps guide nursing practice to check back on the client, ensure that adequate pain relief has been obtained, and also plan nursing activities.*

- Discuss the client's fears of undertreated pain, overdose, and addiction. *Because of the many misconceptions regarding pain and its treatment, education about the ability to control pain effectively and correction of myths about the use of opioids should be included as part of the treatment plan. Addiction is unlikely when clients use opioids for pain management (APS, 2004; McCaffery, Pasero & Portenoy, 2001).* **EBN:** *Clients with cancer pain revealed that many harbored fears and misconceptions regarding the use of analgesics, management of side effects, and risk of addiction (Ward et al, 1993).*

- ▲ When opioids are administered, assess pain intensity, sedation, and respiratory status at regular intervals. Assess sedation and respiratory status at least every 2 hours for the first 24 hours of opioid therapy in opioid-naive clients (those who have not been taking regular daily doses of opioids). Awaken sleeping clients for further assessment if they have an inadequate respiratory rate; shallow, irregular, or noisy (snoring) respirations; or apneic episodes. Decrease the opioid dose immediately if the client is excessively sedated (Pasero, Eksterowicz & McCaffery, 2007). *Opioids may cause respiratory depression because they reduce the responsiveness of carbon dioxide chemoreceptors located in the respiratory centers of the brain. Because even more opioid is required to produce respiratory depression than is required to produce sedation, clients with clinically significant respiratory depression are usually also sedated. Respiratory depression can be prevented by assessing sedation and decreasing the opioid dose when the client is arousable but has difficulty staying awake (Pasero & McCaffery, 2002).*

- Review the client's flow sheet and medication records to determine overall degree of pain relief, side effects, and analgesic requirements during the previous 24 hours. **EBN:** *Systematic tracking of pain was an important factor in improving pain management (Faries et al, 1991).*

- ▲ Administer supplemental opioid doses as ordered to keep pain ratings at or below the comfort-function goal. *An order for as-needed supplementary opioid doses between regular doses is an essential backup (McCaffery & Pasero, 2003; Pasero & McCaffery, 2004).*

- ▲ Obtain prescriptions to increase or decrease opioid doses as needed; base prescriptions on the client's report of pain severity and response to the previous dose in terms of relief, side effects, and ability to perform the activities of recovery. *Nurses should be knowledgeable in pain management have an "as needed" range of opioid doses available to provide appropriate pain relief (APS, 2004b; Pasero, Manworren & McCaffery, 2007).*

- ▲ When the client is able to tolerate oral analgesics, obtain a prescription to change to the oral route; use an equianalgesic chart to determine initial dose. (Refer to the Equianalgesic Chart before this care plan.) *The oral route is preferred because it is the most convenient and cost effective (APS, 2004). The use of equianalgesic doses when switching from one opioid or route of administration to another helps prevent loss of pain control from underdosing and side effects from overdosing (McCaffery, 2003; McCaffery & Pasero, 2003).*

- In addition to administering analgesics, support the client's use of nonpharmacological methods to help control pain, such as distraction, imagery, relaxation, and application of heat and cold. *Cognitive-behavioral strategies can restore the client's sense of self-control, personal efficacy, and active participation in his or her own care (APS, 2004).*

- Teach and implement nonpharmacological interventions when pain is relatively well controlled with pharmacological interventions. *Nonpharmacological interventions should be used to supplement, not replace, pharmacological interventions (APS, 2004).*

▲ Ask the client to describe appetite, bowel elimination, and ability to rest and sleep. Administer medications and treatments to improve these functions. Obtain a prescription for a stool softener plus a peristaltic stimulant to prevent opioid-induced constipation if needed. *Because there is great individual variation in the development of opioid-induced side effects, these side effects should be monitored and prophylactically treated if their development is inevitable (e.g., constipation). Opioids cause constipation by decreasing bowel peristalsis (Plaisance & Ellis, 2002).*

Pediatric

- As with adults, use complementary therapies to supplement, not replace, pharmacological interventions. **EBN:** *Complementary therapies such as relaxation, distraction, hypnotics, art therapy, and imagery may play an important role in holistic pain management (Lassetter, 2006).*
- For the neonate, use oral sucrose for pain of short duration such as heel stick or venipuncture. *Neonates are as sensitive to pain as adults, and premature infants are thought to be highly sensitive. Concentrated (24%) oral sucrose briefly produces analgesia in neonates up to age 6 months (Pasero, 2004). Breastfeeding and supplemental breast milk have been shown to reduce pain behaviors in neonates, but are not as effective as concentrated oral sucrose (Pasero, 2007).*
- Recognize that breastfeeding has been shown to reduce behavioral indicators of pain. *Breastfeeding, however, is not as effective in reducing pain as oral sucrose (Pasero, 2007).*
- Use a topical local anesthetic such as EMLA cream or LMX-4 before performing venipuncture in an infant or child. *Venipuncture pain is often not minor pain to the child experiencing the pain. Nurses are obligated to minimize all kinds of pain (Wong, 2003).*
- For the neonate experiencing moderate to severe pain, use opioid analgesics and anesthetics in appropriate dosages. *Neonates undergoing endotracheal intubation and chest tube placement or other procedures causing pain should receive adequate pain medication (Pasero, 2004).*
- For the young child (age 4 years and older), use the Wong-Baker FACES Scale or the Faces Pain Scale to determine the level of pain present (see Pain: Assessment Guide and Appendix D for examples). **EB:** *The Faces Pain Scale was shown to be valid in 4- to 12-year-olds postoperatively. It was further validated with 600 children age 4 to 5 years receiving immunizations (Wood et al, 2003; Hicks & Lavender, 2001). Children are able to quantify pain optimally by using a self-report pain rating scale at age 8 years (Spagrud, Piira & Von Baeyer, 2003).*

Geriatric

▲ Always take the older client's reports of pain seriously and ensure that the pain is relieved. *In spite of what many professionals and clients believe, pain is not an expected part of normal aging (American Geriatrics Society [AGS], 2002; Herr, 2002).*

- When assessing pain, speak clearly, slowly, and loudly enough for the client to hear, and if the client uses a hearing aid, be sure it is in place; repeat information as needed. Be sure the client can see well enough to read the pain scale (use an enlarged scale) and written materials. *Elders often have difficulty hearing and seeing. Comprehension is improved when instructions are given slowly and clearly and when the client can see visual aids (Herr, 2002).*

- Handle the client's body gently. Allow the client to move at his or her own speed. *Encourage the older adult to relax; reduction of emotional and physical tension and stressors allows the body to respond more effectively.* **EBN:** *Relaxation training had the following clinical benefits as produced in various research studies: decreased anxiety, easing of muscle tension pain, decreased fatigue, increased restful sleep, and helped dissociation from pain (Dossey, 2005).*

▲ Use acetaminophen and nonsteroidal antiinflammatory drugs (NSAIDs) with low gastrointestinal side effect profiles, such as the selective COX-2 selective NSAID celecoxib or the nonselective NSAID naproxen may be the safest, in clients with cardiovascular risk. Watch for side effects such as gastrointestinal and cardiovascular disturbances and renal dysfunction. *Opioids may be safer than NSAIDs in some clients. The lowest effective dose for the shortest period is recommended (AGS, 2002). Elders are at increased risk for gastric and renal toxicity from NSAIDs (Fine, 2004; Hutchinson, 2004; AGS, 2002).*

▲ Avoid or use with caution drugs with a long half-life, such as the NSAID piroxicam (Feldene) and the opioids methadone (Dolophine) and levorphanol (LevoDromoran). *The higher prevalence of renal insufficiency in elders compared with younger persons can result in toxicity from drug accumulation (Fick et al, 2003; AGS, 2002).*

▲ Use opioids with caution in the older client. **EBN:** *Elders are more sensitive to the analgesic effects of opioid drugs because they experience a higher peak effect and a longer duration of pain relief (AGS, 2002). Reduce the initial recommended adult starting opioid dosage by 25% to 50%, especially if the client is frail and debilitated; then increase the dosage by 25% on an individual basis if needed (Ardery et al, 2003).*

▲ Avoid the use of opioids with toxic metabolites, such as meperidine (Demerol) and propoxyphene (Darvon, Darvocet), in older clients. *Meperidine's metabolite, normeperidine, can produce central nervous system irritability, seizures, and even death; propoxyphene's metabolite, norpropoxyphene, can produce central nervous system toxicity. Both metabolites are eliminated by the kidneys, which makes meperidine and propoxyphene particularly poor choices for older clients, many of whom have at least some degree of renal insufficiency (Ardery et al, 2003; Fick et al, 2003; AGS, 2002).*

Multicultural

• Assess for the influence of cultural beliefs, norms, and values on the client's perception and experience of pain. **EB:** *Native American clients may think that asking for pain medication is disrespectful because it implies that healthcare providers do not know what they are doing (Brant, 2001). A recent study of African-American elders found the use of prayer or faith for pain management, care, and prevention was very common (Ibrahim et al, 2004). A representational approach first developed at the University of Wisconsin-Madison School of Nursing offers a flexible framework for nurses to get cancer clients to delve deeply into their own belief systems about health, disease, pain, and so on and to add sound concepts that work for their pain management. The program is called Representational Intervention to Decrease Cancer Pain (RIDcancer-Pain) and has the following six steps:*
  1. *Performing a representational assessment: the client describes beliefs about cancer pain along five dimensions: identity, cause, timeline, consequences, and cure/control*
  2. *Exploring misconceptions, with emphasis on their origins*
  3. *Creating conditions for conceptual change by discussing the limitations of holding beliefs that are misconceptions (i.e., what one loses by maintaining those beliefs)*
  4. *Introducing replacement information*
  5. *Summarizing and discussing benefits of adopting beliefs that are credible replacements*
  6. *Developing a plan and strategies (Ward, Donovan & Gunnarsdottir, in press)*

• Assess for the effect of fatalism on the client's beliefs regarding the current state of comfort. **EBN:** *Fatalistic perspectives, which involve the belief that one cannot control one's own fate, may influence health behaviors in some African-American and Latino populations (Phillips, Cohen & Moses, 1999; Harmon, Castro & Coe, 1996).*

• Assess for pain disparities among racial and ethnic minorities. **EB:** *Racial and ethnic minorities tend to be undertreated for pain compared with non-Hispanic whites (Green et al, 2003).* **EBN:** *Persons from various ethnic and cultural groups vary in their affective response to pain, requests for pain medication, tolerance to pain, and physiological reaction to pain medication (Giger & Davidhizar, 2004; Davidhizar & Giger, 2004.)*

• Incorporate safe and effective folk healthcare practices and beliefs into care whenever possible. *The caregiver is responsible for ensuring that safe and effective pain management is provided. Although support of an individual's healthcare beliefs is recommended, when research does not support the safety or effectiveness of a method or when research does not exist, this should be fully explained to the client (McCaffery, 2002).* **EBN:** *Incorporating folk health care beliefs and practices into pain management care increased compliance with the treatment plan (Juarez, Ferrell & Borneman, 1998).*

• Use a family-centered approach to care. **EBN:** *Involving the family in pain management care increased compliance with the treatment regimen (Juarez, Ferrell & Borneman, 1998).*

• Teach information about pain medications and their side effects and how to work with healthcare providers to manage pain, and encourage clients to use religious faith to cope with pain. **EB:**

Socioeconomically disadvantaged African-American and Hispanic clients benefit from educational inter-ventions on pain that dispel myths about opioids and teach clients to communicate assertively about their pain with their physicians and nurses (Anderson et al, 2002).

- Use culturally relevant pain scales to assess pain in the client. **EBN:** *Clients from minority cultures may express pain differently than clients from the majority culture. The Faces Pain Scale-Revised was shown to be preferred over other self-report pain rating tools in older minority adults (Jowers Ware et al, 2006; Ware et al, 2006) and in Chinese adults (Li, Liu & Herr, 2007). The Oucher scale is available in African-American and Hispanic versions and is used to assess pain in children (Beyers, Denyes & Villarruel, 1992). A variety of pain assessment instruments are available for use with various cultural and ethnic groups, but tools must be evaluated for reliability and validity for and across cultures (Davidhizar & Giger, 2004).*

- Ensure that directions for medication use are available in the client's language of choice and are understood by the client and caregiver. **EB:** *Use of bilingual instructions for medication administra-tion increased compliance with the pain management plan (Juarez, Ferrell & Borneman, 1998). The use of specific phrases in Spanish to assess acute pain in non–English-speaking Hispanic clients helps provide timely pain assessment and management (Collins, Gullette & Schnepf, 2004).*

Home Care

- Develop the treatment plan with the client and caregivers. *Client input into the plan of care im-proves the likelihood of successful management.*
- ▲ Develop a full medication profile, including medications prescribed by all physicians and all over-the-counter medications. Assess for drug interactions. Instruct the client to refrain from mixing medications without physician approval. *Pain medications may significantly affect or be af-fected by other medications and may cause severe side effects. Some combinations of drugs are specifically contraindicated (APS, 2004; Pasero, 2003a).*
- Assess the client's and family's knowledge of side effects and safety precautions associated with pain medications (e.g., use caution in operating machinery when opioids are first taken or dosage has been significantly increased). *The cognitive effects of opioids usually subside within a week of initial dosing or dosage increases. The use of long-term opioid treatment does not appear to affect neuro-psychological performance.* **EB:** *Pain itself may reduce performance on neuropsychological tests more than oral opioid treatment (Sjogren et al, 2000).*
- If medication is administered by using highly technological methods, assess the home for the necessary resources (e.g., electricity) and ensure that responsible caregivers will be available to assist the client with administration.
- ▲ Assess the knowledge base of the client and family with regard to highly technological medica-tion administration. Teach as necessary. Be sure the client knows when, how, and whom to contact if analgesia is unsatisfactory.

Client/Family Teaching

NOTE: To avoid the negative connotations associated with the words *drugs* and *narcotics,* use the term *pain medicine* when teaching clients.

- Provide written materials on pain control such as *Understanding Your Pain: Using a Pain Rating Scale* (McCaffery, Pasero & Portenoy, 2001) (see instructions on the use of pain rating scales) and *Taking Oral Opioid Analgesics* (McCaffery, Pasero & Portenoy, 2004).
- Discuss the various discomforts encompassed by the word *pain* and ask the client to give exam-ples of previously experienced pain. Explain the pain assessment process and the purpose of the pain rating scale. *Clients often have difficulty understanding the concept of pain and describing their pain experience. The use of alternative words and a complete description of the assessment process, includ-ing the use of scales, ensure that an accurate treatment plan is developed (Pasero & McCaffery, 2004).*
- ▲ Teach the client to use the pain rating scale to rate the intensity of past or current pain. Ask the client to set a comfort-function goal by selecting a pain level on the rating scale that makes it easy to perform recovery activities (e.g., turn, cough, deep breathe). If pain is above this level, the client should take action that decreases pain or notify a member of the healthcare team. (See in-formation on teaching clients to use the pain rating scale.) *The use of comfort-function goals pro-vides direction for the treatment plan. Changes are made according to the client's response and achieve-ment of the goals of recovery or rehabilitation (Pasero & McCaffery, 2004).*

• = Independent;   ▲ = Collaborative;   EBN = Evidence-Based Nursing;   EB = Evidence-Based

▲ Demonstrate medication administration and the use of supplies and equipment. If PCA is ordered, determine the client's ability to press the appropriate button. Remind the client and staff that the PCA button is for client use only.

• Reinforce the importance of taking pain medications to keep pain under control. *Teaching clients to stay on top of their pain and prevent it from getting out of control improves the ability to accomplish the goals of recovery (Pasero & McCaffery, 2004).*

• Reinforce that taking opioids for pain relief is not addiction and that addiction is not likely to occur. *The development of addiction when opioids are taken for pain relief is rare (APS, 2004).*

• Demonstrate the use of appropriate nonpharmacological approaches in addition to pharmacological approaches for helping control pain, such as application of heat and/or cold, distraction techniques, relaxation breathing, visualization, rocking, stroking, music listening, and television watching. *Nonpharmacological interventions are used to complement, not replace, pharmacological interventions (APS, 2004).*

evolve See the EVOLVE website for World Wide Web resources for client education.

REFERENCES

American Geriatrics Society: The management of persistent pain in older persons, *J Am Geriatr Soc* 50(6 suppl):S205-S224, 2002.

American Pain Society: *Pain: current understanding of assessment, management and treatments,* www. ampainsoc.org/ce/npc, accessed September 6, 2004.

American Pain Society: *Principles of analgesic use in the treatment of acute pain and cancer pain,* ed 5, Glenville, Ill, 2003.

Anderson KO, Richman SP, Hurley J et al: Cancer pain management among underserved minority outpatients: perceived needs and barriers to optimal control, *Cancer* 94(8):2295-2304, 2002.

Ardery G, Herr KA, Titler MG et al: Assessing and managing acute pain in older adults: a research base to guide practice, *Medsurg Nurs* 12(1):7, 2003.

Bainbridge D, Martin JE, Cheng DC: Patient-controlled versus nurse-controlled analgesia after cardiac surgery—a meta-analysis, *Can J Anaesth* 53(5):492-499, 2006.

Berry PH, Covington ED, Dahl J et al. *Pain: current understanding of assessment, management, and treatment,* Reston, VA, 2006, National Pharmaceutical Council.

Beyers J, Denyes M, Villarruel A: The creation, validation, and continuing development of the Oucher: a measure of pain intensity in children, *J Pediatr Nurs* 7(5):335, 1992.

Brant JM: Cultural implications of pain education, a Native American example, presented at Cancer Pain and Education for Patients and the Public conference, City of Hope National Medical Center, Duarte, CA, October 18, 2001.

Chang AM, Ip WY, Cheung TH: Patient-controlled analgesia versus conventional intramuscular injection: a cost effectiveness analysis, *J Adv Nurs* 46(5):531, 2004.

Collins AS, Gullette D, Schnepf M: Break through language barriers, *Nurs Manag* 35(8):34-36, 2004.

Davidhizar R, Giger J: A nursing review of the literature on pain and culture, *Int Nursing Rev* 51(1):42-54, 2004.

Dossey B: *Holistic nursing: a handbook for practice,* ed 4, Boston, 2005, Jones and Bartlett.

Faries JE, Mills DS, Goldsmith KW et al: Systematic pain records and their impact on pain control, *Cancer Nurs* 14(6):306, 1991.

Fetzer SJ: Reducing venipuncture and intravenous insertion pain with eutectic mixture of local anesthetic: a meta-analysis, *Nurs Res* 51(2):119-124, 2002.

Fick DM, Cooper JW, Wade WE et al: Updating the Beers criteria for potentially inappropriate mediation use in older adults, *Arch Int Med* 163:2716-2724, 2003.

Fine P: Pharmacological management of persistent pain in older patients, *Clin J Pain* 20(4):220-226, 2004.

Giger J, Davidhizar R: *Transcultural assessment: assessment and intervention,* St Louis, 2004, Mosby.

Green CR, Anderson KO, Baker TA et al: The unequal burden of pain: confronting racial and ethnic disparities in pain, *Pain Med* 4(3):277-294, 2003.

Griffie J: Pain control: addressing inadequate pain relief, *Am J Nurs* 103(8):61-63, 2003.

Harmon MP, Castro FG, Coe K: Acculturation and cervical cancer: knowledge, beliefs, and behaviors of Hispanic women, *Women Health* 24(3):37, 1996.

Herr K: Pain assessment in cognitively impaired older adults, *Am J Nurs* 102(12):65, 2002.

Herr K, Coyne P, McCaffery M et al: Pain assessment in the nonverbal patient: position statement with clinical recommendations, *Pain Manage Nurs* 7(2):44-52, 2006.

Hicks MD, Lavender R: Psychosocial practice trends in pediatric oncology, *J Pediatr Oncol Nurs* 18(4):143-153, 2001.

Hutchinson R: Pain control. COX-2-selective NSAIDS: a review and comparison with nonselective NSAIDS, *Am J Nurs* 104(5):16, 2004.

Ibrahim SA, Zhang A, Mercer MB et al: Inner city African-American elderly patients' perceptions and preferences for the care of chronic knee and hip pain: findings from focus groups, *J Gerontol Series A Biol Sci Med Sci* 59(12):1318-1322, 2004.

Jensen MP: The validity and reliability of pain measures in adults with cancer, *J Pain* 4(1):2, 2003.

The Joint Commission on Accreditation of Healthcare Organizations (JCAHO): *2000 Hospital accreditation standards,* Oakbrook Terrace, Ill, 2000, The Joint Commission.

Jowers Ware et al: Evaluation of the revised faces pain scale, verbal descriptor scale, numeric rating scale, and Iowa pain thermometer in older minority adults, *Pain Manag Nurs* 7(3):117-125, 2006.

Juarez G, Ferrell BR, Borneman T: Influence of culture on cancer pain management in Hispanic clients, *Cancer Pract* 6(5):262, 1998.

Layman Young J, Horton FM, Davidhizar R: Nursing attitudes and beliefs in pain assessment and management, *J Adv Nurs* 53(4):412-421, 2006.

Lassetter JH: The effectiveness of complementary therapies on the pain experience of hospitalized children, *J Holist Nurs* 24(3):196-211, 2006.

Li L, Liu X, Herr K: Postoperative pain intensity assessment: a comparison of four scales in Chinese adults, *Pain Med* 8(3):223-234, 2007.

McCaffery M: *Nursing practice theories related to cognition, bodily pain, and man-environment interactions,* Los Angeles, 1968, University of California.

McCaffery M: What is the role of nondrug methods in the nursing care of patients with acute pain? *Pain Management Nursing* 3(3):77-80, 2002.

McCaffery M: Switching from IV to PO, *Am J Nurs* 103(5):62-63, 2003.

McCaffery M, Pasero C: *Pain: clinical manual,* ed 2, St Louis, 1999, Mosby.

McCaffery M, Pasero C: Breakthrough pain, *Am J Nurs* 103(4):83, 2003.

McCaffery M, Pasero C, Portenoy RK: *Understanding your pain: using a pain rating scale,* Chadds Ford, PA, 2001, Endo Pharmaceuticals.

McCaffery M, Pasero C, Portenoy RK: *Understanding your pain: taking oral opioid analgesics,* Chadds Ford, PA, 2004, Endo Pharmaceuticals.

Mersky H, Bogduk N, editors: *Classification of chronic pain,* ed 2, Seattle, 1994, International Association for the Study of Pain (IASP).

Noble KA: What a pain! *J Perianesth Nurs* 21(5):353-356, 2006.

Pasero C: Multimodal analgesia in the PACU, *J Perianesth Nurs* 18(4):265-268, 2003a.

Pasero C: Pain in the critically ill, *J Perianesth Nurs* 18(6):422-425, 2003b.

Pasero C: Pain relief for neonates, *Am J Nurs* 104(5):44, 2004.

Pasero C: Breastfeeding may reduce neonatal procedural pain. Pain assessment in preterm neonates, *Am J Nurs* 107(4):65-66, 2007.

Pasero C, Eksterowicz N, McCaffery M: The nurse's role in pain management. In Sinatra RS, deLeon Cassasola O, Viscusi G et al: *Acute pain management,* New York, 2007, Cambridge University Press.

Pasero C, Manworren RCB, McCaffery M: IV opioid range orders, *Am J Nurs* 107(2):52-59, 2007.

Pasero C, McCaffery M: Monitoring opioid-induced sedation, *Am J Nurs* 102(2):67-68, 2002.

Pasero C, McCaffery M: Comfort-function goals, *Am J Nurs* 104(9):77, 2004.

Pasero C, McCaffery M: Pain in the critically ill, *Am J Nurs* 102(1):59-60, 2002.

Pasero C, McCaffery M: No self-report means no pain intensity, *Am J Nurs* 105(10):50-53, 2005.

Pasero C, McCaffery M: Orthopedic postoperative pain management, *J Peri Anesth Nursing* 22(3): 2007.

Phillips JM, Cohen MZ, Moses G: Breast cancer screening and African American women: fear, fatalism, and silence, *Oncol Nurs Forum* 26(3):561, 1999.

Plaisance L, Ellis JA: Opioid-induced constipation, *Am J Nurs* 102(3):72-73, 2002.

Sjogren P, Olsen AK, Thomsen AB et al: Neuropsychological performance in cancer clients: the role of oral opioids, pain and performance status, *Pain* 86(3):237, 2000.

Spagrud LJ, Piira T, Von Baeyer CL: Children's self-report of pain intensity, *Am J Nurs* 103(12):62-64, 2003.

Vallerand AH: Knowledge of and barriers to pain management in caregivers of cancer patients receiving homecare, *Cancer Nurs* 30(1):31-37, 2007.

Ward S, Donovan H, Gunnarsdottir S et al: A representational intervention to decrease cancer pain (RIDcancerPain), in press.

Ware LJ, Epps CD, Herr K et al: Evaluation of the Revised Faces Pain Scale, Verbal Descriptor Scale, Numeric Rating Scale, and Iowa Pain Thermometer in older minority adults, *Pain Manag Nurs* 7(3):117-125, 2006.

Wong D: Pain control; topical local anesthetics, *Am J Nurs* 103(6):42-45, 2003.

Wood C et al: *Self-assessment by the Faces Pain Scale: revised of immediate post-vaccination pain following administration of Priorix versus MMRII as a second dose in 4 to 6 year old children.* Presented at the Sixth International Symposium on Pediatric Pain, Sydney, Australia, 2003.

P

Chronic Pain   *Chris Pasero, MS, RN-BC, FAAN, and Margo McCaffery, MS, RN-BC, FAAN*

NANDA   Definition

Pain is whatever the experiencing person says it is, existing whenever the person says it does (McCaffery, 1968).

Pain is an unpleasant sensory and emotional experience arising from actual or potential tissue damage or described in terms of such damage (Mersky & Bogduk, 1994); sudden or slow onset of pain of any intensity from mild to severe, constant or recurring, without anticipated or predictable end and a duration of greater than six months (NANDA-I); state in which the individual experiences pain that persists for a period beyond the usual course of acute illness or a reasonable duration for the injury to heal, is associated with a chronic pathological process, or recurs at intervals for months or years.

Defining Characteristics
Subjective

Pain is always subjective and cannot be proved or disproved. The client's report of pain is the most reliable indicator of pain (American Pain Society [APS], 2004). Clients with cognitive abilities who can speak or point should use a pain rating scale (e.g., 0 to 10) to identify their current level of pain intensity (self-report) and determine a comfort-function goal (Pasero & McCaffery, 2004b). Establishment of a comfort-function goal involves assisting clients in selecting a pain rating that will allow them to easily perform identified functional goals (e.g., a pain rating of 3 on a scale of 0 to 10 to work or walk the dog).

• = Independent;   ▲ = Collaborative;   EBN = Evidence-Based Nursing;   EB = Evidence-Based

Objective

Expressions of pain are extremely variable and cannot be used in lieu of self-report. Neither behavior nor vital signs can substitute for the client's self-report (APS, 2004). However, observable responses to pain may be helpful in pain assessment, especially in clients who cannot or will not use a self-report pain rating scale. Observable responses may be loss of appetite or the inability to ambulate, perform ADLs, work, or sleep. Clients may show guarding, self-protective behavior, self-focusing or narrowed focus, distraction behavior ranging from crying to laughing, and muscle tension or rigidity. In sudden severe pain, autonomic responses such as diaphoresis, blood pressure and pulse changes, pupillary dilation, and increase or decrease in respiratory rate and depth may be present but are usually not seen with chronic pain that is relatively stable. A hierarchy of pain measures is recommended for the assessment of pain in clients who cannot report pain: (1) attempt to obtain self report, (2) consider the presence of underlying painful pathology or condition and assume pain is present if appropriate, (3) observe behaviors that may indicate the presence of pain, (4) obtain a proxy (parent, caregiver, or significant other who knows patient very well) report of behaviors that might indicate pain, (5) attempt an analgesic trial whereby a dose of analgesia is administered and any reduction in pain behaviors is noted. From this analgesic trial a pain treatment plan can be developed (Pasero & McCaffery, 2005; Herr et al, 2006). (See Pain: Assessment Guide and Appendix D for specific guidelines.) Clients with chronic or persistent cancer or nonmalignant pain may experience threats to self-image; a perceived lack of options for coping; and worsening helplessness, anxiety, and depression. Chronic pain may affect almost every aspect of the client's daily life, including concentration, work, and relationships.

Related Factors (r/t)

Actual or potential tissue damage; tumor progression and related pathology; diagnostic and therapeutic procedures; central or peripheral nerve injury (neuropathic pain). NOTE: The cause of chronic nonmalignant pain may not be known because pain study is a new science and an area encompassing diverse types of problems.

NOC   Outcomes (Nursing Outcomes Classification)

Suggested Outcomes

Comfort Level, Pain Control, Pain: Disruptive Effects, Pain Level

---

Example NOC Outcome—Pain Level

Pain Level as evidenced by the following indicators: reported pain/Length of pain episodes/Facial expressions of pain/Muscle tension (Rate the outcome and indicators of **Pain Level**: 1 = severe, 2 = substantial, 3 = moderate, 4 = mild, 5 = none [see Section I].)

Client Outcomes

Client Will (Specify Time Frame):

• Use pain rating scale to identify current level of pain intensity, determine comfort/function goal, and maintain a pain diary (if client has cognitive abilities)
• Describe total plan for pharmacological and nonpharmacological pain relief, including how to safely and effectively take medicines and integrate nondrug therapies
• Demonstrate ability to pace self, taking rest breaks before they are needed
• Function on acceptable ability level with minimal interference from pain and medication side effects (if pain is above comfort-function goal, take action that decreases pain or notify a member of healthcare team)
• If cognitively impaired, demonstrate a reduction in pain behaviors, have manageable and tolerable side effects, and perform ADLs satisfactorily

NIC   Interventions (Nursing Interventions Classification)

Suggested NIC Interventions

Analgesic Administration, Pain Management

• = Independent;   ▲ = Collaborative;   EBN = Evidence-Based Nursing;   EB = Evidence-Based

Example NIC Activities—Pain Management
Assure patient attentive analgesic care; Perform a comprehensive assessment of pain, to include location, characteristics, onset and duration, frequency, quality, intensity or severity of pain, and precipitating factors

Nursing Interventions and *Rationales*

▲ Determine whether the client is experiencing pain at the time of the initial interview. If so, intervene at that time to provide pain relief. Assess and document the intensity, character, onset, duration, and aggravating and relieving factors of pain during the initial evaluation of the client. *The initial assessment and documentation provide direction for the pain treatment plan. A comprehensive pain assessment includes all characteristics of the pain that the client can provide. The client's report of the pain is considered the single most reliable indicator of pain (APS, 2004; JCAHO, 2000).*

• Assess pain in a client by using a self-report 0 to 10 numerical pain rating scale, Wong-Baker FACES scale, or Faces Pain Scale (see Pain: Assessment Guide and Appendix D for examples). **EB:** *Single-item ratings of pain intensity are valid and reliable as measures of pain intensity (Jensen, 2003).*

• Question the client regarding pain at frequent intervals, such as while taking vital signs. *Pain assessment is as important as taking vital signs, and the APS suggests applying the concept of pain assessment as the "fifth vital sign" (APS, 2004).*

• Tell the client to report pain location, intensity, and quality when experiencing pain. Assess and document the intensity of pain and discomfort after any known pain-producing procedure, with each new report of pain, and at regular intervals. *Systematic ongoing assessment and documentation provide direction for the pain treatment plan; adjustments are based on the client's response. The client's report of pain is the single most reliable indicator of pain (APS, 2004).*

• Question the client regarding the level of pain that he or she believes is appropriate to achieve a state of comfort and appropriate function. Attempt to keep pain level no higher than that level, preferably much lower. *The pain rating that allows the client to have comfort and appropriate function should be determined; this allows a tangible way to measure outcomes of pain management (Pasero & McCaffery, 2004b; Griffie, 2003).*

• Ask the client to describe past and current experiences with pain and the effectiveness of the methods used to manage the pain, including experiences with side effects, typical coping responses, and the way the client expresses pain. **EBN:** *A study of 270 people with cancer pain revealed that those surveyed had a number of concerns (barriers) that affected their willingness to report pain and use analgesics (Vallerand et al, 2007). Many harbored fears and misconceptions regarding the use of analgesics, management of side effects, and risk of addiction.*

• Describe the adverse effects of unrelieved pain. **EBN and EB:** *Numerous pathophysiological and psychological morbidity factors may be associated with pain (Noble, 2006). One study demonstrated that persistent unrelieved pain suppressed immune function, which can lead to infection, increased tumor growth, and other complications. Analgesics such as opioids and local anesthetics have been shown to block immunosuppression (Page & Ben-Eliyahu, 1997).*

• Ask the client to maintain a diary (if able) of pain ratings, timing, precipitating events, medications, treatments, and steps that work best to relieve pain. **EBN:** *Studies have shown that systematic tracking of pain was an important factor in improving pain management (Schumacher et al, 2002).*

• If the client is cognitively impaired and unable to report pain or use a pain rating scale, assess and document behaviors that might be indicative of pain (e.g., change in activity, loss of appetite, guarding, grimacing, moaning). Use a hierarchy of pain measures to assess pain in clients who cannot report pain: (1) attempt to obtain a self-report, (2) consider the presence of underlying painful pathology or condition and assume pain is present if appropriate, (3) observe behaviors that may indicate the presence of pain, (4) obtain a proxy (parent, caregiver, or significant other who knows client very well) report of behaviors that might indicate pain, (5) attempt an analgesic trial in which a dose of analgesia is administered and any reduction in pain behaviors is noted. Develop a treatment plan based on the analgesic trial (Pasero & McCaffery, 2005). *The absence of behaviors thought to be indicative of pain does not necessarily mean that pain is absent (Herr, 2002; Pasero, 2003b; Pasero & McCaffery, 2002).* **EBN:** *Certain behaviors have been shown to be indicative of pain and can be used to assess pain in clients who cannot use a self-report pain rating tool (e.g., in the cognitively impaired client). The clinician should be aware that pain expression is highly in-*

dividual, and what may be a pain behavior in one client may not be in another. Pain assessment must be individualized (Herr, 2002).

▲ Assume that pain is present and treat accordingly in clients who have a pathological condition or are undergoing a procedure thought to be painful. *Pain is associated with certain pathological conditions (e.g., arthritis) and procedures (e.g., surgery). In the absence of the client's report of pain (e.g., in critically ill or cognitively impaired clients), the clinician should assume that pain is present and treat accordingly (Pasero, 2003b; Pasero & McCaffery, 2002, 2005).*

• Obtain a complete history of medications the client is taking, including over-the-counter medications, or has taken to prevent drug-drug interactions and toxicity problems that can occur when incompatible drugs are combined or when allergies are present. *The history also provides the clinician with an understanding of what medications have been tried and were or were not effective in treating the client's pain (APS, 2004).*

▲ Explore the need for medications from the three classes of analgesic: opioids (narcotics), nonopioids (acetaminophen, nonsteroidal antiinflammatory drugs), and adjuvant medications. For chronic neuropathic pain, consider adjuvant medications that are analgesic, such as anticonvulsants and antidepressants. *The analgesic regimen should include a nonopioid drug around the clock, even if pain is severe enough to require the addition of an opioid (APS, 2004). Some types of pain respond to nonopioid drugs alone. If the pain is not responding, however, consider increasing the dosage or adding an opioid. At any level of pain, analgesic adjuvants may be useful (APS, 2004). Analgesic combinations may enhance pain relief. Combining analgesics can result in acceptable pain relief with lower dosages of each analgesic than would be possible with one analgesic alone. Lower dosages can result in fewer or less-severe side effects (Pasero, 2003a).*

▲ For persistent mild cancer pain, obtain a prescription to administer nonopioid analgesics. *When pain persists or increases, an opioid such as morphine or oxycodone should be added to the nonopioid. If this is not effective, switch to morphine or other single-entity opioids (Pasero & McCaffery, 2004a; Miaskowski et al, 2005).* **EB:** *A multimodal approach combining analgesics that attack different underlying pain mechanisms is recommended for the treatment persistent cancer pain (Miaskowski et al, 2005).*

▲ For persistent chronic nonmalignant pain, discuss the use of opioid analgesics with the healthcare team and obtain a prescription to administer if appropriate. *These agents should be used in clients with chronic nonmalignant pain (e.g., osteoarthritis, rheumatoid arthritis) when other medications and nonpharmacological interventions produce inadequate pain relief and the client's quality of life is affected by the pain (APS, 2004).*

▲ The oral route for pain medication administration is preferred. If the client is receiving parenteral analgesia, use an equianalgesic chart to convert to a controlled release, long-acting oral medication as soon as possible (McCaffery, 2003). (Refer to the Equianalgesic Chart at the start of this section.) *The least invasive route of administration capable of providing adequate pain control is recommended. The oral route is preferred because it is the most convenient and cost effective (McCaffery, 2003).*

▲ Avoid the IM route for administration of pain medication. *The IM route is avoided because of unreliable absorption, pain, and inconvenience (APS, 2003). Repeated IM injections can cause sterile abscesses and fibrosis of muscle and soft tissue (APS, 2003).*

▲ Establish around-the-clock dosing and administer supplemental opioid doses for breakthrough pain as needed to keep pain ratings at or below the comfort-function goal (Pasero & McCaffery, 2004b). *An order for an as-needed breakthrough dose, which is one sixth to one tenth of the total daily opioid dose, is an essential backup because breakthrough pain is common in clients with chronic pain (McCaffery & Pasero, 2003).*

▲ Ask the client to describe appetite and bowel elimination. Always obtain a prescription for a stool softener and a peristaltic stimulant daily to prevent opioid-induced constipation in clients taking regular daily doses of opioids. *Because the development of opioid-induced side effects varies greatly from person to person, clients should be monitored and, if their development is inevitable (e.g., constipation), prophylactically treated. Opioids cause constipation by decreasing bowel peristalsis (Plaisance & Ellis, 2002).*

• Question the client about any disruption in sleep. **EB:** *Clients with low back pain had significant loss of sleep (Marin, Cyhan & Miklos, 2006).*

• Watch for signs of depression in clients with chronic pain, including sleeplessness, not eating, flat affect, statements of depression, or suicidal ideation. **EB:** *Clients with chronic pain had twice* *the rate of suicide than the people without pain (Tang & Crane, 2006). Clients older than 60 years who committed suicide had physical illness (especially pain), breathlessness, and disability (Harwood et al, 2006).*

- Explain to the client the pain management approach that has been ordered, including therapies, medication administration, side effects, and complications. *One of the most important steps toward improved control of pain is a better client understanding of the nature of pain, its treatment, and the role the client needs to play in pain control (APS, 2004).*

- Discuss the client's fears of undertreated pain, addiction, and overdose. *Because of the many misconceptions regarding pain and its treatment, education about the ability to control pain effectively and correction of myths about the use of opioids should be included as part of the treatment plan (McCaffery, Pasero & Portenoy, 2004). Opioid tolerance and physical dependence are expected with long-term opioid treatment and should not be confused with addiction (APS, 2004). Addiction is unlikely when clients use opioids for pain relief (APS, 2003; McCaffery, Pasero & Portenoy, 2004; Miaskowski et al, 2005).* **EBN:** *A survey of 270 people with cancer pain revealed that many harbor fears and misconceptions regarding the use of analgesics, management of side effects, and risk of addiction (Ward et al, 1993).*

- Review the client's pain diary, flow sheet, and medication records to determine the overall degree of pain relief, side effects, and analgesic requirements for an appropriate period (e.g., 1 week). **EBN:** *Systematic tracking of pain was found to be an important factor in improving pain management (Schumacher et al, 2002).*

▲ Obtain prescriptions to increase or decrease analgesic doses when indicated. Base prescriptions on the client's report of pain severity and the comfort-function goal and response to previous dose in terms of relief, side effects, and ability to perform ADLs and comply with the prescribed therapeutic regimen. *Analgesic dosages should be adjusted to achieve pain relief with manageable and tolerable adverse effects (Pasero & McCaffery, 2004b; Pasero, 2003a).*

▲ If opioid dose is increased, monitor sedation and respiratory status for a brief time. *Clients receiving long-term opioid therapy generally develop tolerance to the respiratory depressant effects of these agents (APS, 2003; Miaskowski et al, 2005; Pasero & McCaffery, 2002).*

▲ In addition to the use of analgesics, support the client's use of nonpharmacological methods to help control pain, such as physical therapy, group therapy, distraction, imagery, relaxation, massage, and application of heat and cold. *Cognitive-behavioral strategies can restore the client's sense of self-control, personal efficacy, and active participation in his or her own care (APS, 2004; Miaskowski et al, 2005).*

- Teach and implement nonpharmacological interventions when pain is relatively well controlled with pharmacological means. *Nonpharmacological interventions should be used to supplement, not replace, pharmacological interventions (APS, 2004; Miaskowski et al, 2005).*

- Encourage the client to plan activities around periods of greatest comfort whenever possible. *Pain diminishes activity. Clients find it easier to perform their ADLs and enjoy social activities when they are rested and pain is under control (Pasero & McCaffery, 2004b).*

- Explore appropriate resources for management of pain on a long-term basis (e.g., hospice, pain care center). *Most clients with cancer or chronic nonmalignant pain are treated for pain in outpatient and home care settings. Plans should be made to ensure ongoing assessment of the pain and the effectiveness of treatments in these settings (APS, 2004).*

- If the client has progressive cancer pain, assist the client and family with handling issues related to death and dying. *Peer support groups and pastoral counseling may increase the client's and family's coping skills and provide needed support (APS, 2004).*

- Assist the client and family in minimizing the effects of pain on interpersonal relationships and daily activities such as work and recreation. **EBN:** *Pain can reduce clients' options to exercise control, diminish psychological well-being, and make them feel helpless and vulnerable. Therefore clinicians should encourage active client involvement in effective and practical methods to manage pain (Hitchcock, Ferrell & McCaffery, 1994).*

Pediatric

- For the young child (4 years of age and older) use the Wong-Baker FACES Scale or the Faces Pain Scale to determine the level of pain present. **EB:** *The Faces Pain Scale was shown to be valid using 4- to 12-year-olds postoperatively. It was further validated with 600 children age 4 to 5 years re-*

P

ceiving immunizations (Wood et al, 2003; Hicks et al, 2001). Children are able to quantify pain opti-mally by using a self-report pain rating scale at age 8 years (Spagrud et al, 2003).

- Help children and adolescents learn and use techniques such as relaxation and cognitive-behavioral techniques to handle pain. **EBN:** *Studies have shown that the use of psychological interventions can reduce the frequency and severity of pain in children and adolescents (Eccleston et al, 2002).*

Geriatric

▲ Always take an older client's reports of pain seriously and ensure that the pain is relieved. *Pain is not an expected part of normal aging (AGS, 2002; Herr, 2002). Unrelieved pain can cause decreased cognition, depression, mood disorders, and reduced ADLs (Davis & Srivastava, 2003; Pasero & McCaffery, 2004b).*

- When assessing pain, speak clearly, slowly, and loudly enough for the client to hear. If the client uses a hearing aid, be sure it is in place; repeat information as needed. Be sure the client can see well enough to read the pain scale (use an enlarged scale) and written materials. **EBN:** *Older clients often have difficulty hearing and seeing. Comprehension is improved when instructions are given slowly and clearly and when clients can see visual aids (Herr, 2002).*

- In the absence of the client's report of pain in situations where pain is expected (e.g., anesthe-tized, critically ill, or cognitively impaired client), the clinician should assume pain is present and treat accordingly (Herr, 2002; Pasero, 2003b; Pasero & McCaffery, 2002, 2005).

- Handle the client's body gently. Allow the client to move at his or her own speed. *Elders are par-ticularly susceptible to injury during care activities. Caregivers must be client and expect that older clients will move more slowly than younger clients; they may also perform better and experience less pain when they are allowed to move themselves (McCaffery & Pasero, 1999).*

▲ Use acetaminophen and NSAIDs with low gastrointestinal side effect profiles, such as celecoxib (Celebrex), choline magnesium trisalicylate (Trilisate), and diflunisal (Dolobid). Naproxen may be the best choice for long term treatment. Watch closely for side effects, such as cardiovascular and gastrointestinal disturbances and bleeding and renal problems. *Elders are at increased risk for gastric and renal toxicity from NSAIDs (Davis and Srivastava, 2003; AGS, 2002). Opioid adminis-tration around the clock is preferable to long-term administration of nonselective NSAIDs in the older client because of an increased risk for NSAID adverse effects (Fine, 2004; AGS, 2002).*

▲ Avoid or use with caution drugs with a long half-life, such as the NSAID piroxicam (Feldene) and the opioids methadone (Dolophine) and levorphanol (LevoDromoran). *The higher prevalence of renal insufficiency in elders compared with younger persons can result in toxicity from drug accumula-tion (AGS, 2002; APS, 2004; Fick et al, 2003).*

▲ Use opioids cautiously in the older client with moderate to severe pain unrelieved by NSAIDs. Reduce initial doses by 25% to 50%. After titrating to comfort with a short-acting opioid, switch to an extended-release opioid for persistent pain treatment. **EBN:** *Older clients are more sensitive to the analgesic effects of opioid drugs because they experience a higher peak effect and a longer duration of pain relief (APS, 2003). Reduce the initial recommended adult starting opioid dosage by 25% to 50%, especially if the client is frail and debilitated; then increase the dosage by 25% on an individual basis if needed (Ardery et al, 2003).*

▲ Avoid the use of opioids with toxic metabolites, such as meperidine (Demerol) and propoxy-phene (Darvon, Darvocet), in older clients. *Meperidine's metabolite, normeperidine, can produce central nervous system irritability, seizures, and even death; propoxyphene's metabolite, norpropoxy-phene, can produce central nervous system toxicity. Both metabolites are eliminated by the kidneys, which makes meperidine and propoxyphene particularly poor choices for older clients, many of whom have at least some degree of renal insufficiency (Ardery et al, 2003; Fick et al, 2003).*

▲ Monitor for signs of depression in elders and refer for treatment if needed. **EB:** *A study demon-strated that treatment of depression in elders with arthritis also helped decrease pain and improve func-tional abilities (Lin et al, 2003).*

Multicultural

- Assess for the influence of cultural beliefs, norms, and values on the client's perception and expe-rience of pain. **EB:** *Native-American clients may think that asking for pain medication is disrespectful because it implies that health care providers do not know what they are doing (Brant, 2001). The use of prayer or faith for pain management, care, and prevention was found to be common in African-American elders (Ibrahim et al, 2004).*

• = Independent; ▲ = Collaborative; EBN = Evidence-Based Nursing; EB = Evidence-Based

- A representational approach offers a flexible framework for nurses to get cancer clients to delve deeply into their own belief systems about health, disease, and pain and to add sound concepts that work for their pain management. *The program is called Representational Intervention to Decrease Cancer Pain (RIDcancerPain) and has the following 6 steps:*
  1. *Representational assessment: the client describes beliefs about cancer pain along five dimensions (identity, cause, timeline, consequences, and cure/control)*
  2. *Exploring misconceptions, with emphasis on their origins*
  3. *Creating conditions for conceptual change by discussing the limitations of holding beliefs that are misconceptions (i.e., what one loses by maintaining those beliefs)*
  4. *Introducing replacement information*
  5. *Summarizing and discussing benefits of adopting beliefs that are credible replacements*
  6. *Developing a plan and strategies (Ward et al, in press)*
- Assess for the effect of fatalism on the client's beliefs regarding the current state of comfort. **EBN:** *Fatalistic perspectives, which involve the belief that one cannot control one's own fate, may influence health behaviors in some African-American and Latino populations (Harmon, Castro & Coe, 1996; Phillips, Cohen & Moses, 1999).*
- Assess for pain disparities among racial and ethnic minorities. **EB:** *Racial and ethnic minorities tend to be undertreated for pain when compared with non-Hispanic whites (Green et al, 2003).*
- Incorporate safe and effective folk healthcare practices and beliefs into care whenever possible. *Although support of an individual's healthcare beliefs is recommended, when research does not support the safety or effectiveness of a method or when research does not exist, this should be explained fully to the client (McCaffery, 2002).* **EBN:** *Incorporating folk healthcare beliefs and practices into pain management care increased compliance with the treatment plan (Juarez, Ferrell & Borneman, 1998).*
- Use a family-centered approach to care. **EBN:** *Involving the family in pain management care increased compliance with the treatment regimen (Juarez, Ferrell & Borneman, 1998).*
- Teach information about pain medications and their side effects and how to work with health care providers to manage pain, and encourage the use of religious faith to cope with pain. **EB:** *Socioeconomically disadvantaged African-American and Hispanic clients benefit from educational interventions on pain that dispel myths about opioids and teach clients to communicate assertively about their pain with their physicians and nurses (Anderson et al, 2002).*
- Use culturally relevant pain scales to assess pain in the client. **EBN:** *The Faces Pain Scale-Revised was shown to be preferred over other self-report pain rating tools in older minority adults (Jowers Ware et al, 2006; Ware et al, 2006) and in Chinese adults (Li, Liu & Herr, 2007). Clients from minority cultures may express pain differently than clients from the majority culture. The Oucher Scale is available in African-American and Hispanic versions and is used to assess pain in children (Beyer, Denyes & Villarruel, 1992).*
- Ensure that directions for medication use are available in the client's language of choice and are understood by the client and caregiver. **EB:** *Bilingual instructions for medication administration increased compliance with the pain management plan (Juarez, Ferrell & Borneman, 1998). Using specific phrases in Spanish to assess acute pain in non–English-speaking Hispanic clients helps provide timely pain assessment and management (Collins, Gullette & Schnepf, 2004).*

 Home Care

- Develop the treatment plan with the client and caregivers. *Clients and caregivers will be more likely to follow the treatment plan when their input is considered (McCaffery & Pasero, 1999).*
- ▲ Develop a full medication profile, including medications prescribed by all physicians and all over-the-counter medications. Assess for drug interactions. Instruct the client to refrain from mixing medications without physician approval. *Pain medications may significantly affect or be affected by other medications and may cause severe side effects. Some combinations of drugs are specifically contraindicated.*
- Assess the client's and family's knowledge of side effects and safety precautions associated with pain medications (e.g., use caution if operating machinery when opioids are first taken or dosage has been significantly increased). *The cognitive effects of opioids usually subside within a week of initial dosing or dose increases. The use of long-term opioid treatment does not appear to affect neuropsychological performance.* **EB:** *Pain itself may reduce performance on neuropsychological tests more than oral opioid treatment (Sjogren et al, 2000).*

• = Independent;   ▲ = Collaborative;   EBN = Evidence-Based Nursing;   EB = Evidence-Based

P

▲ Collaborate with the healthcare team (including the client and family) on an ongoing basis to determine an optimal pain control profile. Identify the most effective interventions and the medication administration routes most acceptable to the client and family. *Success in pain control partially depends on the acceptability of the suggested intervention. Acceptability promotes compliance.*

• If medication is administered by highly technological methods, assess the home for necessary resources (e.g., electricity) and ensure that responsible caregivers will be available to help the client with administration. *Some routes of medication administration require special conditions and procedures to be safe and accurate.*

▲ Assess the knowledge base of the client and family for highly technological medication administration. Teach as necessary. Be sure the client knows when, how, and whom to contact if analgesia is unsatisfactory. *Appropriate instruction in the home increases the accuracy and safety of medication administration.*

• Support the client and family in the use of opioid analgesics. *Well-intentioned friends and family may create added stress by expressing judgment or fears regarding the use of opioid analgesics.*

Client/Family Teaching

NOTE: To avoid the negative connotations associated with the words *drugs* and *narcotics*, use the term *pain medicine* when teaching clients.

• Provide written materials on pain control such as *Understanding Your Pain: Using a Pain Rating Scale* (McCaffery, Pasero & Portenoy, 2001; see instructions on the use of a pain rating scale) and *Taking Oral Opioid Analgesics* (McCaffery, Pasero & Portenoy, 2004). *Written materials are provided in addition to verbal instructions so that the client has a reference during treatment.*

• Discuss the various discomforts encompassed by the word pain and ask the client to give examples of previously experienced pain. Explain the pain assessment process and the purpose of the pain rating scale. *Clients often have difficulty understanding the concept of pain and describing their pain experience. The use of alternative words and a complete description of the assessment process, including the use of scales, ensures that an accurate treatment plan is developed (Pasero & McCaffery, 2004b). Teach clients to use the pain rating scale to rate the intensity of past or current pain.*

▲ Ask the client to set a comfort-function goal by selecting a pain level on the rating scale that makes it easy to perform recovery activities (e.g., turn, cough, deep breathe). If pain is above this level, the client should take action that decreases pain or notify a member of the healthcare team. (See information on teaching clients to use the pain rating scale.) *The use of comfort-function goals provides direction for the treatment plan. Changes are made according to the client's response and achievement of the goals of recovery or rehabilitation (Pasero & McCaffery, 2004b).*

• Discuss the total plan for pharmacological and nonpharmacological treatment, including the medication plan for around-the-clock administration and supplemental doses, the maintenance of a pain diary, and the use of supplies and equipment. *Appropriate instruction increases the accuracy and safety of medication administration.*

• Reinforce the importance of taking pain medications to keep pain under control. *Teaching clients to stay on top of their pain and prevent it from getting out of control will improve their ability to perform ADLs and accomplish goals (Pasero & McCaffery, 2004b).*

• Reinforce that taking opioids for pain relief is not addiction and that addiction is highly unlikely. *The development of addiction when opioids are taken for pain relief is rare (APS, 2004; McCaffery, Pasero & Portenoy, 2004).*

• Explain to a client with chronic neuropathic pain the process of taking adjuvant analgesics (e.g., tricyclic antidepressants). *A low dose of adjuvant analgesic is used initially and the dose is increased gradually. Pain relief is delayed, and the adjuvant analgesics must be taken daily. Teaching clients that although the medicine is an antidepressant, it is used for analgesia and not depression will increase understanding of the drug. Comparable teaching should take place when an anticonvulsant is prescribed for analgesia.*

• Suggest the client with cancer try having a massage, with aromatherapy if desired. **EB:** *Both massage and aromatherapy have short-term benefits on psychological well-being for the client with cancer (Fellowes, Barnes & Wilkinson, 2004).*

• Emphasize to the client the importance of pacing himself or herself and taking rest breaks before they are needed. *Clients find they are able to perform their ADLs and achieve goals better when they are rested (Pasero & McCaffery, 2004b).*

• = Independent;   ▲ = Collaborative;   EBN = Evidence-Based Nursing;   EB = Evidence-Based

▲ Demonstrate the use of appropriate nonpharmacological approaches in addition to pharmacological approaches for helping to control pain (e.g., physical therapy, group therapy, distraction, imagery, and application of heat and cold) (Miaskowski et al, 2005).

• Teach and implement nonpharmacological interventions when pain is relatively well controlled with pharmacological means. *Nonpharmacological interventions are used to supplement, not replace, pharmacological interventions (APS, 2004; Miaskowski et al, 2005).*

 See the EVOLVE website for World Wide Web resources for client education.

REFERENCES

American Geriatric Society: The management of persistent pain in older persons, *J Am Geriatr Soc* 50:S205, 1-20, 2002.

American Pain Society: *Principles of analgesic use for the treatment of acute pain and cancer pain,* Glenview, IL, 2003, American Pain Society.

American Pain Society: *Pain: current understanding of assessment, management and treatments,* 2004, www.ampainsoc.org/ce/npc, accessed March 26, 2007.

Anderson KO et al: Cancer pain management among underserved minority outpatients: perceived needs and barriers to optimal control, *Cancer* 94(8):2295-2304, 2002.

Ardery G, Herr KA, Titler MG et al: Assessing and managing acute pain in older adults: a research base to guide practice, *Med-Surg Nurs* 12:1, 2003.

Beyer J, Denyes M, Villarruel A: The creation, validation, and continuing development of the Oucher: a measure of pain intensity in children, *J Pediatr Nurs* 7(5):335, 1992.

Brant JM: *Cultural implications of pain education,* presented at Cancer Pain and Education for Patients and the Public Conference, City of Hope National Medical Center, Duarte, CA, October 18, 2001.

Collins AS, Gullette D, Schnepf M: Break through language barriers, *Nurs Manage* 35(8):34-36, 38, 2004.

Davis MP, Srivastava M: Demographics, assessment and management of pain in the elderly, *Drugs Aging* 20(1):23, 2003.

Eccleston C, Morley S, Williams A et al: Systematic review of randomized controlled trials of psychological therapy for chronic pain in children and adolescents with a subset meta-analysis of pain relief, *Pain* 99(1-2):157-166, 2002.

Fellowes D, Barnes K, Wilkinson S: Aromatherapy and massage for symptom relief in patients with cancer, *The Cochrane Library,* CD002287, 2004.

Fick DM, Cooper JW, Wade WE et al: Updating the Beers criteria for potentially inappropriate mediation use in older adults, *Arch Int Med* 163:2716-2724, 2003.

Fine P: Pharmacological management of persistent pain in older patients, *Clin J Pain* 20(4):220-226, 2004.

Green CR et al: The unequal burden of pain: confronting racial and ethnic disparities in pain, *Pain Med* 4(3):277-294, 2003.

Griffie J: Pain control: addressing inadequate pain relief, *Am J Nurs* 8:62-63, 103, 2003.

Harmon MP, Castro FG, Coe K: Acculturation and cervical cancer: knowledge, beliefs, and behaviors of Hispanic women, *Women Health* 24(3):37, 1996.

Harwood DM, Hawton K, Hope T et al: Life problems and physical illness as risk factors for suicide in older people: a descriptive and case-control study, *Psychol Med* 36(9):1265-1274, 2006.

Herr K: Pain assessment in cognitively impaired older adults, *Am J Nurs* 102(12):65, 66, 68, 2002.

Herr K, Coyne P, McCaffery M et al: Pain assessment in the nonverbal patient: position statement with clinical recommendations, *Pain Manage Nurs* 7(2):44-52, 2006.

Hicks CL et al: The Faces Pain Scale-Revised: toward a common metric in pediatric pain measurement, *Pain* 93(2):173, 2001.

Hitchcock LS, Ferrell BR, McCaffery M: The experience of chronic nonmalignant pain, *J Pain Symptom Manage* 9:312, 1994.

Ibrahim SA et al: Inner city African-American elderly patients' perceptions and preferences for the care of chronic knee and hip pain: findings from focus groups, *J Gerontol A Biol Sci Med Sci* 59(12):1318-1322, 2004.

Jensen MP: The validity and reliability of pain measures in adults with cancer, *J Pain* 4(1):52-55, 2003.

The Joint Commission on Accreditation of Healthcare Organizations (JCAHO): *Hospital Accreditation Standards,* Oakbrook Terrace, IL, 2000, The Commission.

Jowers Ware L et al: Evaluation of the revised faces pain scale, verbal descriptor scale, numeric rating scale, and Iowa pain thermometer in older minority adults. *Pain Manag Nurs* 7(3):117-125, 2006.

Juarez G, Ferrell B, Borneman T: Influence of culture on cancer pain management in Hispanic clients, *Cancer Pract* 6(5):262, 1998.

Li L, Liu X, Herr K: Postoperative pain intensity assessment: a comparison of four scales in Chinese adults, *Pain Med* 8(3):223-234, 2007.

Lin EHB, Katon W, Von Korff M et al: Effect of improving depression care on pain and functional outcomes among older adults with arthritis, *JAMA* 290(18):2428, 2003.

Marin R, Cyhan T, Miklos W: Sleep disturbance in patients with chronic low back pain, *Am J Phys Med Rehabil* 85(5):430-435, 2006.

McCaffery M: *Nursing practice theories related to cognition, bodily pain, and man-environment interactions,* Los Angeles, 1968, University of California.

McCaffery M: What is the role of nondrug methods in the nursing care of patients with acute pain? *Pain Management Nursing* 3(3):77-80, 2002.

McCaffery M: Pain control: switching from IV to PO, *Am J Nurs* 103(5):62-63, 2003.

McCaffery M, Pasero C: *Pain: Clinical manual,* ed 2, St. Louis, 1999, Mosby.

McCaffery M, Pasero C: Breakthrough pain, *Am J Nurs* 103(4):83, 84, 86, 2003.

McCaffery M, Pasero C, Portenoy RK: *Understanding your pain: using a pain rating scale,* Chadds Ford, PA, 2001, Endo Pharmaceuticals.

McCaffery M, Pasero C, Portenoy RK: *Understanding your pain: taking oral opioid analgesics,* Chadds Ford, PA, 2004, Endo Pharmaceuticals.

Mersky H, Bogduk N, editors: *Classification of chronic pain,* ed 2, Seattle, 1994, International Association for the Study of Pain (IASP).

Miaskowski C, Cleary J, Burney R et al: *Guideline for the management of cancer pain in adults and children,* Glenview, IL, 2005, American Pain Society.

Noble KA: What a pain! *J PeriAnesth Nurs* 21(5):353-356, 2006.

Page GG, Ben-Eliyahu S: The immune-suppressive nature of pain, *Semin Oncol Nurs* 13(1):10, 1997.

Pasero C: Multimodal analgesia in the PACU, *J Perianesth Nursing* 18(4):265-268, 2003a.

Pasero C: Pain in the critically ill, *J Perianesth Nursing* 18(6):422-425, 2003b.

Pasero C, McCaffery M: Monitoring opioid-induced sedation, *Am J Nurs* 102(2):67-68, 2002.

Pasero C, McCaffery M: Pain in the critically ill, *Am J Nurs* 102(1):59-60, 2002.

Pasero C, McCaffery M: Controlled-release oxycodone, *Am J Nurs* 104(1):30-32, 2004a.

Pasero, C, McCaffery M: Comfort-function goals, *Am J Nurs* 104(9):77-78, 81, 2004b.

Pasero C, McCaffery M: No self report means no pain intensity, *Am J Nurs* 105(10):50-53, 2005.

Phillips JM, Cohen MZ, Moses G: Breast cancer screening and African American women: fear, fatalism, and silence, *Oncol Nurs Forum* 26(3):561, 1999.

Plaisance L, Ellis JA: Opioid-induced constipation, *Am J Nurs* 102(3):72-73, 2002.

Schumacher KL, Koresawa S, West C et al: The usefulness of a daily pain management diary for outpatients with cancer-related pain, *Oncol Nurs Forum* 29(9):1304, 2002.

Sjogren P et al: Neuropsychological performance in cancer clients: the role of oral opioids, pain and performance status, *Pain* 86: 237, 2000.

Spagrud LJ et al: Children's self-report of pain intensity. The Faces Pain Scale-Revised, *Am J Nurs* 103(12):62-64, 2003.

Tang NK, Crane C: Suicidality in chronic pain: a review of the prevalence, risk factors and psychological links, *Psychol Med* 36(5):575-586, 2006.

Vallerand AH et al: Knowledge of and barriers to pain management in caregivers of cancer patients receiving homecare, *Cancer Nurs* 30(1):31-37, 2007.

Ward S et al: Client-related barriers to management of cancer pain, *Pain* 52:319, 1993.

Ward S, Donovan H, Gunnarsdottir S et al: A representational intervention to decrease cancer pain (RIDcancerPain), in press.

Ware LJ, Epps CD, Hero K et al: Evaluation of the Revised FACES Pain Scale, Verbal Descriptor Scale, Numeric Rating Scale, and Iowa Pain Thermometer in older minority adults, *Pain Manag Nurs* 7(3):117-125, 2006.

Wood C et al: *Self-assessment by the Faces Pain Scale: revised of immediate post vaccination pain following administration of Priorix versus MMRII as a second dose in 4 to 6 year old children,* presented at the Sixth International Symposium on Pediatric Pain, Sydney, Australia, 2003.

Readiness for enhanced Parenting *T. Heather Herdman, RN, PhD*

NANDA Definition

A pattern of providing an environment for children or other dependent person(s) that is sufficient to nurture growth and development and can be strengthened.

P Defining Characteristics

Children or other dependent person(s) express(es) satisfaction with home environment, emotional support of children; evidence of attachment; exhibits realistic expectations of children; expresses willingness to enhance parenting; needs of children are met (e.g., physical and emotional)

NOC Outcomes (Nursing Outcomes Classification)

Suggested NOC Outcomes

Child Development: 1 Month, 2 Months, 4 Months, 6 Months, 12 Months, Preschool, Middle Childhood, Adolescence; Growth; Health-Promoting Behavior; Health-Seeking Behavior; Immunization Behavior; Knowledge: Breastfeeding, Child Physical Safety, Diet, Health Behavior, Health Resources, Infection Control, Medication, Personal Safety; Leisure Participation; Nutritional Status; Parent-Infant Attachment; Parenting Performance; Parenting: Psychosocial Safety; Risk Control; Risk Detection; Role Performance; Safe Home Environment; Self-Esteem

Example NOC Outcome with Indicators
Parenting Performance as evidenced by the following indicators: Provides regular preventive and episodic health care/Stimulates cognitive and social development/Stimulates emotional and spiritual growth/Interacts positively with child/Empathizes with child/Expresses satisfaction with parental role/Expresses positive self-esteem (Rate the outcome and indicators of **Parenting Performance:** 1 = never demonstrated, 2 = rarely demonstrated, 3 = sometimes demonstrated, 4 = often demonstrated, 5 = consistently demonstrated [see Section I].)

Client Outcomes

Client/Family Will (Specify Time Frame):

- Affirm desire to improve parenting skills to further support growth and development of children
- Demonstrate loving relationship with children
- Provide a safe, nurturing environment
- Assess risks in home/environment and takes steps to prevent possibility of harm to children
- Meet physical, psychosocial, and spiritual needs or seek appropriate assistance

NIC   Interventions (Nursing Interventions Classification)

Suggested NIC Interventions

Anticipatory Guidance; Attachment Promotion; Developmental Enhancement: Adolescent, Child; Family Integrity Promotion: Childbearing Family; Infant Care; Newborn Care; Parent Education: Adolescent, Childrearing Family, Infant; Parenting Promotion; Teaching: Infant Stimulation

Example NIC Activities—Parenting Promotion

Assist parents to have realistic expectations appropriate to developmental and ability level of child; Assist parents with role transition and expectations of parenthood

Nursing Interventions and *Rationales*

- Use family-centered care and role modeling for holistic care of families. **EBN:** *Specific techniques of role modeling and reflective practice are suggested as effective approaches to teach the family sensitive care in clinical settings in which families are part of the care environment (Tomlinson et al, 2002).*
- Assess parents' feelings when dealing with a child who has a chronic illness. **EBN:** *Knowing how parents feel about a child's asthma is the first step in helping them manage this common chronic disease (Clark & Chalmers, 2003).*
- Encourage positive parenting: respect for children, understanding of normal development, and use of creative and loving approaches to meet parenting challenges. **EBN:** *Understanding normal development is a first step so that parents can distinguish common behaviors for a given stage of development from "problems" (Ahmann, 2002).*
- Promote low-technology interventions, such as massage and multisensory interventions (maternal voice, eye-to-eye contact, and rocking) to reduce maternal and infant stress and improve mother-infant relationship. **EBN:** *These are strategies aimed at reducing maternal and infant stress and improving the mother-infant relationship (White-Traut, 2004). Incorporating infant massage into a planned parenting enhancement program may promote effective parenting through a special focus on infant stimulation through massage (Porter & Porter, 2004).*
- Provide opportunities for mother-infant skin-to-skin contact (kangaroo care) for preterm infants. **EB:** *The neurodevelopmental profile was more mature for infants receiving kangaroo care (Feldman & Eidelman, 2003).*
- Provide the parent with the opportunity to assist in the newborn's first bath, allowing a flexible bath time. **EBN:** *A flexible bathing time is recommended depending on the characteristics and stability of the newborn and family desires. (Behring, Vezeau & Fink, 2003).*
- When the person who is ill is the parent, use family-centered assessment skills to determine the impact of an adult's illness on the child and then guide the parent through those topics that are most likely to be of concern. **EBN:** *The pediatric nurse, by embracing core principles of openness and honesty and by providing concrete developmental information, can empower parents to support their own children (McCue & Bonn, 2003).*
- ▲ Have family members participate in client conferences that involve all members of the healthcare team. *Conferences allow distribution of information, input by all members at one time, and a decrease in anxiety levels of family members.*
- ▲ Help parents develop realistic expectations of their child's development. **EBN:** *One study demonstrated the potential of parent training and support to alter the style of interactions between parents and their children (Letourneau, 2001).*

P

• = Independent;   ▲ = Collaborative;   EBN = Evidence-Based Nursing;   EB = Evidence-Based

- Provide practical and psychological assistance for parents of clients with psychiatric diagnoses, such as schizophrenia. **EBN:** *Parents may be overloaded with their long-term caring tasks, and provision of practical and psychological assistance can be of benefit (Jungbauer et al, 2003).*

Multicultural

- Assess the influence of cultural beliefs, norms, and values on the client's perception of parenting. **EBN:** *What the client considers normal parenting may be based on cultural perceptions (Leininger & McFarland, 2002).*
- Acknowledge racial and ethnic differences at the onset of care. **EB:** *Acknowledgment of racial and ethnicity issues enhances communication, establishes rapport, and promotes treatment outcomes (D'Avanzo et al, 2001).*
- Clarify parents' feelings, expectations, perceptions, and availability regarding participation in the care of their sick child. **EBN:** *Cultural differences in regard to parent participation in the care of ill or hospitalized children should be considered (Pongjaturawit & Harrigan, 2003).*
- Acknowledge that value conflicts from acculturation stresses may contribute to increased anxiety and significant conflict with children. **EBN:** *Immigrant mothers scored significantly lower on the evaluation of parenting knowledge than U.S.-born mothers (Bornstein & Cote, 2004). Chinese immigrant mothers identified that a larger perceived acculturation gap was associated with more parenting difficulties (Buki et al, 2003).*
- Acknowledge and praise parenting strengths noted. **EBN:** *Such acknowledgment increases trust and fosters a working relationship with the parent (Seideman et al, 1996). Clinicians could explore and support the positive qualities of authoritative parenting in Mexican descent families (Varela et al, 2004).*

Home Care

- The nursing interventions previously described should be used in the home environment with adaptations as necessary.
- ▲ Refer to a parenting program to facilitate learning of parenting skills. **EBN:** *At the end of an 8-week parenting program, parents demonstrated statistically significant reduced levels of clinical anxiety and depression. Parents showed an increase in more positive ratings of personality states, such as not shouting at their children and being more calm and energetic, at the end of the program (Long et al, 2001).*

Client/Family Teaching

- Refer to Client/Family Teaching for **Impaired Parenting** and **Risk for impaired Parenting** for suggestions that may be used with minor adaptations.
- Teach parents home safety: reduction of hot water temperature, proper poison storage, use of smoke alarms, and installation of safety gates for stairs. **EB:** *Counseling and convenient access to reduced-cost products appear to be an effective strategy for promoting children's home safety (Gielen, McDonald & Wilson, 2002).*
- Teach parents and young teens conflict resolution by using a hypothetical conflict solution with and without a structured conflict resolution guide. **EBN:** *Parents and young teens do not use a systematic method of solving disagreements, but with structured guidance the parents and teens are able to resolve conflicts (Riesch et al, 2003).*
- ▲ Refer mothers of children with type 1 diabetes for community support in babysitting, child care, or respite. **EBN:** *Mothers raising young children older than 4 years with type 1 diabetes highlight the importance of identifying family and/or community resources that could reduce some of the tremendous stress and burden of responsibility experienced after a child is diagnosed with diabetes (Sullivan-Bolyai et al, 2003).*
- Support empowerment of parents of children with asthma and other chronic diseases. **EBN:** *Asthma is the most common chronic illness in children and has a significant impact on children and their families. Empowering parents by facilitating their sense of control resulted in increased knowledge and ability to make decisions regarding their child's care (McCarthy et al, 2002; Schuman et al, 1993).*
- Parent training is one of the most effective interventions for behavior problems in young children. **EB:** *Parent training programs can be delivered to the parents alone, to the parents and children in separate group meetings, or to the parents and children together in sessions for at least part of the time.*

• = Independent; ▲ = Collaborative; EBN = Evidence-Based Nursing; EB = Evidence-Based

An overview of findings from research on these programs indicates that these programs have consistent and replicated effects on children's behavior, parents' improved use of effective discipline strategies, and improved family functioning (Cartwright-Hatton, McNally & White, 2005; White, McNally & Cartwright-Hatton, 2003; Lochman, 2000).

- Teach families the importance of monitoring television viewing and limiting exposure to violence. **EBN:** *Media violence can be hazardous to children's health, and studies overwhelmingly point to a causal connection between media violence and aggressive attitudes, values, and behaviors in some children (Muscari, 2002).*

- Consider individual- and/or group-based parenting programs for teenage mothers. **EB:** *Those engaged in individual and/or group parenting programs in the areas of mother-infant interaction, language development, parental attitudes, parental knowledge, maternal mealtime communication, maternal self-confidence, and maternal identity supported positive parenting (Coren & Barlow, 2004).*

- Consider group-based parenting programs for parents of children younger than 3 years with emotional and behavioral problems. **EB:** *A meta-analysis indicated that results favored those engaged in parenting programs in terms of improving the emotional and behavioral adjustment of children younger than 3 years (Barlow & Parsons, 2003).*

- Consider group-based parenting programs for parents with anxiety, depression, and/or low self-esteem. **EB:** *Parenting programs can make a significant contribution to the short-term psychosocial health of mothers and have a potential role to play in the promotion of mental health (Barlow & Coren, 2004).*

- ▲ Refer adolescent parents for comprehensive psychoeducational parenting classes. **EBN:** *A study indicated that a comprehensive psychoeducational parenting group can be effective in changing parenting attitudes and beliefs (Thomas & Looney, 2004).*

- Promotion of better-quality relationships between parents and children is an effective strategy that can lead to enhanced learning. Good-quality parenting leads to improved cognitive and social skills for the children. **EB:** *Research supports that effective early interventions lead to enhanced short-term gains in cognitive and social skills, particularly for children at risk of low educational achievement (National Literary Trust, 2005).*

evolve See the EVOLVE website for World Wide Web resources for client education.

REFERENCES

Ahmann E: Promoting positive parenting: an annotated bibliography, *Pediatr Nurs* 28(4):382, 2002.

Barlow J, Coren E: Parent-training programmes for improving maternal psychosocial health, *Cochrane Database Syst Rev* CD002020, 2004.

Barlow J, Parsons J: Group-based parent-training programmes for improving emotional and behavioral adjustment in 0-3 year old children, *Cochrane Database Syst Rev*, (3):CD003680, 2003.

Behring A, Vezeau TM, Fink R: Timing of the newborn first bath: a replication, *Neonatal Network* 22(1):39, 2003.

Bornstein MH, Cote LR: "Who is sitting across from me?" Immigrant mothers' knowledge of parenting and children's development, *Pediatrics* 114(5):e557-e564, 2004.

Buki LP, Ma TC, Strom RD et al: Chinese immigrant mothers of adolescents: self-perceptions of acculturation effects on parenting, *Cultur Divers Ethnic Minor Psychol* 9(2):127-140, 2003.

Cartwright-Hatton S, McNally D, White C: A new cognitive behavioural parenting intervention for families of young anxious children: a pilot study, *Behav Cognit Psychother* 33:243-247, 2005.

Clark BA, Chalmers KL: Helping parents cope, *Can Nurse* 99(2):19, 2003.

Coren E, Barlow J: Individual and group-based parenting programmes for improving psychosocial outcomes for teenage parents and their children, *Cochrane Database Syst Rev*, CD002964, 2004.

D'Avanzo CE, Naegle MA: Developing culturally informed strategies for substance-related interventions. In Naegle MA, D'Avanzo CE,

editors: *Addictions and substance abuse: strategies for advanced practice nursing*, St Louis, 2001, Mosby.

Feldman R, Eidelman A: Skin-to-skin contact (kangaroo care) accelerates autonomic and neurobehavioral maturation in preterm infants, *Dev Med Child Neurol* 45(4):274, 2003.

Gielen AC, McDonald EM, Wilson ME: Effects of improved access to safety counseling, products, and home visits on parents' safety practices: results of a randomized trial, *Arch Pediatr Adolesc Med* 156(1):33, 2002.

Jungbauer J, Wittmund B, Dietrich S et al: Subjective burden over 12 months in parents of patients with schizophrenia, *Arch Psychiatr Nurs* 17(3):126-134, 2003.

Leininger MM, McFarland MR: *Transcultural nursing: concepts, theories, research and practices*, ed 3, New York, 2002, McGraw-Hill.

Letourneau N: Improving adolescent parent-infant interactions: a pilot study, *J Pediatr Nurs* 16(1):53-62, 2001.

Lochman J: Parent and family skills training in targeted prevention programs for at-risk youth, *J Prim Prev* 21(2):253-265, 2000.

Long A, McCarney S, Smyth G et al: The effectiveness of parenting programmes facilitated by health visitors, *J Adv Nurs* 34(5):611, 2001.

McCarthy MJ, Herbert R, Brimacombe M et al: Empowering parents through asthma education, *Pediatr Nurs* 28(5):465, 2002.

McCue K, Bonn R: Helping children through an adult's serious illness, *Pediatr Nurs* 29(1):47, 2003.

Muscari M: Media violence: advice for parents, *Pediatr Nurs* 28(6):585, 2002.

P

• = Independent;   ▲ = Collaborative;   EBN = Evidence-Based Nursing;   EB = Evidence-Based

National Literacy Trust: *Birth to school study: a longitudinal evaluation of the Peers Early Education Partnership (PEEP) 1998-2005,* 2005, www.literacytrust.org.uk/talktoyourbaby/PEEPstudy2005.html, accessed January 2007.

Pongjaturawit Y, Harrigan R: Parent participation in the care of hospitalized child in Thai and Western cultures, *Issues Compr Pediatr Nurs* 26(3):183-199, 2003.

Porter LS, Porter BO: A blended infant massage-parenting enhancement program for recovering substance-abusing mothers, *Pediatr Nur* 30(5):363-372, 389-390, 401, 2004.

Riesch SK, Gray J, Hoeffs M et al: Conflict and conflict resolution: parent and young teen perceptions, *J Pediatr Health Care* 17(1):22, 2003.

Schuman W, Armstrong FD, Pegelow C et al: Enhanced parenting knowledge and skills in mothers of preschool children with sickle cell disease, *J Pediatr Psychol* 18(5):575-591, 1993.

Seideman RY, Jacobson S, Primeaux M et al: Assessing American Indian families, *MCN Am J Matern Child Nurs* 21(6):274, 1996.

Sullivan-Bolyai S, Deatrick J, Gruppuso P et al: Constant vigilance: mothers' work parenting young children with type 1 diabetes, *J Pediatr Nurs* 18(1):21, 2003.

Thomas DV, Looney SW: Effectiveness of a comprehensive psychoeducational intervention with pregnant and parenting adolescents: a pilot study, *J Child Adolesc Psychiatr Nurs* 17(2):66-77, 2004.

Tomlinson PS, Thomlinson E, Peden-McAlpine C et al: Clinical innovation for promoting family care in paediatric intensive care: demonstration, role modeling and reflective practice, *J Adv Nurs* 38(2):161, 2002.

Varela RE, Vernberg EM, Sanchez-Sosa JJ et al: Parenting style of Mexican, Mexican American, and Caucasian non-Hispanic families: social context and cultural influences, *J Fam Psychol* 18(4):651-657, 2004.

White C, McNally D, Cartwright-Hatton S: Cognitively enhanced parent training, *Behav and Cogn Psychother* 31:99-102, 2003.

White-Traut R: Providing a nurturing environment for infants in adverse situations: multisensory strategies for newborn care, *J Midwifery Womens Health* 49(4 suppl 1):36, 2004.

Impaired Parenting   *T. Heather Herdman, RN, PhD*   **evolve**

NANDA   Definition

Inability of the primary caretaker to create, maintain, or regain an environment that promotes the optimum growth and development of the child.

Defining Characteristics

Infant or Child

Behavioral disorders; failure to thrive; frequent accidents; frequent illness; incidence of abuse; incidence of trauma (e.g., physical and psychological); lack of attachment; lack of separation anxiety; poor academic performance; poor cognitive development; poor social competence; runaway

Parental

Abandonment; child abuse; child neglect; frequently punitive; hostility to child; inadequate attachment; inadequate child health maintenance; inappropriate caretaking skills; inappropriate stimulation (e.g., visual, tactile, auditory); inappropriate child care arrangements; inconsistent behavior management; inconsistent care; inflexibility in meeting needs of child; little cuddling; maternal-child interaction deficit; negative statements about child; poor parent-child interaction; rejection of child; statements of inability to meet child's needs; unsafe home environment; verbalization of inability to control child; verbalization of frustration; verbalization of role inadequacy

Related Factors (r/t)

Infant/Child

Altered perceptual abilities; attention deficit–hyperactivity disorder; developmental delay; difficult temperament; handicapping condition; illness; multiple births; not desired gender; premature birth; separation from parent; temperamental conflicts with parental expectations

Knowledge

Deficient knowledge about child development; deficient knowledge about child health maintenance; deficient knowledge about parenting skills; inability to respond to infant cues; lack of cognitive readiness for parenthood; lack of education; limited cognitive functioning; poor communication skills; preference for physical punishment; unrealistic expectations

• = Independent;   ▲ = Collaborative;   EBN = Evidence-Based Nursing;   EB = Evidence-Based

Physiological

Physical illness

Psychological

Closely spaced pregnancies; depression; difficult birthing process; disability; high number of pregnancies; history of mental illness; history of substance abuse; lack of prenatal care; sleep deprivation; sleep disruption; young parental age

Social

Change in family unit; chronic low self-esteem; father of child not involved; financial difficulties; history of being abused; history of being abusive; inability to put child's needs before own; job problems; lack of family cohesiveness; lack of parental role model; lack of resources; lack of social support networks; lack of transportation; lack of valuing of parenthood; legal difficulties; low socioeconomic status; maladaptive coping strategies; marital conflict; mother of child not involved; single parent; social isolation; poor home environment; poor parental role model; poor problem-solving skills; poverty; presence of stress (e.g., financial, legal, recent crisis, cultural move); relocations; role strain; situational low self-esteem; unemployment; unplanned pregnancy; unwanted pregnancy

NOC Outcomes (Nursing Outcomes Classification)

Suggested NOC Outcomes

Abuse Cessation; Abuse Protection; Abuse Recovery: Emotional; Abusive Behavior Self-Restraint; Child Development (all); Communication; Coping; Family Functioning; Family Integrity; Family Normalization; Family Physical Environment; Family Social Climate; Knowledge: Child Physical Safety; Neglect Recovery; Parent-Infant Attachment; Parenting Performance; Parenting: Psychosocial Safety; Role Performance; Safe Home Environment; Social Support

> #### Example NOC Outcome with Indicators
>
> **Parenting: Psychosocial Safety** as evidenced by the following indicators: Fosters open communication/ Recognizes risk(s) of abuse/Uses strategies to eliminate risk(s) of abuse/Selects appropriate supplemental caregiver(s)/ Uses strategies to prevent high-risk social behaviors/Provides needed level of supervision/Sets clear rules for behavior/ Maintains structure and daily routine in child's life (Rate the outcome and indicators of **Parenting: Psychosocial Safety:** 1 = never demonstrated, 2 = rarely demonstrated, 3 = sometimes demonstrated, 4 = often demonstrated, 5 = consistently demonstrated [see Section I].)

Client Outcomes

Client Will (Specify Time Frame):

- Initiate appropriate measures to develop a safe, nurturing environment
- Acquire and display attentive, supportive parenting behaviors and child supervision
- Identify appropriate strategies to manage a child's inappropriate behaviors
- Identify strategies to protect child from harm and/or neglect and initiate action when indicated

NIC Interventions (Nursing Interventions Classification)

Suggested NIC Interventions

Abuse Protection Support: Child; Attachment Promotion; Caregiver Support; Developmental Enhancement: Adolescent, Child; Environmental Management: Attachment Process; Environmental Management: Family Integrity Promotion; Family Support; Family Therapy; Impulse Control Training; Infant Care; Parent Education: Adolescent, Childrearing Family, Infant; Parenting Promotion; Role Enhancement; Simple Relaxation Therapy; Spiritual Support; Substance Use Prevention, Treatment; Teaching: Infant Stimulation, Toddler Nutrition, Toddler Safety

Example NIC Activities—Family Integrity Promotion
Identify typical family coping mechanisms; Determine typical family relationships for each family; Counsel family members on additional effective coping skills for their own use; Assist family with conflict resolution; Monitor current family relationships; Facilitate a tone of togetherness within and among the family; Encourage family to maintain positive relationships; Refer for family therapy, as indicated

Nursing Interventions and *Rationales*

- Refer to **Readiness for enhanced Parenting** for additional interventions.
- Use the Parenting Risk Scale to assess parenting. **EB:** *One study demonstrated that the Parenting Risk Scale is a reliable and valid measure for the systemic assessment of five key dimensions of parenting (Mrazek, Mrazek & Klinnert, 1995).*
- Examine the characteristics of parenting style and behaviors, including the following: emotional climate at home, attribution of negative traits to the child, failure to support the child's increases in autonomy, type of interaction with the infant or child, competition with the child for attention of spouse/significant other, lack of knowledge or concern about health maintenance or behavioral problems, other behaviors or concerns. **EB:** *Children are at risk for neglect, abuse, and other negative psychosocial outcomes in families with dysfunctions (Mrazek, Mrazek & Klinnert, 1995).*
- ▲ Institute abuse/neglect protection measures if evidence exists of an inability to cope with family stressors or crisis, signs of parental substance abuse are observed, or a significant level of social isolation is apparent. **EBN:** *Maternal difficult life circumstances, psychiatric-mental health symptoms, educational level, maternal experience in the family of origin, and parenting stress explained 74% of the variance in maternal sensitivity and responsiveness of mothers with their toddlers in the laboratory setting (LeCuyer-Maus, 2003).*
- ▲ For a mother with a toddler, assess maternal depression, perceptions of difficult temperament in the toddler, and low maternal self-efficacy. Make appropriate referral. **EBN:** *Negative feelings about oneself and one's child are likely to influence the parent-child relationship negatively (Gross et al, 1994).*
- Appraise the parent's resources and the availability of social support systems. Determine the single mother's particular sources of support, especially the availability of her own mother and partner. Encourage the use of healthy, strong support systems. *Before adequate interventions and education can be initiated, the current support system and concerns must be understood. The mother's partner and her mother are often important sources of support (Zacharia, 1994).*
- Provide education to at-risk parents on behavioral management techniques such as looking ahead, giving good instructions, providing positive reinforcement, redirecting, planned ignoring, and instituting time-outs. **EB:** *These behavioral management techniques are effective approaches for dealing with ineffective parent-child interactions and improving family relationships (Nicholson et al, 2002).*
- Promotion of better-quality relationships between parents and children is an effective strategy that can lead to enhanced learning. Good-quality parenting leads to improved cognitive and social skills for the children. **EB:** *Research supports that effective early interventions lead to enhanced short-term gains in cognitive and social skills, particularly for children at risk of low educational achievement (National Literacy Trust, 2005).*
- Support parents' competence in appraising their infant's behavior and responses. **EBN:** *Parents must be supported and welcomed as active collaborators in their infant's care (Lawhon, 2002).*
- Aim supportive interventions at minimizing parents' experience of strain. *Research supports interventions that lead to parents becoming empowered in their parenthood (Nystrom & Ohrling, 2004).*
- Encourage kangaroo care by parents of preterm infants. **EB:** *Parents have been found to be more sensitive and show more positive affect, touch, and adaptation to infant cues when participating in kangaroo care (Feldman et al, 2002).*
- Model age-appropriate and cognitively appropriate caregiver skills by doing the following: communicating with the child at an appropriate cognitive level of development, giving the child tasks and responsibilities appropriate to age or functional age/level, instituting safety considerations such as the use of assistive equipment, and encouraging the child to perform activities of daily living as appropriate. *These activities illustrate parenting and childrearing skills and behaviors for parents and family (McCloskey & Bulechek, 1992).*

P

• = Independent;   ▲ = Collaborative;   EBN = Evidence-Based Nursing;   EB = Evidence-Based

- Encourage mothers to understand and capitalize on their infants' capacity to interact, particularly in the early months of life. **EBN:** *A study suggested that nurses should routinely assess parent-child interactions in all high-risk, disadvantaged families with very young children (Schiffman, Omar & McKelvey, 2003).*
- ▲ Provide programs for homeless mothers with severe mental illness who have lost physical custody of their children. **EBN:** *Programs for homeless mothers with severe mental illness can effect changes that promote family reunification. Changes in housing, psychosis, substance use, and therapeutic relationships predicated reunification (Hoffman & Rosenheck, 2001).*
- ▲ Provide a recovery program that includes instruction in parenting skills and child development for mothers who are addicted to cocaine. **EBN:** *Women addicted to cocaine who are parenting children need strong encouragement from the healthcare system to begin a recovery program and also gain parenting skills. Lack of parenting knowledge may be a major barrier for them (Coyer, 2003).*

Multicultural

- Acknowledge racial and ethnic differences at the onset of care. **EBN:** *Acknowledgment of racial and ethnicity issues enhances communication, establishes rapport, and promotes treatment outcomes (D'Avanzo et al, 2001; Ludwick & Silva, 2000; Vontress & Epp, 1997).*
- Approach individuals of color with respect, warmth, and professional courtesy. **EBN:** *Instances of disrespect have special significance for individuals of color (D'Avanzo et al, 2001; Vontress & Epp, 1997).*
- Clarify parents' feelings, expectations, perceptions, and availability regarding participation in the care of their sick child. **EBN:** *Cultural differences in regard to parent participation in the care of ill or hospitalized children should be considered (Pongjaturawit & Harrigan, 2003).*
- Use a neutral, indirect style when addressing areas in which improvement is needed, such as a need for verbal stimulation when working with Native-American clients. **EBN:** *Using indirect statements such as "Other mothers have tried . . ." or "I had a client who tried 'X,' and it seemed to work very well" help avoid resentment from the parent (Seideman et al, 1996).*
- Provide support for Chinese families caring for children with disabilities. **EBN:** *The care of children with handicaps strains and violates the Chinese culturally expected order of parental obligations. The following themes emerged: disruptions to natural order, public opinions on what constitutes personhood and ordered bodies, and the establishment of moral reputations linked to shame and blame and the gendered division of parenting (Holroyd, 2003).*
- Validate the client's feelings regarding parenting. **EBN:** *Validation is a therapeutic communication technique that lets the client know that the nurse has heard and understood what was said, and it promotes the nurse-client relationship (Heineken, 1998).*
- Facilitate modeling and role playing to help the family improve parenting skills. **EBN:** *It is helpful for the family and the client to practice parenting skills in a safe environment before trying them in real-life situations (Rivera-Andino & Lopez, 2000).*

Home Care

- The interventions previously described may be adapted for home care use.
- Assess parenting stress at each home visit to provide appropriate support and anticipatory guidance to families of children with a chronic disease. **EB:** *Parents found it difficult to set limits or discipline children with heart disease; older age of the child was associated with higher parenting stress scores (Uzark & Jones, 2003).*
- Assess the single mother's history regarding childhood and partner abuse and current status regarding depressive symptoms, abusive parenting attitudes (lack of empathy, favorable opinion of corporal punishment, parent-child role-reversal, inappropriate expectations). Refer for mental health services as indicated. **EBN:** *History of partner and child abuse predicted higher daily stress, leading to lower self-esteem. The presence of more depressive symptoms and daily stressors was associated with greater anger. Greater anger was associated with lower parental empathy. Partner abuse predicted higher levels of abusive parenting attitudes (Lutenbacher, 2002).*
- ▲ Implement behavioral parent training, including enhancement of skills in child-directed play, effective use of commands, use of discipline measures such as imposing time-outs and providing immediate and natural consequences, problem solving, and communication strategies. **EBN:** *Initial work (Gross, Fogg & Tucker, 1995) and follow-up at 1 year (Tucker et al, 1998) of a behav-*

• = Independent;   ▲ = Collaborative;   EBN = Evidence-Based Nursing;   EB = Evidence-Based

ioral training program for parents showed improvements in maternal self-efficacy and stress reduction and in the quality of maternal-infant interaction. A higher amount of behavioral parent training was associated with fewer maternal critical statements and negative physical behaviors.

Client/Family Teaching

- Consider individual and/or group-based parenting programs for teenage mothers. **EB:** *A systematic review indicated that results favored those engaged in individual and/or group parenting programs in the areas of mother–infant interaction, language development, parental attitudes, parental knowledge, maternal mealtime communication, maternal self-confidence, and maternal identity (Barlow & Coren, 2004).*

- Consider group-based parenting programs for parents of children younger than 3 years with emotional and behavioral problems. **EB:** *A meta-analysis indicated that results favored those engaged (Barlow & Parsons, 2003).*

- ▲ Refer adolescent parents for comprehensive psychoeducational parenting classes. **EBN:** *A study indicated that a comprehensive psychoeducational parenting group can be effective in changing parenting attitudes and beliefs (Thomas & Looney, 2004).*

- Explain individual differences in children's temperaments and compare them with the parents' expectations. Help parents determine and understand the implications of their child's temperament. **EBN:** *Promoting parental understanding of temperament facilitates development of more realistic expectations (Melvin, 1995; McClowry, 1992).*

- Support empowerment of parents of children with asthma and other chronic diseases. **EBN:** *Asthma is the most common chronic illness in children and has a significant impact on children and their families. Empowering parents by facilitating their sense of control resulted in increased knowledge and ability to make decisions regarding their child's care (McCarthy et al, 2002; Lowes & Lyne, 1999; Schuman et al, 1993).*

- Parent training is one of the most effective interventions for behavior problems in young children. **EB:** *Parent training implementation and parental engagement may be improved by the introduction of a cognitive component. Parent training programs can be delivered to the parents alone, to the parents and children in separate group meetings, or to the parents and children together in sessions for at least part of the time. An overview of findings from research on these programs indicates that these programs have consistent and replicated effects on children's behavior, on parents' improved use of effective discipline strategies, and on improved family functioning (Cartwright-Hatton, McNally & White, 2005; White, McNally & Cartwright-Hatton, 2003; Lochman, 2000).*

- Discuss sound disciplinary techniques, which include catching children being good, listening actively, conveying positive regard, ignoring minor transgressions, giving good directions, using praise, and imposing time-outs. *A variety of opinions exist about disciplinary methods. Proper discipline provides children with security, and clearly enforced rules help them learn self-control and social standards. Parenting classes can be beneficial when the parent has had little formal or informal preparation (Herman-Staab, 1994).*

- Encourage positive parenting: respect for children, understanding of normal development, and creative and loving approaches to meet parenting challenges. **EBN:** *Understanding normal development is a first step for parents to distinguish common behaviors for a given stage of development from "problems." Central to positive parenting is developing approaches that can be used in place of anger, manipulation, punishment, and rewards (Ahmann, 2002).*

- Plan parental education directed toward the following age-related parental concerns. Birth to 2 years: transition, sleep, aggression; 3 to 5 years: transition, parent-child relationship, sleep; 6 to 10 years: school, parent-child relationship, divorce; 11 to 18 years: parent-child relationship, divorce, school. *Parents with children of any age may seek basic information about a variety of concerns, which can be anticipated and addressed by providing ongoing information and support (Jones, Maestri & McCoy, 1993).*

- ▲ Initiate referrals to community agencies, parent education programs, stress management training, and social support groups. *The parent needs support to manage angry or inappropriate behaviors. Use of support systems and social services can provide an opportunity to decrease feelings of inadequacy (Baker, 1994; Campbell, 1992).*

- ▲ Provide information regarding available telephone counseling services. *Telephone counseling ser-*

• = Independent; ▲ = Collaborative; EBN = Evidence-Based Nursing; EB = Evidence-Based

vices can provide confidential advice and support to families who might not otherwise have access to help in dealing with behavioral problems and parenting concerns (Jones, Maestri and McCoy, 1993).

- Refer to the care plan for **Delayed Growth and development** and **Impaired parent/child Attachment** for additional teaching interventions.

evolve See the EVOLVE website for World Wide Web resources for client education.

REFERENCES

Ahmann E: Promoting positive parenting: an annotated bibliography, *Pediatr Nurs* 28(4):382, 2002.

Baker NA: Avoid collisions with challenging families, *MCN Am J Matern Child Nurs* 19:97, 1994.

Barlow J, Coren E: Parent-training programmes for improving maternal psychosocial health, *Cochrane Database Syst Rev* (1): CD002020, 2004.

Barlow J, Parsons J: Group-based parent-training programmes for improving emotional and behavioral adjustment in 0-3 year old children, *Cochrane Database Syst Rev* (1):CD003680, 2003.

Campbell JM: Parenting classes: focus on discipline, *J Community Health Nurs* 9:197, 1992.

Cartwright-Hatton S, McNally D, White C: A new cognitive behavioural parenting intervention for families of young anxious children: a pilot study, *Behav Cogni Psychother* 33:243-247, 2005.

Coyer SM: Women in recovery discuss parenting while addicted to cocaine, *MCN Am J Matern Child Nurs* 28(1):45, 2003.

D'Avanzo CE, Naegle MA: Developing culturally informed strategies for substance-related interventions. In Naegle MA, D'Avanzo CE, editors: *Addictions and substance abuse: strategies for advanced practice nursing*, St Louis, 2001, Mosby.

Feldman R, Eidelman AI, Sirota L et al: Comparison of skin-to-skin (kangaroo) and traditional care: parenting outcomes and preterm infant behavior, *Pediatrics* 110(1):16, 2002.

Gross D, Conrad B, Fogg L et al: A longitudinal model of maternal self-efficacy, depression, and difficult temperament during toddlerhood, *Res Nurs Health* 17:207, 1994.

Gross D, Fogg L, Tucker S: The efficacy of parent training for promoting positive parent-toddler relationships, *Res Nurs Health* 18:489, 1995.

Heineken J: Patient silence is not necessarily client satisfaction: communication in home care nursing, *Home Healthc Nurse* 16(2):115, 1998.

Herman-Staab B: Screening, management and appropriate referral for pediatric behavior problems, *Nurs Pract* 19:40, 1994.

Hoffman D, Rosenheck R: Homeless mothers with severe mental illnesses and their children: predictors of family reunification, *Psychiatr Rehabil J* 25(2):163, 2001.

Holroyd EE: Chinese cultural influences on parental caregiving obligations toward children with disabilities, *Qual Health Res* 13(1):4, 2003.

Jones LC, Maestri BO, McCoy K: Why parents use the warm line, *MCN Am J Matern Child Nurs* 18:258, 1993.

Lawhon G: Facilitation of parenting the premature infant within the newborn intensive care unit, *J Perinat Neonatal Nurs* 16(1):71, 2002.

LeCuyer-Maus E: Stress and coping in high-risk mothers: difficult life circumstances, psychiatric-mental health symptoms, education, and experiences in their families of origin, *Public Health Nurs* 20(2):132, 2003.

Lochman J: Parent and family skills training in targeted prevention programs for at-risk youth, *J Prim Prev* 21(2):253-265, 2000.

Lowes L, Lyne P: A normal lifestyle: parental stress and coping in childhood diabetes, *Br J Nurs* 8(3):133-139,1999.

Ludwick R, Silva M: Nursing around the world: cultural values and ethical conflicts, *Online J Issues Nurs,* August 14, 2000, www.nursingworld.org/ojin/ethcol/ethics_4.htm, accessed June 19, 2003.

Lutenbacher M: Relationships between psychosocial factors and abusive parenting attitudes in low-income single mothers, *Nurs Res* 51:158, 2002.

McCarthy MJ, Herbert R, Brimacombe M et al: Empowering parents through asthma education, *Pediatr Nurs* 28(5):465, 2002.

McCloskey JC, Bulechek GM, editors: *Nursing interventions classification (NIC)*, St Louis, 1992, Mosby.

McClowry SG: Temperament theory and research, *Image* 24:319, 1992.

Melvin N: Children's temperament: intervention for parents, *J Pediatr Nurs* 10:152, 1995.

Mrazek DA, Mrazek P, Klinnert M: Clinical assessment of parenting, *J Am Acad Child Adolesc Psychiatry* 34: 272, 1995.

National Literacy Trust: *Birth to school study: a longitudinal evaluation of the Peers Early Education Partnership (PEEP) 1998-2005*, 2005, www.literacytrust.org.uk/talktoyourbaby/PEEPstudy2005.html, accessed January 2007.

Nicholson B, Anderson M, Fox R et al: One family at a time: a prevention program for at-risk parents, *J Couns Dev* 80(3):362, 2002.

Nystrom K, Ohrling K: Parenthood experiences during the child's first year: literature review, *J Adv Nurs* 46(3):319-330, 2004.

Pongjaturawit Y, Harrigan R: Parent participation in the care of hospitalized child in Thai and Western cultures, *Issues Comp Pediatr Nurs* 26(3):183-199, 2003.

Rivera-Andino J, Lopez L: When culture complicates care, *RN* 63(7):47, 2000.

Schiffman RF, Omar MA, McKelvey LM: Mother-infant interaction in low-income families, *MCN Am J Matern Child Nurs* 28(4):246-251, 2003.

Schuman W, Armstrong FD, Pegelow C et al: Enhanced parenting knowledge and skills in mothers of preschool children with sickle cell disease, *J Pediatr Psychol* 18(5):575-591, 1993.

Seideman RY, Jacobson S, Primeaux M: Assessing American Indian families, *MCN Am J Matern Child Nurs* 21(6):274, 1996.

Thomas DV, Looney SW: Effectiveness of a comprehensive psychoeducational intervention with pregnant and parenting adolescents: a pilot study, *J Child Adolesc Psychiatr Nurs* 17(2):66-77, 2004.

Tucker S, Gross D, Fogg L et al: The long-term efficacy of a behavioral parent training intervention for families with 2-year-olds, *Res Nurs Health* 21:199, 1998.

Uzark K, Jones K: Parenting stress and children with heart disease, *J Pediatr Health Care* 17(4):163-168, 2003.

Vontress CE, Epp LR: Historical hostility in the African American client: implications for counseling, *J Multicult Counseling Dev* 25:170, 1997.

White C, McNally D, Cartwright-Hatton S: Cognitively enhanced parent training, *Behav Cogn Psychother* 31:99-102, 2003.

Zacharia R: Perceived social support and social network of low-income mothers of infants and preschoolers: pre-and postparenting program, *J Community Health Nurs* 11:11, 1994.

P

• = Independent; ▲ = Collaborative; EBN = Evidence-Based Nursing; EB = Evidence-Based

Risk for impaired Parenting   *T. Heather Herdman, RN, PhD*

NANDA   Definition

Risk for inability of the primary caretaker to create, maintain, or regain an environment that promotes the optimum growth and development of the child.

Risk Factors

Infant/Child

Altered perceptual abilities; attention deficit–hyperactivity disorder; developmental delay; difficult
temperament; handicapping condition; illness; multiple births; not gender desired; premature birth;
prolonged separation from parent; temperamental conflicts with parental expectation

Knowledge

Deficient knowledge about child development; deficient knowledge about child health maintenance;
deficient knowledge about parenting skills; inability to respond to infant cues; lack of cognitive
readiness for parenthood; low cognitive functioning; low educational level or attainment; poor communication skills; preference for physical punishment; unrealistic expectations of child

Physiological

Physical illness

Psychological

Closely spaced pregnancies; depression; difficult birthing process; disability; high number of pregnancies; history of mental illness; history of substance abuse; sleep deprivation; sleep disruption;
young parental age

Social

Change in family unit; chronic low self-esteem; father of child not involved; financial difficulties;
history of being abused; history of being abusive; inadequate child care arrangements; job problems;
lack of access to resources; lack of family cohesiveness; lack of parental role model; lack of prenatal
care; lack of resources; lack of social support network; lack of transportation; lack of valuing of parenthood; late prenatal care; legal difficulties; low socioeconomic class; maladaptive coping strategies;
marital conflict; mother of child not involved; parent-child separation; poor home environment; poor
parental role model; poor problem-solving skills; poverty; role strain; single parent; situational low self
esteem; social isolation; stress; relocation; unemployment; unplanned pregnancy; unwanted pregnancy

NOC   Outcomes (Nursing Outcomes Classification)

Suggested NOC Outcomes

Abuse Recovery: Emotional, Physical, Sexual; Abusive Behavior Self-Restraint; Caregiver
Emotional Health; Caregiver Stressors; Coping; Parent-Infant Attachment; Parenting Performance;
Risk Control: Unintended Pregnancy; Social Interaction Skills

Example NOC Outcome with Indicators
Parenting Performance as evidenced by the following indicators: Provides for child's physical needs/Interacts positively with child/Expresses realistic expectations of parental role/Exhibits a loving relationship/Expresses satisfaction with parental role (Rate the outcome and indicators of **Parenting Performance:** 1 = not adequate, 2 = slightly adequate, 3 = moderately adequate, 4 = substantially adequate, 5 = totally adequate [see Section I].)

Client Outcomes

Client Will (Specify Time Frame):

* Successfully establish a nurturing parenting role
* Affirm desire to acquire and maintain constructive parenting skills to support infant/child
  growth and development

• = Independent;   ▲ = Collaborative;   EBN = Evidence-Based Nursing;   EB = Evidence-Based

- Maintain appropriate measures to develop a safe, nurturing environment
- Display attentive, supportive parenting behaviors
- Have knowledge of strategies to protect child from harm and/or neglect

NIC   Interventions (Nursing Interventions Classification)

Suggested NIC Interventions

Abuse Protection Support: Child; Attachment Promotion; Caregiver Support; Developmental Enhancement: Adolescent, Child; Environmental Management: Attachment Process; Family Integrity Promotion; Family Support; Family Therapy; Infant Care; Kangaroo Care; Parent Education: Adolescent, Childrearing Family, Infant; Risk Identification: Childbearing Family; Role Enhancement

Example NIC Activities—Kangaroo Care
Determine and monitor parent's level of confidence in caring for infant; Encourage parent to initiate infant care

Nursing Interventions, *Rationales*, and References

Refer to care plans **Readiness for enhanced Parenting** and **Impaired Parenting.**

Risk for Peripheral neurovascular dysfunction   *evolve*

Betty J. Ackley, MSN, EdS, RN

NANDA   Definition

At risk for disruption in circulation, sensation, or motion of an extremity

Risk Factors

Burns; fractures; immobilization; mechanical compression (e.g., tourniquet, cane, cast, brace, dressing, restraint); orthopedic surgery; trauma; vascular obstruction

NOC   Outcomes (Nursing Outcomes Classification)

Suggested NOC Outcomes

Circulation Status, Neurological Status: Spinal Sensory/Motor Function, Tissue Perfusion: Peripheral

Example NOC Outcome with Indicators
Tissue Perfusion: Peripheral as evidenced by the following indicators: Distal peripheral pulses/Sensation/Skin color/Muscle function/Skin integrity/Peripheral edema not present/Localized extremity pain not present (Rate the outcome and indicators of **Tissue Perfusion: Peripheral:** 1 = severely compromised, 2 = substantially compromised, 3 = moderately compromised, 4 = mildly compromised, 5 = not compromised [see Section I].)

Client Outcomes

Client Will (Specify Time Frame):

- Maintain circulation, sensation, and movement of an extremity within client's own normal limits
- Explain signs of neurovascular compromise and ways to prevent venous stasis

● = Independent;   ▲ = Collaborative;   EBN = Evidence-Based Nursing;   EB = Evidence-Based

NIC   Interventions (Nursing Interventions Classification)

Suggested NIC Interventions

Exercise Therapy: Joint Mobility, Peripheral Sensation Management

Example NIC Activities—Peripheral Sensation Management
Monitor for paresthesia: numbness, tingling, hyperesthesia, and hypoesthesia; Monitor for thrombophlebitis and deep vein thrombosis

Nursing Interventions and *Rationales*

- Perform neurovascular assessment every 1 to 4 hours or every 15 minutes as ordered.
- Use the six Ps of assessment:
  - **Pain:** Assess severity (on a scale of 1 to 10), quality, radiation, and relief by medications. *Diffuse pain that is aggravated by passive movement and is unrelieved by medication can be an early symptom of compartment syndrome or a symptom of limb ischemia (Kasirajan & Ouriel, 2002; Walls, 2002).*
  - **Pulses:** Check the pulses distal to the injury. *Check the uninjured side first to establish a baseline for a bilateral comparison. An intact pulse generally indicates a good blood supply to the extremity, although compartment syndrome may be present even if the pulse is intact (Walls, 2002).*
  - **Pallor/Poikilothermia:** Check color and temperature changes below the injury site. Check capillary refill. *If pallor is present, record the level of coldness carefully. A cold, pale, or bluish extremity indicates arterial insufficiency or arterial damage, and a physician should be notified (Bickley & Szilagyi, 2007;Kasirajan & Ouriel, 2002). A reddened, warm extremity may indicate infection (Kasper et al, 2005). Normal capillary refill time is 3 seconds or less (McConnell, 2002).*
  - **Paresthesia** (change in sensation): Check by lightly touching the skin proximal and distal to the injury. Ask if the client has any unusual sensations such as hypersensitivity, tingling, prickling, decreased feeling, or numbness. *Changes in sensation are indicative of nerve compression and damage and can also indicate compartment syndrome (Kasirajan & Ouriel, 2002; Walls, 2002).*
  - **Paralysis:** Ask the client to perform appropriate range-of-motion exercises in the unaffected and then the affected extremity. *Paralysis is a late and ominous symptom of compartment syndrome or limb ischemia (Kasirajan & Ouriel, 2002; Walls, 2002).*
  - **Pressure:** Check by feeling the extremity; note new onset of firmness of the extremity. *With compartment syndrome, the affected area becomes taut and feels firm when touched (Walls, 2002).*
- Monitor the client for symptoms of compartment syndrome evidenced by pain greater than expected, pain with passive movement, decreased sensation, weakness, loss of movement, absence of pulse, and tension in the skin that surrounds the muscle compartment. *These symptoms are not always present and can be difficult to assess. Compartment syndrome is characterized by increased pressure within the muscle compartment, which compromises circulation, viability, and function of tissues (Edwards, 2004; Walls, 2002).*
- Monitor appropriate application and function of corrective device (e.g., cast, splint, traction) every 1 to 4 hours as needed. *An improperly applied device can cause nerve damage, circulatory impairment, or pressure ulcers.*
- Position the extremity in correct alignment with each position change; check every hour to ensure appropriate alignment.
- ▲ Get the client out of bed and mobilize the client as soon as possible after consultation with the physician. *Immobility is a risk factor for DVT; early ambulation can help prevent clot formation (Roman, 2005).*
- ▲ Monitor for signs of DVT, especially in high-risk populations, including persons older than 40 years; persons with immobility or obesity; persons taking estrogen or oral contraceptives; persons with a history of trauma, surgery, or previous DVT; and persons with a cerebrovascular accident, varicose veins, malignancy, or cardiovascular disease. **EBN:** *These are identified risk factors that increase the incidence of DVT and have been validated by a DVT risk scale (Autar, 2003).*

• = Independent;   ▲ = Collaborative;   EBN = Evidence-Based Nursing;   EB = Evidence-Based

▲ Apply graduated compression stockings if ordered; measure carefully to ensure proper fit, removing at least daily to assess circulation and skin condition. **EBN and EB:** *Graduated compression stockings reduced the incidence of DVT in a high-risk orthopedic surgical population and that additional antithrombotic measures, along with stocking use, decreased the incidence even further (Joanna Briggs Institute, 2001). The use of graduated compression stockings, alone or in conjunction with other prevention modalities, prevents DVT in hospitalized clients (Amarigiri & Lees, 2005).*

• Watch for and report signs of DVT as evidenced by pain, deep tenderness, swelling in the calf and thigh, and redness in the involved extremity. Take serial leg measurements of the thigh and leg circumferences. In some clients, a tender venous cord can be felt in the popliteal fossa. Do not rely on Homans' sign. *Thrombosis with clot formation is usually first detected as edema of the involved leg and then as pain. Homans' sign is not reliable (Kasper et al, 2005).*

▲ Help the client perform prescribed exercises every 4 hours as ordered.

• Provide a nutritious diet and adequate fluid replacement. *Good nutrition and sufficient fluids are needed to promote healing and prevent complications.*

Geriatric

• Use heat and cold therapies cautiously. *Elderly clients often have decreased sensation and circulation.*

Home Care

• Assess the knowledge base of the client and family after any institutional care.

• Teach about the disease process and care as necessary. *The length of time of institutional care and teaching may have been too short and insufficient for learning.*

• If risk is related to fractures and cast care, teach the family to complete a neurovascular assessment; it may be performed as often as every 4 hours but is more commonly done two to three times per day. *A risk requiring monitoring more often than every 4 hours for longer than 24 hours indicates a need for hospital-based care.*

• If the fracture is peripheral, position the limb for comfort and change position frequently, avoiding dependent positions for extended periods. *Changes in position enhance circulation.*

▲ Refer to physical therapy services as necessary to establish an exercise program and safety in transfers or mobility within limitations of physical status.

• Establish an emergency plan.

Client/Family Teaching

• Teach the client and family to recognize signs of neurovascular dysfunction and report signs immediately to the appropriate person.

• Emphasize proper nutrition to promote healing.

▲ If necessary, refer the client to a rehabilitation facility for instruction in proper use of assistive devices and measures to improve mobility without compromising neurovascular function.

 See the EVOLVE website for World Wide Web resources for client education.

REFERENCES

Amarigiri SV, Lees TA: Elastic compression stockings for prevention of deep vein thrombosis, *Cochrane Database Syst Rev* (3): CD001484, 2005.

Autar R: The management of deep vein thrombosis: the Autar DVT risk assessment scale re-visited, *J Orthop Nurs* 7(3):114, 2003.

Bickley LS, Szilagyi PG: *Bates' guide to physical examination*, ed 9, Philadelphia, 2007, Lippincott Williams & Wilkins.

Edwards S: Acute compartment syndrome, *Emerg Nurse* 12(3):32, 2004.

Joanna Briggs Institute: Best practice: graduated compression stockings for the prevention of post-operative venous thromboembolism, *EB Pract Inform Sheets Health Profes* 5:2, 2001.

Kasirajan K, Ouriel K: Current options in the diagnosis and management of acute limb ischemia, *Prog Cardiovasc Nurs* 17:1, 2002.

Kasper DL et al: *Harrison's principles of internal medicine*, ed 16, New York, 2005, McGraw-Hill.

McConnell EA: Assessing neurovascular status in a casted limb, *Nursing* 32(9):20, 2002.

Roman M: Deep vein thrombosis: an overview, *Medsurg Matters* 14(1), 2005.

Walls M: Orthopedic trauma, *RN* 65:7, 2002.

• = Independent; ▲ = Collaborative; EBN = Evidence-Based Nursing; EB = Evidence-Based

Risk for Poisoning *Mary Stahle, MSN-NEdu, CEN, RN, and Betty J. Ackley, MSN, EdS, RN*

NANDA Definition

Accentuated risk of accidental exposure to, or ingestion of, drugs or dangerous products in doses sufficient to cause poisoning

Risk Factors

External

Availability of illicit drugs potentially contaminated by poisonous additives; dangerous products placed within reach of children; dangerous products placed within reach of confused individuals; large supplies of drugs in house; medicines stored in unlocked cabinets; medicines stored in unlocked cabinets accessible to confused individuals

Internal

Cognitive difficulties; emotional difficulties; lack of drug education; lack of proper precaution; lack of safety education; reduced vision; verbalization that occupational setting is without adequate safeguards

Related Factors (r/t)

See Risk Factors.

NOC Outcomes (Nursing Outcomes Classification)

Suggested NOC Outcomes

Knowledge: Child Physical Safety, Medication, Personal Safety; Parenting Performance; Risk Control; Risk Control: Alcohol Use, Drug Use; Risk Detection; Safe Home Environment

Example NOC Outcome with Indicators
Risk Control as evidenced by the following indicators: Monitors environmental risk factors/Develops effective risk control strategies (Rate the outcome and indicators of **Risk Control:** 1 = never demonstrated, 2 = rarely demonstrated, 3 = sometimes demonstrated, 4 = often demonstrated, 5 = consistently demonstrated [see Section I].)

Client Outcomes

Client Will (Specify Time Frame):

- Prevent inadvertent ingestion of or exposure to toxins or poisonous substances
- Explain and undertake appropriate safety measures to prevent ingestion of or exposure to toxins or poisonous substances

NIC Interventions (Nursing Interventions Classification)

Suggested NIC Interventions

Environmental Management: Safety, First Aid, Health Education, Medication Management, Surveillance, Surveillance: Safety

Example NIC Activities—Environmental Management: Safety
Identify safety hazards in the environment (i.e., physical, biological, and chemical); Remove hazards from the environment, when possible

Nursing Interventions and *Rationales*

- When a client comes to the hospital with possible poisoning, begin care following the ABCs and administer oxygen if needed. *Poisoning is an emergency and should be treated as such (Broderick,*

• = Independent; ▲ = Collaborative; EBN = Evidence-Based Nursing; EB = Evidence-Based

2004). Nursing assessment should center on ventilation, perfusion, cognition, and elimination. Assess and reassess these areas because changes occur rapidly (Kidd & Stuart, 2000). The primary nurse should call the poison control center to determine definitive treatment quickly (Kidd & Stuart, 2000).

- Obtain a thorough history of what was ingested, how much, and when, and ask to look at the container. Note the client's age, weight, medications, and any medical conditions. *A thorough history is critical to success of treatment (Broderick, 2004).*

- Carefully inspect for signs of ingestion of poisons, including an odor on the breath, a trace of the substance on the clothing, burns or redness around the mouth and lips, as well as signs of confusion, vomiting, or dyspnea. **EB:** *It is important to look for signs of ingestion of poison before initiating treatment because up to 40% of children who present with poisoning have not actually been exposed to the suspected toxin (Hwang, Foot & Eddie, 2003).*

- Note results of toxicology screens, arterial blood gasses, blood glucose levels, and any other ordered laboratory tests. *If information about what was ingested is incomplete or inaccurate, laboratory tests may be needed to determine treatment (Broderick, 2004).*

▲ Initiate any ordered treatment for poisoning quickly. *The goal is to prevent further absorption of the agent; charcoal is most effective if administered in the first hour after ingestion of the poison (Bryant & Singer, 2003).*

- Prevent iatrogenic harm to the hospitalized client by following these guidelines for administering medications:
  ▪ Use at least two methods to identify the client before administering medications or blood products, such as the client's name and medical record number or birth date.
  ▪ When taking verbal or telephone orders, the orders should be written down and then read back for verification to the individual giving the order.
  ▪ Standardize use of abbreviations and eliminate those that are prone to cause errors.
  ▪ Take high-alert medications off the nursing unit, such as potassium chloride. Standardize concentrations of medications such as morphine in PCA pumps.
  ▪ Use only IV pumps that prevent free flow of IV solution when the tubing is taken out of the pump.
  ▪ Identify all the client's current medications on admission to a healthcare facility and ensure that all healthcare staff have access to the information. *Accurate and complete medication reconciliation can prevent numerous prescribing and administration errors (The Joint Commission, 2006). These are the National Patient Safety Goals and are required actions to improve client safety in a hospital or healthcare facility from the Joint Commission (Chai, 2005).*

- Detect possible interactions and cumulative or other adverse effects among prescribed medications, self-administered over-the-counter products, culturally based home treatments, herbal remedies, and foods. *Serious consequences may occur if interactions are not identified; herbal preparations can be toxic.*

Pediatric

▲ Evaluate lead exposure risk and consult the healthcare provider regarding lead screening measures as indicated (public/ambulatory health). *Lead poisoning is one of the most common and preventable types of childhood poisoning today. Assessment of exposure risk and blood level testing are important preventive measures (Kim, Staley & Curtis, 2002).*

- Supply "Mr. Yuk" labels for families with children. *Implementing poisoning prevention program strategies benefits the client and family (Dart & Rumack, 2003). Information on how to obtain "Mr Yuk" labels is available at www.chp.edu/mryuk/05a_mryuk.php.*

- Provide guidance for parents and caregivers regarding age-related safety measures, including the following:
  ▪ Store potentially harmful substances in the original containers with safety closures intact.
  ▪ Recognize that no container is completely childproof.
  ▪ Do not store medications or toxic substances in food containers.
  ▪ Remove poisonous houseplants from the home. Teach children not to put leaves or berries in their mouths.
  ▪ Keep cleaning agents, disinfectants, and other hazardous materials out of sight and out of children's reach; keep them locked up.

- Do not take medications in front of children; children mimic parents' behaviors.
- Do not suggest that medications such as aspirin and children's vitamins are candy.
- If interrupted when using a harmful product, take it with you; children can get into it within seconds.
- Use extreme caution with pesticides and gardening materials close to children's play areas.
- Keep perfume and makeup out of reach of children.

Infants have a high level of hand-to-mouth behavior and ingest anything. Young children may inadvertently ingest poisonous materials, particularly if those materials are thought to be food or a beverage (Broderick, 2004; Dart & Rumack, 2003). **EB:** *A study of poisoning incidences in children in which the child was brought to the emergency department demonstrated that 73% of the parents received no instructions on how to prevent another incidence of poisoning (Demorest et al, 2004).*

- Teach the family to keep the home safe for children by keeping harmful cleaning products and all liquids containing hydrocarbons away from children and using child-resistant packaging as available. *Liquid products that contain more than 10% hydrocarbons (e.g., cosmetics such as hair oils, automotive chemicals, cleaning solvents, or water repellents) are now required to be in child-resistant packaging. When these products enter the lungs inadvertently, they can cause chemical pneumonia and death in children (Barone, 2002).*
- Advise families that syrup of ipecac is no longer recommended to be kept and used in the home. *Syrup of ipecac is not considered effective and can delay or hamper administration of charcoal admixture, which may be more effective (Rudolph et al, 2003). There is a high aspiration potential with these clients. Giving ipecac may delay the administration or reduce the effectiveness of activated charcoal, oral antidotes, and whole bowel irrigation (Ressel, 2004).*

Geriatric

- Caution the client and family to avoid storing medications with similar appearances close to one another (e.g., nitroglycerin ointment near toothpaste or denture creams). *Confusion and visual impairment can place the older person at risk of incorrectly identifying the contents.*
- Place medications in a medication box that indicates when they are to be taken. *Failing eyesight, the use of multiple drugs, and difficulty in remembering whether a medication was taken are among the causes of accidental poisoning in older persons.* **EB:** *A study that reviewed causes of calls to poison information centers by adults older than 50 years demonstrated that most of the calls related to errors in taking drugs, and then adverse drug reactions (Skarupski, Mrvos & Krenzelok, 2004).*
- Remind the older client to store medications out of reach when young children come to visit. *Children are inquisitive and may ingest medicines in containers without safety caps.*
- Perform medication reconciliation on all elderly clients entering the healthcare system as well as on discharge. *Elderly clients do not compare drugs that they have at home with new prescriptions and often take multiple drugs with the same indications, leading to toxicity.*

Home Care

- The interventions previously described may be adapted for home care use.
- Provide the client and/or family with a poison control poster to be kept on the refrigerator or a bulletin board. Ensure that the telephone number for local poison control information is readily available.
- Prepour medications for a client who is at risk of ingesting too much of a given medication because of mistakes in preparation. Delegate this task to the family or caregivers if possible. *Elderly clients who live alone are at greatest risk of poisoning.*
- Identify poisonous substances in the immediate surroundings of the home, such as a garage or barn, including paints and thinners, fertilizers, rodent and bug control substances, animal medications, gasoline, and oil. Label with the name, a poison warning sign, and a poison control center number. Lock out of the reach of children. *Dangerous poisonous substances can be found in areas other than the internal home setting. Curious children are at risk for ingestion when exploring.*
- Identify the risk of toxicity from environmental activities such as spraying trees or roadside shrubs. Contact local departments of agriculture or transportation to obtain material substance data sheets or to prevent the activity in desired areas. *Very young children, women who are of child-bearing age or who are pregnant, and the elderly are at greatest risk.*

- Avoid carbon monoxide poisoning. Instruct the client and family in the importance of using a carbon monoxide detector in the home, having the chimney professionally cleaned each year, having the furnace professionally inspected each year, ensuring that all combustion equipment is properly vented, and installing a chimney screen and cap to prevent small animals from moving into the chimney. *Many deaths each year are attributed to carbon monoxide poisoning. Take these precautions to protect the child and family (Jordan, 2002).*

Multicultural

- Assess housing for pathways of lead poisoning. **EB:** *Minority individuals are more likely to reside in older and substandard housing. Approximately 74% of privately owned, occupied housing units in the United States built before 1980 contain lead-based paint (Centers for Disease Control and Prevention, 2001).*
- Prompt caregivers to take action to prevent lead poisoning. **EB:** *A lead poisoning awareness campaign targeted at ethnic minority parents of preschool-age children respondents reported an increase in steps to prevent lead poisoning after exposure to the campaign (McLaughlin et al, 2004).*
- Inform minority parents of children who present for treatment of a poisoning episode of poisoning prevention education as part of the medical encounter. **EB:** *Research suggests that young children experiencing a first poisoning episode will have a second occurrence and that poisoning prevention education may prevent repeat poisoning occurrence (Demorest et al, 2004).*
- Poison control centers should offer information in bilingual and bicultural manner. **EB:** *Research suggests that poison control centers are underused by low-income minority and Spanish-speaking parents because of lack of knowledge and misconception. A videotape intervention was highly effective in changing knowledge, attitudes, behaviors, and behavioral intentions concerning the poison control center within this population (Kelly et al, 2003; Shepherd et al, 2004).*

Client/Family Teaching

- Counsel the client and family members regarding the following points of medication safety:
  - Avoid sharing prescriptions.
  - Always use good light when preparing medication.
  - Read the label before you open the bottle, after you remove a dose, and again before you give it.
  - Always use child-resistant caps and lock all medications away from your child or confused elder.
  - Give the correct dose. NEVER guess.
  - Do not increase or decrease the dose without calling the physician.
  - Always follow the weight and age recommendations on the label.
  - Avoid making conversions. If the label calls for 2 tsp and you have a dosing cup labeled only with ounces, do not use it.
  - Be sure the physician knows if you are taking more than one medication at a time.
  - Never let young children take medication by themselves.
  - Read and follow labeling instructions on all products; adjust dosage for age.
  - Avoid excessive amounts and/or frequency of doses. ("If a little does some good, a lot should do more.")

  Each year, thousands of adverse drug-related events occur, including poisoning. Poisoning is a major cause of morbidity and mortality (American Academy of Pediatrics, 2002).
- Advise the family to post first-aid charts and poison control center instructions in an accessible location. Poison control center telephone numbers should be posted close to each telephone and the number programmed into cell phones. *A poison control center should always be called immediately before initiating any first-aid measures. The national toll-free number is (800) 222-1222; the agency will connect the caller to the closest poison control center (Broderick, 2004).*
- Advise family when calling the poison control center to do the following:
  - Give as much information as possible, including your name, location, and telephone number, so that the poison control operator can call back in case you are disconnected or to summon help if needed.
  - Give the name of the potential poison ingested and, if possible, the amount and time of in-

gestion. If the bottle or package is available, give the trade name and ingredients if they are listed.

- ■ Be prepared to tell the person the child's height, weight, and age.
- ■ Describe the state of the poisoning victim. Is the victim conscious? Does he or she have any symptoms? What is the person's general appearance, skin color, respiration, breathing difficulties, mental status (alert, sleepy, unusual behavior)? Is the person vomiting? Having convulsions?

Rapid initiation of proper treatment reduces mortality and morbidity rates and decreases emergency department visits and inpatient admissions. Consultation with a poison control center is necessary to assess and treat poisoned clients (Broderick, 2004; Ressel, 2004).

- • Encourage the client and family to take first-aid and other types of safety-related programs. *These programs raise participants' level of emergency preparation.*
- ▲ Initiate referrals to peer group interventions, peer counseling, and other types of substance abuse prevention/rehabilitation programs when substance abuse is identified as a risk factor. **EBN:** *Clients with substance abuse problems are at risk for contact with tainted substances or for overdose. The peer pressure factor is extremely strong for adolescents; rehabilitation programs providing nonpunitive and skill-focused approaches are most effective (Anderson, 1996).*

evolve See the EVOLVE website for World Wide Web resources for client education.

REFERENCES

American Academy of Pediatrics: *Medications: taking medicine correctly,* 2002, www.medem.com/MedLB/article_detaillb_for_printer. cfm?article_ID=ZZZYLAKE03D&sub_cat=27, accessed December 31, 2006.

Anderson NLR: Decisions about substance abuse among adolescents in juvenile detention, *Image J Nurs Sch* 28:65, 1996.

Barone S: Child-resistant packaging, *Consumer Product Safety Review* 6(3):3, 2002.

Broderick M: Pediatric poisoning! *RN* 67(9):37-38, 40-42, 2004.

Bryant S, Singer J: Management of toxic exposure in children, *Emerg Med Clin North Am* 21(1):101, 2003.

Centers for Disease Control and Prevention: Sources and pathways of lead exposure. In *Preventing lead poisoning in young children,* Atlanta, 2001, The Centers for Disease Control and Prevention.

Chai K: Patient safety goals and the impact on the JCAHO survey, *Cinahl Information Systems,* No 2005048933, 2005.

Dart RC, Rumack BA: Poisoning. In Hay WW et al, editors: *Current pediatrics: diagnosis and treatment,* ed 16, New York, 2003, McGraw-Hill.

Demorest RA, Posner JC, Osterhoudt KC et al: Poisoning prevention education during emergency department visits for childhood poisoning, *Pediatr Emerg Care* 20(5):281, 2004.

Hwang CF, Foot CL, Eddie G: The utility of the history and clinical signs of poisoning in childhood: a prospective study, *Ther Drug Monit* 25(6):728, 2003.

The Joint Commission: *Sentinel event alert,* available at http://www.

jointcommission.org/SentinelEvents/SentinelEventAlert/sea_35. htm, January 25, 2006. Accessed April 25, 2007.

Jordan RA: Preventing CO poisoning: carbon monoxide, *Consumer Product Safety Review* 6(3):4, 2002.

Kelly NR, Huffman LC, Mendoza FS et al: Effects of a videotape to increase use of poison control centers by low-income and Spanish-speaking families: a randomized, controlled trial, *Pediatrics* 111(1):21-26, 2003.

Kidd P, Stuart P: Toxicologic conditions. In Kidd P, Stuart P, Fultz J: *Emergency nursing reference,* ed 2, St Louis, 2000, Mosby.

Kim DY, Staley F, Curtis G: Relation between housing age, housing value and childhood blood levels in children in Jefferson County, Ky, *Am J Public Health* 92(5):769, 2002.

McLaughlin TJ, Humphries O Jr, Nguyen T et al: "Getting the lead out" in Hartford, Connecticut: a multifaceted lead-poisoning awareness campaign, *Environ Health Perspect* 112(1):1-5, 2004.

Ressel GW: AAP releases policy statement on poison treatment in the home, *Am Family Physician* 69(3):741, 2004.

Rudolph CD et al: *Rudolph's pediatrics,* ed 21, New York, 2003, McGraw-Hill.

Shepherd G, Larkin GL, Velez LI et al: Language preferences among callers to a regional Poison Center, *Vet Hum Toxicol* 46(2):100-101, 2004.

Skarupski KA, Mrvos R, Krenzelok EP: A profile of calls to a poison information center regarding older adults, *J Aging Health* 16(2):228, 2004.

Post-trauma syndrome   *Michele Walters, RN, MSN, ARNP*

NANDA   **Definition**

Sustained maladaptive response to a traumatic, overwhelming event.

Defining Characteristics

Aggression; alienation; altered mood state; anger and/or rage; anxiety; avoidance; compulsive behavior; denial; depression; detachment; difficulty in concentrating; enuresis (in children); exaggerated

• = Independent;   ▲ = Collaborative;   EBN = Evidence-Based Nursing;   EB = Evidence-Based

startle response; fear; flashbacks; gastric irritability; grieving; guilt; headaches; hopelessness; horror; hypervigilance; intrusive dreams; intrusive thoughts; irritability; neurosensory irritability; nightmares; palpitations; panic attack; psychogenic amnesia; rape; reports feeling numb; repression; shame; substance abuse

Related Factors (r/t)

Abuse (physical and psychosocial); being held prisoner of war; criminal victimization; disasters; epidemics; events outside range of usual human experience; serious accidents (e.g., industrial, motor vehicle); serious injury/threat to self or loved ones; sudden destruction of one's home or community; torture; tragic occurrence involving multiple deaths; wars; witnessing of mutilation/violent death

NOC   Outcomes (Nursing Outcomes Classification)

Suggested NOC Outcomes

Abuse Cessation; Abuse Protection; Abuse Recovery: Emotional, Sexual; Coping; Impulse Self-Control; Self-Mutilation Restraint

Example NOC Outcome with Indicators
Abuse Recovery: Emotional as evidenced by the following indicators: Trauma-induced psychoneurotic behaviors, conduct disorders, and learning difficulties (Rate outcome and indicators of **Abuse Recovery Emotional:** 1 = extensive, 2 = substantial, 3 = moderate, 4 = limited, 5 = none [see Section I].)

Client Outcomes

Client Will (Specify Time Frame):

• Return to pretrauma level of functioning as quickly as possible
• Acknowledge traumatic event and begin to work with the trauma by talking about the experience and expressing feelings of fear, anger, anxiety, guilt, and helplessness
• Identify support systems and available resources and be able to connect with them
• Return to and strengthen coping mechanisms used in previous traumatic event
• Acknowledge event and perceive it without distortions
• Assimilate event and move forward to set and pursue life goals

NIC   Interventions (Nursing Interventions Classification)

Suggested NIC Interventions

Counseling, Support System Enhancement

Example NIC Activities—Counseling
Encourage expression of feelings; Assist patient to identify strengths and reinforce them

Nursing Interventions and *Rationales*

• Observe for a reaction to a traumatic event in all clients regardless of age or sex. **EB:** *Women are more likely to meet the criteria for posttraumatic stress disorder (PTSD), although they are less likely to experience posttraumatic events. Women are more likely than men to experience sexual assault and child sexual abuse but less likely to experience accidents, nonsexual assaults, witness of death injury, disaster, fire, or combat during war (Tolin & Foa, 2006).*
• Provide a safe and therapeutic environment. *This will assist the client in regaining control (Townsend, 2003).*
• Remain with the client and provide support during periods of overwhelming emotions. **EBN:** *The importance of trust was found to be a key element in a nurse-client relationship (Lowenberg, 2003).*

• = Independent;   ▲ = Collaborative;   EBN = Evidence-Based Nursing;   EB = Evidence-Based

- Help the individual try to comprehend the trauma if possible. **EB:** *A stronger sense of coherence as the ability to perceive a stressor as comprehensible, manageable, and meaningful renders the client some-what resilient to symptoms of PTSD (Engelhan, van den Hout & Vheyen, 2003).*
- Use touch with the client's permission (e.g., a hand on the shoulder, holding a hand). **EB:** *TT has been found to reduce tension, confusion, anxiety, and pain and increases quality of life or general well-being (Collinge, Wentworth & Sabo, 2005).*
- Explore and enhance available support systems. **EB:** *Support systems decrease isolation and encourage communication, which may reduce negative affect and enhance the understanding and assimilation of the event (Engelhan et al, 2003).*
- Help the client regain previous sleeping and eating habits. **EBN:** *Associated behavioral symptoms after a traumatic event may include substance abuse, eating disorders, high-risk sexual behavior, suicidality, and revictimization (Seng et al, 2004).*
- ▲ Provide the client pain medication if he or she has physical pain. **EB:** *Pain may act as a proprioceptive trigger, stimulating posttraumatic reactions (Martz, 2004).*
- ▲ Assess the need for pharmacotherapy. **EB:** *Selective serotonin reuptake inhibitors are the medications most commonly prescribed for reexperiencing and avoidance/withdrawal symptoms of PTSD. Selective serotonin reuptake inhibitors and anticonvulsants are the medications most commonly prescribed for hyperarousal, irritability, or paranoia (Rosen et al, 2004).*
- Help the client use positive cognitive restructuring to reestablish feelings of self-worth. **EB:** *Veterans with and without PTSD were found to have temporal fluctuations in self-esteem and negative affect, which are associated with diminished well-being (Kashdan et al, 2006).*
- Provide the means for the client to express feelings through therapeutic drawing. **EBN:** *Expressive techniques such as therapeutic drawing can be used to facilitate the emotional work of coping with chronic trauma or life-threatening events and facilitate a better understanding of the experience to healthcare professionals (Locsin et al, 2003).*
- Encourage the client to return to the normal routine as quickly as possible. *PTSD leads to disruption of normal daily and nighttime routines. Early treatment includes collaboration to develop a plan to establish normal daily routines (Carr, 2004).*
- Talk to and assess the client's social support after a traumatic event. **EB:** *Greater social support is found to be associated with a significantly reduced risk of poor perceived mental health (Coker et al, 2002).*

Pediatric

Refer to nursing care plan **Risk for Post-Trauma syndrome.**

Geriatric

- Carefully screen elderly for signs of PTSD, especially after a disaster. **EB:** *Clients with PTSD are often not recognized or incorrectly diagnosed. Increased knowledge on vulnerability factors for PTSD can facilitate diagnostic procedures and health management in the elderly. Because of age-related changes and associated disease processes, stress reaction in older adults may lead to a deterioration of function and a worsening of existing conditions (Marren & Christianson, 2005).*
- Consider using the Horwitz Impact of Event Scale, which is an appropriate instrument to measure the subjective response to stress in the senior population. *The Impact of Event Scale is recognized as one of the earliest self-report tools developed to assess post-traumatic stress (Marren & Christianson, 2005).*
- Allow the client more time to establish trust and express anger, guilt, and shame about the trauma. Review past coping skills and give the client positive reinforcement for successfully dealing with other life crises. *Clients who have adjusted positively to aging and can put events into proper perspective may adjust to loss more positively.*
- ▲ Monitor the client for clinical signs of depression and anxiety; refer to a physician for medication if appropriate. *Depression in the elderly is underestimated in the United States.*
- Instill hope. *The energy generated by hope can help the elderly cope, overcome obstacles, and maintain normal functioning.*

• = Independent; ▲ = Collaborative; EBN = Evidence-Based Nursing; EB = Evidence-Based

Multicultural

- Assess the influence of cultural beliefs, norms, and values on the client's ability to cope with a traumatic experience. **EBN:** *What the client views as healthy coping may be based on cultural perceptions (Leininger & McFarland, 2002).*
- Acknowledge racial and ethnic differences at the onset of care. **EBN:** *Acknowledgment of race and ethnicity issues enhances communication, establishes rapport, and promotes positive treatment outcomes (D'Avanzo et al, 2001). Black veterans' rate of service connection for PTSD was 43% compared with 56% for other respondents ($P = .003$) even after adjusting for differences in PTSD severity and functional status (Murdoch et al, 2003). Race has been identified as a factor in who receives treatment for trauma (Koenen et al, 2003).*
- Use a family-centered approach when working with Latino, Asian, African-American, and Native-American clients. **EBN:** *Latinos may perceive the family as a source of support, solver of problems, and source of pride. Asian Americans may regard the family as the primary decision maker and influence on individual family members (D'Avanzo et al, 2001). A school-based program using a family approach to treat traumatized immigrant children showed modest decline in trauma-related mental health problems (Kataoka et al, 2003).*
- When working with Asian-American clients, provide opportunities by which the family can save face. **EBN:** *Asian-American families may avoid situations and discussion of issues that they perceive will bring shame on the family unit (D'Avanzo et al, 2001).*
- Validate the client's feelings regarding the trauma. **EBN:** *Validation is a therapeutic communication technique that lets the client know that the nurse has heard and understood what was said, and it promotes the nurse-client relationship (Heineken, 1998).*
- Incorporate cultural traditions as appropriate. **EB:** *Activities such as tundra walks and time with elders were supported in treatment of trauma for the Yup'ik and Cup'ik Eskimo of Southwest Alaska (Mills, 2003).*

Home Care

- ▲ Assess family support and the response to the client's coping mechanisms. Refer the family for medical social services or other counseling as necessary. *Persons who have not shared the client's traumatic experience may have unrealistic expectations about recovery and recovery time. Support may be denied if the client's response to the trauma does not stay within support system expectations.*
- Provide a stable routine of day-to-day activities consistent with pretrauma experience. Do not force a new routine on the client. *Resuming a pretrauma routine can be reassuring to the client and can help place the trauma in perspective. Imposing an undesired routine can further isolate the client.*
- ▲ Assess the impact of the trauma on significant others (e.g., a father may have to take over his partner's parenting responsibility after she has been raped and injured). Provide empathy and caring to significant others. Refer for additional services as necessary. *Traumatic events can pose a crisis for both significant others and the involved client. Trying to help parents with PTSD implement a behavioral program for their children is likely to lead to a failed experience. Parents with PTSD should be offered an opportunity to undergo treatment for their own PTSD (Carr, 2004).*

Client/Family Teaching

- Explain to the client and family what to expect the first few days after the traumatic event and in the future. *Knowing what to expect can minimize much of the anxiety that accompanies a traumatic response.*
- Teach positive coping skills and avoidance of negative coping skills. *Cognitive coping skills teach the individual to challenge fearful or threatening cognitions and appraise anxiety-evoking situations in less-threatening ways (Carr, 2004).*
- Teach stress reduction methods such as deep breathing, visualization, meditation, and physical exercise. Encourage their use especially when intrusive thoughts or flashbacks occur. **EB:** *After a traumatic event, clients may be tempted to cope maladaptively with their overwhelming emotions, which can establish unhealthy patterns for the future (Lang et al, 2003).*

• = Independent;   ▲ = Collaborative;   EBN = Evidence-Based Nursing;   EB = Evidence-Based

- Encourage other healthy living habits of proper diet, adequate sleep, regular exercise, family activities, and spiritual pursuits. *A wide range of preventive, educational, and supportive interventions for trauma survivors are used. Despite this, research is lacking to prove their effectiveness (Schnurr & Green, 2004).*
- ▲ Refer the client to peer support groups. **EB:** *Peer support decreases the sense of social isolation and enhances knowledge, which may reduce the negative effects and enhance the understanding and assimilation of the event (Engelhan et al, 2003).*
- Instruct the family in ways to be helpful to and supportive of the traumatized person. Emphasize the importance of listening and being there. Also emphasize that no magic phrases are capable of easing the person's emotional suffering.
- ▲ Consider the use of complementary and alternative therapies. **EB:** *Evidence suggests that Sudarshan kriya yoga is potentially beneficial as a low-risk adjunct treatment for stress, anxiety, PTSD, depression, and stress-related medical illnesses (Brown & Gerbarg, 2005).*

evolve See the EVOLVE website for World Wide Web resources for client education.

REFERENCES

Brown RP, Gerbarg PL: Sudarshan kriya yogic breathing in the treatment of stress, anxiety, and depression: Part II—clinical applications and guidelines, *J Altern Complement Med* 11(4):711-717, 2005.

Carr A: Interventions for post-traumatic stress disorder in children and adolescents, *Pediatr Rehab* 7(4):231-244, 2004.

Coker A, Smith P, Thompson M et al: Social support protects against the negative effects of partner violence on mental health, *J Womens Health Gend Based Med* 11:465-476, 2002.

Collinge W, Wentworth R, Sabo S: Integrating complementary therapies into community mental health practice: an exploration, *J Alt Complement Med* 11(3):569-574, 2005.

D'Avanzo CE, Naegle MA: Developing culturally informed strategies for substance-related interventions. In Naegle MA, D'Avanzo CE, editors: *Addictions and substance abuse: strategies for advanced practice nursing,* St Louis, 2001, Mosby.

Engelhan I, van den Hout M, Vheyen J: The sense of coherence in early pregnancy and crisis support and posttraumatic stress after pregnancy loss: a prospective study, *Behav Med* 29:80-84, 2003.

Heineken J: Patient silence is not necessarily client satisfaction: communication in home care nursing, *Home Healthc Nurse* 16(2):115, 1998.

Kashdan TB, Uswatte G, Steger MF et al: Fragile self-esteem and affective instability in posttraumatic stress disorders, *Behav Res Ther* 44(11):1609-1619, 2006.

Kataoka SH, Stein BD, Jaycox LH et al: A school-based mental health program for traumatized Latino immigrant children, *J Am Acad Child Adolesc Psychiatry* 42(3):311-318, 2003.

Koenen KC, Goodwin R, Struening E et al: Posttraumatic stress disorder and treatment seeking in a national screening sample, *J Trauma Stress* 16(1):5-16, 2003.

Lang A, Rodgers C, Laffaye C et al: Sexual trauma, posttraumatic stress disorder, and health behavior, *Behav Med* 28:150-158, 2003.

Leininger MM, McFarland MR: *Transcultural nursing: concepts, theories, research and practices,* ed 3, New York, 2002, McGraw-Hill.

Locsin R, Barnard A, Matua A et al: Surviving Ebola: understanding experience through artistic expression, *Int Nurs Rev* 50:156-166, 2003.

Lowenberg J: The nurse-client relationship in a stress management clinic, *Holist Nurs Pract* 17(2):99-109, 2003.

Marren J, Christianson S: Horowitz's Impact of Event Scale: an assessment of post traumatic stress in older adults, *Medsurg Nurs* 14(5):329-330, 2005.

Martz E: Death anxiety as a predictor of posttraumatic stress levels among individuals with spinal cord injuries, *Death Stud* 28:1-17, 2004.

Mills PA: Incorporating Yup'ik and Cup'ik Eskimo traditions into behavioral health treatment, *J Psychoactive Drugs* 35(1):85-88, 2003.

Murdoch M, Hodges J, Cowper D et al: Racial disparities in VA service connection for posttraumatic stress disorder disability, *Med Care* 41(4):536-549, 2003.

Rosen CS, Chow HC, Finney JF et al: VA practices patterns and practice guidelines for treating posttraumatic stress disorder, *J Traum Stress* 17(3):213-222, 2004.

Schnurr PP, Green BL: Understanding relationships among trauma, post-traumatic stress disorder, and health outcomes, *Adv Mind Body Med* 20(1):18-29, 2004.

Seng J, Low L, Sparbel K et al: Abuse-related post-traumatic stress during the childbearing year, *J Adv Nurs* 46(6):604-613, 2004.

Tolin DF, Foa EB: Sex differences in trauma and posttraumatic stress disorder: a quantitative review of 25 years of research, *Psychol Bull* 132(6):959-992, 2006.

Townsend M: *Psychiatric mental health nursing: concepts of care*, ed 4, Philadelphia, 2003, F.A. Davis.

Risk for Post-trauma syndrome   *Michele Walters, RN, MSN, ARNP*

NANDA   Definition

At risk for sustained maladaptive response to a traumatic, overwhelming event.

Risk Factors

Diminished ego strength; displacement from home; duration of event; exaggerated sense of responsibility; inadequate social support; nonsupportive environment; occupation (e.g., police, fire, rescue, corrections, emergency department, mental health worker); perception of event; survivor's role in the event

NOC   Outcomes (Nursing Outcomes Classification)

Suggested NOC Outcomes

Abuse Cessation, Abuse Protection, Abuse Recovery: Emotional, Aggression Self-Control, Anxiety Self-Control, Coping, Grief Resolution, Sleep

Example NOC Outcome with Indicators
Abuse Recovery: Emotional as evidenced by the following indicator: Trauma-induced psychoneurotic behaviors, conduct disorders, and learning difficulties (Rate outcome and indicators of **Abuse Recovery: Emotional:** 1 = extensive, 2 = substantial, 3 = moderate, 4 = limited, 5 = none [see Section I].)

Client Outcomes

Client Will (Specify Time Frame):

- Identify symptoms associated with PTSD and seek help
- Identify the event in realistic, cognitive terms
- State that he or she is not to blame for the event

NIC   Interventions (Nursing Interventions Classification)

Suggested NIC Interventions

Counseling, Support System Enhancement

Example NIC Activities—Counseling
Encourage expression of feelings; Assist patient to identify strengths and reinforce them

Nursing Interventions and *Rationales*

- Assess for PTSD in a client who has chronic illness, anxiety, or personality disorder; was a witness to serious injury or death; or experienced sexual molestation. **EB:** *PTSD has emerged as the most common anxiety disorder in women. There are also high rates of PTSD in chronically ill and psychiatric clients (Yen et al, 2002). Women are more likely than men to meet the criteria for PTSD, although they are less likely to have experienced posttraumatic events (Tolin & Foa, 2006).*
- Consider the use of a self-reported screening questionnaire. **EB:** *Client self-reported screening questionnaires are efficient ways to assess for PTSD (National Center for PTSD, 2007).*
- Assess for ongoing symptoms of dissociation, avoidant behavior, hypervigilance, and reexperiencing. **EB:** *A study of acute stress disorder as a predictor of PTSD identified these symptoms as being 79% predictable of subsequent PTSD cases (Brink, 2004).*
- Assess for past experiences with traumatic events. **EB:** *As individuals become accustomed to traumatic situations, they can develop stress inoculation and acquire coping skills. This is supported by previous research suggesting that prolonged exposure results in habituation (Ronen, Gahav & Appel, 2004).*

• = Independent;   ▲ = Collaborative;   EBN = Evidence-Based Nursing;   EB = Evidence-Based

- Consider screening for PTSD in a client who is a high user of medical care. **EB:** *Traumatic stress is associated with increased health complaints, health services utilization, morbidity, and mortality (National Center for PTSD, 2007).*
- ▲ Provide peer support to contact co-workers experiencing trauma to remind them that others in the organization are concerned about their welfare. *Peer supporters are not counselors. Their tasks include contacting co-workers to remind them that others in the organization are concerned about their welfare, providing the opportunity to discuss the incident, and assessing for the need for further post-trauma services (Post Trauma Resources, 2001).*
- Provide posttrauma debriefings. Effective posttrauma coping skills are taught, and each participant creates a plan for his or her recovery. During the debriefing, the facilitators assess participants to determine their needs for further services in the form of posttrauma counseling. For maximal effectiveness, the debriefing should occur within 2 to 5 days of the incident. *Current treatment strategies for PTSD involve a combination of posttrauma debriefing, education, pharmacotherapy, and psychotherapy (Guess, 2006).*
- Provide posttrauma counseling. Counseling sessions are extensions of debriefings and include continued discussion of the traumatic event and posttrauma consequences and the further development of coping skills. *Immediate posttrauma responses cannot be prevented. Long-term problems can develop if posttrauma consequences are not managed. Current treatment strategies for PTSD involve a combination of posttrauma debriefing, education, pharmacotherapy, and psychotherapy (Guess, 2006).*
- Instruct the client to use the following critical incident stress management techniques:

Things to Try: Critical Incident Stress Debriefing

- Within the first 24 to 48 hours, engaging in periods of appropriate physical exercise alternated with relaxation to alleviate some of the physical reactions.
- Structure your time; keep busy.
- You are normal and are having normal reactions; do not label yourself as "crazy."
- Talk to people; talk is the most healing medicine.
- Be aware of numbing the pain with overuse of drugs or alcohol; you do not need to complicate the stress with a substance abuse problem.
- Reach out; people do care.
- Maintain as normal a schedule as possible.
- Spend time with others.
- Help your co-workers as much as possible by sharing feelings and checking out how they are doing.
- Give yourself permission to feel rotten and share your feelings with others.
- Keep a journal; write your way through those sleepless hours.
- Do things that feel good to you.
- Realize that those around you are under stress.
- Do not make any big life changes.
- Do make as many daily decisions as possible to give you a feeling of control over your life (e.g., if someone asks you what you want to eat, answer the person even if you are not sure).
- Get plenty of rest.
- Reoccurring thoughts, dreams, or flashbacks are normal; do not try to fight them because they will decrease over time and become less painful.
- Eat well-balanced and regular meals (even if you do not feel like it).

The critical incident stress debriefing process is specifically designed to prevent or mitigate the development of PTSD among emergency services professions. Critical incident stress debriefing interventions are especially directed toward the mitigation of posttraumatic stress reactions (International Critical Incident Stress Foundation, 2007).

- Assess for a history of life-threatening illness such as cancer and provide appropriate counseling. *The physical and psychological impact of having a life-threatening disease, undergoing cancer treatment, and living with recurring threats to physical integrity and autonomy constitute traumatic experiences for many cancer clients (National Cancer Institute, 2007).*

Pediatric

- Children with cancer should continue to be assessed for PTSD into adulthood. **EBN:** *In children surviving childhood cancer, PTSD symptoms may continue to emerge into young adulthood (Meeske et al, 2001).*
- Provide protection for a child who has witnessed violence or who has had traumatic injuries. Help the child acknowledge the event and express grief over the event. The children in Iraq are particularly vulnerable. **EB:** *Violence-exposed adolescents reporting parental alcohol or drug use had the highest rates of psychiatric diagnoses (Hanson et al, 2006). There is an urgent need to address the needs of all children in Iraq by means of preventive programs such as life skills education and care programs within the school setting (Razokhi et al, 2006).*
- Assess for a medical history of anxiety disorders. **EB:** *The conditional risk for PTSD was increased for youth with anxiety disorders (Breslau, Lucia & Alvarado, 2006).*
- Consider implementation of a school-based program for children to decrease PTSD after catastrophic events. **EBN:** *The Catastrophic Stress Intervention was implemented after Hurricane Hugo to decrease mental stress by increasing the children's understanding of stress and enhancing their self-efficacy and social support, thus decreasing the symptoms of PTSD (Hardin et al, 2002).*

Geriatric/Multicultural

- Refer to the care plan for **Post-trauma syndrome.**

Home Care

- ▲ Assess the client's ability to meet primary needs of shelter, nourishment, and safety. Refer to medical social services, state departments of human services, or other organizations as appropriate. *Clients in need of primary life requirements are unable to master a higher level of coping.*
- Identify other losses or stressors that may affect coping ability (e.g., role or relationship changes, deaths). *The presence of other stressors can compound the risk of posttrauma stress response and ineffective coping.*
- ▲ Assess the family's response to the client's risk. Refer the family to medical social services, mental health services, or support groups as necessary. Provide nursing support. *Individuals in the client's support systems may not understand or be able to cope with the risk involved in selected occupations or the response to selected traumatic events in the client's experience. This is a barrier to the provision of immediate and ongoing support to the client.*
- ▲ If the client is on medication, assess its effectiveness and the client's compliance with the regimen. Identify who administers the medication. *Clients with diminished ego strength may have difficulty adhering to a medication regimen.*
- Help the client in the home identify and establish daily patterns that have meaning for the client. *Daily patterns provide the client and support system with structure, stability, and a point of reference for perspective development.*
- For a client who is displaced from the home, identify internal values that can be maintained while the client is displaced, such as respite, contact with specific persons, and honesty. *Maintaining internal values reinforces ego strength, supports dignity, and promotes hope. NOTE: Hope should not be misconstrued to mean that a client displaced from the home can return home if this is not possible.*
- ▲ Encourage the client to verbalize feelings of risk and trauma to therapeutic staff or other supportive persons. Refer to medical social services or mental health/support group services as appropriate. *Expressing feelings validates client feelings, fears, and needs. Professional support systems may be a necessary substitute for inadequate personal support systems on a temporary basis.*
- ▲ Evaluate the client's response to a traumatic or critical event. If screening warrants, refer to a therapist for counseling/treatment. *A review of psychological debriefing has concluded that little evidence exists to support its use. Early intervention recommendations are to assess the need for sustained treatment, provide psychological first aid, and provide education about trauma and information about treatment resources. Recommendations for secondary prevention of PTSD include education, anxiety management, cognitive restructuring, exposure, and relapse prevention (Litz et al, 2002).*
- Refer to the care plan for **Post-trauma syndrome.**

P

• = Independent;   ▲ = Collaborative;   EBN = Evidence-Based Nursing;   EB = Evidence-Based

Client/Family Teaching

- Instruct family and friends to use the following critical incident stress management techniques (International Critical Incident Stress Foundation, 2007):
    - Listen carefully.
    - Spend time with the traumatized person.
    - Offer your assistance and a listening ear, even if the person has not asked for help.
    - Help the person with everyday tasks such as cleaning, cooking, caring for the family, and minding children.
    - Give the person some private time.
    - Do not take the individual's anger or other feelings personally, and do not tell the person that he or she is "lucky it wasn't worse"; such statements do not console traumatized people. Instead, tell the person that you are sorry such an event has occurred and you want to understand and assist him or her.
- Teach the client and family to recognize symptoms of PTSD and seek treatment when the client does the following (McDermott & Cvitanovich, 2000):
    - Relives the traumatic event by thinking or dreaming about it often.
    - Is unsettled or distressed in other areas of his or her life such as in school, at work, or in personal relationships.
    - Avoids any situation that might cause him or her to relive the trauma.
    - Demonstrates a certain amount of generalized emotional numbness.
    - Shows a heightened sense of being on guard.
- Provide education to explain that acute stress disorder symptoms are normal reactions that are likely to resolve. Instruct to seek help if the symptoms persist. **EB:** *This assists in identifying the client who is in need of a referral for treatment of PTSD (Winston et al, 2002).*

evolve See the EVOLVE website for World Wide Web resources for client education.

REFERENCES

Breslau N, Lucia VC, Alvarado GF: Intelligence and other predisposing factors in exposure to trauma and posttraumatic stress disorder: a follow-up study at age 17 years, *Arch Gen Psychiatry* 63(11):1238-1242, 2006.

Brink E: Acute stress disorder as a predictor of post-traumatic stress disorder in physical assault victims, *J Interpers Violence* 19(6):709-726, 2004.

Guess KF: Posttraumatic stress disorder: early detection is key, *Nurse Pract* 31(3):26-35, 2006.

Hanson RF, Self-Brown S, Fricker-Elhai A et al: Relations among parental substance use, violence exposure and mental health: the national survey of adolescents, *Addict Behav* 31(11):1988-2001, 2006.

Hardin SB, Weinrich S, Weinrich M et al: Effects of a long-term psychosocial nursing intervention on adolescents exposed to catastrophic stress, *Issues Ment Health Nurs* 23(6):537, 2002.

International Critical Incident Stress Foundation: *Critical incident stress information, signs and symptoms,* www.icisf.org/CIS.html, accessed January 4, 2007.

Litz BT, Gray MJ, Bryant RA et al: Early intervention for trauma: current status and future direction, *Clin Psychol Sci Pract* 9:112, 2002.

McDermott BM, Cvitanovich A: Posttraumatic stress disorder and emotional problems in children following motor vehicle accidents: an extended case series, *Aust N Z J Psychiatry* 34:446, 2000.

Meeske KA, Ruccione K, Globe DR et al: Posttraumatic stress, quality of life, and psychological distress in young adult survivors of childhood cancer, *Oncol Nurs Forum* 28(3):481, 2001.

National Cancer Institute: *Posttraumatic stress disorder,* www.cancer.gov/cancerinfo/pdq/supportivecare/post-traumatic-stress/HealthProfessional, accessed January 4, 2007.

National Center for PSTD: *Screening for PTSD in primary care settings,* www.ncptsd.va.gov/publications/assessment, accessed January 4, 2007.

Post Trauma Resources: *Tools for an unsafe world,* 2001, www.post-trauma.com/tools.htm, accessed January 4, 2007.

Razokhi A, Taha I, Taib N et al: Mental health of Iraqi children, *Lancet* 368(9538):838-839, 2006.

Ronen T, Gahav G, Appel N: Adolescent stress responses to a single acute stress and to continuous external stress: terrorist attacks, *J Loss Trauma* 8:261-282, 2004.

Tolin DF, Foa EF: Sex differences in trauma and posttraumatic stress disorder: a quantitative review of 25 years of research, *Psychol Bull* 132(6):959-992, 2006.

Winston F, Kassam-Adams N, Vivarelli-O'Neill C et al: Acute stress disorder in children and their parents after pediatric traffic injury, *Pediatrics* 109(6):e90, 2002.

Yen S, Shea MT, Battle CL et al: Traumatic exposure and posttraumatic stress disorder in borderline, schizotypal, avoidant, and obsessive-compulsive personality disorders: findings from the collaborative longitudinal personality disorders study, *J Nerv Ment Dis* 190(8):510, 2002.

• = Independent; ▲ = Collaborative; EBN = Evidence-Based Nursing; EB = Evidence-Based

Readiness for enhanced Power   *Margaret Lunney, RN, PhD, and Marie Giordano, MS, RN*

NANDA   Definition

A pattern of participating knowingly in change that is sufficient for well-being and can be strengthened

Defining Characteristics

Expresses readiness to enhance awareness of possible changes to be made; freedom to perform actions for change; identification of choices that can be made for change; involvement in creating change; knowledge for participation in change; participation in choices for daily living and health; power

NOC   Outcomes (Nursing Outcomes Classification)

Suggested NOC Outcomes

Health Beliefs: Perceived Control, Participation in Health Care Decisions, Personal Autonomy

Example NOC Outcome with Indicators
Health Beliefs: Perceived Control as evidenced by the following indicators: Belief that own actions and decisions control health outcomes/ Perceived responsibility for health decisions/Efforts at gathering information (Rate the outcome and indicators of **Health Beliefs: Perceived Control:** 1 = very weak, 2 = weak, 3 = moderate, 4 = strong, 5 = very strong [see Section I].)

Client Outcomes

Client Will (Specify Time Frame):

- Evaluate power resources
- Identify perceptions of control
- Select options to support health
- Seek assistance as needed
- Participate with health providers in relation to health issues and concerns

NIC   Interventions (Nursing Interventions Classification)

Suggested NIC Interventions

Mutual Goal Setting, Self-Esteem Enhancement, Self Responsibility Facilitation

Example NIC Activities—Mutual Goal Setting
Encourage the identification of specific life values; Identify with patient the goals of care; Assist the patient in examining available resources to meet goals

Nursing Interventions and *Rationales*

- Support and enhance the client's inherent power. **EBN:** *A nursing theory of power as knowing participation in change was derived from Martha Rogers' conceptual framework, the* Science of Unitary Human Beings *(Barrett, 1990). Extensive research findings have demonstrated that people have power, and power is associated with determinants of health (Barrett & Caroselli, 1998; Caroselli & Barrett, 1998). A conclusion from this body of research is that health providers should support and enhance the inherent power of the people they serve. Shearer and Reed, in a reformulation of empowerment, showed that power and empowerment can be compatible concepts (2004). Funnell (2004) also described empowerment as helping people discover and use their own innate ability or power.*
- Focus on the positive aspects of power rather than the prevention of powerlessness. **EBN:** *Numerous studies conducted during development of the health promotion model show that promotion differs from prevention and requires a positive rather than negative approach (Pender, Murdaugh & Parsons, 2006).*

• = Independent;   ▲ = Collaborative;   EBN = Evidence-Based Nursing;   EB = Evidence-Based

- Follow the client's agenda. **EBN:** *Following the client's agenda was identified as the fist step of client empowerment in a focus group study with 28 parish nurses (Weis, Schank & Matheus, 2006).*
- Develop partnerships with clients for shared power. **EBN:** *In a quasiexperimental study with two groups, one that was involved in a client-centered approach that relied on client's autonomy, active participation, and collaborative care (n = 73) and the other that received traditional medical services to manage diabetes (n = 35), the intervention group reported higher quality of life and improved diabetic outcomes when compared with the control group (Pibernik-Okanovic et al, 2003). In a historical review of clients' roles, power and subjective choice in healthcare services in the United Kingdom, it was determined that the culture of medicine and health care is changing to a view of client power and decision making (McGregor, 2006). This perspective was also a conclusion of a literature review on trust, choice, and power in mental health (Langharne & Priebe, 2006).*
- Listen with intent. **EBN:** *In a study that tested a model for nurse-client partnership, the Self Care TALK model, listening with intent (similar to Active Listening described in the NIC) conveyed presence and connection (Leenerts & Teel, 2006). In a focus group study with 28 parish nurses, presence and listening was identified as important components of client empowerment (Weis, Schank & Matheus, 2006).*
- Affirm emotions. **EBN:** *In the Leenerts & Teel (2006) study, affirming the client's emotions and the nurse exhibiting emotional responsiveness demonstrated empathy and resulted in deeper nurse-client discussions toward the achievement of partnership.*
- Help the client create images that support and sustain self-care, such as identification of people or events that provided encouragement and meaning. **EBN:** *The creation of self-care images supported mutual goal setting and helped clients build meaning in relation to self-care (Leenerts & Teel, 2006). For example, in a qualitative analysis by an advanced practice nurse of how she helped her parents promote self-care, she compared discussing health concerns with familiar situations, such as asking how her father (a mechanic) would know what was wrong with customers' cars. Her father recognized that without information from his customers, he could not know how to fix their cars; this helped him create images of the need to work collaboratively with health providers (Guinn, 2004).*
- Collaborate with the person to identify resources to put a plan into action. **EBN:** *In a survey of 24,609 adult Americans, aged 19 to 69 years, collaborative care was associated with better control of many disease risk factors as well as the treatment of effects of pain and emotional problems (Wasson et al, 2006). Planning enactment is the last step in the Leenerts and Teel (2006) model for building partnerships with clients. Connections and linkages to resources were identified by 28 parish nurses as a source of client empowerment (Weis et al, 2006).*
- Assess the meaning of health-related issues to the person. **EBN:** *Understanding the meaning of events was shown to be an important power resource (n = 12 Chinese clients with cancer) (Mok, 2001). In an analysis of eight studies (N = 4663) of power beliefs, perceived behavioral control, and health-related intentions, power beliefs had a significant direct relation with health-related intentions such as health promotion (Godin, Gagne & Sheeran, 2004). In a concept analysis of empowerment with frail elderly, reflection on the meaning of events was identified as an essential component of empowerment (Hage & Lorensen, 2005).*
- Facilitate the person's trust in self and others. **EBN:** *In a correlational study of 189 men and women who were randomly selected from a national mailing list, there was a positive correlation of trust and power (r = .49, P <.001) (Wright, 2004).*
- Help the client mobilize social supports. **EBN:** *In a correlational study of 92 women recruited from a community clinic, perceived social support was significantly related to health empowerment (Shearer, 2004).*
- Identify and support beliefs of power and perceptions of behavioral control. **EB:** *In an integration of eight studies related to perceived behavioral control with a total of 4663 adults, the overall findings supported that power beliefs related to power intention and perceived behavioral control partially mediated power beliefs and intentions (Godin, Gagne & Sheeran, 2004).*
- Promote optimal level of functioning. **EBN:** *In a study of 12 menopausal women, every woman perceived that her body and mind were empowered by regular exercise (Jeng et al, 2004).*
- Change organizational and management patterns to support clients' power. **EB:** *Organizational support of clients' power and participation in all phases of health care has been increasingly recognized as a good marketing strategy for the achievement of positive health outcomes (Powers & Bendall, 2003).*

• = Independent;   ▲ = Collaborative;   EBN = Evidence-Based Nursing;   EB = Evidence-Based

Home Care

- Above interventions may be adapted for home care use.
- ▲ Work with families to support the power of individual family members. **EBN:** *Families have opportunities to support the power of individual family members and are important resources for individual power (Wright & Leahey, 2005).*

 Client/Family Teaching

- When conducting any client or family teaching, support the client's power by working in partnership to identify learning needs, learning styles, health literacy, and desired objectives and content. **EBN:** *In numerous studies related to client education, working in partnership to enhance power was associated with positive learning outcomes (Redman, 2007).*

  See the EVOLVE website for World Wide Web resources for client education.

REFERENCES

Barrett EAM: A measure of power as knowing participation in change. In Strickland OL, Waltz CF, editors: *Measurement of nursing outcomes. Vol 4, Measuring client self care and coping skills,* New York, 1990, Springer.

Barrett EAM, Caroselli C: Methodological ponderings related to the Power as Knowing Participation in Change Tool, *Nurs Sci Q* 11(1):17-22, 1998.

Caroselli C, Barrett EAM: A review of the power as knowing participation in change literature, *Nurs Sci Q* 11(1):9-16, 1998.

Funnell MM: Patient empowerment, *Crit Care Nurs Q* 27(2):201-204, 2004.

Godin G, Gagne C, Sheeran P: Does perceived behavioural control mediate the relationship between power beliefs and intention? *Br J Health Psychol* 9:557-568, 2004.

Guinn MJ: A daughter's journey promoting geriatric self care: promoting positive health care interactions, *Geriatr Nurs* 25:267-271, 2004.

Hage AM, Lorensen M: A philosophical analysis of the concept empowerment: the fundament of an education-programme to the frail elderly, *Nurs Philos* 6:235-246, 2005.

Jeng C, Yang S, Chang P et al: Menopausal women: perceiving continuous power through the experience of regular exercise, *J Clin Nurs* 13:447-454, 2004.

Langharne R, Priebe S: Trust, choice and power in mental health: a literature review, *Soc Psychiatry Psychiatr Epidemiol* 41:843-852, 2006.

Leenerts MH, Teel CS: Relational conversation as method for creating partnerships: pilot study, *J Adv Nurs* 54:467-476, 2006.

McGregor S: Review: roles, power and subjective choice. *Patient Educ Couns* 60:5-9, 2006.

Mok E: Empowerment of cancer patients: from a Chinese perspective, *Nurs Ethics* 8(1):69-76, 2001.

Pender NJ, Murdaugh CL, Parsons MA: *Health promotion in nursing practice,* ed 5, Stamford, CT, 2006, Appleton & Lange.

Pibernik-Okanovic M, Prasek M, Poljicanin-Filipovic T et al: Effects of an empowerment-based psychosocial intervention on quality of life and metabolic control in type 2 diabetic patients, *Patient Educ Couns* 52:193-199, 2003.

Powers TL, Bendall D: Improving health outcomes through patient empowerment, *J Hosp Mark Public Relations* 15(1):45-59, 2003.

Redman BK: *The practice of patient education: a case study approach,* ed 10, St Louis, 2007, Mosby.

Shearer NB: Relationships of contextual and relational factors to health empowerment in women, *Res Theory Nurs Pract Int J* 18(4):357-370, 2004.

Shearer NBC, Reed PG: Empowerment: reformulation of a non-Rogerian concept, *Nurs Sci Q,* 17(3):253-259, 2004.

Wasson JH, Johnson DJ, Benjamin R et al: Patients report positive impacts of collaborative care, *J Ambul Care Manage* 29:199-206, 2006.

Weis D, Schank MJ, Matheus R: The process of empowerment: a parish nurse perspective, *J Holist Nurs* 24(1):17-24, 2006.

Wright BW: Trust and power in adults: an investigation using Rogers' science of unitary human beings, *Nurs Sci Q* 17(2):139-146, 2004.

Wright LM, Leahey M: *Nurses and families: a guide to family assessment and interventions,* ed 4, Philadelphia, 2005, F.A. Davis.

P

Powerlessness   *Kathleen L. Patusky, PhD, APRN-BC*   **evolve**

NANDA   Definition

Perception that one's own actions will not significantly affect an outcome; perceived lack of control over current situation or immediate happening

Defining Characteristics

Low

Expressions of uncertainty about fluctuating energy levels; passivity

Moderate

Anger; dependence on others that may result in irritability; does not defend self-care practices when challenged; does not monitor progress; expressions of dissatisfaction over inability to perform previous tasks/activities; expressions of doubt regarding role performance; expressions of frustration over inability to perform previous tasks/activities; fear of alienation from caregivers; guilt; inability to seek information regarding care; nonparticipation in care when opportunities are provided; nonparticipation in decision making when opportunities are provided; passivity; reluctance to express true feelings; resentment

Severe

Apathy; depression over physical deterioration; verbal expressions of having no control (e.g., over self-care, situation, outcome)

Related Factors (r/t)

Healthcare environment; illness-related regimen; interpersonal interactions; lifestyle of helplessness

NOC   Outcomes (Nursing Outcomes Classification)

Suggested NOC Outcomes

Depression Self-Control; Health Beliefs; Health Beliefs: Perceived Ability to Perform, Perceived Control, Perceived Resources; Participation in Health Care Decisions

Example NOC Outcome with Indicators
Health Beliefs: Perceived Control as evidenced by the following indicators: Perceived responsibility for health decisions/Beliefs that own decisions and actions control health outcomes (Rate the outcome and indicators of **Health Beliefs: Perceived Control:** 1 = very weak belief, 2 = weak belief, 3 = moderately strong belief, 4 = strong belief, 5 = very strong belief [see Section I].)

Consider using one of the measures of powerlessness that are available for general and specific client groups:
- Spreitzer's Psychological Empowerment Questionnaire (Boudrias, Gaudreau & Laschinger, 2004)
- Personal Progress Scale—Revised, tested with women (Johnson, Worell & Chandler, 2005)
- Life Situation Questionnaire—Powerlessness subscale, tested with stroke caregivers (Larson et al, 2005)
- Making Decisions Scale, tested in clients with mental illness (Hansson & Bjorkman, 2005)

Client Outcomes

Client Will (Specify Time Frame):

- State feelings of powerlessness and other feelings related to powerlessness (e.g., anger, sadness, hopelessness)
- Identify factors that are uncontrollable

• = Independent;   ▲ = Collaborative;   EBN = Evidence-Based Nursing;   EB = Evidence-Based

- Participate in planning and implementing care; make decisions regarding care and treatment when possible
- Ask questions about care and treatment
- Verbalize hope for the future and sense of participation in planning and implementing care

NIC   Interventions (Nursing Interventions Classification)

Suggested NIC Interventions

Cognitive Restructuring, Complex Relationship Building, Mutual Goal Setting, Self-Esteem Enhancement, Self-Responsibility Facilitation

Example NIC Activities—Self-Responsibility Facilitation
Encourage independence but assist patient when unable to perform; Assist patient to identify areas in which they could readily assume more responsibility

Nursing Interventions and *Rationales*

NOTE: Before implementation of interventions in the face of client powerlessness, nurses should examine their own philosophies of care to ensure that control issues or lack of faith in client capabilities will not bias the ability to intervene sincerely and effectively. **EBN:** *Nurses and other healthcare professionals may feel that they, rather than clients, should make medical decisions, or profess a support of client empowerment that they find difficult to implement (Ko & Muecke, 2006; Paliadelis et al, 2005).*

- Observe for factors contributing to powerlessness (e.g., immobility, hospitalization, unfavorable prognosis, lack of support system, misinformation about situation, inflexible routine, chronic illness). **EBN:** *The essence of ill health is powerlessness, involving the sense of being imprisoned by circumstances (because of limited choices and abilities) and emotional suffering (Strandmark, 2004). Multiple client situations have been associated with powerlessness, including chronic disorders (Dzurec, Hoover & Fields, 2002), cancer (Rydahl-Hansen, 2005), and domestic violence (Hyden, 2005), particularly when client perceptions are invalidated or ignored.*
- Assess for **ineffective Therapeutic regimen management** or **Noncompliance.** Be alert to client behaviors that attempt to assert power, even if they seem confrontational. Help clients channel their behaviors in an effective manner. **EBN:** *Strategies women have used to regain control over uncertain illness trajectories included exiting (changing healthcare providers when dissatisfied), noncompliance (when medical advice did not seem to make sense), confrontation (especially when clients' perspectives were questioned or ignored), persuasion/insistence, making demands, and demonstrative distancing (refusing to participate in discussion) (Asbring & Narvanen, 2004).*
- Assess the client's locus of control related to his or her health. **EB:** *An external locus of control can negatively influence clients' perception of their power over a health situation, and religious faith may be a component of personal control beliefs (Sparks, Peterson & Tangenberg, 2005).*
- Establish a therapeutic relationship with the client by spending one-on-one time with him or her, assigning the same caregiver, keeping commitments (e.g., saying, "I will be back to answer your questions in the next hour"), providing encouragement and support, and being empathetic. **EBN:** *Clients reported as empowering the support of family members, friends, and healthcare providers (Bolse et al, 2005) and believed they had to seek out nursing care as a means of alleviating powerlessness (Shattell, 2005).*
- Encourage the client to share his or her beliefs, thoughts, and expectations about his or her illness. *The Health Belief Model identifies perceptions and expectations about disease, including perceived barriers and perceived susceptibility to disease, as powerful predictors of clients' motivation in taking action to prevent disease and participate in self-care management (Pender, Murdaugh & Parsons, 2005).*
- Have the client assist in planning care whenever possible (e.g., determining what time to bathe, taking pain medication before uncomfortable procedures, expressing food and fluid preferences). Document specifics in the care plan. *Self-regulation and self-care management promote feelings of*

P

self-efficacy, increasing confidence about managing chronic illness (Lorig et al, 2001). **EBN:** *Cancer clients made use of the Internet to self-manage symptoms and empower decision making (Dickerson et al, 2006).*

- Help the client specify the health goals he or she would like to achieve, prioritizing those goals with regard to immediate concerns and identifying actions that will achieve the goals. Goals may need to be small to be attainable (e.g., dangle legs at bedside for 2 days, then sit in chair 10 minutes for 2 days, then walk to window). *People need goals that have value for them; the discrepancy between these goals and reality motivates action to reduce the discrepancy. Goals must be realistic and achievable; otherwise, the inability to perceive progress will increase hopelessness and powerlessness (Pender, Murdaugh & Parsons, 2005).*

- Support clients' efforts to regain control of their lives by learning everything they can about their illnesses and treatment regimen. **EB:** *Acquiring knowledge about their illnesses or treatment regimens helped clients regain a sense of control, whether the condition was chronic fatigue syndrome or fibromyalgia (Asbring & Narvanen, 2004), ventilator-dependence (Johnson, 2004), or diabetes (Panja, Starr & Colleran, 2005; Siminerio, Piatt & Zgibor, 2005).*

- Encourage the client in goal-directed activities that promote a sense of accomplishment, especially regular exercise. *Goal direction enhances self-efficacy, an important antecedent of empowerment (Finfgeld, 2004; Fitzsimons & Fuller, 2002).* **EBN:** *In a study of menopausal women, regular exercise promoted a sense of self-fulfillment and an increasing sense of power (Jeng, Yang & Chang, 2004).*

- Recognize the client's need to experience a sense of reciprocity in dealing with others. Negotiate actions that the client can contribute to the caregiving partnership with both family and nurse (e.g., have the client prepare a cup of tea for the nurse during visits if the client is able). **EBN:** *Ill or injured individuals made attempts to exchange what skills they could for physical care in attempts to gain a feeling of equity (Dewar, 2001). For older adults, a lack of reciprocity (equitable exchange) was associated with depression, although older adults receiving home care services seemed to have adjusted to the lack of reciprocity (Patusky, 2000).*

- Allow time for questions (15 to 20 minutes each shift). Have the client write down questions, and encourage the client to record a summary of answers received if desired or practicable or provide written material that reinforces answers. *Encouraging the client to write down questions and answers emphasizes the importance of client input and nurses' willingness to attend to that input.* **EB:** *Women reported the experiences of not being listened to, loss of privacy and dignity, and loss of day-to-day control—in short, powerlessness (Polimeni & Moore, 2002).* **EBN:** *For clients experiencing a first-time hospitalization, powerlessness was found to result from lack of staff support (in the form of not being listened to) and lack of information about their illness or medical treatment (Blockley, 2003).*

- Encourage the client to take control of as many ADLs as possible; keep the client informed of all care that will be given. Keep items the client uses and needs, such as a urinal, tissues, telephone, and television controls, within reach. *Choice in ADLs such as eating, sleeping, and grooming contributes to a sense of control. Clients are more amenable to therapy if they know what to expect and can perform some tasks independently. Dependence can be alleviated by fostering an expectation of control over activities, which leads to the development of a sense of mastery (Faulkner, 2001).*

- Give realistic and sincere praise for accomplishments. *Frequent positive reinforcement helps clients feel successful and competent, especially when it is immediate and is used to balance feedback about errors (Pender, Murdaugh & Parsons, 2005).*

- While the client's perspective is paramount, family members' powerlessness in assisting with client care must also be addressed to enhance family support. **EB:** *Family members of clients with mental illness or traumatic brain injury have identified empowerment as an important factor in their ability to cope with client behavior and care needs (Gavois, Paulsson & Fridlund, 2006; Leith, Phillips & Sample, 2004; Sjoblom, Pejlert & Asplund, 2005).*

- In evaluating outcomes implemented to address powerlessness, look to changes in the client, changes in relationships with others, and changes in behavior. **EBN:** *In response to interventions, clients achieve increased self-confidence and self-esteem; improved relationships with families and friends as well as with healthcare providers; and the ability to make healthier choices for themselves (Falk-Rafael, 2001).*

- Refer to the care plans for **Hopelessness** and **Spiritual distress.**

• = Independent; ▲ = Collaborative; EBN = Evidence-Based Nursing; EB = Evidence-Based

Pediatric

Two key issues that lead to powerlessness for children and their families are hospitalization and peer victimization or bullying.

- Encourage emotional expression through processes that are appropriate to the child's level of development. **EBN:** *Qualitative analysis of play therapy using expressive arts allowing hospitalized children free self-expression revealed a theme of powerlessness as well as the ability of expressive arts to facilitate the child's communication (Wikstrom, 2005).*
- Recognize that a sense of powerlessness can prevent children and adolescents from reporting peer victimization. Be supportive, encourage disclosure without pressure, and help the child or adolescent problem solve options to deal with their stressors. **EBN:** *Pregnant teens reported family, partner, and gang violence that they had not mentioned to healthcare providers, with powerlessness as a theme (Renker, 2006).* **EB:** *Disclosure of bullying was found to be inhibited by perceived powerlessness, with active listening and validation recommended as approaches (Mishna & Aleggia, 2005).*
- Provide instruction and visual aids to family members so they may better understand a child's illness and how the family members can help. **EBN:** *New mothers found instruction on child care to be empowering, helping them to be independent, increasing their confidence, and using their strengths (Aston et al, 2006).* **EB:** *Family members of a child with acquired brain injury who were new to medical and special education systems benefited from videos and informational booklets that addressed the child's needs (Forsyth et al, 2005).*

Geriatric

In addition to the above interventions as appropriate:

- Initiate focused assessment questioning and education regarding syndromes common in the elderly. **EBN:** *Studies indicate that disease management programs led by nurses have a positive effect on the perception of powerlessness, loneliness, and disease management (Murchie et al, 2004).*
- Assess for the presence of elder abuse. Initiate referral to Adult Protective Services and help client regain a sense of safety and control. *Older adults who need assistance are particularly vulnerable to feelings of powerlessness and dependence on caregivers.* **EB:** *Psychosocial assessment, relationship building, and empowerment were important in helping abused elders gain independence and control over their daily lives (Dayton, 2005).*
- Explore feelings of powerlessness—the feeling that the client's behavior will not affect outcomes. **EBN:** *Older adults who engaged in effective strategies to control their health problems had fewer depressive symptoms, particularly in the presence of acute physical symptoms (Wrosch, Schulz & Heckhausen, 2002).*
- Explore personality resources and inner strengths that the client has used in the past. Incorporate these into the treatment plan. **EBN:** *Although resources and strengths cultivated by older adults over the years often go unrecognized, they contribute to the older adult's sense of coherence (perception that life is meaningful, comprehensible, and manageable) and have been shown to optimize quality of life in older women with chronic health problems (Nesbitt & Heidrich, 2000).*
- Establish therapeutic relationships by listening; participate with the client in generating choices and incorporate his or her statement of limitations. **EBN:** *An individualized approach to health promotion, providing education that will support the individual client's needs, creates a partnership relationship that permits the nurse to enhance self-care practices of the older adult and thereby promote self-care ability and activity (Leenerts, Teel & Pendleton, 2002; Resnick, 2001).*
- ▲ Monitor the use of alternative therapies but do not intervene unless the therapy interacts negatively with the existing therapeutic regimen. Ensure that all healthcare providers involved with the client are aware of the alternative therapies being used. *Older women in particular may use alternative therapies learned in their roles as mothers, midwives, and shamans. Familiarity with these alternatives to a patriarchal medical model can increase control over health and enhance prevention and self-care (Gaylord, 1999).*
- Instruct caregivers in effective means of managing the behavior of clients with dementia. **EBN:** *Dementia caregivers reported a dichotomy between feeling powerless, with their lives in chaos, versus feeling capable, gaining control and confidence over their abilities to respond to client behaviors (Graneheim et al, 2005).*

P

• = Independent; ▲ = Collaborative; EBN = Evidence-Based Nursing; EB = Evidence-Based

Multicultural

- Assess the influence of cultural beliefs, norms, and values on the client's feelings of powerlessness. **EBN:** *Older Chinese adults who had fallen reported powerlessness, fear, and care seeking (Kong et al, 2002). Elderly Taiwanese men with heart trouble identified powerlessness as arising from lacking choice in living arrangements, having no control over discomfort, being unable to obtain care and companionship from families and friends, failing to get medical information about their disease and treatment options, or expecting deteriorating health and receiving no assistance (Shih et al, 2000).* **EBN:** *When 58 African-American and Latino homeless women were given social support and taught to build skills, health outcomes improved (Hatton & Kaiser, 2004).* **EBN:** *African-American women gained energy and decreased depression scores when a closed group using meditative exercise with culturally specific scenarios was used (Kohn et al, 2002).*

- Assess the effect of fatalism on the client's expression of powerlessness. *Fatalistic perspectives, which involve the belief that one cannot control one's own fate, may influence health behaviors in some African-American, Latino, and Native-American populations (Green et al, 2004; Ramirez et al, 2002).*

- Encourage spirituality as a source of support to decrease powerlessness. *African Americans and Latinos may identify spirituality, religiousness, prayer, and church-based approaches as coping resources (Samuel-Hodge et al, 2000).*

- Validate the client's feelings regarding the impact of health status on current lifestyle. **EBN:** *Powerlessness among diabetics was reported as a concern of African-American clients (Blanchard et al, 1999).* **EBN:** *When 326 African-American women gained knowledge of breast cancer risk and screening and breast self-examination proficiency, breast self-examination skills scores significantly increased (Wood, Duffy & Carner, 2002).*

- For inner-city clients, help the client redefine behaviors as ways of coping with a hostile environment and reconnecting with community supports. **EBN:** *Powerlessness among inner-city African Americans can arise in reaction to inner-city environments, poverty, and racism. Strategies that involve redefining behavior and reconnecting to the community promote empowerment (Dancy et al, 2001).*

- Use an empowerment approach when working with African-American women. **EB:** *Three strategies of empowerment for working with African-American women caregivers were identified as (1) raising critical group consciousness through storytelling, (2) teaching concrete problem-solving skills, and (3) teaching advocacy skills and mobilizing resources (Chadiha et al, 2004).* **EBN:** *By providing women-focused intervention of culturally enriched content founded in empowerment theory and feminism/skills training relative to HIV risk, African-American woman gained independence and increased personal power and control over behavioral choices (Wechsberg et al, 2004).*

Home Care

- Include an initial and ongoing assessment and evaluation of potential abuse and neglect. Photograph evidence of abuse or neglect when possible. *Victims of abuse perceive themselves to be powerless to change the situation. Long-term abuse and neglect of the elderly by the spouse or other family member is often hidden until home care personnel are actively involved.*

- ▲ If neglect or abuse is suspected, identify an emergency plan that addresses the problem immediately, ensures client safety, and includes a report to the appropriate authorities. *Client safety is a nursing priority. An emergency plan should address either immediate removal to a safe environment or identification of appropriate steps to take in the event of abuse, and the securing of resources for anticipated action (e.g., telephone is accessible, bag is packed, alternative living arrangements are available). Reporting abuse is a legal requirement of healthcare workers.*

- Develop a therapeutic relationship in the home setting that respects the client's domain. **EBN:** *Effective home care empowers and makes vulnerable both nurse and client (Spiers, 2002).*

- Develop a written contract with the client that designates what care will be given and who has responsibility for care elements. Focus should be on care that is controlled by the client. Enable the client to develop his or her own resources actively. *A written contract reassures the client that the designation of control of care will be honored.*

- Empower the client by encouraging the client to guide specifics of care such as wound care procedures and dressing and grooming details. Confirm the client's knowledge and document in the

---

• = Independent; ▲ = Collaborative; EBN = Evidence-Based Nursing; EB = Evidence-Based

chart that the client is able to guide procedures. Document in the home and in the chart the preferred approach to procedures. Orient the family and caregivers to the client's role. **EBN:** *Negotiation, reciprocity, shared decision making, creation of opportunities, and effective information and support are key elements of empowerment in the home (Houston & Cowley, 2002).*

- Identify the client's concerns and implement interventions to address the consequences of disability in clients with medical illness. **EB:** *In clients with cancer being cared for at home, primary factors influencing vulnerability to depression and suicide were identified as real or feared loss of autonomy and independence, concerns about being a burden on others, hopelessness about their condition, and fear of suffering (Filiberti et al, 2001).*

- Enhance self-efficacy by creating an environment that supports physical activities; provide support in the form of encouragement, anticipatory guidance, sharing of how others perform, and realistic assessment of the client's abilities. **EBN:** *Increasing self-efficacy in clients with heart failure can decrease symptomatology and improve quality of life (Borsody et al, 1999).*

- Respect the client's choices regarding desired assistance. Identify knowledge deficits and provide education to ensure that the client's choice is accurately informed. **EBN:** *The client may identify a problem but choose not to receive help at this time. Assessment is an opportunity to discuss health needs, not a condition for treatment (Houston & Cowley, 2002).*

- Assess the affective climate within the family and family support system, including other caregivers. Instruct the family in appropriate expectations of the client and in the specifics of the client's illness. Encourage the family and client in efforts toward educating friends and co-workers regarding appropriate expectations for the client. **EBN:** *Recognize that clients with an illness requiring extensive physical assistance may become caught in a dilemma; they may be dependent on others for assistance, but that very dependence may hamper their ability to respond naturally within the relationship or require that caregivers meet certain standards. Abuse is also a possibility (Curry, Hassouneh-Phillips & Johnston-Silverberg, 2001).* Refer to care plan for **Risk for other-directed Violence.** *Clients experiencing a catastrophic illness or injury felt distressed by family members' or friends' comments that indicated a lack of understanding of the illness experience (Dewar, 2001).*

- Evaluate the powerlessness of caregivers to ensure they continue their ability to care for the client. Provide assistance using interventions from this care plan. **EB:** *In next of kin of clients with cancer receiving palliative home care, powerlessness and helplessness were reported regarding client's suffering, fading away, and next of kin's feeling of inadequacy (Milberg, Strang & Jakobsson, 2004).*

- Be aware of and assist clients with potential needs for help in negotiating the healthcare system. **EB:** *Among individuals with disabilities, powerlessness may arise as a response to failures of the system to provide needed services (Helgøy, Ravneberg & Solvang, 2003).*

▲ Refer for homemaker or psychiatric home healthcare services for respite, client reassurance, and implementation of a therapeutic regimen. *Respite care decreases caregiver stress. The presence of caring individuals is reassuring to both the client and caregivers, especially during periods of client anxiety or depression.*

- Explain all relevant symptoms, procedures, treatments, and expected outcomes. **EBN:** *In a study of clients' perceptions of their health care, clients who expressed powerlessness described a lack of knowledge and information about treatment strategies (Nordgren & Fridlund, 2001).*

- Provide written instructions for treatments and procedures for which the client will be responsible. *A written record provides a concrete reference so that the client and family can clarify any verbal information that was given. People tend to forget half of what they hear within a few minutes, so nurses should supplement oral instructions with written material (Wong, 1992).*

- Continually assess the client for signs of inappropriate exercise of self-care. Confront such applications of self-care; instruct the client in the dangers that inappropriate care may present and in alternatives for care that would be more effective. **EBN:** *Clients often attempt to implement treatment on their own (e.g., through the use of previous prescribed medications, home remedies, or over-the-counter medication) and may not be aware that they are misjudging a need for professional services or selecting less-than-optimal treatment options (Edwardson & Dean, 1999).*

- Teach stress reduction, relaxation, and imagery. Many audio recordings are available on relaxation and meditation. Assist the client with relaxation based on the client's preference indicated in the initial assessment. *These techniques can restore power in the client by allowing the client to*

P

learn how to control the autonomic nervous system and other physiological mechanisms (Johnson, Dahlen & Roberts, 1997). Relaxation techniques, desensitization, and guided imagery can help clients cope, increase their control, and allay anxiety (Narsavage, 1997).

- Teach cognitive-behavioral activities, such as active problem solving, reframing (reappraising the situation from a different perspective), or thought stopping (in response to a negative thought, such as picturing a large stop sign and replacing the image with a prearranged positive alternative). Teach the client to confront his or her own negative thought patterns (cognitive distortions). *Through cognitive-behavioral interventions, clients become more aware of their cognitive choices in adopting and maintaining their belief systems, thereby exercising greater control over their own reactions (Hagerty & Patusky, 2003).*

- Help the client practice assertive communication techniques. **EBN:** *Clients with conditions such as quadriplegia need to be assertive so that they can direct their care and be as independent as possible (Bach & McDaniel, 1993).*

- Role play (e.g., say, "Tell me what you are going to ask your doctor"). *Role playing is the most commonly used technique in assertiveness training. It deconditions the anxiety that arises from interpersonal encounters by allowing the client to practice how he or she might respond in a given situation.*

- Identify the strengths of the caregiver and efforts to gain control of unpredictable situations. Help the caregiver stay connected with a client who may be behaving differently than usual to make life as routine as possible, help the client set goals and sustain hope, and allow the client space to experience progress. **EBN:** *Identifying positive caregiver responses to the client's illness assists the caregiver in tolerating his or her own feelings of powerlessness. Family members of persons with severe mental illness have found it helpful to work at staying connected to the person with mental illness, finding a role that they can feel comfortable with, and helping the relative move forward (Rose, 1998).*

- ▲ Refer the client to support groups, pastoral care, or social services. *There is an assignment of power in the imparting of advice (Bonhote, Romano-Egan & Cornwell, 1999). These services help decrease levels of stress, increase levels of self-esteem, and reassure clients that they are not alone.*

evolve See the EVOLVE website for World Wide Web resources for client education.

REFERENCES

Asbring P, Narvanen A: Patient power and control: a study of women with uncertain illness trajectories, *Qual Health Res* 14(2):226, 2004.

Aston M, Meagher-Stewart D, Sheppard-Lemoin D et al: Family health nursing and empowering relationships, *Ped Nurs* 32:61, 2006.

Bach C, McDaniel R: Quality of life in quadriplegic adults: a focus group study, *Rehabil Nurs* 18:364, 1993.

Blanchard MA, Rose LE, Taylor J et al: Using a focus group to design a diabetes education program for an African American population, *Diabetes Educ* 25(6):917, 1999.

Blockley C: Experiences of first time hospitalisation for acute illness, *Nurs Prax N Z* 19(2):19, 2003.

Bolse K, Hamilton G, Flanagan J et al: Ways of experiencing the life situation among United States patients with an implantable cardioverter-defibrillator: a qualitative study, *Prog Cardiovasc Nurs* 20(1):4, 2005.

Bonhote K, Romano-Egan J, Cornwell C: Altruism and creative expressions in a long-term older adult psychotherapy group, *Issues Ment Health Nurs* 20(6):603, 1999.

Borsody JM, Courtney M, Taylor K et al: Using self-efficacy to increase physical activity in patients with heart failure, *Home Healthc Nurs* 17:113, 1999.

Boudrias J, Gaudreau P, Laschinger HKS: Testing the structure of psychological empowerment: does gender make a difference? *Educ Psychol Meas* 64:861, 2004.

Chadiha LA, Adams P, Biegel DE et al: Empowering African American women informal caregivers: a literature synthesis and practice strategies, *Soc Work* 49(1):97-108, 2004.

Curry MA, Hassouneh-Phillips D, Johnston-Silverberg A: Abuse of women with disabilities: an ecological model and review, *Violence Against Women* 7(1):60, 2001.

Dancy BL, McCreary L, Daye M et al: Empowerment: a view of two low-income African-American communities, *J Natl Black Nurses Assoc* 12(2):49, 2001.

Dayton C: Elder abuse: the social worker's perspective, *Clin Gerontol* 28:135, 2005.

Dewar A: Protecting strategies used by sufferers of catastrophic illness and injuries, *J Clin Nurs* 19:600, 2001.

Dickerson SS, Boehmke M, Ogle C et al: Seeking and managing hope: patients' experiences using the Internet for cancer care, *Oncology Nurs Forum* 33:E8, 2006.

Dzurec LC, Hoover PM, Fields J: Acknowledging unexplained fatigue of tired women, *J Nurs Scholarsh* 34:41, 2002.

Edwardson SR, Dean KJ: Appropriateness of self-care responses to symptoms among elders: identifying pathways of influence, *Res Nurs Health* 22:329, 1999.

Falk-Rafael AR: Empowerment as a process of evolving consciousness: a model of empowered caring, *Adv Nurs Sci* 24(1):1, 2001.

Faulkner M: The onset and alleviation of learned helplessness in older hospitalized people, *Aging Ment Health* 5:379, 2001.

Filiberti A, Ripamonti C, Totis A et al: Characteristics of terminal cancer patients who committed suicide during a home palliative care program, *J Pain Symptom Manage* 22:544, 2001.

Finfgeld DL: Empowerment of individuals with enduring mental health problems: results from concept analyses and qualitative investigations, *Adv Nurs Sci* 27(1):44, 2004.

• = Independent;   ▲ = Collaborative;   EBN = Evidence-Based Nursing;   EB = Evidence-Based

Fitzsimons S, Fuller R: Empowerment and its implications for clinical practice in mental health: a review, *J Ment Health* 11(5): 481, 2002.

Forsyth RJ, Kelly TP, Wicks B et al: "Must try harder?" A family empowerment intervention for acquired brain injury, *Ped Rehab* 8(2):140, 2005.

Gavois H, Paulsson G, Fridlund B: Mental health professional support in families with a member suffering from severe mental illness: a grounded theory model, *Scand J Caring Sci* 20:102, 2006.

Gaylord S: Alternative therapies and empowerment of older women, *J Women Aging* 11(2-3):29, 1999.

Graneheim UH, Isaksson U, Ljung IP et al: Balancing between contradictions: the meaning of interaction with people suffering from dementia and "behavioral disturbances," *Intl J Aging Hum Devel* 60(2):145, 2005.

Green BL, Lewis RK, Wang MQ et al: Powerlessness, destiny, and control: the influence on health behaviors of African Americans, *J Community Health* 29(1):15-27, 2004.

Hagerty B, Patusky K: Mood disorders: depression and mania. In Fortinash KM, Holoday-Worret PA, editors: *Psychiatric mental health nursing,* ed 3, St Louis, 2003, Mosby.

Hansson L, Bjorkman T: Empowerment in people with a mental illness: reliability and validity of the Swedish version of an empowerment scale, *Scand J Caring Sci* 19:32, 2005.

Hatton D, Kaiser L: Methodological and ethical issues emerging from pilot testing an intervention with women in a transitional shelter, *West J Nurs Res* 26(1):129-136, 2004.

Helgoy I, Ravneberg B, Solvang P: Service provision for an independent life, *Disability Soc* 18(4):471, 2003.

Houston AM, Cowley S: An empowerment approach to needs assessment in health visiting practice, *J Clin Nurs* 11:640, 2002.

Hyden M: "I must have been an idiot to let it go on": Agency and positioning in battered women's narratives of leaving, *Fem Psychol* 15:169, 2005.

Jeng C, Yang S, Chang P: Menopausal women: perceiving continuous power through the experience of regular exercise, *J Clin Nurs* 13:447, 2004.

Johnson DM, Worell J, Chandler RK: Assessing psychological health and empowerment in women: The Personal Progress Scale Revised, *Women Health* 41(1):109, 2005.

Johnson LH, Dahlen R, Roberts SL: Supporting hope in congestive heart failure patients, *Dimens Crit Care Nurs* 16(2):65, 1997.

Johnson P: Reclaiming the everyday world: how long-term ventilated patients in critical care seek to gain aspects of power and control over their environment, *Intensive Crit Care Nurs* 20:190, 2004.

Ko NY, Muecke MA: Prevailing discourses among AIDS care professionals about childbearing by couples with HIV in Taiwan, *AIDS Care* 18(1):82, 2006.

Kohn L, Oden T, Munoz R et al: Adapted cognitive behavioral group therapy for depressed low-income African American women, *Community Ment Health J* 38(6):497-504, 2002.

Kong KS, Lee FK, Mackenzie AE et al: Psychosocial consequences of falling: the perspective of older Hong Kong Chinese who had experienced recent falls, *J Adv Nurs* 37:234, 2002.

Larson J, Franzen-Dahlen J, Billing E et al: Spouse's life situation after partner's stroke: psychometric testing of a questionnaire, *J Adv Nurs* 52:300, 2005.

Leenerts MH, Teel CS, Pendleton MK: Building a model of self-care for health promotion in aging, *J Nurs Scholarsh* 34:355, 2002.

Leith KH, Phillips L, Sample PL: Exploring the service needs and experiences of persons with TBI and their families: The South Carolina experience, *Brain Inj* 18:1191, 2004.

Lorig KR, Ritter P, Stewart AL et al: Chronic disease self-management program: 2-year health status and health care utilization outcomes, *Med Care* 39:1217, 2001.

Milberg A, Strang P, Jakobsson M: Next of kin's experience of powerlessness and helplessness in palliative home care, *Support Care Cancer* 12:120, 2004.

Mishna F, Aleggia R: Weighing the risks: a child's decision to disclose peer victimization, *Child Schools* 27:218, 2005.

Murchie P, Campbell N, Ritchie LD et al: Effects of secondary prevention clinics on health status in patients with coronary heart disease: 4 year follow-up randomized trial in primary care, *Fam Pract* 21(5):567-574, 2004.

Narsavage GL: Promoting function in clients with chronic lung disease by increasing their perception of control, *Holist Nurs Pract* 12(1):17, 1997.

Nesbitt BJ, Heidrich SM: Sense of coherence and illness appraisal in older women's quality of life, *Res Nurs Health* 23:25, 2000.

Nordgren S, Fridlund B: Patients' perceptions of self-determination as expressed in the context of care, *J Adv Nurs* 35(1):117, 2001.

Paliadelis P, Cruickshank M, Wainohu D et al: Implementing family-centred care: an exploration of the beliefs and practices of paediatric nurses, *Austr J Adv Nurs* 23(1):31, 2005.

Panja S, Starr B, Colleran KM: Patient knowledge improves glycemic control: Is it time to go back to the classroom? *J Invest Med* 53:264, 2005.

Patusky KL: *Event-generated dependence and its psychological sequelae in older adults,* doctoral dissertation, Ann Arbor, MI, 2000, University of Michigan.

Pender NJ, Murdaugh CL, Parsons MA: *Health promotion in nursing practice,* ed 5, Upper Saddle River, NJ, 2005, Prentice-Hall.

Polimeni A, Moore S: Insights into women's experiences of hospital stays: perceived control, powerlessness and satisfaction, *Behav Change* 19(1):52, 2002.

Ramirez JR, Crano WD, Quist R et al: Effects of fatalism and family communication on HIV/AIDS awareness variations in American and Anglo parents and children, *AIDS Educ Prev* 14(1):29, 2002.

Renker PR: Perinatal violence assessment: teenagers' rationale for denying violence when asked, *JOGNN* 35(1):56, 2006.

Resnick B: Motivating older adults to engage in self-care, *Pat Care Nurs Pract* 4:13, 2001.

Rose LE: Gaining control: family members relate to persons with severe mental illness, *Res Nurs Health* 21:363, 1998.

Rydahl-Hansen S: Hospitalized patients experienced suffering in life with incurable cancer, *Scand J Caring Sci* 19:213, 2005.

Samuel-Hodge CD, Headen SW, Skelly AH et al: Influences on day-to-day self-management of type 2 diabetes among African American women: spirituality, the multi-caregiver role, and other social context factors, *Diabetes Care* 23(7):928, 2000.

Shattell M: Nurse bait: strategies hospitalized patients use to entice nurses within the context of the interpersonal relationship, *Issues Ment Health Nurs* 26:205, 2005.

Shih SN, Shih FJ, Chen CH et al: The forgotten faces: the lonely journey of powerlessness experienced by elderly single Chinese men with heart disease in Taiwan, *Geriatr Nurs* 21:254, 2000.

Siminerio LM, Piatt G, Zgibor JC: Implementing the chronic care model for improvements in diabetes care and education in a rural primary care practice, *Diabetes Educ* 31:225, 2005.

Sjoblom L, Pejlert A, Asplund K: Nurses' view of the family in psychiatric care, *J Clin Nurs* 14:562, 2005.

Sparks A, Peterson NA, Tangenberg K: Belief in personal control among low-income African American, Puerto Rican, and European American single mothers, *Affilia J Women Soc Work* 20:401, 2005.

Spiers JA: The interpersonal contexts of negotiating care in home care nurse-patient interactions, *Qual Health Res* 12:1033, 2002.

Strandmark M: Ill heath is powerlessness: a phenomenological study about worthlessness, limitations and suffering, *Scand J Caring Sci* 18:135, 2004.

• = Independent; ▲ = Collaborative; EBN = Evidence-Based Nursing; EB = Evidence-Based

Wechsberg WM, Lam WK, Zule WA et al: Violence, homelessness, and HIV risk among crack-using African-American women, *Subst Use Misuse* 38:671-701, 2003.

Wikstrom B: Communicating via expressive arts: the natural medium of self-expression for hospitalized children, *Ped Nurs* 31:480, 2005.

Wong M: Self-care instructions: do patients understand educational materials? *Focus Crit Care* 19:47, 1992.

Wood R, Duffy M, Morris S et al: The effect of an education intervention on promoting breast self-examination in older African-American and Caucasian women, *Oncol Nurs Forum* 29(7):1081-1090, 2002.

Wrosch C, Schulz R, Heckhausen J: Health stresses and depressive symptomatology in the elderly: the importance of health engagement control strategies, *Health Psychol* 21:340, 2002.

Risk for Powerlessness   *Kathleen L. Patusky, PhD, APRN-BC*

NANDA   Definition

At risk for perceived lack of control over a situation and/or one's ability to significantly affect an outcome

Risk Factors (r/t)

Physiological

Acute injury; aging; dying; illness; progressive debilitating disease process (e.g., spinal cord injury, multiple sclerosis)

Psychosocial

Absence of integrality (e.g., essence of power); chronic low self-esteem; deficient knowledge (e.g., of illness or healthcare system); disturbed body image; inadequate coping patterns; lifestyle of dependency; situational low self-esteem

NOC   Outcomes (Nursing Outcomes Classification)

Suggested NOC Outcomes

Depression Self-Control; Health Beliefs; Health Beliefs: Perceived Ability to Perform, Perceived Control, Perceived Resources; Participation in Health Care Decisions

Example NOC Outcome with Indicators
Health Beliefs: Perceived Control as evidenced by the following indicators: Perceived responsibility for health decisions/Belief that own decisions and actions control health outcomes (Rate the outcome and indicators of **Health Beliefs: Perceived Control:** I = very weak, 2 = weak, 3 = moderate, 4 = strong, 5 = very strong [see Section I].)

Client Outcomes

Client Will (Specify Time Frame):

*   State feelings of powerlessness and other feelings related to powerlessness (e.g., anger, sadness, hopelessness)
*   Identify factors that are uncontrollable
*   Participate in planning and implementing care; make decisions regarding care and treatment when possible
*   Ask questions about care and treatment
*   Verbalize hope for the future and sense of participation in planning and implementing care

NIC   Interventions (Nursing Interventions Classification)

Suggested NIC Interventions

Cognitive Restructuring, Complex Relationship Building, Mutual Goal Setting, Self-Esteem Enhancement, Self-Responsibility Facilitation

• = Independent;   ▲ = Collaborative;   EBN = Evidence-Based Nursing;   EB = Evidence-Based

Example NIC Activities—Self-Responsibility Facilitation
Encourage independence but assist patient when unable to perform; Assist patients to identify areas in which they could readily assume more responsibility

Nursing Interventions, *Rationales*, and References

See the care plan for **Powerlessness**.

Ineffective Protection   *Gail B. Ladwig, MSN, CHTP, RN*

NANDA   Definition

Decrease in ability to guard self from internal or external threats such as illness or injury.

Defining Characteristics

Altered clotting; anorexia; chilling; cough; deficient immunity; disorientation; dyspnea; fatigue; immobility; impaired healing; insomnia; itching; maladaptive stress response; neurosensory alteration; perspiring; pressure ulcers; restlessness; weakness

Related Factors (r/t)

Abnormal blood profiles (e.g., leukopenia, thrombocytopenia, anemia, coagulation); alcohol abuse; cancer; drug therapies (e.g., antineoplastic, corticosteroid, immune, anticoagulant, thrombolytic); extremes of age; immune disorders; inadequate nutrition; treatments (e.g., surgery, radiation)

NOC   Outcomes (Nursing Outcomes Classification)

Suggested NOC Outcomes

Health-Promoting Behavior, Blood Coagulation, Endurance, Immune Status

P

Example NOC Outcome with Indicators
Immune Status as evidenced by the following indicators: Recurrent infections not present/Tumors not present/ Gastrointestinal function/Respiratory function/Weight loss not present/Body temperature/Absolute WBC (Rate the outcome and indicators of **Immune Status**: 1 = severely compromised, 2 = substantially compromised, 3 = moderately compromised, 4 = mildly compromised, 5 = not compromised [see Section I].)

Client Outcomes

Client Will (Specify Time Frame):

- Remain free of infection
- Remain free of any evidence of new bleeding
- Explain precautions to take to prevent infection
- Explain precautions to take to prevent bleeding

NIC   Interventions (Nursing Interventions Classification)

Suggested NIC Interventions

Bleeding Precautions, Infection Control, Infection Protection

• = Independent;   ▲ = Collaborative;   EBN = Evidence-Based Nursing;   EB = Evidence-Based

Example NIC Activities—Infection Protection Control
Monitor for systemic and localized signs and symptoms of infection; Inspect skin and mucous membranes for redness, extreme warmth, or drainage

Nursing Interventions and *Rationales*

- Take temperature, pulse, and blood pressure (e.g., every 1 to 4 hours). *Prospective surveillance study for nosocomial infection on hematology-oncology units should include fever of unknown origin as the single most common and clinically important entity (Engelhart et al, 2002). Changes in vital signs can indicate the onset of bleeding or infection.*
- ▲ Observe nutritional status (e.g., weight, serum protein and albumin levels, muscle mass, usual food intake). Work with the dietitian to improve nutritional status if needed. All clients diagnosed with HIV should have a dietary consult. **EB:** *Nutrient status is an important factor contributing to immune competence; undernutrition impairs the immune system (Calder & Kew, 2002).* **EBN:** *Nutrition complications of HIV infection, including wasting syndrome, nutrient deficiencies, and metabolic complications, have been well documented over the last 25 years (Coyne-Meyers & Trombley, 2004).*
- Observe the client's sleep pattern; if altered, see Nursing Interventions and Rationales for **Disturbed Sleep patterns.**
- Determine the amount of stress in the client's life. If stress is uncontrollable, see Nursing Interventions and Rationales for **Ineffective Coping.** *Uncontrolled stress depresses immune system function (Carter, 1993).*

Prevention of Infection

- Refer to care plan **Risk for Infection.**
- ▲ Monitor for and report any signs of infection (e.g., fever, chills, flushed skin, drainage, edema, redness, abnormal laboratory values, and pain) and notify the physician promptly. *The immune system is stimulated with the onset of infection, which results in classic signs of infection (Quadri & Brown, 2000).* **EBN:** *In many cases, changes in hematological parameters may be the initial sign of an occult infectious or inflammatory disorder (Szymanski, 2001).*
- ▲ If the client's immune system is depressed, notify the physician of elevated temperature, even in the absence of other symptoms of infection. *Clients with depressed immune function are unable to mount the usual immune responses to the onset of infection; fever may be the only sign of infection. A neutropenic client with fever represents an absolute medical emergency (Burney, 2000; Quadri & Brown, 2000).*
- If white blood cell count is severely decreased (i.e., absolute neutrophil count of <1000/mm^3), initiate the following precautions:
  - Take vital signs every 4 hours.
  - Complete a head-to-toe assessment twice daily, including inspection of oral mucosa, invasive sites, wounds, urine, and stool; monitor for onset of new reports of pain.
  - Avoid any invasive procedures, including catheterization, injections, or rectal or vaginal procedures. *Infectious agents can invade when a treatment damages the skin or mucous membranes, which are natural barriers against infection (Flyge, 1993).*
- Consider warming the client before elective surgery. **EBN:** *In clients undergoing elective hernia repair, varicose vein surgery, or breast surgery, preoperative warming with a local device or a warm air blanket reduced the incidence of wound infection after surgery (Borbasi & Brougham, 2002). Normothermia is associated with low postoperative infection rates (Leeper, 2006)*
- ▲ Administer granulocyte growth factor therapy as ordered. *Myeloid growth factors for granulocytes are more useful for preventing than for treating neutropenic infections in cancer clients (Glaspy, 2000). Clinical trials suggest that granulocyte macrophage colony-stimulating factor shortens the duration of mucositis and diarrhea, stimulating dendritic cells, preventing infection, acting as an adjuvant vaccine agent, and facilitating antitumor activity (Buchsel et al, 2002).*
- Take meticulous care of all invasive sites; use chlorhexidine gluconate for cleansing. **EBN:** *Use of chlorhexidine gluconate for vascular catheter site care reduced catheter-related bloodstream infections and*

• = Independent;   ▲ = Collaborative;   EBN = Evidence-Based Nursing;   EB = Evidence-Based

catheter colonization more than use of povidone iodine (Chaiyakunapruk et al, 2002; Young, Commiskey & Wilson 2006).

- Provide frequent oral care. *The effects of chemotherapy or radiation leave the mouth inflamed; combined with immunosuppression, this can result in stomatitis. Good oral care can help prevent this complication (Dose, 1995).*
▲ Refer for prophylactic medication to prevent oral candidiasis. **EB:** *Drugs absorbed or partially absorbed from the gastrointestinal tract prevent oral candidiasis in the client receiving treatment for cancer (Worthington, Clarkson & Eden, 2007).*
▲ Refer for appropriate prophylactic antifungal treatment and avoid pathogen exposure (through air filtration, regular hand hygiene, avoidance of plants and flowers). *Practical measures can be taken to avoid exposing the client to fungi (Maertens, Vrebos & Boogaerts, 2001).* **EB:** *IV amphotericin B is the only antifungal agent for which there is evidence suggesting that its use might reduce mortality (Gotzsche & Johansen, 2002).*
- Have the client wear a mask when leaving the room. **EB:** *To prevent nosocomial pulmonary aspergillosis during hospital construction, neutropenic clients with hematological malignancy were required to wear high-efficiency filtering masks when leaving their rooms (Raad et al, 2002).*
- Limit and screen visitors to minimize exposure to contagion.
- Help the client bathe daily.
- Practice food safety; a neutropenic diet may not be necessary (www.foodsafety.gov). *No clear evidence exists that the neutropenic diet makes a difference in overall rates of infection (Demille et al, 2006).*
▲ Ensure that the client is well nourished. Provide food with protein and consider vitamin supplements. If appetite is suppressed, institute a dietary referral. Keep track of serum albumin levels as well as transferrin and prealbumin levels. **EB:** *Levels of the visceral proteins (albumin, transferrin, and prealbumin) are an indirect measure of nutritional status (Calder & Kew, 2002).*
- Refer to care plan **Readiness for enhanced Nutrition** for additional interventions.
- Help the client to cough and practice deep breathing regularly. Maintain an appropriate activity level.
- Obtain a private room for the client. Use high-energy particulate air filters if available and appropriate. Protective isolation is not recommended. Recognize that cotton cover gowns may not be effective in decreasing infection. **EB:** *High-risk clients, especially those with prolonged granulocytopenia or organ transplants, should be cared for in hospital units with HEPA-filtered air (Safdar, Crnich & Maki, 2005).* **EBN:** *The routine use of cotton cover gowns in the care of neutropenic clients found that the rates of infection were no different than when cover gowns were not used (Kenny & Lawson, 2000). Abandoning protective isolation combined with increased hygienic measures in nursing of clients with severe neutropenia does not increase the risk of infections (Mank & van der Lelie, 2003).*
▲ Watch for signs of sepsis, including change in mental status, fever, shaking, chills, and hypotension. If present, notify the physician promptly. *Change in mental status, fever, shaking, chills, and hypotension are indicators of sepsis (Flyge, 1993).*

Pediatric

- Suggest kangaroo care, frequent and exclusive or nearly exclusive breastfeeding, and early discharge from hospital for low birth weight infants. **EBN:** *Kangaroo care appears to reduce severe infant morbidity without any serious deleterious effect reported (Conde-Agudelo et al, 2003).*
- Treat postoperative fever in pediatric oncology clients promptly. **EBN:** *A postoperative fever in immunocompromised pediatric clients indicates infection and may lead to complications if not treated promptly (Chang, Hendershot & Colapinto, 2006).*
- For hand hygiene with low birth weight infants, use alcohol hand rub and gloves. **EBN:** *The introduction of the alcohol hand rub and glove protocol was associated with a 2.8-fold reduction in the incidence of late-onset systemic infection and a significant decrease in the incidence of methicillin-resistant* Staphylococcus aureus *septicemia and necrotizing enterocolitis in very low birth weight infants (Ng et al, 2004).*

Geriatric

- If not contraindicated, promote exercise to strengthen the immune system in the elderly. **EB:**

Adults age 62 years and older suggest that lifestyle factors, including exercise, may influence immune response to influenza immunization. The practice of regular, vigorous exercise was associated with enhanced immune response after influenza vaccination in older adults (Kohut et al, 2002; Phillips et al, 2007).

- Give elderly clients with imbalanced nutrition a nutritional supplement to enhance immune function. **EB:** *Consumption of this complete liquid nutritional supplement may have a beneficial effect on antibody response to influenza vaccination in the elderly population (Wouters-Wesseling et al, 2002).*
- Refer to the care plan for **Risk for Infection** for more interventions related to the prevention of infection.

Prevention of Bleeding

- Monitor the client's risk for bleeding; evaluate results of clotting studies and platelet counts. *Laboratory studies give a good indication of the seriousness of the bleeding disorder.*
- Watch for hematuria, melena, hematemesis, hemoptysis, epistaxis, bleeding from mucosa, petechiae, and ecchymoses. *These types of bleeding can be detected in a bleeding disorder (Ellenberger, Hass & Cundiff, 1993; Paschall, 1993).*
- ▲ Give medications orally or IV only; avoid giving them IM, subcutaneously, or rectally (Shuey, 1996). Apply pressure for a longer time than usual to invasive sites such as venipuncture or injection sites. *Additional pressure is needed to stop bleeding of invasive sites in clients with bleeding disorders.*
- Take vital signs often; watch for changes associated with fluid volume loss. *Excessive bleeding causes decreased blood pressure and increased pulse and respiratory rates.*
- Monitor menstrual flow if relevant; have the client use pads instead of tampons. *Menstruation can be excessive in clients with bleeding disorders. Use of tampons can increase trauma to the vagina.*
- Have the client use a moistened toothette or a very soft child's toothbrush instead of an adult toothbrush. Have the client use alcohol-free dental products and avoid flossing. *These actions help prevent trauma to the oral mucosa, which could result in bleeding (Shuey, 1996).*
- Ask the client either not to shave or to use an electric razor only. *This helps prevent any unnecessary trauma that could result in bleeding (Shuey, 1996).*
- To decrease risk of bleeding, avoid administering salicylates or nonsteroidal antiinflammatory drugs (NSAIDs) if possible. *Salicylates and NSAIDs can cause gastrointestinal bleeding; salicylates interfere with platelet function and can increase bleeding.*

Home Care

- Some of the interventions previously described may be adapted for home care use.
- ▲ Consider institution of a nurse-administered mobile care unit for monitoring anticoagulant therapy. **EBN:** *Establishment of anticoagulation therapy management clinics led to improvements in quality of care in terms of improved control of international normalized ratio and reduced complications (Gill & Landis, 2002).*
- ▲ For terminally ill clients, teach and institute all of the aforementioned noninvasive precautions that maintain quality of life. Discuss with the client, family, and physician the consequences of contracting infection. Determine which precautions do not maintain quality of life and should not be used (e.g., physical assessment twice daily, multiple vital sign assessments). *Multiple assessments and other invasive procedures are recovery-based, cure-focused activities. The client and physician must agree on an approach to care for the client's remaining life.*

Client/Family Teaching

Depressed Immune Function

- Teach precautions to take to decrease the chance of infection (e.g., avoiding uncooked fruits and vegetables, using appropriate self-care, ensuring a safe environment).
- Teach the client and family how to take a temperature. Encourage the family to take the client's temperature between 3 PM and 7 PM at least once daily. *For most people, the difference between high and low values throughout the day is approximately 2.0° F (1.1° C) (97° to 99° F [36.1° to 37.2° C]), with the lowest value typically occurring in the early morning hours (2 AM to 5 AM) and the highest values commonly occurring in the evening (7 PM to 10 PM) (Round-the-Clock Systems, 2003).*

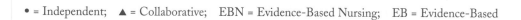

• = Independent;   ▲ = Collaborative;   EBN = Evidence-Based Nursing;   EB = Evidence-Based

- Teach the client to avoid crowds and contact with persons who have infections. Teach the need for good nutrition, avoidance of stress, and adequate rest to maintain immune system function. *Client education to increase nutrition, manage stress, and perform self-care can reduce the risk of neutropenic infection (Carter, 1993).*

Bleeding Disorder

▲ Teach the client to wear a medical alert bracelet and notify all healthcare personnel of the bleeding disorder. *Emergency identification schemes such as medical alert bracelets use emblems that alert healthcare professionals to potential problems and can ensure appropriate and prompt treatment (Morton et al, 2002).*

▲ Teach the client and family the signs of bleeding, precautions to take to prevent bleeding, and action to take if bleeding begins. Caution the client to avoid taking over-the-counter medications without the permission of the physician. Medications containing salicylates can increase bleeding.

- Teach the client to wear loose-fitting clothes and avoid physical activity that might cause trauma.

 See the EVOLVE website for World Wide Web resources for client education.

REFERENCES

Borbasi S, Brougham L: Warming clients before clean surgery reduced the incidence of postoperative wound infection, *Evid Based Nurs* 5(2):48, 2002.

Buchsel PC, Forgey A, Grape FB et al: Granulocyte macrophage colony-stimulating factor: current practice and novel approaches, *Clin J Oncol Nurs* 6(4):198, 2002.

Burney KY: Tips for timely management of febrile neutropenia, *Oncol Nurs Forum* 27(4):617, 2000.

Calder PC, Kew S: The immune system: a target for functional foods? *Br J Nutr* 88(suppl 2):S165, 2002.

Carter LW: Influences of nutrition and stress on people at risk for neutropenia: nursing implications, *Oncol Nurs Forum* 20(8):1241, 1993.

Chaiyakunapruk N, Veenstra DL, Lipsky BA et al: Chlorhexidine compared with povidone-iodine solution for vascular catheter-site care: a meta-analysis, *Ann Intern Med* 136(11):792, 2002.

Chang A, Hendershot E, Colapinto K: Minimizing complications related to fever in the postoperative pediatric oncology patient, *J Pediatr Oncol* 23(2):75-81, 2006.

Conde-Agudelo A, Diaz-Rossello JL, Belizan JM: Kangaroo mother care to reduce morbidity and mortality in low birthweight infants, *Cochrane Database Syst Rev* (2):CD002771, 2003.

Coyne-Meyers K, Trombley LE: A review of nutrition in human immunodeficiency virus infection in the era of highly active antiretroviral therapy, *Nutr Clin Pract* 19(4):340-355, 2004.

Demille D, Deming P, Lupinacci P et al: The effect of the neutropenic diet in the outpatient setting: a pilot study, *J Pediatr Hematol Oncol* 28(3):126-133, 2006.

Dose AM: The symptom experience of mucositis, stomatitis, and xerostomia, *Semin Oncol Nurs* 11:248, 1995.

Ellenberger BJ, Hass L, Cundiff L: Thrombotic thrombocytopenia purpura: nursing during the acute phase, *Dimens Crit Care Nurs* 12:58, 1993.

Engelhart S, Glasmacher A, Exner M et al: Surveillance for nosocomial infections and fever of unknown origin among adult hematology/oncology patients, *Infect Control Hosp Epidemiol* 23(5):244, 2002.

Flyge HA: Meeting the challenge of neutropenia, *Nursing* 23(7):60, 1993.

Gill JM, Landis MK: Benefits of a mobile, point-of-care anticoagulation therapy management program, *Joint Comm J Qual Improv* 28(11):625, 2002.

Glaspy JA: Hematologic supportive care of the critically ill cancer patient, *Semin Oncol* 27(3):375, 2000.

Gotzsche PC, Johansen HK: Routine versus selective antifungal administration for control of fungal infections in patients with cancer, *Cochrane Database Syst Rev* (2):CD000026, 2002.

Kenny H, Lawson E: The efficacy of cotton cover gowns in reducing infection in nursing neutropenic patients: an evidence-based study, *Int J Nurs Pract* 6(3):135, 2000.

Kohut ML, Cooper MM, Nickolaus MS et al: Exercise and psychosocial factors modulate immunity to influenza vaccine in elderly individuals, *J Gerontol A Biol Sci Med Sci* 57(9):M557, 2002.

Leaper D: Effects of local and systemic warming on postoperative infections, *Surg Infect (Larchmt)* 7(suppl 2):S101-S103, 2006.

Maertens J, Vrebos M, Boogaerts M: Assessing risk factors for systemic fungal infections, *Eur J Cancer Care (Engl)* 10(1):56, 2001.

Mank A, van der Lelie H: there still an indication for nursing patients with prolonged neutropenia in protective isolation? An evidence-based nursing and medical study of 4 years experience for nursing patients with neutropenia without isolation, *Eur J Oncol Nurs* 7(1):17-23, 2003.

Morton L, Murad S, Omar RZ et al: Importance of emergency identification schemes, *Emerg Med J* 19(6):584-586, 2002.

Ng PC, Wong HL, Lyon DJ et al: Combined use of alcohol hand rub and gloves reduces the incidence of late onset infection in very low birthweight infants, *Arch Dis Child Fetal Neonatal Ed* 89(4):F336-F340, 2004.

Paschall FE: Thrombotic thrombocytopenic purpura: the challenges of a complex disease process, *AACN Clin Issues* 4:655, 1993.

Phillips AC, Burns VE, Lord JM: Stress and exercise: getting the balance right for aging immunity, *Exerc Sport Sci Rev* 35(1):35-39, 2007.

Quadri TL, Brown AE: Infectious complications in the critically ill patient with cancer, *Semin Oncol* 27(3):335, 2000.

Raad I, Hanna H, Osting C et al: Masking of neutropenic patients on transport from hospital rooms is associated with a decrease in nosocomial aspergillosis during construction, *Infect Control Hosp Epidemiol* 23(1):41, 2002.

Round-the-Clock Systems: *Circadian rhythms,* www.matrices.com/Workplace/Learning/sw.circadian.html, accessed April 5, 2005.

Safdar N, Crnich C, Maki D: The pathogenesis of ventilator-associated pneumonia: its relevance to developing effective strategies for prevention, *Respir Care* 50(6):725-741, 2005.

Shuey KM: Platelet-associated bleeding disorders, *Semin Oncol Nurs* 12(1):15, 1996.

Szymanski N: Infection and inflammation in dialysis patients: impact on laboratory parameters and anemia. Case study of the anemic patient, *Nephrol Nurse J* 28(3):337, 2001.

Worthington HV, Clarkson JE, Eden OB: Interventions for preventing oral candidiasis for patients with cancer receiving treatment, *Cochrane Database Syst Rev* (1):CD003807, 2007.

Wouters-Wesseling W, Rozendaal M, Snijder M et al: Effect of a complete nutritional supplement on antibody response to influenza vaccine in elderly people, *J Gerontol A Biol Sci Med Sci* 57(9):M563, 2002.

Young E, Commiskey M, Wilson SJ: Translating evidence into practice to prevent central venous catheter-associated bloodstream infections: a systems-based intervention, *Am J Infect Control* 34(8):503-506, 2006.

Pruritus *Betty Ackley, MSN, EdS, RN*

Definition (NOTE: This is not a NANDA-I Diagnosis)

State in which an individual experiences an uncomfortable itching sensation in response to a noxious stimulus

Defining Characteristics

Verbalization of itching sensation; observed behaviors of itching; irritated skin from scratching

Related Factors (r/t)

Reaction to irritants, including allergies, dry skin, chronic illness, stress; medication side effect

NOC Outcomes (Nursing Outcomes Classification)

Suggested NOC Outcomes

Comfort Level, Symptom Control

Example NOC Outcome with Indicators
Comfort Level as evidenced by the following indicators: Physical well-being/Symptom control (Rate the outcome and indicators of **Comfort Level:** 1 = not at all satisfied, 2 = somewhat satisfied, 3 = moderately satisfied, 4 = very satisfied, 5 = completely satisfied [see Section I].)

Client Outcomes

Client Will (Specify Time Frame):

- State he or she is comfortable
- State that his or her itching is relieved to an acceptable level
- Explain methods to decrease itching
- Have intact skin

NIC Interventions (Nursing Interventions Classification)

Suggested NIC Interventions

Pruritus Management, Distraction, Environmental Management: Comfort, Medication Administration, Music Therapy, Progressive Muscle Relaxation, Pruritus Management, Simple

• = Independent;   ▲ = Collaborative;   EBN = Evidence-Based Nursing;   EB = Evidence-Based

Guided Imagery, Simple Massage, Simple Relaxation Therapy, Skin Care: Topical Treatments, Touch

Example NIC Activities—Pruritus Management
Apply medicated creams and lotions, as appropriate; Instruct patient to limit bathing to once or twice a week, as appropriate

Nursing Interventions and *Rationales*

- Perform a complete assessment to determine the cause of pruritus (e.g., dry skin, contact with irritating substance, medication side effect, insect bite, infection, healing burns, underlying systemic disease). *The cause of pruritus helps direct treatment. Pruritus may be caused by serious illnesses such as renal failure, liver failure, malignancy, or diabetes as well as by dry skin and various skin conditions. Treatment should be individualized (Yosipovitch & Hundley, 2004; Tomson & Burrows, 2006).*
- Implement soaks with cool or cold washcloths or offer cool baths if appropriate. **EB:** *Some clients report that bathing with cool or cold water can depress the itching sensation (Yosipovitch et al, 2002). Bathing with salts may improve skin barrier protection and have an emollient effect. Baking soda, colloidal oatmeal (with and without oil), and bath oils may also be comforting. A study with an experimental irritant design demonstrated reduced transepidermal water loss and improved skin water capacitance with the use of sea water and water containing sodium chloride (NaCl) and potassium chloride (KCl) (Yoshizawa et al, 2001). A study comparing postburn itching in individuals showering with either a 5% colloidal oatmeal and liquid paraffin combination or a plain liquid paraffin bath oil found the colloidal oatmeal and oil combination significantly more effective (Matheson, Clayton & Muller, 2001).*
- ▲ Apply topical agents as ordered to decrease itching. Include cooling agents, topical anesthetics, topical antihistamines, capsaicin, and topical corticosteroids. *These treatments can help decrease the itching sensation (Yosipovitch & Hundley, 2004).*
- Recognize that a common cause of itching is dry skin (xerosis), especially in the elderly, during winter months, and in people who take frequent baths or showers with hot water (Moses, 2003; Tagami et al, 2006).
- Apply creams or ointments to keep the skin well hydrated immediately after bathing. At times it may be necessary to use both a heavy ointment followed by an oil to adequately moisturize the skin. *Hydrating the skin helps restore the skin barrier function of skin and is generally the first step to treat itching (Yosipovitch & Hundley, 2004). For hydrating the skin, ointments are most effective, then creams; least effective are lotions (Barr, 2006).* **EB:** *A study demonstrated that aloe vera extracts were effective in increasing skin hydration (Dal'Belo, Gaspar & Campos, 2006). A study of clients with pruritus demonstrated that Aveeno skin relief moisturizing lotion was effective in decreasing itching and improving the condition of the skin (Pacifico et al, 2005). Daily application of moisturizers can have the persistent clinical effect of relieving dry skin (Tabata et al, 2000).*
- Keep the client's fingernails short; have the client wear mitts if necessary. *Scratching with fingernails can excoriate the area and increase skin damage and risk of cellulitis (Sherman, 2001).*
- Leave pruritic area open to the air if possible. *Covering the area with a nonventilated dressing can increase itching sensation and warmth in the area.*
- Cleanse the body using nonallergenic, low-pH cleansing agents on the perineum and axilla; avoid use of regular soap. *Many soaps can be irritating to the skin and increase the itching sensation (Yosipovitch & Hundley, 2004).*
- Use behavior modification to help reduce self-injury caused by scratching and improve quality of life. *Incorporating a behavioral model for care using a habit reversal technique into nursing care plans for clients with atopic eczema has been advocated (Buchanan, 2001).*
- ▲ Advocate altering or substituting medications if pruritus is potentially a side effect of the current medication regimen.
- Assess for sleep disturbances. **EB:** *One study found that a majority of clients reported difficulty falling asleep and that itching was more frequent at night (Yosipovitch et al, 2002).*

P

• = Independent;   ▲ = Collaborative;   EBN = Evidence-Based Nursing;   EB = Evidence-Based

▲ Consult the physician for appropriate medications to relieve itching. Be aware of current research regarding medications best suited to relieving the pruritus associated with different causes. **EB and EBN:** *Many medications are potentially useful for pruritic conditions (Buchanan, 2001). Medications such as topical steroids or antihistamines can be helpful (Buchanan, 2001). Antihistamines are not always effective, but the sedative effects of sedation may be useful at bedtime (Toomey & Biddle, 2006).*

Multicultural

• Assess black skin for ashy appearance for signs of dry skin. **EBN:** *Black skin and the skin of other people of color will appear ashy as a result of the flaking off of the top layer of the epidermis (Smith & Burns, 1999; Jackson, 1998).*
• Encourage the use of lanolin-based lotions for African-American clients with dry skin. **EBN:** *Vaseline may clog the pores and cause cellulitis or other skin problems (Jackson, 1998).*
• Offer hair oil and lanolin-based lotion for dry scalp and skin. **EBN:** *Black skin seems to produce less oil than lighter-colored skin; therefore African Americans may use more lubricants as a normal part of skin hygiene (Smith & Burns, 1999).*
• Use soap sparingly if the skin is dry. **EBN:** *Black skin tends to be dry, and soap exacerbates this condition (Jackson, 1998).*

Client/Family Teaching

• Teach techniques to alleviate dry skin:
  ■ Decrease time in the shower or bath.
  ■ Add oil to the bathwater.
  ■ Use lukewarm water only.
  ■ Apply emollients immediately after bathing to slightly damp skin to "seal in" the moisture.
  ■ Use low-pH cleansers; wash in essential areas only.
  ■ Use a humidifier to put more moisture in the air in winter (Yosipovitch & Hundley, 2004; Barr, 2006).
• Teach techniques to deal with itching sensation:
  ■ Keep skin well hydrated with emollients and good fluid intake.
  ■ Use rubbing, massage, pressure, or vibration for scratching when itching is severe and irrepressible.
  ■ Wear cool clothing and keep the ambient temperature cooler.
  ■ Avoid hot or spicy foods, hot liquids, and alcohol, which can stimulate the histamine response resulting in itching.
  ■ Keep fingernails short (Yosipovitch & Hundley, 2004).
• Teach techniques to use when the client is uncomfortable, including relaxation techniques, guided imagery, hypnosis, and music therapy. *Interventions such as progressive muscle relaxation, guided imagery, hypnosis, and music therapy can effectively decrease the itching sensation.*
• Teach the client and the family correct application or administration of prescribed medications or therapies.
▲ Instruct the client to see the primary care practitioner if itching persists and no cause is found. *Itching can be a symptom of many conditions, including chronic diseases (Yosipovitch & Hundley, 2004).*

REFERENCES

Barr JE: Skin matters: impaired skin integrity in the elderly, *Ostomy Wound Manag* 52(5):22-28, 2006.

Buchanan PI: Behavior modification: a nursing approach for young children with atopic eczema, *Dermatol Nurs* 13(1):15-18, 21-23, 2001.

Dal'Belo SE, Gaspar LR, Campos M: Moisturizing effect of cosmetic formulations containing Aloe vera extract in different concentra-

tions assessed by skin bioengineering techniques, *Skin Res Technol* 12(4):241-246, 2006.

Jackson F: The ABC's of black hair and skin care, *ABNF J* 9(5):100-104, 1998.

Matheson JD, Clayton J, Muller MJ: The reduction of itch during burn wound healing, *J Burn Care Rehabil* 22(1):76-81, 2001.

Moses S: Pruritus, *Am Fam Physician* 68(6):1135-1144, 2003.

Pacifico A et al: Clinical trial on Aveeno skin relief moisturizing lotion in patients with itching accompanied by skin lesions and xerosis, *J Apply Res* 5(2):325-330, 2005.

Smith W, Burns C: Managing the hair and skin of African-American pediatric patients, *J Pediatr Health Care* 13(2):72-78, 1999.

Tagami H, Kobayashi H, O'goshi K et al: Atopic xerosis: employment of noninvasive biophysical instrumentation for the functional analyses of the mildly abnormal stratum corneum and for the efficacy assessment of skin care products, *J Cosmet Dermatol* 5(2):140-149, 2006.

Tomson N, Burrows N: Pruritis: causes and management, *Geriatr Med*, 36(7):35-41, 2006.

Tabata N, O'Goshi K, Zhen YX et al: Biophysical assessment of persis-tent effects of moisturizers after their daily applications: evaluation of corneotherapy, *Dermatology* 200(4):308-313, 2000.

Toomey M, Biddle C: Itching, the "little" big problem as an orphan symptom, *AANA J* 74(5):379-384, 2006.

Yoshizawa Y, Tanojo H, Kim SJ et al: Sea water or its components alter experimental irritant dermatitis in man, *Skin Res Technol* 7(1):36-39, 2001.

Yosipovitch G, Hundley JL: Practical guidelines for relief of itch, *Dermatol Nurs* 16(4):325-329, 2004.

Yosipovitch G, Goon AT, Wee J et al: Itch characteristics in Chinese patients with atopic dermatitis using a new questionnaire for the assessment of pruritus, *Int J Dermatol* 41(4):212-216, 2002.

Rape-trauma syndrome   *Mary Shoemaker, RN, MSN, SANE*

NANDA   Definition

Sustained maladaptive response to forced, violent sexual penetration against the victim's will and consent

Defining Characteristics

Aggression; agitation; anger; anxiety; change in relationships; confusion; denial; dependence; depression; disorganization; dissociative disorders; embarrassment; fear; guilt; helplessness; humiliation; hyperalertness; impaired decision making; loss of self-esteem; mood swings; muscle spasms; muscle tension; nightmares; paranoia; phobias; physical trauma; powerlessness; revenge; self-blame; sexual dysfunction; shame; shock; sleep disturbances; substance abuse; suicide attempts; vulnerability

Related Factors (r/t)

Rape

NOC   Outcomes (Nursing Outcomes Classification)

Suggested NOC Outcomes

Abuse Cessation; Abuse Protection; Abuse Recovery: Emotional, Sexual; Coping; Impulse Self-Control; Self-Mutilation Restraint

Example NOC Outcome with Indicators
Abuse Recovery: Sexual as evidenced by the following indicators: Acknowledgment of right to disclose abusive situation/Expression of right to have been protected from abuse (Rate the outcome and indicators of **Abuse Recovery: Sexual:** 1 = none, 2 = limited, 3 = moderate, 4 = substantial, 5 = extensive [see Section I].)

Client Outcomes

Client Will (Specify Time Frame):

• Share feelings, concerns, and fears
• Recognize that the rape or attempt was not client's own fault

R

- State that, no matter what the situation, no one has the right to assault another
- Describe medical/legal treatment procedures and reasons for treatment
- Report absence of physical complications or pain
- Identify support people and be able to ask them for help in dealing with this trauma
- Function at same level as before crisis, including sexual functioning
- Recognize that it is normal for full recovery to take a minimum of 1 year

NIC   Interventions (Nursing Interventions Classification)

Suggested NIC Interventions

Counseling, Rape-Trauma Treatment

Example NIC Activities—Rape-Trauma Treatment Counseling
Explain rape protocol and obtain consent to proceed through protocol; Implement crisis intervention counseling

Nursing Interventions and *Rationales*

- Observe the client's responses, including anger, fear, self-blame, sleep pattern disturbances, and phobias.
- Monitor the client's verbal and nonverbal psychological state (e.g., crying, hand wringing, avoidance of interactions or eye contact with staff, silence, and denial). **EB:** *This study demonstrates that individuals respond in a variety of ways to violence and trauma (Carlson, 2005).*
- ▲ Stay with (or have a trusted person stay with) the client initially. If a law enforcement interview is permitted, provide support by staying with the client, but only at the client's request. **EBN:** *Allow the client to make the decision about whom the client wishes to have present during any interviews or examinations to allow a return of control to the client (Ledray, 1998a).*
- Explain the entire medical/legal examination to the client before beginning any procedures. **EBN:** *Explain to the client that the injuries or symptoms may require hospitalization and that the care provider in the hospital will be aware of their special needs. (Sommers & Buschur, 2004).* **EBN:** *This returns control to the client. Explain that a speculum examination will be performed for the purpose of identifying any injury and collecting evidence (Hutson, 2002).*
- Do not wait for the client to ask questions; explain everything you are doing, clarify why it must be done, and describe when and where you will touch. *Eye contact is very important because it helps the client feel worthy and alive (Ruckman, 1992).*
- ▲ Observe for signs of physical injury as you are asking the client to undress and collecting the client's clothing for evidence. Ask the client where it hurts without asking leading questions. Do not ask specific questions but allow the client to give you a history of the sexual assault in the client's own words. If the examiner needs further clarification, ask the client to point to areas that were injured or touched. Inform the client that photographs of any injuries are necessary for forensic evidence. Obtain specific written permission for photographs to be taken and released to law enforcement personnel. **EBN:** *The aforementioned non-leading questions are recommended. Do not ask questions that could indicate to the defense attorney and the jury that the examiner was leading the client and may have influenced the client's report of the assault (Ledray, 1998b).*
- Documentation of a sexual assault examination is critical to evidentiary reports. It is important to document the client's exact description of the assault and then to collect evidence and photographs that validate the history the client reports. **EBN:** *Evidence collection kits prepared by sexual assault nurse examiners (SANEs) are more accurate and complete when compared with evidence collection kits prepared by non-SANE nurses and physicians (Sievers, Murphy & Miller, 2003).*
- It is also very important for the examiner not to offer any opinions in the documentation about whether or not the assault occurred according to the physical findings. **EBN:** *These opinions should be offered to the legal system only when they are requested for prosecution (Ledray, 1998b).*
- ▲ Document a one- or two-sentence summary of what happened. The chief complaint of the client reporting sexual assault should always be listed as "reported sexual assault"; obtaining the

---

• = Independent;   ▲ = Collaborative;   EBN = Evidence-Based Nursing;   EB = Evidence-Based

details of the sequence of events is the police officer's job. **EBN:** *The chief complaint of the client reporting sexual assault should always be listed as "reported sexual assault" (Hutson, 2002).*

- Encourage the client to verbalize feelings. *Individuals at risk for developing long-term problems after an assault should be identified during the initial assessment (Sadler et al, 2000).*
- Escort the client to the treatment room immediately to remove the client from the general population; do not question the client in the triage area. Close curtains and door, and avoid other interruptions during contact with the client (e.g., telephone calls, absence from the room, outside stimuli such as radios). **EB and EBN:** *This not only serves the client but also allows for the accurate collection and preservation of evidence (Ledray, 1999; McGregor, Du Mont & Myhr, 2002).*
- ▲ Provide a sexual assault response team (SART) that includes a SANE, rape counseling advocate, and representative of law enforcement. **EBN:** *The quality of care the client receives from "first responders" may determine the client's willingness to continue with long-term treatment (Ledray, 1998a). The importance of SANE examination for sexual assault victims is stressed for well-being for victims (Patterson, Campbell & Townsend, 2006).*
- ▲ The rape crisis center advocate should be part of the SART and respond when the SANE responds. *Because advocates are better trained and prepared to talk to clients of acute sexual assault, they are usually more successful in encouraging further follow-up than are the medical/nursing staff.* **EB:** *Trained professionals working together within the care setting ensures that survivors and their families' needs are met (Preston, 2003).*
- Provide items for self-care after examination (e.g., for cleansing the vaginal and rectal area). **EBN:** *Many facilities provide items for personal hygiene (i.e., shampoo, soap, toothbrush, toothpaste, new underwear, and outer clothing to replace those secured for evidential purposes) (Hutson, 2002).*
- ▲ Most states provide sexual assault evidence collection kits that have been reviewed by the SART members to provide adequate evidence for analysis by the forensic laboratory. Explain to the client that all or some of the client's clothing may be kept for evidential purposes. **EBN:** *If the client arrives at the medical facility with the evidentiary clothing already in a bag, explain to the client that you will notify law enforcement personnel to pick it up directly from the client (Hutson, 2002).*
- ▲ Discuss the possibility of pregnancy and sexually transmitted diseases (STDs) and the treatments available. *Most clients prefer to prevent pregnancy rather than face the possibility of terminating it in the future. The risk of human immunodeficiency virus (HIV) exposure is a special concern to rape victims; the nurse should bring up this issue and inform the client of locations and schedules for HIV testing.*
- ▲ Encourage the client to report the rape to a law enforcement agency. **EBN:** *Reporting is an issue separate from prosecution; if victims report, they will not be forced to appear as a witness (Ledray, 1992).*
- Discuss the client's support system. Involve the support system if appropriate and if the client grants permission. **EB:** *Significant others are coping with their own responses to the trauma and may be incapable of supporting the victim (Mackey et al, 1992).*
- ▲ Obtaining blood alcohol levels or levels of any drug should be discussed thoroughly with the medical director of your facility and the SART members. *Often alcohol or drug levels are used to prove that the client was unable to give consent for sexual contact. However, often levels are used by defense attorneys to destroy the client's credibility (Hutson, 2002).*

Geriatric

- Build a trusting relationship with the client. **EBN:** *Recognize the attitudes and values of an older generation; stigmatization may cause victims to view themselves with disgust and shame (Delorey & Wolf, 1993).*
- ▲ Explain reporting and encourage the client to report. **EB and EBN:** *Older rape victims have reported having a greater fear that people will find out about their rape than have younger women (Tyra, 1993).* **EB:** *Timely reporting, although important, should not determine whether a client receives appropriate medical care. Clients requesting medical treatment, prophylactic antibiotics, and contraception should be treated the same whether they report the incident to the police or not (Schei et al, 2003).*
- Observe for psychosocial distress (e.g., memory impairment, sleep disturbances, regression, changes in bodily functions). *Exacerbation of a chronic illness may be a major consequence of sexual assault.*

• = Independent;   ▲ = Collaborative;   EBN = Evidence-Based Nursing;   EB = Evidence-Based

▲ All examinations should be done on the elderly as they would be done on any adult client after sexual assault. Evidence should be collected, and consent for collection, photography, and law enforcement contact should be obtained as in all cases. Special attention should be given to the explanation of the genital examination, especially as it relates to the use of a speculum. **EBN:** *Because of the altered levels of awareness in the elderly, it is important for members of the SART to evaluate the client's ability to give informed consent (Hutson, 2002).*

• Modify the rape protocol to promote comfort for the geriatric client. Consider positioning female clients with pillows rather than stirrups and consider using a smaller speculum. *Aging results in decreased muscle tone and thinning of the vaginal wall.*

• Assess for mobility limitations and cognitive impairment. *Elicit information from family or caregivers to verify the client's level of functioning before sexual assault.*

• Respect the client's need for privacy. *Older clients may be reluctant to have their children or younger family members present during the examination and treatment; give clients a choice.*

▲ Consider arrangements for temporary housing. *Most sexual assaults of older clients occur in the home (or nursing home).* **EBN:** *Older age increases the powerlessness of a person, especially if the individual is isolated as a result of living alone. Physical injury can have a much greater effect on older victims, and they may experience a compound reaction because they are older. Sexual violence against an older woman is a reflection of antiage and antiwoman attitudes (Delorey & Wolf, 1993).*

Male Rape

• Reactions to male rape are often either disbelief or an assumption that the man who was raped is gay. **EBN:** *Most women are aware of the possibility that they may be raped, but many men are not. The care required is very similar to the care of women who have been raped (Laurent, 1993).*

Multicultural

• Assess for the influence of cultural beliefs, norms, and values on the client's ability to cope with the trauma of the rape experience. **EBN:** *What the client views as healthy coping may be based on cultural perceptions (Leininger & McFarland, 2002).*

• Assess to determine if physically abused women are also victims of sexual assault. **EB:** *Sexual assault is experienced by most physically abused women and associated with significantly higher levels of post-traumatic stress disorder (PTSD) compared with women physically abused only. The risk of reassault is decreased if contact is made with health or justice agencies (McFarlane et al, 2005).* **EBN:** *The nurse's awareness of the impact of trauma and abuse on psychological health can facilitate more appropriate assessment and support during maternity care (Mezey et al, 2005). Rape is more likely to occur in certain ethnic minority and socially disadvantaged groups than in other groups. The incidence of rape varies with race and ethnicity. Women who are raped are likely to be African-American women who have been raped by African-American men. Of the number of rapes, 65% occur at night (between the hours of 8 PM and 4 PM, 43% occur near the victim's home, and 15% occur at a friend's house. Although a greater number of women report "stranger rape," the incidence of acquaintance rape (date rape) and domestic violence rape is greatly underreported (Giger & Davidhizar, 2004).*

• Provide opportunities by which the family and individual can save face when working with Asian-American clients. **EBN:** *Asian-American families may avoid situations and discussion of issues that they perceive will bring shame on the family unit (D'Avanzo et al, 2001).*

• Assure the client of confidentiality. **EBN:** *Many Indo-Chinese women will not discuss rape if they think that other staff members, their families, their husbands, or their community may find out (Mollica & Lavelle, 1988).*

• Validate the client's feelings regarding the rape and allow the client to tell his or her rape story. **EBN:** *Interventions should reaffirm therapeutic strategies that emphasize effective listening, based on speech styles appropriate to the cultural experiences of the women in question (Bletzer & Koss, 2004).*

• A culturally sensitive approach should be part of the training of all SARTs and members of SARTs. *Compassion and familiarity in a care plan will allow all care providers to provide a comfortable environment for the client (McCleary, 1994).*

Home Care

• Some of the interventions described previously may be adapted for home care use.

- Interact with the client supportively and nonjudgmentally; this supports the client's self-worth. *Rape victims usually experience a loss of self-worth.*
- Assist the client with realistically assessing the home setting for safety and/or selecting a safe environment in which to live. *Rape clients may be unable to make a realistic assessment of home safety both immediately after the rape and during long-term recovery.*
- ▲ Ensure that the client has a support system in place for long-term support. Instruct the family that recovery may take a long time. Refer for medical social work services to assist in setting up a support system if necessary. Refer for counseling if necessary. *The long-term response to rape (up to 4 years) requires ongoing support for the client to reorganize and reintegrate.*
- ▲ Make sure that physical symptoms from the rape or other physical conditions are followed up. Follow-up should include a visit to the primary care physician or the local health department in 3 to 4 weeks for repeat pregnancy testing and STD testing. Explain to the client that additional medication may be necessary for the treatment of STDs or pregnancy (Ohio Chapter of the International Association of Forensic Nurses [IAFN], 2002). *Stress response to rape can precipitate reemergence of other physical conditions that may be ignored because of the rape.*
- ▲ If the client is homebound, refer for psychiatric home healthcare services for client reassurance and implementation of a therapeutic regimen. *Psychiatric home care nurses can address issues relating to the client's rape-trauma syndrome. Behavioral interventions in the home can help the client to participate more effectively in the treatment plan (Patusky, Rodning & Martinez-Kratz, 1996).*

Client/Family Teaching

- ▲ Provide information on prophylactic antibiotic therapy, hepatitis B vaccination, and tetanus prophylaxis for nonimmunized clients with trauma. *Prophylactic treatment for STDs should be provided as part of the initial examination (Ohio Chapter of the IAFN, 2002).*
- Discharge instructions should be written out for the client. *Anxiety can hamper comprehension and retention of information; repeat instructions and provide them in a written form.*
- Give instructions to significant others. *Significant others need many of the same supportive and caring interventions as the client; suggest that they too might benefit from counseling.*
- Explain the purpose of the "morning-after pill." *The morning-after pill (norgestrel [Ovral]) often prevents pregnancy and is used only in emergencies. It must be taken within 72 hours (3 days) of sexual contact to be effective. It will not cause a miscarriage if the client is already pregnant, but it could harm the fetus.*
- ▲ Explain the potential for common side effects related to treatment with norgestrel, such as breast swelling or nausea and vomiting. (Call the emergency department if the client vomits within 1 hour of taking the pill because the pill may need to be taken again.) (Discuss any issues about prophylactic medications at the follow-up visit in 3 to 4 weeks.) It may take 3 to 30 days for the menstrual period to start; if menstruation has not begun in 30 days, contact a physician.
- ▲ Explain the potential for severe side effects related to treatment with norgestrel, such as severe leg or chest pain, trouble breathing, coughing up of blood, severe headache or dizziness, and trouble seeing or talking.
- Advise the client to call or return if new problems develop. *Physical injuries may not be recognized because of the client's emotional numbness during the initial examination or because the client may have forgotten or not understood some of the instructions.*
- Discuss practical lifestyle changes within the client's control to reduce the risk of future attacks. *A client's financial situation may limit some options, such as moving to another home. Provide other alternatives such as keeping doors locked, checking the car before getting in, not walking alone at night, keeping someone informed of whereabouts, asking someone to check if the client has not arrived at a destination within a reasonable amount of time, keeping lights on in an entryway, having keys in hand when approaching the car or house, and having a remote key entry car or garage.*
- ▲ Teach the client to use self-defense techniques to surprise an attacker and create an opportunity to run for help. Refer the client to a self-defense school.
- Teach the client appropriate outlets for anger. Encourage the significant other to direct anger at the event and the attacker, not at the client.
- Emphasize the vulnerability of the client and ensure that reactions are appropriate for the victim of sexual assault. *Females are at higher risk for depression than males, and the risk is significantly higher between the ages of 18 and 44 (Mackey et al, 1992).*

R

NOTE: Post traumatic stress disorder has a high probability of being a psychological sequela to rape. Research demonstrated two effective treatments for improvement of PTSD in rape victims—prolonged exposure and stress inoculation training (Foa et al, 1991). Prolonged exposure involves reliving the rape experience by imagining it as vividly as possible, describing it aloud in the present tense, taping this description, and listening to the tape at least once daily. Stress inoculation training uses breathing exercises to diminish anxiety and instruction in coping skills, thought stopping, cognitive restructuring, self-dialogue, and role playing. Research suggests that a combination of both treatments may provide the optimal effect.

evolve See the EVOLVE website for World Wide Web resources for client education.

REFERENCES

Bletzer KV, Koss MP: Narrative constructions of sexual violence as told by female rape survivors in three populations of the southwestern United States: scripts of coercion, scripts of consent, *Med Anthropol* 23(2):113-156, 2004.

Carlson BE: The most important things learned about violence and trauma in the past 20 years, *J Interpers Violence*, 20(1):119-126, 2005.

D'Avanzo CE, Naegle MA: Developing culturally informed strategies for substance-related interventions. In Naegle MA, D'Avanzo CE, editors: *Addictions and substance abuse: strategies for advanced practice nursing*, St. Louis, 2001, Mosby.

Delorey C, Wolf KA: Sexual violence and older women, *AWHONNS Clin Issues Perinat Womens Health Nurs* 4:173, 1993.

Foa EB, Rothbaum BO, Riggs DS et al: Treatment of posttraumatic stress disorder in rape victims: a comparison between cognitive-behavioral procedures and counseling, *J Consult Clin Psychol* 59(5):715, 1991.

Giger J, Davidhizar R: *Transcultural nursing: assessment and intervention,* ed 4, St. Louis, 2004, Mosby.

Hutson L: Development of sexual assault nurse examiner programs, *Nurs Clin North Am* 37(1):79-88, 2002.

Laurent C: Male rape, *Nurs Times* 89(6):18, 1993.

Ledray LE: Sexual assault: clinical issues. IAFN Sixth Annual Scientific Assembly highlights, *J Emerg Nurs* 25(1):63, 1999.

Ledray L: Sexual assault: clinical issues. SANE development and operation guide, *J Emerg Nurs* 24(2):197, 1998a.

Ledray L: Sexual assault: clinical issues. SANE expert and factual testimony, *J Emerg Nurs* 24(3):284, 1998b.

Ledray L: The sexual assault nurse clinician: a 15-year experience in Minneapolis, *J Emerg Nurs* 18(3):217, 1992.

Leininger MM, McFarland MR: *Transcultural nursing: concepts, theories, research and practices*, ed 3, New York, 2002, McGraw-Hill.

Mackey T, Sereika SM, Weissfeld LA et al: Factors associated with long-term depressive symptoms of sexual assault victims, *Arch Psychiatr Nurs* 6(1):10-25, 1992.

McCleary PH: Female genitalia mutilation and childbirth: a case report, *Birth* 21(4):221, 1994.

McFarlane J, Malecha A, Watson K et al: Intimate partner sexual assault against women: frequency, health consequences, and treatment outcomes, *Obstet Gynecol* 105(1):99-108, 2005.

McGregor MJ, Du Mont J, Myhr TL: Sexual assault forensic medical examination: is evidence related to successful prosecution? *Ann Emerg Med* 39(6):639-647, 2002.

Mezey G, Bacchus L, Bewley S et al: Domestic violence, lifetime trauma and psychological health of childbearing women, *BJOG* 112(2):197-204, 2005.

Mollica RF, Lavelle J: Southeast Asian refugees. In Comas-Diaz L, Griffith EEH, editors: *Clinical guidelines in cross-cultural mental health*, New York, 1988, John Wiley and Sons.

Ohio Chapter of the International Association of Forensic Nurses: *The Ohio adolescent and adult sexual assault nurse examiner training manual*, Cleveland, 2002, Ohio Office of the Attorney General.

Patterson D, Campbell R, Townsend SM: Sexual Assault Nurse Examiner (SANE) program goals and patient care practices, *J Nurs Scholarsh* 38(2):180-186, 2006.

Patusky KL, Rodning C, Martinez-Kratz M: Clinical lessons in psychiatric home care: a case study approach, *J Home Health Case Manag* 9:18, 1996.

Preston L: The sexual assault nurse examiner and the rape crisis center advocate: a necessary partnership, *Top Emerg Med* 3:244-246, 2003.

Ruckman LM: Rape: how to begin the healing, *Am J Nurs* 92(9):48-51, 1992.

Sadler AG, Booth BM, Nielson D et al: Health-related consequences of physical and sexual violence: women in the military, *Obstet Gynecol* 96(3):473-480, 2000.

Schei B, Sidenius K, Lundvall L et al: Adult victims of sexual assault: acute medical response and police reporting among women consulting a center for victims of sexual assault, *Acta Obstet Gynecol Scand* 82(8):750-752, 2003.

Sievers V, Murphy S, Miller JJ: Sexual assault evidence collection more accurate when completed by sexual assault nurse examiners: Colorado's experience, *J Emerg Nurs* 29(6):511-514, 2003.

Sommers M, Buschur C: Injury in women who are raped: what every critical care nurse needs to know, *Dimens Crit Care Nurs* 23(2):62-68, 2004.

Tyra PA: Older women: victims of rape, *J Gerontol Nurs* 19(5):7-12, 1993.

R

• = Independent; ▲ = Collaborative; EBN = Evidence-Based Nursing; EB = Evidence-Based

Rape-trauma syndrome: compound reaction   *Mary Shoemaker, RN, MSN, SANE*

NANDA   Definition

Forced violent sexual penetration against the victim's will and consent. The trauma syndrome that develops from this attack or attempted attack includes an acute phase of disorganization of victim's lifestyle and a long-term process of reorganization of lifestyle.

Defining Characteristics

Change in lifestyle (e.g., changes in residence, dealing with repetitive nightmares and phobias, seeking family support, seeking social network support in long-term phase); emotional reaction (e.g., anger, embarrassment, fear of physical violence and death, humiliation, revenge, self-blame in acute phase); multiple physical symptoms (e.g., gastrointestinal irritability, genitourinary discomfort, muscle tension, sleep pattern disturbance in acute phase); reactivated symptoms of previous conditions (e.g., physical illness, psychiatric illness in acute phase); substance abuse (acute phase)

Related Factors (r/t)

To be developed

NOC   Outcomes (Nursing Outcomes Classification)

Suggested NOC Outcomes

Abuse Cessation, Abuse Protection, Abuse Recovery: Emotional, Sexual, Coping, Impulse Self-Control, Self-Mutilation Restraint

Example NOC Outcome with Indicators
Abuse Recovery: Sexual as evidenced by the following indicators: Acknowledgment of right to disclose abusive situation/Expression of right to have been protected from abuse (Rate the outcome and indicators of **Abuse Recovery: Sexual:** 1 = none, 2 = limited, 3 = moderate, 4 = substantial, 5 = extensive [see Section I].)

Client Outcomes

Client Will (Specify Time Frame):

* Share feelings, concerns, and fears
* Recognize that the rape or attempt was not client's own fault
* State that, no matter what the situation, no one has the right to assault another
* Describe medical/legal treatment procedures and reasons for treatment
* Report absence of physical complications or pain
* Identify support people and be able to ask them for help in dealing with this trauma
* Function at same level as before crisis, including sexual functioning
* Recognize that it is normal for full recovery to take a minimum of 1 year

NIC   Interventions (Nursing Interventions Classification)

Suggested NIC Interventions

Counseling, Rape-Trauma Treatment

Example NIC Activities—Counseling
Encourage expression of feelings; Assist patient to identify strengths, and reinforce these

Nursing Interventions and *Rationales*

* Refer to the care plans for **Rape-trauma syndrome, Powerlessness, Ineffective Coping, Dysfunctional Grieving, Anxiety, Fear, Risk for self-directed Violence,** and **Sexual dysfunction**.

• = Independent;   ▲ = Collaborative;   EBN = Evidence-Based Nursing;   EB = Evidence-Based

Geriatric

- A new subgroup of rape victims resides in nursing homes. Treatment is necessary. *Nursing home victims can suffer both compound and silent rape trauma (Burgess, Dowdell & Prentky, 2000).*

Risk for Compound Reaction

- See the care plan for **Rape-trauma syndrome.**

Home Care

- ▲ If the client has pursued psychiatric counseling, monitor and encourage attendance. *Reliving the rape experience and the accompanying feelings is painful. The client may need additional support to continue.*
- ▲ If the client is receiving medication, assess the client's knowledge of its purpose, side effects, and interactions with medications for other diagnoses. Monitor for effectiveness, side effects, and interactions. *Ongoing stress may leave the client overwhelmed and less able to cope with the impact of changing medical status.*
- ▲ Establish an emergency plan including use of hotlines. Contract with the client to use the emergency plan. Roleplay using the hotlines. *Having an emergency plan reassures the client and decreases the risk of suicide.*
- • For other home care and hospice considerations, refer to the care plan for **Rape-trauma syndrome.**

Client/Family Teaching

- • Teach the client what reactions to expect during the acute and long-term phases: acute phase-anger, fear, self-blame, embarrassment, vengeful feelings, physical symptoms, muscle tension, sleeplessness, stomach upset, genitourinary discomfort; long-term phase-changes in lifestyle or residence, nightmares, phobias, seeking of family and social network support. *Of assessed rape victims, 16.5% were diagnosed with post-traumatic stress disorder (PTSD) an average of 17 years after the assault (Mackey et al, 1992).* **EB:** *Past experiences of sexual assault/abuse and current age have an effect on whether or not the client identifies the current incident to be a rape or sexual assault (Kahn et al, 2003).*
- ▲ Encourage psychiatric consultation if the client is suicidal, violent, or unable to continue activities of daily living (ADLs). *Rape victims are four times more likely than the general population to attempt suicide, which is an 8.7% higher rate than that of nonrape victims (Mackey et al, 1992).*
- ▲ Discuss any of the client's current stress-relieving medications that may result in substance abuse. *Following massive trauma, neurotransmitters are depleted at the synapse level, which is associated with long-term depression and numbing (Mackey et al, 1992).*

evolve See the EVOLVE website for World Wide Web resources for client education.

REFERENCES

Burgess AW, Dowdell EB, Prentky RA: Sexual abuse of nursing home residents, *J Psychosoc Nurs Ment Health Serv* 38(6):10-18, 2000.

Kahn AS, Jackson J, Kully C et al: Calling it rape: differences in experiences of women who do or do not label their sexual assault as rape, *Psychol Women Q* 27(3):233, 2003.

Mackey T, Sereika SM, Weissfeld LA et al: Factors associated with long-term depressive symptoms of sexual assault victims, *Arch Psychiatr Nurs* 6(1):10-25, 1992.

Rape-trauma syndrome: silent reaction   *Mary Shoemaker, RN, MSN, SANE*

NANDA   Definition

Forced violent sexual penetration against the victim's will and consent. The trauma syndrome that develops from this attack or attempted attack includes an acute phase of disorganization of the victim's lifestyle and a long-term process of reorganization of lifestyle.

• = Independent;   ▲ = Collaborative;   EBN = Evidence-Based Nursing;   EB = Evidence-Based

Defining Characteristics

Abrupt changes in relationships with men; increase in nightmares; increased anxiety during interview (e.g., blocking of associations, long periods of silence, minor stuttering, physical distress); no verbalization of the occurrence of rape; pronounced changes in sexual behavior; sudden onset of phobic reactions

Related Factors (r/t)

To be developed

NOC Outcomes (Nursing Outcomes Classification)

Suggested NOC Outcomes

Abuse Cessation, Abuse Protection, Abuse Recovery: Emotional, Sexual, Coping, Impulse Self-Control, Self-Mutilation Restraint

Example NOC Outcome with Indicators
Abuse Recovery: Emotional as evidenced by the following indicators: Demonstration of confidence/ Demonstration of self-esteem (Rate the outcome and indicators of **Abuse Recovery: Emotional:** 1 = none, 2 = limited, 3 = moderate, 4 = substantial, 5 = extensive [see Section I].)

Client Outcomes

Client Will (Specify Time Frame):

- Resume previous level of relationships with significant others
- State improvement in sleep and fewer nightmares
- Express feelings about and discuss the rape
- Return to usual pattern of sexual behavior
- Remain free of phobic reactions

Refer to the care plan for **Rape-trauma syndrome.**

NIC Interventions (Nursing Interventions Classification)

Suggested NIC Interventions

Counseling, Support System Enhancement

Example NIC Activities—Counseling
Encourage expression of feelings; Assist patient to identify strengths, and reinforce these

R

Nursing Interventions and *Rationales*

- Refer to the care plans for **Rape-trauma syndrome, Powerlessness, Ineffective Coping, Dysfunctional Grieving, Anxiety, Fear, Risk for self-directed Violence, Sexual dysfunction,** and **Impaired verbal Communication.**
- Observe for disruptions in relationships with significant others. *Poorly adjusted clients may elicit nonsupportive behavior from others or perceive the actions of others in a negative way.*
- Monitor for signs of increased anxiety (e.g., silence, stuttering, physical distress, irritability, unexplained crying spells).
- Focus on the client's coping strengths. **EB:** *By letting go of negative attitudes and beliefs, the person returns to a more responsible existential position and an improved quality of life (Ventegodt et al, 2005).*
- Observe for changes in sexual behavior. *Sexual assertiveness can be an emotional asset by increasing feelings of anger and diminishing feelings of sadness that are respectively related to assertive and diplomatic responding (Nurius et al, 2004).*

• = Independent;   ▲ = Collaborative;   EBN = Evidence-Based Nursing;   EB = Evidence-Based

- Identify phobic reactions to persons or objects in the environment (e.g., strangers, doorbells, groups of people, knives).
- Provide support by listening when the client is ready to talk. **EB:** *Close friends are the most common confidants (Smith et al, 2000).*
- Remain with an anxious client even if the client is silent. Use gentle speech and actions; move slowly. **EBN:** *The importance of examination of sexual assault victims by a sexual assault nurse examiner (SANE) is stressed for well-being for victims. (Patterson, Campbell & Townsend, 2006).*
- Evaluate somatic complaints. *Women are at higher risk for depression than men (Mackey et al, 1992).*

Geriatric

- A new subgroup of rape victims resides in nursing homes. Treatment is necessary. **EBN:** *Nursing home victims can suffer both compound and silent rape trauma (Burgess, Dowdell & Prentky, 2000).*
- Refer to the care plan for **Rape-trauma syndrome.**

Multicultural

- Allow the client to tell his or her rape story without probing. **EBN:** *Interventions should reaffirm therapeutic strategies that emphasize effective listening, based on speech styles appropriate to the cultural experiences of the women in question (Bletzer & Koss, 2004).*

Home Care

Refer to the care plan for **Rape-trauma syndrome.**

Client/Family Teaching

▲ Refer the client to a sexual assault counselor. Long-term counseling may be necessary. **EB:** *Empowerment interventions should address risk factors in combination. This prevention strategy better reflects women's lives and can increase women's awareness and management of these factors (Nurius et al, 2004).*
- Refer to the care plan for **Rape-trauma syndrome.**

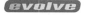 See the EVOLVE website for World Wide Web resources for client education.

REFERENCES

Bletzer KV, Koss MP: Narrative constructions of sexual violence as told by female rape survivors in three populations of the southwestern United States: scripts of coercion, scripts of consent, *Med Anthropol* 23(2):113-156, 2004.

Burgess AW, Dowdell EB, Prentky RA: Sexual abuse of nursing home residents, *J Psychosoc Nurs Ment Health Serv* 38(6):10-18, 2000.

Mackey T, Sereika SM, Weissfeld LA et al: Factors associated with long-term depressive symptoms of sexual assault victims, *Arch Psychiatr Nurs* 6(1):10-25, 1992.

Nurius PS, Norris J, Macy RJ et al: Women's situational coping with acquaintance sexual assault: applying an appraisal-based model, *Violence Against Women* 10:450-478, 2004.

Patterson D, Campbell R, Townsend SM: Sexual Assault Nurse Examiner (SANE) program goals and patient care practices, *J Nurs Scholarsh* 38(2):180-186, 2006.

Smith DW, Letourneau EJ, Saunders BE et al: Delay in disclosure of childhood rape: results from a national survey, *Child Abuse Negl* 24(2):273-287, 2000.

Ventegodt S, Kandel I, Neikrug S et al: Clinical holistic medicine: holistic treatment of rape and incest trauma, *Sci World J* 5:288-297, 2005.

Impaired Religiosity   *Lisa Burkhart, PhD, MPH, RN*

NANDA   **Definition**

Impaired ability to exercise reliance on beliefs and/or participate in rituals of a particular faith tradition

Defining Characteristics

Difficulty adhering to prescribed religious beliefs and rituals (e.g., religious ceremonies, dietary regulations, clothing, prayer, worship/religious services, private religious behaviors/reading religious

• = Independent;   ▲ = Collaborative;   EBN = Evidence-Based Nursing;   EB = Evidence-Based

material/media, holiday observances, meetings with religious leaders); expresses emotional distress because of separation from faith community; expresses a need to reconnect with previous belief patterns; expresses a need to reconnect with previous customs; questions religious belief patterns; questions religious customs

Related Factors (r/t)

Developmental and Situational: Aging; end-stage life crises; life transitions
Physical: Illness; pain
Psychological: Anxiety; fear of death; ineffective coping; ineffective support; lack of security; personal crisis; use of religion to manipulate
Sociocultural: Cultural barriers to practicing religion; environmental barriers to practicing religion; lack of social integration; lack of sociocultural interaction
Spiritual: Spiritual crises; suffering
NOTE: The DDC recognizes that the term *religiosity* may be culture specific; however, the term is useful in the U.S. and is well-supported in the U.S. literature.

NOC   Outcomes (Nursing Outcomes Classification)

Suggested NOC Outcomes

Client Satisfaction: Cultural Needs Fulfillment

Example NOC Outcome with Indicators
Client Satisfaction: Cultural Needs Fulfillment as evidenced by the following indicators: Respect for religious beliefs/Respect for cultural health behaviors/Incorporation of cultural beliefs in health teaching/Respect for personal values (Rate outcome and indicators of **Client Satisfaction: Cultural Needs Fulfillment**: 1 = not at all satisfied, 2 = somewhat satisfied, 3 = moderately satisfied, 4 = very satisfied, 5 = completely satisfied [see Section I].)

Client Outcomes

Client Will (Specify Time Frame):

- Express satisfaction with the ability to express religious practices
- Express satisfaction with access to religious materials and rituals
- Demonstrate balance between religious practices and healthy lifestyles
- Avoid high-risk, controlling religious relationships that inflict physical, sexual, or emotional harm and/or exploitation

NIC   Interventions (Nursing Interventions Classification)

Suggested NIC Interventions

Abuse Protection Support: Religious Culture Brokerage, Religious Addiction Prevention, Religious Ritual Enhancement

Example NIC Activities—Religious Ritual Enhancement
Encourage the use of and participation in religious rituals and practices that are not detrimental to health

Nursing Interventions and *Rationales*

- Identify client's concerns regarding religious expression. **EB:** *Religiousness and spirituality predict greater social support, fewer depressive symptoms, better cognitive function, greater cooperativeness, and better physical functioning (Koenig, George & Titus, 2004). Many clients would like to be asked about their religious beliefs during an office visit and feel their physician should be aware of their religious beliefs (MacLean et al, 2003). Religious salience is associated with being satisfied by one's health care*

• = Independent;   ▲ = Collaborative;   EBN = Evidence-Based Nursing;   EB = Evidence-Based

(Benjamin, 2006). **EBN:** *Most nurse practitioners do not believe religious practices hinder health (Stranahan, 2001). Individuals who have a religious faith tend to use that tradition in times of stress, but individuals without a religious faith do not turn to religion during times of stress (McGrath, 2003). Nurses commonly support religious beliefs and practices and a cultural approach that integrates non-mainstream religious practices in care (Narayanasamy & Owens, 2001).*

- Encourage and/or coordinate the use of and participation in usual religious rituals or practices that are not detrimental to health. **EB:** *Religiosity is associated with more social support, fewer depressive symptoms, higher cognitive status, more cooperativeness, and better physical health (Koenig, George & Titus, 2004).* **EBN:** *Church attendance and reading the Bible are rated highly in promoting spiritual well-being among battered women (Humphreys, 2000). Religious rites and rituals (e.g., ministering, offering communion, laying on of hands, and anointing) support clients spiritually (Tuck, Wallace & Pullen, 2001). Helping a client incorporate religious rites and rituals can enhance meaning in life and promote a sense of connectedness with a faith community and/or a higher power (Lauver, 2000).*

- Encourage the use of prayer or meditation as appropriate. **EB:** *College students who participated in a religious spiritual mediation exercise experienced significantly less anxiety and more positive mood, spiritual health, and spiritual experiences and higher pain tolerance (Wachholtz & Pargament, 2005). Spiritual interventions (including prayer and scripture reading) may help in weight loss (Reicks, Mills & Henry, 2004).* **EBN:** *Themes of spiritual coping mechanisms in chronically ill clients include reaching out to God in the belief and faith that help will be forthcoming, feeling connected to God through prayer, meaning and purpose, strategy of privacy, and connectedness with others (Narayanasamy, 2004).*

- Determine family's religious practices and encourage use of religious practices (if used) to help cope with loss. **EB:** *Religious faith and spirituality assist survivors in coping with life's challenges after the loved one is gone (Keeley, 2004).*

- Coordinate or provide transportation to worship site, particularly for the elderly and in meeting the needs of the disabled or ill. **EB:** *Widows and widowers who participate in organized religion demonstrate higher levels of psychological well-being (Fry, 2001). Religion is a protective factor in depression for African-American women who live in poor urban areas (van Olphen et al, 2003). Religiousness was associated with perceived well-being and fewer psychiatric symptoms in a sample of mentally ill individuals (Corrigan et al, 2003).* **EBN:** *Survivors of child abuse identified spiritual connection as a positive value to cope with negative experiences, church as a location for accessing God and communing with others, and a growing relationship to the natural world and the body (Hall, 2003).*

- ▲ Identify individuals at risk for an excessive dependence upon religion, religious leaders, or religious practices. **EB:** *Religious beliefs may be strengthened during crisis only if the subject has a history of religious beliefs (McGrath, 2003). Self-identified lesbians diagnosed with cancer identified spirituality as important in life and illness journey, but religion could be a barrier (Varner, 2004).*

- ▲ Refer to religious leader, professional counseling, or support group as needed. **EBN:** *The number one need expressed by hospitalized clients of all denominations and faiths was for their pastor/rabbi/spiritual advisor to not abandon them. For those who did not belong to a religious/spiritual group, the number one need was at least to be asked about some type of religious/spiritual preference (Moller, 1999).*

Geriatric

- Promote established religious practices in the elderly. **EB:** *Religious belief has been associated with higher levels of well-being and lower levels of depression and suicide (Van Ness & Larson, 2002). Widows and widowers who participate in organized religion demonstrate higher levels of psychological well-being (Fry, 2001). Older women who had not experienced a recent loss or terminal illness identified a need to feel connected, spiritual questioning, existential angst, thoughts about death and dying, and reliance on organized religion as important. Those who relied on religion don't experience the other themes (Moremen, 2005).* **EBN:** *Older Caucasian and African-American women associate religious coping strategies with healthcare utilization (Ark et al, 2006).*

Multicultural

• Promote religious practices that are culturally appropriate. **EB:** *African-American women living in an urban area who pray less often may report a greater number of depressive symptoms with social support mediating the positive relationship (van Olphen et al, 2003). African Americans and Latinos may identify spirituality, religiousness, prayer, and church-based approaches as coping resources (Samuel-Hodge et al, 2000).* **EBN:** *How the client copes with spiritual distress may be based on cultural perceptions (Leininger & McFarland, 2002). Older Caucasian and African-American women associate religious coping strategies with health care utilization. African-American women may use more religious coping strategies than Caucasian women (Ark et al, 2006). Hispanic women may draw strength from spiritual and religious resources (Dingley & Roux, 2003). African-American women living in an urban area who pray less often report a greater number of depressive symptoms with social support mediating the positive relationship (van Olphen et al, 2003).*

evolve See the EVOLVE website for World Wide Web resources for client education.

REFERENCES

Ark PD, Hull PC, Husaini BA et al: Religiosity, religious cooing styles, and health service use, *J Gerontol Nurs* 32(8):20-29, 2006.

Benjamin MR: Does religion influence patient satisfaction? *Am J Health Behav* 30(1):85-91, 2006.

Corrigan P, McCorkle B, Schell B et al: Religion and spirituality in the lives of people with serious mental illness, *Community Ment Health J* 39(6):487-499, 2003.

Dingley C, Roux G: Inner strength in older Hispanic women with chronic illness, *J Cult Divers* 10(1):11-22, 2003.

Fry PS: The unique contribution of key existential factors to the prediction of psychological well-being of older adults following spousal loss, *Gerontologist* 41(1):69-81, 2001.

Hall JM: Positive self-transitions in women child abuse survivor, *Issues Ment Health Nurs* 24(6-7):647-666, 2003.

Humphreys J: Spirituality and distress in sheltered battered women, *J Nurs Scholarsh* 32(3):273-278, 2000.

Keeley MP: Final conversations: survivors' memorable messages concerning religious faith and spirituality, *Health Commun* 16(1):87-104, 2004.

Koenig HG, George LK, Titus P: Religion, spirituality, and health in medically ill hospitalized older patients, *J Am Geriatr Soc* 52(4):554-562, 2004.

Lauver D: Commonalities in women's spirituality and women's health, *Adv Nurs Sci* 22(3):76-88, 2000.

Leininger MM, McFarland MR: *Transcultural nursing: concepts, theories, research and practices,* ed 3, New York, 2002, McGraw-Hill.

MacLean, CD, Susi B, Phifer N et al: Patient preference for physician discussion and practice of spirituality: results from a multicenter patient survey, *J Gen Intern Med* 18(1):38-43, 2003.

McGrath P: Religiosity and the challenge of terminal illness, *Death Studies,* 27(10):881-899, 2003.

Moller MD: Meeting spiritual needs on an inpatient unit, *J Psychosoc Nurs Ment Health Serv* 37(11):5-10, 1999.

Moremen RD: What is the meaning of life? Women's spirituality at the end of life span, *Omega* 50(4):309-330, 2005.

Narayanasamy A: Spiritual coping mechanisms in chronic illness: a qualitative study, *J Clin Nurs* 12(1):116-117, 2004.

Narayanasamy A, Owens J: A critical incident study of nurses' responses to the spiritual needs of their patients, *J Adv Nurs* 33(4):446-455, 2001.

Reicks M, Mills J, Henry H: Qualitative study of spirituality in a weight loss program: contribution to self-efficacy and locus of control, *J Nutr Educ Behav* 36(1):13-19, 2004.

Samuel-Hodge CD, Headen SW, Ingram AF et al: Influences on day-to-day self-management of type 2 diabetes among African American women: spirituality, the multi-caregiver role, and other social context factors, *Diabetes Care* 23(7):928-933, 2000.

Stranahan S: Spiritual perception, attitudes about spiritual care, and spiritual care practices among nurse practitioners, *West J Nurs Res* 23(1):90-104, 2001.

Tuck I, Wallace D, Pullen L: Spirituality and spiritual care provided by parish nurses, *West J Nurs Res* 23(5):144-162, 2001.

Van Ness PH, Larson DB: Religion, senescence, and mental health: the end of life is not the end of hope, *Am J Geriatr Psychiatry* 10(4):386-397, 2002.

van Olphen J, Schulz A, Israel B et al: Religious involvement, social support, and health among African-American women on the east side of Detroit, *J Gen Intern Med* 18(7):549-557, 2003.

Varner A: Spirituality and religion among lesbian women diagnosed with cancer: a qualitative study, *J Psychosoc Oncol* 22(1):75-89, 2004.

Wachholtz AB, Pargament KI: Is spirituality a critical ingredient of meditation? Comparing the effects of spiritual meditation, secular meditation, and relaxation on spiritual, psychological, cardiac, and pain outcomes, *J Behav Med* 28(4):367-384, 2005.

Readiness for enhanced Religiosity   *Lisa Burkhart, PhD, MPH, RN*

NANDA   Definition

Ability to exercise reliance on beliefs and/or participate in rituals of a particular faith tradition

Defining Characteristics

Expresses desire to strengthen religious belief patterns that had provided comfort in the past; expresses desire to strengthen religious belief patterns that had provided religion in the past; expresses desire to strengthen religious customs that had provided comfort in the past; expresses desire to strengthen religious customs that had provided religion in the past; questions belief patterns that are harmful; questions customs that are harmful; rejects belief patterns that are harmful; rejects customs that are harmful; requests assistance expanding religious options; request for assistance to increase participation in prescribed religious beliefs (e.g., religious ceremonies, dietary regulations/rituals, clothing prayer, worship/religious services, private religious behaviors, reading religious materials/media, holiday observances); requests forgiveness; requests meeting with religious leaders/facilitators; requests reconciliation; requests religious experiences; requests religious materials

NOTE: The DDC recognizes that the term *"religiosity"* may be culture specific; however, the term is useful in the U.S. and is well-supported in the U.S. literature.

Related Factors (r/t)

Health Seeking Behaviors to express one's chosen faith tradition or to reject harmful belief patterns and customs

NOC   Outcomes (Nursing Outcomes Classification)

Suggested NOC Outcomes

Client Satisfaction: Cultural Needs Fulfillment, Spiritual Health

Example NOC Outcome with Indicators
Client Satisfaction: Cultural Needs Fulfillment as evidenced by the following indicators: Respect for religious beliefs/Respect for cultural health behaviors/Incorporation of cultural beliefs in health teaching/Respect for personal values (Rate outcome and indicators of **Client Satisfaction: Cultural Needs Fulfillment:** 1 = not at all satisfied, 2 = somewhat satisfied, 3 = moderately satisfied, 4 = very satisfied, 5 = completely satisfied [see Section I].)

Client Outcomes

Client Will (Specify Time Frame):

- Express satisfaction with an enhanced ability to express religious practices
- Express satisfaction with access to religious materials and rituals
- Demonstrate balance between religious practices and healthy lifestyles
- Avoid high-risk, controlling religious relationships that inflict physical, sexual, or emotional harm and/or exploitation

NIC   Interventions (Nursing Interventions Classification)

Suggested NIC Interventions

Cultural Brokerage, Religious Ritual Enhancement, Spiritual Growth Facilitation

Example NIC Activities—Religious Ritual Enhancement
Encourage the use of and participation in religious rituals and practices that are not detrimental to health

R

• = Independent;   ▲ = Collaborative;   EBN = Evidence-Based Nursing;   EB = Evidence-Based

Nursing Interventions and *Rationales*

See care plan for **Impaired Religiosity.**

Pediatric

- Provide spiritual care for children based on developmental level. *When nurses are comfortable providing spiritual care, they can implement numerous spiritual care activities and interventions to meet the spiritual needs of the child and family. After determining the child's spiritual beliefs and spiritual needs, a plan of care is developed based on the child's developmental age (Elkins & Cavendish, 2004).*
  - **Infants:** Have the same nurse care for the child on a daily basis. Encourage holding, cuddling, rocking, playing with, and singing to the infant. *Continuity of care will promote the establishment of trust because nurses provide much of the needed ongoing support. The infant who is ill or dying still needs to be sung to, talked to, played with, held, cuddled, and rocked (Elkins & Cavendish, 2004).*
  - **Toddlers:** Provide consistency in care and familiar toys, music, stories, clothing blankets, pillows, and any other individual object of contentment. Schedule home religious routines into the plan of care and support home routines regarding good and bad behavior. *The importance of consistency in care and routine with this age group cannot be overemphasized. The nurse should support parents' home routines during hospitalization as much as possible and encourage them to continue to have the same expectations regarding good and bad behavior. If particular religious routines are carried out at certain times of the day, the nurse should schedule them in the care plan (Elkins & Cavendish, 2004).*
  - **School-age children and adolescents:** Encourage both groups to express their feelings regarding spirituality. Ask them, "Do you wish to pray and what do want to pray about?" Offer age-appropriate complimentary therapies such as music, art, videos, and connectedness with peers through cards, letters, and visits. *School-age children and adolescents should be encouraged to express their feelings, concerns, and needs regarding spirituality. For adolescents, nurses need to accept their beliefs and wishes even if they are different from their caregiver's. The nurse needs to facilitate the child's participation in religious rituals and spiritual practices. Referrals to clergy and other spiritual support may be necessary (Elkins & Cavendish, 2004).*

REFERENCE

Elkins M, Cavendish R: Developing a plan for pediatric spiritual care,
   Holist Nurs Pract 18(4):179-184, 2004.

R

Risk for impaired Religiosity   *Lisa Burkhart, PhD, MPH, RN*

NANDA   Definition

At risk for an impaired ability to exercise reliance on religious beliefs and/or participate in rituals of a particular faith tradition

Related Factors (r/t)

Developmental: Life transitions
Environmental: Barriers to practicing religion; lack of transportation
Physical: Hospitalization; illness; pain
Psychological: Depression; ineffective caregiving; ineffective coping; ineffective support; lack of security
Sociocultural: Cultural barrier to practicing religion; lack of social interaction; social isolation
Spiritual: Suffering
NOTE: The DDC recognizes that the term "religiosity" may be culture specific; however, the term is useful in the U.S. and is well-supported in the U.S. literature.

NOC   Outcomes (Nursing Outcomes Classification)

Suggested NOC Outcomes

Client Satisfaction: Cultural Needs Fulfillment, Spiritual Health

Example NOC Outcome with Indicators
Client Satisfaction: Cultural Needs Fulfillment as evidenced by the following indicators: Respect for religious beliefs/Respect for cultural health behaviors/Incorporation of cultural beliefs in health teaching/Respect for personal values (Rate outcome and indicators of **Client Satisfaction: Cultural Needs Fulfillment:** 1 = not at all satisfied, 2 = somewhat satisfied, 3 = moderately satisfied, 4 = very satisfied, 5 = completely satisfied [see Section I].)

Client Outcomes

Client Will (Specify Time Frame):

* Express satisfaction with the ability to express religious practices
* Express satisfaction with access to religious materials and rituals
* Demonstrate balance between religious practices and healthy lifestyles
* Avoid high-risk, controlling religious relationships that inflict physical, sexual, or emotional harm and/or exploitation

NIC   Interventions (Nursing Interventions Classification)

Suggested NIC Interventions

Abuse Protection: Religious, Cultural Brokerage, Religious Addiction Prevention, Religious Ritual Enhancement

Example NIC Activities—Religious Ritual Enhancement
Encourage the use of and participation in religious rituals and practices that are not detrimental to health

Nursing Interventions and *Rationales*

See care plan for **Impaired Religiosity.**

R

Relocation stress syndrome   *Rebecca A. Johnson, PhD, RN*

NANDA   Definition

Physiological and/or psychosocial disturbances that result from transfer from one environment to another

Defining Characteristics

Temporary and/or permanent move; voluntary and/or involuntary move; aloneness, alienation, or loneliness; depression; anxiety (e.g., separation); sleep disturbance; withdrawal; anger; loss of identity, self-worth, or self-esteem; increased verbalization of needs, unwillingness to move or concern over relocation; increased physical symptoms/illness (e.g., gastrointestinal disturbance, weight change); dependency; insecurity; pessimism; frustration; worry; fear

Related Factors (r/t)

Unpredictability of experience/isolation from family/friends; passive coping; language barrier; decreased health status; impaired psychosocial health; past, concurrent, and recent losses; feeling of powerlessness; lack of adequate support system/group; lack of predeparture counseling

• = Independent;   ▲ = Collaborative;   EBN = Evidence-Based Nursing;   EB = Evidence-Based

NOC   Outcomes (Nursing Outcomes Classification)

Suggested NOC Outcomes

Anxiety Self-Control, Child Adaptation to Hospitalization, Coping, Depression Level, Depression Self-Control, Loneliness Severity, Psychosocial Adjustment: Life Change, Quality of Life

Example NOC Outcome with Indicators
Anxiety Self-Control as evidenced by the following indicators: Seeks information to reduce anxiety/Plans coping strategies for stressful situations/Uses effective coping strategies/Uses relaxation techniques to reduce anxiety/Maintains social relationships/Maintains adequate sleep/Controls anxiety response (Rate the outcome and indicators of **Anxiety Self-Control:** 1 = never demonstrated, 2 = rarely demonstrated, 3 = sometimes demonstrated, 4 = often demonstrated, 5 = consistently demonstrated [see Section I].)

Client Outcomes

Client Will (Specify Time Frame):

- Recognize and know the name of at least one staff member
- Express concern about move when encouraged to do so during individual contacts
- Carry out activities of daily living (ADLs) in usual manner
- Maintain previous mental and physical health status (e.g., nutrition, elimination, sleep, social interaction)

NIC   Interventions (Nursing Interventions Classification)

Suggested NIC Interventions

Anxiety Reduction, Coping Enhancement, Discharge Planning, Hope Instillation, Self-Responsibility Facilitation

Example NIC Activities—Anxiety Reduction
Stay with patient to promote safety and reduce fear; Provide objects that symbolize safeness

Nursing Interventions and *Rationales*

- Begin relocation planning as early in the decision process as possible. **EB:** *Having a well-organized plan for the move with support and advocacy through the process may reduce anxiety (Jackson et al, 2000a, 2000b; Talerico, 2004).*
- Obtain a history, including the reason for the move, the client's usual coping mechanisms, history of losses, and family support for the client. A history helps the nurse determine the amount of support needed and appropriate interventions to decrease relocation stress.
- Identify to what extent the client can participate in the relocation decisions and advocate for this participation. **EBN:** *Older adults with poor mental functioning may be less able to be involved in the decisions and more vulnerable to disempowerment by others (Dwyer, 2005; Popejoy, 2005).*
- Assess family members' perceptions of clients' ability to participate in relocation decisions. **EB:** *Family members' and healthcare providers' perceptions of older adults' physical functioning may block elders' decision-making participation (Nolan & Dellesega, 2000).*
- Consider the clients' and families' cultural and ethnic values as much as possible when choosing roommates, foods, and other aspects of care. **EBN:** *Nurses need to be aware of the differences in values and practices of different cultures and ensure they give culturally appropriate care that is respectful of elders and family caregivers' beliefs about elder care (Caron & Bowers, 2003; Johnson & Tripp-Reimer, 2001a, 2001b).*
- Promote clear communication between all participants in the relocation process. **EBN:** *Case studies revealed the importance of using integrated approach to planning with clear communication among practitioners (LeClerc & Wells, 2001).*

R

- = Independent;   ▲ = Collaborative;   EBN = Evidence-Based Nursing;   EB = Evidence-Based

- Observe the following procedures if the client is being transferred to an extended care facility or assisted living facility:
  - Facilitate the client's participation in decisions and choice of placement and arrange a preadmission visit if possible. *Honoring relocation control beliefs may smooth relocation (Oswald & Wahl, 2004) and may help reduce mortality (Thorson & Davis, 2000).* **EB:** *Research has shown a link between the loss of independence with transfer to a nursing home and depression (Loeher et al, 2004).*
  - If the client cannot visit the new facility, arrange for a visit or telephone call by a member of the staff to welcome the client and show a videotape or at least provide pictures of the new care facility.
  - Have a familiar person accompany the client to the new facility. *This lessens client and family anxiety, confusion, and dissatisfaction.*
  - Recommend that the caregiver write a journal of thoughts and feelings regarding the relocation of their loved one. *Writing has been found to improve physical and emotional health among caregivers of older adults (Dellasega & Haagen, 2004).*
- Validate the caregiver's feelings of difficulty with deciding to relocate a loved one to a different environment. *This is a distressing experience, and caregivers feel responsible.*
- Identify previous routines for ADLs. Try to maintain as much continuity with the previous schedule as possible. *Continuity of routines has been shown to be a crucial factor in positively influencing adjustment to a new environment (Kao, Travis & Acton, 2004).*
- Bring in familiar items from home (e.g., pictures, clocks, afghans).
- Establish the way the client would like to be addressed (Mr., Mrs., Miss, first name, nickname). *Calling clients by the desired name shows respect.*
- Thoroughly orient the client and the family to the new environment and routines; repeat directions as needed. *The stress of the move may interfere with the client's ability to remember directions. A progressive introduction and orientation for both the client and the family should be done (Kao, Travis & Acton, 2004).*
- Spend one-to-one time with the client. Allow the client to express feelings and convey acceptance of them; emphasize that the client's feelings are real and individual and that it is acceptable to be sad or angry about moving. *Expressing feelings can help the client deal with the change and facilitate grief work that accompanies loss of independence (Tracy & DeYoung, 2004).*
- Assign the same staff members to the client if compatible with client; maintain consistency in the personnel the client interacts with. *Consistency hastens adjustment and increases quality of care (Iwasiw et al, 2003).*
- Ask the client to state one positive aspect of the new living situation each day. *Helping the client focus on the positive aspects of the move can help change attitude and reframe the situation in a positive fashion.*
- Monitor the client's health status and provide appropriate interventions for problems with social interaction, nutrition, sleep, new onset of infection, or elimination problems. **EB and EBN:** *Health problems may appear first as declines in ADLs (e.g., bathing, eating, dressing) (Chen & Wilmoth, 2004). Morbidity and mortality outcomes for elders are similar between assisted living and nursing home (Pruchno & Rose, 2000). Clients who moved showed lower natural killer cell immunity 1 month after moving than was shown by a control group of elderly who did not move (Lutgendorf et al, 1999). Older adults who were relocated had lower natural killer cell cytotoxicity than those who did not move, but the clients generally recovered normal immune function by 3 months (Lutgendorf et al, 2001).*
- If the client is being transferred within a facility, have staff members from the new unit visit the client before transfer.
- Work with the caregivers & family members helping them deal with stages of "making the best of it," "making the move," and "making it better." **EBN:** *A study demonstrated that relatives of clients entering a nursing home can work in partnership with healthcare staff to ease the transition for their loved one more effectively (Davies & Nolan, 2004).*
- If a client is being transferred from the intensive care unit (ICU), have previous staff make occasional visits until the client is comfortable in the new surroundings. Ensure that the family is told relevant information. **EBN:** *Leaving the ICU staff may be the most negative component of*

transfer (McKinney & Deeny, 2002). A review of the literature in this area demonstrated that infor-mation needs were most important to families of clients transferred out of ICU (Mitchell, Courtney & Coyer, 2003).

- Watch for coping problems (e.g., withdrawal, regression, angry behavior, impaired sleeping, refusal to eat, flat affect) and intervene immediately. **EB:** *Research has shown a link between the loss of independence with transfer to a nursing home and depression (Loeher et al, 2004).*
- Encourage the client to express grief for the loss of the old situation; explain that it is normal to feel sadness over change and loss. **EB:** *Older adults in long-term care grieve loss of home, possessions, and independence (Pilkington, 2005).*
- Encourage the client to participate in care as much as possible and make own decisions when possible (e.g., placement of the bed, choice of roommate, bathing routines).
- Make an effort to accommodate the client. *Having choices helps prevent feelings of powerlessness that may lead to depression.* **EB:** *Research showed that residents who viewed the nursing home move negatively after 3 months felt powerless, vulnerable, and isolated (Iwasiw et al, 2003).*

Pediatric

- Provide support for a child and family who must relocate to be near a transplant center. **EBN:** *Recognizing the unique needs of parents who must relocate for a child's transplantation procedure sup-ports the delivery of individualized nursing care and the effective allocation of program resources (Stubblefield & Murray, 2002).*
- Encourage child to verbalize concerns in divorce situations when they and/or a parent relocate. **EB:** *Relocation of a parent in divorce has been linked with children's financial concerns, hostility toward parents, views of parents as not socially supportive, and poorer self-perceived health (Braver, Ellman & Fabricius, 2003).*
- If the client is an adolescent, try to avoid a move in the middle of the school year, find a new-comers' club for the adolescent to join, and refer for counseling if needed. *Most adolescents who relocate suffer a brief period of loss of companionship and intimacy with close friends (Vernberg, Greenhoot & Biggs, 2006).*
- Assess adolescents' perceptions of their acceptance by peers. **EB:** *Poor perceptions of peer acceptance have been related to less initiation of social interactions in new settings (Aikins, Bierman & Parker, 2005).*

Geriatric

- Monitor the need for transfer and transfer only when necessary. **EB:** *Older adults often experience loss of function after relocation (Chen & Wilmoth, 2004), and relocation may even cause death (Thorson & Davis, 2000).*
- Implement discharge planning early so that it is not rushed. **EBN:** *Early discharge planning en-hanced elders' information levels and decreased their concerns (Kleinpell, 2004).*
- Protect the client from injuries such as falls. *Older adults who fell were more likely to be admitted to a nursing home (Seematter-Bagnoud et al, 2006). Having one fall increases the likelihood of additional falls (Quadri et al, 2005).*
- After the transfer, determine the client's mental status. *Document and observe for any new onset of confusion. Confusion can follow relocation because of the overwhelming stress and sensory overload.*
- ▲ Facilitate visits from companion animals. **EB:** *A randomized trial of 6 weeks of animal-assisted therapy (dog visits) decreased loneliness among nursing home residents (Banks & Banks, 2002).*
- Encourage reminiscence of happy times. **EB:** *Nine weeks of group reminiscence therapy enhanced self-esteem among 24 nursing home residents in a two-group, nonrandomized study (Chao et al, 2006).*
- ▲ Refer for music therapy. **EBN:** *One case study indicated that music therapy may facilitate a resident's adjustment to life in a long-term-care facility (Kydd, 2001).*
- Monitor neuroleptic prescriptions. **EB:** *A cohort study showed that 60% of older adults admitted to nursing homes were prescribed these drugs (most commonly Haloperidol) and 10% in doses over recom-mended levels within 100 days of admission (Bronskill et al, 2004).*

Client/Family Teaching

- Teach family members and remind direct care staff about relocation stress syndrome. Encourage

R

• = Independent;   ▲ = Collaborative;   EBN = Evidence-Based Nursing;   EB = Evidence-Based

them to monitor for signs of the syndrome. **EBN:** *Relocation Stress Syndrome begins to ease at approximately 4 weeks after the move (Hodgson et al, 2004).*
- Help significant others learn how to support the client in the move by setting up a schedule of visits, arranging for holidays, bringing familiar items from home, and establishing a system for contact when the client needs support.

evolve See the EVOLVE website for World Wide Web resources for client education.

REFERENCES

Aikins JW, Bierman KL, Parker JG: Navigating the transition to junior high school: the influence of pre-transition friendship and self-system characteristics, *Soc Dev* 14:42-60, 2005.

Banks M, Banks W: The effects of animal-assisted therapy on loneliness in an elderly population in long-term care facilities, *J Gerontol A Biol Sci Med Sci* 57A(7):M428-M432, 2002.

Braver SL, Ellman IM, Fabricius WV: Relocation of children after divorce and children's best interests: new evidence and legal considerations, *J Fam Psychol* 17(2):206-219, 2003.

Bronskill SE, Anderson GM, Sykora K et al: Neuroleptic drug therapy in older adults newly admitted to nursing homes: incidence, dose, and specialist contact, *J Am Geriatr Soc* 52(5):749-755, 2004.

Caron CD, Bowers BJ: Deciding whether to continue, share, or relinquish caregiving: caregiver views, *Qual Health Res* 13(9):1252-1271, 2003.

Chao S, Lui H, Wu C et al: Effects of group reminiscence therapy on depression, self-esteem and life satisfaction of elderly nursing home residents, *J Nurs Res* 14(1):36-45, 2006.

Chen PC, Wilmoth J: The effects of residential mobility on ADL and IADL limitations in the very old living in the community, *J Gerontol B Soc Sci* 59B(3):S164-S172, 2004.

Davies S, Nolan M: Making the move: relatives' experiences of the transition to a care home, *Health Soc Care Comm* 12(6):517, 2004.

Dellasega C, Haagen B: A different kind of caregiving support group, *J Psychosoc Nurs Ment Health Serv* 42(8):46-55, 2004.

Dwyer S: Older people and permanent care: whose decision? *Br J Soc Work* 35:1081-1092, 2005.

Hodgson N, Freedman V, Granger D et al: Biobehavioral correlates of relocation in the frail elderly: salivary cortisol, affect, and cognitive function, *J Am Geriatr Soc* 52(11):1856-1862, 2004.

Iwasiw C, Goldenberg D, Bol N et al: Resident and family perspectives: the first year in a long-term care facility, *J Gerontol Nurs* 29(1):45, 2003.

Jackson B, Swanson C, Hicks LE et al: Bridge of continuity from hospital to nursing home—Part I: a proactive approach to reduce relocation stress syndrome in the elderly, *Continuum* 20(1):3-8, 2000a.

Jackson B, Swanson C, Hicks LE et al: Bridge of continuity from hospital to nursing home—Part II: reducing relocation stress syndrome—an interdisciplinary guide, *Continuum* 20(1):9-14, 2000b.

Johnson RA, Tripp-Reimer T: Aging, ethnicity & social support: a review—part 1, *J Gerontol Nurs,* 27(6):15-21, 2001a.

Johnson RA, Tripp-Reimer T: Relocation among ethnic elders: a review—part 2, *J Gerontol Nurs,* 27(6):22-27, 2001b.

Kao HF, Travis SS, Acton GJ: Relocation to a long-term care facility: working with patients and families before, during, and after, *J Psychos Nurs Ment Health Serv* 42(3):10, 2004.

Kleinpell R: Randomized trial of an intensive care-based early discharge planning intervention for critically ill elderly patients, *Am J Crit Care* 13:335-345, 2004.

Kydd P: Using music therapy to help a client with Alzheimer's disease adapt to long-term care, *Am J Alzheimers Dis Other Demen* 16(2):103, 2001.

LeClerc M, Wells DL: Process evaluation of an integrated model of discharge planning, *Can J Nurs Leadersh* 14(2):19-26, 2001.

Loeher KE, Bank AL, MacNeill SE et al: Nursing home transition and depressive symptoms in older medical rehabilitation patients, *Clin Gerontol* 27(1/2):59-70, 2004.

Lutgendorf SK, Reimer TT, Harvey JH et al: Effects of housing relocation on immunocompetence and psychosocial functioning in older adults, *J Gerontol A Biol Sci Med Sci* 56(2):M97, 2001.

Lutgendorf SK, Vitaliano PP, Tripp-Reimer T et al: Sense of coherence moderates the relationship between life stress and natural killer cell activity in healthy older adults, *Psychol Aging* 14(4):552, 1999.

McKinney AA, Deeny P: Leaving the intensive care unit: a phenomenological study of the patients' experience, *Intens Crit Care Nurs* 18(6):320, 2002.

Mitchell ML, Courtney M, Coyer F: Understanding uncertainty and minimizing families' anxiety at the time of transfer from intensive care, *Nurs Health Sci* 5(3):207, 2003.

Nolan M, Dellesega C: 'I feel I've let him down': supporting family carers during long-term care placement for elders, *J Adv Nurs* 31(4):759-767, 2000.

Oswald F, Wahl HW: Housing and health in later life, *Rev Environ Health,* 19(3-4):223-252, 2004.

Pilkington FB: Grieving a loss: the lived experience for elders residing in an institution, *Nurs Sci Q,* 18(3):233-242, 2005.

Popejoy L: Health related decision making by older adults and their families: how clinicians can help, *J Gerontol Nurs* 13(9):12-18, 2005.

Pruchno R, Rose M: The effect of long-term care environments on health outcomes, *Gerontologist* 40(4):422-428, 2000.

Quadri P, Tettamanti M, Bernasconi S et al: Lower limb function as predictor of falls and loss of mobility with social repercussions one year after discharge among elderly inpatients, *Aging Clin Exper Res* 17(2):82-89, 2005.

Seematter-Bagnoud L, Wietlisbach V, Yersin B et al: Healthcare utilization of elderly persons hospitalized after a noninjurious fall in a Swiss academic medical center, *J Am Geriatr Soc* 54(6):891-897, 2006.

Stubblefield C, Murray RL: Waiting for lung transplantation: family experiences of relocation, *Pediatr Nurs* 28(5):501, 2002.

Talerico KA: Relocation to a long-term care facility: working with patients and families before, during, and after, *J Psychosoc Nurs* 42(3):10-16, 2004.

Thorson JA, Davis RE: Relocation of the institutionalized aged, *J Clin Psychol* 56(1):131, 2000.

Tracy JP, DeYoung S: Moving to an assisted living facility: exploring the transitional experience of elderly individuals, *J Gerontol Nurs* 30(10):26, 2004.

Vernberg E, Greenhoot A, Biggs B: Intercommunity relocation and adolescent friendships: who struggles and why? *J Consult Clin Psychol* 74(3):511-523, 2006.

R

Risk for Relocation stress syndrome   *Betty J. Ackley, MSN, EdS, RN*

NANDA   Definition

At risk for physiological and/or psychosocial disturbances that result from transfer from one environment to another

Risk Factors

Decreased health status; feelings of powerlessness; lack of adequate support system; lack of predeparture counseling; losses; moderate to high degree of environmental change; moderate mental competence; move from one environment to another; passive coping; unpredictability of experiences

NOC   Outcomes (Nursing Outcomes Classification)

Suggested NOC Outcomes

Anxiety Self-Control, Child Adaptation to Hospitalization, Coping, Loneliness Severity, Psychosocial Adjustment: Life Change, Quality of Life

Example NOC Outcome with Indicators
Anxiety Self-Control as evidenced by the following indicators: Seeks information to reduce anxiety/Plans coping strategies for stressful situations/Uses effective coping strategies/Uses relaxation techniques to reduce anxiety/Maintains social relationships/Maintains adequate sleep/Controls anxiety response (Rate the outcome and indicators of **Anxiety Self-Control:** 1 = never demonstrated, 2 = rarely demonstrated, 3 = sometimes demonstrated, 4 = often demonstrated, 5 = consistently demonstrated [see Section I].)

Client Outcomes, Nursing Interventions and *Rationales,* Client/Family Teaching

Refer to the care plan for **Relocation stress syndrome.**

Ineffective Role performance   *Gail B. Ladwig, MSN, CHTP, RN*

R

NANDA   Definition

Patterns of behavior and self-expression that do not match the environmental context, norms, and expectations

Defining Characteristics

Altered role perceptions; anxiety; change in capacity to resume role; change in other's perception of role; change in self-perception of role; change in usual patterns of responsibility; deficient knowledge; depression; discrimination; domestic violence; harassment; inadequate adaptation to change; inadequate confidence; inadequate coping; inadequate external support for role enactment; inadequate motivation; inadequate opportunities for role enactment; inadequate role competency; inadequate self-management; inadequate skills; inappropriate developmental expectations; pessimism; powerlessness; role ambivalence; role conflict; role confusion; role denial; role dissatisfaction; role overload; role strain; system conflict; uncertainty

Related Factors (r/t)

Knowledge

Inadequate role model; inadequate role preparation (e.g., role transition, skill rehearsal, validation); lack of education; lack of role model; unrealistic role expectations

• = Independent;   ▲ = Collaborative;   EBN = Evidence-Based Nursing;   EB = Evidence-Based

Physiological

Body image alteration; cognitive deficits; depression; fatigue; low self-esteem; mental illness; neurological defects; pain; physical illness; substance abuse

Social

Conflict; developmental level; domestic violence; inadequate role socialization; inadequate support system; inappropriate linkage with the healthcare system; job schedule demands; lack of resources; lack of rewards; low socioeconomic status; stress; young age

NOC   Outcomes (Nursing Outcomes Classification)

Suggested NOC Outcomes

Coping, Psychosocial Adjustment: Life Change, Role Performance

Example NOC Outcome with Indicators
Role Performance as evidenced by the following indicators: Ability to meet role expectations/Knowledge of role transition periods/Reported strategies for role change(s) (Rate the outcome and indicators of **Role Performance:** 1 = not adequate, 2 = slightly adequate, 3 = moderately adequate, 4 = substantially adequate, 5 = totally adequate [see Section I].)

Client Outcomes

Client Will (Specify Time Frame):

• Identify realistic perception of role
• State personal strengths
• Acknowledge problems contributing to inability to carry out usual role
• Accept physical limitations regarding role responsibility and consider ways to change lifestyle to accomplish goals associated with role performance
• Demonstrate knowledge of appropriate behaviors associated with new or changed role
• State knowledge of change in responsibility and new behaviors associated with new responsibility
• Verbalize acceptance of new responsibility

NIC   Interventions (Nursing Interventions Classification)

Suggested NIC Intervention

Role Enhancement

Example NIC Activities—Role Enhancement
Assist patient to identify behaviors needed for role development; Assist patient to identify positive strategies for managing role changes

Nursing Interventions and *Rationales*

Social

• Ask the client direct questions regarding new roles and how the health care system can help him or her continue in roles. **EBN:** *The best practice with regard to communication in palliative care could be achieved by using a sensitive assessment of how each client chooses to cope with his or her situation rather than a uniform approach to care (Dean, 2002).*
• Allow the client to express feelings regarding the role change. **EBN:** *Cancer affects men's role as a father, change in self-image as a man and as a parent. This consists of gaining control, balancing emotions, subjective well-being, being open or not toward the family, and challenges in family life and to family well-being (Elmberger & Bolund, 2002).*

• = Independent;   ▲ = Collaborative;   EBN = Evidence-Based Nursing;   EB = Evidence-Based

- Reinforce the client's strengths and internalized values. **EB:** *Participants in this study whose intentions were more aligned with their moral norm were more likely to perform healthy behaviors (driving within speed limit, applying universal precautions, exercising, not smoking) (Godin, Conner & Sheeran, 2005).*
- Have the client make a list of strengths that are needed for the new role. Acknowledge which strengths the client has and which strengths need to be developed. Work with the client to set goals for desired role. **EBN:** *Adversity can be an opportunity to focus on strengths and nurture resiliency. Clients should not subscribe to "victim" labels. Resilience should be celebrated (Engel, 2007).*
- Support the client's religious practices. **EB:** *The majority of well-conducted studies found that higher levels of religious involvement are positively associated with indicators of psychological well-being (life satisfaction, happiness, positive affect, and higher morale) and with less depression, suicidal thoughts and behavior, drug/alcohol use/abuse (Moreira-Almeida, Neto & Koenig, 2006).*

Physiological

- ▲ Identify ways to compensate for physical disabilities (e.g., have a ramp built to provide access to house, put household objects within the client's reach from wheelchair) and provide technological assistance when available. **EB:** *Among people with disability, use of assistive technology was associated with use of fewer hours of personal assistance (Hoenig, Taylor & Sloan, 2003).*
- Refer to the care plans for **Readiness for enhanced family Coping, Readiness for enhanced Decision Making, Impaired Home maintenance, Impaired Parenting, Risk for Loneliness, Readiness for enhanced community Coping, Readiness for enhanced Self-Care,** and **Ineffective Sexuality patterns.**

Pediatric

- Assist new parents to adjust to changes in workload associated with childbirth. **EB:** *Expectant parents in this study anticipated increase in workload after childbirth. Work increases were greater for women than for men (Gjerdingen, 2000; Gjerdingen & Center, 2003).*
- Assist parents in coping with infants with colic, a condition common in infants. **EBN:** *Even though nursing interventions do not cure infant colic, the amount of crying may be reduced and life made easier for the families if the parents are offered help in coping with the situation (Helseth, 2002).*
- ▲ Refer to home health agency for home visits when there is an infant who has excessive crying. **EBN:** *Almost every aspect of family life was disrupted when there was an infant who cried excessively, resulting in strained relationships, feelings of guilt, and concerns about losing control. A health visitor needs to visit frequently, stay for a prolonged period, demonstrate engagement with the family and its difficulties, and impart specific messages with conviction and sincerity (Long & Johnson, 2001).*
- Provide parents with coping skills when the role change is associated with a critically ill child. **EBN:** *Results from mothers who received the Creating Opportunities for Parent Empowerment (COPE) program indicate the need to educate parents regarding their children's responses as they recover from critical illness and how they can assist their children in coping with the stressful experience (Melnyk, Feinstein & Fairbanks, 2006).*
- ▲ Assist families how to manage day-to day needs of a child with cerebral palsy (CP). Teach family members to value the small things children do, connect with other families, locate community resources, and understand the short- and long-term needs of the child. **EB:** *In families of children with CP, strategies for optimizing caregiver physical and psychological health include supports for behavioral management and daily functional activities as well as stress management and self-efficacy techniques. These data support clinical pathways that require biopsychosocial frameworks that are family centered (Raina et al, 2005).*
- ▲ Consider the use of media-based behavioral treatments for children with behavioral disorders. **EB:** *Behaviors problems in children are quite common. For straightforward cases, media-based interventions may be enough to make clinically significant changes in a child's behavior. Media-based therapies appear to have both clinical and economic implications for the treatment of children with behavioral problems (Montgomery, 2005).*

R

• = Independent;   ▲ = Collaborative;   EBN = Evidence-Based Nursing;   EB = Evidence-Based

Geriatric

▲ Provide support for grandparents raising grandchildren. **EBN:** *Most grandparents raising grand-children reported that their health was compromised (Gibbons & Jones, 2003).*

• Provide support for spouses and families of clients with strokes. **EB:** *In this study three roles of spouses are described: (i) the role of caregiver, (ii) the role of client, and (iii) the role of family member: A family-centered approach is indicated in which the strengths and needs of all family members are addressed, including the client with the stroke (Visser-Meily et al, 2006).*

▲ Support the client's religious beliefs and activities and provide appropriate spiritual support persons. **EB:** *Usually the positive impact of religious involvement on mental health is more robust among people under stressful circumstances (the elderly and those with disability and medical illness) (Moreira-Almeida, Neto & Koenig, 2006).*

• Encourage the use of humor by family caregivers to describe their role reversal. **EB:** *This study suggested that humor is a useful communication tool for family caregivers in that it releases nervous energy (Bethea, Travis & Pecchioni, 2000).*

• Explore community needs after assessing the client's strengths. Encourage elders to participate in volunteer programs. **EB:** *Engagement in social and generative activities has benefits for the well-being of older adults; programs such as Experience Corps Baltimore provide a social model for health promotion for older adult volunteers in public schools (Martinez et al, 2006).*

▲ Refer to appropriate support groups for adjustment to role changes. **EBN:** *Healthcare professionals should provide information on Parkinson's disease symptom management, identify appropriate resources to reduce caregiver burden, and use of support groups (Edwards & Scheetz, 2002).* **EBN:** *Significant differences were found for distress levels and quality of life, with the mutual support group having greater improvements than the control group for dementia family caregivers (Fung & Chien, 2002).*

▲ Refer to therapy to improve memory for clients with Alzheimer's disease. **EB:** *The available evidence shows that alternative and innovative ways of memory rehabilitation for Alzheimer's clients can indeed be clinically effective or pragmatically useful with a great potential for use within the new culture of a more graded and proactive type of Alzheimer's disease care (De Vreese et al, 2001).* **EB:** *Facing an inevitable decline, persons with early-stage dementia and their care partners found it helpful to talk with one another and with peers in the same circumstances about the disease and its effects in this memory club (Zarit et al, 2004).*

Multicultural

• Assess for the influence of cultural beliefs, norms, values, and expectations on the individual's role. **EBN:** *The individual's role may be based on cultural perceptions (Leininger & McFarland, 2002).*

• Assess for conflicts between the caregiver's cultural role obligations and competing factors like employment or school. **EBN:** *Mexican immigrant children provide essential help to their families, including translating, interpreting, and caring for siblings (Orellana, 2003). A recent study found that African-American caregivers experienced a wide range of caregiver role strain (Wallace Williams, Dilworth-Anderson & Goodwin, 2003).*

• Negotiate with the client regarding the aspects of their role that can be modified and still honor cultural beliefs. **EBN:** *Give and take with the client will lead to culturally congruent care (Leininger & McFarland, 2002).*

• Encourage family to use support groups or other service programs to assist with role changes. **EBN:** *Studies indicate that minority families of clients with dementia use few support programs even though these programs could have a positive impact on caregiver well-being (Cox, 1999).*

Home Care

• Above interventions may be adapted for home care use.

▲ Offer a referral to medical social services to assist with assessing the short- and long-term impacts of role change. *Social workers may assist clients with life care planning (Rice, Hicks & Wiehe, 2000).*

• = Independent;   ▲ = Collaborative;   EBN = Evidence-Based Nursing;   EB = Evidence-Based

Client/Family Teaching

- Provide educational materials to family members on client behavior management plus caregiver stress-coping management. **EB:** *Brief primary care interventions as described above may be effective in reducing caregiver distress and burden in the long-term management of the dementia client (Burns et al, 2003).*
- Help the client identify resources for assistance in caring for a disabled or aging parent (e.g., adult day care). **EBN:** *The wives of men with chronic obstructive pulmonary disease (COPD) in this phenomenological study were dissatisfied with their lack of recreation, as well as support from friends, families, and healthcare providers (Bergs, 2002).*
- ▲ Refer to appropriate community agencies to learn skills for functioning in the new or changed role (e.g., vocational rehabilitation, parenting classes, hospice, respite care). **EB:** *Program Without Walls (PWW) is a person-centered, community-based approach for state rehabilitation counselors to provide vocational rehabilitation (VR) services to people with traumatic brain injury (TBI). This study demonstrated that the PWW showed promise as a systems change effort to improve VR services for people with TBI (O'Neill et al 2004).*

evolve See the EVOLVE website for World Wide Web resources for client education.

REFERENCES

Bergs D: "The Hidden Client"—women caring for husbands with COPD: their experience of quality of life *J Clin Nurs* 11(5):613, 2002.

Bethea LS, Travis SS, Pecchioni L: Family caregivers' use of humor in conveying information about caring for dependent older adults, *Health Commun* 12(4):361, 2000.

Burns R, Nichols LO, Martindale-Adams J et al: Primary care interventions for dementia caregivers: 2-year outcomes from the REACH study, *Gerontologist* 43(4):547-555, 2003.

Cox C: Race and caregiving: patterns of service use by African American and white caregivers of persons with Alzheimer's, *J Gerontol Soc Work* 32(2):5, 1999.

De Vreese LP, Neri M, Fioravanti M et al: Memory rehabilitation in Alzheimer's disease: a review of progress, *Int J Geriatr Psychiatry* 16(8):794, 2001.

Dean A: Talking to dying clients of their hopes and needs, *Nurs Times* 98(43):34, 2002.

Edwards NE, Scheetz PS: Predictors of burden for caregivers of patients with Parkinson's disease, *J Neurosci Nurs* 34(4):184, 2002.

Elmberger E, Bolund C: Men with cancer. Changes in attempts to master the self-image as a man and as a parent, *Cancer Nurs* 25(6):477, 2002.

Engel B: Eagle soaring: the power of the resilient self, *J Psychosoc Nurs Ment Health Serv* 45(2):44-49, 2007.

Fung WY, Chien WT: The effectiveness of a mutual support group for family caregivers of a relative with dementia, *Arch Psychiatr Nurs* 16(3):134, 2002.

Gibbons C, Jones TC: Kinship care: health profiles of grandparents raising their grandchildren, *J Fam Soc Work* 7(1):1-14, 2003.

Gjerdingen D: Expectant parents' anticipated changes in workload after the birth of their first child, *J Fam Pract* 49(11):993, 2000.

Gjerdingen DK, Center BA: First-time parents' prenatal to postpartum changes in health, and the relation of postpartum health to work and partner characteristics, *J Am Board Fam Pract* 16(4):304-311, 2003.

Godin G, Conner M, Sheeran P: Bridging the intention-behavior 'gap': the role of moral norm, *Br J Soc Psychol,* 44(Pt 4):497-512, 2005.

Helseth S: Help in times of crying: nurses' approach to parents with colicky infants, *J Adv Nurs* 40(3):267-274, 2002.

Hoenig H, Taylor DH Jr, Sloan FA: Does assistive technology substitute for personal assistance among the disabled elderly? *Am J Public Health* 93(2):330-337, 2003.

Leininger MM, McFarland MR: *Transcultural nursing: concepts, theories, research and practices,* ed 3, New York, 2002, McGraw-Hill.

Long T, Johnson M: Living and coping with excessive infantile crying, *J Adv Nurs* 34(2):155, 2001.

Martinez IL, Frick K, Glass TA et al: Engaging older adults in high impact volunteering that enhances health: recruitment and retention in The Experience Corps Baltimore, *J Urban Health* 83(5):941-953, 2006.

Melnyk BM, Feinstein N, Fairbanks E: Two decades of evidence to support implementation of the COPE program as standard practice with parents of young unexpectedly hospitalized/critically ill children and premature infants, *Pediatr Nurs* 32(5):475-481, 2006.

Montgomery M: Media-based behavioral treatments for behavioral disorders in children, *Cochrane Database Syst Rev* (1):CD002206, 2005.

Moreira-Almeida A, Neto FL, Koenig HG: Religiousness and mental health: a review, *Rev Bras Psiquiatr* 28(3):242-250, 2006.

O'Neill JH, Zuger RR, Fields A et al: The Program Without Walls: innovative approach to state agency vocational rehabilitation of persons with traumatic brain injury, *Arch Phys Med Rehabil* 85(4 Suppl 2):S68-S72, 2004.

Orellana MF: Responsibilities of children in Latino immigrant homes, *New Dir Youth Dev* (100):25-39, 2003.

Raina P, O'Donnell M, Rosenbaum P et al: The health and well-being of caregivers of children with cerebral palsy, *Pediatrics* 115(6):e626-e636, 2005.

Rice J, Hicks PB, Wiehe V: Life care planning: a role for social workers, *Soc Work Health Care* 31(1):85, 2000.

Visser-Meily A, Post M, Gorter JW et al: Rehabilitation of stroke patients needs a family-centered approach, *Disabil Rehabil* 28(24):1557-1561, 2006.

Wallace Williams S, Dilworth-Anderson P, Goodwin PY: Caregiver role strain: the contribution of multiple roles and available resources in African-American women, *Aging Ment Health* 7(2):103-112, 2003.

Zarit SH, Femia EE, Watson J et al: Memory Club: a group intervention for people with early-stage dementia and their care partners, *Gerontologist* 44(2):262-269, 2004.

R

Readiness for enhanced Self-Care   *Barbara Kraynyak Luise, RN, EdD*

NANDA   Definition

A pattern of performing activities for oneself that helps to meet health-related goals and can be strengthened

Defining Characteristics

Expresses desire to enhance independence in monitoring life; expresses desire to enhance independence in maintaining health; expresses desire to enhance independence in maintaining personal development; expresses desire to enhance independence in maintaining well-being; expresses desire to enhance knowledge of strategies for self-care; expresses desire to enhance responsibility for self-care; expresses desire to enhance self-care

Related Factors (r/t)

To be developed.

NOC   Outcomes (Nursing Outcomes Classification)

Suggested NOC Outcomes

Adherence Behavior, Health Seeking Behavior, Information Processing, Knowledge: Decision Process, Health Behavior, Health Promotion, Participation in Health Care Decisions, Self-Care Status

Example NOC Outcome with Indicators
Adherence Behavior as evidenced by the following indicators: Asks health-related questions when indicated/ Seeks health-related information from a variety of sources/Uses strategies to maximize health/Performs self-screening/ Performs self-monitoring of health status (Rate the outcome and indicators of **Adherence Behavior:** 1 = never demonstrated, 2 = rarely demonstrated, 3 = sometimes demonstrated, 4 = often demonstrated, 5 = consistently demonstrated.)

Client Outcomes

Client Will (Specify Time Frame):

- Assess current level of self-care activities as acceptable
- Express the need or desire to enhance level of self-care
- Seek out health-related information as needed
- Identify strategies to enhance self-care
- Perform appropriate interventions as needed
- Monitor level of self-care
- Evaluate effectiveness of self-care interventions at regular intervals

NIC   Interventions (Nursing Interventions Classification)

Suggested NIC Interventions

Active Listening, Consultation, Coping Enhancement, Energy Management, Family Integrity Promotion, Hope Instillation, Learning Facilitation, Multidisciplinary Care Conference, Mutual Goal Setting, Self-Care Assistance, Self-Esteem Enhancement, Self-Respect Facilitation, Spiritual Growth Facilitation, Support System Enhancement, Teaching: Decision Process, Individual

Example NIC Activities—Self-care Assistance
Encourage patient to perform normal activities of daily living to level of ability

• = Independent;   ▲ = Collaborative;   EBN = Evidence-Based Nursing;   EB = Evidence-Based

Nursing Interventions and *Rationales*

- Assess client's current level of self-care. *Assessment is the critical first step of the nursing process; the remainder of the nursing process rests on this foundation (Wilkinson & VanLeuven, 2007). Self-care is an adult's continuous contribution to his or her own continued existence, health, and well-being. It is voluntary and guided by principles that give direction to actions (Orem, 2001).*
- Educate clients that enhanced self-care is an achievable, desirable, and positive life goal. *Persons must know how to distinguish good or desirable from bad or undesirable, and know why it is beneficial to choose to attain the good or desirable (Orem, 2001).*
- Promote trust and enhanced communication between clients and their healthcare provider. **EBN:** *Respect for an individual is a necessary condition for clients' experience of participation (Eldh, Ekman & Ehnfors, 2006).* **EB:** *Client attachment style is significantly associated with desired self-management and outcomes (Ciechanowski et al, 2004).* **EB:** *Women and youth require empowerment in asking medical professionals about HIV/AIDS; medical professionals should be sensitized to provide safe and comfortable environments so that such dialogues can take place (Takahashi et al, 2006).*
- Promote opportunities for spiritual care and growth. **EBN:** *Spiritual care needs are unique to each individual, and the provision of spiritual care can be an expectation in today's healthcare system. Clients may use their spirituality to make decisions, guide actions, and to accept, reorder, and transcend life events. Many use prayer as a spiritual practice; many practices have a special meaning and fulfill spiritual needs (Cavendish et al, 2006). Through interventions that promote spiritual growth, nurses may be able to improve a client's self-care agency, resulting in the practice of health-promoting self-care behaviors and the outcomes of health (Callaghan, 2003).*
- Increase social support and family involvement. **EBN:** *Self-care behaviors are often necessary to prevent repeated hospitalization and to promote positive health outcomes in heart failure clients. Heart failure clients who lived alone were less likely to ask for help during episodes of shortness of breath, were less likely to contact the doctor when they noticed symptoms, and were more likely to consume food with high sodium content, such as canned foods and frozen entrees. Knowledge was also related to self-care (Artinian et al, 2002).* **EB:** *Physical activity and exercise are critical factors in the management of arthritis. To help increase activity, interventions should include strategies to increase self-efficacy, such as acknowledging the attainment of performance goals and having subjects interact with other subjects with arthritis who have been successful in increasing physical activity (Greene et al, 2006). In the "Aging Gracefully" program, expert clinicians observed that participants benefited greatly from socializing and that nurses can promote the self-care and ultimately the independence of older adults by establishing and implementing these types of programs (Gerson et al, 2004).*
- Identify what information clients will need to enhance self-care activities and provide educational opportunities as needed. **EBN:** *Chemotherapy often causes serious side effects in clients, and self-care behaviors are often used to manage these ill effects. Teaching effective self-care behaviors via audiotapes enhances clients' independence, comfort, control, and quality of life (Williams & Schreier, 2004).* **EBN:** *Self-care is a challenge that clients face in the long-term management of HIV/AIDS. They develop symptom self-care strategies primarily from their experiences, learning from family, friends, and community resources. Identifying sources of self-care information were healthcare providers, self, personal networks, and communities (Chou et al, 2004).* **EB:** *Although cardiovascular disease is the leading cause of death among women in the United States, national studies indicate that women have less awareness and knowledge about heart disease than others. Information message frames significantly increase knowledge, self-efficacy and intervention efficacy beliefs, and behavioral intentions with women who are at risk for the development of heart disease (Scott & Curbow, 2006).*
- As needed, promote a wide range of intervention strategies to enhance self-care, such as client empowerment, early intervention, and hope instillment. *Medication self-care is a vital daily activity that must be done safely by older adults so they can remain independent. Empowering clients to ask the right questions, such as whether a medication is cost effective, therapeutically effective, and as safe as possible will help older adults and their caregivers to become informed consumers (Miller, 2004). When persons engage in self-care or other forms of deliberate action, they must have essential powers that are activated through stimuli (Denyes, Orem & Sozwiss, 2001).* **EBN:** *Elderly men and those with fewer comorbid illnesses were most successful at heart-failure self-care. Persons with few symptoms had greater*

S

treatment adherence, but at three months the best predictor of self-care was early intervention (Chriss et al, 2004). **EBN:** *The attitude of nurses toward clients and their families was associated with self-efficacy. Carefully listening to clients and understanding their hopes is important in helping them to have hope in life until the end and to be able to live the way they wish (Ueno, Kaneko & Okamura, 2006).* **EB:** *Optimistic chronically ill clients do not tend to have a biased perception of their health status, and positive efficacy expectancies appear to encourage self-care behaviors six months later (Ridder, Fournier & Bensing, 2004).*

- Evaluate the effectiveness of all self-care activities, and intervene or adjust as needed. *Regulatory requirements for engagement in self-care change during the life cycle and with human and environmental conditions (Denyes, Orem & Sozwiss, 2001). In individuals, self-care must be learned. When self-care deficits arise, they may result from an individual's limitations or the lack of effectiveness of self-care (Orem, 2001).*

Pediatrics

- Assess and evaluate a child's level of self-care and adjust strategies as needed. *Caring for or doing for are appropriate interventions for nursing young infants or children. Guiding and supporting older children in their self-care actions is appropriate. Nurses should help adolescents to develop beneficial self-care practices (Orem, 2001).* **EBN:** *Parents of children with asthma needed to be able to detect, interpret, and monitor meaningful symptoms to adequately control them. When barriers exist for enhanced self-care activities, treatment in an emergency room is the consequence even if the parents are well intended (Cox & Taylor, 2005).*

- ▲ Assist families to engage in and maintain social support networks. **EBN:** *Children with cancer are competent agents, performing many practices in the area of universal and developmental self-care requisites (Moore & Beckwitt, 2004).* **EBN:** *Improved caregiver-child relationship suggests participation in an internet support group as soon as possible for primary caregivers of a child with special healthcare needs (Baum, 2004).* **EBN:** *Both social support and self-esteem have been linked to positive health practices. Social support is a powerful variable in positive health practices in adolescents; self-esteem is not as powerful a variable in positive health practices in this group of early adolescents (Yarcheski, Mahon & Yarcheski, 2003).*

- Encourage activities that support or enhance spiritual care. **EBN:** *Spiritual growth is significantly related to an adolescent's initiation and responsibility for self-care. With spiritual growth came the adolescent's assumption of responsibilities for self-care (Callaghan, 2005).* **EBN:** *When opportunities that enhance spiritual growth are explicated from research, nurses can assess and intervene to promote positive health outcomes. A spectrum of life events can promote a spiritual response leading to spiritual enhancement (Cavendish et al, 2000). Every child is born with an intrinsic spiritual essence that can be enhanced. Nurses must realize that a child's spirituality can effect their health and illness states. For an infant, the needs for love and trust, intrinsically related to spiritual care, must be addressed. School-aged children can play, attend religious services, and receive visits from clergy (Elkins & Cavendish, 2004).*

Multicultural

- Identify cultural beliefs, values, lifestyle practices, and problem-solving strategies when assessing clients' level of self-care. *Self-care needs are not inborn. Activities of self-care are learned according to one's cultural way of life. Hence, there are many variations in self-care practice (Orem, 2001). For common minor illnesses, many people use self-care with medicines, vitamins, herbs, exercise, or foods that they believe have healing powers. Many self-care practices are handed down from generation to generation. When self-care measures do not work, only then will people turn to professional or folk healing systems (Andrews & Boyle, 2003). As nurses we need to be aware of our client's health beliefs, practice-related folklore, and ethnocultural knowledge. Health promotion and protection practices can range from seeing a physician to wearing a clove of garlic around one's neck (Spector, 2004).*

- Enhance cultural knowledge by seeking out information regarding different cultural or ethnic groups. *To provide culturally competent and appropriate care, nurses need to skillfully and artfully use transcultural knowledge. The transcultural nurse must be guided by acquired knowledge in the assessment, diagnosis, planning, implementation, and evaluation of the client's needs, based on culturally relevant information (Giger & Davidhizar, 2004). Cultural self-assessment is the first step in providing*

S

culturally competent care. Through self-assessment one can overcome ethnocentric tendencies and cultural stereotypes that often lead to prejudice and discrimination against members of certain groups (Andrews & Boyle, 2003).

- Recognize the impact of culture on self-care behaviors. **EB:** *Self-care practices play a critical role in the management of chronic illness, yet little is known about the self-care practices of chronically ill African Americans or how lack of access to health care affects health care. Self-care practices are culturally based; the cultural component of self-care has been underemphasized, and self-care strategies to maximize chronic illness management have not been realized for people who lack access to health care (Becker, Gates & Newsom, 2004).* **EB:** *In noting the factors that influence self-efficacy in HIV risk reduction among Asian and Pacific Islanders, variations in reported self-efficacy for female respondents are explained by acculturation, comfort in asking medical practitioners about HIV/AIDS, and to a lesser degree such variables as age, education, and HIV knowledge (Takahashi et al, 2006).*
- Provide culturally competent care. *Culturally competent care implies that within the delivered care the provider understands and attends to the total context of the client's situation. It is a complex combination of knowledge, attitude, and skills (Spector, 2004). Cultural competence is a continuous process of awareness, knowledge, skill, interaction, and sensitivity that is demonstrated among those who render care and the services they provide (Giger & Davidhizar, 2004).*

Home Care

- The nursing interventions described previously can be used in the home care setting with adaptation as needed.
- Identify discharge planning needs. *One of the first components of home care nursing is self-care. As more health care is provided outside of the acute care setting, clients and family must assume responsibility for their own care. Discharge planning helps to prevent problems by ensuring continuity of care (Hunt, 2005).*
- ▲ Make appropriate referrals as needed to enhance self-care activities. *Referrals can be made to another person, organization, or provider to ensure that appropriate and timely information is shared so that needs are met and care is coordinated (Hunt, 2005). When clients must become involved in highly technical care, such as when parents participate in or completely provide continuous care for their child at home, nurses must carefully determine how these parents can be assisted without harm to them or their child (Orem, 2001).*
- Assess the need for financial assistance. *Financial assessments and options to reduce the cost of home care while continuing to provide quality care need to be explored with every child and family. Based on insurance coverage, home care services may be fully covered, partially covered, or limited (Hunt, 2005).*
- ▲ Provide an interdisciplinary approach to health care. *Many specialized services can be provided in the home health setting, such as physical therapy, occupational therapy, and nutrition counseling. Interdisciplinary collaboration promotes continuity of care, and professionals who work in home care are in a unique setting where they can truly work together to accomplish a client's healthcare goals (Stanhope & Lancaster, 2006).*
- Evaluate regularly if enhanced self-care is attainable in the home setting. *Home health agencies monitor closely the care they deliver to their clients. All agencies are accountable to their clients, their families, their reimbursement sources, and to themselves regarding the level of care that they provide (Stanhope & Lancaster, 2006).*

Client/Family Teaching

- Teach clients how to regularly assess their level of self-care
- Instruct clients that a variety of interventions may be needed to enhance self-care
- Help clients to understand that enhanced self-care is an achievable goal
- Empower clients
- Teach clients about the decision-making process and self-care activities needed to manage their illness state and promote well being
- Continuously stress that all self-care activities must be regularly evaluated to ensure that enhanced levels of self-care can be maintained

S

REFERENCES

Andrews M, Boyle J: *Transcultural concepts in nursing care,* ed 4, Philadelphia, 2003, Lippincott Williams & Wilkins.

Artinian N, Magnan M, Sloan M et al: Self-care behaviors among patients with heart failure, *Heart Lung* 31(3):161-172, 2002.

Baum L: Internet parent support groups for primary caregivers of a child with special health care needs, *Pediatr Nurs* 30(5):381-401, 2004.

Becker G, Gates R, Newsom E: Self-care among chronically ill African Americans: culture, health disparities, and health insurance status, *Am J Public Health* 94(12):2066-2073, 2004.

Callaghan D: Health promoting self-care behaviors, self-care, self-efficacy, and self-care agency, *Nurs Sci Q* 16(3):247-254, 2003.

Callaghan D: The influence of spiritual growth on adolescents' initiative and responsibility for self-care, *Pediatr Nurs* 31(2):91-97, 2005.

Cavendish R, Konecny L, Naradovy L et al: Patients' perceptions of spirituality and the nurse as a spiritual care provider, *Holist Nurs Pract* 20(1):41-47, 2006.

Cavendish R, Luise B, Home K et al: Opportunities for enhanced spirituality relevant to well adults, *Int J Nurs Lang Classif* 11(4):151-163, 2000.

Chou F, Holzemer W, Portillo C et al: Self-care strategies and sources of information for HIV/AIDS symptom management, *Nurs Res* 53(5):332-339, 2004.

Chriss P, Sheposh J, Carlson B et al: Predictors of successful heart failure self-care maintenance in the first three months after hospitalization, *Heart Lung* 33(6):345-353, 2004.

Ciechanowski P, Russo J, Katon W et al: Influence of patient attachment style on self-care and outcomes in diabetes, *Psychosom Med* 66:720-728, 2004.

Cox K, Taylor S: Orem's self-care deficit nursing theory: pediatric asthma as exemplar, *Nurs Sci Q* 18(3):249-257, 2005.

Denyes M, Orem D, Sozwiss G: Self-care: a foundational science, *Nurs Sci Q* 14(1):48-54, 2001.

Eldh A, Ekman I, Ehnfors M: Conditions for patient participation and non-participation in health care, *Nurs Ethics* 13(5):503-514, 2006.

Elkins M, Cavendish R: Developing a plan for pediatric spiritual care, *Holist Nurs Pract* 14(4):179-184, 2004.

Gerson L, Dorsey C, Berg J et al: Enhancing self-care in community dwelling older adults, *Geriatr Nurs* 25(5):272-276, 2004.

Giger J, Davidhizar R: *Transcultural nursing,* ed 4, St Louis, 2004, Mosby.

Greene B, Haldeman G, Kaminski A et al: Factors affecting physical activity behavior in urban adults with arthritis who are predominantly African-American and female, *Phys Ther* 86(4):510-519, 2006.

Hunt R: *Introduction to community based nursing,* ed 3, Philadelphia, 2005, Lippincott Williams & Wilkins.

Miller C: Teaching older adults medication self-care, *Geriatr Nurs* 25(5):318-319, 2004.

Moore J, Beckwitt A: Children with cancer and their parents: self-care and dependent-care practices, *Issues Compr Pediatr Nurs* 27:1-17, 2004.

Orem D: *Nursing concepts of practice,* ed 6, St Louis, 2001, Mosby.

Ridder D, Fournier M, Bensing J: Does optimism affect symptom report in chronic disease? What are its consequences for self-care behavior and physical functioning, *J Psychosom Res* 56:341-350, 2004.

Scott L, Curbow B: The effect of message frames and CVD risk factors on behavioral outcomes, *Am J Health Behav* 30(6):582-597, 2006.

Spector R: *Cultural diversity in health and illness,* ed 6, Upper Saddle River, NJ, 2004, Prentice Hall.

Stanhope M, Lancaster J: *Foundations of nursing in the community,* ed 2, St Louis, 2006, Mosby.

Takahashi L, Magalong M, DeBell P et al: HIV and AIDS in suburban Asian and Pacific Islander communities: factors influencing self-efficacy in HIV risk reduction, *AIDS Educ Prev* 18(6):529-545, 2006.

Ueno K, Kaneko F, Okamura H: Factors associated with self-efficacy of terminally ill cancer patients, *Am J Hosp Palliat Care* 8(3):147-154, 2006.

Wilkinson J, VanLeuven K: *Fundamentals of nursing,* Philadelphia, 2007, FA Davis.

Williams S, Schreier A: The effects of education in managing side effects in women receiving chemotherapy for treatment of breast cancer, *Oncol Nurs Forum* 31(1):16-23, 2004.

Yarcheski T, Mahon N, Yarcheski A: Social support, self-esteem, and positive health practices of early adolescents, *Psychol Rep* 92:99-103, 2003.

S

Bathing/hygiene Self-care deficit   Linda S. Williams, MSN, RNBC

NANDA   Definition

Impaired ability to perform or complete bathing/hygiene activities for oneself

Defining Characteristics

Inability to access bathroom; inability to dry body; inability to get bath supplies; inability to obtain water source; inability to regulate bath water; inability to wash body

• = Independent;   ▲ = Collaborative;   EBN = Evidence-Based Nursing;   EB = Evidence-Based

Related Factors (r/t)

Cognitive impairment; decreased motivation; environmental barriers; inability to perceive body part; inability to perceive spatial relationship; musculoskeletal impairment; neuromuscular impairment; pain; perceptual impairment; severe anxiety; weakness
NOTE: Specify level of independence using a standardized functional scale.

NOC   Outcomes (Nursing Outcomes Classification)

Suggested NOC Outcomes

Self-Care: Activities of Daily Living (ADL), Bathing, Hygiene

Example NOC Outcome with Indicators
Self-Care: Activities of Daily Living (ADL) as evidenced by the following indicators: Bathing/Hygiene (Rate outcome and indicators of **Self-Care: Activities of Daily Living (ADL):** 1 = severely compromised, 2 = substantially compromised, 3 = moderately compromised, 4 = mildly compromised, 5 = not compromised [see Section I].)

Client Outcomes

Client Will (Specify Time Frame):

• Remain free of body odor and maintain intact skin
• State satisfaction with ability to use adaptive devices to bathe
• Use methods to bathe safely with minimal difficulty
• Bathe with assistance of caregiver as needed and report sense of dignity is maintained
• Bathe with assistance of caregiver as needed without exhibiting defensive (aggressive) behaviors

NIC   Interventions (Nursing Interventions Classification)

Suggested NIC Interventions

Self-Care Assistance: Bathing/Hygiene

Example NIC Activities—Self-Care Assistance: Bathing/Hygiene
Determine amount and type of assistance needed; Consider the culture of the patient when promoting self-care activities; Provide assistance until patient is fully able to assume self-care

Nursing Interventions and *Rationales*

• Establish the goal of client's bathing as being a pleasant experience, especially for cognitively impaired clients, without the symptoms of unmet needs—hitting, biting, kicking, screaming, resisting—and plan for client preferences in timing, type and length of bathing, water temperature, and with silence or music. **EBN:** *Sensations that make bathing pleasant should be used for everyone to avoid behaviors that are symptoms of unpleasant bathing, which are often due to pain (Rader et al, 2006).*
• Use and teach client-centered bathing: foster development of an understanding relationship with client, plan for client's comfort and preferences, personalize care, show respect in communications, critically think to solve issues that arise, and use a gentle approach. **EBN:** *Focusing on the client rather than the task of bathing results in greater comfort and fewer aggressive (defensive) behaviors (Hoeffer et al, 2006).*
• Ask the client for input on bathing habits and cultural bathing preferences. **EB:** *Creating opportunities for guiding personal care honors long-standing routines, increases control, and makes bath time more pleasant for client and caregiver (Perlmutter & Camberg, 2004).*
• Develop a bathing care plan based on the client's own history of bathing practices that addresses skin needs, self-care needs, client response to bathing, and equipment needs. *Bathing is a healing*

S

rite and should be a comforting experience that concentrates on the client's needs, rather than being a routinely scheduled task (Rasin & Barrick, 2004).

- Individualize bathing by identifying the function of bathing (e.g., odor, urine removal), frequency required to achieve function, and best bathing form (e.g., towel bathing, tub, shower) to meet client preferences, preserve client dignity, make bathing a soothing experience, and reduce client aggression. **EB:** *Client behaviors labeled as aggressive are likely defensive behavior that results from being threatened or anxious and increases with shower (especially) and tub bathing. Towel bathing increases privacy and eliminates need to move the client to central bathing area; therefore it is a more soothing experience than either showering or tub bathing (Perimutter & Camberg, 2004).*
- Bathe cognitively impaired or older adult clients before bedtime. *Bathing a cognitively impaired client in the evening helps improve symptoms of dementia (Deguchi et al, 1999). An evening bath helps older adult clients sleep better (Kanda, Tochihara & Ohnaka, 1999).*
- Provide pain relief measures, such as ice packs, heat, and analgesics for sore joints 45 minutes before bathing; move extremities slowly and carefully; and inform the client before movements associated with pain. These movements include walking; transferring to a new location; moving joints; and washing genitals, face, and between toes and under arms. Have the client wash painful areas, recognize indicators of pain, and apologize for any pain caused. **EBN:** *Pain relief and client participation reduces discomfort, preserves dignity, and gives a sense of control (Rader et al, 2006).*
- Consider environmental and human factors that may limit bathing ability, such as bending to get into the tub, reaching for bathing items, grasping faucets, and lifting oneself. Adapt environment by placing items within easy reach, lowering faucets, and using a hand held shower. *Environmental factors affect task performance. Function can be improved based on engineering principles that adapt environmental factors to the meet the client's capabilities.*
- Use a comfortable padded shower chair with foot support, (or adapt a chair: pad it with towels/washcloths, cover the cold back with dry towels, and cover the arms with foam pipe insulation). **EBN:** *Unpadded shower chairs with large openings and no foot support contribute to pain by allowing clients to sink into the opening with their feet unsupported. The client's feet may become discolored from impaired foot circulation (Rader et al, 2006).*
- Provide privacy. Have only one trusted, consistent caregiver assist with bathing, encourage a traffic-free bathing area, and post privacy signs. *The client perceives less privacy if more than one caregiver participates or if bathing takes place in a central bathing area in a high-traffic location that allows staff to enter freely during care (Calkins, 2005).* **EBN:** *Consistent caregiver allows development of a relationship and understanding of client's bathing wishes and needs (Rader et al, 2006).*
- Ensure bathing assistance preserves client dignity through conveyance of honor and recognition of the deservedness of respect and esteem of all persons, regardless of their dependency and infirmity. **EB:** *Needing assistance with bathing, being hospitalized, and having pain, were among the most significant issues fracturing a sense of the terminally ill client's dignity, which resulted in a higher desire for death and loss of will to live (Chochinov et al, 2002).*
- If the client is bathing alone, place the assistance call light within reach. *A readily available signaling device promotes safety and provides reassurance for the client.*
- Keep the client warmly covered. *Clients, especially older adults or terminally ill clients who are prone to hypothermia, may experience evaporative cooling during and after bathing, which produces an unpleasant cold sensation.*
- For cognitively impaired clients, avoid upsetting factors associated with bathing: instead of using the terms *bath, shower,* or *wash,* use comforting words, such as *warm, relaxing,* or *massage.* Start at the client's feet and bathe upward; bathe the face last after washing hands and using a clean cloth. Use a beautician/barber or wash hair at another time to avoid water dripping in the face. **EBN:** *Some words are associated with unpleasant bathing experiences, whereas others convey a pleasant bathing experience. Starting with the face or hair is distressing, because water drips on the face and the head becomes cold and wet (Rader et al, 2006).*
- Use towel bathing especially when other forms of bathing are distressing to client. Bathe client in bed using no-rinse soap, a bath blanket, and warm towels to keep the client covered the entire time. Warm and moisten towels/washcloths with no rinse soap and place in plastic bags to keep

S

them warm. Use warm, moist towels to massage large areas (front, back) and one washcloth for facial areas and another one for genital areas. No rinsing or drying is needed. **EBN:** *Towel bathing is a gentle experience, reducing aggression and bathing time (Hoeffer et al, 2006).* **EBN:** *Using nondetergent, no-rinse cleansers reduces skin tears, bathing time, and skin dryness without compromising hygiene (Burch & Coggins, 2003).*

- For shower bathing, use client-centered techniques: allow client to have choices, keep client covered with towels and cleanse under the towels, use no-rinse products, use favorite bathing items, and use a hand-held shower with adjustable spray. **EBN:** *Covering the client is an easy means to maintain dignity, reduce embarrassment, and keep the client warm and unexposed without increasing bathing time (Rader et al, 2006). Use of sensory channels to stimulate memory with favorite items may help foster understanding of bathing and self-care.*
- Allow the client to participate as able in bathing. Smile and provide praise for accomplishments in a relaxed manner. **EB:** *Improved communication decreases aggression during bathing and individualizes care (Perimutter & Camberg, 2004).*
- Inspect skin condition during bathing. *Towel bathing facilitates inspection of skin to detect skin problems.*

Geriatric

- Assess for grieving resulting from loss of function. *Grief resulting from loss of function can inhibit relearning of self-care.*
- Develop the client's muscle strength building plan through exercising and walking to build the client's physiological capacity and prevent decline in ADLs. **EB:** *Maintaining independence in ADLs is vital to a sense of dignity and autonomy (Taylor et al, 2003).*
- Emphasize how the client experiences the bathing setting with a secondary focus on ways the environment can support the caregiver. *Recognizing and supporting cognitive, emotional, psychological, spiritual, and physical needs of individuals should be reflected in spaces where the most personal care—such as bathing—is provided, which demonstrates the quality of a care setting (Calkins, 2005).*
- ▲ Design the bathing environment for comfort: *Visual.* Reduce clutter and use partitions to hide equipment storage. Laminate and put artwork or decorative objects in bather's view, or place cue cards to bathing process (wall, ceiling, shower). Stand or sit in bather's position to experience what he/she sees. Decrease glare from tiles, white walls, and artificial lights. Use contrasting colors and soft but adequate lighting on a dimming switch for adjustment. *Bathing rooms are sterile, institutional, and frightening spaces filled with unfamiliar equipment—tubs with sides that open up and look like they might swallow you, or gurneys with arms that look like construction cranes. Overhead lights can be bright and shine into the bather's eyes. Glare can cause visual discomfort, especially in clients with visual changes or cataracts (Calkins, 2005).*
- Arrange the bathing environment to promote sensory comfort: *Auditory.* Reduce noise of voices and water. Do not allow traffic into bathing room. Add fabric to absorb sound (three to four times the width of the opening for sound absorbing folds). Play soft music. *Noise discomfort can result from high-echo tiled walls, loud voices, and running water. Traffic can compromise privacy. Absorb negative sounds, and add positive sounds through music (Calkins, 2005).*
- Design the bathing environment for comfort: *Tactile.* Use heat lamps or radiant heat panels to keep the room warm. Use powder-coated grab bars in decorative colors with nonslip grip. Provide a soft rug to stand on. Ensure that flooring is not slippery (a high coefficient of friction, ideally above 80, is desired and obtained through flooring coatings). *If the caregiver is warm to the point of sweating, room temperature is about right for an older person being bathed. Appealing, stable grab bars are needed for balance. Preventing the floor from becoming slippery from water is essential (Calkins, 2005).*
- When bathing a cognitively impaired client, have all bathing items ready for the client's needs before bathing begins. *Injury often occurs when a cognitively impaired client is left alone while forgotten items are obtained.*
- Teach caregivers to use behaviors that validate the client's feelings, reassure the client, and segment tasks. Teach them to explain the care process while bathing clients with Alzheimer's disease. **EBN:** *Caregivers should work to make bathing more therapeutic for individuals with Alzheimer's disease (Somboontanont et al, 2004).*

S

- Train caregivers bathing clients with dementia to avoid behaviors that can trigger assault: confrontational communication, invalidation of the resident's feelings, failure to prepare a resident for a task, initiating shower spray or touch during bathing without verbal prompts beforehand, washing the hair/face, speaking disrespectfully to the client, and hurrying the pace of the bath. **EBN:** *During bathing, assaults (defensive behavior) by nursing home residents with dementia are frequently triggered by caregiver actions that startle, frighten, hurt, or upset the resident. This might happen when caregivers spray water on a resident without warning or when they touch a resident's feet, axilla, or perineum, possibly due to the startle reflex (Somboontanont et al, 2004).*
- Limit total body bathing using tepid water to once a week; provide a towel bath at other times. **EBN**: *Frequent bathing and using hot water promotes skin dryness (Rader et al, 2006).*
- Test water temperature before use with a thermometer. *With assistive bathing, temperature changes are not felt by the person controlling them (Fathers, 2004).*
- Use a gentle touch when bathing a client; avoid vigorous scrubbing motions. *Aging skin is thinner, more fragile, and less able to withstand mechanical friction than younger skin.*
- Teach caregiver to use gentle massage for frail older adult clients during bathing. *Gentle massage is desired by clients to reduce pain or agitation (Perlmutter & Camberg, 2004).*
- Add hydrating bath oils to tub bath water 15 minutes after the client immerses in water. *If bath oil is placed in the water before the client's skin is moistened, the skin is coated with oil rather than being hydrated.*
- Allow the client or caregiver adequate time to complete the bathing activity. *Significant aging increases the time required to complete a task; therefore older persons with a self-care deficit require more time to complete a task and do so comfortably.*

 Home Care

- If in a typical bathing setting for the client, assess the client's ability to bathe self via direct observation using physical performance tests for ADLs. *Observation of bathing performed in an atypical bathing setting may result in false data. Use of a physical performance test compensates to provide more accurate ability data.*
- ▲ Request referrals for occupational and physical therapy if client has difficulty showering or getting into a tub. **EBN:** *Interdisciplinary team member's assessment of a client's functional abilities increases the client's mastery of self-care tasks by identifying aids, such as grab bars or bath seat, that allow client to participate in the task more easily (Rader et al, 2006).*
- ▲ Based on functional assessment and rehabilitation capacity, refer for home health aide services to assist with bathing and hygiene. *Support by home health aides preserves the energy of the client and provides respite for caregivers.*
- Recommend use of a water temperature–sensing shower valve to prevent scalding. *Older or disabled people have slower reflexes to respond to hot water and may be unable to regulate water temperature. Yet they may be left unattended. Water at 130° F takes 20 seconds to produce a first-degree burn; at 135°-140° F, exposure for 5-6 seconds causes third-degree burns (Fathers, 2004).*
- Turn down temperature of hot water heater. **EBN:** *Prevent accidental scalding by reducing the thermostat on the water heater (Gerdner, Buckwalter & Reed 2002).*
- Show caregiver a videotape of caregiver self-care activities (organizing the day, talking when frustrated, taking time for self, and talking to a nonjudgmental person) followed by a discussion. **EBN:** *Videotape intervention and discussion can model self-care activities and buffer caregiver stress (Clark & Lester, 2000).*
- Cue cognitively impaired clients in the steps of hygiene. *Cognitively impaired clients can successfully participate in many activities with cueing, and participation in self-care can enhance their self-esteem.*
- Respect the preference of terminally ill clients to refuse or limit hygiene care. *Maintaining hygiene, even with assistance, may require excessive energy demands from terminally ill clients. Pain from touch or movement may be intractable and unresolved by medication.*
- If a terminally ill client requests hygiene care, make an extra effort to meet the request and provide care when the client and family will most benefit (e.g., before visitors arrive, at bedtime, in the early morning). *When desired, improved hygiene greatly boosts the morale of terminally ill clients.*

S

• = Independent;   ▲ = Collaborative;   EBN = Evidence-Based Nursing;   EB = Evidence-Based

Client/Family Teaching

- Teach the client and family how to use adaptive devices for bathing (e.g., long-handled brushes, soap-on-a-rope, washcloth mitt, wall bars, tub bench, padded shower chair, commode chair without pan), and teach bathing techniques that promote safety and prevent burns (e.g., getting into tub before filling it with water if a temperature sensor valve is used; testing water with a thermometer; emptying water before getting out; using an antislip mat, wall-grab bars, and tub bench). *Adaptive devices can provide independence, safety, and speed. Burns can be prevented with the use of water temperature-sensor valve (Fathers, 2004).* **EB:** *Follow-up teaching in the home increases device use and safety of bathing (Chiu & Man, 2004).*
- Teach the client and family an individualized bathing routine that includes a frequency schedule, privacy, skin inspection, no-rinse products, skin lubricants, chill prevention, and bathing options, such as sponge or towel. **EBN:** *Families and caregivers who are taught methods to meet the client's bathing needs can increase the client's satisfaction with the bathing experience in a quicker, easier, and less anxious manner (Rader et al, 2006).*

evolve See the EVOLVE website for World Wide Web resources for client education.

REFERENCES

Burch S, Coggins T: No rinse, one step bed bath: the effects on the occurrence of skin tears in a long-term care setting, *Ostomy Wound Manage* 49(1):64, 2003.

Calkins M: Designing bathing rooms that comfort, *Nurs Homes* 54(1):54-55, 2005.

Chiu C, Man D: The effect of training older adults with stroke to use home-based assistive devices, *OTJR* 24(3):113-120, 2004.

Chochinov H, Hack T, Hassard T et al: Dignity in the terminally ill: a cross-sectional, cohort study, *Lancet* 360(9350):2026-2030, 2002.

Clark M, Lester J: The effect of video-based interventions on self-care, *West J Nurs Res* 22(8):895, 2000.

Deguchi A, Nakamura S, Yoneyama S et al: Improving symptoms of senile dementia by a night time spa bathing, *Arch Gerontol Geriatr* 29(3):267, 1999.

Fathers B: Bathing safety for the elderly and disabled, *Nurs Homes* 53(9):50-52, 2004.

Gerdner LA, Buckwalter KC, Reed D: Impact of a psychoeducational intervention on caregiver response to behavioral problems, *Nurs Res* 51(6):363, 2002.

Hoeffer B, Amann Talerico K, Rasin J et al: Assisting cognitively impaired nursing home residents with bathing: effects of two bathing interventions on caregiving, *Gerontologist* 46(4):524-532, 2006.

Kanda K, Tochihara Y, Ohnaka T: Bathing before sleep in the young and in the elderly, *Eur J Appl Physiol* 80:71, 1999.

Perimutter J, Camberg L: Better bathing for residents with Alzheimer's, *Nurs Homes* 53(4):40-42, 2004.

Rader J, Barrick AL, Hoeffer B et al: The bathing of older adults with dementia: easing the unnecessarily unpleasant aspects of assisted bathing, *Am J Nurs* 106(4):4-49, 2006.

Rasin J, Barrick AL: Bathing patients with dementia, *Am J Nurs* 104(3):30-34, 2004.

Somboontanont W, Sloane P, Floyd F et al: Assaultive behavior in Alzheimer's disease: identifying immediate antecedents during bathing, *J Gerontol Nurs* 30(9):22-29, 2004.

Taylor L, Whittington F, Hollingsworth C et al: A comparison of functional outcomes following a physical activity intervention for frail older adults in personal care homes, *J Geriatr Phys Ther* 26(1):7-11, 2003.

S

Dressing/grooming Self-care deficit   Linda S. Williams, MSN, RNBC

NANDA   **Definition**

Impaired ability to perform or complete dressing and grooming activities for self

Defining Characteristics

Inability to choose clothing; inability to put clothing on lower body; inability to maintain appearance at a satisfactory level; inability to pick up clothing; inability to put clothing on upper body; inability to put on shoes; inability to put on socks; inability to remove clothes; inability to use assistive devices; inability to use zippers; impaired ability to fasten clothing; impaired ability to obtain clothing; impaired ability to put on necessary items of clothing; impaired ability to take off necessary items of clothing

• = Independent;   ▲ = Collaborative;   EBN = Evidence-Based Nursing;   EB = Evidence-Based

Related Factors (r/t)

Cognitive impairment; decreased motivation; discomfort; environmental barriers; fatigue; musculo-skeletal impairment; neuromuscular impairment; pain perceptual impairment; severe anxiety; weakness

NOTE: Specify level of independence using a standardized functional scale.

NOC Outcomes (Nursing Outcomes Classification)

Suggested NOC Outcomes

Self-Care: Activities of Daily Living (ADL), Dressing, Hygiene, Grooming

Example NOC Outcome with Indicators
Self-Care: Dressing as evidenced by the following indicators: Gets clothing from drawer and closet/Puts clothing on upper body and lower body (Rate outcome and indicators of **Self-Care: Dressing:** 1 = severely compromised, 2 = substantially compromised, 3 = moderately compromised, 4 = mildly compromised, 5 = not compromised [see Section I].)

Client Outcomes

Client Will (Specify Time Frame):

• Dress and groom self to optimal potential
• Use adaptive devices to dress and groom
• Explain and use methods to enhance strengths during dressing and grooming
• Dress and groom with assistance of caregiver as needed

NIC Interventions (Nursing Interventions Classification)

Suggested NIC Interventions

Self-Care Assistance: Dressing/Grooming

Example NIC Activities—Self-Care Assistance: Dressing/Grooming
Be available for assistance in dressing, as necessary; Reinforce efforts to dress self; Maintain privacy while the patient is dressing

Nursing Interventions and *Rationales*

S

• Observe the client's ability to dress and groom self through direct observation and from the client/caregiver report, noting specific deficits and their causes. **EB:** *Presence of a chronic disease alters dressing routines, and understanding these routines can allow development of energy conservation methods for dressing to increase activity tolerance and promote self-care (Poole & Cordova, 2004).* **EB:** *Older adults with cerebral palsy often lost the ability to dress themselves, whereas other skill performance remained (Strauss et al, 2004).*
• Assess client for symptoms of general weakness, arm paralysis, and fatigue for planning methods to promote self-care in dressing. **EB:** *General weakness, arm paralysis, and fatigue were reported to be main causes of being unable to dress oneself (Leveille, Fried & Guralnik, 2002).*
• Determine the client's personal preferences for dressing and grooming to maintain autonomy, personal routine, and quality of life of older client by using the Self-maintenance Habits and Preferences in Elderly (SHAPE) questionnaire and focus on items most preferred by the client. **EB:** *The SHAPE questionnaire measures a client's customary daily routines to plan for personal preferences in dressing and grooming. It is used to assist the client with self-care through continuity of client's past and present practices (Cohen-Mansfield & Jensen 2007).*
• Encourage older clients to dress and groom rather than completing the tasks for them. *Performing self-care helps maintain independence and prevents functional decline, which is a common complication of hospitalization for older adults (Graf, 2006).*

• = Independent; ▲ = Collaborative; EBN = Evidence-Based Nursing; EB = Evidence-Based

- Consider and remove environmental barriers and human factors that may limit dressing/grooming ability, such as having to reach for clothes or grooming aids in closets or drawers. Help the client arrange clothing and grooming devices within easy reach. Installing turntables, closet rods, or drawers between eye and hip level is helpful. **EB:** *Reducing barriers to improve client's capabilities can improve function (Stark, 2004).*
- Ask the client for input on clothing choices and how to increase the ease of dressing. **EB:** *The physical and sociocultural environments of nursing homes created more obstacles for older residents to overcome to participate in their care than if they had remained in their homes (Sacco-Peterson & Borell, 2004).*
- ▲ Request referrals for occupational and physical therapy. **EB:** *Clients with a stroke who had occupational therapy regained more independence in ADLs over 8 weeks than those that did not have therapy (Landi et al, 2006).*
- ▲ Provide medication for pain 45 minutes before dressing and grooming as needed. *Upper and lower extremity pain symptoms were the most commonly reported causes of difficulty with dressing, so relieving pain can promote participation in self-care (Leveille, Fried & Guralnik, 2002).*
- Provide privacy and limit the number of people/caregivers in the room. **EBN:** *Privacy conveys respect and increases dressing ability (Beck et al, 1997).*
- Select clothing in larger sizes; clothing with elastic waistbands, wide sleeves, and pant legs; dresses that open down the back (for wheelchair-bound women), and clothing with Velcro fasteners or larger buttons. *Simplifying clothing facilitates dressing for those with impaired mobility.*
- Use adaptive dressing and grooming equipment as needed (e.g., long-handled brushes, grasping devices, Velcro closures, zipper pulls, button hooks, elastic shoelaces, large buttons, soap-on-a-rope, suction holders). *Adaptive devices increase self-care and safety, and decrease exertion.*
- Lay clothing out in the order that it will be put on by the client. Dress bottom half, then top half of body. **EBN:** *Simplifying dressing tasks increases self-care ability (Beck et al, 1997).*
- Encourage the client to dress appropriately for time of day. Perform dressing and grooming activities in a consistent sequence each day. *An established routine of waking and dressing provides a sense of normalcy and increases motivation to perform self-care.*
- Teach caregivers to see dressing as an opportunity to promote independence for clients who are able and as a time to increase social talk for others. **EB:** *The dressing process should not be viewed as a race for efficiency but rather a time for social interaction that reduces isolation and loneliness by allowing residents to experience social contact, exercise, and independence (Cohen-Mansfield et al, 2006).*
- Teach Certified Nursing Assistants to use graduated verbal prompting for clients with dementia to complete dressing task and provide positive reinforcement immediately for accomplished steps of task. **EB:** *Client independence in dressing increased and range of motion improved when CNAs were taught to use graduated verbal prompting to allow client to participate in the dressing task (Engleman, Mathews & Altus, 2002).*
- For clients with dementia, maintain a specific routine for dressing to prevent increase in dressing time required. **EBN:** *Stage of dementia does not affect time required for dressing or undressing, unless caregivers failed to keep to a specific routine (Kobayashi & Yamamoto, 2004).*
- Encourage participation; guide the client's hand through task if necessary. **EBN:** *Experiencing the normal process of a task through guided practice facilitates optimal relearning (Beck et al, 1997).*
- If the client does not groom self, sit side by side with the client, put your hand over the client's hand, support the client's elbow with your other hand, and help the client comb his or her hair. *This technique increases client mobility, range of motion, and independence (Pedretti, 1996).*
- Nurture personal attributes, such as humor, positive attitude, faith, and hope, and control of stress for clients with multiple sclerosis. **EBN:** *For those with multiple sclerosis, personal attributes intervene between emotional distress and ADL functioning by decreasing a stress appraisal response (Gulick, 2001).*
- Allow clients with a spinal cord injury to maximize control over activities and teach them how to direct their caregivers. **EB:** *Those with a spinal cord injury who were responsible for directing their caregivers felt more self-control, reported greater satisfaction with care and life, had better physical health, and had fewer social handicaps (Chase, Cornille & English, 2000).*
- If the client has had a cerebrovascular accident (CVA) with hemiparesis, consider use of constraint-induced movement therapy (CIMT), where the functional extremity is purposely

constrained and the client is forced to use the involved extremity. *Constraint therapy is estimated to benefit about half of people who had a CVA (Barker, 2005).* **EB:** *The plasticity of the brain allows it to rewire and reroute neural connections to take up the work of the injured area of the brain (National Institute of Neurological Disorders and Stroke, 2005).*

Geriatric

- Assess for grieving resulting from loss of function. *Grief resulting from loss of function can inhibit relearning of self-care tasks.*
- ▲ Provide medication for pain if needed, and plan activities to prevent fatigue before dressing/grooming. **EBN:** *Level of functioning is increased for older adults with chronic medical conditions if pain and fatigue are controlled (Bennett et al, 2002).*
- Assess tasks the client can complete, noting areas of independence and difficulty to make adaptations. **EBN:** *Some steps of a task can be performed independently, but certain dressing tasks are reported as most difficult: tying shoelaces, fastening pants, and buttoning shirts; difficult grooming tasks are applying toothpaste and combing hair at the top and back of the head (Johnson et al, 1992).*
- Allow the client or caregiver adequate time to complete dressing (e.g., do not insist that the client is dressed at an early hour). *Significant aging increases the time required to complete a task; older adult clients with a self-care deficit require more time than others to complete a task.*
- ▲ Request referral for older women with cardiac disease to rehabilitation programs for strength training. *Older women with coronary heart disease demonstrated that an intense resistance-training program improved their performance with dressing and other daily activities (Ades et al, 2003).*

Home Care

- Involve the client in planning of informal care and provide access to health professionals and financial support for the care. **EBN:** *This study demonstrated that to maintain self-care in dressing/grooming it is important to have continuity between past and present practices. The staff needs to be aware of and sensitive to an individual's preferences and prior routines (Cohen-Mansfield & Jensen, 2007).*
- ▲ Based on functional assessment and rehabilitation capacity, refer for home health services for rehabilitation and to assist with dressing and grooming. **EB:** *Rehabilitative care results in greater functional abilities, a greater likelihood of being able to remain in the home, fewer emergency room visits, and shorter home care (Tinetti et al, 2002).*
- Have caregivers view a videotape showing caregiver self-care activities (organizing the day, talking when frustrated, taking time for self, and talking to a nonjudgmental person) followed by a discussion. **EBN:** *Videotape intervention and discussion can model self-care activities and buffer caregiver stress (Clark & Lester, 2000).*
- Cue cognitively impaired clients in steps of dressing and grooming. *Cognitively impaired clients can participate successfully in many activities with cueing, and participation in self-care can enhance their self-esteem.*
- Respect the preference of the terminally ill client to refuse dressing and limit grooming. *Dressing and grooming, even with assistance, may require excessive energy from the terminally ill. Pain when touched or moved may be intractable and unresolved by medication.*
- If terminally ill clients request dressing and grooming, make an extra effort to meet the request and provide care when the client and family will most benefit (e.g., before visitors, in early morning). *When desired, dressing and grooming are a great boost to the morale of terminally ill clients and their families.*
- Maintain the temperature of the home at a comfortable level when dressing a terminally ill client. *Terminally ill clients may have difficulty with thermoregulation, which will add to the energy demand or decrease comfort during hygiene activities.*

Client/Family Teaching

- Teach the client to dress the affected side first, then the unaffected side. *Dressing the affected side first allows for easier manipulation of clothing.*
- Teach the simplest step in a task until mastered, and then proceed to more complicated steps. Give praise. **EBN:** *Simplifying dressing and grooming tasks that consist of many small steps promotes mastery (Beck et al, 1997).*

• = Independent;   ▲ = Collaborative;   EBN = Evidence-Based Nursing;   EB = Evidence-Based

- Teach the client how to use adaptive devices for dressing and grooming. *Adaptive devices can provide independence and safety and promote speed (Ryan & Cole, 2003).*

evolve   See the EVOLVE website for World Wide Web resources for client education.

REFERENCES

Ades P, Savage P, Cress M et al: Resistance training on physical performance in disabled older female cardiac patients, *Med Sci Sports Exerc* 35(8):1265-1270, 2003.

Barker E: New hope for stroke patients, *RN* 68(2):38, 2005.

Beck C, Heacock P, Mercer SO et al: Improving dressing behavior in cognitively impaired nursing home residents, *Nurs Res* 46(3):126, 1997.

Bennett JA, Stewart AL, Kayser-Jones J et al: The mediating effect of pain and fatigue on level of functioning in older adults, *Nurs Res* 51(4):254, 2002.

Chase B, Cornille T, English R: Life satisfaction among persons with spinal cord injuries, *J Rehabil* 66(3):14-20, 2000.

Clark M, Lester J: The effect of video-based interventions on self-care, *West J Nurs Res* 22(8):895, 2000.

Cohen-Mansfield J, Creedon MA, Malone T et al: Dressing of cognitively impaired nursing home residents: description and analysis, *Gerontologist* 46(1):89-96, 2006.

Cohen-Mansfield J, Jensen B: Dressing and grooming: preferences of community-dwelling older adults, *J Gerontol Nurs* 33(2):31-39, 2007.

Engleman K, Mathews R, Altus D: Restoring dressing independence in persons with Alzheimer's disease: a pilot study, *Am J Alzheimers Dis Other Demen* 17(1):37-43, 2002.

Graf C: Functional decline in hospitalized older adults, *Am J Nurs* 106(1):58-67, 2006.

Gulick E: Emotional distress and activities of daily living functioning in persons with multiple sclerosis, *Nurs Res* 50(3):147, 2001.

Johnson PA, Stone MA, Larson AM et al: Applying nursing diagnosis and nursing process to activities of daily living and mobility, *Geriatric Nurs* 13:25, 1992.

Kobayashi N, Yamamoto M: Impact of the stage of dementia on the time required for bathing-related care: a pilot study in a Japanese nursing home, *Int J Nurs Stud* 41(7):767-774, 2004.

Landi F, Cesari M, Onder G et al: Effects of an occupational therapy program on functional outcomes in older stroke patients, *Gerontology* 52(2):85-91, 2006.

Leveille SG, Fried L, Guralnik JM: Disabling symptoms: what do older women report? *J Gen Intern Med* 17(10): 766-773, 2002.

National Institute of Neurological Disorders and Stroke: *Stroke: hope through research,* available at http://www.ninds.nih.gov/disorders/stroke/stroke.htm. Accessed April 24, 2007.

Pedretti LW: *Occupational therapy: practice skills for physical dysfunction,* ed 4, St Louis, 1996, Mosby.

Poole J, Cordova J: Dressing routines in women with chronic disease: a pilot study, *N Z J Occup Ther* 51(1):30-35, 2004.

Ryan L, Cole M: Reaching your goals: low-tech patient aids can make all the difference in performing daily activities, *Rehab Manag* 16(7):42, 44-46, 2003.

Sacco-Peterson M, Borell L: Struggles for autonomy in self-care: the impact of the physical and socio-cultural environment in a long-term care setting, *Scand J Caring Sci* 18(4):376-386, 2004.

Stark S: Removing environmental barriers in the homes of older adults with disabilities improves occupational performance, *OTJR* 24(1):32, 2004.

Strauss D, Ojdana K, Shavelle R et al: Decline in function and life expectancy of older persons with cerebral palsy, *NeuroRehabilitation* 19(1):69-78, 2004.

Tinetti, ME, Baker D, Gallo WT et al: Evaluation of restorative care vs usual care for older adults receiving an acute episode of home care, *JAMA* 287(16):2098-2105, 2002.

Feeding Self-care deficit   *Linda S. Williams, MSN, RNBC*

S

NANDA   **Definition**

Impaired ability to perform or complete feeding activities

Defining Characteristics

Inability to bring food from a receptacle to the mouth; inability to chew food; inability to complete a meal; inability to get food onto utensil; inability to handle utensils; inability to ingest food in a socially acceptable manner; inability to ingest food safely; inability to ingest sufficient food; inability to manipulate food in mouth; inability to open containers; inability to pick up cup or glass; inability to prepare food for ingestion; inability to swallow food; inability to use assistive device

Related Factors (r/t)

Cognitive impairment; decreased motivation; discomfort; environmental barriers; fatigue; musculoskeletal impairment; neuromuscular impairment; pain; perceptual impairment; severe anxiety; weakness

NOTE: Specify level of independence using a standardized functional scale.

• = Independent;   ▲ = Collaborative;   EBN = Evidence-Based Nursing;   EB = Evidence-Based

NOC   Outcomes (Nursing Outcomes Classification)

Suggested NOC Outcomes

Self-Care: Activities of Daily Living (ADL), Eating

Example NOC Outcome with Indicators
Self-Care: Eating as evidenced by the following indicators: Opens containers/Uses utensils/Completes a meal (Rate the outcome and indicators of **Self-Care: Eating**: 1 = severely compromised, 2 = substantially compromised, 3 = moderately compromised, 4 = mildly compromised, 5 = not compromised [see Section I].)

Client Outcomes

Client Will (Specify Time Frame):

• Feed self safely
• State satisfaction with ability to use adaptive devices for feeding
• Use assistance with feeding when necessary (caregiver)

NIC   Interventions (Nursing Interventions Classification)

Suggested NIC Interventions

Self-Care Assistance: Feeding

Example NIC Activities—Self-Care Assistance: Feeding
Provide adaptive devices to facilitate the client's feeding self (e.g., long handles, handle with large circumference, or small strap-on utensils), as needed; Provide frequent cueing and close supervision as appropriate

Nursing Interventions and *Rationales*

• Assess the client's ability to feed self and note specific deficits. *Functional assessment provides ADL task analysis data for matching the client's ability to feed self with caregiver's level of assistance (Van Ort & Phillips, 1995).*
• Ask the client for input on methods to facilitate eating and feeding (e.g., cultural foods, other food and fluid preferences developed during a lifetime), and provide four entrée choices, including ethnic choice. **EBN:** *Using client input on preferences individualizes client care (Evans, Crogan & Schultz, 2005).*
▲ Consult speech-language pathologist for individualized feeding care plans. **EB:** *Speech-language pathologists design feeding plans to feed clients adequate nutrition in a safe, dignified manner (Pelletier, 2004).*
▲ Request referral for occupational and physical therapy; request a dietician. **EB:** *Clients with a stroke who had occupational therapy regained more independence in ADLs over 8 weeks than those that did not have therapy (Landi et al, 2006).*
• Use any necessary adaptive feeding equipment (e.g., rocker knives, plate guards, suction mats, built-up handles on utensils, scoop dishes, large-handled cups). *Adaptive devices increase independence.*
• Before feeding the client with brain trauma or dementia, provide oral hygiene: for dry mouth, give tart or sour foods/fluids before meals; give proteolytic enzymes before meals if thick oral secretions are a problem. **EB:** *Oral hygiene stimulates saliva flow and taste, and tart/sour foods stimulate saliva production (Ramritu et al, 2000).*
• Position the client with brain trauma or dementia for feeding: help the client sit upright with hips and knees flexed, feet supported, trunk and head in midline position, and head slightly flexed with chin down; for an immobilized client in bed, use high Fowler's position and support the head and neck with neck slightly flexed; for a client with unilateral paralysis, tilt the head slightly to unaffected side and rotate the head toward the affected side. **EBN:** *Gravity*

S

• = Independent;   ▲ = Collaborative;   EBN = Evidence-Based Nursing;   EB = Evidence-Based

assists with swallowing, and aspiration is decreased when the client is sitting upright (Ramritu et al, 2000).

- Provide small portions of favorite foods, one entrée at a time, at proper serving temperature, with unnecessary items and utensils removed. **EBN:** *Food intake is increased when the meal appeals to the client and is simplified to avoid distraction for those with brain trauma or dementia (Ramritu et al, 2000).*
- To increase oral intake, use a feeding assistance intervention protocol: individual assistance, proper positioning, dining location preferences, and meal tray substitutions; use graduated prompting to enhance self-feeding ability as needed: (1) social stimulation and encouragement, (2) nonverbal cueing, (3) verbal cueing, (4) physical guidance, and (5) full physical assistance. **EB:** *Individualized nutritional care increased client daily oral intake for 90% of participants when one or both of the feeding assistance intervention protocols was used or the between-meal snack was included (Simmons & Schnelle, 2004).*
- To increase oral intake, include between-meal snacks three times a day alone or if intake is not increased 15% with the feeding assistance intervention protocol (discussed previously) delivered to the client on a movable cart with a variety of food/fluid choices. **EB:** *Individualized nutritional care increased client daily oral intake for 90% of participants when one or both of the feeding assistance intervention protocols was used or the between-meal snack was included (Simmons & Schnelle, 2004).*
- The caregiver should sit beside the client (on the client's unaffected side) at eye level. *Sitting at eye level with the client increases eye contact and promotes a relaxed atmosphere that increases the amount of food consumed (Holzapfel et al, 1996).*
- Presentation of feeding: provide ½-1 teaspoon of solid food or 10-15 mL of liquid at a time; wait until client has swallowed prior food/liquid. **EBN:** *Feeding a small volume is the best practice for clients with brain trauma or dementia (Ramritu et al, 2000).* **EB:** *Feeding large volumes and feeding quickly occurred commonly because caregivers lacked knowledge that this could exacerbate dysphagia and increase the risk of health problems (Pelletier, 2004).*
- Provide the client with a pleasant, quiet meal environment with no distractions. **EBN:** *Food intake is increased when the client can concentrate on eating (Ramritu et al, 2000).*
- Keep the environment free of toileting devices and odors, avoid painful procedures before meals, remove lids from tray, and provide clean utensils for separate courses. *Attention to the aesthetics of feeding increases food intake (Kayser-Jones & Schell, 1997).*
- Do not mix different foods together when assisting the client with eating. *Mixing foods together decreases client dignity and reduces appeal of food, decreasing food intake (Kayser-Jones & Schell, 1997).*
- Encourage the client to keep food on the unaffected side of mouth with a rocking motion to deposit the food, if applicable. **EBN:** *Keeping food away from the affected side of the mouth prevents pocketing of food (Ramritu et al, 2000).*
- Be prepared to intervene if choking occurs; have suction equipment readily available and know the Heimlich maneuver. **EBN:** *Dysphagia increases the risk of choking (Ramritu et al, 2000).*
- For clients with conditions such as Parkinson's disease or myasthenia gravis, ensure that their medications are given so that peak drug action occurs during meal times. **EBN:** *Peak action of medications promotes safety in eating and self-care ability (Ramritu et al, 2000).*
- ▲ Clients who have had a stroke should continue rehabilitation efforts long-term to achieve optimal functioning. **EBN:** *Client improvement may continue 6 months or longer after a stroke (Cavanagh et al, 2002).*
- If client has had a cerebrovascular accident (CVA) with hemiparesis, consider use of constraint-induced movement therapy (CIMT), where the functional extremity is purposely constrained and the client is forced to use the involved extremity. *Constraint therapy is estimated to benefit about half of people who have had a CVA (Barker, 2005).* **EB:** *The plasticity of the brain allows the brain to rewire and reroute neural connections to take up the work of the injured area of the brain (National Institute of Neurological Disorders and Stroke, 2004).*
- If the client does not feed self, sit side by side with the client, put your hand over the client's hand, support the client's elbow with your other hand, and help the client feed self. *This feeding technique increases client mobility, range of motion, and independence, and clients often eat more food (Pedretti, 1996).*
- Provide oral hygiene after every meal and check for pocketing of food. **EB:** *The incidence of pneumonia is reduced when clients receive oral care after every meal (Yoneyama et al, 2002).*

S

● = Independent;   ▲ = Collaborative;   EBN = Evidence-Based Nursing;   EB = Evidence-Based

Geriatric

- Provide nutrition care that honors the individual client and enhances rather than detracts from each client's quality of life. *Principles to guide quality assurance for nutrition in nursing homes include meeting quality-of-life and nutrient needs of clients and implementing processes to provide high-quality nutrition care (Castellanos, 2004).*
- Use aromatherapy to increase appetite and pleasure in eating. *Making food pleasant and home-like helps prevent weight loss and maintains client independence (Pfeiffer et al, 2005).*
- ▲ Implement Hospital Elder Life Program, a model of care to prevent functional and cognitive decline of older persons during hospitalization. *The Hospital Elder Life Program successfully prevents cognitive and functional decline in at-risk older clients (Inouye et al, 2000).*
- ▲ Implement the Wellspring model, which advocates education and empowerment of CNAs to solve problems without direct administrative oversight. **EB:** *Feeding techniques of nursing assistants can be improved with use of the Wellspring model (Stone et al, 2002).*
- ▲ Ensure CNAs know the signs/symptoms of dysphagia, such as choking, coughing, oral/chewing problems, throat clearing, wet voice, gurgling voice, or pneumonia; if any of these are exhibited during feeding, report them promptly. **EB:** *CNAs who were knowledgeable of symptoms and who indicated they would report them did not acknowledge or report symptoms during feeding other than to generally feed clients slower or with smaller volumes (Pelletier, 2004).*
- ▲ Seek CNA input on feeding concerns during discussion of possible actions and share techniques that are beneficial to specific clients. **EB:** *Collaborative communication may result in better feeding practices, because CNAs will feel that their concerns are heard (Pelletier, 2004).*
- ▲ Ensure CNA feeding training includes the need to decrease command statements to clients being fed and instead offer encouraging statements. **EB:** *Improved intake and enjoyment during meals may occur with this type of communication (Pelletier, 2004).*
- ▲ Suggest that CNAs learn 3-5 personal details about their client during the feeding. **EB:** *CNA communication skills while feeding and a client's psychosocial needs may increase by requiring the learning of personal data (Pelletier, 2004).*
- ▲ Provide medication for pain before meals if needed, and plan activities to prevent fatigue before meals. **EBN:** *Level of functioning is increased for older adults with chronic medical conditions if pain and fatigue are controlled (Bennett et al, 2002).*
- Upon admission to long-term care, assess and maintain documentation about eating and nutrition (include weight) for clients who have had a stroke. **EBN:** *Clients who have had a stroke may have multiple nutritional deficits that require early and ongoing assessment to enable appropriate care and promotion of health (Kumlien & Axelsson, 2002).*
- Serve meals family style, with food in serving bowls and an empty plate to be filled by the client. **EBN:** *Institutional practices foster "excess disability," with eating often the first skill to go; serving meals family style rather than on prepared meal plates allows selecting food and portion size, self-serving, passing serving bowls, selecting seconds, and engaging socially. An added benefit is that less staff time is needed to prepare plates (Altus, Engelman & Mathews, 2002).*
- Obtain and incorporate the client's view of the agency's food selection and presentation into agency food service. **EBN:** *Using the FoodEx-LTC, a 44-item questionnaire that measures food and food service satisfaction, can be used to promote the resident's enjoyment and increase nutritional intake of food (Evans & Crogan, 2005).*
- ▲ Ensure adequate staffing at meal times. **EBN:** *Short staffing results in decreased time for feeding, which contributes to reduced nutritional intake (Crogan et al, 2001).*
- Choose soft foods rather than liquids, or use dietary thickeners. *Choking occurs more easily with clear liquids than with solid or soft foods (Ramritu et al, 2000).*
- Assess for intolerance to food texture and, if found, reverse food texture pattern as tolerated, progressing finally to the texture stage of thick liquids. *Clients with dementia lose the ability to tolerate texture-pattern reverses from regular to soft to mechanical soft to mechanical soft with chopped meat to puree to thick liquids. Pocketing of food is seen, along with statements of choking and spitting of food (Boylston et al, 1995).*
- Provide finger foods for clients with Alzheimer's disease and place the food in their hands as needed to cue. **EB:** *Finger foods increase independence and reduce the need for dietary supplements (Jean, 1997).*

S

• = Independent;   ▲ = Collaborative;   EBN = Evidence-Based Nursing;   EB = Evidence-Based

- Provide a dignified assisted dining experience: create a home-like dining room; provide leisurely pace, which allows the client with dentures adequate time to chew; and support choices and independence. **EB:** *Assisted dining can be a dignified experience based on the environment and individualization of feeding (Ruigrok & Sheridan, 2006).*
- Provide emotionally neutral, nonverbal cues to improve table-sitting behavior if the client rises from table early; for example, place a firm hand on the dominant shoulder, indicating that the client should sit. **EBN:** *Wanderers often receive positive social engagement from staff when they leave the table early, so emotionally neutral behavior-extinguishing cues are useful to increase table sitting and food intake (Beattie & Algase, 2002).*

Home Care

- ▲ Based on functional assessment and rehabilitation capacity, refer for home health aide services to assist with feeding. *Support by home health aides preserves the energy of the client and provides respite for caregivers.*
- Cue cognitively impaired clients when feeding them. *Cognitively impaired clients can participate successfully in many activities with cueing. Participation in self-care can enhance the self-esteem of cognitively impaired clients.*
- Respect the preference of terminally ill clients to refuse nutrition or assistance with eating. Refer to the care plans for **Imbalanced Nutrition: less than body requirements** and **Impaired Swallowing.**
- If a terminally ill client requests nutrition, take special care to provide foods and assistive devices that protect the client from aspiration, minimize energy requirements, and meet the client's taste preferences. *Terminally ill clients have altered taste and other sensations, which affect their willingness to eat or to invest time or energy in eating.*

Client/Family Teaching

- Teach the client how to use adaptive devices. *Adaptive devices increase independence.*
- Teach the client with hemianopsia to turn the head so that the plate is in the line of vision. *Compensation for hemianopsia is done by turning the head to place items in the line of vision (Needham, 1993).*
- Teach visually impaired clients to locate foods according to numbers on a clock. *Clients can locate desired foods based on a clock reference.*
- Teach the caregiver feeding techniques that prevent choking (e.g., sitting beside the client on the unaffected side, feeding the client slowly, checking food temperature, providing fluid between bites, establishing a method to communicate readiness for next bite, limiting conversation while chewing). *Caregivers should use techniques during eating to prevent choking.*

evolve   See the EVOLVE website for World Wide Web resources for client education.

REFERENCES

Altus DE, Engelman KK, Mathews RM: Using family-style meals to increase participation and communication in persons with dementia, *J Gerontol Nurs* 28(9):47, 2002.

Barker E: New hope for stroke patients, *RN* 68(2):38, 2005.

Beattie E, Algase D: Improving table-sitting behavior of wanderers, *J Gerontol Nurs* 28(10):6, 2002.

Bennett JA, Stewart AL, Kayser-Jones J et al: The mediating effect of pain and fatigue on level of functioning in older adults, *Nurs Res* 51(4): 254, 2002.

Boylston E, Ryan C, Brown C et al: Increase oral intake in dementia patients by altering food texture, *Am J Alzheimers Dis Other Demen* 10(6):37, 1995.

Castellanos V: Food and nutrition in nursing homes, *Generations* 28(3):65-71, 2004.

Cavanagh S, Hogan K, Fairfax J et al: Assessing cognitive function after stroke using the FIM instrument, *J Neurosci Nurs* 34(2):99, 2002.

Crogan NL, Shultz JA, Adams CE et al: Barriers to nutrition care for nursing home residents, *J Gerontol Nurs* 27(12):25, 2001.

Evans BC, Crogan NL: Using the FoodEx-LTC to assess institutional food service practices through nursing home residents' perspectives on nutrition care, *J Gerontol A Biol Sci Med Sci,* 60(1):125-128, 2005.

Evans BC, Crogan NL, Schultz JA: The meaning of mealtimes: connection to the social world of the nursing home, *J Gerontol Nurs* 31(2):11-17, 2005.

Holzapfel SK, Ramirez RF, Layton MS et al: Feeder position and food and fluid consumed by nursing home residents, *J Gerontol Nurs* 22(4):6, 1996.

Inouye SK, Bogardus, Jr, ST, Baker DI et al: The Hospital Elder Life Program: a model of care to prevent cognitive and functional decline in older hospitalized patients, *J Am Geriatr Soc* 48(12):1697, 2000.

Jean LA: "Finger food menu" restores independence in dining. *Health Care Food Nutr Focus* 14(1):4-6, 1997.

S

• = Independent;   ▲ = Collaborative;   EBN = Evidence-Based Nursing;   EB = Evidence-Based

Kayser-Jones J, Schell E: The mealtime experience of a cognitively impaired elder: ineffective and effective strategies, *J Gerontol Nurs* 23(7):33, 1997.

Kumlien S, Axelsson K: Stroke patients in nursing homes: eating, feeding, nutrition and related care, *J Clin Nurs* 11(4):498, 2002.

Landi F, Cesari M, Onder G et al: Effects of an occupational therapy program on functional outcomes in older stroke patients, *Gerontology* 52(2):85-91, 2006.

National Institute of Neurological Disorders and Stroke: *Stroke: hope through research*, available at www.ninds.nih.gov/disorders/stroke/stroke.htm. Accessed April 24, 2007.

Needham J: *Gerontological nursing: a restorative approach*, Albany, NY, 1993, Delmar.

Pedretti LW: *Occupational therapy: practice skills for physical dysfunction*, ed 4, St Louis, 1996, Mosby.

Pelletier C: What do certified nurse assistants actually know about dysphagia and feeding nursing home residents? *Am J Speech Lang Pathol* 13(2):99-113, 2004.

Pfeiffer NA, Rogers DA, Roseman MR et al: What's new in long-term care dining? *N C Med J* 66(4):287-291, 2005.

Ramritu P, Finlayson K, Mitchell A et al: *Identification and nursing management of dysphagia in individuals with neurological impairment*, Adelaide, South Australia, 2000, The Joanna Briggs Institute for Evidence Based Nursing and Midwifery. Available at http://www.joannabriggs.edu.au, accessed February 4, 2007.

Ruigrok J, Sheridan L: Life enrichment programme; enhanced dining experience, a pilot project, *Int J Health Care Qual Assur Inc Leadersh Health Serv* 19(4-5):420-429, 2006.

Simmons S, Schnelle J: Individualized feeding assistance care for nursing home residents: staffing requirements to implement two interventions, *J Gerontol A Biol Sci Med Sci* 59(9):M966-M973, 2004.

Stone R, Reinhard S, Bowers B et al: *Evaluation of the Wellspring model for improving nursing home quality*, Washington, DC, 2002, The Commonwealth Fund.

Van Ort S, Phillips L: Nursing interventions to promote functional feeding, *J Gerontol Nurs* 21:6, 1995.

Yoneyama T, Yoshida M, Ohrui T et al: Oral care reduces pneumonia in older patients in nursing homes, *J Am Geriatr Soc* 50:430-433, 2002.

Toileting Self-care deficit   *Linda S. Williams, MSN, RNBC*

NANDA   Definition

Impaired ability to perform or complete own toileting activities

Defining Characteristics

Inability to carry out proper toilet hygiene; inability to flush toilet or commode; inability to get to toilet or commode; inability to manipulate clothing for toileting; inability to rise from toilet or commode; inability to sit on toilet or commode

Related Factors (r/t)

Cognitive impairment; decreased motivation; environmental barriers; fatigue; impaired mobility status; impaired transfer ability; musculoskeletal impairment; neuromuscular impairment; pain; perceptual impairment; severe anxiety; weakness

NOC   Outcomes (Nursing Outcomes Classification)

Suggested NOC Outcomes

Self-Care: Activities of Daily Living (ADLs), Toileting

Example NOC Outcome with Indicators
Self-Care: Toileting as evidenced by the following indicators: Responds to full bladder and urge to have a bowel movement in a timely manner/Gets to and from toilet (Rate the outcome and indicators of **Self-Care: Toileting:** 1 = severely compromised, 2 = substantially compromised, 3 = moderately compromised, 4 = mildly compromised, 5 = not compromised [see Section I].)

Client Outcomes

Client Will (Specify Time Frame):

• Remain free of incontinence and impaction with no urine or stool on skin
• State satisfaction with ability to use adaptive devices for toileting
• Explain and use methods to be safe and independent in toileting

• = Independent;   ▲ = Collaborative;   EBN = Evidence-Based Nursing;   EB = Evidence-Based

NIC   Interventions (Nursing Interventions Classification)

Suggested NIC Interventions

Environmental Management, Self-Care Assistance: Toileting

Example NIC Activities—Self-Care Assistance: Toileting
Assist patient to toilet/commode/bedpan/fracture pan/urinal at specified intervals; Institute a toileting schedule, as appropriate

Nursing Interventions and *Rationales*

- Provide privacy. *Lack of privacy may contribute to incontinence (MacDonald & Butler, 2007).*
- Assess ability to toilet; note specific deficits. *Functional assessment provides analysis data for ADL tasks for use in goal and intervention planning (Lekan-Rutledge, 2004).*
- Assess the client's usual bowel and bladder toileting patterns and the terminology used for toileting. *Individuals develop a unique pattern of toileting over time for faster, normal elimination.*
- Observe cause of inability to toilet independently (see Related Factors). Self-care requires multisystem competence. *Restorative program planning is specific to problems that interfere with self-care.*
- Ask the client for input on toileting methods and timing and how to better provide toileting activity assistance. **EBN:** *Client's task performance may be affected by a loss of individual control due to frustration from not being able to anticipate timing of care events, an inability to predict if nurse or client would perform tasks, and perception that nurse permission is necessary before performing a task (Brubaker, 1996).*
- Assess barriers to implementation of a toileting program. **EBN:** *Barriers to successful implementation of toileting programs can include extra physical/cognitive demands on staff, perceived workload increase, lack of value to staff, and lack of incentives (Mather & Bakas, 2002). Additionally, inadequate communication, lack of ownership, belief that incontinence is part of aging, and unwillingness to alter routine affect implementation (Mueller & Cain, 2002).*
- Make assistance call button readily available to the client and answer call light promptly. *To decrease incontinence and promote safety, the client needs rapid access to toileting facilities.*
- Use any necessary assistive toileting equipment (e.g., raised toilet seat, bedside commode, suction mats, spill-proof urinals, support rails next to toilet, toilet safety frames, Sanifems [allows a woman to void standing], fracture bedpans, long-handled toilet paper holders). *Adaptive devices promote independence and safety (Lekan-Rutledge, 2004).*
- If a client's voiding patterns are consistent, place them on an individualized toileting schedule that is documented and allows the client to use the toilet/commode. **EBN:** *Scheduled toileting improves bowel and bladder hygiene, skin care, and client dignity and reduces frustration, agitation, and violence toward staff (Frantz et al, 2003).*
- Develop toileting schedule using clocks, written schedules, or verbal prompting as cues for the client, and provide assistance at scheduled times. **EBN:** *Toileting schedules convey continence is valued, and help maintain continence (Eustice, Roe & Patterson, 2000).*
- Schedule toileting to occur when the defecation urge is strongest or voiding is likely (e.g., in the morning, every 2 hours, after meals, at bedtime). Assist the client until self-care ability increases. *The defecation urge is strongest in the morning or within 1 hour after eating a meal or drinking a warm beverage. Approximately 50–75 mL of urine is produced hourly, and the urge to void occurs when 200 mL has accumulated.* **EBN:** *Medications (e.g., laxatives), briefs, linens, and enema use can be reduced with a scheduled toileting program (Engst et al, 2004).*
- Keep toilet paper and hand-washing items within easy reach of the client. Provide prompt skin care and linen changes after incontinence episodes. *The presence of urine or stool on the skin leads to skin breakdown (Gray, Ratliff & Donovan, 2002).*

Geriatric

- Assess the client's functional ability to manipulate clothing for toileting, and if necessary modify clothing with Velcro fasteners and elastic waists. *For clients with impaired dexterity or weakness,*

S

• = Independent;   ▲ = Collaborative;   EBN = Evidence-Based Nursing;   EB = Evidence-Based

wearing dresses, athletic bottoms, or skirts with a stretch waistband make it easier to use the toilet than wearing clothing with buttons and zippers (Lekan-Rutledge, 2004).

- Monitor clients with dementia for behavioral toileting cues (e.g., pacing, restlessness, fidgeting) and assist with prompt toileting, or use an individualized scheduled toileting for memory-impaired older adults. **EBN:** *An individual toileting schedule helps prevent incontinence in moderately cognitively impaired elders (Jirovec & Templin, 2001).*

▲ Remove barriers to toileting, support client's cultural beliefs, and preserve dignity. **EB:** *The physical and sociocultural environments in long-term care required older clients to overcome greater physical and cognitive challenges to maintain their participation, autonomy, and dignity in toileting than if they were at home (Sacco-Peterson & Borell, 2004; Kincade et al, 2003).*

▲ Include regular exercise and a walking program in plan of care. **EB:** *Regular exercise improves functional abilities in clients in long-term care (de Carvalho & Filho, 2004).*

▲ Assist client (especially frail older clients) to exercise (walk 2 minutes, push wheelchair, sit-stand repetitions) for several minutes every time he or she gets up to toilet. **EBN:** *Trunk function training (strength, range of motion, balance) can increase bed/chair rising abilities (Alexander et al, 2000).*

▲ Implement Hospital Elder Life Program, a model of care to prevent functional and cognitive decline of older persons during hospitalization. **EB:** *The Hospital Elder Life Program successfully prevents cognitive and functional decline in at-risk older clients (Inouye et al, 2000).*

- After hip fracture, focus on hospital-based multidisciplinary interventions and discharge planning. **EBN:** *The inability to recover ADL function, including toileting, 1 year postfracture in older adults can be predicted by the inability to independently walk outdoors before the fracture, so discharge planning should focus on methods to promote functional recovery (Lin & Chang, 2004).*

- Provide a small footstool in front of the toilet or commode. *Elevating the knees above the hips increases intraabdominal pressure, which facilitates elimination in elderly persons with weak abdominal muscles.*

- Avoid the use of indwelling catheters if possible, and use condom catheters in men without dementia. **EB:** *Using a condom catheter rather than an indwelling urinary catheter can reduce infection or death, especially in men without dementia (Saint, Kaufman & Rodgers, 2006).*

 ### Home Care

▲ Request referral for occupational and physical therapy to identify barriers and suggest strategies for safe toileting. **EB:** *A multicomponent intervention targeting modifiable environmental and behavioral factors results in life quality improvements in community-dwelling older people, especially for toileting (Gitlin et al, 2006).*

▲ Based on functional assessment and rehabilitation capacity, refer for home health aide services to assist with toileting. *Support by home health aides preserves the energy of the client and provides respite for caregivers.*

▲ Avoid the use of medications that place undue toileting stress on the client who is terminally ill.

▲ Provide pain medication for terminally ill clients 20-45 minutes before toileting in anticipation of possible pain (e.g., in coordination with a bowel stimulation program). See the care plan for **Constipation.** *Pain from touch or movement may be intractable and not resolved by medication, but medication may decrease the pain enough to allow limited movement and passing of stool.*

▲ Consider use of an indwelling catheter for terminally ill clients in too much pain to move when hygiene and skin integrity are difficult to maintain. *The goal of hospice care is to promote comfort and dignity in the dying process.*

 ### Client/Family Teaching

- Teach the client and family about bladder control and how to toilet the client with adaptive and safety devices. **EBN:** *Older clients want to learn about bladder control (Palmer & Newman, 2006).*

- Have the family install a toilet seat of a contrasting color. **EBN:** *Visualization of the toilet is aided by installing a toilet seat of a contrasting color (Gerdner, Buckwalter & Reed, 2002).*

- Prepare the client for toileting needs by teaching the action of medications, such as diuretics. *Medications that promote elimination require prompt responses to toileting needs.*

- Help the visually impaired client to develop a plan for locating bathrooms in new environments. *Clients with visual impairments may find locating bathrooms in unfamiliar settings difficult.*

 See the EVOLVE website for World Wide Web resources for client education.

• = Independent;   ▲ = Collaborative;   EBN = Evidence-Based Nursing;   EB = Evidence-Based

REFERENCES

Alexander N, Galecki L, Nyquist M et al: Chair and bed rise performance in ADL-impaired congregate housing residents, *J Am Geriatr Soc* 48(5):526-533, 2000.

Brubaker B: Self care in nursing home residents, *J Gerontol Nurs* 22(7):22, 1996.

de Carvalho B, Filho W: Effect of an exercise program on functional performance of institutionalized elderly, *J Rehabil Res Dev* 41(5):659-68, 2004.

Engst C, Chhokar R, Robinson D et al: Implementation of a scheduled toileting program in a long term care facility, *AAOHN J* 52(10):427-435, 2004.

Eustice S, Roe B, Patterson J: Prompted voiding for the management of urinary incontinence in adults, *Cochrane Database Syst Rev* (2): CD002113, 2000

Frantz R, Xakellis G Jr, Harvey P et al: Implementing an incontinence management protocol in long-term care: clinical outcomes and costs, *J Gerontol Nurs* 29(8):46-53, 2003.

Gerdner LA, Buckwalter KC, Reed D: Impact of a psychoeducational intervention on caregiver response to behavioral problems, *Nurs Res* 51(6):363, 2002.

Gitlin LN, Winter K, Dennis MP et al: A randomized trial of a multicomponent home intervention to reduce functional difficulties in older adults, *J Am Geriatr Soc* 54(5):809-816, 2006.

Gray M, Ratliff C, Donovan A: Perineal skin care for the incontinent patient, *Adv Skin Wound Care*, 15:170-179, 2002.

Inouye SK, Bogardus ST Jr, Baker DI et al: The Hospital Elder Life Program: a model of care to prevent cognitive and functional decline in older hospitalized patients, *J Am Geriatr Soc* 48(12):1697, 2000.

Jirovec MM, Templin T: Predicting success using individualized scheduled toileting for memory-impaired elders at home, *Res Nurs Health* 24:1, 2001.

Kincade JE, Boyington AR, Lekan-Rutledge D et al: Bladder management in adult care homes: review of a program in North Carolina, *J Gerontol Nurs* 29(10):30-36, 2003.

Lekan-Rutledge D: Urinary incontinence strategies for frail elderly women, *Urol Nurs* 24(4):281-283, 287-302, 2004.

Lin P, Chang S: Functional recovery among elderly people one year after hip fracture surgery, *J Nurs Res* 12(1):72-82, 2004.

MacDonald CD, Butler L: Silent no more: elderly women's stories of living with urinary incontinence in long-term care, *J Gerontol Nurs* 33(1):14, 2007.

Mather K, Bakas T: Nursing assistants' perceptions of their ability to provide continence care, *Geriatr Nurs* 23(2):76-81, 2002.

Mueller C, Cain H: Comprehensive management of urinary incontinence through quality improvement efforts, *Geriatr Nurs* 23(2):82-87, 2002.

Palmer M, Newman D: Bladder control: educational needs of older adults, *J Gerontol Nurs* 32(1):28-32, 2006.

Sacco-Peterson M, Borell L: Struggles for autonomy in self-care: the impact of the physical and socio-cultural environment in a long-term care setting, *Scand J Caring Sci* 18(4):376-386, 2004.

Saint S, Kaufman S, Rodgers M: Condom versus indwelling urinary catheters: a randomized trial, *J Am Geriatr Soc* 54(7):1055-1061, 2006.

Readiness for enhanced Self-concept   *Gail B. Ladwig, MSN, CHTP, RN*

NANDA   Definition

A pattern of perceptions or ideas about the self that is sufficient for well-being and can be strengthened

Defining Characteristics

Accepts limitations; accepts strengths; actions are congruent with verbal expression; expresses confidence in abilities; expresses satisfaction with body image; expresses satisfaction with personal identity; expresses satisfaction with role performance; expresses satisfaction with sense of worthiness; expresses satisfaction with thoughts about self; expresses willingness to enhance self-concept

Related Factors (r/t)

To be developed.

NOC   Outcomes (Nursing Outcomes Classification)

Suggested NOC Outcome

Self-Esteem

Example NOC Outcome with Indicators
Self-Esteem as evidenced by the following indicators: Verbalizations of self-acceptance/Open communication/ Confidence level/Description of pride in self (Rate the outcome and indicators of **Self-Esteem:** 1 = never positive, 2 = rarely positive, 3 = sometimes positive, 4 = often positive, 5 = consistently positive [see Section I].)

• = Independent;   ▲ = Collaborative;   EBN = Evidence-Based Nursing;   EB = Evidence-Based

S

Client Outcomes

Client Will (Specify Time Frame):

- State willingness to enhance self-concept
- State satisfaction with thoughts about self, sense of worthiness, role performance, body image, and personal identity
- Demonstrate actions that are congruent with expressed feelings and thoughts
- State confidence in abilities
- Accept strengths and limitations

NIC   Interventions (Nursing Interventions Classification)

Suggested NIC Intervention

Self-Esteem Enhancement

Example NIC Activities—Self-Esteem Enhancement
Encourage patient to identify strengths; Assist patient in setting realistic goals to achieve higher self-esteem

Nursing Interventions and *Rationales*

- Assess and support activities that promote self-concept developmentally. **EB:** *High self-esteem is associated with high academic achievement, involvement in sport and physical activity, and development of effective coping and peer pressure resistance skills (King, Vidourek & Davis, 2002).* **EBN:** *Social support, self-esteem, and optimism were all positively related to positive health practices (McNicholas, 2002).*
- ▲ Refer to nutritional and exercise programs to support weight loss **EB:** *Changes in weight using a community wellness center with exercise and nutrition information resulted in body satisfaction and an increase in the physical self-concept scale (Annesi, 2007).*
- ▲ Clients with cancer often use massage therapy as an adjunct treatment. *Safe and effective massage therapy to clients with cancer only is achieved when the client, healthcare providers, and licensed massage therapist (LMT) collaborate effectively (Gecsedi, 2002).*
- ▲ Support establishing a church-based community health promotion programs (CBHPPs) with the following key elements: partnerships, positive health values, availability of services, access to church facilities, community-focused interventions, health behavior change, and supportive social relationships. *CBHPPs, health promotion professionals, and churches can be dynamic partners (Peterson, Atwood & Yates, 2002).*
- ▲ For clients who have had breast surgery and need a prosthesis, provide the appropriate prosthesis before the client leaves the health care facility. *A diagnosis of breast cancer carries enormous implications for the client in terms of physical and psychological health. For this reason, it is vital that nurses respond sensitively to these needs and assist women to cope with the changes in body image and have the appropriate knowledge to fit the soft breast prosthesis (Keeton & McAloon, 2002).*

Pediatric

- ▲ Consider the development of a Healthy Kids mentoring program that has four components: (1) relationship building, (2) self-esteem enhancement, (3) goal setting, and (4) academic assistance (tutoring). Mentors met with students twice each week for 1½ hours each session on school grounds. During each meeting, mentors devoted time to each program component. **EB:** *The Healthy Kids Mentoring Program results indicated students' overall self-esteem, school connectedness, peer connectedness, and family connectedness were significantly higher at posttest than at pretest (King, Vidourek & Davis, 2002). Results of this study suggest that healthy adolescent development includes positive resources from important others (e.g., parents, schools, and communities) (Youngblade et al, 2007).*
- ▲ Assess and provide referrals to mental health professionals for clients with unresolved worries associated with terrorism. **EBN:** *The National Association of Pediatric Nurse Practitioners (NAPNAP) initiated a new national campaign entitled Keep Your Children/Yourself Safe and Secure (KySS). Interventions are urgently needed to assist children and teens in coping with the multitude of stressors related to growing up in today's society (Melnyk et al, 2002).*

• = Independent;   ▲ = Collaborative;   EBN = Evidence-Based Nursing;   EB = Evidence-Based

▲ Provide an alternative school-based program for pregnant and parenting teenagers. **EBN:** *The girls who attended this program developed close relationships with their peers and teachers. Many of them experienced academic success for the first time and reported that pregnancy and impending motherhood motivated them to do better in school (Spear, 2002).*

 ### Geriatric

▲ Encourage clients to consider a Web-based support program when they are in a caregiving situation. **EBN:** *In this study of caregivers of clients with stroke, the caregivers came together and provided support for each other via a Web-based support program (Pierce, Steiner & Govoni, 2004).*

▲ Consider a strength, mobility, balance, and endurance training program. **EB:** *This pilot study indicates that a physical training program may improve functional capacity for institutionalized elderly persons with multiple diagnoses (Rydwik, Frandin & Akner, 2005).*

 ### Multicultural

• Carefully assess each client and allow families to participate in providing care that is acceptable based on the client's cultural beliefs. **EBN:** *The results of this study contribute to the essential knowledge about culturally sensitive nursing practices. An understanding of client suffering that is shaped by traditional cultural values helps nurses communicate empathy in a culturally sensitive manner to facilitate the therapeutic relationship and clinical outcomes (Hsiao et al, 2006).*

• Provide support for health-promoting behaviors and self-concept for clients from diverse cultures. **EBN:** *In this convenience sample, regression analyses demonstrated that the internalization racial identity stage and self-esteem contributed to the variance in health-promoting lifestyles (Johnson, 2002).*

• Refer to the care plans **Disturbed Body image**, **Readiness for enhanced Coping**, **Chronic low Self-esteem**, and **Readiness for enhanced Spiritual well-being.**

 ### Home Care

• Previously discussed interventions may be used in the home care setting.

evolve   See the EVOLVE website for World Wide Web resources for client education.

REFERENCES

Annesi JJ: Relations of changes in exercise self-efficacy, physical self-concept, and body satisfaction with weight changes in obese white and African American women initiating a physical activity program, *Ethn Dis* 17(1):19-22, 2007.

Gecsedi RA: Massage therapy for patients with cancer, *Clin J Oncol Nurs* 6(1):52, 2002.

Hsiao FH, Klimidis S, Minas H et al: Cultural attribution of mental health suffering in Chinese societies: the views of Chinese patients with mental illness and their caregivers, *J Clin Nurs* 15(8):998-1006, 2006.

Johnson RL: The relationships among racial identity, self-esteem, sociodemographics, and health-promoting lifestyles, *Res Theory Nurs Pract* 16(3):193-207, 2002.

Keeton S, McAloon L: The supply and fitting of a temporary breast prosthesis, *Nurs Stand* 16(41):43, 2002.

King K, Vidourek R, Davis B: Increasing self-esteem and school connectedness through a multidimensional mentoring program, *J Sch Health* 72(7):294, 2002.

McNicholas SL: Social support and positive health practices, *West J Nurs Res* 24(7):772, 2002.

Melnyk BM, Feinstein NF, Tuttle J et al: Mental health worries, communication, and needs in the year of the U.S. terrorist attack: national KySS survey findings, *J Pediatr Health Care* 16(5):222, 2002.

Peterson J, Atwood JR, Yates B: Key elements for church-based health promotion programs: outcome-based literature review, *Public Health Nurs* 19(6):401, 2002.

Pierce LL, Steiner V, Govoni AL: Caregivers dealing with stroke pull together and feel connected, *J Neurosci Nurs* 36(1):32-39, 2004.

Rydwik E, Frandin K, Akner G: Physical training in institutionalized elderly people with multiple diagnoses—a controlled pilot study. *Arch Gerontol Geriatr* 40(1):29-44, 2005.

Spear HJ: Reading, writing, and having babies: a nurturing alternative school program, *J Sch Nurs* 18(5):293, 2002.

Youngblade LM, Theokas C, Schulenberg J et al: Risk and promotive factors in families, schools, and communities: a contextual model of positive youth development in adolescence, *Pediatrics* 119(suppl 1): S47-S53, 2007.

S

Chronic low Self-esteem   *Judith R. Gentz, RN, CS, NP*

NANDA   Definition

Long-standing negative self-evaluation/feelings about self or self-capabilities

Defining Characteristics

Dependent on others' opinions; evaluates self as unable to deal with events; exaggerates negative feedback about self; excessively seeks reassurance; expressions of guilt; expressions of shame; frequent lack of success in life events; hesitant to try new things/situations; indecisive; lack of eye contact; nonassertive; overly conforming; passive; rejects positive feedback about self; self-negating verbalization

Related Factors (r/t)

To be developed.

NOC   Outcomes (Nursing Outcomes Classification)

Suggested NOC Outcomes

Self-Esteem

Example NOC Outcome with Indicators
Demonstrates improved **Self-Esteem** as evidenced by the following indicators: Verbalizations of acceptance of self and limitations/Open communication (Rate the outcome and indicators of **Self-Esteem**: 1 = never positive, 2 = rarely positive, 3 = sometimes positive, 4 = often positive, 5 = consistently positive [see Section I].)

Client Outcomes

Client Will (Specify Time Frame):

- Demonstrate improved ability to interact with others (e.g., maintains eye contact, engages in conversation, expresses thoughts/feelings)
- Verbalize increased self-acceptance through positive self-statements about self
- Identify personal strengths, accomplishments, and values
- Identify and work on small, achievable goals
- Improve independent decision-making and problem-solving skills

NIC   Interventions (Nursing Interventions Classification)

Suggested NIC Intervention

Self-Esteem Enhancement

Example NIC Activities—Self-Esteem Enhancement
Encourage patient to identify strengths; Assist in setting realistic goals to achieve higher self-esteem

Nursing Interventions and *Rationales*

- Actively listen to and respect the client. **EBN:** *Listening and nurturing are important aspects of care (George, 2002).*
- Assess the client's environmental and everyday stressors, including physical health concerns and the potential of abusive relationships. **EBN:** *High everyday stress and a history of abuse in relationships are associated with low self-esteem and depressive symptoms (Lutenbacher, 2002).*
- Assess existing strengths and coping abilities, and provide opportunities for their expression and recognition. *Supporting a client's beliefs and self-reflection and helping them cope can affect self-esteem (Räty & Gustaffson, 2006).*

S

• = Independent;   ▲ = Collaborative;   EBN = Evidence-Based Nursing;   EB = Evidence-Based

- Reinforce the personal strengths and positive self-perceptions that a client identifies. **EBN:** *Clients with low self-esteem need to have their existence and value confirmed (Räty & Gustaffson, 2006).*
- Identify client's negative self-assessments. **EBN:** *Body-esteem and self-esteem are significantly related to one another (Limb, 2006).*
- Encourage realistic and achievable goal setting and resources and identify impediments to achievement. **EBN:** *This promotes self-acceptance, which is associated with psychological well-being (Macinnes, 2006).*
- Demonstrate and promote effective communication techniques; spend time with the client. **EBN:** *Presence and caring during communication is important (Sundin, Jansson & Norberg, 2002).*
- Encourage independent decision making by reviewing options and their possible consequences with client. **EBN:** *Decision-making capacity is vital to a sense of autonomy (Hickman, 2004).*
- Assist client to challenge negative perceptions of self and performance. *Reduction in negative thinking will increase self-esteem.*
- Use failure as an opportunity to provide valuable feedback. *This allows clients to change expectations of what would happen given the reality of what did happen (Pierce & Hicks, 2001).*
- Promote maintaining a level of functioning in the community. **EBN:** *Community involvement (volunteering) increased self-esteem among women living in poverty (Messias, DeJong & McLoughlin, 2005).*
- Assist client with evaluating the effect of family and peer group on feelings of self-worth. **EB:** *Self-esteem is related to events that enhance social support and interpersonal relationships (Drew & Mabry, 2004).*
- Support socialization and communication skills. **EBN:** *Social support increases the client's ability to cope with problems (Beebe, 2002).*
- Encourage journal/diary writing as a safe way of expressing emotions. **EBN:** *Journal writing prompts mood elevating activities and reduces reactive depression (Smith, Leenerts & Gajewski, 2003).*

Geriatric

- Support client in identifying and adapting to functional changes. **EBN:** *Changes in physical well-being decrease emotional resources to cope with stress/grief (Talerico, 2003).*
- Use reminiscence therapy to identify patterns of strength and accomplishment. *Identifying strengths and accomplishments counteracts pervasive negativity.*
- Encourage participation in peer group activities. **EBN:** *Withdrawal and social isolation are detrimental to feelings of self-worth (Stuart-Shor et al, 2003).*
- Encourage activities in which a client can support/help others. **EBN:** *Helping others increases self-esteem in older adults (Krause & Shaw, 2000).*

Multicultural

- Assess for the influence of cultural beliefs, norms, and values on the client's sense of self-esteem. **EBN:** *How the client values self may be based on cultural perceptions (Giger & Davidhizar, 2004). Asian-American youths demonstrate lower levels of self-esteem than their non-Asian peers (Rhee, Chang & Rhee, 2003).*
- Assess for evidence of client financial strain. **EB:** *A recent study of Mexican origin individuals showed that financial strain was associated with cognitive self-esteem (Angel et al, 2003).*
- Assess for drug and alcohol use in individuals with low self-esteem. **EB:** *Among Mexican-American female adolescents, poor self-confidence predicts higher levels of alcohol use (Swaim & Wayman, 2004).*
- Validate the client's feelings regarding ethnic or racial identity. **EBN:** *Individuals with strong ethnic affiliation have higher levels of self-esteem than others (Greig, 2003).*

S

Home Care

- Assess a client's immediate support system/family for relationship patterns and content of communication. *Knowledge of client relationships helps the nurse to individualize care.*
- Encourage the client's family to provide support and feedback regarding client value or worth. *The family is a socially significant cultural group that generates behavior, defines roles, and promotes values.*

• = Independent;   ▲ = Collaborative;   EBN = Evidence-Based Nursing;   EB = Evidence-Based

▲ Refer to medical social services to assist the family in pattern changes that could benefit the client. *The best nursing plan may be to access specialty services for the client and family.*

▲ If a client is involved in counseling or self-help groups, monitor and encourage attendance. Help the client identify the value of group participation after each group encounter. *Discussion about group participation clarifies and reinforces group feedback and support.*

▲ If a client is taking prescribed psychotropic medications, assess for knowledge of medication side effects and reasons for taking medication. Teach as necessary. *Understanding the medical regimen supports compliance.*

▲ Assess medications for effectiveness and side effects and monitor client for compliance. *Clients with poor ego strength may have difficulty adhering to a medication regimen. Clients who experience negative side effects are less likely than others to adhere to medication regimen.*

Client/Family Teaching

▲ Refer to community agencies for psychotherapeutic counseling
▲ Refer to psychoeducational groups on stress reduction and coping skills
▲ Refer to self-help support groups specific to needs

 See the EVOLVE website for World Wide Web resources for client education.

REFERENCES

Angel RJ, Frisco M, Angel JL et al: Financial strain and health among elderly Mexican-origin individuals, *J Health Soc Behav* 44(4):536-551, 2003.

Beebe LH: Problems in community living identified by people with schizophrenia, *J Psychosoc Nurs Ment Health Serv* 40(2):38, 2002.

Drew L, Mabry J: Predictors of positive life events: self-esteem and positive affect, *Gerontologist* 44(1):230, 2004.

George TB: Care meanings, expressions and experiences of those with chronic mental illness, *Arch Psychiatr Nurs* 16(1):25, 2002.

Giger JN, Davidhizar RE: *Transcultural nursing; Assessment and Intervention,* ed 4, St Louis, 2004, Mosby Year Book.

Greig R: Ethnic identity development: implications for mental health in African-American and Hispanic adolescents, *Issues Ment Health Nurs* 24(3):317-331, 2003.

Hickman SE: Honoring resident autonomy in long-term care, *J Psychosoc Nurs Ment Health Serv* 42(1):12, 2004.

Krause N, Shaw BA: Giving social support to others: socioeconomic status and self-esteem in late life, *J Gerontol B Psychol Sci Soc Sci* 55(6):S323, 2000.

Limb M: A study investigating the relationships between self-esteem and body-esteem in adult males and females undergoing limb reconstruction procedures, *J Orthop Nurs* 10(1):15, 2006.

Lutenbacher M: Relationships between psychosocial factors and abusive parenting attitudes in low-income single mothers, *Nurs Res* 51(3):158, 2002.

Macinnes DL: Self-esteem and self-acceptance: an examination into

their relationship and their effect on psychological health, *J Psychiatr Ment Health Nurs* 13(5):483, 2006.

Messias D, DeJong M, McLoughlin K: Being involved and making a difference: empowerment and well-being among women living in poverty, *J Holist Nurs* 23:70-88, 2005.

Pierce P, Hicks F: Patient decision-making behavior: an emerging paradigm for nursing science, *Nurs Res* 50(5):267, 2001.

Räty L, Gustaffson B: Emotions in relation to healthcare encounters affecting self-esteem, *J Neurosci Nurs* 38(1):42, 2006.

Rhee S, Chang J, Rhee J: Acculturation, communication patterns, and self-esteem among Asian and Caucasian American adolescents, *Adolescence* 38(152):749-768, 2003.

Smith CE, Leenerts MH, Gajewski BJ: A systematically tested intervention for managing reactive depression, *Nurs Res* 52(6):401, 2003.

Stuart-Shor EM, Buselli EF, Carroll DL et al: Are psychosocial factors associated with the pathogenesis and consequences of cardiovascular disease in the elderly? *J Cardiovasc Nurs* 18(3):169, 2003.

Sundin K, Jansson L, Norberg A: Understanding between care providers and patients with stroke and aphasia: a phenomenological hermeneutic inquiry, *Nurs Inq* 9(2):93, 2002.

Swaim RC, Wayman JC: Multidimensional self-esteem and alcohol use among Mexican American and White non-Latino adolescents: concurrent and prospective effects, *Am J Orthopsychiatry* 74(4):559-570, 2004.

Talerico K: Grief and older adults: differences, issues, and clinical approaches, *J Psychosoc Nurs Ment Health Serv* 41(7):12, 2003.

Situational low Self-esteem *Judith R. Gentz, RN, CS, NP*

NANDA Definition

Development of a negative perception of self-worth in response to a current situation (specify)

Defining Characteristics

Evaluation of self as unable to deal with situations or events; expressions of helplessness; expressions of uselessness; indecisive behavior; nonassertive behavior; self-negating verbalizations; verbally reports current situational challenge to self-worth

• = Independent;   ▲ = Collaborative;   EBN = Evidence-Based Nursing;   EB = Evidence-Based

Related Factors (r/t)

Behavior inconsistent with values; developmental changes; disturbed body image; failures; functional impairment; lack of recognition; loss rejections; social role changes

NOC   Outcomes (Nursing Outcomes Classification)

Suggested NOC Outcomes

Decision Making, Self-Esteem

Example NOC Outcome with Indicators
Demonstrates **Self-Esteem** as evidenced by the following indicators: Verbalizations of acceptance of self and limitations/Open communication (Rate the outcome and indicators of **Self-Esteem:** 1 = never positive, 2 = rarely positive, 3 = sometimes positive, 4 = often positive, 5 = consistently positive [see Section I].)

Client Outcomes

Client Will (Specify Time Frame):

- State effect of life events on feelings about self
- State personal strengths
- Acknowledge presence of guilt and not blame self if an action was related to another person's appraisal
- Seek help when necessary
- Demonstrate self-perceptions are accurate given physical capabilities
- Demonstrate separation of self-perceptions from societal stigmas

NIC   Interventions (Nursing Interventions Classification)

Suggested NIC Interventions

Self-Esteem Enhancement

Example NIC Activities—Self-Esteem Enhancement
Encourage patient to identify strengths; Assist in setting realistic goals to achieve higher self-esteem

Nursing Interventions and *Rationales*

- ▲ Assess the client for signs and symptoms of depression and potential for suicide and/or violence. If present, immediately notify the appropriate personnel of symptoms. See care plans for **Risk for other-directed Violence** and **Risk for Suicide.** *Nursing plays a vital role in assessing safety issues, managing the clients, and supervising other staff (Barloon, 2003).*
- Actively listen to, demonstrate respect for, and accept client. **EBN:** *Encounters between client and caregivers affect the client's emotional status and well being (Räty & Gustafsson, 2006).*
- Assist in the identification of problems and situational factors that contribute to problems, offering options for resolution. **EBN:** *Clients often expect professionals to recommend remedies to problems and need encouragement to participate in selecting treatment options (Pierce & Hicks, 2001).*
- Mutually identify strengths, resources, and previously effective coping strategies. **EBN:** *Knowledgeable clients make better decisions regarding their health care (Pierce & Hicks, 2001).*
- Have client list strengths. **EBN:** *Clients were found to use a variety of self-care strategies, medication management techniques, and emotional supports to alleviate symptoms of chronic heart failure (CHF) (Bennett et al, 2000).*
- Accept client's own pace in working through grief or crisis situations. *Maladjustment to loss or change can have detrimental effects on the entire concept of self (Drench, 1994).*
- Accept the client's own defenses in dealing with the crisis. *Decision-making behaviors adapt and change with time and experience (Pierce & Hicks, 2001).*

S

• = Independent;   ▲ = Collaborative;   EBN = Evidence-Based Nursing;   EB = Evidence-Based

- Assess for unhealthy coping mechanisms, such as substance abuse. *More than 50% of clients with mental illness also have substance abuse, and low self-esteem increases the risk further (NAMI online fact sheet, 2004).*
- Provide information about support groups of people who have common experiences or interests. **EB:** *Social support and healthy interpersonal relationships foster improved mental and physical health (Drew & Mabry, 2004).*
- Teach the client mindfulness techniques to cope more effectively with strong emotional responses. **EBN:** *Development of mindfulness strategies increased resolution of internal conflicts (Horton-Deutsch & Horton, 2003).*
- Support problem-solving strategies but discourage decision making when in crisis. **EBN:** *Uncertainty is a significant negative predictor of resourcefulness (Dirsken, 2000).*
- Assess the client's environmental and everyday stressors, including evidence of abusive relationships. **EBN:** *High everyday stressors and a history of abuse in relationships are associated with low self-esteem and depression (Lutenbacher, 2002).*
- Encourage objective appraisal of self and life events and challenge negative or perfectionist expectations of self. **EB:** *Positive life events improve self-esteem and positive affect (Drew & Mabry, 2004).*
- Provide psychoeducation to client and family. **EBN:** *Knowledge provides empowerment, which will increase self-esteem (Merrell, 2001).*
- Validate confusion when feeling ill but looking well. **EBN:** *Validation of emotions is related to a client's experience of caring (Räty & Gustafsson, 2006).*
- Acknowledge the presence of societal stigma. Teach management tools. **EBN:** *Stigma was reported as a major influence on whether depressed and/or suicidal clients sought treatment (Raingruber, 2002).*
- Validate the effect of negative past experiences on self-esteem and work on corrective measures. *People with low self-esteem have a need to be affirmed regarding their value (Räty & Gustaffson, 2006).*
- See care plan for **Chronic low Self-esteem.**

Geriatric and Multicultural

- See care plan for **Chronic low Self-esteem.**

Home Care

- Establish an emergency plan and contract with the client for its use. *Having an emergency plan is reassuring to the client. Establishing a contract validates the worth of the client and provides a caring link between the client and society.*
- Access supplies that support a client's success at independent living.
- See care plan for **Chronic low Self-esteem.**

Client/Family Teaching

- Assess the person's support system (family, friends, and community) and involve them if desired.
- Educate client and family regarding the grief process. *Understanding this process normalizes responses of sadness, anger, guilt, and helplessness.*
- Teach client and family that the crisis is temporary. *Knowing that the crisis is temporary provides a sense of hope for the future.*
- ▲ Refer to appropriate community resources or crisis intervention centers.
- ▲ Refer to resources for handicap and/or disability services.
- ▲ Refer to illness-specific consumer support groups.
- ▲ Refer to self-help support groups specific to needs.

evolve   See the EVOLVE website for World Wide Web resources for client education.

REFERENCES

Barloon LF: Legal aspects of psychiatric nursing, *Nurs Clin North Am* 38(1):9, 2003.

Bennett SJ, Cordes DK, Westmoreland G et al: Self-care strategies for symptom management in patients with chronic heart failure, *Nurs Res* 49(3):139-145, 2000.

Dirsken SR: Predicting well-being among breast cancer survivors, *J Adv Nurs* 32 (4):937, 2000.

Drench ME: Changes in body image secondary to disease and injury, *Rehabil Nurs* 19:31, 1994.

Drew L, Mabry J: Predictors of positive life events: self-esteem and positive affect, *Gerontologist* 44(1):230, 2004.

Horton-Deutsch S, Horton S: Mindfulness: overcoming intractable conflict, *Arch Psychiatr Nurs* 17(4):186, 2003.

Lutenbacher M: Relationships between psychosocial factors and abu-

• = Independent;   ▲ = Collaborative;   EBN = Evidence-Based Nursing;   EB = Evidence-Based

sive parenting attitudes in low-income single mothers, *Nurs Res* 51(3):158, 2002.

Merrell J: Social support for victims of domestic violence, *J Psychosoc Nurs* 39(11):30, 2001.

NAMI online fact sheet: *Dual disorders and integrated treatment*, available at http://www.nami.org/Content/ContentGroups/E-News/20023/April_20022/NAMI_Submits_Comments_on_Upcoming_SAMHSA_Report_on_Co-Occurring_Mental_Illness_and_Substance_Abuse_D.htm. Accessed April 24, 2007.

Pierce P, Hicks F: Patient decision-making behavior: an emerging paradigm for nursing science, *Nurs Res* 50(5):267, 2001.

Raingruber B: Client and provider perspectives regarding the stigma of and non-stigmatizing interventions for depression, *Arch Psychiatr Nurs* 16(5):201, 2002.

Räty L, Gustafsson B: Emotions in relation to healthcare encounters affecting self-esteem, *J Neurosci Nurs* 38(1):42, 2006.

Risk for situational low Self-esteem   *Judith R. Gentz, RN, CS, NP*

NANDA   Definition

At risk for developing negative perception of self-worth in response to a current situation (specify)

Risk Factors

Behavior inconsistent with values; decreased control over environment; developmental changes; disturbed body image; failures; functional impairment; history of abandonment; history of abuse; history of learned helplessness; history of neglect; lack of recognition; loss; physical illness; rejections; social role changes; unrealistic self-expectations

NOC   Outcomes (Nursing Outcomes Classification)

Suggested NOC Outcomes

Decision Making, Self-Esteem

Example NOC Outcome with Indicators
Demonstrates **Self-Esteem** as evidenced by the following indicators: Verbalizations of self-acceptance/Acceptance of self-limitations/Open communication (Rate the outcome and indicators of **Self-Esteem:** 1 = never positive, 2 = rarely positive, 3 = sometimes positive, 4 = often positive, 5 = consistently positive [see Section I].)

Client Outcomes

Client Will (Specify Time Frame):

- State accurate self-appraisal
- Demonstrate the ability to self-validate
- Demonstrate the ability to make decisions independent of primary peer group
- Express effects of media on self-appraisal
- Express influence of substances on self-esteem
- Identify strengths and healthy coping skills
- State life events and change as influencing self-esteem

NIC   Interventions (Nursing Interventions Classification)

Suggested NIC Intervention

Self-Esteem Enhancement

Example NIC Activities—Self-Esteem Enhancement
Encourage patient to identify strengths; Assist in setting realistic goals to achieve higher self-esteem

S

• = Independent;   ▲ = Collaborative;   EBN = Evidence-Based Nursing;   EB = Evidence-Based

Nursing Interventions and *Rationales*

- Identify environmental and/or developmental factors that increase risk for low self-esteem, especially in children/adolescents, to make needed referrals. **EBN:** *Self-esteem enhancement programs can improve self-esteem in school-age children (Dalgas-Pelish, 2006).*
- Assess the client's previous experiences with health care and coping with illness to determine the level of education and support needed. **EBN:** *Experienced clients report needing a different level of support than inexperienced clients (Edwards et al, 2001).*
- Assess for low and negative affect (expression of feelings). **EBN:** *Self-esteem is more closely associated with affect than self-acceptance is (Macinnes, 2006).*
- Encourage client to maintain highest level of community functioning. **EBN:** *Community volunteerism supports improved self-esteem (Messias, DeJong & McLoughlin, 2005).*
- Treat the client with respect and as an equal to maintain positive self-esteem. **EBN:** *Clients with higher self-esteem need to be confirmed as being equal with care providers (Räty & Gustaffson, 2006).*
- Help the client to identify the resources and social support network available at this time. **EBN:** *Greater resourcefulness positively affects feelings of self-worth (Dirksen, 2000).*
- Assess for unhealthy coping mechanisms, such as substance abuse. *More than 50% of people with mental illness also have substance abuse, and low self-esteem increases the risk further (NAMI online fact sheet, 2004).*
- Encourage the client to find a self-help or therapy group that focuses on self-esteem enhancement. **EBN:** *Group therapy provides a safe place for feeling exploration, validation, positive role models, and gaining knowledge (Merrell, 2001).*
- Teach the client mindfulness techniques to cope with strong emotional responses and to prevent decreases in self-esteem. **EBN:** *Mindfulness strategies increase resolution of internal conflict and promote relaxation (Horton-Deutsch & Horton, 2003).*
- Encourage the client to create a sense of competence through short-term goal setting and goal achievement. **EB:** *Sense of competence is related to global self-esteem (Willoughby et al, 2000).*
- ▲ Assess the client for symptoms of depression and anxiety. Refer to specialist as needed. *Prompt and effective treatment can prevent exacerbation of symptoms or safety risks.*
- Teach client a systematic problem-solving process. *Crisis provides an opportunity for effective change in coping skills.*
- See care plans for **Disturbed personal Identity** and **Situational low Self-esteem.**

Geriatric

- Help the client to identify age-related and/or developmental factors that may be affecting self-esteem. *Self-esteem levels vary with the normal aging process and tend to decrease with older age (Dietz, 1996).*
- Assist the client in life review and identifying positive accomplishments. *Life review is a developmental task that increases a person's sense of peace and serenity.*
- Help client to establish a peer group and structured daily activities. *Social isolation and lack of structure increase a client's sense of feeling lost and worthless.*

Home Care

- Assess current environmental stresses and identify community resources. *Accessing resources to help decrease environmental stress will increase the client's ability to cope.*
- Encourage family members to acknowledge and validate the client's strengths. *Validation allows the client to increase self-reliance and to trust personal decisions.*
- Assess the need for establishing an emergency plan. *Openly assessing safety risks increases the client's sense of limits, boundaries, and safety.*
- See care plans for **Situational low Self-esteem** and **Chronic low Self-esteem.**

Client/Family Teaching

- ▲ Refer the client/family to community-based self-help and support groups.
- ▲ Refer the client to educational classes on stress management, relaxation training, and so on.
- ▲ Refer the client to community agencies that offer support and environmental resources.

 See the EVOLVE website for World Wide Web resources for client education.

• = Independent;   ▲ = Collaborative;   EBN = Evidence-Based Nursing;   EB = Evidence-Based

REFERENCES

Dalgas-Pelish P: Effects of a self-esteem intervention program on school-aged children, *Pediatr Nurs* 32(4):241, 2006.

Dietz BE: The relationship of aging to self-esteem: the relative effects of maturation and role accumulation, *Int J Aging Hum Dev* 3:43, 1996.

Dirkson SR: Predicting well being among breast cancer survivors, *J Adv Nurs* 4:32, 2000.

Edwards J, Mulherin D, Ryan S et al: The experience of patients with rheumatoid arthritis admitted to the hospital, *Arthritis Care Res* 45:1-7, 2001.

Horton-Deutsch S, Horton S: Mindfulness: overcoming intractable conflict, *Arch Psychiatr Nurs* 17(4):186, 2003.

Macinnes DL: Self-esteem and self-acceptance: an examination into their relationship and their effect on psychological health, *J Psychiatr Ment Health Nurs* 13(5):483, 2006.

Merrell J: Social support for victims of domestic violence, *J Psychosoc Nurs Ment Health Serv* 39(11):30, 2001.

Messias D, DeJong M, McLoughlin K: Being involved and making a difference: empowerment and well-being among women living in poverty, *J Holist Nurs* 23(1):66, 2005.

NAMI online fact sheet: *Dual disorders and integrated treatment*, available at http://www.nami.org/Content/ContentGroups/E-News/20023/April_20022/NAMI_Submits_Comments_on_Upcoming_SAMHSA_Report_on_Co-Occurring_Mental_Illness_and_Substance_Abuse_D.htm. Accessed April 24, 2007.

Räty L, Gustaffson B: Emotions in relation to healthcare encounters affecting self-esteem, *J Neurosci Nurs* 38(1):42, 2006.

Willoughby C, Polatajko H, Currado C et al: Measuring the self-esteem of adolescents with mental health problems: theory meets practice, *Can J Occup Ther* 67(4):230, 2000.

Self-mutilation   *Kathleen L. Patusky, PhD, APRN-BC*

NANDA   Definition

Deliberate self-injurious behavior causing tissue damage with the intent of causing nonfatal injury to attain relief of tension

Defining Characteristics

Abrading; biting; constricting a body part; cuts on body; hitting; ingestion of harmful substances; inhalation of harmful substances; insertion of object into body orifice; picking at wounds; scratches on body; self-inflicted burns; severing

Related Factors (r/t)

Adolescence; autistic individual; battered child; borderline personality disorder; character disorder; childhood illness; childhood sexual abuse; childhood surgery; depersonalization; developmentally delayed individual; dissociation; disturbed body image; disturbed interpersonal relationships; eating disorders; emotionally disturbed; family alcoholism; family divorce; family history of self-destructive behaviors; feels threatened with loss of significant relationship; history of inability to plan solutions; history of inability to see long-term consequences; history of self-injurious behavior; impulsivity; inability to express tension verbally; incarceration; ineffective coping; irresistible urge to cut/damage self; isolation from peers; labile behavior; lack of family confidant; living in nontraditional setting (e.g., foster, group institutional care); low self-esteem; mounting tension that is intolerable; needs quick reduction of stress; negative feelings (e.g., depression, rejection, self-hatred, separation anxiety, guilt, depersonalization); peers who self-mutilate; perfectionism; poor communication between parent and adolescent; psychotic state (e.g., command hallucinations); sexual identity crisis; substance abuse; unstable body image; unstable self-esteem; use of manipulation to obtain nurturing relationship with others; violence between parental figures

NOC   Outcomes (Nursing Outcomes Classification)

Suggested NOC Outcomes

Aggression Self-Control, Distorted Thought Self-Control, Impulse Self-Control, Mood Equilibrium, Risk Detection, Self-Mutilation Restraint

Example NOC Outcome with Indicators
Self-Mutilation Restraint as evidenced by the following indicators: Refrains from gathering means for self-injury/Seeks help when feeling urge to injure self/Upholds contract not to harm self/Maintains self-control without supervision/Refrains from injuring self (Rate the outcome and indicators of **Self-Mutilation Restraint:** 1 = never demonstrated, 2 = rarely demonstrated, 3 = sometimes demonstrated, 4 = often demonstrated, 5 = consistently demonstrated [see Section I].)

• = Independent;   ▲ = Collaborative;   EBN = Evidence-Based Nursing;   EB = Evidence-Based

Client Outcomes

Client Will (Specify Time Frame):

- Have injuries treated
- Refrain from further self-injury
- State appropriate ways to cope with increased psychological or physiological tension
- Express feelings
- Seek help when having urges to self-mutilate
- Maintain self-control without supervision
- Use appropriate community agencies when caregivers are unable to attend to emotional needs

NIC Interventions (Nursing Interventions Classification)

Suggested NIC Interventions

Active Listening, Anger Control Assistance, Behavior Management: Self-Harm, Calming Technique, Environmental Management: Safety, Limit Setting, Mood Management, Mutual Goal Setting, Risk Identification, Self-Responsibility Facilitation

Example NIC Activities—Behavior Management: Self-Harm

Anticipate trigger situations that may prompt self-harm and intervene to prevent it; Teach and reinforce patient for effective coping behaviors and appropriate expression of feelings

Nursing Interventions and *Rationales*

NOTE: Before implementation of interventions in the face of self-mutilation, nurses should examine their own emotional responses to incidents of self-harm to ensure that interventions will not be based on countertransference reactions. **EBN:** *Emergency department nurses encountering individuals who self-mutilate showed that nurses may experience negative feelings toward such clients (McAllister et al, 2002).*

▲ Provide medical treatment for injuries. Use careful aseptic technique when caring for wounds. Care for the wounds in a matter-of-fact manner. *A significant impediment to wound healing is infection. A matter-of-fact approach avoids promoting inappropriate attention-getting behavior and may decrease repetition of behavior.*

• Assess for risk of suicide or other self-damaging behaviors. **EB:** *Although self-mutilation should not be viewed simply as failed suicide, it is a significant indicator of suicide risk (Guertin et al, 2001; Milnes, Owens & Blenkiron, 2002). A study of suicide attempters showed that individuals who mutilate themselves are at greater risk for suicide than those who do not (Stanley et al, 2001). They may also engage in other self-damaging behaviors, including substance abuse or eating disorders (Favaro, Ferrara & Santonastaso, 2007).* Refer to the care plan for **Risk for Suicide.**

• Assess for signs of depression, anxiety, and impulsivity. *These behaviors are identified in clients with a history of self-mutilation (Stanley et al, 2001).*

• Assess for presence of hallucinations. Ask specific questions such as, "Do you hear voices that other people do not hear? Are they telling you to hurt yourself?" *Command hallucinations occurring with schizophrenia or brief psychotic episodes may direct the client to hurt himself or herself, or others (Kress, 2003). Acknowledging that the client may hear something that others do not may open up communication and help establish trust. The presence of hallucinations may also indicate use of specific medications (i.e., antipsychotics) that can reduce the hallucinations more effectively than antianxiety medications.*

▲ Assure the client that he or she will not be alone and will be safe during hallucinations. Provide referrals for medication. *Hallucinations can be very frightening; therefore clients need reassurance that they will not be left alone.*

▲ Assess for the presence of medical disorders, mental retardation, medication effects, or psychiatric disorders that may include self-mutilation. Initiate referral for evaluation and treatment as appropriate. **EB:** *Self-mutilation has been reported as a presenting symptom with medical disorders, such as the genetic Lesch–Nyhan syndrome (multiple types of behaviors; Robey et al, 2003); and as a be-*

S

havior initiated or aggravated by medications, such as certain serotonin reuptake inhibitors (skin picking; Denys, van Megen & Westenberg, 2003) or amphetamines (genital mutilation; Israel & Lee, 2002). (Additional relevant research: Myers & Nguyen, 2001; Zafeiriou et al, 2004; Vogel & Anderson, 2002).

▲ Case finding and referral by school nurses for psychological or psychiatric treatment is critical. *Treatment includes starting therapy and medications, increasing coping skills, facilitating decision-making, encouraging positive relationships, and fostering self esteem (McDonald, 2006).*

• Monitor the client's behavior, using 15-minute checks at irregular times so that the client does not notice a pattern. *When lack of control exists, client safety is an important issue and close observation is essential. Avoiding a pattern prevents clients from being self-abusive when they know a care-giver will not be present.*

• Establish trust. *Establishing trust appears to be the most critical component of assessing and treating the client who self-mutilates (Derouin & Bravender, 2004; Machoian, 2001).*

• Recognize that self-mutilation may serve a variety of functions for the person. *Self-mutilation may help with the regulation of dysphoric affect, the expression of emotions, or coping with dissociative states (Paris, 2005).*

• Be extremely cautious about touching the client when he or she is experiencing an abreaction (reenactment of precipitating trauma). Sometimes physically holding a client is necessary to prevent self-injury. *Even well-intentioned or consoling touching may further upset the client. A therapist who is attempting to be consoling should always ask abreacting clients whether they may be touched. Clients may initially refuse, but they generally appreciate the offer (Weber, 2002).*

• Assess the client's ability to enter into a no-suicide contract. Secure a written or verbal contract from the client to notify staff when experiencing the desire to self-mutilate. *Discussing feelings of self-harm with a trusted person provides relief for the client. A contract gets the subject out in the open and places some of the responsibility for safety with the client. Some clients are not appropriate for a contract: those under the influence of drugs or alcohol or unwilling to abstain from substance use, and those who are isolated or alone without assistance to keep the environment safe (Hauenstein, 2002). If the client will not contract, the risk of suicide should be considered higher. The lack of willingness for self-disclosure has been shown to discriminate the serious suicide attempter from clients with suicidal ideation or mild attempts (Apter et al, 2001).* **EBN:** *Contracting is a common practice in the psychiatric care setting. Self-harm is not prevented by contracts (Drew, 2001).*

▲ Use a collaborative approach for care. *A collaborative approach to care is more helpful to the client.*

▲ Refer for medication, such as clozapine. **EB:** *In a study of seven subjects known to have a personality disorder and severe self-mutilation, there was a statistically significant reduction in incidents of self-mutilation with the use of medication (Chengappa et al, 1999).*

▲ Consider partial hospitalization with individual and group therapy. **EB:** *Psychoanalytically oriented partial hospitalization is superior to standard psychiatric care for clients with borderline personality disorder. These clients had a decrease in self-mutilation (Bateman & Fonagy, 1999).*

• Refer to the care plan for **Risk for Self-mutilation** for additional information.

Home Care and Client/Family Teaching

See the care plan for **Risk for Self-mutilation.**

evolve   See the EVOLVE website for World Wide Web resources for client education.

REFERENCES

Apter A, Horesh N, Gothelf D et al: Relationship between self-disclosure and serious suicidal behavior, *Compr Psychiatry* 42(1):70, 2001.

Bateman A, Fonagy P: Effectiveness of partial hospitalization in the treatment of borderline personality disorder: a randomized controlled trial, *Am J Psychiatry* 156(10):1563, 1999.

Chengappa KN, Ebeling T, Kang JS et al: Clozapine reduces severe self-mutilation and aggression in psychotic patients with borderline personality disorder, *J Clin Psychiatry* 60(7):477, 1999.

Denys D, van Megen HG, Westenberg HG: Emerging skin-picking

behaviour after serotonin reuptake inhibitor treatment in patients with obsessive-compulsive disorder: possible mechanisms and implications for clinical care, *J Psychopharmacol* 17(1):127, 2003.

Derouin A, Bravender T: Living on the edge: the current phenomenon of self-mutilation in adolescents, *MCN Am J Matern Child Nurs* 29(1):12, 2004.

Drew BL: Self-harm behavior and no-suicide contracting in psychiatric inpatient settings, *Arch Psychiatr Nurs* 15:99, 2001.

Favaro A, Ferrara S, Santonastaso P: Self-injurious behavior in a community sample of young women: relationship with childhood abuse

• = Independent;   ▲ = Collaborative;   EBN = Evidence-Based Nursing;   EB = Evidence-Based

and other types of self-damaging behaviors, *J Clin Psychiatry* 68:122, 2007.

Guertin T, Lloyd-Richardson E, Spirito A et al: Self-mutilative behavior in adolescents who attempt suicide by overdose, *J Am Acad Child Adolesc Psychiatry* 40(9):1062, 2001.

Hauenstein EJ: Case finding and care in suicide: children, adolescents, and adults. In Boyd MA, editor: *Psychiatric nursing: contemporary practice,* ed 2, Philadelphia, 2002, Lippincott Williams & Wilkins.

Israel JA, Lee K: Amphetamine usage and genital self-mutilation, *Addiction* 97:1213, 2002.

Kress VEW: Self-injurious behaviors: assessment and diagnosis, *J Counsel Develop* 81(4):490, 2003.

Machoian L: Cutting voices: self-injury in three adolescent girls, *J Psychosoc Nurs Ment Health Serv* 39(11):22, 2001.

McAllister M, Creedy D, Moyle W et al: Nurses' attitudes towards clients who self-harm, *J Adv Nurs* 40(5):578, 2002.

McDonald C: Self-mutilation in adolescents, *J Sch Nurs* 22:193, 2006.

Milnes D, Owens D, Blenkiron P: Problems reported by self-harm patients. Perception, hopelessness, and suicidal intent, *J Psychosom Res* 53:819, 2002.

Myers WC, Nguyen M: Autocastration as a presenting sign of incipient schizophrenia, *Psychiatr Serv* 52(5):685, 2001.

Paris J: Understanding self-mutilation in borderline personality disorder, *Harv Rev Psychiatry* 13:179, 2005.

Robey KL, Reck JF, Giacomini KD et al: Modes and patterns of self-mutilation in persons with Lesch-Nyhan disease, *Dev Med Child Neurol* 45:167, 2003.

Stanley B, Gameroff MJ, Michalsen V et al: Are suicide attempters who self-mutilate a unique population? *Am J Psychiatry* 158(3):427, 2001.

Vogel LC, Anderson CJ: Self-injurious behavior in children and adolescents with spinal cord injuries, *Spinal Cord* 40:666, 2002.

Weber MT: Triggers for self-abuse: a qualitative study, *Arch Psychiatr Nurs* 16:118, 2002.

Zafeiriou DI, Vargiami E, Economou M et al: Self-mutilation and mental retardation: clues to congenital insensitivity to pain with anhidrosis, *J Pediatr* 144:284, 2004.

Risk for Self-mutilation   *Kathleen L. Patusky, PhD, APRN-BC*

NANDA   Definition

At risk for deliberate self-injurious behavior causing tissue damage with the intent of causing nonfatal injury to attain relief of tension

Risk Factors

Adolescence; autistic individuals; battered child; borderline personality disorders; character disorders; childhood illness; childhood sexual abuse; childhood surgery; depersonalization; developmentally delayed individuals; dissociation; disturbed body image; disturbed interpersonal relationships; eating disorders; emotionally disturbed child; family alcoholism; family divorce; family history of self-destructive behaviors; feels threatened with loss of significant relationship; history of inability to plan solutions; history of inability to see long-term consequences; history of self-injurious behavior; impulsivity; inability to express tension verbally; inadequate coping; incarceration; irresistible urge to damage self; isolation from peers; living in nontraditional setting (e.g., foster group, or institutional care); loss of control over problem-solving situations; low self-esteem; loss of significant relationship(s); mounting tension that is intolerable; needs quick reduction of stress; negative feelings (e.g., depression, rejection, self-hatred, separation anxiety, guilt); peers who self-mutilate; perfectionism; psychotic state (e.g., command hallucinations); sexual identity crisis; substance abuse; unstable self-esteem; use of manipulation to obtain nurturing relationship with others; violence between parental figures

NOC   Outcomes (Nursing Outcomes Classification)

Suggested NOC Outcomes

Aggression Self-Control, Distorted Thought Self-Control, Impulse Self-Control, Mood Equilibrium, Risk Detection, Self-Mutilation Restraint

Example NOC Outcome with Indicators
Self-Mutilation Restraint as evidenced by the following indicators: Refrains from gathering means for self-injury/Seeks help when feeling urge to injure self (Rate the outcome and indicators of **Self-Mutilation Restraint:** 1 = never demonstrated, 2 = rarely demonstrated, 3 = sometimes demonstrated, 4 = often demonstrated, 5 = consistently demonstrated [see Section I].)

S

• = Independent;   ▲ = Collaborative;   EBN = Evidence-Based Nursing;   EB = Evidence-Based

Client Outcomes

Client Will (Specify Time Frame):

- Refrain from self-injury
- Identify triggers to self-mutilation
- State appropriate ways to cope with increased psychological or physiological tension
- Express feelings
- Seek help when having urges to self-mutilate
- Maintain self-control without supervision
- Use appropriate community agencies when caregivers are unable to attend to emotional needs

NIC   Interventions (Nursing Interventions Classification)

Suggested NIC Interventions

Active Listening, Anger Control Assistance, Behavior Management: Self-Harm, Counseling, Environmental Management: Safety, Limit Setting, Mood Management, Mutual Goal Setting, Risk Identification, Self-Responsibility Facilitation

Example NIC Activities—Behavior Management: Self-Harm
Anticipate trigger situations that may prompt self-harm and intervene to prevent it; Teach and reinforce patient for effective coping behaviors and appropriate expression of feelings

Nursing Interventions and *Rationales*

- Refer to the care plan for **Self-mutilation**
- Assessment data from the client and family members may have to be gathered at different times; allowing a family member or trusted friend with whom the client is comfortable to be present during the assessment may be helpful. *Self-mutilation sometimes occurs if clients have been victims of abuse. Clients or family members may be more willing to disclose the presence of abuse if greater privacy is afforded them. Presence of a trusted family member or friend may help clients to respond more comfortably to the interview situation.*
- Assess for risk factors of self-mutilation, including categories of psychiatric disorders (particularly borderline personality disorder, psychosis, eating disorders, autism); psychological precursors (e.g., low tolerance for stress, impulsivity, perfectionism); psychosocial dysfunction (e.g., presence of sexual abuse, divorce or alcoholism in the family, manipulative behavior to gain nurturing, chaotic interpersonal relationships); coping difficulties (e.g., inability to plan solutions or see long-term consequences of behavior); personal history (e.g., childhood illness or surgery, past self-injurious behavior); and peer influences (e.g., friends who mutilate, isolation from peers). *These risk factors have been associated with self-mutilation.* **EB:** *An analysis of variables associated with self-mutilation found that self-mutilators were more likely to have a history of physical or psychological abuse, or eating disorder; they were currently more depressed and dissociated (Turell & Armsworth, 2003). Persons with borderline personality disorder who initiate self-harm as children will have the most serious course (Zanarini et al, 2005).*
- Assess for co-occurring disorders that require response, specifically childhood abuse, substance abuse, and suicide attempts. **EB:** *A relationship has been found between self-mutilating behavior, substance abuse, childhood abuse, alexithymia, and suicide attempts (Evren & Evren, 2005). Long-term glue sniffing has been associated with violent behavior and/or self mutilation (Shu & Tsai, 2003). Self-mutilation was found more often in drug-dependent than alcohol-dependent persons (Evren, Kural & Cakmak, 2006).*
- Assess family dynamics and the need for family therapy and community supports. *Treatment generally focuses on increasing support for the client, improving family communication, and enhancing the client's sense of control over the environment (Derouin & Bravender, 2004).*
- Assess for a possible genetic disorder that results in severe and involuntary self-mutilation. *Hallmark symptoms of Lesch-Nyhan syndrome include severe lip or finger biting. Lesch-Nyhan syndrome is a rare X-linked recessive genetic disorder generally found in men (Robey et al, 2003).*

S

• = Independent;   ▲ = Collaborative;   EBN = Evidence-Based Nursing;   EB = Evidence-Based

- Be alert to other risk factors of self-mutilation in clients with psychosis, including acute intoxication, dramatic changes in body appearance, preoccupation with religion and sexuality, and anticipated or perceived object loss. **EB:** *A client with bipolar disorder who self-mutilated presented with command auditory hallucinations (Green, Knysz & Tsuang, 2000).*
- Monitor clients with obsessive-compulsive disorder for possible self-mutilation. *Clients with high levels of obsessive-compulsive symptoms may self-mutilate (McKay, Kulchycky & Danyko, 2000).*
- Assess clients who have issues with gender identity or men who were molested as children for possible self-mutilation. *Clients attending gender dysphoria clinics were at risk for self-mutilation (Wylie, 2000).* **EB:** *Another study of men who experienced child sexual abuse found that all forms of sexual molestation were predictive of self-harming behavior (King, Coxell & Mezey, 2002).*
- Maintain ongoing surveillance of the client and environment. Monitor the client's behavior, using 15-minute checks at irregular times so that the client does not notice a pattern. *When lack of control exists, client safety is an important issue and close observation is essential. Not following a pattern prevents clients from being self-abusive when they know a caregiver will not be present.*
- When the client is experiencing extreme anxiety, use one-to-one staffing. Offer activities that will serve as a distraction. **EBN:** *The presence of a trusted individual may calm fears about personal safety. Distraction was reported by self-abusing women as one way of preventing a self-injury episode (Weber, 2002).*
- Implement active listening and early intervention. **EBN:** *In one study, adolescent girls with a history of trauma found that cutting themselves communicated psychological distress when others would not listen to their verbal grievances; but self-mutilation lead to a pattern of self-harm when intervention was not forthcoming (Machoian, 2001).*
- ▲ Refer to mental health counseling. Multiple therapeutic modalities are available for treatment. **EBN:** *Solution-focused brief therapy has been shown to be an effective treatment option for reducing repetitive self-harm (Wiseman, 2003).*
- When working with self-mutilative clients who have borderline personality disorder, develop an effective therapeutic relationship by avoiding labeling, seeking to understand the meaning of the self-mutilation, and advocating for adequate opportunities for care. **EBN:** *Persons with borderline personality disorder experience being labeled rather than diagnosed, leading to a sense of being marginalized and potentially mistreated; having self-mutilation viewed as deliberate attempts to manipulate others rather than a means of controlling emotional pain; and having limited access to care when healthcare providers conclude nothing will help and clients should "help themselves" (Moffat, 1999; Nehls, 1999).*
- When working with self-mutilative clients with a diagnosis of a Cluster B Personality Disorder (borderline, antisocial, narcissistic, or histrionic), carefully assess suicidal ideation. **EB:** *Suicide attempters who also had a history of self-mutilation tended to be more depressed, anxious, and impulsive than those who did not self-mutilate. They tended to underestimate the lethality of their suicide attempt; as a result, clinicians could unintentionally underestimate the suicide risk (Stanley et al, 2001).*
- Maintain a consistent relational distance from the client with borderline personality disorder who self-mutilates: neither too close nor too distant, neither rewarding unacceptable behavior nor trying to control or avoid the client. *Clients with borderline personality disorder recreate the chaos of their previous relationships in dealing with healthcare providers. Clients fear that they will be overwhelmed by or abandoned in relationships, and their reactions can change rapidly. The most effective posture is one that is consistent, allowing clients to react as they need to, while assuring clients that they will not be abandoned.*
- Inform the client of expectations for appropriate behavior and consequences within the unit. Emphasize that the client must comply with the rules. Contract with the client for no self-harm. Give positive reinforcement for compliance and minimize attention paid to disruptive behavior while setting limits. *Clients benefit from clear guidance regarding behavioral expectations and consequences, providing much-needed structure. It is important to reinforce appropriate behavior to encourage repetition. The unit serves as a microcosm of the client's outside world, so adherence to social norms within the unit models adherence upon discharge, while providing the client with staff support to learn appropriate coping skills and alternative behaviors.*
- Clients need to learn to recognize distress as it occurs and express it verbally rather than as a physical action against the self. *Self-mutilation serves to act out feeling states that the client cannot*

S

express or process. Such acts may attempt to relieve pain or punish the self. Therapy helps the client to articulate emotions and needs (Derouin et al, 2004).

- Assist the client to identify the motives/reasons for self-mutilation that have been perceived as positive. *Self-mutilation serves the following functions: releasing tension, returning to reality, regaining control of some aspect of self, expressing forbidden anger, escaping self-hatred associated with incest, aiming to decrease alienation from or influence others, relieving pressure from multiple personalities, and achieving sexual gratification. The sight of blood provides emotional release, and the pain and the blood stop feelings of emptiness. The client must learn alternative ways of securing these gains if they are to give up self-mutilation (McAllister, 2001).*
- Help the client identify cues that precede impulsive behavior. **EB:** *Dialectical behavior therapy (DBT) was found to be superior to non-DBT treatment in reducing self-mutilation among individuals with borderline personality disorder (Verheul et al, 2003).* **EBN:** *The DBT technique of behavioral chain analysis was found to reduce self-harm behaviors by processing events that precipitate self-mutilation (Alper & Peterson, 2001).*
- Give praise when the client identifies urges and delays self-destructive behavior. *Delaying destructive behavior and increasing awareness of urges to be self-destructive should both be acknowledged as progress.*
- Assist clients to identify ways to sooth themselves and generate hopefulness when faced with painful emotions. **EBN:** *Women with a history of childhood abuse may not have developed the internal ability to comfort themselves, or self-soothe, resulting in neurobiological disruptions that lead to self-harm as a means of relieving pain (Gallop, 2002). Generating hopefulness is an important self-comforting intervention (Weber, 2002).*
- Reinforce alternative ways of dealing with depression and anxiety, such as exercise, engaging in unit activities, or talking about feelings. *A study testing response to exercise, treatment with sertraline, or both found that the exercise-only group experienced the lowest depression levels, with the benefit of exercise continuing after the intervention period (Babyak et al, 2000).*
- Keep the environment safe; remove all harmful objects from the area. Use of unbreakable glass is recommended for the client at risk for self-injury. *Client safety is a nursing priority. Unbreakable glass would eliminate this type of injury.*
- Encourage the client to seek out care providers to talk with as the urge to harm oneself occurs. Develop a positive therapeutic relationship. *When the client seeks out staff, he or she is exercising self-responsibility and self-care management.* **EBN:** *Even with a contract in place, clients are reassured that staff really do want to help. Self-abusing women have reported that caring relationships have kept them from hurting themselves, and that feeling comforted, supported, and believed would be helpful (Weber, 2002).*
- Anticipate trigger situations and intervene to assist the client in applying alternatives to self-mutilation. *When triggers occur, client stress level may obstruct ability to apply new learning. Assistance facilitates the ability to practice new skills in real situations.*
- Reduce or eliminate use of caffeine, alcohol, and street drugs. *Caffeine can increase anxiety, which may trigger self-mutilation. Alcohol and street drugs alter mood and increase impulsivity while decreasing inhibitions (Derouin et al, 2004).*
- If self-mutilation does occur, use a calm, nonpunitive approach. Whenever possible, assist the client to assume responsibility for consequences (e.g., dress self-inflicted wound). Refer to the care plan for **Self-mutilation.** *This approach does not promote inappropriate attention-getting behavior, may decrease repetition of behavior, and reinforces self-responsibility and self-care management.*
- If the client is unable to control self-mutilation behavior, provide interactive supervision, not isolation. *Isolation and deprivation take away individuals' coping abilities and place them at risk for self-harm. Implementing seclusion for clients who have injured themselves in the past may actually facilitate self-injury. Clients are extraordinarily resourceful at identifying environmental objects with which to self-mutilate.*
- ▲ Refer for medication, such as clozapine. **EB:** *In a study of seven subjects known to have a personality disorder and severe self-mutilation, there was a statistically significant reduction in incidents of self-mutilation with use of medication (Chengappa et al, 1999).*
- Involve the client in planning their care and problem solving, and emphasize that the client makes choices. **EB:** *Problem solving is a way to gain better emotional control by assisting clients with*

seeing the connection between problems and emotions. Problem-solving therapy with self-mutilators indicates that the therapy significantly decreases depression, hopelessness, and perceived problems (Townsend et al, 2001). Individuals who self-mutilate were found to use more problem avoidance behaviors and to perceive that they had less control over problem-solving options (Haines & Williams, 2003).

▲ Involve the client in group therapy. *Through interaction with others, group members learn to identify patterns of behavior that were acquired from painful past events. The past is not trivialized but acknowledged as leading to patterns that now influence all interactions.*

▲ Use group therapy to exchange information about methods of coping with loneliness, self-destructive impulses, and interpersonal relationships as well as housing, employment, and health-care system issues directly and noninterpretively. *The group's focus should be here and now, supportive and psychoeducative, while providing a comforting level of structure.*

▲ Refer to protective services if evidence of abuse exists. *It is the nurse's legal responsibility to report abuse.*

▲ Discharge planning: provide follow-up to ensure clients attend mental health appointments. *Only a small fraction of people who present in general health care settings with self-mutilation actually follow through with mental health specialist appointments (Tobin et al, 2001).*

• Monitor the client for self-harm impulses that may progress to suicidal ideation. *Self-mutilation is a significant indicator of suicide risk (Guertin et al, 2001; Milnes, Owens & Blenkiron, 2002).*

 ## Pediatrics

• Be aware of increasing incidence of self-mutilation, especially among teens and young adults. *The developmental stressors of adolescence, along with depression, may increase the incidence of self-mutilation (Derouin et al, 2004).* **EBN:** *Teens who self-mutilate may be academically and socially successful, high-achieving, and outgoing, managing to hide evidence of problems or ineffective coping skills (Machoian, 2001).*

• Conduct a thorough physical examination, being alert for superficial scars that may be patterned, although in most cases scabbing or infection is not evident. *Apart from obvious sites, evidence of cutting or burning may be hidden in such areas as the axilla, abdomen, inner thighs, feet, and under breasts (Derouin et al, 2004).*

• Maintaining a therapeutic relationship with teens requires explicit assurances of confidentiality, consistency of clinical routines, and a nonjudgmental communication style. *Even adolescents younger than age 18 years need assurances that confidentiality will be maintained unless there is a serious risk of harm to themselves or others (Bravender, 2002). However, teens of all ages should be advised that parental notification will be made to ensure the teen's safety and to implement a treatment plan (Derouin et al, 2004).*

• Attend to behavioral clues of self-mutilation; a brief self-report assessment can be useful. *Self-mutilators can exhibit mood swings, low self-esteem, poor impulse control, anxiety, self-disappointment, or an inability to identify positive elements in their lives (Machoian, 2001). The American Medical Association's Guidelines for Adolescent Preventive Services (GAPS) can be helpful, and is available at www.ama-assn.org/ama/pub/category/2280.html (Derouin et al, 2004).*

• Assess for the presence of an eating disorder or substance abuse. Attend to the themes that preoccupy teens with eating disorders who self-mutilate. **EB:** *Self-mutilation was shown to be more common among adolescents with dependence issues (drug abuse and eating disorders) (Bolognini et al, 2003). The thought processes of adolescents with eating disorders were found to center on feeling undeserving of receiving help, feeling helpless and hopeless in dealing with the eating disorder itself, having difficulty with recognizing and expressing feelings, feeling ambivalent about treatment, and mistrusting healthcare providers (Manley & Leichner, 2003).*

• Evaluate for suicidal ideation/suicide risk. Refer to the care plan for **Risk for Suicide** for additional information. **EB:** *Adolescents who attempted suicide by overdose admitted to some method of self-mutilation. The self-mutilators were significantly more likely than non–self-mutilators to be diagnosed with oppositional defiant disorder, major depression, and dysthymia, and had higher scores on measures of hopelessness, loneliness, anger, risk taking, and alcohol use (Guertin et al, 2001).*

• Be aware that there is not complete overlap between self-mutilation and suicidal behavior. The motivation may be different (coping with difficult feelings rather than ending life), and the method is usually different. **EB:** *In one study, about half of the participants reported both attempted suicide and self-mutilation; the other half reported no overlap in types of acts (Bolognini et al, 2003).*

- Use treatment approaches detailed previously, with modifications as appropriate for this age group.

Geriatric

- Provide hand or back rubs and calming music when elderly clients experience anxiety. **EBN:** *In a study of older adults in nursing homes, calming music and hand massage were found to soothe agitation for up to 1 hour. No additional benefit was found from combining the two interventions (Remington, 2002).*
- Provide soft objects for elderly clients to hold and manipulate when self-mutilation occurs as a function of delirium or dementia. Apply mitts, splints, helmets, or restraints as appropriate. *Delirious or demented clients may unconsciously scratch or pick at themselves. Soft objects may provide a substitute object to pick at; mitts or restraints may be necessary if the client is unable to exercise self-restraint.*
- Older adults who show self-destructive behaviors should be evaluated for dementia. **EB:** *In a study of nursing home residents, self-destructive behaviors were common and more likely related to dementia than to depression (Draper et al, 2002).*

Home Care

- Communicate degree of risk to family/caregivers; assess the family and caregiving situation for ability to protect the client and to understand the client's self-mutilative behavior. Provide family and caregivers with guidelines on how to manage self-harm behaviors in the home environment. *Client safety between home visits is a nursing priority. Appropriate family/caregiver support is important to the client. Appropriate support will only be forthcoming if all parties understand the basis of the behavior and how to respond to it.*
- Establish an emergency plan, including when to use hotlines and 911. Develop a contract with the client and family for use of the emergency plan. Role play access to the emergency resources with the client and caregivers. *Having an emergency plan reassures the client and caregivers and promotes client safety. Contracting gives guided control to the client and enhances self-esteem.*
- Assess the home environment for harmful objects. Have family remove or lock objects as able. *Client safety is a nursing priority.*
- ▲ If client behaviors intensify, institute an emergency plan for mental health intervention. *The degree of disturbance and the ability to manage care safely at home determines the level of services needed to protect the client.*
- ▲ Refer for homemaker or psychiatric home healthcare services for respite, client reassurance, and implementation of therapeutic regimen. *Responsibility for a person at high risk for self-mutilation provides high caregiver stress. Respite decreases caregiver stress. The presence of caring individuals is reassuring to both the client and caregivers, especially during periods of client anxiety. A client with self-mutilative behavior, especially if accompanied by depression, can benefit from the interventions described previously, modified for the home setting.*
- ▲ If the client is on psychotropic medications, assess client and family knowledge of medication administration and side effects. Teach as necessary. *Knowledge of the medical regimen promotes compliance and promotes safe use of medications.*
- ▲ Evaluate the effectiveness and side effects of medications. *Accurate clinical feedback improves physician ability to prescribe an effective medical regimen specific to client needs.*

Client/Family Teaching

- Explain all relevant symptoms, procedures, treatments, and expected outcomes for self-mutilation that is illness based (e.g., borderline personality disorder, autism). *By increasing knowledge and adapting new behaviors, clients learn that they have some control over their health (Hennessy-Harstad, 1999).*
- Assist family members to understand the complex issues of self-mutilation. Provide instruction on relevant developmental issues and on actions parents can take to avoid media that glorify self-

S

harm behaviors. *Family members need to understand the behaviors they are dealing with, receive positive reinforcement that will promote their patience and perseverance, and know that they can take positive action to remove media triggers for self-mutilation (Derouin et al, 2004).*

- Provide written instructions for treatments and procedures for which the client will be responsible. *A written record provides a concrete reference so that the client and family can clarify any verbal information that was given.*
- Instruct the client in coping strategies (assertiveness training, impulse control training, deep breathing, progressive muscle relaxation). *Clients who self-mutilate have difficulty dealing with stress and painful emotions, which serve as triggers to self-harm. Once clients are able to identify these triggers, they need to learn how to respond to them more effectively through assertiveness, impulse control, or relaxation, as appropriate.*
- Role play (e.g., say, "Tell me how you will respond if someone ignores you"). *Role playing is the most commonly used technique in assertiveness training. It deconditions the anxiety that arises from interpersonal encounters by allowing the client to practice how they might respond in a given situation. Anxiety levels tend to be higher in situations that are unfamiliar.*
- Teach cognitive-behavioral activities, such as active problem solving, reframing (reappraising the situation from a different perspective), or thought-stopping (in response to a negative thought, picture a large stop sign and replace the image with a prearranged positive alternative). Teach the client to confront his or her own negative thought patterns (or cognitive distortions), such as catastrophizing (expecting the very worst), dichotomous thinking (perceiving events in only one of two opposite categories), or magnification (placing distorted emphasis on a single event). *Cognitive-behavioral activities address clients' assumptions, beliefs, and attitudes about their situations, fostering modification of these elements to be as realistic and optimistic as possible. Through cognitive-behavioral interventions, clients become more aware of their cognitive choices in adopting and maintaining their belief systems, thereby exercising greater control over their own reactions (Hagerty & Patusky, 2007; Sinclair et al, 1998).*
- ▲ Provide the client and family with phone numbers of appropriate community agencies for therapy and counseling. *Continuous follow-up care should be implemented; therefore the method to access this care must be given to the client.*
- ▲ Give the client positive things on which to focus by referring to appropriate agencies for job-training skills or education. *Alternative coping skills and the means to access them are essential for continued good mental health.*

evolve See the EVOLVE website for World Wide Web resources for client education.

REFERENCES

Alper G, Peterson SJ: Dialectical behavior therapy for patients with borderline personality disorder, *J Psychosoc Nurs Ment Health Serv* 39(10):38, 52, 2001.

Babyak M, Blumenthal JA, Herman S et al: Exercise treatment for major depression: maintenance of therapeutic benefit at 10 months, *Psychosom Med* 62:633, 2000.

Bolognini M, Plancherel B, Laget J et al: Adolescents' self-mutilation: relationship with dependent behaviour, *Swiss J Psychol* 62(4):241, 2003.

Bravender T: *Adolescent medicine,* Monograph ed. No. 279, Laewood, Kan, 2002, American Academy of Family Physicians.

Chengappa KN, Ebeling T, Kang JS et al: Clozapine reduces severe self-mutilation and aggression in psychotic patients with borderline personality disorder, *J Clin Psychiatry* 60(7):477, 1999.

Derouin A, Bravender T: Living on the edge: the current phenomenon of self-mutilation in adolescents, *MCN Am J Matern Child Nurs* 29(1):12, 2004.

Draper B, Brodaty H, Lee-Fay L et al: Self-destructive behaviors in nursing home residents, *J Am Geriatr Soc* 50(2):354, 2002.

Evren C, Evren B: Self-mutilation in substance-dependent patients and relationship with childhood abuse and neglect, alexithymia and temperament and character dimensions of personality, *Drug Alcohol Depend* 80(1):15-22, 2005.

Evren C, Kural S, Cakmak D: Clinical correlates of self-mutilation in Turkish male substance-dependent inpatients, *Psychopathology* 39:248, 2006.

Gallop R: Failure of the capacity for self-soothing in women who have a history of abuse and self-harm, *J Am Psychiatr Nurses Assoc* 8:20, 2002.

Green CS, Knysz W, Tsuang MT: A homeless person with bipolar disorder and a history of serious self-mutilation, *Am J Psychiatry* 157:1392, 2000.

Guertin T, Lloyd-Richardson E, Spirito A et al: Self-mutilative behavior in adolescents who attempt suicide by overdose, *J Am Acad Child Adolesc Psychiatry* 40(9):1062, 2001.

Hagerty B, Patusky K: Mood disorders: depression and mania. In Fortinash KM, Holoday-Worret PA, editors: *Psychiatric mental health nursing,* ed 4, St Louis, 2007, Mosby.

Haines J, Williams CL: Coping and problem solving of self-mutilators, *J Clin Psychol* 59(10):1097, 2003.

Hennessy-Harstad EB: Empowering adolescents with asthma to take control through adaptation, *J Pediatr Health Care* 13:273, 1999.

King M, Coxell A, Mezey G: Sexual molestation of males: associations with psychological disturbance, *Br J Psychiatry* 181:153, 2002.

Machoian L: Cutting voices: self-injury in three adolescent girls, *J Psychosoc Nurs Ment Health Serv* 39(11):22, 2001.

• = Independent; ▲ = Collaborative; EBN = Evidence-Based Nursing; EB = Evidence-Based

Manley RS, Leichner P: Anguish and despair in adolescents with eating disorders: helping to manage suicidal ideation and impulses, *Crisis* 24(1):32, 2003.

McAllister MM: In harm's way: a postmodern narrative inquiry, *J Psychiatr Ment Health Nurs* 8:391, 2001.

McKay D, Kulchycky S, Danyko S: Borderline personality and obsessive-compulsive symptoms, *J Personal Disord* 14(1):57, 2000.

Milnes D, Owens D, Blenkiron P: Problems reported by self-harm patients. Perception, hopelessness, and suicidal intent, *J Psychosom Res* 53:819, 2002.

Moffat C: Wound care. Self-inflicted wounding. I. Psychosomatic concepts and physical conditions, *Br J Community Nurs* 4:502, 1999.

Nehls N: Borderline personality disorder: the voice of patients, *Res Nurs Health* 22:285, 1999.

Remington R: Calming music and hand massage with agitated elderly, *Nurs Res* 51:317, 2002.

Robey KL, Reck JF, Giacomini KD et al: Modes and patterns of self-mutilation in persons with Lesch-Nyhan disease, *Dev Med Child Neurol* 45:167, 2003.

Shu L, Tsai S: Long-term glue sniffing: report of six cases, *Intl J Psychiatry Med* 33:163, 2003.

Sinclair VG, Wallston KA, Dwyer KA et al: Effects of a cognitive-behavioral intervention for women with rheumatoid arthritis, *Res Nurs Health* 21:315, 1998.

Stanley B, Gameroff MJ, Michalsen V et al: Are suicide attempters who self-mutilate a unique population? *Am J Psychiatry* 158(3): 427, 2001.

Tobin MJ, Clarke AR, Buss R et al: From efficacy to effectiveness: managing organizational change to improve health services for young people with deliberate self harm behaviour, *Aust Health Rev* 24:143, 2001.

Townsend E, Hawton K, Altman DG et al: The efficacy of problem-solving treatments after deliberate self-harm: meta-analysis of randomized controlled trials with respect to depression, hopelessness and improvement in problems, *Psychol Med* 31:979, 2001.

Turell SC, Armsworth MW: A log-linear analysis of variables associated with self-mutilation behaviors of women with histories of child sexual abuse, *Violence Against Women* 9:487, 2003.

Verheul R, Van den Bosch LMC, Koeter MWJ et al: Dialectical behaviour therapy for women with borderline personality disorder, *Br J Psychiatry* 182:135, 2003.

Weber MT: Triggers for self-abuse: a qualitative study, *Arch Psychiatr Nurs* 16:118, 2002.

Wiseman S: Brief intervention: reducing the repetition of deliberate self-harm, *Nurs Times* 99:35, 2003.

Wylie KR: Suction to the breasts of a transsexual male, *J Sex Marital Ther* 26(4):353, 2000.

Zanarini MC, Frankenburg FR, Hennen J et al: The McLean Study of Adult Development (MSAD): overview and implications of the first six years of prospective follow-up, *J Personal Disord* 19:524, 2005.

Disturbed Sensory perception (specify: visual, auditory, kinesthetic, gustatory, tactile, olfactory)   *Sheryl Sommer, PhD, RN, and Betty J. Ackley, MSN, EdS, RN*

NANDA   ### Definition

Change in the amount or patterning of incoming stimuli accompanied by a diminished, exaggerated, distorted, or impaired response to such stimuli

Defining Characteristics

Change in behavior pattern; change in problem-solving abilities; change in sensory acuity; change in usual response to stimuli; disorientation; hallucinations; impaired communication; irritability; poor concentration; restlessness; sensory distortions

Related Factors (r/t)

Altered sensory integration; altered sensory reception; altered sensory transmission; biochemical imbalance; electrolyte imbalance; excessive environmental stimuli; insufficient environmental stimuli; psychological stress

S

NOC   ### Outcomes (Nursing Outcomes Classification) for Disturbed Sensory Perception: Visual

Suggested NOC Outcomes

Body Image, Cognitive Orientation, Sensory Function: Vision, Vision Compensation Behavior

Example **NOC** Outcome with Indicators
Vision Compensation Behavior as evidenced by the following indicators: Uses adequate light for activity being performed/Wears eyeglasses correctly/Uses vision assistive devices/Uses computer assistive devices/Uses support services for low-vision (Rate the outcome and indicators of **Vision Compensation Behavior**: 1 = never demonstrated, 2 = rarely demonstrated, 3 = sometimes demonstrated, 4 = often demonstrated, 5 = consistently demonstrated [see Section I].)

• = Independent;   ▲ = Collaborative;   EBN = Evidence-Based Nursing;   EB = Evidence-Based

NOC   Outcomes (Nursing Outcomes Classification) for Disturbed Sensory Perception: Auditory

Suggested NOC Outcomes

Cognitive Orientation, Communication: Receptive, Distorted Thought Self-Control, Hearing Compensation Behavior

Example NOC Outcome with Indicators
Hearing Compensation Behavior as evidenced by the following indicators: Monitors symptoms of hearing deterioration/Positions self to advantage hearing/Reminds others to use techniques that advantage hearing/Eliminates background noise/Uses sign language/Uses lip reading/Uses closed captioning for television viewing/Uses hearing assistive devices/Uses hearing aid(s) correctly/Cares for internal hearing assistive devices correctly/Cares for external hearing assistive devices correctly/Uses support services for hearing impaired (Rate the outcome and indicators of **Hearing Compensation Behavior:** 1 = never demonstrated, 2 = rarely demonstrated, 3 = sometimes demonstrated, 4 = often demonstrated, 5 = consistently demonstrated [see Section I].)

Client Outcomes

Client Will (Specify Time Frame):

- Demonstrate understanding by a verbal, written, or signed response
- Demonstrate relaxed body movements and facial expressions
- Explain plan to modify lifestyle to accommodate visual or hearing impairment
- Remain free of physical harm resulting from decreased balance or a loss of vision, hearing, or tactile sensation
- Maintain contact with appropriate community resources

NIC   Interventions (Nursing Interventions Classification)

Suggested NIC Interventions

Cognitive Stimulation, Communication Enhancement: Hearing Deficit, Visual Deficit, Environmental Management

Example NIC Activities—Communication Enhancement: Visual Deficit
Identify yourself when you enter the patient's space; Build on patient's remaining vision, as appropriate

Nursing Interventions and *Rationales*

S

Visual—Loss of Vision

- Identify name and purpose when entering the client's room. *Identification when entering the room helps the client feel secure and decreases social isolation.*
- Orient to time, place, person, and surroundings. Provide a radio or talking books. *These actions help the client remain oriented and provide sensory stimulation.*
- Keep doors completely open or closed. Keep furniture out of path to bathroom and do not rearrange furniture. *Consistency in placement of furniture and doors aids in location and decreases chances of injury (Houde & Huff, 2003).*
- Feed the client at mealtimes if blindness is temporary.
- Keep side rails up using half rails, maintain bed in a low position, keep call light readily available, and designate client a Fall Risk. **EB:** *Clients with visual impairment have increased risk for sustaining a fractured hip from a fall (Ivers et al, 2000).*
- Converse with and touch the client frequently during care if frequent touch is within the client's cultural norm. *Appropriate touch can decrease social isolation.*
- Walk the client by having the client grasp the nurse's elbow and walk partly behind the nurse.

• = Independent;   ▲ = Collaborative;   EBN = Evidence-Based Nursing;   EB = Evidence-Based

- Walk a frightened or confused client by having the client put both hands on the nurse's shoulders; the nurse backs up in desired direction while holding the client around the waist. *These methods help the client feel secure and ensure safety.*
- Keep call light button within client's reach, and check location of call light button before leaving the room.
- ▲ For a blind client, consider referring to a clinic for use of a blind mobility aid device that uses ultrasound. *These devices can be helpful to the blind client to increase acuity to the environment and movement of objects in the environment (Bitjoka & Pourcelot, 1999).*
- Ensure access to eyeglasses or magnifying devices as needed.
- Pay attention to the client's emotional needs. Encourage expression of feelings and expect grieving behavior. *Blind people grieve the loss of vision and experience a loss of identity and control over their lives.* **EB:** *Both psychotherapy and antidepressants are efficacious and may indirectly improve function among older people with vision loss (Casten, Rovner & Edmonds, 2002). An emotion-focused group of people with macular degeneration was only minimally effective in decreasing depression, but the problem-focused group of people with macular degeneration resulted in more problem solving (Wahl et al, 2006).*
- ▲ Refer to optometrist, ophthalmologist, or specialist in vision loss for vision care if needed. **EB:** *Photodynamic therapy for neovascular age-related changes is effective in preventing vision loss (Wormald et al, 2005).*

Auditory—Hearing Loss

- Keep background noise to a minimum. Turn off television and radio when communicating with the client. If the environment is noisy, take the client to a private room and shut the door. *Background noise significantly interferes with hearing in the hearing-impaired client (Sommer & Sommer, 2002). Adults who are deaf or hard of hearing suggested that minimizing background noise could improve communication (Iezzoni et al, 2004). Communication failure between health professionals and hearing-impaired clients is common (King, 2004).*
- Stand or sit directly in front of the client when communicating. Make sure adequate light is on your face, avoid chewing gum or covering the mouth or face with your hands while speaking, establish eye contact, and use nonverbal gestures. *These measures make it easier for the client to read lips and see nonverbal communication, which is a large component of all communication (Sommer & Sommer, 2002).*
- Speak distinctly in lower voice tones if possible. Do not overenunciate or shout at the client. *In many kinds of hearing loss, clients lose the ability to hear higher-pitched tones but can still hear lower-pitched tones. Overenunciating makes it difficult to read lips. Shouting makes the words less clear and may be painful (Jupiter & Spiver, 1997). Communication failure between health professionals and clients is common (King, 2004).*
- State the topic of conversation before beginning the conversation; make it clear when you change conversation topics. *This helps give the client a clear context for interpreting what you are speaking about (Sommer & Sommer, 2002).*
- Verify that the client understands critical information by asking the client to repeat the information back. *Hearing-impaired clients will often smile or nod when asked if they understand to avoid embarrassment; asking them to repeat the information back is the only way to verify they understand what is being said (Sommer & Sommer, 2002).*
- If necessary, provide a communication board or personnel who know sign language. *Healthcare institutions are required to provide and pay for qualified interpreters under the Americans with Disabilities Act; an interpreter can be found through the Registry of Interpreters for the Deaf (Sommer & Sommer, 2002).*
- Prepare pictures or diagrams depicting rests or procedures; have books with relevant pictures available for more detailed discussions. *The use of visual aids can improve communication (Iezzoni et al, 2004).*
- ▲ Refer to appropriate resources, such as a speech and hearing clinic; audiologist; or ear, nose, and throat physician. Refer children early for help. *Hearing loss can be treated with medical or surgical interventions or use of a hearing aid. Research demonstrates the positive effects of early diagnosis and intervention on the social and cognitive development of hearing-impaired children (Meadow-Orlans et al, 1997).*

S

- Encourage the client to wear a hearing aid if available. **EB:** *A large study demonstrated that hearing-impaired persons who wore hearing instruments, compared with those who did not, were more socially active; experienced more interpersonal warmth and less interpersonal negativity; communicated more effectively; had less self-criticism, frustration, anger, and depression; and had better health (Kochkin & Rogin, 2000).*
- Avoid inserting an intravenous cannula in the deaf client's hands. **EBN:** *Inserting an intravenous cannula in the deaf client's hands can impede the client's hand movement for sign language communication (Casey, 1995).*
- ▲ Refer to hearing clinics.
- Observe emotional needs and encourage expression of feelings. *Hearing impairments may cause frustration, anger, fear, and self-imposed isolation.*
- For **Disturbed Sensory perception: kinesthetic, tactile,** see the care plan for **Risk for Injury** or **Risk for Falls.** For **Disturbed Sensory perception: olfactory, gustatory,** see the care plan for **Imbalanced Nutrition: less than body requirements.**

Pediatric

- ▲ Test hearing of infants and begin treatment/therapy early as needed. *Early treatment of a hearing loss can decrease the effects of a hearing loss on social, emotional, and academic development of a child (Smith, Bale & White, 2005).*
- For classroom learning, ensure that ambient noise is minimized and devices are used to decrease reverberation in the environment. *For the hearing-impaired child, it is important that background noise is minimized and reverberation is controlled to increase the child's ability to hear and learn (Boothroyd, 2004; Crandell et al, 2004).*
- Recommend the child use a frequency-modulated system along with a hearing aid in school. **EB:** *For classroom learning, use of a frequency-modulated system in combination with a personal hearing aid substantially improved speech recognition (Anderson & Goldstein, 2004).*
- ▲ Refer the child to a specialist who uses a Language Wizard/Player with Baldi, a computer-animated tutor for teaching vocabulary. **EB:** *A study demonstrated that use of the computer system resulted in excellent retention of learned words 4 weeks after the end of the experiment (Massaro & Light, 2004).*

Geriatric

- Keep environment quiet, soothing, and familiar. Use consistent caregivers. *These measures are comforting to older adults and help decrease confusion.*
- If the client has a sensory deprivation, encourage family to provide appropriate sensory stimulation with music, voices, photographs, touch, and familiar smells.
- Increase the amount of light in the environment for elderly eyes; ensure it is nonglare lighting. *Increased lighting can help compensate for some of the visual changes of aging, including reduced visual acuity, reduced contrast sensitivity, and reduced color discrimination (Boyce, 2003).*
- Determine the origin of vision loss. If it is vision loss from a stroke, watch for hemianopia. *Clients who have dominant (left) hemisphere injury usually have deficits in the visual field on the right. Clients with nondominant (right) hemisphere injury may also have visual field deficits. Encourage clients to scan the environment by turning the head from side to side. Also assess for visual spatial misconception. Clients may underestimate distances and bump into doors and become confused.*
- ▲ Refer to low-vision clinics, or the Independent Living Program, which is designed for older individuals who are blind to help maintain independence (Houde & Huff, 2003). *Clients with vision loss should be referred to clinics early, preferably before vision is gone, for help dealing with the loss* **EB:** *A research study demonstrated that mobility function improved after blind rehabilitation training for a group of older veterans (Kuyk et al, 2004). Another study found that clients using the Independent Living Program were highly satisfied with the quality, timeliness of services, and help in accomplishing independent living goals (Moore et al, 2006).*
- For a hearing impairment in older adults, use the Hearing Handicap Inventory for the Elderly (HHIE-S) to determine how individuals perceive the emotional and social problems associated with a hearing loss. **EB:** *The HHIE-S is a valid and reliable questionnaire to predict social and emotional effects of hearing loss (Demers, 2001). The HHIE-S is a valid and reliable instrument for screening of hearing loss (Yueh et al, 2003).*

• = Independent;   ▲ = Collaborative;   EBN = Evidence-Based Nursing;   EB = Evidence-Based

- If the client has a hearing or vision loss, work with the client to ensure contact with others and to strengthen the social network. **EBN and EB:** *Severe loneliness can accompany vision loss in older clients from self-imposed isolation (Foxall et al, 1992). Loss of hearing has a negative effect on psychosocial function, with occurrence of loneliness and increased rate of depression (Wallhagen, Strawbridge & Kaplan, 2001; Wallhagen, 2002; Mullins, 2004).*

Home Care

- The previously listed interventions are applicable in the home care setting.

Client/Family Teaching
Low Vision

- Teach the client how to use a lighted magnification device to increase the ability to read text or see details.
- Teach the client to put a sheet of yellow acetate over text to make the text more visible. *An alternative method is to highlight the text with a green or yellow highlighter (Beaver & Mann, 1995).*
- Put red, yellow, or orange identifiers on important items that need to be seen, such as a red strip at the edge of steps, red behind a light switch, or a red dot on a stove or washing machine to indicate how far to turn knob. **EB:** *Color cues can improve the legibility of the environment and increase the ability to target objects quickly (Cooper, 1999).*
- Use a watch or clock that verbally tells time and a phone with large numbers and emergency numbers programmed into it.
- Teach blind clients new eating techniques, such as associating food on a plate with hours on a clock, so that the client can identify the location of foods.
- Use low-vision aids, including magnifying devices for near vision, telescopes for seeing objects at a distance, a closed-circuit television that magnifies print, and guides for writing checks and envelopes. *Low vision aids can improve vision in clients with limited sight (Derrington, 2002).*
- Teach the client with vision loss to do the following:
  - Use a magnifying mirror to shave or apply makeup. Use an electric razor only.
  - Put personal care products in brightly colored pump containers (red, yellow, or orange) for identification.
  - Use tactile clues, such as safety pins or buttons placed in hems, to help client match clothing.
  - Use prefilled medication organizers with large lettering or three-dimensional (3D) markers.
  These methods can help maintain the independence of the client (McGrory, Remington & Secrest, 2004).
- Increase lighting in the home to help vision in the following ways:
  - Ensure adequate illumination of the entire home, adding light fixtures and increasing wattage of existing bulbs as needed.
  - Decrease glare where light reflects on shiny surfaces by moving or covering reflective object.
  - Use nonglare wax on the floor.
  - Use motion-sensitive lights that come on automatically when a person enters the room for nighttime use.
  - Add indoor strip or "runway" type of lighting to baseboards.
  Visual acuity can be improved by taking steps to overcome age-related changes to vision (Slay, 2002).
  EB: *Illumination can increase mobility in clients with age-related macular degeneration (Kuyk & Elliott, 1999).*

Hearing Loss

- Suggest installation of such devices as ring signalers for the telephone and doorbell, sensors that detect an infant's cry, alarm clocks that vibrate the bed, and closed caption decoders for television sets. Other helpful devices include telephone amplifiers, speakerphones, pocket talker personal listening system, and FM and infrared amplification systems that connect directly to a TV or audio output jack. Also available is a telecommunication device—a typewriter keyboard with an alphanumeric display that allows the hearing-impaired person to send typed messages over the telephone line; software and modems are available that allow a home computer to be used in this fashion. Use of hearing ear dogs, which are specially trained to alert their owners to specific

S

sound, may also be helpful. *These devices and the dogs can improve communication and increase safety for the hearing-impaired client (Zazove et al, 2004).*

- Teach the client to avoid excessive noise at work and at home and wear hearing protection when necessary. Any noise that hurts the ears or is above 90 decibels is excessive. *Hearing loss from excessive noise is common and preventable (Lusk, 2002; Smith, Bale & White, 2005).*

 See the EVOLVE website for World Wide Web resources for client education.

REFERENCES

Anderson KL, Goldstein H: Speech perception benefits of FM and infrared devices to children with hearing aids in a typical classroom, *Lang Speech Hear Serv Sch* 35(2):169, 2004.

Beaver KA, Mann WC: Overview of technology for low vision, *Am J Occup Ther* 49:913, 1995.

Bitjoka L, Pourcelot L: New blind mobility aid devices based on the ultrasonic Doppler effect, *Int J Rehabil Res* 22(3):227, 1999.

Boothroyd A: Room acoustics and speech perception, *Semin Hear* 25(2):155, 2004.

Boyce PR: Lighting for the elderly, *Technol Disabil* 15(3):165, 2003.

Casey JD: Seeing deafness in a new light, *Can Nurse* 91(2):51-54, 1995.

Casten RJ, Rovner BW, Edmonds SE: The impact of depression in older adults with age-related macular degeneration, *J Vis Impair Blind* 96(6):399, 2002.

Cooper BA: The utility of functional colour cues: seniors' views, *Scand J Caring Sci* 13(3):186, 1999.

Crandell CC, Kreisman BM, Smaldino JJ et al: Room acoustics intervention efficacy measures, *Semin Hear* 25(2):201-206, 2004.

Demers K: Best practices in nursing care to older adults: hearing screening, *J Gerontol Nurs* 27(11):8, 2001.

Derrington D: Aids to low vision, *Nurs Res Care* 4:5, 2002.

Foxall MJ, Barron CR, Von Dollen K et al: Predictors of loneliness in low vision adults, *West J Nurs Res* 14(1):86-99, 1992.

Houde SC, Huff MA: Age-related vision loss in older adults: a challenge for gerontological nurses, *J Gerontol Nurs* 29(4):25, 2003.

Iezzoni L, O'Day B, Killeen M et al: Communicating about health care: observations from persons who are deaf or hard of hearing, *Ann Intern Med* 140(5):356-363, 2004.

Ivers RQ, Norton R, Cumming RG et al: Visual impairment and risk of hip fracture, *Am J Epidemiol* 152(7):633-639, 2000.

Jupiter T, Spiver V: Perception of hearing loss and hearing handicap on hearing aid use by nursing home residents: geriatric nursing, *Am J Care Aging* 18(5):201, 1997.

King A: Hearing and the elderly: a simple cure, *Geriatr Med* 34(6):9, 2004.

Kochkin W, Rogin CM: Quantifying the obvious: the impact of hearing instruments on quality of life, *Hearing Rev* 7:1, 2000.

Kuyk T, Elliott JL: Visual factors and mobility in persons with age-related macular degeneration, *J Rehabil Res Dev* 36(4):303, 1999.

Kuyk T, Elliott JL, Wesley J et al: Mobility function in older veterans improves after blind rehabilitation, *J Rehabil Res Dev* 41(3A):337-346, 2004.

Lusk SL: Preventing noise-induced hearing loss, *Nurs Clin North Am* 37(2):257, 2002.

Massaro DW, Light J: Improving the vocabulary of children with hearing loss, *Volta Rev* 104(3):141, 2004.

McGrory A, Remington R, Secrest JA: Optimizing the functionality of clients with age-related macular degeneration, *Rehabil Nurs* 29(3):90, 2004.

Meadow-Orlans KP, Mertens DM, Sass-Lehrer MA et al: Support services for parents and their children who are deaf or hard of hearing. A national survey, *Am Ann Deaf* 142(4): 278-288, 1997.

Moore JE, Steinman BA, Giesen JM et al: Functional outcomes and consumer satisfaction in the Independent Living Program for Older Individuals who are blind, *J Vis Impair Blind* 100(5):285-294, 2006.

Mullins T: Depression in older adults with hearing loss, *ASHA Leader* 9(1):12, 2004.

Slay DH: Home-based environmental lighting assessments for people who are visually impaired: developing techniques and tools, *J Vis Impair Blind* 96:2, 2002.

Smith RJ, Bale JF, White KR: Sensorineural hearing loss in children, *Lancet* 365(9462):879, 2005.

Sommer SK, Sommer NW: When your patient is hearing impaired, *RN* 65(12):28, 2002.

Wahl H, Kammerer A, Holz F et al: Psychosocial intervention for age-related macular degeneration: a pilot project. *J Vis Impair Blind* 100(9):533-545, 2006.

Wallhagen MI: Hearing impairment, *Annu Rev Nurs Res* 20:341, 2002.

Wallhagen MI, Strawbridge WJ, Kaplan GA: Five-year impact of hearing impairment on physical functioning, mental health and social relationships, *Br Soc Audiol News* 32:9, 2001.

Wormald R, Evans J, Smeeth L et al: Photo dynamic therapy for neovascular age-related macular degeneration, *Cochrane Database Syst Rev* (4):CD002030, 2005.

Yueh B, Shapiro N, MacLean CH et al: Screening and management of adult hearing loss in primary care, *JAMA* 289(15):1976-1985, 2003.

Zazove P et al: Deaf persons and computer use, *Am Ann Deaf* 148(5):376, 2004.

S

Sexual dysfunction   *Elaine E. Steinke, PhD, RN*

NANDA   Definition

The state in which an individual experiences a change in sexual function during the sexual response phases of desire, excitation, and/or orgasm, which is viewed as unsatisfying, unrewarding, or inadequate

• = Independent;   ▲ = Collaborative;   EBN = Evidence-Based Nursing;   EB = Evidence-Based

Defining Characteristics

Actual limitations imposed by disease; actual limitations imposed by therapy; alterations in achieving perceived sex role; alterations in achieving sexual satisfaction; change of interest in others; change of interest in self; inability to achieve desired satisfaction; perceived alteration in sexual excitation; perceived deficiency of sexual desire; perceived limitations imposed by disease; perceived limitations imposed by therapy; seeking confirmation of desirability; verbalization of problem

Related Factors (r/t)

Absent role models; altered body function (e.g., pregnancy, recent childbirth, drugs, surgery, anomalies, disease process, trauma, radiation); altered body structure (e.g., pregnancy, recent childbirth, surgery, anomalies, disease process, trauma, radiation); biopsychosocial alteration of sexuality; ineffectual role models; lack of privacy; lack of significant other; misinformation or lack of knowledge; physical abuse; psychosocial abuse (e.g., harmful relationships); values conflict; vulnerability

NOC Outcomes (Nursing Outcomes Classification)

Suggested NOC Outcomes

Abuse Recovery: Sexual, Physical Aging, Risk Control: Sexually Transmitted Diseases (STDs), Sexual Functioning, Sexual Identity

Example NOC Outcome with Indicators

Sexual Functioning as evidenced by the following indicators: Expresses comfort with sexual expression/Expresses comfort with body/Expresses sexual interest (Rate the outcome and indicators of **Sexual Functioning**: 1 = never demonstrated, 2 = rarely demonstrated, 3 = sometimes demonstrated, 4 = often demonstrated, 5 = consistently demonstrated [see Section I].)

Client Outcomes

Client Will (Specify Time Frame):

- Identify individual cause of sexual dysfunction
- Identify stressors that contribute to dysfunction
- Discuss alternative, satisfying, and acceptable sexual practices for self and partner
- Identify the degree of sexual interest by the patient and partner
- Adapt sexual technique as needed to cope with sexual problems
- Discuss with partner concerns about body image and sex role

NIC Interventions (Nursing Interventions Classification)

Suggested NIC Intervention

Sexual Counseling

Example NIC Activities—Sexual Counseling

Provide privacy and ensure confidentiality; Discuss necessary modifications in sexual activity, as appropriate; Provide referral/consultation with other members of the healthcare team, as appropriate

Nursing Interventions and *Rationales*

- Gather the client's sexual history, noting normal patterns of functioning and the client's vocabulary. **EBN:** *Healthcare professionals in urologic, gynecologic, and family practice offices and clinics are in key roles to identify females experiencing sexual dysfunction (Brassil & Keller, 2002).* **EBN:** *Documentation of sexual function after all local treatments, including prostate brachytherapy, may help to clarify the cause of treatment-induced erectile dysfunction (ED) (Stipetich et al, 2002).*
- Assess duration of sexual dysfunction and explore potential causes such as medications, medical problems, or psychosocial issues. Evaluate if sexual dysfunction may be related to either psycho-

logical or medical causes. **EB:** *New onset sexual dysfunction may be related to prescription and non-prescription medications as one cause, while sexual dysfunction of longer duration may be related to a disease process, and can be a symptom of cardiovascular disease (Billups, 2005).* **EB:** *The most common sexual problems reported in a general practice were erectile failure and loss of desire for men and loss of desire and failure in orgasmic response for women (Nazareth, Boynton & King, 2003).*

- Assess for history of sexual abuse. **EB:** *In Australian women, 23% recalled past abuse and 12% recalled multiple episodes of abuse. Women who had been abused had lower scores on sexual satisfaction and frequency (Howard, O'Neill & Travers, 2006).*

- Determine the client's and partner's current knowledge and understanding. **EB:** *This survey indicated that in clinical practice and for those who have a partner, sexual disabilities and distress caused by them should be regarded from the partner relationship perspective (Fugl-Meyer & Fugl-Meyer, 2002).* **EB:** *Including couples in counseling improved overall male distress and male and female global sexual function at 3 months after treatment for prostate carcinoma (Canada et al, 2005).*

- Assess and provide treatment for sexual dysfunction. Involve the person's partner in the process. Consider pharmacologic and nonpharmacologic interventions. **EB:** *Of equal value—and necessity—is the involvement of the man's partner in both the assessment and treatment processes of ED. Nonpharmacologic interventions should be considered as means to support and augment the effects of phosphodiesterase type 5 (PDE-5) inhibitors (Dunn, 2004).* **EB:** *Improved exercise tolerance and coronary dilatation occurred for those taking PDE-5 inhibitors. The safety profile of the drugs is excellent (Carson, 2005).* **EB:** *Post-menopausal women taking valsartan for hypertension reported positive improvements in sexual desire, changes in sexual behavior, and sexual fantasies (Fogari et al, 2004).*

- Observe for stress and anxiety as possible causes of dysfunction. **EBN:** *Sexual dysfunction can be attributed to many psychological factors. Anxiety is often high with cardiac illness, and decreased sexual satisfaction has been shown to heighten anxiety among myocardial infarction clients (Steinke & Wright, 2006).* **EB:** *Clients with implantable cardioverter defibrillators (ICD) report fear of ICD discharge with sexual activity, and 44% avoided sexual encounters (Steinke, 2003).* **EBN:** *General anxiety and sexual anxiety were related in a sample of heart failure clients and healthy elders, and sexual self-concept, sexual anxiety, sexual self-efficacy, younger age, and marital status predicted sexual activity (Steinke, Wright & Moser, 2006).*

- Assess for depression as a possible cause of sexual dysfunction. Sexual problems and depression are common in chronic disease and those with chronic pain. **EBN:** *Global depression and sexual depression have been linked (Steinke, Wright & Moser, 2006).* **EB:** *For women with advanced breast cancer, one-third had a diagnosis of depression, affecting quality of life and with the potential of affecting sexual function (Grabsch et al, 2006).*

- Observe for grief related to loss (e.g., amputation, mastectomy, ostomy). *A change in body image often precedes sexual dysfunction (see care plan for* **Disturbed Body image***).* **EB:** *An integrative review of 13 studies revealed that up to one-half of women with prophylactic mastectomy suffered a negative effect on body image and changes in sexuality (McGaughey, 2006).* **EB:** *Among sexually active women, body image problems were associated with mastectomy and possible reconstruction, hair loss from chemotherapy, concern with weight gain/loss, poorer mental health, and decreased self-esteem (Fobair et al, 2006). Survivors of breast cancer report that issues of body image, sexuality, and partner communication are rarely addressed by traditional healthcare providers (Anllo, 2000). (Additional relevant research: Burwell et al, 2006.)*

- Explore physical causes such as diabetes, arteriosclerotic heart disease, arthritis, benign prostatic hypertrophy, drug or medication side effects, or smoking (males). **EB:** *Erectile dysfunction (ED) is an early manifestation of arteriosclerosis and precedes systemic vascular disease as a result of endothelial dysfunction, a paradigm shift from the belief that ED occurred only as a result of cardiovascular disease or treatment (Billups, 2005).* **EBN:** *Research has demonstrated that the symptoms of rheumatoid arthritis can negatively impact on a client's sexuality (Ryan & Wylie, 2005).* **EB:** *Studies reveal the detrimental effect of smoking on erectile function in males and sexual dysfunction in females, both in U.S. and international samples, and particularly when combined with other risk factors (Addis et al, 2005; Barqawi et al, 2005; Lam et al, 2006; Moreira et al, 2006; Oksuz & Malhan, 2006; Russell, Khandheria & Nehra, 2004; Zitzmann, Faber & Nieschlag, 2006).*

- Provide privacy and be verbally and nonverbally nonjudgmental. *Privacy is important to ensure*

S

confidentiality. To facilitate communication, it is also vital that the nurse clarify personal values and remain nonjudgmental (Steinke, 2005).

- Provide privacy to allow sexual expression between the client and partner (e.g., private room, "Do Not Disturb" sign for a specified length of time). *The hospital setting has little opportunity for privacy, so the nurse must ensure that it is available.*
- Explain the need for the client to share concerns with partner. **EBN:** *The partner should be involved in the assessment, diagnosis, client education, counseling, and choice of treatment for long-term treatment to be successful, unless the informed client is unwilling (Dorey, 2001).*
- Validate the client's feelings, let the client know that he or she is normal, and correct misinformation. **EB:** *Because men see the primary care physician's office as a natural and expected place in which to address issues of sexual health, those healthcare professionals who are prepared to initiate discussion of ED can offer clients and their partners the possibility of effective and enduring treatment success and the restoration of a satisfying relationship (Dunn, 2004).*
- ▲ Refer to appropriate medical providers for consideration of medication for premature ejaculation, erectile dysfunction, or orgasmic problems. **EB:** *The clients with premature ejaculation treated with citalopram showed significantly greater improvement compared with the clients receiving placebo (Atmaca et al, 2002).* **EB:** *Reduced or absent orgasm, erectile dysfunction, and ejaculatory disturbances were noted for up to 2 years after treatment for testicular cancer (Nazareth, Lewin & King, 2001).* **EB:** *Phosphodiesterase-5 inhibitors are safe and effective in those with chronic stable coronary disease (Jackson, 2005).*
- ▲ Refer women for possible pharmacologic intervention when sexual dysfunction is present. **EB:** *For women with sexual dysfunction, pharmacotherapy may augment desire, arousability, and genital congestion, and lessen the pain of chronic dyspareunia (Basson, 2004).*

Geriatric

- ▲ Carefully assess the sexuality needs of the elderly client and refer for counseling if needed. **EB:** *Older adults face several barriers to sexual expression. Because sexual issues are seldom volunteered, questions regarding sexuality and intimacy may have to be raised by the clinician, who can help his or her clients with sexual expression by providing appropriate assessment and counseling (Messinger-Rapport, Sandhu & Hujer, 2003).*
- Carefully assess sexual functioning needs of clients with dementia and provide privacy for them and their spouse. **EBN:** *Although women with dementia are particularly vulnerable to abuse, for some, if not most, sexual activity between loving spouses may be morally permissible even when one partner has dementia and cannot consent (Lingler, 2003).*
- Teach about normal changes that occur with aging: Female—reduction in vaginal lubrication, decrease in the degree and speed of vaginal expansion, reduction in duration and resolution of orgasm. Male—increase in time required for erection, increase in erection time without ejaculation, less firm erection, decrease in volume of seminal fluid, increase in time before another erection can occur (12-24 hours). **EBN:** *The older adult experiences a number of physiologic changes; however, these changes are gradual and vary from person to person (Salzman, 2006).* **EBN:** *Erectile dysfunction may affect 1 in 10 men as they age (Sounes, 2001).*
- ▲ Suggest the following to enhance sexual functioning: Female—use water-based vaginal lubricant, increase foreplay time, avoid direct stimulation of the clitoris if painful (clitoris may be exposed because of atrophy of the labia), practice Kegel exercises (alternately contracting and relaxing the muscles in the pelvic area), urinate immediately after coitus to prevent irritation of the urethra and bladder, and consult with a physician about use of systemic estrogen therapy or topical estrogen cream. Male—have female partner try a new coital position by bending her knees and placing a pillow under her hips to elevate pelvis (will more easily accommodate a partially erect penis); massage penis down using pressure at base, which puts pressure on major blood vessel and keeps blood in the penis; ask the female partner to push the penis into the vagina herself and flex her vaginal muscles that have been strengthened by Kegel exercises. If one of the partners has a protruding abdomen, experiment to find a position that allows the penis to reach the vagina (e.g., have woman lie on her back with legs apart and knees sharply bent while the man places himself over her with his hips under the angle formed by the raised knees). **EBN:** *The management of sexual problems in older adults should be guided by the same principles irrespective of*

S

• = Independent;   ▲ = Collaborative;   EBN = Evidence-Based Nursing;   EB = Evidence-Based

age. Both partners should take part in therapy. A preliminary medical and social history may suggest contributing factors (Tallis, 2003).

- Explore various sexual gratification alternatives (e.g., caressing, sharing feelings) with the client and partner. *Many satisfying alternatives are available for expressing sexual feelings. The many losses associated with aging leave the elderly with special needs for love and affection.*
- Discuss the difference between sexual function and sexuality. *All individuals possess sexuality from birth to death, regardless of the changes that occur over the life span.*
- ▲ If prescribed, instruct clients with chronic pain to take the pain medication prior to sexual activity. Nitroglycerine can be used for anginal pain, if prescribed. *Pain inhibits satisfying sexual activity.*
- See care plan for **Ineffective Sexuality pattern.**

Multicultural

- Assess for the influence of cultural beliefs, norms, and values on the client's perceptions of normal sexual functioning. **EBN:** *What the client considers normal sexual functioning may be based on cultural perceptions (Leininger & McFarland, 2002). Hasidic (ultraorthodox) Jews believe that male ejaculation must be vaginally contained. This belief will influence choice of interventions for certain sexual dysfunctions (Ribner, 2004). Most research on the sexual health of ethnic minority populations is typically focused on preventive sexual health without examination of the racial or ethnic aspects of sexual health (Lewis, 2004).*
- Discuss with the client those aspects of sexual health/lifestyle that remain unchanged by his or her health status. **EBN:** *Aspects of the client's life that are valuable to him or her should be understood and preserved without change (Leininger & McFarland, 2002).*
- Validate the client's feelings and emotions regarding the changes in sexual behavior. **EBN:** *Validation lets the client know the nurse has heard and understands what was said, and it promotes the nurse-client relationship (Heineken, 1998).* **EBN:** *A study of African-American men treated for prostate cancer with prostatectomy or radiation found more positive attitudes than did Caucasian men toward seeking help for sexual problems and were more likely to report seeking past help and intending to seek future help (Jenkins et al, 2004).*

Home Care

- Previously discussed interventions may be adapted for home care use.
- Identify specific sources of concern about sexual activity. Provide reassurance and instruction on appropriate expectations as indicated. **EBN:** *Heart transplantation client and spouses reported large improvements in sexual function after transplant (Bohachick et al, 2001).* **EBN:** *A descriptive study of heart failure clients found a positive relationship between the 6-minute walk test and client levels of sexual function (Jaarsma et al, 1996).* **EBN:** *An intervention with female myocardial infarction clients revealed that women had fewer symptoms and less concern about sexual activity after participating in the intervention (Varvaro, 2000).*
- Help the client and significant other to identify a place and time in the home and daily living for privacy to share sexual or relationship activity. If necessary, help the client to communicate the need for privacy to other family members. Consider periodic escapes to desirable surroundings. *The home setting can be one that affords little, if any, privacy without conscious effort on the part of members of the home.*
- Confirm that physical reasons for dysfunction have been addressed. Encourage participation in support groups or therapy if appropriate. **EBN:** *Alterations in physical appearance can significantly influence people's perceptions of their sexual identities, attractiveness, and worthiness. Clients with lung cancer receiving chemotherapy may need sexual counseling (Schwartz & Plawecki, 2002).*
- Reinforce or teach the client about sexual functioning, alternative sexual practices, and necessary sexual precautions. Update teaching as the client status changes. **EBN:** *The experiences of couples living with prostate cancer demonstrated a need for information and support. Both men and spouse-caregivers felt unprepared to manage treatment effects (Harden et al, 2002).* **EBN:** *A link between sexual self-esteem and sexual function was noted in a study of women post-pancreas and kidney transplant, although the majority had some difficulty with sexual function (Muehrer, Keller & Powwattana, 2006).*

• = Independent;   ▲ = Collaborative;   EBN = Evidence-Based Nursing;   EB = Evidence-Based

Client/Family Teaching

- Provide accurate information for clients concerning sexual activity after a myocardial infarction (MI); consider use of a videotape. **EBN:** *Clients had insufficient information about their future sexual functioning after an MI. Unnecessary limitations in sexual activities and mistakes in the reorganization of activities, such as resumption of sexual activity and frequency and positions of sexual intercourse, were identified (Akdolun & Terakye, 2001).* **EBN:** *Significant improvements in knowledge were found in clients who had a videotape to view at home on return to sexual activity. This intervention provides an alternative method for education to facilitate recovery post-MI (Steinke & Swan, 2004).*
- Teach the client and partner about condom use, for those at risk. **EB:** *A study of HIV seropositive and seronegative women revealed condom use by 68% of sexually active women, and those with HIV were more likely to use a condom (Wilson et al, 2003).*
- Teach the client that sexual activity can be resumed in 1 to 2 weeks after an uncomplicated MI (ACC/AHA, 2004). Also discuss being well rested, reporting any cardiac warning signs, using foreplay to determine tolerance for sexual activity, not using alcohol or eating heavy meals prior to sex, and having sex with a familiar partner and in the usual setting to decrease any stress the couple might feel. **EB:** *If this can be done without shortness of breath or other symptoms, then the client is ready to begin pre-established levels of sexual activity (Papadopoulos, 1991).* **EB:** *Sexual activity can be discussed in the context of other usual activities, comparing the energy expenditure for each as compared to sexual activity. The average energy expenditure for sex with a long-standing partner is 2.5 metabolic equivalent levels (METs) with the partner on top and 3.3 METs with the man on top, similar to walking at a moderate pace or doing a household chore like washing floors (Cheitlin, 2005).*
- Provide written educational materials that address sexual issues for clients and families of clients with implantable cardiac defibrillators (ICDs). **EBN:** *Addressing the fears and concerns related to sexual function of ICD clients and partners is an essential aspect of rehabilitation and recovery. Study results suggest a need for written client education tools specific to sexual issues for clients and partners, as well as educational resources for health professionals (Steinke, 2003).*
- ▲ Refer to appropriate community resources, such as a clinical specialist, family counselor, or sexual counselor. If appropriate, include both partners in the discussion. **EB:** *Changes in the sexual relationship were described in the context of the effects of having interstitial cystitis and the centrality of maintaining relationships. Participation in support groups has a healing potential related to the woman's desire to maintain independence and to help others with the disease (Webster, 1997).*
- Teach vaginal dilation to prevent stenosis. Inform the client to expect a bit of spotting after first session of intercourse. **EB:** *Women who had pelvic radio therapy, the use of vaginal dilators to prevent the development of vaginal stenosis is supported (Denton & Maher, 2003).*
- Teach how drug therapy affects sexual response (e.g., the possible side effects and the need to report them). **EB:** *Sexual dysfunction induced by selective serotonin reuptake inhibitors (SSRIs) affects 30% to 50% or more of individuals who take these drugs for depression (Keltner, McAfee & Taylor, 2002).*
- Teach the importance of diabetic control and its effect on sexuality to clients with insulin-dependent diabetes. **EBN:** *Sexual functioning may be changed by alterations in glucose levels, infections that affect comfort during sexual intercourse, changes in vaginal lubrication and penile erection, and changes in sexual desire and arousal (Lemone, 1993).*
- ▲ Refer for medical advice for ED that lasts longer than 2 months or is recurring. *ED can be treated, and underlying causes need to be investigated (Mayo Foundation for Medical Education and Research, 2003).*
- Teach the following interventions to decrease the likelihood of ED: limit or avoid the use of alcohol, stop smoking, exercise regularly, reduce stress, get enough sleep, deal with anxiety or depression, and see doctor for regular checkups and medical screening tests. **EB:** *These interventions may prevent or improve symptoms of ED (Guay, 2005; Mayo Foundation for Medical Education and Research, 2003).*
- ▲ Refer for medication to treat ED if necessary. **EB:** *The PDE-5 inhibitors are now widely used in selected clients (Jackson, 2005).* **EB:** *Sildenafil use is effective and well tolerated in clients with olanzapine-induced ED (Atmaca, Kuloglu & Tezcan, 2002).* **EB:** *In this prospective, parallel-group, randomized, double-blind, placebo-controlled trial, sildenafil effectively improved erectile function and*

S

• = Independent;   ▲ = Collaborative;   EBN = Evidence-Based Nursing;   EB = Evidence-Based

other aspects of sexual function in men with sexual dysfunction associated with the use of SSRI antidepressants (Nurnberg et al, 2003).

- Teach specifics if the client has a stoma: do not substitute the stoma for an anus. *If a stoma is abused in this way, it can become traumatized and need further surgery (Taylor, 1994).*
- See Geriatric Interventions if a problem with erection is associated with stoma surgery.

evolve See the EVOLVE website for World Wide Web resources for client education.

REFERENCES

Addis IB, Ireland CC, Vittinghoff E et al: Sexual activity and function in postmenopausal women with heart disease, *Obstet Gynecol* 106:121-127, 2005.

Akdolun N, Terakye G: Sexual problems before and after myocardial infarction: patients' needs for information, *Rehabil Nurs* 26(4):152, 2001.

Anllo LM: Sexual life after breast cancer, *J Sex Marital Ther* 26(3):241, 2000.

Antman EM, Anbe DT, Armstrong PW et al: ACC/AHA guidelines for the management of patients with ST-elevation in myocardial infarction: a report of the American College of Cardiology/American Heart Association Task Force on Practice Guidelines, *Circulation* 110(9):e82-e292, 2004.

Atmaca M, Kuloglu M, Tezcan E: Sildenafil use in patients with olanzapine-induced erectile dysfunction, *Int J Impot Res* 14(6): 547-549, 2002.

Atmaca M, Kuloglu M, Tezcan E et al: The efficacy of citalopram in the treatment of premature ejaculation: a placebo-controlled study, *Int J Impot Res* 14(6):502-505, 2002.

Barqawi A, O'Donnell C, Kumar R et al: Correlation between LUTS (AUA-SS) and erectile function (SHIM) in an age-matched racially diverse mail population: data from the Prostate Cancer Awareness Week (PCAW), *Int J Impot Res* 17:370-374, 2005.

Basson R: Pharmacotherapy for sexual dysfunction in women, *Expert Opin Pharmacother* 5(5):1045-1059, 2004.

Billups K: Sexual dysfunction and cardiovascular disease: integrative concepts and strategies, *Am J Cardiol* 96(suppl):57M-61M, 2005.

Bohachick P, Reeder S, Taylor MV et al: Psychosocial impact of heart transplantation on spouses, *Clin Nurs Res* 10(1):6, 2001.

Brassil DF, Keller M: Female sexual dysfunction: definitions, causes, and treatment, *Urol Nurs* 22(4):237, 284; quiz 245, 248, 2002.

Burwell SR, Case LD, Kaelin C et al: Sexual problems in younger women after breast cancer surgery, *J Clin Oncol* 24:2815-2821, 2006.

Canada A, Neese L, Sui D et al: Pilot intervention to enhance sexual rehabilitation for couples after treatment for localized prostate carcinoma, *Cancer* 104:2689-2700, 2005.

Carson C III: Cardiac safety in clinical trials of phosphodiesterase 5 inhibitors, *Am J Cardiol* 96(suppl):37M-41M, 2005.

Cheitlin MD: Sexual activity and cardiac risk, *Am J Cardiol* 96(suppl):24M-28M; 2005.

Denton AS, Maher EJ: Interventions for the physical aspects of sexual dysfunction in women following pelvic radiotherapy, *Cochrane Database Sys Rev* (1):CD003750, 2003.

Dorey G: Partners' perspective of erectile dysfunction: literature review, *Br J Nurs* 10(3):187, 2001.

Dunn ME: Restoration of couple's intimacy and relationship vital to reestablishing erectile function, *J Am Osteopath Assoc* 104(3):S6-S10, S16, 2004.

Fobair P, Stewart SL, Chang S et al: Body image and sexual problems in young women with breast cancer, *Psychooncology* 15:579-594, 2006.

Fogari R, Preti P, Zoppi A et al: Effect of valsartan and atenolol on sexual behavior in hypertensive postmenopausal women, *Am J Hypertens* 17:77-81, 2004.

Fugl-Meyer K, Fugl-Meyer AR: Sexual disabilities are not singularities, *Int J Impot Res* 14(6):487, 2002.

Grabsch B, Clarke DM, Love A et al: Psychological morbidity and quality of life in women with advanced breast cancer: a cross-sectional study, *Palliat Support Care* 4(1):47-56, 2006.

Guay AT: Relation of endothelial cell function to erectile dysfunction: implications for treatment, *Am J Cardiol* 96(suppl):52M-56M, 2005.

Harden J, Schafenacker A, Northouse L et al: Couples' experiences with prostate cancer: focus group research, *Oncol Nurs Forum* 29(4):701, 2002.

Heineken J: Patient silence is not necessarily client satisfaction: communication in home care nursing, *Home Healthc Nurse* 16(2):115, 1998.

Howard JR, O'Neill S, Travers C: Factors affecting sexuality in older Australian women: sexual interest, sexual arousal, relationships and sexual distress in older Australian women, *Climacteric* 9:355-367, 2006.

Jaarsma T, Dracup K, Walden J et al: Sexual function in patients with advanced heart failure, *Heart Lung* 25:262-270, 1996.

Jackson G: Hemodynamic and exercise effects of phosphodiesterase 5 inhibitors, *Am J Cardiol* 96(suppl):32M-36M, 2005.

Jenkins R, Schover LR, Fouladi RT et al: Sexuality and health-related quality of life after prostate cancer in African-American and white men treated for localized disease, *J Sex Marital Ther* 30(2):79-93, 2004.

Keltner NL, McAfee KM, Taylor CL: Mechanisms and treatments of SSRI-induced sexual dysfunction, *Perspect Psychiatr Care* 38(3):111, 2002.

Lam TH, Abdullah AS, Ho LM et al: Smoking and sexual dysfunction in Chinese males: findings from men's health survey, *Int J Impot Res* 18:364-369, 2006.

Leininger MM, McFarland MR: *Transcultural nursing: concepts, theories, research and practices,* ed 3, New York, 2002, McGraw-Hill.

Lemone P: Human sexuality in adults with insulin-dependent diabetes mellitus, *Image* 25:101, 1993.

Lewis LJ: Examining sexual health discourses in a racial/ethnic context, *Arch Sex Behav* 33(3):223-234, 2004.

Lingler JH: Ethical issues in distinguishing sexual activity from sexual maltreatment among women with dementia, *J Elder Abuse Neglect* 15(2):85-102, 2003.

Mayo Foundation for Medical Education and Research: *Erectile dysfunction.* Available at http://www.mayoclinic.com/health/erectile-dysfunction/DS00162, accessed November 18, 2003.

McGaughey A: Body image after bilateral prophylactic mastectomy: an integrative literature review, *J Midwifery Womens Health* 51(6):e45-e49, 2006.

Messinger-Rapport BJ, Sandhu SK, Hujer ME: Sex and sexuality: is it over after 60? *Clin Geriatr* 11(10):45-55, 2003.

S

Moreira ED Jr, Kim SC, Glasser D et al: Sexual activity, prevalence of sexual problems, and associated help-seeking patterns in men and women aged 40-80 years in Korea: data from the Global Study of Sexual Attitudes and Behaviors (GSSAB), *J Sex Med* 3(2):201-211, 2006.

Muehrer RJ, Keller ML, Powwattana A: Sexuality among women recipients of a pancreas kidney transplant, *West J Nurs Res* 28:137-150, 2006.

Nazareth I, Boynton P, King M: Problems with sexual function in people attending London general practitioners: cross sectional study, *BMJ* 327:423-428, 2003.

Nazareth I, Lewin J, King M: Sexual dysfunction after treatment for testicular cancer: a systematic review, *J Psychosomatic Res* 51:735-743, 2001.

Nurnberg HG, Hensley PL, Gelenberg AJ et al: Treatment of antidepressant-associated sexual dysfunction with sildenafil: a randomized controlled trial, *JAMA* 289(1):56, 2003.

Oksuz E, Malhan S: Prevalence and risk factors for female sexual dysfunction in Turkish women, *J Urol* 175:654-658, 2006.

Papadopoulos C: Sex and the cardiac patient, *Med Aspects Hum Sexuality* 24:55, 1991.

Ribner D: Ejaculatory restrictions as a factor in the treatment of Haredi (Ultraorthodox) Jewish couples, *Arch Sex Behav* 33(3):303-308, 2004.

Russell ST, Khandheria Bk, Nehra A: Erectile dysfunction and cardiovascular disease, *Mayo Clin Proc* 79:782-794, 2004.

Ryan S, Wylie E: An exploratory survey of the practice of rheumatology nurses addressing the sexuality of patients with rheumatoid arthritis, *Musculoskeletal Care*, 3(1):44-53, 2005.

Salzman B: Myths and realities of aging, *Care Manage J* 7(3)141-150, 2006.

Schwartz S, Plawecki HM: Consequences of chemotherapy on the sexuality of patients with lung cancer, *Clin J Oncol Nurs* 6(4):212, 2002.

Sounes P: Providing nursing care for erectile dysfunction, *Prof Nurse* 16(9):1374-1376, 2001.

Steinke EE: Intimacy needs and chronic illness: strategies for sexual counseling and self-management, *J Gerontol Nurs* 31(5):40-50, 2005.

Steinke EE: Sexual concerns of patients and partners after an implantable cardioverter defibrillator, *Dimen Crit Care Nurs* 22(2):89-96, 2003.

Steinke EE, Swan JH: Effectiveness of a videotape for sexual counseling after myocardial infarction, *Res Nurs Health* 27(4):269-280, 2004.

Steinke EE, Wright DW: The role of sexual satisfaction, age, and cardiac risk factors in the reduction of post-MI anxiety, *Eur J Cardiovasc Nurs* 5:190-196, 2006.

Steinke EE, Wright DW, Moser DK: Sexual self-concept, anxiety, and self-efficacy predict sexual activity in heart failure and healthy elders, *Circulation* 114(18)II-703, 2006.

Stipetich RL, Abel LJ, Blatt HJ et al: Nursing assessment of sexual function following permanent prostate brachytherapy for patients with early-stage prostate cancer, *Clin J Oncol Nurs* 6(5):271, 2002.

Tallis R: *Geriatric medicine and gerontology*, ed 6, Oxford, UK, 2003, Churchill Livingstone, 1140-1142.

Taylor P: Beating the taboo, stoma and sexual difficulty, *Nurs Times* 90:51, 1994.

Varvaro F: Family role and work adaptation in MI women, *Clin Nurs Res* 9:339-351, 2000.

Webster DC: Recontextualizing sexuality in chronic illness: women and interstitial cystitis, *Health Care Women Int* 18(6):575, 1997.

Wilson T, Koenig L, Ickovics J et al: Contraception use, family planning, and unprotected sex: few differences among HIV-infected and uninfected postpartum women in four US states, *J Acquir Immune Defic Syndr* 33:608-613, 2003.

Zitzmann M, Faber S, Nieschlag E: Association of specific symptoms and metabolic risks with serum testosterone in older men, *J Clin Endocrinol Metab* 91:4335-4343, 2006.

Ineffective Sexuality pattern   *Elaine E. Steinke, PhD, RN*

S

NANDA   Definition

Expressions of concern regarding own sexuality

Defining Characteristics

Alteration in relationship with significant other; alterations in achieving perceived sex role; conflicts involving values; reported changes in sexual activities; reported changes in sexual behaviors; reported difficulties in sexual activities; reported difficulties in sexual behaviors; reported limitations in sexual activities; reported limitations in sexual behaviors

Related Factors (r/t)

Absent role model; conflicts with sexual orientation or variant preferences; fear of acquiring a sexually transmitted disease; fear of pregnancy; impaired relationship with a significant other; ineffective role model; knowledge/skill deficit about alternative responses to health-related transitions, altered body function or structure, illness, or medical treatment; lack of privacy; lack of significant other

NOC Outcomes (Nursing Outcomes Classification)

Suggested NOC Outcomes

Abuse Recovery: Sexual, Body Image, Child Development: Middle Childhood/Adolescence, Risk Control: Sexually Transmitted Diseases (STDs), Risk Control: Unintended Pregnancy, Role Performance, Self-Esteem

Example NOC Outcome with Indicators
Risk Control: Sexually Transmitted Diseases (STD) as evidenced by the following indicators: Acknowledges individual risk for STD; Uses methods to control STD transmission (Rate the outcome and indicators of **Risk Control: Sexually Transmitted Diseases (STD):** 1 = never demonstrated, 2 = rarely demonstrated, 3 = sometimes demonstrated, 4 = often demonstrated, 5 = consistently demonstrated [see Section I].)

Client Outcomes

Client Will (Specify Time Frame):

- State knowledge of difficulties, limitations, or changes in sexual behaviors or activities
- State knowledge of sexual anatomy and functioning
- State acceptance of altered body structure or functioning
- Describe acceptable alternative sexual practices
- Identify importance of discussing sexual issues with significant other
- Describe practice of safe sex with regard to pregnancy and avoidance of STDs

NIC Interventions (Nursing Interventions Classification)

Suggested NIC Intervention

Sexual Counseling

Example NIC Activities—Sexual Counseling
Provide privacy and ensure confidentiality; Provide information about sexual functioning, as appropriate

Nursing Interventions and *Rationales*

- Refer to the care plan **Sexual dysfunction** for additional interventions.
- After establishing rapport or therapeutic relationship, give the client permission to discuss issues dealing with sexuality. Ask the client specifically, "Have you been or are you concerned about functioning sexually because of your health status?" *The history may also give a strong indication of the cause of the problem and will help ascertain what the person and his or her partner are expecting from treatment. Men may find it difficult or embarrassing to discuss such an intimate subject, so the health professional must be open and nonjudgmental with excellent communication skills (Ashford, 2003). Start with more general questions and then ask those that are more personal. Discuss exercise recommendations and then discuss sex as another form of exercise. Recognize that some older adults may not be sexually active at the present time, but may want information for future reference (Steinke, 2005).*
- Encourage the client to discuss concerns with his or her partner. *Carefully assess a client's sexuality. A sexual relationship may be heterosexual or homosexual, and nurses must not lose sight of this (Silenzio, 2003). A daily walk together is an ideal time to discuss sexual concerns, while increasing the client's strength and stamina and promoting health (Steinke, 2005).*
- Assess psychosocial function such as anxiety, depression, and low self-esteem. **EBN:** *Psychosocial function was a powerful predictor of information needs at 6 months and at 1 year, including the need for sexual information among those who had coronary bypass or coronary angioplasty (Kattainen, Merilainen & Jokela, 2004).*
- Discuss alternative sexual expressions for altered body functioning or structure. Closeness and

S

• = Independent;   ▲ = Collaborative;   EBN = Evidence-Based Nursing;   EB = Evidence-Based

touching are other forms of expression. *Recognize that the meaning of sex and sexuality is individually defined, with some engaging in sexual intercourse, while others may prefer touching, holding one another, or kissing (Steinke, 2005). Extensive touching, hugging, holding, huddling, and cuddling in intimate (committed, close, and prolonged) relationships is important couple and family therapy (L'Abate, 2001).*

- Some clients choose masturbation for sexual release. **EB:** *Staff who worked with clients with intellectual disability identified more training and clear policy guidelines as the two means of increasing their confidence in dealing with issues of client sexuality such as masturbation (McConkey & Ryan, 2001).*
- If mutual masturbation is a choice of expression, provide latex gloves. *Latex gloves prevent possible exposure to infection through cuts on hands (Tucker et al, 1996).*
- The following are *guidelines for sexual activity* for clients who have had total hip replacement (THR) surgery:
  - Do not bend the affected leg more than 90 degrees at the hip. When lying on your back, do not turn or roll your affected leg toward the other leg. Do not turn the toes of the affected leg inward. When lying on your side, keep both legs separated with pillows between them. Do not let your knees touch and do not let the toes of your affected leg turn downward.
- The following are **recommended sexual positions** for clients who have had THR surgery:
  1. **Bottom position for the male or female client:** Place one or two pillows under your affected thigh for support and comfort and to reduce friction on your skin, which may still be healing. Keep the toes of your affected leg pointed upward and slightly outward—but never inward.
  2. **Top position for male clients only:** Do not bend your affected hip more than 90 degrees while getting into position. Keep your affected leg out to the side with your toes pointed slightly outward. (Female clients: Do not assume this position because it will require that you bend more than 90 degrees at the hip.)
  3. **Side-lying position for the male client:** Lie on your unaffected side. Both you and your partner should face the same direction. You should be behind your partner in a "spooning" position. Your partner should place at least two pillows between her legs and your affected leg should rest on top of hers during intercourse. Do not bend your affected leg more than 90 degrees, and do not let the toes of your affected leg dangle or turn downward.
  4. **Side-lying position for the female client:** Lie on your unaffected side and place enough pillows between your legs to support the affected leg. Make sure the affected leg does not drop off the pillows during intercourse. Your partner should assume the spooning position behind you. Do not bend your affected hip more than 90 degrees, and do not let the toes of your affected leg turn downward.
  - *Caution:* If you dislocate your hip during sexual intercourse, you will experience pain, your affected leg will appear shorter, and your foot will turn inward. Lie down, do not move, and tell your partner to call an ambulance.
  - *The goal of rehabilitation after THR is to sustain and, if possible, increase clients' ability to function, including sexual function. Addressing issues about sexual activity should therefore be made a part of the standard instructions given to THR clients on how to protect the new hip (Rogers, 2003).*
- The following are suggestions to be used for those who have had a myocardial infarction (MI):
  - Sexual activity can be resumed in about 1 week to 10 days for those who had an uncomplicated MI. Sex should occur in familiar surroundings, in a comfortable room temperature, with the usual partner, and when well rested to minimize any cardiac stress. Heavy meals or alcohol should be avoided for 2 to 3 hours before sexual activity. Clients should choose the most comfortable position, one that minimizes any stress they may feel. *Anal sex stimulates the vagus nerve and is accompanied by slowed heart rate and rhythm and coronary blood flow; therefore, further evaluation by the physician may be needed before anal sex can be resumed (Steinke, 2005).*
- The following are suggestions for those with an implantable cardioverter defibrillator (ICD):
  - Assure the client and partner that fears about being shocked during sexual activity are normal. Sex can be resumed after the ICD is placed as long as strain on the implant site is avoided. If the ICD does discharge with sexual activity, the client should stop and rest and later notify the physician that the device fired so that it can be evaluated whether changes in the device settings are needed. The client should be instructed to report any dyspnea, chest

S

pain, or dizziness with sexual activity. *Partners are often fearful and overprotective of the client, and some have noted sensations when the client's ICD fired, though not harmful to the partner (Steinke, 2003, 2005).*

- The following are suggestions for those with chronic lung disease:
  - Sexual activity should be planned when energy level is highest and using positions that minimize shortness of breath, such as a semi-reclining position. *Planning sexual activity when the medications may be at their peak effectiveness may also be helpful. An oxygen cannula can be used, if prescribed, to provide oxygen before, during, or after sex (Steinke, 2005).*

Pediatric

- Provide age-appropriate information for adolescents regarding human immunodeficiency virus (HIV) or the acquired immunodeficiency syndrome (AIDS) and sexual behavior. **EB:** *Attempts should be made to make HIV education more relevant for teens so that they use the information they have when making decisions about safer sexual behavior (Hoppe, Graham & Wilsdon, 2004).* **EBN:** *Pregnant adolescents and young mothers are vulnerable to acquiring HIV/AIDS through sexual transmission because they lack the resources, social status, and power to protect themselves (Lesser, Oakes & Koniak-Griffin, 2003).*
- Provide support for the client's chosen ways to cope with HIV or AIDS. **EBN:** *Female adolescents infected with HIV/AIDS revealed that the most often used coping strategies identified by the adolescents were listening to music, thinking about good things, making your own decisions, being close to someone you care about, sleeping, trying on your own to deal with problems, eating, watching television, daydreaming, and praying (Lewis & Brown, 2002).*

Geriatric

- Carefully assess the sexuality needs of the elderly client and refer for counseling if needed. *Being a sexual being and having sexual feelings are part of what it is to be a human being—there are no age limits to enjoying a healthy sex life and having the ability to love and be loved (Peate, 2004). The ability to form satisfying social relationships and to be intimate with others, including building strong emotional intimate connections, contributes to adaptation and successful aging (Fleming, 2001; Kingsberg, 2000; Steinke, 2005).* **EB:** *Older adults often maintain moderate to strong interest and many remain sexually active, although decline in frequency of sexual activity may occur (Avis, 2000).*
- Explore possible changes in sexuality related to health status, menopause, and medications. **EB:** *Men report changes in sexual activity related to poor health, medications, and erectile dysfunction, while women report that menopause affects their interest and desire. Women often do not have an available sexual partner (Avis, 2000). In a study of older Australian women, few reported low relationship satisfaction and sexual distress, although higher levels of distress were noted among younger women and those with partners (Howard, O'Neill & Travers, 2006).*
- Allow the client to verbalize feelings regarding loss of sexual partner or significant other. Acknowledge problems such as disapproval of children, lack of available partner for women, and environmental variables that make forming new relationships difficult. *After a loss of this magnitude, elderly persons often find that forming new relationships is difficult. Privacy is also a problem (Shell & Smith, 1994).*
- Provide a milieu that allows for discussion of sexual issues and a higher level of sexual satisfaction. Allow couples to room together and bring in double beds from home. Place signs on the door to ensure privacy. *Sexuality among adults in long-term care facilities is a difficult issue for staff to address (Lantz, 2004).* **EBN:** *Assess client's sexual concerns and perceptions of sexuality. For cognitively impaired older adults who have lost social inhibitions, it is important for staff not to overreact, to provide privacy, and to redirect the behavior if needed (Steinke, 1997).*
- Provide clients with the following information:
  - Exercise, such as walking, swimming, cycling, and riding a stationary bike will help control flabby thighs and weak musculature and make people feel more sexually attractive.
  - Overindulgence in food or alcohol can affect sexual activity (see care plan for **Imbalanced Nutrition: more than body requirements**).
  - Resting and sleeping on a firm mattress may augment sexual desire.
  - Femininity and masculinity are still important.

- ▪ Pay attention to cleanliness, skin care, and clothing.
- ▪ Change the environment, and experiment with position changes.

Because the majority of the elderly population maintains sexual interest, desire, and functioning, these interventions may be helpful during the rehabilitation process. Older adults may exercise aerobically 3 to 5 times a week for 15 to 30 minutes depending on physical status and treatment regimen (Steinke & Bergen, 1986).

- • See care plan for **Sexual dysfunction.**

Multicultural

- • Assess for the influence of cultural beliefs, norms, and values on client's perceptions of normal sexual behavior. **EBN:** *What the client considers normal sexual behavior may be based on cultural perceptions (Leininger & McFarland, 2002). Religion may also influence one's perception of sexual behavior (Lazoritz & McDermott, 2002). Common cultural beliefs and behaviors of South Asian Indian clients around sexuality include the role of the individual client's duty to society, the client's sense of place in society, lack of formal sexual education, prearranged marriages, little premarital contraceptive education, and the dominance of the husband in contraceptive decisions (Fisher, Bowman & Thomas, 2003).*

Home Care

- • Previously discussed interventions may be adapted for home care use. Also see care plan for **Sexual dysfunction.**
- • Help the client and significant other to identify a place and time in the home and daily living for privacy in sharing sexual or relationship activity. If necessary, help the client to communicate the need for privacy to other family members. Consider periodic escapes to desirable surroundings. *The home setting can be one that affords little, if any, privacy without a conscious effort made by members of the home.*
- • Confirm that physical reasons for dysfunction have been addressed. Encourage participation in support groups or therapy if appropriate. **EB:** *Clients express embarrassment at continuing medical intervention or participation in groups once they are back in the community and know that peers may judge their activities (Lundquist & Ojehagen, 2001).*
- • Reinforce or teach about sexual functioning, alternative sexual practices, and necessary sexual precautions. Update teaching as client status changes. *If the client or significant other has received information during an institutional stay, other stressors may have made the information a temporarily low priority or may have impaired learning. Depending on the cause for dysfunction, the client may experience changing status or feelings about the problem.*

Client/Family Teaching

- ▲ Refer to appropriate community agencies (e.g., certified sex counselor, Reach to Recovery, Ostomy Association). **EBN:** *Sexuality concerns should be addressed with all clients undergoing ostomy placement (Sprunk & Alteneder, 2000).*
- • Provide information regarding self-care and sexuality for the woman who has cancer and her partner. **EBN:** *Couples may hesitate to change their routines. Providing this kind of information in a sensitive way often gives permission to change (Shell & Smith, 1994).*
- ▲ Sexuality education is important to all populations, whether hearing or deaf, sighted or blind, disabled or not disabled. Discuss contraceptive choices. Refer to appropriate health professional (e.g., gynecologist, nurse practitioner [NP]). *The spread of myths, opinions, and stereotypes can be reduced by correctly educating children. Sexuality education enables an individual to make the most appropriate decisions to advance his or her sexual and interpersonal health (Getch et al, 2001).*
- • Teach safe sex to all clients including the elderly, which includes using latex condoms, washing with soap immediately after sexual contact, not ingesting semen, avoiding oral-genital contact, not exchanging saliva, avoiding multiple partners, abstaining from sexual activity when ill, and avoiding recreational drugs and alcohol when engaging in sexual activity. Adherence to antiretroviral therapy is important. **EB:** *Predictors of nonadherence to antiretroviral therapy include lack of trust between the health professional and the client, active drug and alcohol use, mental illness such as depression, lack of client education about medications, and unreliable access to medical care. To increase adherence to medications and to support viral suppression, assess emotional and practical life supports;*

assist in determining ways to fit medications into daily routines and stress the importance of taking all doses; discuss that less than optimal adherence leads to resistance; and urge client to keep clinic appointments (US Department Health & Human Services, 2006). **EBN:** *Interventions that focus on self-efficacy are most likely to reduce anxiety related to condom use, increase positive perceptions about condoms, and increase the likelihood of adopting condom use behaviors (Dilorio et al, 2000).* **EB:** *Older adults can and will acquire new information regarding AIDS-related information when it is presented to them (Falvo & Norman, 2004). (Additional resource: Centers for Disease Control, 2006.)*

evolve See the EVOLVE website for World Wide Web resources for client education.

REFERENCES

Ashford L: Erectile dysfunction, *J Pract Nurs* 25(1):18-19, 23-24, 26-27, 2003.

Avis N: Sexual function and aging in men and women: community and population-based studies, *J Gender-Specific Med* 3(2):37-41, 2000.

Centers for Disease Control (CDC): Incorporating HIV prevention into the medical care of persons living with HIV, in CDC: *Provisional Procedural Guidance for Community-Based Organizations,* 2006. Available at: http://www.cdc.gov/hiv/topics/prev_prog/ahp/resources/guidelines/pro_guidance.pdf. Accessed November 19, 2006.

Dilorio C, Dudley WN, Soet J et al: A social cognitive-based model for condom use among college students, *Nurs Res* 49(4):208, 2000.

Falvo N, Norman S: Never too old to learn: the impact of an HIV/AIDS education program on older adults' knowledge, *Clin Gerontol* 27(1/2):103-117, 2004.

Fisher JA, Bowman M, Thomas T: Issues for South Asian Indian patients surrounding sexuality, fertility, and childbirth in the US health care system, *J Am Board Fam Pract* 16(2):151-155, 2003.

Fleming JM: Successful again. In MO Hogstel, editor: *Gerontology: nursing care for the older adult,* Albany, NY, 2001, Delmar, p 148.

Getch YQ, Branca DL, Fitz-Gerald D et al: A rationale and recommendations for sexuality education in schools for students who are deaf, *Am Ann Deaf* 146(5):401-404, 2001.

Hoppe MJ, Graham L, Wilsdon A: Teens speak out about HIV/AIDS: focus group discussions about risk and decision-making, *J Adolesc Health* 35(4):345-346, 2004.

Howard JR, O'Neill S, Travers C: Factors affecting sexuality in older Australian women: sexual interest, sexual arousal, relationships and sexual distress in older Australian women, *Climacteric* 9:355-367, 2006.

Kattainen E, Merilainen P, Jokela V: CABG and PTCA patients' expectations of informational support in health-related quality of life themes and adequacy of information at 1-year follow-up, *Eur J Cardiovasc Nurs* 3:149-163, 2004.

Kingsberg SA: The psychological impact of aging on sexuality and relationships, *J Women's Health Gender-Based Med* 9(Suppl 1):S33-S38, 2000.

L'Abate L: Hugging, holding, huddling and cuddling (3HC): a task prescription in couple and family therapy, *J Clin Activities Assignments Handouts Psychother Pract* 1(1):5, 2001.

Lantz MS: Consenting adults: sexuality in the nursing home, *Clin Geriatr* 12(6):33-36, 2004.

Lazoritz S, McDermott RT: Adolescent sexuality, cultural sensitivity and the teachings of the Catholic Church, *J Reprod Med* 47(8):603, 2002.

Leininger MM, McFarland MR: *Transcultural nursing: concepts, theories, research and practices,* ed 3, New York, 2002, McGraw-Hill.

Lesser J, Oakes R, Koniak-Griffin D: Vulnerable adolescent mothers' perceptions of maternal role and HIV risk, *Health Care Women Int* 24(6):513-528, 2003.

Lewis CL, Brown SC: Coping strategies of female adolescents with HIV/AIDS, *ABNF J* 13(4):72, 2002.

Lundquist G, Ojehagen A: Childhood sexual abuse: an evaluation of a two-year group therapy in adult women, *Eur Psychiatry* 16(1):64, 2001.

McConkey R, Ryan D: Experiences of staff in dealing with client sexuality in services for teenagers and adults with intellectual disability, *J Intell Disabil Res* 45(1):83, 2001.

Peate I: Sexuality and sexual health promotion for the older person, *Br J Nurs* 13(4):188-193, 2004.

Rogers D: New meaning for safe sex, *RN* 66(1):38-42, 2003.

Shell J, Smith C: Sexuality and the older person with cancer, *Oncology* 21:553, 1994.

Silenzio VMB: Anthropological assessment for culturally appropriate interventions targeting men who have sex with men, *Am J Pub Health* 93(6):867-871, 2003.

Sprunk E, Alteneder RR: The impact of an ostomy on sexuality, *Clin J Oncol Nurs* 4(2):85, 2000.

Steinke, EE: Intimacy needs and chronic illness, *J Gerontol Nurs* 31(5):40-50, 2005.

Steinke EE: Sexual concerns of patients and partners after an implantable cardioverter defibrillator, *Dimens Crit Care Nurs* 22(2):89-96, 2003.

Steinke EE: Sexuality in aging: implications for nursing home staff, *J Contin Educ Nurs* 28(2):59-63, 1997.

Steinke EE, Bergen MB: Sexuality and aging, *J Gerontol Nurs* 12(6):6-10, 1986.

Tucker M et al: *Patient care standards: collaborative practice planning,* ed 6, St Louis, 1996, Mosby.

US Department of Health and Human Services: *Guidelines for the use of antiretroviral agents in HIV-1-infected adults and adolescents,* 2006, p. 25, available at http://aidsinfo.nih.gov/contentfiles/AdultandAdolescentGL.pdf. Accessed April 25, 2007.

Impaired Skin integrity   *Sharon Baranoski, MSN, DAPWCA, RN*   **evolve**

NANDA   Definition

Altered epidermis and/or dermis

Defining Characteristics

Destruction of skin layers; disruption of skin surface; invasion of body structures

Related Factors (r/t)

External

Chemical substance; extremes in age; humidity; hyperthermia; hypothermia; mechanical factors (e.g., friction, shearing forces, pressure, restraint); medications; moisture; physical immobilization; radiation

Internal

Changes in fluid status; changes in pigmentation; changes in turgor; developmental factors; imbalanced nutritional state (e.g., obesity, emaciation); immunological deficit; impaired circulation; impaired metabolic state; impaired sensation; skeletal prominence

NOC   Outcomes (Nursing Outcomes Classification)

Suggested NOC Outcomes

Tissue Integrity: Skin and Mucous Membranes, Wound Healing: Primary Intention, Secondary Intention

> ### Example NOC Outcome with Indicators
>
> **Tissue Integrity: Skin and Mucous Membranes** will be intact as evidenced by the following indicators: Skin intactness/Skin lesions not present/Tissue perfusion/Skin temperature (Rate the outcome and indicators of **Tissue Integrity: Skin and Mucous Membranes:** 1 = severely compromised, 2 = substantially compromised, 3 = moderately compromised, 4 = mildly compromised, 5 = not compromised [see Section I].)

Client Outcomes

Client Will (Specify Time Frame):

- Regain integrity of skin surface
- Report any altered sensation or pain at site of skin impairment
- Demonstrate understanding of plan to heal skin and prevent reinjury
- Describe measures to protect and heal the skin and to care for any skin lesion

NIC   Interventions (Nursing Interventions Classification)

Suggested NIC Interventions

Incision Site Care, Pressure Ulcer Care, Skin Care: Topical Treatments, Skin Surveillance, Wound Care

> ### Example NIC Activities—Pressure Ulcer Care
>
> Monitor color, temperature, edema, moisture, and appearance of surrounding skin; Note characteristics of any drainage

Nursing Interventions and *Rationales*

- Assess site of skin impairment and determine cause (e.g., acute or chronic wound, burn, dermatological lesion, pressure ulcer, skin tear). **EB:** *The cause of the wound must be determined before ap-*

• = Independent;   ▲ = Collaborative;   EBN = Evidence-Based Nursing;   EB = Evidence-Based

propriate interventions can be implemented. This will provide the basis for additional testing and evaluation to start the assessment process (Baranoski & Ayello, 2003).

- Determine that skin impairment involves skin damage only (e.g., partial-thickness wound, stage I or stage II pressure ulcer). The following classification system is for pressure ulcers:
  - Stage I: Observable pressure-related alteration of intact skin with indicators as compared with the adjacent or opposite area on the body that may include changes in one or more of the following: skin temperature (warmth or coolness), tissue consistency (firm or boggy feel), and/or sensation (pain, itching). The ulcer appears as a defined area of persistent redness in lightly pigmented skin, whereas in darker skin tones, the ulcer may appear with persistent red, blue, or purple hues (National Pressure Ulcer Advisory Panel [NPUAP], 1998).
  - Stage II: Partial-thickness skin loss involving epidermis or dermis superficial ulcer that appears as an abrasion, blister, or shallow crater (NPUAP, 1998).
  - NOTE: For wounds deeper into subcutaneous tissue, muscle, or bone (stage III or stage IV pressure ulcers), see the care plan for **Impaired Tissue integrity.**
- Monitor site of skin impairment at least once a day for color changes, redness, swelling, warmth, pain, or other signs of infection. Determine whether the client is experiencing changes in sensation or pain. Pay special attention to high-risk areas such as bony prominences, skinfolds, the sacrum, and heels. *Systematic inspection can identify impending problems early (Ayello & Braden, 2002).*
- Monitor the client's skin care practices, noting type of soap or other cleansing agents used, temperature of water, and frequency of skin cleansing.
- Individualize plan according to the client's skin condition, needs, and preferences. **EBN:** *Avoid harsh cleansing agents, hot water, extreme friction or force, or cleansing too frequently (Panel for the Prediction and Prevention of Pressure Ulcers in Adults, 1992; Wound, Ostomy, and Continence Nurses Society [WOCN] 2003).*
- Monitor the client's continence status, and minimize exposure of skin impairment and other areas of moisture from incontinence, perspiration, or wound drainage. **EBN:** *Moisture from incontinence contributes to pressure ulcer development by macerating the skin (WOCN, 2003).*
- ▲ If the client is incontinent, implement an incontinence management plan to prevent exposure to chemicals in urine and stool that can strip or erode the skin. Refer to a continence care specialist, urologist, or gastroenterologist for incontinence assessment (WOCN, 2003). **EB:** *Implementing an incontinence prevention plan with the use of a skin protectant or a cleanser protectant can significantly decrease skin breakdown and pressure ulcer formation (Clever et al, 2003; Fantl et al, 1996; Warshaw et al, 2002).*
- For clients with limited mobility, use a risk assessment tool to systematically assess immobility-related risk factors (Ayello & Braden, 2002). *A validated risk assessment tool such as the Norton or Braden scale should be used to identify clients at risk for immobility-related skin breakdown (Ayello & Braden, 2002).* **EB:** *Targeting variables (such as age and Braden Scale Risk Category) can focus assessment on particular risk factors (e.g., pressure) and help guide the plan of prevention and care (Panel for the Prediction and Prevention of Pressure Ulcers in Adults, 1992; WOCN, 2003; Young et al, 2002).*
- Do not position the client on site of skin impairment. If consistent with overall client management goals, turn and position the client at least every 2 hours. Transfer the client with care to protect against the adverse effects of external mechanical forces such as pressure, friction, and shear.
- Evaluate for use of specialty mattresses, beds, or devices as appropriate. Maintain the head of the bed at the lowest possible degree of elevation to reduce shear and friction, and use lift devices, pillows, foam wedges, and pressure-reducing devices in the bed *(WOCN Clinical Practice Guideline series 2, 2003; Panel for the Prediction and Prevention of Pressure Ulcers in Adults, 1992).*
- ▲ Implement a written treatment plan for topical treatment of the site of skin impairment. *A written plan ensures consistency in care and documentation (Baranoski & Ayello, 2003; Maklebust & Sieggreen, 2001).*
- ▲ Select a topical treatment that will maintain a moist wound-healing environment and that is balanced with the need to absorb exudate. **EBN:** *Choose dressings that provide a moist environment, keep periwound skin dry, and control exudate and eliminate dead space (WOCN, 2003).*
- Avoid massaging around the site of skin impairment and over bony prominences. *Research suggests that massage may lead to deep-tissue trauma (Panel for the Prediction and Prevention of Pressure Ulcers in Adults, 1992).*

• = Independent;   ▲ = Collaborative;   EBN = Evidence-Based Nursing;   EB = Evidence-Based

▲ Assess the client's nutritional status. Refer for a nutritional consult and/or institute dietary supplements as necessary. *Optimizing nutritional intake, including calories, fatty acids, protein, and vitamins, is needed to promote wound healing (Russell, 2001).* **EB:** *The benefit of nutritional evaluation and intensive nutritional support in clients at risk for and with pressure ulcers is not supported by rigorous clinical trials. Despite this lack of evidence, NPUAP (2006) endorses the application of reasonable nutritional assessment and treatment for clients at risk for and with pressure ulcers.*

• Identify the client's phase of wound healing (inflammation, proliferation, maturation) and stage of injury. *Accurate understanding of tissue status combined with knowledge of underlying diagnoses and product validity provide a basis for determining appropriate treatment objectives. No single wound dressing is appropriate for all phases of wound healing (Ovington, 1999).*

Home Care

• Some of the interventions described previously may be adapted for home care use.
• Instruct and assist the client and caregivers in how to change dressings and maintain a clean environment. Provide written instructions and observe them completing the dressing change.
• Educate client and caregivers on proper nutrition, signs and symptoms of infection, and when to call the agency and/or physician with concerns.
▲ It may be beneficial to initiate a consultation in a case assignment with a wound, ostomy, continence (WOC) nurse (or wounds specialist) to establish a comprehensive plan for complex wounds.

Client/Family Teaching

• Teach skin and wound assessment and ways to monitor for signs and symptoms of infection, complications, and healing. *Early assessment and intervention help prevent serious problems from developing.*
▲ Teach the client why a topical treatment has been selected. **EBN:** *The type of dressing needed may change over time as the wound heals and/or deteriorates (WOCN, 2003).*
▲ If consistent with overall client management goals, teach how to turn and reposition at least every 2 hours. **EB:** *If the goal of care is to keep a client (e.g., terminally ill client) comfortable, turning and repositioning may not be appropriate (Krasner, Rodeheaver & Sibbald, 2001; Panel for the Prediction and Prevention of Pressure Ulcers in Adults, 1992).*
• Teach the client to use pillows, foam wedges, and pressure-reducing devices to prevent pressure injury. **EB:** *The use of effective pressure-reducing seat cushions for elderly wheelchair users significantly prevented sitting-acquired pressure ulcers (Geyer et al, 2001).*

 See the EVOLVE website for World Wide Web resources for client education.

REFERENCES

Ayello EA, Braden B: How and why to do pressure ulcer risk assessment, *Adv Skin Wound Care* 15(3):125, 2002.

Baranoski S, Ayello EA, editors: *Wound care essentials: practice principles,* Springhouse, Penn, 2003, Lippincott, Williams & Wilkins.

Clever K, Smith G, Bowser C et al: Evaluating the efficacy of a uniquely delivered skin protectant and its effect on the formation of sacral/buttock pressure ulcers, *Ostomy Wound Manag* 48(12):60, 2002.

Fantl JA et al: *Urinary incontinence in adults: acute and chronic management,* Clinical Practice Guideline No 2, 1996 Update, Agency for Health Care Policy and Research, Pub No 96, Rockville, Md, 1996, Public Health Service, US Department of Health and Human Services.

Geyer MJ, Brienza DM, Karg P et al: A randomized control trial to evaluate pressure-reducing seating cushions for elderly wheelchair users, *Adv Skin Wound Care* 14(3):120, 2001.

Krasner D, Rodeheaver G, Sibbald RG: *Chronic wound care: a clinical source book for healthcare professionals,* ed 3, Wayne, Penn, 2001, HMP Communications.

Maklebust J, Sieggreen M: *Pressure ulcers: guidelines for prevention and nursing management,* ed 3, Springhouse, Penn, 2001, Springhouse.

National Pressure Ulcer Advisory Panel (NPUAP): What is the role of nutritional support for patients in the prevention and treatment of

pressure ulcers? Frequently asked questions, 2006, available at http://www.npuap.org/faq.htm. Accessed April 25, 2007.

Ovington L: Dressings and adjunctive therapies: AHCPR guidelines revisited, *Ostomy Wound Manag* 45(suppl 1A):94S-106S, 1999.

Panel for the Prediction and Prevention of Pressure Ulcers in Adults: *Pressure ulcers in adults: prediction and prevention,* Clinical Practice Guideline No 3, Agency for Health Care Policy and Research, Pub No 92, Rockville, MD, 1992, Public Health Services, US Department of Health and Human Services.

Russell L: The importance of patients' nutritional status in wound healing, *Br J Nurs* 10(6):542, 544-549, 2001.

Warshaw E, Nix D, Kula J et al: Clinical and cost effectiveness of a cleanser protectant lotion for treatment of perineal skin breakdown in low-risk patients with incontinence, *Ostomy Wound Manag* 48(6):44, 2002.

Wound, Ostomy, and Continence Nurses Society: *Guideline for prevention and management of pressure ulcers. WOCN clinical practice guideline series no 2,* Glenview, Ill, 2003, The Society.

Young J, Nikoletti S, McCaul K et al: Risk factors associated with pressure ulcer development at a major Western Australia teaching hospital from 1998 to 2000, *J Wound Ostomy Continence Nurs* 29(5):234, 2002.

S

Risk for impaired Skin integrity *Sharon Baranoski, MSN, DAPWCA, RN*

NANDA Definition

At risk for skin being adversely altered

Risk Factors

External

Chemical substance; excretions and/or secretions; extremes of age; humidity; hyperthermia; hypothermia; mechanical factors (e.g., shearing forces, pressure, restraint); moisture; physical immobilization; radiation

Internal

Alterations in skin turgor (change in elasticity); altered circulation; altered metabolic state; altered nutritional state (e.g., obesity, emaciation); altered pigmentation; altered sensation; developmental factors; immunological deficit; medication; psychogenetic, immunological factors; skeletal prominence
NOTE: Risk should be determined by the use of a risk assessment tool (e.g., Norton scale, Braden scale).

NOC Outcomes (Nursing Outcomes Classification)

Suggested NOC Outcomes

Immobility Consequences: Physiological, Tissue Integrity: Skin and Mucous Membranes

Example NOC Outcome with Indicators
Tissue Integrity: Skin and Mucous Membranes will be intact as evidenced by the following indicators: Skin intactness/Skin lesions not present/Tissue perfusion/Skin temperature (Rate the outcome and indicators of **Tissue Integrity: Skin and Mucous Membranes:** I = severely compromised, 2 = substantially compromised, 3 = moderately compromised, 4 = mildly compromised, 5 = not compromised [see Section I].)

Client Outcomes

Client Will (Specify Time Frame):

- Report altered sensation or pain at risk areas
- Demonstrate understanding of personal risk factors for impaired skin integrity
- Verbalize a personal plan for preventing impaired skin integrity

NIC Interventions (Nursing Interventions Classification)

Suggested NIC Interventions

Positioning: Pressure Management, Pressure Ulcer Care, Pressure Ulcer Prevention, Skin Surveillance

Example NIC Activities—Pressure Ulcer Care
Monitor color, temperature, edema, moisture, and appearance of surrounding skin; Note characteristics of any drainage

Nursing Interventions and *Rationales*

- Monitor skin condition at least once a day for color or texture changes, dermatological conditions, or lesions. Determine whether the client is experiencing loss of sensation or pain. *Systematic inspection can identify impending problems early (Ayello & Braden, 2002; Krasner, Rodeheaver & Sibbald, 2001).*
- Identify clients at risk for impaired skin integrity as a result of immobility, chronological age,

• = Independent;   ▲ = Collaborative;   EBN = Evidence-Based Nursing;   EB = Evidence-Based

malnutrition, incontinence, compromised perfusion, immunocompromised status, or chronic medical condition, such as diabetes mellitus, spinal cord injury, or renal failure. **EB:** *These client populations are known to be at high risk for impaired skin integrity (Maklebust & Sieggreen, 2001; Stotts & Wipke-Tevis, 2001). Targeting variables (such as age and Braden Scale Risk Category) can focus assessment on particular risk factors (e.g., pressure) and help guide the plan of prevention and care (Young et al, 2002).*

- Monitor the client's skin care practices, noting type of soap or other cleansing agents used, temperature of water, and frequency of skin cleansing. *Individualize plan according to the client's skin condition, needs, and preferences (Baranoski, 2000).*
- Avoid harsh cleansing agents, hot water, extreme friction or force, or too-frequent cleansing (Panel for the Prediction and Prevention of Pressure Ulcers in Adults, 1992).
- ▲ Monitor the client's continence status and minimize exposure of the site of skin impairment and other areas to moisture from incontinence, perspiration, or wound drainage. If the client is incontinent, implement an incontinence management plan to prevent exposure to chemicals in urine and stool that can strip or erode the skin; refer to a physician (e.g., continence care specialist, urologist, gastroenterologist) for an incontinence assessment (Fantl et al, 1996; Wound, Ostomy, and Continence Nurses Society [WOCN], 2003). **EB:** *Implementing an incontinence prevention plan with the use of a skin protectant or a cleanser protectant can significantly decrease skin breakdown and pressure ulcer formation (Clever et al, 2002; Warshaw et al, 2002).*
- For clients with limited mobility, monitor condition of skin covering bony prominences. *Pressure ulcers usually occur over bony prominences, such as the sacrum, coccyx, trochanter, and heels, as a result of unrelieved pressure between the prominence and support surface (Maklebust & Sieggreen, 2001; WOCN, 2003).*
- Use a risk assessment tool to systematically assess immobility-related risk factors. *A validated risk assessment tool such as the Norton or Braden scale should be used to identify clients at risk for immobility-related skin breakdown (Ayello & Braden, 2002; Panel for the Prediction and Prevention of Pressure Ulcers in Adults, 1992; Sussman & Bates-Jensen, 1998).*
- Implement a written prevention plan. **EB:** *A written plan ensures consistency in care and documentation (Baranoski & Ayello, 2003; Maklebust & Sieggreen, 2001).* **EBN:** *Implementing a prevention protocol can significantly reduce costs and incidence of skin breakdown and pressure ulcers in the long-term care setting (Lyder et al, 2002).*
- If consistent with overall client management goals, turn and position the client at least every 2 hours. Transfer the client with care to protect against the adverse effects of external mechanical forces (e.g., pressure, friction, shear) (WOCN, 2003).
- Evaluate for use of specialty mattresses, beds, or devices as appropriate (Fleck, 2001; Geyer et al, 2001). *If the goal of care is to keep the client (e.g., a terminally ill client) comfortable, turning and repositioning may not be appropriate. Maintain the head of the bed at the lowest possible degree of elevation to reduce shear and friction and use lift devices, pillows, foam wedges, and pressure-reducing devices in the bed (Krasner, Rodeheaver & Sibbald, 2001; Panel for the Prediction and Prevention of Pressure Ulcers in Adults, 1992; WOCN, 2003).*
- Avoid massaging over bony prominences. *Research suggests that massage may lead to deep-tissue trauma (Panel for the Prediction and Prevention of Pressure Ulcers in Adults, 1992; WOCN, 2003).*
- ▲ Assess the client's nutritional status; refer for a nutritional consult, and/or institute dietary supplements. **EB:** *The benefit of nutritional evaluation and intensive nutritional support in clients at risk for or with pressure ulcers is not supported by rigorous clinical trials. Despite this lack of evidence, the National Pressure Ulcer Advisory Panel (NPUAP) (2006) endorses the application of reasonable nutritional assessment and treatment for clients at risk for and with pressure ulcers.*

Geriatric

- Limit number of complete baths to two or three per week, and alternate them with partial baths. Use a tepid water temperature (between 90° and 105° F) for bathing. **EB:** *Excessive bathing, especially in hot water, depletes aging skin of moisture and increases dryness. The ability to retain moisture is decreased in aging skin due to diminished amounts of dermal proteins. One of the most common age-related changes to the skin is damage to the stratum corneum (Baranoski, 2000; Baranoski & Ayello, 2003).*
- Use lotions and moisturizers to prevent skin from drying out, especially in the winter (Sibbald &

Cameron, 2001). *Avoid skin care products that contain allergens such as lanolin, latex, and dyes (Sibbald & Cameron, 2001).*

- Increase fluid intake within cardiac and renal limits to a minimum of 1500 mL per day. *Dry skin is caused by loss of fluid; increasing fluid intake hydrates the skin.*
- Increase humidity in the environment, especially during the winter, by using a humidifier or placing a container of water on a warm object. *Increasing the moisture in the air helps keep moisture in the skin (Sibbald & Cameron, 2001).*

Home Care

- Assess caregiver vigilance and ability. *In a limited study of the Braden Scale, caregiver vigilance and ability were recognized as potentially significant variables for determining the risk of developing pressure sores (Ramundo, 1995).*
- Initiate a consultation in a case assignment with a wound care specialist or wound, ostomy, and continence (WOC) nurse to establish a comprehensive plan as soon as possible.
- See the care plan for **Impaired Skin integrity.**

Client/Family Teaching

- Teach the client skin assessment and ways to monitor for impending skin breakdown. *Early assessment and intervention help prevent the development of serious problems.* **EB:** *Basic elements of a skin assessment are assessment of temperature, color, moisture, turgor, and intact skin (Baranoski & Ayello, 2003).*
- If consistent with overall client management goals, teach how to turn and reposition the client at least every 2 hours. **EB:** *If the goal of care is to keep the client (e.g., a terminally ill client) comfortable, turning and repositioning may not be appropriate (Panel for the Prediction and Prevention of Pressure Ulcers in Adults, 1992).*
- Teach the client to use pillows, foam wedges, and pressure-reducing devices to prevent pressure injury (Krasner & Sibbald, 1999; WOCN, 2003). **EB:** *The use of effective pressure-reducing seat cushions for elderly wheelchair users significantly prevented sitting-acquired pressure ulcers (Geyer et al, 2001).*

evolve See the EVOLVE website for World Wide Web resources for client education.

REFERENCES

Ayello EA, Braden B: How and why to do pressure ulcer risk assessment, *Adv Skin Wound Care* 15(3):125, 2002.

Baranoski S: Skin tears: the enemy of frail skin, *Adv Skin Wound Care* 13(3 Pt 1):123-126, 2000.

Baranoski S, Ayello EA: Skin an essential organ. In Baranoski S, Ayello EA, editors: *Wound care essentials: practice principles,* Springhouse, Penn, 2003, Lippincott, Williams & Wilkins.

Clever K, Smith G, Bowser C et al: Evaluating the efficacy of a uniquely delivered skin protectant and its effect on the formation of sacral/buttock pressure ulcers, *Ostomy Wound Manag* 48(12):60-67, 2002.

Fantl JA et al: *Urinary incontinence in adults: acute and chronic management,* Clinical Practice Guideline No 2, 1996 Update, Agency for Health Care Policy and Research, Pub No 96, Rockville, Md, 1996, Public Health Service, US Department of Health and Human Services.

Fleck C: Support surfaces: criteria and selection. In Krasner D, Rodeheaver G, Sibbald RG, editors: *Chronic wound care: a clinical source book for healthcare professionals,* ed 3, Wayne, Penn, 2001, HMP Communications.

Geyer MJ, Brienza DM, Karg P et al: A randomized control trial to evaluate pressure-reducing seating cushions for elderly wheelchair users, *Adv Skin Wound Care* 14(3):120, 2001.

Krasner D, Rodeheaver G, Sibbald RG: Advanced wound caring for a new millennium. In Krasner D, Rodeheaver G, Sibbald RG, editors: *Chronic wound care: a clinical source book for healthcare professionals,* ed 3, Wayne, Penn, 2001, HMP Communications.

Krasner, Sibbald: Moving beyond the AHCPR guidelines: wound care evolution over the last five years, *Ostomy Wound Manag* 45(1A): 1ss, 1999.

Lyder CH, Shannon R, Empleo-Frazier O et al: A comprehensive program to prevent pressure ulcers in long-term care: exploring costs and outcomes, *Ostomy Wound Manage* 48(4):52, 2002.

Maklebust J, Sieggreen M: *Pressure ulcers: guidelines for prevention and nursing management,* ed 3, Springhouse, Penn, 2001, Springhouse.

National Pressure Ulcer Advisory Panel (NPUAP): What is the role of nutritional support for patients in the prevention and treatment of pressure ulcers? Frequently asked questions 2006, available at http://www.npuap.org/faq.htm. Accessed April 25, 2007.

Panel for the Prediction and Prevention of Pressure Ulcers in Adults: *Pressure ulcers in adults: prediction and prevention,* Clinical Practice Guideline No 3, Agency for Health Care Policy and Research, Pub No 92, Rockville, Md, 1992, Public Health Service, US Department of Health and Human Services.

Ramundo J: Reliability and validity of the Braden Scale in the home care setting, *J Wound Ostomy Cont Nurs* 22:3, 1995.

Sibbald RG, Cameron J: Dermatological aspects of wound care. In Krasner D, Rodeheaver G, Sibbald RG, editors: *Chronic wound care:*

S

a clinical source book for healthcare professionals, ed 3, Wayne, Penn, 2001, HMP Communications.

Stotts NA, Wipke-Tevis D: Co-factors in impaired wound healing. In Krasner D, Rodeheaver G, Sibbald RG, editors: *Chronic wound care: a clinical source book for healthcare professionals,* ed 3, Wayne, Penn, 2001, HMP Communications.

Sussman C, Bates-Jensen BM: *Wound care: a collaborative practice manual for physical therapists and nurses,* Gaithersburg, Md, 1998, Aspen.

Warshaw E, Nix D, Kula J et al: Clinical and cost effectiveness of a

cleanser protectant lotion for treatment of perineal skin breakdown in low-risk patients with incontinence, *Ostomy Wound Manag* 48(6):44, 2002.

Wound, Ostomy, and Continence Nurses Society: *Guideline for prevention and management of pressure ulcers. WOCN clinical practice guideline series no 2,* Glenview, Ill, 2003, The Society.

Young J, Nikoletti S, McCaul K et al: Risk factors associated with pressure ulcer development at a major Western Australia teaching hospital from 1998 to 2000, *J WOCN* 29(5):234, 2002.

Sleep deprivation   *Judith A. Floyd, PhD, RN, and Jean D. Humphries, MSN, RN*

NANDA   Definition

Prolonged periods without sleep (sustained natural, periodic suspension of relative consciousness)

Defining Characteristics

Acute confusion; agitation; anxiety; apathy; combativeness; daytime drowsiness; decreased ability to function; fatigue; fleeting nystagmus; hallucinations; hand tremors; heightened sensitivity to pain; inability to concentrate; irritability; lethargy; listlessness; malaise; perceptual disorders (e.g., disturbed body sensation, delusions, feeling afloat); restlessness; slowed reaction; transient paranoia

Related Factors (r/t)

Aging-related sleep stage shifts; dementia; familial sleep paralysis; idiopathic central nervous system hypersomnolence; inadequate daytime activity; narcolepsy; nightmares; on-sleep inducing parenting practices; periodic limb movement (e.g., restless leg syndrome, nocturnal myoclonus); prolonged discomfort (e.g., physical, psychological); prolonged use of pharmacologic or dietary antisoporifics; sleep apnea; sleep-related enuresis; sleep-related painful erections; sleep terror; sleep walking; sundowner's syndrome; sustained circadian asynchrony; sustained environmental stimulation; sustained inadequate sleep hygiene; sustained uncomfortable sleep environment

NOC   Outcomes (Nursing Outcomes Classification)

Suggested NOC Outcomes

Rest, Sleep, Symptom Severity

Example NOC Outcome with Indicators
Sleep as evidenced by the following indicators: Hours of sleep/Sleep pattern/Sleep quality/Sleep efficiency/Feels rejuvenated after sleep/Napping appropriate for age (Rate the outcome and indicators of **Sleep:** 1 = severely compromised, 2 = substantially compromised, 3 = moderately compromised, 4 = mildly compromised, 5 = not compromised [see Section I].)

Client Outcomes

Client Will (Specify Time Frame):

- Wake up less frequently during night
- Awaken refreshed and be less fatigued during day
- Fall asleep without difficulty
- Verbalize plan that provides adequate time for sleep
- Identify actions that can be taken to improve quality of sleep

NIC   Interventions (Nursing Interventions Classification)

Suggested NIC Intervention

Sleep Enhancement

• = Independent;   ▲ = Collaborative;   EBN = Evidence-Based Nursing;   EB = Evidence-Based

Example NIC Activities—Sleep Enhancement
Monitor/record patient's sleep pattern and number of sleep hours; Encourage patient to establish a bedtime routine to facilitate transition from wakefulness to sleep allows for adequate amounts of sleep; Adjust environment to promote sleep

Nursing Interventions and *Rationales*

- Obtain a sleep-wake history, including work and other scheduled activities, history of sleep problems, changes in sleep with present illness, and use of medications and stimulants. *Assessment of sleep behavior and patterns are an important part of any health status examination (Landis, 2002).*

- Ask the client to keep a sleep-wake diary for several weeks, which includes bedtime, rise time, number of awakenings, naps, and scheduled daytime events that may be depriving the client of adequate sleep time. *Often the client can find the cause of the sleep deprivation when the pattern of sleeping is examined (Pagel et al, 1997). A sleep diary is a necessary component of a behavioral assessment of sleep problems (Landis, 2002).*

- ▲ Assess for underlying physiological illnesses causing sleep loss (e.g., cardiovascular, pulmonary, gastrointestinal, hyperthyroidism, nocturia occurring with benign hypertrophic prostatitis or pain). *Symptomatology of disease states can cause insomnia (Sateia et al, 2000).*

- ▲ Assess level of anxiety. If the client is anxious, use relaxation techniques. See further Nursing Interventions and Rationales for **Anxiety. EBN and EB:** *The use of relaxation techniques to promote sleep in people with chronic insomnia has been shown to be effective (Floyd, Falahee & Fhobir, 2000; Johnson, 1991b; Morin, Culbert & Schwartz, 1994).*

- ▲ Assess for signs of depression: depressed mood state, flat affect, statements of hopelessness, poor appetite. Refer for counseling/treatment as appropriate. *Many symptoms associated with sleep deprivation probably arise from central nervous system hyperarousal in the depressed client (Sateia et al, 2000).*

- ▲ Assess the client for other symptoms of bipolar disorder (mania, hypomania). Refer for mental health services as indicated. *Sleep loss is part of the syndrome of bipolar disorder. Resumption of a normal sleep pattern is unlikely unless the underlying bipolar disorder is treated (Morris, 2003).*

- ▲ Monitor for presence of nocturnal symptoms of restless leg syndrome with uncomfortable restless sensations in legs that occur before sleep onset or during the night. In addition, monitor for nocturnal panic attacks, presence of headaches, or gastroesophageal reflux disease. Refer for treatment as appropriate. *Numerous nocturnal events and symptoms can contribute to sleep loss (Sateia et al, 2000).*

- Assess and then evaluate the client's medication, diet, and caffeine intake. Look for hidden sources of caffeine, such as over-the-counter medications. *Difficulty sleeping can be a side effect of medications such as bronchodilators; caffeine can also interfere with sleep (Benca, 2005).* **EB:** *Caffeine use after 2 PM is associated within poor sleep (Ellis, Hampson & Cropley, 2002).*

- ▲ Provide pain relief shortly before bedtime, and position the client comfortably for sleep. *Clients have reported that uncomfortable positions and pain are common factors in sleep loss (Sateia et al, 2000).*

- ▲ Monitor for presence of sleep disordered breathing as evidenced by loud snoring with periods of apnea, or other sleep disorders such as restless leg syndrome or periodic limb movement disorder. Refer to an accredited sleep disorder center. *Up to 15% of all chronic poor sleep is associated with breathing disturbances (Sateia et al, 2000). Polysomnography evaluation is recommended if a sleep disorder exists (Epstein & Bootzin, 2002).*

- Keep environment quiet for sleeping (e.g., avoid use of intercoms, lower the volume on radio and television, keep beepers on nonaudio mode, anticipate alarms on intravenous [IV] pumps, talk quietly on unit). *Attention to environmental sources of noise can eliminate or reduce them (Barr, 1993).* **EBN:** *Healthy volunteers exposed to recorded critical care noise levels experienced poor quality sleep (Topf, Bookman & Arand, 1996). Excessive noise disrupts sleep (Floyd, 1999). Quiet time increased sleep duration in hospitalized adults (Olson et al, 2001).*

- Use soothing sound generators with sounds of the ocean, rainfall, or waterfall to induce sleep, or use "white noise" such as a fan to block out other sounds. Also consider the use of earplugs. **EBN:** *Ocean sounds promoted sleep for a group of postoperative open-heart surgery clients (Williamson, 1992). Earplugs have been found to decrease the effects of simulated intensive care unit noise on sleep (Wallace et al, 1999).*

S

• = Independent;   ▲ = Collaborative;   EBN = Evidence-Based Nursing;   EB = Evidence-Based

- Encourage the client to use soothing music to facilitate sleep. **EBN:** *Music results in better sleep quality, longer sleep duration, greater sleep efficiency, shorter sleep latency, less sleep disturbance, and less daytime dysfunction (Lai & Good, 2005).*

Geriatric

- Assess if the client has a physiological problem that could result in sleep loss such as pain, cardiovascular disease, pulmonary disease, neurological problems such as dementia, or urinary problems. *Sleep disturbances in the elderly may represent a complex interaction of age-related changes and pathological causes (Sateia et al, 2000).*
- Assess urinary elimination patterns. Have the client decrease fluid intake in the evening, and instruct that diuretics are taken early in the morning. *Many elderly people void during the night. Increasing water intake at night or taking diuretics late in the day increases nocturia, which results in sleep loss (Avidan, 2005).*
- ▲ If the client is waking frequently during the night with periods of apnea or increased leg movement, consider the presence of sleep apnea problems or periodic leg movements disorder and refer to a sleep clinic for evaluation. *Sleep apnea and periodic limb movement disorders interfere more with sleep as clients age (Floyd, 2002).*
- Assist the client with taking a warm bath in the evening. **EBN:** *Passive heating by using a warm bath has been shown to increase deep sleep in the elderly (Dorsey et al, 1996).*
- Help the client recognize that changes in length of sleep occur with aging. *Client may not be able to sleep for 8 hours as when younger, and more frequent awakening is part of the aging process (Floyd, 2002).*
- Help client recognize that increasing age is associated with changes both in the nature and duration of sleep complaints. **EB:** *Only two studies report that older adults with insomnia reveal a greater problem with sleep maintenance. The prevalence of apnea increases significantly with age; other risk factors include being male, snoring, and being obese. Community-based studies have indicated this is common among older adults, affecting approximately 24% of those over 65 (Espie, 2001).*

Home Care

- Interventions discussed above may be adapted for home care use.
- Have the client or caregiver maintain a diary describing evening and nighttime activity, light, and noise levels in the home. Assess diary for potential areas of intervention to decrease interference with nighttime sleep. *Details about the home sleep environment may yield clues to factors leading to sleep deprivation in the home (e.g., excessive noise or light in the sleep environment, the needs of minor children, sleeping arrangements) (Floyd, 2002).*
- ▲ In the presence of a psychiatric disorder, refer for psychiatric home healthcare services for client reassurance and implementation of therapeutic regimen. **EBN:** *Psychiatric home care nurses can address issues relating to the client's sleep deprivation and bipolar disorder. Behavioral interventions in the home can assist the client to participate more effectively in treatment plan (Patusky et al, 1996).*

Client/Family Teaching

- Encourage the client to avoid coffee and other caffeinated foods and liquids and to avoid eating large high-protein or high-fat meals close to bedtime. *Caffeine intake increases the time it takes to fall asleep and increases awake time during the night (Evans & Rogers, 1994).*
- Advise the client to avoid use of alcohol or hypnotics to induce sleep. Avoid alcohol ingestion 4 to 6 hours before bedtime. *Sleep induced by alcohol is often disrupted later in the night (Epstein & Bootzin, 2002).*
- Encourage the client to develop a bedtime ritual that includes quiet activities such as reading, television, or crafts. **EBN:** *The use of a bedtime routine has been shown to be effective in inducing and maintaining sleep in a population of older women (Johnson, 1991a).*
- Teach the following sleep hygiene guidelines for improving sleep habits:
  - Go to bed only when sleepy.
  - When awake in the middle of the night, go to another room, do quiet activities, and go back to bed only when sleepy.
  - Use the bed only for sleeping.
  - Avoid afternoon and evening naps.

• = Independent;   ▲ = Collaborative;   EBN = Evidence-Based Nursing;   EB = Evidence-Based

- Get up at the same time every morning.
- Recognize that not everyone needs 8 hours of sleep.
- Do not associate lulls in performance with sleeplessness; sleeplessness should not be blamed for everything that goes wrong during the day.

EB: *These guidelines on sleep hygiene have been shown to effectively improve quality of sleep (Morin et al, 2005; Morin, Culbert & Schwartz, 1994).*

evolve   See the EVOLVE website for World Wide Web resources for client education.

REFERENCES

Avidan AY: Sleep in the geriatric patient population, *Semin Neurol* 25(1):52-63, 2005.

Barr WJ: Noise notes: working smart, *Am J Nurs* 93:16, 1993.

Benca RM: Diagnosis and treatment of chronic insomnia: a review, *Psychiatr Serv* 56(3):332-343, 2005.

Dorsey CM, Lukas SE, Teicher MH et al: Effects of passive body heating on the sleep of older female insomniacs, *J Geriatr Psychiatry Neurol* 9(2):83, 1996.

Ellis J, Hampson SE, Cropley M: Sleep hygiene or compensatory sleep practices: an examination of behaviours affecting sleep in older adults, *Psychol Health Med* 7(2):156-161, 2002.

Epstein DR, Bootzin RR: Insomnia, *Nurs Clin North Am* 37(4):611-631, 2002.

Espie CA: The clinical effectiveness of cognitive behavior therapy for chronic insomnia: implementation and evaluation of a sleep clinic in general medical practice, *Behav Resp Ther* 39:45-60, 2001.

Evans BD, Rogers AE: 24-hour sleep/wake patterns in healthy elderly persons, *Appl Nurs Res* 7(2):75-83, 1994.

Floyd JA: Sleep and aging, *Nurs Clin North Am* 37(4):719-731, 2002.

Floyd JA: Sleep promotion in adults, *Annu Rev Nurs Res* 17:27-56, 1999.

Floyd JA, Falahee ML, Fhobir RH: Creation and analysis of a computerized database of interventions to facilitate adult sleep, *Nurs Res* 49(4):236-241, 2000.

Johnson JE: A comparative study of the bedtime routines and sleep of older adults, *J Community Health Nurs* 8(3):129-136, 1991a.

Johnson JE: Progressive relaxation and the sleep of older noninstitutionalized women, *Appl Nurs Res* 4(4):165-170, 1991b.

Lai HL, Good M: Music improves sleep quality in older adults, *J Adv Nurs* 49(3):234-244, 2005.

Landis CA: Sleep and methods of assessment, *Nurs Clin North Am* 37(4):583-597, 2002.

Morin C, Beaulieu-Bonneau S, LeBlanc M et al: Self-help treatment for insomnia: a randomized controlled trial, *Sleep* 28(1):1319-1327, 2005.

Morin CM, Culbert JP, Schwartz SM: Nonpharmacological interventions for insomnia: a meta-analysis of treatment efficacy, *Am J Psychiatry* 151(8):1172-1180, 1994.

Morris CM: Managing depression in primary care, *Physician Assist* 27(1):20, 2003.

Olson, DM, Borel CO, Laskowitz DT et al: Quiet time: a nursing intervention to promote sleep in neurocritical care units, *Am J Crit Care* 10(2):74, 2001.

Pagel JF et al: How to prescribe a good night's sleep, *Patient Care* 31(4):87, 1997.

Patusky KL et al: Clinical lessons in psychiatric home health care: a case study approach, *Home Healthc Manag Pract* 9(1):8, 1996.

Sateia MJ, Doghramji K, Hauri PJ et al: Evaluation of chronic insomnia. An American Academy of Sleep Medicine review, *Sleep* 23(2):243, 2000.

Topf M, Bookman M, Arand D: Effects of critical care unit noise on the subjective quality of sleep, *J Adv Nurs* 24(3):545-551, 1996.

Wallace CJ, Robins J, Alvord LS et al: The effect of earplugs on sleep measures during exposure to simulated intensive care unit noise, *Am J Crit Care* 8(4):210-219, 1999.

Williamson J: The effect of ocean sounds on sleep after coronary artery bypass graft surgery, *Am J Crit Care* 1(1):91, 1992.

S Readiness for enhanced Sleep   Judith A. Floyd, PhD, RN, and Jean D. Humphries, MSN, RN

NANDA   Definition

A pattern of natural, periodic suspension of consciousness that provides adequate rest, sustains a desired lifestyle, and can be strengthened

Defining Characteristics

Amount of sleep is congruent with developmental needs; expresses a feeling of being rested after sleep; expresses willingness to enhance sleep; follows sleep routines that promote sleep habits; occasional use of medications to induce sleep

NOC   Outcomes (Nursing Outcomes Classification)

Suggested NOC Outcomes

Personal Well-Being, Rest, Sleep

• = Independent;   ▲ = Collaborative;   EBN = Evidence-Based Nursing;   EB = Evidence-Based

Example NOC Outcome with Indicators
Sleep as evidenced by the following indicators: Hours of sleep/Sleep pattern/Sleep quality/Sleep efficiency/Feels rejuvenated after sleep/Napping appropriate for age (Rate the outcome and indicators of **Sleep:** 1 = severely compromised, 2 = substantially compromised, 3 = moderately compromised, 4 = mildly compromised, 5 = not compromised [see Section I].)

Client Outcomes

Client Will (Specify Time Frame):

- Awaken naturally, feeling refreshed, and is not fatigued during day
- Fall asleep without difficulty
- Verbalize plan to implement sleep promotion routines

NIC   Interventions (Nursing Interventions Classification)

Suggested NIC Intervention

Sleep Enhancement

Example NIC Activities—Sleep Enhancement
Determine patient's sleep/activity pattern; Adjust environment and promote sleep/Encourage patient to establish a bedtime routine to facilitate transition from wakefulness to sleep

Nursing Interventions and *Rationales*

- Obtain a sleep history including bedtime routines, sleep patterns, and use of medications and stimulants. *Assessment of sleep behavior and patterns is an important part of any health status examination (Landis, 2002).*
- Determine level of anxiety. If the client is anxious, use relaxation techniques. See further Nursing Interventions and Rationales for **Anxiety. EBN and EB:** *The use of relaxation techniques to promote sleep in people with chronic insomnia has been shown to be effective (Floyd, Falahee & Fhobir, 2000, Johnson, 1991b; Morin, Culbert & Schwartz, 1994).*
- Assess the client's medication, diet, and caffeine intake. Evaluate for hidden sources of caffeine, such as over-the-counter medications. **EB:** *Difficulty sleeping can be a side effect of medications such as bronchodilators; caffeine can also interfere with sleep (Benca, 2005). Caffeine use after 2 PM is associated within poor sleep (Ellis, Hampson & Cropley, 2002).*
- Provide interventions before bedtime to assist with sleep (e.g., quiet time to allow the mind to slow down, carbohydrates such as crackers). *Simple measures can increase quality of sleep. Carbohydrates cause release of the neurotransmitter serotonin, which helps induce and maintain sleep (Somer, 1999).*
- Provide a back massage before bedtime. **EBN:** *Use of a back massage has been shown effective for promoting relaxation, which likely leads to improved sleep (Richards et al, 2003).*
- Initiate nonpharmacologic interventions for improved sleep: control of disturbing environmental stimuli, sleep restriction, increasing sunlight exposure, acupuncture, and cognitive and educational interventions to address dysfunctional attitudes about sleep. **EBN and EB:** *Nonpharmacologic interventions have been shown to improve sleep efficiency and continuity, increase satisfaction with sleep pattern, while reducing hypnotic usage (Morin, Mimeault & Gagne, 1999; Woodward, 1999). Nursing interventions have been directed at making environments conducive to sleep, relaxing the client, or entraining the circadian sleep-wake cycle (Floyd, 1999).*

 ### Geriatric

- Ask the client to keep a sleep diary for several weeks, which includes bedtime, rise time, number of awakenings, naps, and energy-using activities. *A sleep-wake diary is a necessary component of a behavioral assessment of sleep problems (Landis, 2002).*

S

• = Independent;   ▲ = Collaborative;   EBN = Evidence-Based Nursing;   EB = Evidence-Based

- Instruct the client in expectations for normal sleep. Elicit expectations for sleep, previous sleep patterns; correct misconceptions that influence emotional responses to deviation from expectations. *The elderly person may be unduly concerned by normal age-related changes in sleep patterns (i.e., lighter sleep and occasional awakenings may be misconstrued as sleep disorders). Reassurance may ease concerns (Woodward, 1999).* **EBN:** *As people age, increased time is needed to fall asleep; frequency of waking after sleep onset increases; length of waking after sleep onset increases (which may be related to unrecognized sleep apnea); and nighttime sleep amount tends to decrease (Floyd et al, 2000).*
- Encourage the client to develop a bedtime ritual that includes quiet activities such as reading, television, or crafts. **EBN:** *The use of a bedtime routine has been shown to be effective in inducing and maintaining sleep in a population of older women (Johnson, 1991a).*
- Encourage the client to take a warm bath in the evening. **EBN and EB:** *Passive heating by using a warm bath has been shown to increase deep sleep in the elderly (Dorsey et al, 1996; Liao, 2002).*
- Encourage the client to use soothing music to facilitate sleep. **EBN:** *Music results in better sleep quality, longer sleep duration, greater sleep efficiency, shorter sleep latency, less sleep disturbance, and less daytime dysfunction (Lai & Good, 2005).*
- Assess urinary elimination patterns. The client should decrease fluid intake in the evening and diuretics should be administered early in the morning unless contraindicated. *Many elderly people awaken to void during the night. Increasing water intake at night or taking diuretics late in the day increases nocturia, which results in disrupted sleep (Avidan, 2005).*
- Encourage social activities. Help elderly get outside for increased light exposure and to enjoy nature. *Exposure to natural light and social interactions influence the circadian rhythms that control sleep (Labyak, 2002).*
- Increase daytime physical and social activity. Encourage walking as the client is able. **EBN:** *Increasing activity during the day is effective in promoting sleep (Richards et al, 2001).* **EB:** *Research focusing on older adults suggested significant sleep benefits resulting from exercise (Lichstein & Morin, 2000).*
- Recommend avoidance of hypnotics and alcohol to induce sleep. Avoid alcohol ingestion 4 to 6 hours before bedtime. *Long-term use of hypnotics can induce a drug-related insomnia. Alcohol also disrupts sleep and can exacerbate sleep apnea (Evans & Rogers, 1994). Sleep induced by alcohol is often disrupted later in the night (Epstein & Bootzin, 2002).* **EB:** *In nonalcoholic sleepers, bedtime alcohol use decreased sleep latency but increased wakefulness during the latter part of the sleep period (Roehrs & Roth, 1997).*
- Reduce daytime napping in the late afternoon; limit naps to short intervals as early in the day as possible. *The majority of elderly nap during the day (Evans & Rogers, 1994). Avoiding naps in the late afternoon makes it easier to fall asleep at night.* **EBN:** *Naps longer than 50 minutes were associated with increased nighttime awakening (Floyd, 1995).* **EB:** *Napping short intervals early in the day enhanced cognitive and psychomotor performance (Campbell, Murphy & Stauble, 2005).*

Client/Family Teaching

- Teach somatic and cognitive relaxation techniques to induce the relaxation response and facilitate sleep. **EBN and EB:** *The use of relaxation techniques to promote sleep in people with chronic insomnia has been shown to be effective (Floyd, Falahee & Fhobir, 2000; Johnson, 1991b; Morin, Culbert & Schwartz, 1994).*
- Teach the following guidelines for good sleep hygiene to improve sleep habits:
  - Go to bed only when sleepy.
  - When awake in the middle of the night, go to another room, do quiet activities, and go back to bed only when sleepy.
  - Use the bed only for sleeping.
  - Avoid afternoon and evening naps.
  - Get out of bed at the same time every morning.
  - Recognize that not everyone needs 8 hours of sleep.
  - Move the alarm clock away from the bed so that it cannot be seen.
  - Do not associate lulls in performance with sleeplessness; sleeplessness should not be blamed for everything that goes wrong during the day.

• = Independent;   ▲ = Collaborative;   EBN = Evidence-Based Nursing;   EB = Evidence-Based

EB: *These guidelines on sleep hygiene have been shown to effectively improve quality of sleep (Benca, 2005; Morin, Culbert & Schwartz, 1994).*

Home Care

- Interventions discussed above may be adapted for home care use.
- ▲ Assess the conduciveness of the home environment for both the caregivers and the care recipient's sleep. *Many factors in the home environment can promote or interfere with the sleep readiness of clients/family members (Floyd, 1999).* **EBN:** *Activities of family members have been found to be a major disrupter of sleep in the home (Floyd, 1993).*

 See the EVOLVE website for World Wide Web resources for client education.

REFERENCES

Avidan AY: Sleep in the geriatric patient population, *Semin Neurol* 25(1):52-63, 2005.

Benca RM: Diagnosis and treatment of chronic insomnia: a review, *Psychiatr Serv* 56(3):334-343, 2005.

Campbell SS, Murphy PJ, Stauble TN: Effects of a nap on nighttime sleep and waking function in older subjects, *J Am Geriatr Soc* 53(1):48-53, 2005.

Dorsey CM, Lukas SE, Teicher MH et al: Effects of passive body heating on the sleep of older female insomniacs, *J Geriatr Psychiatry Neurol* 9(2):83-90, 1996.

Ellis J, Hampson SE, Cropley M: Sleep hygiene or compensatory sleep practices: an examination of behaviours affecting sleep in older adults, *Psychol Health Med* 7(2):157-161, 2002.

Epstein DR, Bootzin RR: Insomnia, *Nurs Clin North Am* 37(4):611-631, 2002.

Evans BD, Rogers AE: 24-hour sleep/wake patterns in healthy elderly persons, *Appl Nurs Res* 7(2):75-83, 1994.

Floyd JA: Another look at napping in the older adult, *Geriatr Nurs* 16:136, 1995.

Floyd JA: Sleep promotion in adults, *Annu Rev Nurs Res* 17:27, 1999.

Floyd JA: The use of across-method triangulation in the study of sleep concerns in healthy older adults, *ANS* 16(2):70, 1993.

Floyd JA, Falahee ML, Fhobir RH: Creation and analysis of a computerized database of interventions to facilitate adult sleep, *Nurs Res* 49(4):236-241, 2000.

Floyd JA, Medler SM, Ager JW et al: Age-related changes in initiation and maintenance of sleep: a meta-analysis, *Res Nurs Health* 23(2):106-117, 2000.

Johnson JE: A comparative study of the bedtime routines and sleep of older adults, *J Community Health Nurs* 8(3):129-136, 1991a.

Johnson JE: Progressive relaxation and the sleep of older noninstitutionalized women, *Appl Nurs Res* 4(4):165-170, 1991b.

Labyak S: Sleep and circadian schedule disorders, *Nurs Clin North Am* 37(4):599-610, 2002.

Lai HL, Good M: Music improves sleep quality in older adults, *J Adv Nurs* 49(3):234-244, 2005.

Landis CA: Sleep and methods of assessment, *Nurs Clin North Am* 37(4):583-597, 2002.

Liao WC: Effects of passive body heating on body temperature and sleep regulation in the elderly: a systematic review, *Int J Nurs Stud* 39(8):803-810, 2002.

Lichstein KL, Morin, CM: *Treatment of late-life insomnia*, Thousand Oaks, Calif, 2000, Sage Publications.

Morin C, Culbert JP, Schwartz SM: Nonpharmacological interventions for insomnia: a meta-analysis of treatment efficacy, *Am J Psychiatry* 151(8):1172-1180, 1994.

Morin CM, Mimeault V, Gagne A: Nonpharmacological treatment of late-life insomnia, *J Psychosom Res* 46(2):103-116, 1999.

Richards K, Nagel C, Markie M et al: Use of complementary and alternative therapies to promote sleep in critical ill patients, *Crit Care Nurs Clin North Am* 15(3):329-340, 2003.

Richards KC, Sullivan SC, Phillips RL et al: The effect of individualized activities on the sleep of nursing home residents who are cognitively impaired: a pilot study, *J Gerontol Nurs* 27(9):30-37, 2001.

Roehrs T, Roth T: Hypnotics, alcohol, and caffeine: relation to insomnia. In Pressman MR, Orr WC, editors: *Understanding sleep: the evaluation and treatment of sleep disorders*, Washington, DC, 1997, American Psychological Association.

Somer E: *Food and mood: the complete guide to eating well and feeling your best*, ed 2, New York, 1999, Henry Holt.

Woodward M: Insomnia in the elderly, *Aust Fam Physician* 28(7):653-658, 1999.

S

Impaired Social interaction   *Gail B. Ladwig, MSN, CHTP, RN*

NANDA   Definition

Insufficient or excessive quantity or ineffective quality of social exchange

Defining Characteristics

Discomfort in social situations; dysfunctional interaction with others; family report of changes in interaction (e.g., style, pattern); inability to communicate a satisfying sense of social engagement (e.g., belonging, caring, interest, or shared history); inability to receive a satisfying sense of social engagement (e.g., belonging, caring, interest, or shared history); use of unsuccessful social interaction behaviors

---

• = Independent;   ▲ = Collaborative;   EBN = Evidence-Based Nursing;   EB = Evidence-Based

Related Factors (r/t)

Absence of significant others; communication barriers; deficit about ways to enhance mutuality (e.g., knowledge, skills); disturbed thought processes; environmental barriers; limited physical mobility; self-concept disturbance; sociocultural dissonance; therapeutic isolation

NOC   Outcomes (Nursing Outcomes Classification)

Suggested NOC Outcomes

Child Development: Middle Childhood, Adolescence, Play Participation, Role Performance, Social Interaction Skills, Social Involvement

Example NOC Outcome with Indicators
Social Involvement as evidenced by the following indicator: Interacts with close friends, neighbors, family members, and members of work groups (Rate the outcome and indicators of **Social Involvement:** 1 = never demonstrated, 2 = rarely demonstrated, 3 = sometimes demonstrated, 4 = often demonstrated, 5 = consistently demonstrated [see Section I].)

Client Outcomes

Client Will (Specify Time Frame):

• Identify barriers that cause impaired social interactions
• Discuss feelings that accompany impaired and successful social interactions
• Use available opportunities to practice interactions
• Use successful social interaction behaviors
• Report increased comfort in social situations
• Communicate, state feelings of belonging, demonstrate caring and interest in others
• Report effective interactions with others

NIC   Interventions (Nursing Interventions Classification)

Suggested NIC Intervention

Socialization Enhancement

Example NIC Activities—Socialization Enhancement
Encourage patience in developing relationships; Help patient increase awareness of strengths and limitations in communicating with others

S

Nursing Interventions and *Rationales*

• Consider using a self rating scale to assess social functioning. *Social functioning is an important dimension to assess.* **EB:** *This scale seems to be a valuable instrument for the monitoring of social functioning in psychiatric clients. It sets up the expectation of change and allows reality testing of clients' and therapists' beliefs about the presence of progress or not and to identify if therapy is working on this specific outcome domain (Zanello et al, 2006).*
• Monitor the client's use of defense mechanisms, and support healthy defenses (e.g., the client focuses on present and avoids placing blame on others for personal behavior). **EBN:** *Solution-focused techniques have been demonstrated to be beneficial. Therapy focuses on client's present and future, capitalizing on the strengths and resources of the client and significant others around them (Bowles, 2002; University of Central Lancashire Department of Nursing, 2003).*
• Spend time with the client. **EBN:** *Being truly present was listed as one behavior that demonstrated caring (Melnechenko, 2003; Yonge & Molzahn, 2002).*
• Use active listening skills, including assessment and clarification of the client's verbal and non-verbal responses and interactions. **EBN:** *The best practice with regard to communication in palliative*

• = Independent;   ▲ = Collaborative;   EBN = Evidence-Based Nursing;   EB = Evidence-Based

care could be achieved by using a sensitive assessment of how each client chooses to cope with his or her situation rather than by adopting a uniform approach to care (Dean, 2002; Lunney, 2006).

- Encourage social support for clients with visual impairments. **EB:** *Research on Dutch adolescents with visual impairments indicates that social support, especially the support of peers, is important to adolescents with visual impairments (Kef, 2002).*
- Identify client strengths. Have the client make a list of strengths and refer to it when experiencing negative feelings. He or she may find it helpful to put the list on a note card to carry at all times. **EBN:** *Extra stress is reduced by positive thinking (Makinen et al, 2000).*
- Have group members support each other in a group setting. **EB:** *The data in this study of clients suffering from schizophrenia suggest that each client, given enough time and support, can increase his or her own level of maturation and functioning in a group setting (Sigman & Hassan, 2006).*
- Model appropriate social interactions. Give positive verbal and nonverbal feedback for appropriate behavior (e.g., make statements such as, "I'm proud that you made it to work on time and did all the tasks assigned to you without saying that your supervisor was picking on you"; make eye contact). If not contraindicated, touch the client's arm or hand when speaking. **EBN:** *Shared feelings increased communication with stroke and aphasia clients without words (Sundin, Jansson & Norberg, 2000).*
- Use role playing to increase social skills. **EB:** *Role playing has been demonstrated to increase social functioning with clients with schizophrenia (Bellack, Brown & Thomas-Lohrman, 2006).*
- Use client-centered humor as appropriate. **EBN:** *This study demonstrated that client-initiated humor is important for increasing the client-caregiver communication and creating a supportive humanistic atmosphere for client care (Adamle & Turkoski, 2006).*
- ▲ Consider use of animal therapy; arrange for visitation. **EBN:** *Equine-facilitated psychotherapy, although not a new idea, is a little-known experiential intervention that offers the opportunity to achieve healing (Vidrine et al, 2002).*
- Consider the use of the Internet to promote socialization. **EBN:** *Use of the Internet was effective in providing social support and education for isolated rural women with chronic illness (Hill & Weinert, 2004).*
- ▲ Refer client for behavioral interventions (life skills program) to increase social skills. **EB:** *A commercially available, facilitator-administered or self-administered behavioral training product can have significant beneficial effects on psychosocial well-being in a healthy community sample (Kirby et al, 2006).*
- Refer to care plans for **Risk for Loneliness** and **Social isolation** for additional interventions.

Pediatric

- Provide computers and the Internet access to children with chronic disabilities that limit socialization. **EB:** *Parents who had a child with Duchenne's muscular dystrophy and were provided with a personal computer and e-mail and Internet connectivity indicated that social isolation was felt to have been reduced, and an occupation, interest, and enjoyment provided for the boys and their families (Soutter, Hamilton & Russell, 2004).*
- ▲ Consider use of RAP therapy (therapy using rap music) in groups to advance social skills of urban adolescents. **EB:** *Findings were unequivocally in favor of the RAP therapy as a tool for advancing pro-social behavior in three adolescent groups: violent offenders, status offenders, and a control condition of high school students with no criminal history (DeCarlo & Hockman, 2003).*

Geriatric

- Avoid assuming that social isolation is normal for elderly clients. **EBN:** *Socialization is important throughout the life span. It provides a mode for enhancing a person's quality of life (Gosline, 2003).*
- ▲ Assess the client's potential or actual sensory problems with hearing and vision and make appropriate referrals if a problem is identified. **EB:** *Sensory problems are common experiences within the older U.S. population, and there is substantial difficulty sustaining social participation activities (Crews & Campbell, 2004).*
- Monitor for depression, a particular risk in the elderly. *Age and its associated losses may cause formerly socially active people to be alone. Loneliness contributes to depression and social withdrawal (Warren, 1993).*
- Encourage group physical activity, such as aerobics or stretching and toning. *These activities de-*

S

creased loneliness in former sedentary adults *(McAuley et al, 2000)*. **EB:** *Where appropriate, the development of sport and physical activity opportunities for service users should be considered by mental health professionals (Carter-Morris & Faulkner, 2003).*

- Have clients reminisce. **EBN:** *Through the process of reminiscence, older adults can actively evaluate life experiences and explore the meaning of memorable events (Harrand & Bollstetter, 2000).*
- Refer to care plans for **Risk for Loneliness** and **Social isolation** for additional interventions.

Multicultural

- Refer to care plan **Social isolation** for additional interventions.
- Assess for the effect of racism on the client's perceptions of social interactions. **EB:** *Accumulated experiences of racial discrimination by African-American women constitute an independent risk factor for preterm delivery (Collins et al, 2004).*
- Approach individuals of color with respect, warmth, and professional courtesy. **EBN:** *Physicians engaged in less client-centered communication with African-American clients than with Caucasian clients (Johnson et al, 2004). Minorities were significantly more likely to report being treated with disrespect or being looked down upon in the client-provider relationship (Blanchard & Lurie, 2004).*
- Validate the client's feelings regarding social interaction. **EBN:** *Research suggests that an increased risk of health pessimism among African-American adults is due in part to race differences in the perception of interpersonal maltreatment (Boardman, 2004).*
- Use interpreters as needed. **EB:** *Primary care nurses act as gatekeepers to interpreting services (Gerrish et al, 2004).*

Home Care

- Previously discussed interventions may be adapted for home care use.
- ▲ Assess family and living environment for social dynamics. Refer for medical social services to assist with family dynamics if appropriate. *The family is a socially significant cultural group that generates behavior, defines roles, and promotes values.*
- Suggest that the client avoid contact with negative persons. *Negative interactions reinforce undesired patterns.*
- ▲ Refer to or support involvement with supportive groups and counseling. **EB:** *Cognitive behavioral group therapy was effective for social phobia in this group of 11 adolescent girls (Hayward et al, 2000). Group settings provide the opportunity to practice new skills (Alfano & Rowland, 2006).*

Client/Family Teaching

- ▲ Refer to appropriate social agencies for assistance (e.g., family therapy, self-help groups, crisis intervention), especially individuals who are seriously ill. **EB:** *Intensive psychotherapy may be most applicable to severely ill clients with bipolar disorder, whereas briefer treatments may be adequate for less severely ill clients (Miklowitz, 2006).*

S See the EVOLVE website for World Wide Web resources for client education.

REFERENCES

Adamle K, Turkoski B: Responding to patient-initiated humor: guidelines for practice, *Home Healthc Nurse* 24(10):638-644, 2006.

Alfano CM, Rowland JH: Recovery issues in cancer survivorship: a new challenge for supportive care, *Cancer J* 12(5):432-443, 2006.

Bellack AS, Brown CH, Thomas-Lohrman S: Psychometric characteristics of role-play assessments of social skill in schizophrenia, *Behav Ther* 37(4):339-352, 2006.

Blanchard J, Lurie N: R-E-S-P-E-C-T: patient reports of disrespect in the health care setting and its impact on care, *J Fam Pract* 53(9):721-730, 2004.

Boardman JD: Health pessimism among black and white adults: the role of interpersonal and institutional maltreatment, *Soc Sci Med* 59(12):2523-2533, 2004.

Bowles N: A solution-focused approach to engagement in acute psychiatry, *Nurs Times* 98(48):26-27, 2002.

Carter-Morris P, Faulkner G: A football project for service users: the role of football in reducing social exclusion, *J Ment Health Promot* 2(1):7, 2003.

Collins JW Jr, David RJ, Handler A et al: Very low birthweight in African American infants: the role of maternal exposure to interpersonal racial discrimination, *Am J Public Health* 94(12):2132-2138, 2004.

Crews JE, Campbell VA: Vision impairment and hearing loss among community-dwelling older Americans: implications for health functioning, *Am J Pub Health* 94(5):823-829, 2004.

Dean A: Talking to dying patients of their hopes and needs, *Nurs Times* 98(43):34-35, 2002.

• = Independent;   ▲ = Collaborative;   EBN = Evidence-Based Nursing;   EB = Evidence-Based

DeCarlo A, Hockman E: RAP therapy: a group work intervention method for urban adolescents, *Soc Work Groups* 26(3):45-59, 2003.

Gerrish K, Chau R, Sobowale A et al: Bridging the language barrier: the use of interpreters in primary care nursing, *Health Soc Care Community* 12(5):407-413, 2004.

Gosline MB: Client participation to enhance socialization for frail elders, *Geriatr Nurs* 24(5):286-289, 2003.

Harrand AG, Bollstetter JJ: Developing a community-based reminiscence group for the elderly, *Clin Nurse Spec* 14(1):17, 2000.

Hayward C, Varady S, Albano AM et al: Cognitive-behavioral group therapy for social phobia in female adolescents: results of a pilot study, *J Am Acad Child Adolesc Psychiatry* 39(6):721, 2000.

Hill WG, Weinert C: An evaluation of an online intervention to provide social support and health education, *Comput Inform Nurs* 22(5):282-288, 2004.

Johnson RL, Roter D, Powe NR et al: Patient race/ethnicity and quality of patient-physician communication during medical visits, *Am J Public Health* 94(12):2084-2090, 2004.

Kef S: Psychosocial adjustment and the meaning of social support for visually impaired adolescents, *J Visual Impair Blind* 96(1):22, 2002.

Kirby ED, Williams VP, Hocking MC et al: Psychosocial benefits of three formats of a standardized behavioral stress management program, *Psychosom Med* 68(6):816-823, 2006.

Lunney M: Stress overload: a new diagnosis, *Int J Nurs Terminol Classif* 17(4):165-175, 2006.

Makinen S, Suominen T, Lauri S: Self-care in adults with asthma: how they cope, *J Clin Nurs* 9(4):557, 2000.

McAuley E, Blissmer B, Marquez DX et al: Social relations, physical activity, and well-being in older adults, *Prev Med* 31(5):608, 2000.

Melnechenko KL: To make a difference: nursing presence, *Nurs Forum* 38(2):18-24, 2003.

Miklowitz DJ: An update on the role of psychotherapy in the management of bipolar disorder. *Curr Psychiatry Rep* 8(6):498-503, 2006.

Sigman M, Hassan S: Benefits of long-term group therapy to individuals suffering schizophrenia: a prospective 7-year study, *Bull Menninger Clin* 70(4):273-282, 2006.

Soutter J, Hamilton N, Russell P: The golden freeway: a preliminary evaluation of a pilot study advancing information technology as a social intervention for boys with Duchenne muscular dystrophy and their families, *Health Soc Care Community* 12(1): 25-33, 2004.

Sundin K, Jansson L, Norberg A: Communicating with people with stroke and aphasia: understanding through sensation without words, *J Clin Nurs* 9(4):481, 2000.

University of Central Lancashire: Department of Nursing: *Solution focused interventions* (NU3307), available at www.uclan.ac.uk/courses/factsheets/health/nursing/3284.pdf. Accessed January 18, 2003.

Vidrine M, Owen-Smith P, Faulkner P et al: Equine-facilitated group psychotherapy: applications for therapeutic vaulting, *Ment Health Nurs* 23(6):587, 2002.

Warren BJ: Explaining social isolation through concept analysis, *Arch Psychiatr Nurs* 7:270, 1993.

Yonge O, Molzahn A: Exceptional nontraditional caring practices of nurses, *Scand J Caring Sci* 16(4):399, 2002.

Zanello A, Weber Rouget B, Gex-Fabry M et al: Validation of the QFS measuring the frequency and satisfaction in social behaviours in psychiatric adult population, *Encephale* 32(1 Pt 1):45-59, 2006.

Social isolation *Gail B. Ladwig, MSN, CHTP, RN*

NANDA Definition

Aloneness experienced by the individual and perceived as imposed by others and as a negative or threatening state

Defining Characteristics

Objective

Absence of supportive significant other(s); developmentally inappropriate behaviors; dull affect; evidence of handicap (e.g. physical, mental) exists in a subculture; illness; meaningless actions; no eye contact; preoccupation with own thoughts; projects hostility; repetitive actions; sad affect; seeks to be alone; shows behavior unaccepted by dominant cultural group; uncommunicative; withdrawn

Subjective

Developmentally inappropriate interests; experiences feelings of differences from others; expresses feelings of aloneness imposed by others; expresses feelings of rejection; expresses values unacceptable to the dominant cultural group; inability to meet expectations of others; inadequate purpose in life; insecurity in public

Related Factors (r/t)

Alterations in mental status; alterations in physical appearance; altered state of wellness; factors contributing to the absence of satisfying personal relationships (e.g., delay in accomplishing developmental tasks); immature interests; inability to engage in satisfying personal relationships; inadequate personal resources; unaccepted social behavior; unaccepted social values

• = Independent; ▲ = Collaborative; EBN = Evidence-Based Nursing; EB = Evidence-Based

NOC Outcomes (Nursing Outcomes Classification)

Suggested NOC Outcomes

Loneliness Severity, Mood Equilibrium, Personal Well-Being, Play Participation, Social Interaction Skills, Social Involvement, Social Support

Example NOC Outcome with Indicators
Social Involvement as evidenced by the following indicator: Interacts with close friends, neighbors, family members, and members of work groups (Rate the outcome and indicators of **Social Involvement:** 1 = never demonstrated, 2 = rarely demonstrated, 3 = sometimes demonstrated, 4 = often demonstrated, 5 = consistently demonstrated [see Section I].)

Client Outcomes

Client Will (Specify Time Frame):

* Identify feelings of isolation
* Practice social and communication skills needed to interact with others
* Initiate interactions with others; set and meet goals
* Participate in activities and programs at level of ability and desire
* Describe feelings of self-worth

NIC Interventions (Nursing Interventions Classification)

Suggested NIC Intervention

Socialization Enhancement

Example NIC Activities—Socialization Enhancement
Encourage patience in developing relationships; Help patient increase awareness of strengths and limitations in communicating with others

Nursing Interventions and *Rationales*

* Establish a therapeutic relationship by being emotionally present and authentic. *Being emotionally present and authentic fosters growth in relationships and decreases isolation (Jordan, 2000).* **EBN:** *Being truly present was listed as one behavior that demonstrated caring (Yonge & Molzahn, 2002).*
* Observe for barriers to social interaction (e.g., illness; incontinence; decreasing ability to form relationships; lack of transportation, money, support system, or knowledge). **EBN:** *Causes of social isolation may be different for each individual; therefore adequate information must be gathered so that appropriate interventions can be planned (Badger, 1990).*
* Note risk factors (e.g., membership in ethnic/cultural minority, chronic physiological or psychological illness or deformities, advanced age). **EBN:** *Clients with these risk factors may be at risk for social isolation. Young adults with mental illness identify social isolation as their main concern (Mostafanejad, 2006).*
* Discuss causes of perceived or actual isolation. **EBN:** *The individual's experience of illness; the circumstances of everyday living that influence quality of life; and emotions, fears, and concerns all have a bearing on the way illness is managed (Anderson, 1991).*
* Establish trust one on one and then gradually introduce the client to others. Allow the client opportunities to introduce issues and to describe his or her daily life. **EBN:** *Individualization of care, or tailoring of care, involves taking into account the client's individuality and allowing that individuality to determine interpersonal approaches and health-illness management actions (Brown, 1994).*
* ▲ Promote social interactions. Support the expression of feelings. Consider the use of music therapy. **EB:** *Music plays role in accessing emotion (Clements-Cortes, 2004).*
* Involve clients in writing specific outcomes, such as identifying what is most important from their viewpoint and lifestyle. **EBN:** *Women diagnosed with early breast cancer state the importance of*

S

making decisions for medical treatment is a mandatory step in designing customized decision support (Budden et al, 2003).

- Provide positive reinforcement when the client seeks out others. **EBN:** *Receiving instrumental social support, such as practical help, advice, and feedback, significantly contributes to positive well-being (White et al, 1992).*
- Help the client identify appropriate diversional activities to encourage socialization. *Active participation by the client is essential for behavioral changes.*
- Encourage physical closeness (e.g., use touch) if appropriate. **EBN:** *Touch helps with integration and fosters social relatedness. Tactile stimulation benefits the older adult's psychological well-being (Jamison, 1997).*
- Identify available support systems and involve these individuals in the client's care. **EBN:** *Clients cope more successfully with stressful life events if they have support (White, 1992).*
- ▲ Refer clients to support groups. **EB:** *Clients who are victims of domestic violence often endure social isolation imposed by significant others and benefit from support groups (Larance & Porter, 2004).*
- Encourage liberal visitation for a client who is hospitalized or in an extended care facility. **EB:** *Visits from those in an emotionally close network were associated with perceived support, and this was associated with a decrease in depression (Oxman & Hull, 2001).*
- Help the client identify role models and others with similar interests. *Sometimes the client needs someone to model the appropriate behavior.*
- See the care plan for **Risk for Loneliness.**

Pediatric

- ▲ Refer obese adolescents for diet, exercise, and psychosocial support. *Obese teens in this study reported shame and social isolation related to their obesity (Sjoberg, Nilsson & Leppert, 2005).*
- See the care plan for **Risk for Loneliness.**

Geriatric

- Assess physical and mental status to establish a firm basis for planning social activities. **EBN:** *Socialization is important throughout the life span. It provides a mode for enhancing a person's quality of life. Older adults living alone and with spouses continue to desire social interaction at levels similar to their participation in earlier life stages (Gosline, 2003).*
- ▲ Assess for hearing deficit. Provide aids and use adaptive techniques. **EB:** *The odds of demonstrating auditory processing abnormality for average older participants increased by 4% to 9% per year of age. Men were approximately twice as likely as women to demonstrate this abnormality (Golding et al, 2006). Declines in speech understanding in noise and central auditory processing are common in the growing population of older women (Garstecki & Erler, 2001).*
- ▲ Involve client in goal setting and planning activities. Have them write down five activities in which they would like to participate. **EBN:** *Frail older adults, involved in participation of goal setting and planning of social activities enhanced both their anticipation and their participation in the activities (Gosline, 2003).*
- ▲ Involve nonprofessionals in activities, projects, and goal setting with the client. Practice interdisciplinary management for unit-based activities: engaging in arts and crafts projects, sewing, watching videos, reading large-print books, reading magazines, playing games, playing musical instruments, and using assistive listening devices. **EBN:** *Nursing assistants are commonly concerned about the social support of residents; therefore they can be a valuable resource for generating intervention ideas—alterations in job descriptions would be required (Windriver, 1993).* **EBN:** *In a study of the use of calming music and hand massage, physically nonaggressive behaviors decreased during each of the interventions (Remington, 2002).*
- Offer the client a choice of activities and persons with whom to sit and socialize. Introductions to strangers may need to be repeated several times. **EBN:** *A recognized intervention for loneliness is to provide opportunities and assistance for making choices, setting goals, and making decisions. Cognitively impaired clients may require several repetitions (Windriver, 1993).*
- Put clients in groups according to activity preferences, abilities, age, life situations, personal and cultural characteristics, and social networks. **EBN:** *Positive social interactions are enhanced by the aforementioned interventions (Windriver, 1993).*
- Develop and display a seating chart for the common areas of each personal care unit and develop

S

a process for both identifying needed changes and executing them promptly. **EBN:** *Personality factors that are difficult to predict affect the success of social groupings (Windriver, 1993).*

- Provide physical activity, either aerobic or stretching and toning. **EB:** *Physical activity increased social support in a group of older, formerly sedentary adults (McAuley et al, 2000).*
- Provide music with active participation, such as drum and rhythm circles. **EBN:** *There is no active participation for many residents when the music programs they experience are limited to attendance at concerts and sing-alongs. Drum circles and rhythm circles actively involve residents, even those who are cognitively impaired (Rozon, Hagens & Martin, 2004).*
- Consider the use of simulated presence therapy (see the care plan for **Hopelessness**). **EBN:** *Simulated presence therapy appears to be the most effective therapy for treating social isolation (Woods & Ashley, 1995).*
- ▲ Refer to programs such as Foster Grandparents and Senior Companions. **EB:** *Social programs help increase contact with peers and decrease isolation. Programs to alleviate emotional isolation should focus on attachment loss (Dugan & Kivett, 1994).*
- Consider using computers and the Internet to alleviate or reduce loneliness and social isolation. **EBN:** *Participants age 65 years and older living alone used the computer to combat loneliness (Clark, 2002). Internet use was found to decrease loneliness and depression significantly, while perceived social support and self-esteem increased significantly (Shaw & Gant, 2002).*

Multicultural

- Acknowledge racial/ethnic differences at the onset of care. **EBN:** *Acknowledgment of race/ethnicity issues will enhance communication, establish rapport, and promote positive treatment outcomes (D'Avanzo et al, 2001).*
- Assess for the influence of cultural beliefs, norms, and values on the client's perception of social activity and relationships. **EBN:** *What the client considers normal social interaction may be based on cultural perceptions (Leininger & McFarland, 2002).*
- Approach individuals of color with respect, warmth, and professional courtesy. **EBN:** *Instances of disrespect and lack of caring have special significance for individuals of color and may impede efforts to increase social outlets (D'Avanzo et al, 2001).*
- Assess personal space needs, communication styles, acceptable body language, attitude toward eye contact, perception of touch, and paraverbal messages when communicating with the client. **EBN:** *Nurses need to consider these aspects when interpreting verbal and nonverbal messages (Purnell, 2000). Native-American clients may consider avoiding direct eye contact to be a sign of respect and asking questions to be rude and intrusive (Seideman et al, 1996).*
- Use a family-centered approach when working with Latino, Asian-American, African-American, and Native-American clients. **EBN:** *Latinos may perceive the family as source of support, solver of problems, and source of pride. Asian Americans may regard the family as the primary decision maker and primary influence on individual family members (D'Avanzo et al, 2001).*
- Promote a sense of ethnic attachment. **EBN:** *Older Korean clients with strong ethnic attachments had higher levels of social involvement than others (Kim, 1999).*
- Validate the client's feelings regarding social isolation. **EBN:** *Validation lets the client know that the nurse has heard and understood what was said, and it promotes the nurse-client relationship (Heineken, 1998). A study of African-American men found a sense of family in the AIDS dedicated nursing home, making it potentially a valuable source of needed social support, which decreased social isolation (Fields & Jemmot, 2003).*
- ▲ Assist refugees who are relocated to access health care; support their connections with cultural, social, and religious groups. *Sub-Saharan refugees in Australia are isolated when they relocate and do not know where or how to seek healthcare services (Sheikh-Mohammed et al, 2006).*

Home Care

- The interventions described previously may be adapted for home care use.
- Confirm that the home setting has a telephone. Obtain one if necessary for medical safety. If the client lives alone, set up a Lifeline safety system that requires the client to answer the telephone. *The telephone can be used to achieve continuity of care and successful client-family interaction (Skinner, 2001).*

• = Independent;   ▲ = Collaborative;   EBN = Evidence-Based Nursing;   EB = Evidence-Based

- Consider the use of the computer and Internet to decrease isolation. **EBN:** *Pregnant women on home bed rest for preterm labor stated that their participation in a virtual online peer support group was valuable and beneficial in helping them to cope with the hardships of bed rest (Adler & Zarchin, 2002). Homebound older adults found that the Internet and e-mail were excellent sources of support and enjoyment (Nahm & Resnick, 2001).* **EB:** *These studies demonstrated computer social support for rural women with chronic illness. The women declared the computer-based social support to have positive effects (Hill, Weinert & Cudney, 2006).*

▲ Assess options for living that allow the client privacy but not isolation (e.g., boarding home, congregate living, assertive community treatment programs). **EB:** *Adults with schizophrenia described their relationships with other mental health clients in primarily positive terms, yet several participants expressed dissatisfaction and desired greater integration into mainstream social networks (Angell, 2003).*

▲ Assist clients to interact with neighbors in the community when they move to supported housing. *Without the personal contact between the mentally ill person and the neighbors, there may be a risk that the integration will fail (Hogberg, Magnusson & Lutzen, 2006).*

Client/Family Teaching

- Teach role playing (practicing communication skills in specific situations). **EB:** *Role playing may help clients develop social interaction skills and identify feelings associated with their isolation.*

▲ Encourage the client to initiate contacts with self-help groups, counselors, and therapists. **EBN:** *If adjustment is to be successful and maintained, management of a chronic illness cannot occur in isolation; it requires a complex interaction of resources (White, 1992).*

- Provide information to the client about senior citizen services, house sharing, pets, day care centers, churches, and community resources. **EBN:** *The well-documented negative effect of social isolation suggests that clients without confidants and supportive others must be referred to alternative sources, such as cardiac rehabilitation programs, support groups, and community agencies (McCauley, 1995).*

▲ Refer socially isolated caregivers to appropriate support groups as well. *Identification and recognition of the overwhelming task of caregiving are needed so that caregivers do not suffer in silence (Bergman-Evans, 1994). (See the care plan for* **Caregiver role strain.***)*

evolve   See the EVOLVE website for World Wide Web resources for client education.

REFERENCES

Adler CL, Zarchin YR: The "virtual focus group": using the Internet to reach pregnant women on home bed rest, *J Obstet Gynecol Neonatal Nurs* 31(4):418, 2002.

Anderson JM: Immigrant women speak of chronic illness: the social construction of the devalued self, *J Adv Nurs* 16:710, 1991.

Angell B: Contexts of social relationship development among assertive community treatment clients, *Ment Health Serv Res* 5(1):13, 2003.

Badger VT: Men with cardiovascular diseases and their spouses: coping, health and marital adjustment, *Arch Psychiatr Nurs* 4:319, 1990.

Bergman-Evans BF: Alzheimer's and related disorders: loneliness, depression, and social support of spousal caregivers, *J Gerontol Nurs* 20:6, 1994.

Brown S: Communication strategies used by an expert nurse, *Clin Nurs Res* 3(1):43, 1994.

Budden LM, Pierce PF, Hayes BA et al: Australian women's prediagnostic decision-making styles, relating to treatment choices for early breast cancer treatment, *Res Theory Nurs Pract* 17(2):117-136, 2003.

Clark DJ: Older adults living through and with their computers, *Comput Inform Nurs* 20(3):117, 2002.

Clements-Cortes A: The use of music in facilitating emotional expression in the terminally ill, *Am J Hosp Palliat Care* 21(4):255-260, 2004.

D'Avanzo CE, Naegle MA: Developing culturally informed strategies for substance-related interventions. In Naegle MA, D'Avanzo CE,

editors: *Addictions and substance abuse: strategies for advanced practice nursing,* St Louis, 2001, Mosby.

Dugan E, Kivett V: The importance of emotional and social isolation to loneliness among very old rural adults, *Gerontologist* 34:340, 1994.

Fields SD, Jemmott LS: The love and belonging healthcare needs of HIV infected African-American men upon admission to an AIDS dedicated nursing home, *J Natl Black Nurses Assoc* 14(1):38-44, 2003.

Garstecki DC, Erler SF: Personal and social conditions potentially influencing women's hearing loss management, *Am J Audiol* 10:2, 2001.

Golding M, Taylor A, Cupples L et al: Odds of demonstrating auditory processing abnormality in the average older adult: the Blue Mountains Hearing Study, *Ear Hear* 27(2):129-138, 2006.

Gosline MB: Client participation to enhance socialization for frail elders, *Geriatr Nurs* 24(5):286-289, 2003.

Heineken J: Patient silence is not necessarily client satisfaction: communication in home care nursing, *Home Healthc Nurse* 16(2):115, 1998.

Hill W, Weinert C, Cudney S: Influence of a computer intervention on the psychological status of chronically ill rural women: preliminary results, *Nurs Res* 55(1):34-42, 2006.

Hogberg T, Magnusson A, Lutzen K: Living by themselves? Psychiatric nurses' views on supported housing for persons with severe and

S

persistent mental illness, *J Psychiatr Ment Health Nurs* 13(6):735-741, 2006.

Jamison M: Failure to thrive in older adults, *J Gerontol Nurs* 23(2):13, 1997.

Jordan JV: The role of mutual empathy in relational/cultural therapy, *J Clin Psychol* 56(8):1005, 2000.

Kim O: Mediation effect of social support between ethnic attachment and loneliness in older Korean immigrants, *Res Nurs Health* 22(2):169, 1999.

Larance LY, Porter ML: Observations from practice: support group membership as a process of social capital formation among female survivors of domestic violence, *J Interpers Violence* 19(6):676-690, 2004.

Leininger MM, McFarland MR: *Transcultural nursing: concepts, theories, research and practices,* ed 3, New York, 2002, McGraw-Hill.

McAuley E, Blissmer B, Marquez DX et al: Social relations, physical activity, and well-being in older adults, *Prev Med* 31(5):608, 2000.

McCauley K: Assessing social support in patients with cardiac disease, *J Cardiovasc Nurs* 10:73, 1995.

Mostafanejad K: Reducing the isolation of young adults living with a mental illness in rural Australia, *Int J Ment Health Nurs* 15(3):181-188, 2006.

Nahm ES, Resnick B: Homebound older adults' experiences with the Internet and e-mail, *Comput Nurs* 19(6):257, 2001.

Oxman TE, Hull JG: Social support and treatment response in older depressed primary care patients, *J Gerontol B Psychol Sci Soc Sci* 56(1):P35, 2001.

Purnell L: A description of the Purnell model for cultural competence, *J Transcult Nurs* 11(1):40, 2000.

Remington R: Calming music and hand massage with agitated elderly, *Nurs Res* 51(5):317, 2002.

Rozon L, Hagens C, Martin LS: Music programs that create a sense of community: music therapy for even the most severe cognitively impaired resident, *Can Nurs Home* 15(1):57-59, 2004.

Seideman RY, Jacobson S, Primeaux M et al: Assessing American Indian families, *MCN Am J Matern Child Nurs* 21(6):274, 1996.

Shaw LH, Gant LM: In defense of the Internet: the relationship between Internet communication and depression, loneliness, self-esteem, and perceived social support, *Cyberpsychol Behav* 5(2):157, 2002.

Sheikh-Mohammed M, Macintyre CR, Wood NJ et al: Barriers to access to health care for newly resettled sub-Saharan refugees in Australia, *Med J Aust* 85(11-12):594-597, 2006.

Sjoberg RL, Nilsson KW, Leppert J: Obesity, shame, and depression in school-aged children: a population-based study, *Pediatrics* 116(3): e389-e92, 2005.

Skinner D: Intimacy and the telephone, *Caring* 20(2):28, 2001.

White NE, Richter JM, Fry C: Coping, social support, and adaptation to chronic illness, *West J Nurs Res* 14(2):211-224, 1992.

Windriver W: Social isolation: unit-based activities for impaired elders, *J Gerontol Nurs* 19:15, 1993.

Woods P, Ashley J: Simulated presence therapy: using selected memories to manage problem behaviors in Alzheimer's disease patients, *Geriatr Nurs* 16:9, 1995.

Yonge O, Molzahn A: Exceptional nontraditional caring practices of nurses, *Scand J Caring Sci* 16(4):399, 2002.

Chronic Sorrow   *Betty J. Ackley, MS, EdS, RN*

NANDA   Definition

Cyclical, recurring, and potentially progressive pattern of pervasive sadness experienced (by parent, caregiver, individual with chronic illness or disability) in response to continual loss throughout the trajectory of an illness or disability

Defining Characteristics

Expresses feelings of sadness (e.g., periodic, recurrent); expresses feelings that interfere with ability to reach highest level of personal well-being; expresses feelings that interfere with ability to reach highest level of social well-being; expresses negative feelings (e.g., anger, being misunderstood, confusion, depression, disappointment, emptiness, fear, frustration, guilt, helplessness, hopelessness, loneliness, low self-esteem, being overwhelmed, recurring loss, self-blame)

Related Factors (r/t)

Death of a loved one; crises in management of the illness; crises related to developmental stages; experiences chronic disability (e.g., physical or mental); experiences chronic illness (e.g., physical or mental); missed milestones; missed opportunities; unending caregiving

NOC   Outcomes (Nursing Outcomes Classification)

Suggested NOC Outcomes

Acceptance: Health Status, Depression Level, Depression Self-Control, Grief Resolution, Hope, Mood Equilibrium

• = Independent;   ▲ = Collaborative;   EBN = Evidence-Based Nursing;   EB = Evidence-Based

---

Example NOC Outcome with Indicators

Grief Resolution with plans for a positive future as evidenced by the following indicators: Resolves feelings about loss/Verbalizes acceptance of loss/Describes meaning of the loss or death/Reports decreased preoccupation with loss/Expresses positive expectations about the future (Rate the outcome and indicators of **Grief Resolution:** 1 = never demonstrated, 2 = rarely demonstrated, 3 = sometimes demonstrated, 4 = often demonstrated, 5 = consistently demonstrated [see Section I].)

Client Outcomes

Client Will (Specify Time Frame):

- Express appropriate feelings of guilt, fear, anger, or sadness
- Identify problems associated with sorrow (e.g., changes in appetite, insomnia, nightmares, loss of libido, decreased energy, alteration in activity levels)
- Seek help in dealing with grief-associated problems
- Plan for future one day at a time
- Function at normal developmental level

NIC   Interventions (Nursing Interventions Classification)

Suggested NIC Interventions

Grief Work Facilitation, Grief Work Facilitation: Perinatal Death

---

Example NIC Activities—Grief Work Facilitation

Encourage the patient to verbalize memories of loss, both past and current; Assist to identify personal coping strategies

---

Nursing Interventions and *Rationales*

- Assess the client's degree of sorrow. Use the Burke/NCRS Chronic Sorrow Questionnaire for the individual or caregiver as appropriate. *This questionnaire is designed to determine the occurrence of chronic sorrow, cues that trigger sorrow, coping strategies, and factors that direct healthcare personnel to deal with the sorrowful client or caregiver (Hainsworth, Eakes & Burke, 1994; Hobdell, 2004).*
- Identify problems of eating and sleeping; ensure that basic human needs are being met. **EBN:** *One study indicated that bereaved individuals, irrespective of whether they had counseling for grief resolution, had a moderate risk for poor nutrition. The implication is that food issues need to be included in grief resolution interventions (Johnson, 2002).*
- Spend time with the client and family. **EB:** *The main suggestion in a study of families who have a child with a chronic illness and are facing loss in their lives was the provision of an empathetic presence (Langridge, 2002).*
- Develop a trusting relationship with the client by using empathetic therapeutic communication techniques. **EB:** *An empathetic person who takes the time to listen, offers support and reassurance, recognizes and focuses on feelings, and appreciates the uniqueness of each individual and family is helpful to clients experiencing chronic sorrow (Eakes, Burke & Hainsworth, 1998).*
- Help the client to understand that sorrow may be ongoing. No timetable exists for grieving, despite popular thought. *After loss, life is characterized by good times and bad times when sorrow is triggered by events.* **EBN:** *Studies have demonstrated that feelings of sadness, guilt, anger, frustration, and fear occur periodically throughout the lives of people experiencing chronic loss resulting in chronic sorrow (Eakes, Burke & Hainsworth, 1998). In an analysis of 85 mourners' narratives, the most prominent theme was feeling the absence of the decedent (Gamino, Hogan & Sewell, 2002).*
- Help the client recognize that, although sadness will occur at intervals for the rest of his or her life, it will become bearable. *In time the client may develop a relationship with grief that is lifelong but livable, and as much filled with comfort as it is with sorrow (Moules et al, 2007). The sadness associated with chronic sorrow is permanent, but as the grief resolves there can be times of satisfaction*

S

• = Independent;   ▲ = Collaborative;   EBN = Evidence-Based Nursing;   EB = Evidence-Based

Example NOC Outcome with Indicators
Spiritual Health as evidenced by the following indicators: Quality of faith, hope/Meaning and purpose in life/ Connectedness with inner self, others/Interaction with others to share thoughts, feelings, and beliefs (Rate the outcome and indicators of **Spiritual Health:** 1 = severely compromised, 2 = substantially compromised, 3 = moderately compromised, 4 = mildly compromised, 5 = not compromised [see Section I].)

Client Outcomes

Client Will (Specify Time Frame):

- Express sense of connectedness with self, others, arts, music, literature, or power greater than oneself
- Express meaning and purpose in life
- Express sense of hope in the future
- Express ability to forgive
- Express acceptance of health status
- Discuss personal response to dying
- Discuss personal response to grieving

NIC   Interventions (Nursing Interventions Classification)

Suggested NIC Interventions

Active Listening, Forgiveness Facilitation, Grief Work Facilitation, Hope Inspiration, Humor, Music Therapy, Presence, Referral, Reminiscence Therapy, Self Awareness Enhancement, Simple Guided Imagery, Simple Massage, Simple Relaxation Therapy, Spiritual Support, Therapeutic Touch, Touch

Example NIC Activities—Spiritual Support
Encourage the use of spiritual resources, if desired; Be available to listen to individual's feelings

Nursing Interventions and *Rationales*

- Observe the client for loss of meaning, purpose, and hope in life. **EBN:** *It is important for health-care providers to identify and assess for spiritual needs (Greasley, Chiu & Gartland, 2001). Spirituality is associated with meaning and purpose in life and hope (Burkhart & Solari-Twadell, 2001). Spirituality has a significant negative correlation with depression and meaning and peace (Nelson et al, 2002). Individuals in crisis express strong spiritual beliefs (McGrath, 2003). Spirituality is used to derive meaning in the life experience (Ferrell et al, 2003). Spiritual well-being is a better predictor than depression for end-of-life clients in terms of hopelessness and suicidal ideation (McClain, Rosenfeld & Breitbart, 2003). Connectedness is an important theme in hope with stroke survivors; spiritual connectedness is a factor in hope-related patterns (Bays, 2001). One of the most prevalent spiritual needs is finding meaning (Taylor, 2006).*
- Respect the client's beliefs; avoid imposing your own spiritual beliefs on the client. Be aware of your own belief systems and accept the client's spirituality. Allow for self-disclosure. Promote a sense of love, caring, and compassion. **EBN:** *Love, caring, and compassion are interpersonal values that promote spiritual care (Greasley, Chiu & Gartland, 2001). One of the most prevalent spiritual needs was giving love to others (Taylor, 2006).*
- Monitor and promote supportive social contacts. **EBN:** *Social supports are positively correlated with spiritual well-being (Coyle, 2002). Spirituality is associated with social inclusion in individuals with mental illness (Corrigan et al, 2003). Spirituality significantly correlates with social functioning (Coleman, 2003). Spirituality was an important theme in final conversations with loved ones (Keeley, 2004).*
- Integrate family into spiritual practices as appropriate. **EBN:** *Undergirding strong families, promoting healing from abusive family situations, and maintaining relationships with ancestors are important in spirituality promotion (Banks-Wallace & Parks, 2004). Women who had just completed the*

S

• = Independent;   ▲ = Collaborative;   EBN = Evidence-Based Nursing;   EB = Evidence-Based

diagnostic process of breast cancer found their personal strength and connection to God or their spiritual beliefs were important and, when overwhelmed, sought out loved ones for support and diversion (Logan, Hackbusch-Pinto & De Grasse, 2006).

▲ Refer the client to a support group or counseling. **EB:** *Counseling significantly lowers mortality rates (Fawzy et al, 1993; Richardson et al, 1990).* **EBN:** *Battered women participated in spiritual discussion and other practices once a week (Humphreys, 2000). Among these sheltered battered women, spirituality may be associated with greater internal resources that buffer distressing feelings and calm the mind. Cultivating relationships that promote transformation, empowerment, and healing promotes spiritual well-being (Lauver, 2000).*

• Coordinate or encourage attending spiritual retreats, courses, or programming. **EB:** *Improved spiritual well-being is associated with decreased coronary stenosis (Morris, 2001). Clients with advanced cancer who participated in a cancer care and rehabilitation project, which included home visits and interventions from nurse practitioners, correlate religious belief and measures of religious activity and connections positively with satisfaction with life and negatively with pain (Yates et al, 1981).*

• Be physically present and actively listen to the client. **EBN:** *Being present and actively listening to the client promotes nurse-client connectedness and helps the client feel valued (Lauver, 2000). Listening and presence support clients spiritually (Tuck, Wallace & Pullen, 2001). Nurses commonly support spiritual needs by assisting client to search for meaning and purpose in life situation (Narayanasamy & Owens, 2001).*

• Support meditation, guided imagery, therapeutic touch, journaling, relaxation, and involvement in art, music, or poetry. Support outdoor activities. **EBN:** *There is a significant correlation between spiritual activities and emotional distress and quality of life for HIV-positive African-American women (Sowell et al, 2000). Guided imagery supports clients spiritually (Tuck et al, 2001). Spirituality includes connectedness with art, music, literature, and nature (Burkhart & Solari-Twadell, 2001).*

▲ Offer or suggest visits with spiritual and/or religious advisors. **EBN:** *The primary need for hospitalized clients was for their pastor/rabbi/spiritual advisor to not abandon them. For those who did not belong to a religious/spiritual group, the primary need was at least to be asked about some type of religious/spiritual preference (Moller, 1999). Religious beliefs are strengthened during crisis only if the subject has a history of religious beliefs; all subjects expressed strong spiritual beliefs, as defined in terms of meaning and purpose in life (McGrath, 2003).*

• Help the client make a list of important and unimportant values. **EBN:** *Nurses implement values clarification to support clients spiritually (Tuck et al, 2001). Spirituality is associated with empowerment in individuals with mental illness (Corrigan et al, 2003).*

• Assist the client in identifying and creating his or her own meaningful experiences.

• Help the client develop skills to deal with illness or lifestyle changes. Include the client in care planning. **EBN:** *Meaningful experiences promote spiritual well-being (Lauver, 2000). Spirituality accounts for 28% of the variance of psychological well-being (Fry, 2003). One of the most prevalent spiritual needs is finding meaning (Taylor, 2006). Spirituality is associated with empowerment in individuals with mental illness (Corrigan et al, 2003).*

• If the client is comfortable with touch, hold the client's hand or place a hand gently on the client's arm. **EBN:** *Touch supports clients spiritually (Tuck et al, 2001).*

• Help the client find a reason for living and be available for support. Promote hope. **EB:** *Hopelessness is correlated with higher cardiac death and reinfarction (Pratt, Ford & Crum, 1996).* **EBN:** *Instilling hope is a common strategy to promote spiritual well-being (Baldacchino & Draper, 2001). Spirituality is associated in hope with individuals with mental illness (Corrigan et al, 2003). For breast cancer survivors, spirituality has significant correlation with hope (Gibson & Parker, 2003). Connectedness is an important theme in hope for stroke survivors; spiritual connectedness is a factor in hope-related patterns (Bays, 2001). There are four themes of spiritual expression: relationships, that which uplifts, spiritual practice, and having hope. Spiritual expression was facilitated by individualized spiritual care. Nurses play an important role in the provision of spiritual care within a hospice setting (Tan, Braunack-Mayer & Beilby, 2005). For breast cancer survivors, spiritual health correlates with more hope and sense of coherence (Gibson & Parker, 2003). Clients with cancer and their caregivers identify one of most prevalent spiritual needs as keeping a positive perspective (Taylor, 2006).*

• Listen to the client's feelings about suffering and/or death. Be nonjudgmental and allow time for grieving. **EBN:** *Individuals at end-of-life, particularly hospice clients, view spirituality as a central*

S

---

theme when coping with disease and treatment (Davidhizar, Bechtel & Cosey, 2000; McGrath, 2003; Keeley, 2004; Tan, Braunack-Mayer & Beilby, 2005), as do people with HIV (Denzin, 1989), cancer (Ferrell et al, 2003; Logan, Hackbusch-Pinto & De Grasse, 2006), chronic renal failure (Walton, 2002), and stroke (Bays, 2001).

- Provide appropriate religious materials, artifacts, or music as requested. **EBN:** *Church attendance and reading the Bible were rated highly in promoting spiritual well-being among battered women (Humphreys, 2000). Helping a client incorporate religious rites and rituals can enhance meaning in life and promote a sense of connectedness with a faith community and/or a higher power (Lauver, 2000). Religious rites and rituals (e.g., ministering, offering communion, laying on of hands, and anointing) support clients spiritually (Tuck et al, 2001). Individuals who have a history of religious beliefs turn to those beliefs in crisis (McGrath, 2003).*

- Promote forgiveness. **EBN:** *Forgiveness is rated as an important part of spirituality among battered women (Humphreys, 2000). Parish nurses promote forgiveness (Tuck et al, 2001). Undergraduate college students identified forgiveness associated with less physical and psychological distress (Younger et al, 2004).*

- Provide privacy or a "sacred space." **EBN:** *Sacred spaces promote spiritual well-being by enhancing a sense of connectedness with self and/or others (Lauver, 2000).*

- Allow time and a place for prayer. **EB:** *Intercessory prayer improved clinical outcomes in coronary bypass clients (Byrd, 1988).* **EBN:** *Prayer is highly rated in promoting spiritual well-being (Humphreys, 2000). Parish nurses indicate that prayer supports clients spiritually (Tuck et al, 2001). Meaning in life and prayer significantly predicted the variance of symptom distress in adults with non–small cell lung cancer (Meraviglia, 2004). Breast cancer survivors associate spiritual well-being with less symptom distress (Manning-Walsh, 2005). Women with breast cancer who use prayer more often find that spiritual health and prayer correlate with more meaning in life and psychological well-being and less physical symptom distress (Meraviglia, 2006). Chronically ill clients determine spiritual coping mechanisms as reaching out to God in the belief and faith that help will be forthcoming, feeling connected to God through prayer, meaning and purpose, strategy of privacy, and connectedness with others (Narayanasamy, 2002). Former runaway and homeless youth include spiritual practice as important in coping, which included prayer and participation in traditional and nontraditional religious practices (Williams & Lindsey, 2005). One of the most prevalent spiritual needs is understanding or relating to God (Taylor, 2006). Spiritual interventions (including prayer and scripture reading) help in weight loss (Reicks, Mills & Henry, 2004).*

- Encourage the use of humor, as appropriate, to promote spiritual well-being. **EBN:** *Breast cancer survivors indicate that humor promotes spirituality and helps them to find meaning and purpose in life (Johnson, 2002).*

Geriatric

- Discuss personal definitions of spiritual wellness with the client. **EBN:** *Those geriatric outpatients who rate themselves in good health report significantly higher levels of spirituality, controlling for functional health, race, and ethnicity (Daaleman, Perera & Studenski, 2004). Nurses identify client needs in older clients by assessing religious beliefs and practice (prayer), absolution, seeking connection, comfort and reassurance, healing or searching for meaning or purpose (Narayanasamy, 2006; Narayanasamy et al, 2004).*

- Identify the client's past sources of spirituality. Help the client explore his or her life and identify those experiences that are noteworthy. Clients may want to read the Bible or other religious text or have it read to them. **EBN:** *Religious belief has been associated with higher levels of well-being and lower levels of depression and suicide (Van Ness & Larson, 2002). Spirituality among adults living in retirement housing estates in Britain has a small significant correlation with psychological well-being, personal growth, and positive relations with others, and spirituality. It reduces the negative effects of frailty (Kirby, Coleman & Daley, 2004).*

Multicultural

- Assess for the influence of cultural beliefs, norms, and values on the client's ability to cope with spiritual distress. **EBN:** *How the client copes with spiritual distress may be based on cultural perceptions (Cesario, 2001; Leininger & McFarland, 2002).*

• = Independent;   ▲ = Collaborative;   EBN = Evidence-Based Nursing;   EB = Evidence-Based

- Acknowledge the value conflicts from acculturation stresses that may contribute to spiritual distress. **EBN:** *Challenges to traditional beliefs are anxiety provoking and can produce distress (Charron, 1998).*
- Encourage spirituality as a source of support. **EBN:** *African Americans and Latinos may identify spirituality, religiousness, prayer, and church-based approaches as coping resources (Banks-Wallace & Parks, 2004; Dingley & Roux, 2003; Simoni, Frick & Huang, 2006).*
- Validate the client's spiritual concerns and convey respect for his or her beliefs. **EBN:** *Validation is a therapeutic communications technique that lets the client know the nurse has heard and understood what was said (Heineken, 1998).*

 Home Care

- All of the nursing interventions described previously apply in the home setting.

evolve See the EVOLVE website for World Wide Web resources for client education.

REFERENCES

Baldacchino D, Draper P: Spiritual coping strategies: a review of the nursing research literature, *J Adv Nurs* 34(6):833-841, 2001.

Banks-Wallace J, Parks L: It's all sacred: African American women's perspectives on spirituality, *Issues Ment Health Nurs* 25(1):25-45, 2004.

Bays CL: Older adults' description of hope after a stroke, *Rehabil Nurs* 26(1):18-27, 2001.

Burkhart L, Solari-Twadell PA: Spirituality and religiousness: differentiating the diagnoses through a review of the nursing literature, *Nurs Diagn* 12(2):45-54, 2001.

Byrd RC: Positive therapeutic effects of intercessory prayer in a coronary care unit population, *South Med J* 81:826, 1988.

Cesario S: Care of the Native American woman: strategies for practice, education, and research, *J Gynecol Neonatal Nurs* 30(1):13, 2001.

Charron HS: Anxiety disorders. In Varcarolis EM, editor: *Foundations of psychiatric mental health nursing*, ed 3, Philadelphia, 1998, Saunders.

Coleman CL: Spirituality and sexual orientation: relationship to mental well-being and functional health status, *J Adv Nurs* 43(5):457-464, 2003.

Corrigan P, McCorkle B, Schell B et al: Religion and spirituality in the lives of people with serious mental illness, *Community Ment Health J* 39(6):487-499, 2003.

Coyle J: Spirituality and health: towards a framework for exploring the relationship between spirituality and health, *J Adv Nurs* 37(6):589-597, 2002.

Daaleman TP, Perera S, Studenski SA: Religion, spirituality, and health status in geriatric outpatients, *Ann Fam Med* 2(1):49-53, 2004.

Davidhizar R, Bechtel G, Cosey E: Hospital extra: the spiritual needs of hospitalized patients, *Am J Nurs* 25:282-289, 2000.

Denzin N: *Interpretive interactionism*, Newbury Park, Calif, 1989, Sage.

Dingley C, Roux G: Inner strength in older Hispanic women with chronic illness, *J Cult Divers* 10(1):11-22, 2003.

Fawzy FI, Fawzy NW, Hyun CS et al: Malignant melanoma: effects of an early structured psychiatric intervention, coping, and affective state on recurrence and survival 6 years later, *Arch Gen Psychiatr* 50(9):681-689, 1993.

Ferrell BR, Smith SL, Juarez G et al: Meaning of illness and spirituality in ovarian cancer survivors, *Oncol Nurs Forum* 30(2):249-257, 2003.

Fry PS: The unique contribution of key existential factors to the prediction of psychological well-being of older adults following spousal loss. *Gerontologist* 41(1):69-81, 2003.

Gibson LMR, Parker V: Inner resources as predictors of psychological well-being in middle-income African American breast cancer survivors, *Cancer Control* 10(5):52-58, 2003.

Greasley P, Chiu LF, Gartland RM: The concept of spiritual care in mental health nursing, *J Adv Nurs* 33(5):629-637, 2001.

Heineken J: Patient silence is not necessarily client satisfaction: communication in home care nursing, *Home Healthc Nurse* 16(2):115, 1998.

Humphreys J: Spirituality and distress in sheltered battered women, *J Nurs Scholarsh* 32(3):273-278, 2000.

Johnson P: The use of humor and its influences on spirituality and coping in breast cancer survivors, *Oncol Nurs Forum* 29(4):691-695, 2002.

Keeley MP: Final conversations: Survivors' memorable messages concerning religious faith and spirituality, *Health Commun* 16(1):87-104, 2004.

Kirby SE, Coleman PG, Daley D: Spirituality and well-being in frail and nonfrail older adults, *J Gerontol B Psychol Sci Soc Sci* 59(3): P123-P129, 2004.

Lauver DR: Commonalities in women's spirituality and women's health, *ANS Adv Nurs Sci* 22(3):76-88, 2000.

Leininger MM, McFarland MR: *Transcultural nursing: concepts, theories, research and practices*, ed 3, New York, 2002, McGraw-Hill.

Logan J, Hackbusch-Pinto R, De Grasse CE: Women undergoing breast diagnostics: the lived experience of spirituality, *Oncol Nurs Forum* 33(1):121-126, 2006.

Manning-Walsh JK: Psychospiritual well-being and symptom distress in women with breast cancer, *Oncol Nurs Forum* 32(3):E56-E62, 2005.

McClain CS, Rosenfeld B, Breitbart W: Effect of spiritual well-being on end-of-life despair in terminally-ill cancer patients *Lancet* 361(9369):1603-1607, 2003.

McGrath P: Religiosity and the challenge of terminal illness, *Death Stud* 27(10):881-899, 2003.

Meraviglia M: Effects of spirituality in breast cancer survivors, *Oncol Nurs Forum* 33(1):E1-E7, 2006.

Meraviglia MG: The effects of spirituality on well-being of people with lung cancer, *Oncol Nurs Forum* 31(1):89-94, 2004.

Moller MD: Meeting spiritual needs on an inpatient unit, *J Psychosoc Nurs Ment Health Serv* 37(11):5, 1999.

Morris EL: The relationship of spirituality to coronary heart disease, *Altern Ther Health Med* 7(5):96-98, 2001.

Narayanasamy A: The impact of empirical studies of spirituality and culture on nurse education, *J Clin Nurs* 15:840-851, 2006.

Narayanasamy A: Spiritual coping mechanisms in chronic illness, *Br J Nurs* 11:1461-1470, 2002.

S

Narayanasamy A, Clisset P, Annasamy S et al: A qualitative study of nurses' responses to the spiritual needs of older people, *J Adv Nurs* 48:6-16, 2004.

Narayanasamy A, Owens J: A critical incident study of nurses' responses to the spiritual needs of their patients, *J Adv Nurs* 33(4):446-455, 2001.

Nelson CJ, Rosenfeld B, Breitbart W et al: Spirituality, religion, and depression in the terminally ill, *Psychosomatics* 43(3):213-220, 2002.

Pratt LA, Ford DE, Crum RM: Coronary heart disease/myocardial infarction: depression, psychotropic medication, and risk of myocardial infarction: prospective data from the Baltimore ECA follow-up, *Circulation* 94(12):3123-3129, 1996.

Reicks M, Mills J, Henry H: Qualitative study of spirituality in a weight loss program: contribution to self-efficacy and locus of control, *J Nutrit Educ Beh* 36(1):13-19, 2004.

Richardson JL, Zarnegar Z, Bisno B et al: Psychosocial status at initiation of cancer treatment and survival, *J Psychosom Res* 34(2):189-201, 1990.

Simoni JM, Frick PA, Huang B: A longitudinal evaluation of a social support model of medication adherence among HIV-positive men and women on antiretroviral therapy, *Health Psychol* 25(1):74-81, 2006.

Sowell R, Moneyham L, Hennessy M et al: Spiritual activities as a resistance resource for women with human immunodeficiency virus, *Nurs Res* 49(2):73-82, 2000.

Tan HM, Braunack-Mayer A, Beilby J: The impact of the hospice environment on patient spiritual expression, *Oncol Nurs Forum* 32(5):1049-1055, 2005.

Taylor EJ: Prevalence and associated factors of spiritual needs among patients with cancer and family caregivers, *Oncol Nurs Forum* 33(4):729-735, 2006.

Tuck I, Wallace D, Pullen L: Spirituality and spiritual care provided by parish nurses, *West J Nurs Res* 23(5):441-453, 2001.

Van Ness PH, Larson DB: Religion, senescence, and mental health: the end of life is not the end of hope, *Am J Geriatr Psychiatr* 10:386, 2002.

Walton J: Finding a balance: a grounded theory study of spirituality in hemodialysis patients, *Nephrol Nurs J* 29(5):447-457, 2002.

Williams NR, Lindsey E: Spirituality and religion in the living of runaway and homeless youth: coping with adversity, *J Relig Spiritual Soc Work* 24(4):19-38, 2005.

Yates JW, Chalmer BJ, St James P et al: Religion in patients with advanced cancer, *Med Pediatr Oncol* 9(2):121-128, 1981.

Younger JW, Piferi RL, Jobe RL et al: Dimensions of forgiveness: the views of laypersons, *J Soc Pers Relat* 21(6):837-855, 2004.

Risk for Spiritual distress   Lisa Burkhart, PhD, MPH, RN

NANDA   Definition

At risk for an impaired ability to experience and integrate meaning and purpose in life through connectedness with self, others, art, music, literature, nature, and/or a power greater than oneself

Risk Factors

Developmental: Life changes
Environmental: Environmental changes; natural disasters
Physical: Chronic illness; physical illness; substance abuse
Psychosocial: Anxiety; blocks to experiencing love; change in religious rituals; change in spiritual practices; cultural conflict; depression; inability to forgive; loss; low self-esteem; poor relationships; racial conflict; separated support systems; stress

NOC   Outcomes (Nursing Outcomes Classification)

Suggested NOC Outcomes

Acceptance: Health Status, Dignified Life Closure, Health Beliefs, Hope, Grief Resolution, Quality of Life, Spiritual Health, Suffering Severity

Example NOC Outcome with Indicators
Spiritual Health as evidenced by the following indicators: Quality of faith, hope/Meaning and purpose in life/ Connectedness with inner self, others/Interaction with others to share thoughts, feelings, and beliefs (Rate the outcome and indicators of **Spiritual Health:** 1 = extremely compromised, 2 = substantially compromised, 3 = moderately compromised, 4 = mildly compromised, 5 = not compromised [see Section I].)

Client Outcomes

Client Will (Specify Time Frame):

• Express sense of connectedness with self, others, arts, music, literature, or power greater than oneself

- Express meaning and purpose in life
- Express sense of optimism and hope in the future
- Express ability to forgive
- Express desire to discuss health state and integrate care in lifestyle
- Discuss personal response to dying
- Discuss personal response to grieving
- Express satisfaction with life circumstances

NIC   Interventions (Nursing Interventions Classification)

Suggested NIC Interventions

Active Listening, Forgiveness Facilitation, Grief Work Facilitation, Hope Inspiration, Humor, Music Therapy, Presence, Referral, Reminiscence Therapy, Self-Awareness Enhancement, Simple Guided Imagery, Simple Massage, Simple Relaxation Therapy, Spiritual Support, Therapeutic Touch, Touch

Example NIC Activities—Spiritual Support
Encourage the use of spiritual resources, if desired; Be available to listen to individual's feelings

Nursing Interventions, *Rationales*, and References

Refer to care plan for **Spiritual distress.**

Readiness for enhanced Spiritual well-being   *Lisa Burkhart, PhD, MPH, RN*

NANDA   Definition

Ability to experience and integrate meaning and purpose in life through connectedness with self, others, art, music, literature, nature, and/or a power greater than oneself that can be strengthened

Defining Characteristics

Connections to self: Expresses desire for enhanced acceptance; expresses desire for enhanced coping; expresses desire for enhanced courage; expresses desire for enhanced forgiveness of self; expresses desire for enhanced hope; expresses desire for enhanced joy; expresses desire for enhanced love; expresses desire for enhanced meaning in life; expresses desire for enhanced purpose in life; expresses desire for enhanced satisfying philosophy of life; expresses desire for enhanced surrender; expresses lack of serenity (e.g., peace); meditation

Connections with others: Provides service to others; requests forgiveness of others; requests interactions with significant others; request interactions with spiritual leaders

Connections with art, music, literature, nature: Displays creative energy (e.g., writing, poetry, singing); listens to music; reads spiritual literature; spends time outdoors

Connections with power greater than self: Expresses awe; expresses reverence; participates in religious activities; prays; reports mystical experiences

NOC   Outcomes (Nursing Outcomes Classification)

Suggested NOC Outcomes

Acceptance: Health Status, Adherence Behavior, Caregiver Emotional Health, Caregiver-Patient Relationship, Caregiver Well-Being, Comfort Level, Coping, Dignified Life Closure, Endurance, Family Integrity, Grief Resolution, Health Beliefs, Health-Promoting Behavior, Hope, Knowledge: Health Behavior, Leisure Participation, Personal Well-Being, Psychosocial Adjustment: Life Change, Quality of Life, Self-Esteem, Social Involvement, Spiritual Health

S

Example NOC Outcome with Indicators
Hope as evidenced by the following indicators: Expresses expectation of a positive future/Expresses faith, optimism, belief in self and others, meaning in life, and inner peace (Rate the outcome and indicators of **Hope:** 1 = never demonstrated, 2 = rarely demonstrated, 3 = sometimes demonstrated, 4 = often demonstrated, 5 = constantly demonstrated [see Section I].)

Client Outcomes

Client Will (Specify Time Frame):

- Express hope
- Express sense of meaning and purpose in life
- Express peace and serenity
- Express acceptance
- Express surrender
- Express forgiveness of self and others
- Express satisfaction with philosophy of life
- Express joy
- Express courage
- Describe being able to cope
- Describe use of spiritual practices
- Describe providing service to others
- Describe interaction with spiritual leaders, friends, and family
- Describe appreciation for art, music, literature, and nature

NIC   Interventions (Nursing Interventions Classification)

Suggested NIC Interventions

Active Listening, Emotional Support, Forgiveness Facilitation, Meditation Facilitation, Mutual Goal Setting, Presence, Religious Ritual Enhancement, Spiritual Growth Facilitation, Spiritual Support, Values Clarification

Example NIC Activities—Spiritual Support
Encourage the use of spiritual resources, if desired; Be available to listen to individual's feelings

Nursing Interventions and *Rationales*

S

- Perform a spiritual assessment that includes the client's relationship with God, meaning and purpose in life, religious affiliation, and any other significant beliefs. **EBN:** *Meaning and purpose in life are associated with spirituality (Burkhart & Solari-Twadell, 2001). Spiritual well-being offers some protection against end-of-life despair (McClain, Rosenfeld & Breitbart, 2003). Women with cancer view a developmental process of spirituality and responses to the diagnosis, treatment, and survival of cancer as a paradox of finding meaning in a belief system but having that belief system challenged as they cope with cure and recurrence (Halstead & Hull, 2001). Clinicians have assisted in the co-creation of sacred spaces where women can connect with themselves and each other (Banks-Wallace & Parks, 2004).*
- Be present for the client. **EBN:** *Presencing is effective not only for clients who are dying or in severe pain but also for those who are experiencing spiritual or emotional discomfort (Taylor, 2002). Presence of others is a theme in spirituality for individuals receiving hemodialysis (Walton, 2002).*
- Listen actively to the client. **EBN:** *Listening and presence are the most frequently used interventions (Tuck, Wallace & Pullen, 2001). Listening is an element of presencing (Taylor, 2002). Engaging in discussions related to spirituality promotes psychological well-being (Gibson & Parker, 2003).*
- Encourage the client to pray, setting the example by praying with and for the client. **EBN:** *Frequent prayer is associated with high mental scores regardless of age and gender (Meisenhelder &*

• = Independent;   ▲ = Collaborative;   EBN = Evidence-Based Nursing;   EB = Evidence-Based

Chandler, 2000). Prayer is considered an adjunct therapy in some critical care settings (Holt-Ashley, 2000). Shared prayer can be one of the deepest forms of communication (Shelly, 2000). Parish nurses reported prayer to be the intervention used most frequently with clients (Tuck, Wallace & Pullen, 2001). Prayer is associated with coping in persons with cancer (Taylor & Outlaw, 2002). Prayer and spiritual study can promote psychological well-being (Gibson & Parker, 2003). Prayer is associated with higher psychological well-being (Meraviglia, 2004; Meraviglia, 2006).

- Encourage spiritual meditation exercises. **EB:** *College students revealed that a spiritual mediation exercise significantly decreased anxiety and increased positive mood, spiritual health, spiritual experiences, and pain tolerance (Wachholtz & Paragment, 2005).*

▲ Coordinate or encourage attending spiritual retreats or courses. **EB:** *Controlled study pre-post test design showed that students who attended a spirituality course significantly increased their spiritual well-being (Bethel, 2004). Controlled study pre-post test and 6-month follow-up design with individuals who participated in a cardiac rehabilitation program revealed a significant increase in well-being, meaning in life, and decreased anger (Kennedy, Abbott & Rosenberg, 2002). Clients with coronary artery disease who meditated had a significant decrease in coronary stenosis (Morris, 2001).*

- Promote hope. **EBN:** *Stroke survivors participating in a stroke support group identified connectedness as an important theme in hope; spiritual connectedness was a factor in hope-related patterns (Bays, 2001). Older adults in a suburban senior center correlated spiritual health with more well-being and hope (Davis, 2005). Ovarian cancer survivors identified spirituality as useful in deriving meaning in the life experience. Spiritual themes that emerged were purpose in survivorship, hopefulness, and awareness of mortality (Ferrell et al, 2003). Hospice residents identified four themes of spiritual expression: relationships, that which uplifts, spiritual practice, and having hope. Spiritual expression was facilitated by individualized spiritual care. Nurses play an important role in the provision of spiritual care within a hospice setting (Tan, Braunack-Mayer & Beilby, 2005).*

- Encourage clients to reflect on what is meaningful to them in life. **EBN:** *Individuals with musculoskeletal disorders identified spirituality as a component of perceived health. Themes in the health model included reflection, interaction and connection, strength of identity, and bearable pain (Faull et al, 2004).*

- Encourage involvement in group religious practices. **EBN:** *Socialization and support found through participation in personal and/or group religious practices may decrease feelings of withdrawal and isolation (Baldacchino & Draper, 2001). Incorporating Bibles and other religious material can promote psychological well-being (Gibson & Parker, 2003).*

- Encourage increased quality of life through social support and family relationships. **EBN:** *Quality of life was potentially related to social support; physical, social, and functional well-being; and appraisal-focused coping in persons living with HIV (Tuck, McCain and Elswick, 2001.) Spirituality is an important theme in final conversations with loved ones (Keeley, 2004). In African-American men and women living with HIV/AIDS, spirituality significantly correlated with social functioning (Coleman, 2003). African-American women identified spirituality as an important resource for dealing with health crises. Functions included assisting women to negotiate health crises, undergirding strong families, promoting healing from abusive family situations, and maintaining relationships with ancestors (Banks-Wallace & Parks, 2004). Hospice residents identified four themes of spiritual expression: relationships, that which uplifts, spiritual practice, and having hope. Spiritual expression was facilitated by individualized spiritual care. Nurses play an important role in the provision of spiritual care within a hospice setting (Tan, Braunack-Mayer & Beilby, 2005). Older adults in rural geriatric communities identified emerging themes of transitions as integration of spirituality, faith, family, and health (Congdon & Magilvy, 2001).*

- Encourage volunteerism. **EBN:** *Individuals receiving hemodialysis identified spirituality as including faith; presence of God, others, community and nature; receiving help; and giving back/helping others (Walton, 2002).*

- Assist the client in identifying religious or spiritual beliefs that encourage integration of meaning and purpose in the client's life. **EBN:** *Beliefs were identified as an important theme that enhanced spirituality (Cavendish et al, 2001). Religious and/or spiritual beliefs were presented as important in interviews conducted with focus groups of users, caregivers, and mental health nursing professionals (Greasely, Chiu and Gartland, 2001). Chronically ill clients determined spiritual coping mechanisms as reaching out to God in the belief and faith that help will be forthcoming, feeling connected to*

S

God through prayer, meaning and purpose, strategy of privacy, and connectedness with others (Narayanasamy, 2002). Hispanic women drew strength from spiritual and religious resources (Dingley & Roux, 2003). Adult women survivors of child abuse identified spiritual connection as a positive value to cope with negative experiences, church as a location for accessing God and communing with others, and a growing relationship to the natural world and the body (Hall, 2003).

• Encourage the client to engage regularly in bibliotherapy. *Reading spiritually uplifting materials, including sacred writings, enhances well-being (Taylor, 2002). Incorporating the Bible and other religious reading material can promote psychological well-being (Gibson & Parker, 2003). Participants in a weight loss program identified spiritual interventions (including prayer and scripture reading) as helping in weight loss (Reicks, Mills & Henry, 2004).*

• Support involvement in expressive art. **EBN:** *Sculpture, painting, knitting, and dance are all forms of expressive art that can boost the spirit (Taylor, 2002).*

• Support the use of humor by the client. **EBN:** *Humor promotes coping in breast cancer survivors (Johnson, 2002).*

• Encourage the client to practice forgiveness. **EBN:** *Battered women rate forgiveness as an important part of spirituality (Humphreys, 2000). Parish nurses promoted forgiveness (Tuck, Wallace & Pullen, 2001).*

• Support the client in contemplating, viewing, and/or experiencing nature. **EBN:** *Nature was a theme in spirituality for individuals receiving hemodialysis (Walton, 2002).*

• Encourage expressions of spirituality. **EBN:** *African Americans and Latinos may identify spirituality, religiousness, prayer, and church-based approaches as coping resources (Samuel-Hodge et al, 2000). Chronically ill clients determined spiritual coping mechanisms as reaching out to God in the belief and faith that help will be forthcoming, feeling connected to God through prayer, meaning and purpose, strategy of privacy, and connectedness with others (Narayanasamy, 2002).*

• Encourage integration of spirituality in healthy lifestyle choices. **EBN:** *Participants in a weight loss program identified changes in eating behaviors, self-reported changes in food purchasing and preparation, self-reported changes made when eating out, self-efficacy, and central locus of control (Reicks, Mills & Henry, 2004). College students correlated higher spiritual health with less marijuana and alcohol use (Ellermann & Reed, 2001). Descriptive study of high school students correlated spiritual health with better self-care initiative and responsibility (Callaghan, 2005).*

• Validate the client's spiritual concerns and convey respect for his or her beliefs. *Validation lets the client know that the nurse has heard and understood what was said (Stuart & Laraia, 2001).* **EBN:** *Presence and use of inner resources in creating a therapeutic environment can promote psychological well-being (Gibson & Parker, 2003).*

▲ Help the client participate in religious rites or obtain spiritual guidance. **EBN:** *Retreats increase spirituality, well-being, meaning in life, confidence in handling problems, and decreased tendency to become angry (Kennedy, Abbott & Rosenberg, 2002).*

• Assist the client in developing spirituality. List the most valuable qualities he or she can bring from within, the circumstances most helpful for unfolding these qualities, and the ways of incorporating these circumstances into the client's lifestyle. **EBN:** *Receiving help and giving help was a theme in spirituality for individuals receiving hemodialysis (Walton, 2002).*

Geriatrics

• Refer to the care plan for **Spiritual distress.**

Multicultural

• Assess for the influence of cultural beliefs, norms, and values on the client's perceptions of spirituality. **EBN:** *The client's expressions of spirituality may be based on cultural perceptions (Stuart & Laraia, 2001). African-American women identified spirituality as an important resource for dealing with health crises. Functions included assisting women to negotiate health crises, undergirding strong families, promoting healing from abusive family situations, and maintaining relationships with ancestors (Banks-Wallace & Parks, 2004).*

• Encourage expressions of spirituality. **EBN:** *African Americans and Latinos may identify spirituality, religiousness, prayer, and church-based approaches as coping resources (Banks-Wallace & Parks*

S

2004; Samuel-Hodge et al, 2000). A qualitative study of five Hispanic women showed that they drew strength from spiritual and religious resources (Dingley & Roux, 2003).

- Validate the client's spiritual concerns and convey respect for his or her beliefs. **EBN:** A *qualitative study of 25 African-American women in five focus groups identified clinicians as assisting in the co-creation of sacred spaces where women can connect with themselves and each other (Banks-Wallace & Parks, 2004).*

 Home Care

- All of the nursing interventions mentioned previously apply in the home setting.
- Refer the client to parish nurses. **EBN:** *Parish nurses are experienced registered nurses committed to helping people meet the health needs of the mind, body, and spirit (Stewart, 2000).*

evolve See the EVOLVE website for World Wide Web resources for client education.

REFERENCES

Baldacchino D, Draper P: Spiritual coping strategies: a review of the nursing research literature, *J Adv Nurs* 34(6):833-841, 2001.

Banks-Wallace J, Parks L: It's all sacred: African American women's perspectives on spirituality, *Issues Ment Health Nurs* 25(1):25-45, 2004.

Bays CL: Older adults' description of hope after a stroke, *Rehabil Nurs* 26(1):18-27, 2001.

Bethel JC: Impact of social work spirituality courses on student attitudes, values, and spiritual wellness, *J Relig Spirituality Soc Work* 23(4):27-45, 2004.

Burkhart L, Solari-Twadell A: Spirituality and religiousness: differentiating the diagnosis through a review of the literature, *Nurs Diagn* 12(2):45, 2001.

Callaghan DM: The influence of spiritual growth on adolescents' initiative and responsibility for self-care, *Pediatr Nurs* 31(2):91-95, 2005.

Cavendish R, Luise BK, Bauer M et al: Recognizing opportunities for spiritual enhancement in young adults: *Nurs Diagn* 12(3):77, 2001.

Coleman CL: Spirituality and sexual orientation: relationship to mental well-being and functional health status, *J Adv Nurs* 43(5):457-464, 2003.

Congdon JG, Magilvy JK: Themes of rural health and aging from a program of research, *Geriatr Nurs* 22(5):234-238, 2001.

Davis B: Mediators of the relationship between hope and well-being in older adults, *Clin Nurs Res* 14(3):253-272, 2005.

Dingley C, Roux G: Inner strength in older Hispanic women with chronic illness, *J Cult Divers* 10(1):11-22, 2003.

Ellerman CR, Reed PG: Self-transcendence and depression in middle-age adults, *West J Nurs Res* 23(7):698-713, 2001.

Faull K, Hills MD, Cochrane G et al: Investigation of health perspectives of those with physical disabilities: the role of spirituality as a determinant of health, *Disabil Rehabil* 26(3):129-144, 2004.

Ferrell BR, Smith SL, Juarez G et al: Meaning of illness and spirituality in ovarian cancer survivors, *Oncol Nurs Forum* 30(2):249-257, 2003.

Gibson LMR, Parker V: Inner resources as predictors of psychological well-being in middle-income African American breast cancer survivors, *Cancer Control* 10(5):52-58, 2003.

Greasley P, Chiu LF, Gartland RM: The concept of spiritual care in mental health nursing, *J Adv Nurs* 33:629, 2001.

Hall JM: Positive self-transitions in women child abuse survivors, *Issues Ment Health Nurs* 24:647-666, 2003.

Halstead MR, Hull M: Struggling with paradoxes: the process of spiritual development in women with cancer, *Oncol Nurs Forum* 28(10):1534-1544, 2001.

Holt-Ashley M: Nurses pray: use of prayer and spirituality as comple-

mentary therapy in the intensive care setting, *AACN Clin Issues* 11(1):60, 2000.

Humphreys J: Spirituality and distress in sheltered battered women, *Image: J Nurs Sch* 32:273, 2000.

Johnson P: The use of humor and its influences on spirituality and coping in breast cancer survivors, *Oncol Nurs Forum* 29(4):691-695, 2002.

Keeley MP: Final conversations: survivors' memorable messages concerning religious faith and spirituality, *Health Commun* 16(1):87-104, 2004.

Kennedy JE, Abbott RA, Rosenberg BS: Changes in spirituality and well-being in a retreat program for cardiac patients, *Alt Ther Health Med* 8(4):64-73, 2002.

McClain CS, Rosenfeld B, Breitbart W: Effect of spiritual well-being on end-of-life despair in terminally-ill cancer patients, *Lancet* 361(9369):1603-1607, 2003.

Meisenhelder JB, Chandler EN: Prayer and health outcomes in church lay leaders, *West J Nurs Res* 22:706, 2000.

Meraviglia MG: The effects of spirituality in breast cancer survivors, *Oncol Nurs Forum* 31(1):E1-E7, 2006.

Meraviglia MG: The effects of spirituality on well-being of people with lung cancer, *Oncol Nurs Forum* 31(1):89-94, 2004.

Morris EL: The relationship of spirituality to coronary heart disease, *Alt Ther Health Med* 7(5):96-98, 2001.

Narayanasamy A: Spiritual coping mechanisms in chronic illness, *Br J Nurs* 11:1461-1470, 2002.

Reicks M, Mills J, Henry H: Qualitative study of spirituality in a weight loss program: contribution to self-efficacy and locus of control, *J Nutr Educ Behav* 36(1):13-19, 2004.

Samuel-Hodge CD, Headen SW, Ingram AF et al: Influences on day-to-day self-management of type 2 diabetes among African American women: spirituality, the multi-caregiver role, and other social context factors, *Diabetes Care* 23(7):928, 2000.

Shelly J: *Spiritual care: a guide for caregivers,* Downers Grove, Ill, 2000, InterVarsity Press.

Stewart LE: Parish nursing: renewing a long tradition of caring, *Gastroenterol Nurs* 23(3):116, 2000.

Stuart GW, Laraia MT: Therapeutic nurse-patient relationship. In Stuart GW, Laraia MT, editors: *Principles and practice of psychiatric nursing,* St Louis, 2001, Mosby, p 30.

Tan HM, Braunack-Mayer A, Beilby J: The impact of the hospice environment on patient spiritual expression, *Oncol Nurs Forum* 32(5):1049-1055, 2005.

Taylor E: *Spiritual care: nursing theory, research and practice,* Upper Saddle River, NJ, 2002, Prentice Hall.

S

Taylor EJ, Outlaw FH: Use of prayer among persons with cancer, *Holist Nurs Pract* 16(3):46-60, 2002.

Tuck I, McCain NL, Elswick RK: Spirituality and psychosocial factors in persons living with HIV, *J Adv Nurs* 33(6):776, 2001.

Tuck I, Wallace D, Pullen L: Spirituality and spiritual care provided by parish nurses, *West J Nurs Res* 23:144, 2001.

Wachholtz AB, Pargament KI: Is spirituality a critical ingredient of meditation? Comparing the effects of spiritual meditation, secular meditation, and relaxation on spiritual, psychological, cardiac, and pain outcomes, *J Behav Med* 28(4):367-384, 2005.

Walton J: Finding a balance: a grounded theory study of spirituality in hemodialysis patients, *Nephrol Nurs J* 29(5):447-457, 2002.

Stress overload   *Margaret Lunney, RN, PhD, and June M. Como, RN, MSA, MS, CCRN, CCNS*

NANDA   Definition

Excessive amounts and types of demands that require action

Defining Characteristics

Demonstrates increased feelings of anger; demonstrates increased feelings of impatience; expresses a feeling of pressure; expresses a feeling of tension; expresses difficulty in functioning; expresses increased feelings of anger; expresses increased feelings of impatience; expresses problems with decision making; reports negative impact from stress (e.g., physical symptoms, psychological distress, feeling of "being sick" or of "going to get sick"); reports situational stress as excessive (e.g., rates stress level as 7 or above on a 10-point scale)

Related Factors (r/t)

Inadequate resources (e.g., financial, social, education/knowledge level); intense, repeated stressors (e.g., family violence, chronic illness, terminal illness); multiple coexisting stressors (e.g., environmental threats, demands); physical threats, demands; social threats, demands

NOC   Outcomes (Nursing Outcomes Classification)

Suggested NOC Outcomes

Anxiety Level, Caregiver Stressors, Stress Level

> **Example NOC Outcome with Indicators**
>
> **Stress Level** as evidenced by the following indicators: elevated blood pressure, restlessness, emotional outbursts, anxiety, diminished attention to detail (Rate the outcome and indicators of **Stress Level:** 1 = severe, 2 = substantial, 3 = moderate, 4 = mild, 5 = none [see Section I].)

Client Outcomes

Client Will (Specify Time Frame):

* Review the amounts and types of stressors in daily living
* Identify stressors that can be modified or eliminated
* Mobilize social supports to facilitate lower stress levels
* Reduce stress levels through use of relaxation techniques and other strategies

NIC   Interventions (Nursing Interventions Classification)

Suggested NIC Interventions

Active Listening, Anger Control Assistance, Anxiety Reduction, Aroma Therapy, Counseling, Crisis Intervention, Emotional Support, Family Integrity Promotion, Presence, Support System Enhancement

S

• = Independent;   ▲ = Collaborative;   EBN = Evidence-Based Nursing;   EB = Evidence-Based

Example NIC Activities—Support System Enhancement
Assess psychological response to situation and availability of support system; Determine adequacy of social networks; Explain to concerned others how they can help; Refer to a self-help group, as appropriate; Provide services in a caring and supportive manner

Nursing Interventions and *Rationales*

- Assess for stress overload during vulnerable life events. **EBN:** *Assessment of critical care stressors was needed because the nurses' and clients' perceptions of the stressors differed from one another (So & Chan, 2004). More than half of women who experienced psychological distress after treatment for gynecological cancer had four or more concerns or worries; the clients who had access to a clinical nurse specialist had significantly fewer worries (Booth, Beaver & Kitchener, 2005). Parents whose deceased children had received stem cell transplants experienced higher levels of anxiety and stress than the parents whose deceased children had not received stem cell transplants (Drew et al, 2005).* **EB:** *Early interventions to reduce stressors could improve quality of life or prevent a significant decrease in quality of life in women who had breast cancer surgery (Golden-Kreutz et al, 2005). Individuals with a history of major depressive disorders (MDD) maintained a lower level of response to uncontrollable stress than those without a history of MDD (Ilgen & Hutchinson, 2005).*
- Listen actively to descriptions of stressors and the stress response. **EBN:** *Having an opportunity to speak about stressors is helpful in dealing with stress overload (Lunney & Myszak, 1997). Listening engenders trust and trust is the first step in the process of helping clients to reduce the psychological distress of stress overload (Ridner, 2004).*
- In younger adult women, assess interpersonal stressors. **EB:** *Daily stressors related to interpersonal relations are associated with physical symptoms in younger but not older adult women (Mallers, Almeida & Neupert, 2005).*
- Categorize stressors as modifiable or nonmodifiable. **EBN:** *Removing or minimizing some stressors, changing responses to stressors, and modifying the long-term effects of stress are all actions that can assist those with diabetes and stress (Lloyd, Smith & Weinger, 2005).*
- Help clients modify or mitigate stressors identified as modifiable. **EBN:** *In a review of stress, stress response and health, problem-based coping strategies, information gathering, planning, and taking action were considered as important to reduce high stress (Motzer & Hertig, 2004). There are numerous possible strategies to modify stressors, including time management, improved organizational skills, problems solving, changing perceptions of stress, breathing, relaxation techniques, visual imagery, soothing rituals (Motzer & Hertig, 2004; Lloyd, Smith & Weinger, 2005).*
- Help clients distinguish between short-term stressors and chronic stressors. **EBN:** *The short-term stressor of college examinations had no negative effects on health and, in fact, had positive effects on students' achievements (Sarid et al, 2004). Help clients focus on the positive aspects of stressors, disengage from some stressors, and seek social support.* **EBN:** *These emotion-based coping strategies supplement and support problem-based coping strategies (Motzer & Hertig, 2004).* **EB:** *High stress does not necessarily have negative effects on health (Nielsen et al, 2005). Disengagement is recommended when women experience the stress of having abusive partners (Eby, 2004). Social support is a critical dimension of health and health promotion and serves as a buffer in the stress response (Pender, Murtaugh & Parsons, 2006).*
- Provide information as needed to reduce stress responses to acute and chronic illnesses. **EBN:** *Information helps reduce the number of stressors (Harwood et al, 2005).*
- Explore possible therapeutic approaches such as cognitive behavior therapy, biofeedback, neurofeedback, pharmacologic agents, and complementary and alternative therapies. **EBN:** *These types of therapies decrease the sympathetic nervous system response to stress (Scollan-Koliopoulos, 2005). Neurofeedback promotes optimum functioning of the central nervous system, induces relaxation, and supports healthy balance, flexibility, and resilience (Brown, 2007). Adults who had experienced hospitalizations of at least 5 days said that spirituality strengthened their coping ability (Cavendish et al, 2006).*
- Help the client to reframe his or her perceptions of some of the stressors. **EB:** *Male policemen who were engaged in active and reappraisal coping showed better functioning (Diong et al, 2005).*
- Assist the client to mobilize social supports for dealing with recent stressors. **EB:** *Social support moderates the impact of recent but not chronic life stress on physical symptom reporting (Cropley & Steptoe, 2005).*

S

- = Independent;   ▲ = Collaborative;   EBN = Evidence-Based Nursing;   EB = Evidence-Based

Pediatric

- With children, nurses should work with parents to help them to reduce children's stressors. **EB**: *A comprehensive review of research on stress and coping in childhood showed that parents can have profound effects on reducing the stressors of childhood (Power, 2004).* **EBN:** *School-related stressors are one of the most significant sources of stress overload (Ryan-Wenger et al, 2005).*
- Help children to manage their feelings related to self-concept. **EBN:** *Events that affected self-concept were shown to be significant stressors for children (Ryan-Wenger et al, 2005).*
- Help children to deal with bullies and other sources of violence in schools and neighborhoods. **EBN:** *Violence in schools and neighborhoods has significant effects on children's stress. Children can be taught how to deal with bullies (Ryan-Wenger, Sharrer & Campbell, 2005).*
- Help young children to identify and mitigate the experience of "feeling sick." **EBN:** *"Feeling sick" is described most often as a stressor. This was related to children's lack of knowledge and experience with illnesses (Taxis et al, 2004).*
- Help children to manage the complexities of chronic illnesses. **EBN:** *Teenagers who had recently been diagnosed with diabetes described high levels of stress that often related to the complexities of managing the illness (Davidson et al, 2004).*

Geriatric

- Assess for chronic stress with older adults and provide a variety of stress relief techniques. *With advancing age, stressors are more likely to be chronic and may have negative effects on memory and cognitive decline; thus chronic stressors should be reduced through a variety of strategies (Vondras et al, 2005).*
- Encourage social support for older adults. *Stressors in highly valued roles affect physical health only when there is insufficient emotional support from social networks (Krause, 2004).*

Multicultural

- Review cultural beliefs and acculturation level in relation to perceived stressors. **EB:** *Multidimensional assessment of acculturation and acculturative stress in Hispanics "has the potential to provide a richer characterization of the individual" (Thoman & Suris, 2004). Such characterizations may lend themselves to a better understanding of stress overload factors. A conclusion from a conceptual analysis of stress and coping was that perceptions of stress are culturally derived (Keil, 2004).*
- Assess families for whether they experience high stress or low stress. **EBN:** *High stress in Lebanese families, often related to war and other community-based factors, was associated with family health (Farhood, 2004).*
- Support social connectedness among cultural groups. **EBN:** *High social connectedness was associated with low stress in children (Taxis et al, 2004).*

Home Care

- The above interventions may be adapted for home care use.
- Develop community-based programs for stress management as needed for groups with increased risk of stress overload (e.g., firefighters, policeman, military personnel, nurses). **EB:** *Some situations have higher risks of stress overload. Stress management interventions may prevent or modify the experience of stress overload (McNulty, 2005).*
- Support and encourage neighborhood stability. **EB:** *A "significant proportion of health differentials across neighborhoods is due to disparate stress levels across [Detroit] neighborhoods" and neighborhood stability was a buffer to reduce the negative effects of high stress (Boardman, 2004).*

Client/Family Teaching

- Diagnose the possibility of stress overload before teaching.
- Establish readiness for learning.
- Provide manageable amounts of information at the appropriate educational level.
- Evaluate the need for additional teaching and learning experiences.

 See the EVOLVE website for World Wide Web resources for client education.

REFERENCES

Boardman JD: Stress and physical health: the role of neighborhoods as mediating and moderating mechanisms, *Soc Sci Med* 58(12):2473-2483, 2004.

Booth K, Beaver K, Kitchener H: Women's experiences of information, psychological distress and worry after treatment for gynaecological cancer, *Patient Educ Couns* 56(2):225-232, 2005.

Brown V: *KARMA or DHARMA: three acronyms that can clarify the core of neurofeedback training, at least in Neurocare.* Paper presented at Conference on Future Health, January 2007, Palm Springs, Calif.

Cavendish R, Naradovy L, Como J et al: Patients' perceptions of spirituality and the nurse as a spiritual care provider, *Holistic Nurs Pract* 20:41-47, 2006.

Cropley M, Steptoe A: Social support, life events and physical symptoms: a prospective study of chronic and recent life stress in men and women, *Psychol Health Med* 10:317-325, 2005.

Davidson M, Penney ED, Muller B et al: Stressors and self-care challenges faced by adolescents living with type 1 diabetes, *Appl Nurs Res* 2:72-80, 2004.

Diong SM, Bishop GD, Enkelmann HC et al: Anger, stress, coping, social support and health: modeling the relationships, *Psychol Health* 20:467-495, 2005.

Drew D, Goodenough B, Maurice L et al: Parental grieving after a child dies from cancer: is stress from stem cell transplant a factor? *Int J Palliat Nurs* 11:266-273, 2005.

Eby KK: Exploring the stressors of low-income women with abusive partners: understanding their needs and developing effective community responses, *J Fam Violence* 19(4):221-232, 2004.

Farhood LF: The impact of high and low stress on the health of Lebanese families, *Res Theory Nurs Pract* 18(2-3):197-212, 2004.

Golden-Kreutz DM, Thorton LM, Wells-Di Gregorio S et al: Traumatic stress, perceived global stress, and life events: prospectively predicting quality of life in breast cancer patients, *Health Psychol* 24(3):288-296, 2005.

Harwood L, Locking-Cusolito H, Spittal J et al: Preparing for hemodialysis: patient stressors and responses, *Nephrol Nurs J* 32(3):295-303, 2005.

Ilgen MA, Hutchinson KE: A history of major depressive disorder and the response to stress, *J Affect Disord* 86(2-3):143-150, 2005.

Keil RMK: Coping and stress: a conceptual analysis, *J Adv Nurs* 45(6):659-665, 2004.

Krause N: Stressors arising in highly valued roles, meaning in life, and the physical health status of older adults, *J Gerontol Soc Sci* 59b: S287-S297, 2004.

Lloyd C, Smith J, Weinger K: Stress and diabetes: a review of the links, *Diabetes Spectr* 18(2):121-127, 2005.

Lunney M, Myszak C: Abstract: stress overload: a new diagnosis. In Rantz MH, LeMone P, editors: *Classification of nursing diagnoses: proceedings of the twelfth conference, North American Nursing Diagnosis Association* (pp 190-191), Glendale, Calif, 1997, CINAHL Information Systems.

Mallers MH, Almeida DM, Neupert SD: Women's daily physical health symptoms and stressful experiences across adulthood, *Psychol Health* 20:389-403, 2005.

McNulty PAF: Reported stressors and health care needs of active duty Navy personnel during three phases of deployment in support of the war in Iraq, *Mil Med* 170:530-535, 2005.

Motzer SA, Hertig V: Stress, stress response and health, *Nurs Clin North Am* 39:1-17, 2004.

Nielsen NR, Zhang ZF, Kristensen TS et al: Self-reported stress and risk of breast cancer, *BMJ* 331(7516):548-550, 2005.

Pender NJ, Murtaugh CL, Parsons MA: *Health promotion in nursing practice,* ed 5, Upper Saddle River, NJ, 2006, Prentice Hall.

Power TG.: Stress and coping in childhood: the parents' role, *Parenting: Sci Pract* 4:271-317, 2004.

Ridner SH.: Psychological distress: concept analysis, *J Adv Nurs* 45:536-545, 2004.

Ryan-Wenger NA, Sharrer VW, Campbell KK: Changes in children's stressors over the past 30 years, *Pediatr Nurs* 31(4):282-291, 2005.

Sarid O, Anson O, Yaari A et al: Academic stress, immunological reaction, and academic performance among students of nursing and physiotherapy, *Res Nurs Health* 27:370-377, 2004.

Scollan-Koliopoulos M: Managing stress response to control hypertension in type 2 diabetes, *Nurse Pract* 30(2):46-49, 2005.

So HM, Chan DSK: Perceptions of stressors by patients and nurses of critical care units in Hong Kong, *Int J Nurs Stud* 4:77-84, 2004.

Taxis JC, Rew L, Jackson K et al: Protective resources and perceptions of stress in a multi-ethnic sample of school-age children, *Pediatr Nurs* 30:477-487, 2004.

Thoman LV, Suris A: Acculturation and acculturative stress as predictors of psychological distress and quality-of-life functioning in Hispanic psychiatric patients, *Hispanic J Behav Sci* 26(3):293-311, 2004.

Vondras DD, Powless MR, Olson AK et al: Differential effects of everyday stress on the episodic memory test performances of young, mid-life, and older adults, *Aging Ment Health* 9(1):60-70, 2005.

S

Risk for Suffocation   *Nadine M. Aktan, MS, RN, APN-C, and Betty Ackley, MSN, EdS, RN*

NANDA   ## Definition

Accentuated risk of accidental suffocation (inadequate air available for inhalation)

Risk Factors

External

Discarding refrigerators without removing doors; eating large mouthfuls of food; hanging a pacifier around infant's neck; household gas leaks; inserting small objects into airway; leaving children unattended in water; low-strung clothesline; pillow placed in infant's crib; playing with plastic bags; propped bottle placed in infant's crib; smoking in bed; use of fuel-burning heaters not vented to outside; vehicle warming in closed garage

• = Independent;   ▲ = Collaborative;   EBN = Evidence-Based Nursing;   EB = Evidence-Based

Internal

Cognitive difficulties; disease process; emotional difficulties; injury process; lack of safety education; lack of safety precautions; reduced motor abilities; reduced olfactory sensation

Suggested NOC Outcomes

Knowledge: Child Physical Safety, Personal Safety, Parenting: Adolescent Physical Safety, Early/Middle Childhood Physical Safety, Infant/Toddler Physical Safety, Risk Control, Risk Detection, Safe Home Environment, Substance Addiction Consequences

> **Example NOC Outcome with Indicators**
>
> **Knowledge: Child Physical Safety** as evidenced by the following indicators: Description of methods to prevent choking on objects/Description of appropriate activities for child's developmental level/Description of first aid techniques (Rate the outcome and indicators of **Knowledge: Child Physical Safety:** 1 = none, 2 = limited, 3 = moderate, 4 = substantial, 5 = extensive [see Section I].)

Client Outcomes

Client Will (Specify Time Frame):

- Explain and undertake appropriate measures to prevent suffocation
- Demonstrate correct techniques for emergency rescue maneuvers (e.g., Heimlich maneuver, rescue breathing, cardiopulmonary resuscitation [CPR]) and describe situations that require them

Suggested NIC Interventions

Aspiration Precautions, Environmental Management: Safety, Infant Care, Positioning, Security Enhancement, Surveillance, Surveillance: Safety, Teaching: Infant Safety

> **Example NIC Activities—Environmental Management: Safety**
>
> Identify safety hazards in the environment (i.e., physical, biological, and chemical); Remove hazards from the environment, when possible

Nursing Interventions and *Rationales*

- Identify hospitalized clients at particular risk for suffocation, including the following:
  - Clients with altered levels of consciousness
  - Infants or young children
  - Clients with developmental delays
  - Clients with mental illness, especially schizophrenia

  Institute safety measures such as proper positioning and feeding precautions. See the care plans for **Risk for Aspiration** *and* **Impaired Swallowing** *for additional interventions. Vigilance and special protective measures are necessary for clients at greater risk for suffocation.* **EB:** *Mental health clients have an increased incidence of choking and suffocation incidents (Corcoran & Walsh, 2003).*

 Pediatric

- Counsel families on the following:
  - Follow general safety practices such as not smoking in bed, not smoking during pregnancy, not smoking in the presence of an infant, properly disposing of large appliances, using properly functioning heating systems and ventilation, having functional smoke and carbon monoxide detectors, and opening garage doors when warming up a car.
  - Position infants on their back to sleep; do not position them in the prone position. **EB:** *Research has demonstrated that the prone position for sleeping infants is a risk factor for sudden*

S

• = Independent;   ▲ = Collaborative;   EBN = Evidence-Based Nursing;   EB = Evidence-Based

*infant death syndrome (SIDS) (Li et al, 2003; Malloy & Freeman, 2004). Population studies have demonstrated a striking trend in decreased incidence of SIDS since parents have been taught to **not** place infants in the prone position (Ponsonby, Dwyer & Cochrane, 2002).*

- Avoid use of loose bedding such as blankets and sheets for sleeping. If blankets are used, they should be tucked in around the crib mattress so the infant's face is less likely to become covered by bedding. "One strategy is to make up the bedding so that the infant's feet are able to reach the foot of the crib with the blankets tucked in around the crib mattress and reaching only the level of the infant's chest" (American Academy of Pediatrics, 2000, p. 650). **EB:** *Infants placed in environments not specifically designed for them, such as sofa or an adult bed, have an increased risk of dying suddenly and unexpectedly (Kemp et al, 2000).*

- Teach parents not to sleep with an infant, especially if alcohol or medications/illicit drugs are used by the parents. **EB:** *Parents who were under the influence of alcohol or illicit drugs or were smoking were more likely to have a SIDS result (James, Klenka & Manning, 2003). Mothers who consumed three or more alcoholic drinks in the past 24 hours increased the risk of SIDS when bed sharing with an infant (Carpenter et al, 2004).*

- Assess for signs and symptoms of abuse such as Munchausen syndrome by proxy (MSBP). **EB:** *Suffocation in MSBP is one important differential diagnosis in suspected cases of SIDS (Vennemann et al, 2005).*

- Conduct risk factor identification, noting special circumstances in which preventive or protective measures are indicated. Note the presence of environmental hazards, including the following:
  - Plastic bags (e.g., dry cleaner's bags, bags used for mattress protection)
  - Cribs with slats wider than 2⅜ inches
  - Ill-fitting crib mattresses that can allow the infant to become wedged between the mattress and crib
  - Pillows in cribs
  - Abandoned large appliances such as refrigerators, dishwashers, or freezers
  - Clothing with cords or hoods that can become entangled
  - Bibs, pacifiers on a string, drapery cords, pull-toy strings

  Suffocation by airway obstruction is a leading cause of death in children younger than 6 years of age. Families need to be taught child protection.

- Counsel families to not serve these foods to the child younger than 4 years of age: hot dogs, popcorn, nuts, pretzels, chips, peanut butter, chunks of meat, hard pieces of fruit or vegetables, raisins, whole grapes, hard candies, marshmallows (Single Parent Central, 2005). *Hot dogs are the most common item associated with fatal choking incidences in children (Behrman, Kliegman & Jenson, 2004).* **EB:** *Children between the ages of 4 and 36 months of age are at risk for suffocation by hollow, semi-rigid hemispherical/ellipsoidal objects through suction formation and complete airway obstruction (Nakamura, Pollack-Nelson & Chidekel, 2003).*

- Provide information to parents about obtaining the "No-choke Test Tube" (no-choke tubes are sold at stores that sell baby items) or using a toilet paper roll: if an object fits in the tube or the roll, it is too small to give to a child (Single Parent Central, 2005). **EB:** *Rigid items that are of a spherical or cylindrical shape can cause upper airway occlusion (Nakamura, Pollack-Nelson & Chidekel, 2003). Accidental suffocation can result from the aspiration of a foreign body with airway occlusion (Bajanowski et al, 2005).*

- Stress water and pool safety precautions, including vigilant, uninterrupted parental supervision. *An intense drive for exploration combined with a lack of awareness of danger makes drowning a threat to small children. A child's high center of gravity and poor coordination make buckets and toilets a threat because a child looking inside can fall over and become lodged (Behrman, Kliegman & Jenson, 2004). Pools should be surrounded completely by fencing that is difficult to climb and that does not allow direct access to the house, and gates should have self-closing latches (Schnitzer, 2006).*

- Underscore the necessity of not allowing children to play with or near electric garage doors and of keeping garage door openers out of the reach of young children. *Children close to the ground may not be large enough to trigger reversal mechanisms on the door and may become trapped.*

- For adolescents, watch for signs of depression that could result in suicide by suffocation. **EB:** *For adolescents 10 to 19 years of age, suffocation by hanging is the second most common method of suicide (Centers for Disease Control and Prevention [CDC], 2004).*

S

Geriatric

- Assess the status of the swallow reflex. Offer appropriate foods and beverages accordingly. *The elderly, especially those receiving antipsychotic medications, have an increased incidence of choking.*
- Observe the client for pocketing of food in the side of the mouth; remove food as needed.
- Position the client in high Fowler's position when eating and for 1 hour afterward. *Elderly clients may be at risk for suffocation that results from dysphagia.*
- Use care in pillow placement when positioning frail elderly clients who are on bed rest. *Frail elderly clients are at risk for suffocation if the head becomes lodged against pillows and the client cannot reposition them because of weakness.*

Home Care

- Assess the home for potential safety hazards in systems that are not likely to be fixed (e.g., faulty pilot lights or gas leaks in gas stoves, carbon monoxide release from heating systems, kerosene fumes from portable heaters). Assist the family in having these areas assessed and making appropriate safety arrangements (e.g., installing detectors, making repairs). *Assessment and correction of system problems prevent accidental suffocation.*

Client/Family Teaching

- ▲ Recommend that families who are seeking day care or in-home care for children, geriatric family members, or at-risk family members with developmental or functional disabilities inspect the environment for hazards and examine the first aid preparation and vigilance of providers. *Many working families must trust others to care for family members.*
- ▲ Involve family members in learning and practicing rescue techniques, including treatment of choking and lack of breathing, as well as CPR. Initiate referral to formal training classes. *Family members need adequate preparation to deal with emergency situations and should take part in the American Heart Association Basic Lifesaving Course or the American Red Cross Infant/Child CPR Course (CDC, 2002).*

evolve See the EVOLVE website for World Wide Web resources for client education.

REFERENCES

American Academy of Pediatrics, Task Force on Infant Sleep Position and Sudden Infant Death Syndrome: Changing concepts of sudden infant death syndrome: implications for infant sleeping environment and sleep position (RE9946), *Pediatrics* 105(3):650, 2000.

Bajanowski T, Vennemann B, Bohnert M et al: Unnatural causes of sudden unexpected deaths initially thought to be SIDS, *Int J Legal Med* 119:213-216, 2005.

Behrman RE, Kliegman RM, Jenson HB: *Nelson textbook of pediatrics*, ed 17, Philadelphia, 2004, Saunders.

Carpenter RG, Irgens LM, Blair PS et al: Sudden unexplained infant death in 20 regions in Europe: case control study, *Lancet* 363(9404):185, 2004.

Centers for Disease Control and Prevention (CDC): Methods of suicide among persons aged 10-19 years—United States, 1992-2001, *MMWR Morb Mort Wkly Rep* 53(22):471, 2004.

Centers for Disease Control and Prevention (CDC): Nonfatal choking-related episodes among children—United States, 2001, *MMWR Morb Mort Wkly Rep* 51(42):945-948, 2002.

Corcoran E, Walsh D: Obstructive asphyxia: a cause of excess mortality in psychiatric patients, *Ir J Psychol Med* 20(3):88-90, 2003.

James C, Klenka H, Manning D: Sudden infant death syndrome: bed sharing with mothers who smoke, *Arch Dis Child* 88(2):112, 2003.

Kemp JS, Unger B, Wilkens D et al: Unsafe sleep practices and an analysis of bed-sharing among infants dying suddenly and unexpectedly:

results of a 4-year, population-based, death scene investigation study of SIDS and related deaths, *Pediatrics* 106(3):E41, 2000.

Li DK, Petitti DB, Willinger M et al: Infant sleeping position and the risk of sudden infant death syndrome in California, 1997-2000, *Am J Epidemiol* 157(5):446, 2003.

Malloy MH, Freeman DH: Age at death, season, and day of death as indicators of the effect of the back to sleep program on sudden infant death syndrome in the United States, 1992-1999, *Arch Pediatr Adolesc Med* 158(4):359-365, 2004.

Nakamura S, Pollack-Nelson C, Chidekel A: Suction-type suffocation incidents in infants and toddlers, *Pediatrics* 111(1):12-16, 2003.

Ponsonby A, Dwyer T, Cochrane JL: Population trends in sudden infant death syndrome, *Semin Perinatol* 26(4):296, 2002.

Ponsonby AL, Dwyer T, Couper D et al: Association between use of a quilt and sudden infant death syndrome: case-control study, *BMJ* 316(7126):195, 1998.

Schnitzer PG: Prevention of unintentional childhood injuries, *Am Fam Physician* 74(11):1864-1869, 2006.

Single Parent Central: *Preventing choking in young children.* Available at http://library.adoption.com/Child-Safety/Preventing-Choking-in-Young-Children/article/2724/1.html, accessed March 1, 2007.

Vennemann B, Bajanowski T, Karger B et al: Suffocation and poisoning—the hard hitting side of Munchausen syndrome by proxy, *Int J Legal Med* 119:98-102, 2005.

• = Independent;   ▲ = Collaborative;   EBN = Evidence-Based Nursing;   EB = Evidence-Based

Risk for Suicide   *Kathleen L. Patusky, PhD, APRN-BC*

NANDA   **Definition**

At risk for self-inflicted, life-threatening injury

Related Factors (r/t)

Behavioral

Buying a gun; changing a will; giving away possessions; history of prior suicide attempt; impulsiveness; making a will; marked changes in attitude; marked changes in behavior; marked changes in school performance; stockpiling medicines; sudden euphoric recovery from major depression

Demographic

Age (e.g., elderly, young adult males, adolescents); divorced; male gender; race (e.g., Caucasian, Native American); widowed

Physical

Chronic pain; physical illness; terminal illness

Psychological

Childhood abuse; family history of suicide; gay or lesbian youth; guilt; psychiatric illness/disorder (e.g., depression, schizophrenia, bipolar disorder); substance abuse

Situational

Adolescents living in nontraditional settings (e.g., juvenile detention center, prison, half-way house, group home); economic instability; institutionalization; living alone; loss of autonomy; loss of independence; presence of gun in home; relocation; retired

Social

Cluster suicides; disciplinary problems; disrupted family life; grief; helplessness; hopelessness; legal problems; loneliness; loss of important relationship; poor support systems; social isolation

Verbal

States desire to die; threats of killing oneself

NOC   **Outcomes (Nursing Outcomes Classification)**

Suggested NOC Outcomes

Depression Level, Distorted Thought Self-Control, Impulse Self-Control, Loneliness Severity, Mood Equilibrium, Risk Detection, Self-Mutilation Restraint, Suicide Self-Restraint

S

Example NOC Outcome with Indicators

Suicide Self-Restraint as evidenced by the following indicators: Expresses feelings/Seeks help when feeling self-destructive/Verbalizes suicidal ideas/Controls impulses (Rate the outcome and indicators of **Suicide Self-Restraint:** 1 = never demonstrated, 2 = rarely demonstrated, 3 = sometimes demonstrated, 4 = often demonstrated, 5 = consistently demonstrated [see Section I].)

Client Outcomes

Client Will (Specify Time Frame):

- Not harm self
- Maintain connectedness in relationships
- Disclose and discuss suicidal ideas if present; seek help
- Express decreased anxiety and control of impulses
- Talk about feelings; express anger appropriately

• = Independent;   ▲ = Collaborative;   EBN = Evidence-Based Nursing;   EB = Evidence-Based

- Refrain from using mood-altering substances
- Obtain no access to harmful objects
- Yield access to harmful objects
- Maintain self-control without supervision

NIC   Interventions (Nursing Interventions Classification)

Suggested NIC Interventions

Anxiety Reduction, Coping Enhancement, Crisis Intervention, Delusion Management, Mood Management, Substance Use Prevention, Suicide Prevention, Support System Enhancement, Surveillance

Example NIC Activities—Suicide Prevention
Determine presence and degree of suicidal risk; Encourage patient to seek out care providers to talk as urge to harm self occurs

Nursing Interventions and *Rationales*

NOTE: Before implementation of interventions in the face of suicidal behavior, nurses should examine their own emotional responses to incidents of suicide to ensure that interventions will not be based on countertransference reactions. **EBN:** *Medical nurses reported that they could not understand why people harm themselves, and they felt they did not have the skills to deal with suicidal clients (Valente & Saunders, 2004).*

- Assess for suicidal ideation when the history reveals the following: depression, substance abuse, and other psychiatric disorders; bipolar disorder, schizophrenia, panic disorder, dissociative disorder, eating disorder, antisocial personality disorder; attempted suicide, current or past; recent stressful life events (divorce and/or separation, relocation, problems with children); recent unemployment; recent bereavement; chronic pain or physical illness; childhood physical or sexual abuse; gay, lesbian, or bisexual gender orientation; family history of suicide. *Clinicians should be alert for suicide when the aforementioned factors are present in asymptomatic persons (American Psychiatric Association, 2005).* **EB:** *32% of successful suicides had contact with mental health services in the preceding year, 75% had contact with primary care providers. Primary care providers could be effective in preventing suicide, particularly among older adults and women (Luoma, Martin & Pearson, 2002).* **EB:** *First episode psychosis is a particular risk factor for suicide; early intervention has been shown to be helpful (Gonzalez-Pinto et al, 2007; Power et al, 2003). (Additional relevant research: Franko et al, 2004; Lambert, 2003; Pies, 2004; Pompili et al, 2004).*
- Assess medical clients and clients with chronic illnesses for their perception of health status. **EB:** *Clients with chronic pain, medical problems, and depression expressed suicidal ideation (Cooper et al, 2005). Medical clients who perceived their health to be poor or who were in chronic pain were significantly more likely to report current suicidal ideation (Tang & Crane, 2006).*
- Use brief self-report measures to improve clinical management of at-risk cases. The client may complete screening instruments such as the Center for Epidemiological Studies Depression Scale (CES-D), which indicates degree of depressed mood, or the Beck Suicide Intent Scale, which identifies a strong intent to die. **EBN:** *The Nurses' Global Assessment of Suicide Risk (NGASR) has been developed, and preliminary support for its use, especially by novice clinicians, has been reported (Cutcliffe & Barker, 2004).* **EB:** *The Suicide Assessment Checklist (SAC) has demonstrated strengths as part of a thorough protocol in evaluating suicidal risk (Rogers, Lewis & Subich, 2002). There was a significant decrease in assessment errors of suicide risk when brief self-report measures were used (Brown et al, 2003).*
- ▲ Assess the client's ability to enter into a no-suicide contract. Contract (verbally or in writing) with the client for no self-harm; recontract at appropriate intervals. *Discussing feelings of self-harm with a trusted person provides relief for the client. A contract gets the subject out in the open and places some of the responsibility for safety with the client. If the client will not contract, the risk of suicide should be considered higher.* **EB:** *The lack of willingness to self-disclose has been shown to discriminate*

S

• = Independent;   ▲ = Collaborative;   EBN = Evidence-Based Nursing;   EB = Evidence-Based

the serious suicide attempter from the client with suicidal ideation or the mild attempter (Apter et al, 2001). **EBN:** *Note: Although contracting is a common practice in psychiatric care settings, research has suggested that self-harm is not prevented by contracts (Drew, 2001). Thorough, ongoing assessment of suicide risk is necessary, whether or not the client has entered into a no-self-harm contract. Contracts may not be appropriate in community settings (Farrow, 2003).*

- Be alert for warning signs of suicide: making statements such as, "I can't go on," "Nothing matters anymore," "I wish I were dead"; becoming depressed or withdrawn; behaving recklessly; getting affairs in order and giving away valued possessions; showing a marked change in behavior, attitudes, or appearance; abusing drugs or alcohol; suffering a major loss or life change. *Suicide is rarely a spontaneous decision. In the days and hours before people kill themselves, clues and warning signs usually appear (Befrienders International, 2003).*

- Take suicide notes seriously. Consider themes of notes in determining appropriate interventions. **EB:** *A theme of "apology/shame" was present in suicide notes, suggesting that alternative solutions to dilemmas may have been welcomed. Cognitive therapy techniques, particularly problem solving, would be useful (Foster, 2003).*

- Question family members regarding the preparatory actions mentioned. *Clinicians should be alert for suicide when these factors are present in asymptomatic persons (American Psychiatric Association, 2005).*

- Determine the presence and degree of suicidal risk. A number of questions will elicit the necessary information: Have you been thinking about hurting or killing yourself?, How often do you have these thoughts and how long do they last? Do you have a plan? What is it? Do you have access to the means to carry out that plan? How likely is it that you could carry out the plan? Are there people or things that could prevent you from hurting yourself? What do you see in your future a year from now? Five years from now? What do you expect would happen if you died? What has kept you alive up to now? *Using the acronym SAL, the nurse can evaluate the client's suicide plan for its Specificity (how detailed and clear is the plan?), Availability (does the client have immediate access to the planned means?), and Lethality (could the plan be fatal, or does the client believe it would be fatal?). Assessment of reasons for living is another important part of evaluating suicidal clients (Malone et al, 2000).*

- ▲ Observe, record, and report any changes in mood or behavior that may signify increasing suicide risk and document results of regular surveillance checks. *Suicidal ideation often is not continuous; it may decrease, then increase in response to negative thinking or exposure to stressors (e.g., family visits). Documentation of surveillance will alert all members of the healthcare team to changes in the client's potential risk for suicide so they may be prepared to respond in the event of suicidal behavior.*

- Develop a positive therapeutic relationship with the client; do not make promises that may not be kept. *Clients will speak of their suicidal ideation more readily if they feel a connection with the nurse. Be aware that some clients may offer to self-disclose if the nurse will promise not to tell anyone what they have said. Clarify with the client that anything they share will be communicated only to other staff but that secrets cannot be kept.*

- ▲ Refer for mental health counseling and possible hospitalization if evidence of suicidal intent exists, which may include evidence of preparatory actions (e.g., obtaining a weapon, making a plan, putting affairs in order, giving away prized possessions, preparing a suicide note).

- Assign a hospitalized client to a room located near the nursing station. *Close assignment increases ease of observation and availability for a rapid response in the event of a suicide attempt.*

- Search the newly hospitalized client and the client's personal belongings for weapons or potential weapons and hoarded medications during the inpatient admission procedure, as appropriate. Remove dangerous items. *Clients intent on suicide may bring the means with them. Action is necessary to maintain a hazard-free environment and client safety.*

- Place the client in the least restrictive environment that allows for the necessary level of observation. Assess suicidal risk at least daily. *Close observation of the client is necessary for safety as long as intent remains high. Suicide risk should be assessed at frequent intervals to adjust suicide precautions and limitations on the client's freedom of movement and to ensure that restrictions continue to be appropriate.*

- Increase surveillance of a hospitalized client at times when staffing is predictably low (e.g., staff meetings, change of shift report, periods of unit disruption). *Clients who remain intent on suicide will be watchful of periods when staff surveillance lessens to permit completion of a suicide plan.*

S

- Consider strategies to decrease isolation and opportunity to act on harmful thoughts (e.g., use of a sitter). **EBN:** *Clients have reported feeling safe and having their hope restored in response to close observation (Bowers & Park, 2001).*
- Explain suicide precautions and relevant safety issues to the client and family (e.g., purpose, duration, behavioral expectations, and behavioral consequences). **EBN:** *Suicide precautions may be viewed as restrictive. Clients have reported the loss of privacy as distressing (Bowers & Park, 2001).*
- ▲ Refer for treatment and participate in the management of any psychiatric illness or symptoms that may be contributing to the client's suicidal ideation or behavior. *Psychiatric disorders have been associated with suicidal behavior. Symptoms of the disorder may require treatment with antidepressant, antipsychotic, or antianxiety medications.*
- ▲ Verify that the client has taken medications as ordered (e.g., conduct mouth checks after medication administration). *The client may attempt to hoard medications for a later suicide attempt.*
- ▲ Maintain increased surveillance of the client whenever use of an antidepressant has been initiated or the dose increased. Antidepressant medications take anywhere from 2 to 6 weeks to achieve full efficacy. *During that period the client's energy level may increase, although the depression has not yet lifted, which increases the potential for suicide.*
- Limit access to windows and exits unless locked and shatterproof, as appropriate. *Suicidal behavior may include attempts to jump out of windows or to escape the unit to find other means of suicide (e.g., gaining roof access for a jump). Hospitals should ensure that exits are secure.*
- Monitor the client during the use of potential weapons (e.g., razor, scissors). *Clients with suicidal intent may take advantage of any opportunity to harm themselves.*
- Involve the client in treatment planning and self-care management of psychiatric disorders. *Self-care management promotes feelings of self-efficacy (Lorig et al, 2001), particularly for clients with depression (Ellis, 2004). Suicidal ideation may occur in response to a sense of hopelessness, a sense that the client has no control over life circumstances. The more clients participate in their own care, the less powerless and hopeless they feel. Refer to the care plan for* **Powerlessness.**
- Explore with the client all circumstances and motivations related to the suicidality. Listen to the client's own views on his or her problems. **EB:** *Primary reasons for suicide attempts were found to be feelings of loneliness and mental illness/psychological problems. Men more often cited socioeconomic problems, whereas women more often reported psychological problems and interpersonal relationship difficulties. A high number of suicide attempters were never married/single, with poor social networks and depressive symptoms. Hopelessness was associated with a wish to die and escape motives (Skogman & Ojehagen, 2003a, 2003b).*
- Explore with the client all perceived consequences that could act as a barrier to suicide (e.g., effect on family, religious beliefs). **EBN:** *The most common barrier to suicide is consequences to family members (Bell, 2000).*
- Avoid repeated discussion of the client's suicide history by keeping discussion oriented to the present and future. *Clients under stress have difficulty focusing their thoughts, which leads to a sense of being overwhelmed by problems. Focusing on the present and future helps the client to address problem solving with regard to current stressors, while avoiding secondary gain from idealizing past behavior.*
- ▲ Discuss plans for dealing with suicidal ideation in the future (e.g., how to identify precipitating factors, whom to contact, where to go for help, how to respond to desire for self-harm). *Clients are supported in self-care management when they are helped to identify actions they can take if suicidal ideation recurs.*
- ▲ Assist the client in identifying a network of supportive persons and resources (e.g., clergy, family, care providers). *Clients who are suicidal often feel alienated from others and benefit from actions that facilitate support of the client by family and friends.*
- ▲ Refer family members and friends to local mental health agencies and crisis intervention centers if the client has suicidal ideation or a suspicion of suicidal thoughts exists. *Clients at risk should receive evaluation and help (American Psychiatric Association, 2005).*
- ▲ Consider outpatient commitment or an overnight psychiatric observation program for an actively suicidal client. *Involuntary outpatient commitment can improve treatment, reduce the likelihood of hospital readmission, and reduce episodes of violent behavior in persons with severe psychiatric illnesses (Torrey & Zdanowicz, 2001). Overnight psychiatric observation followed by outpatient referral also can be an effective alternative to traditional hospitalization without leading to an increase in suicide gestures or attempts (Francis et al, 2000).*

S

• = Independent;   ▲ = Collaborative;   EBN = Evidence-Based Nursing;   EB = Evidence-Based

- Cognitive behavioral techniques help the client to modify thinking styles that promote depression, hopelessness, and a belief that suicide is a valid means of escaping the current situation. *Suicide has been shown to be associated with constriction in cognitive style, leading to decreased problem solving and information processing (Sheehy & O'Connor, 2002).* **EBN:** *Cognitive behavioral techniques and the promotion of problem-solving skills, combined with the therapeutic relationship, have been posited as key interventions when dealing with the hopelessness inherent to suicidal ideation (Collins & Cutcliffe, 2003).*
- Group interventions can be useful to address recurrent suicide attempts. **EB:** *Group therapy was shown to decrease suicidality (Burns et al, 2005).*
- ▲ If imminent suicide is suspected or an attempt has occurred, call for assistance and do not leave the client alone. *Client and staff safety will be served by assistance in the response. The client may attempt additional self-harm if left alone.*
- ▲ With the client's consent, facilitate family-oriented crisis intervention. *Family-oriented crisis intervention can clarify stresses and allow assessment of family dynamics.* **EB:** *Families of suicidal clients were considered more dysfunctional than families of clients with no history of attempted suicide (McDermut et al, 2001).*
- ▲ Involve the family in discharge planning (e.g., illness/medication teaching, recognition of increasing suicidal risk, client's plan for dealing with recurring suicidal thoughts, community resources). *Suicidal clients often are ambivalent about hurting themselves; they may not want to die so much as to escape an intolerable situation. Consequently they often leave clues about their state of mind. Family members can learn to respond to clues early, support the treatment regimen, and encourage the client to initiate the emergency plan.*
- ▲ Before discharge from the hospital, ensure that the client has a supply of ordered medications, has a plan for outpatient follow-up, understands the plan or has a caregiver able and willing to follow the plan, and has the ability to access outpatient treatment. *Clients may be discharged before they have recovered substantial functional ability and may have difficulty concentrating on the plan for follow-up. They may need the assistance of others to ensure that prescriptions are filled, that they attend appointments, or that they have transportation to the outpatient care setting.* **EB:** *Nonresponse to treatment of depression has been associated with the clinical factor of suicidal ideation, socioeconomic factors (unemployment) not usually addressed by medical intervention, and medication nonadherence (Sherbourne et al, 2004).*
- ▲ In the event of successful suicide, refer the family to a therapy group for survivors of suicide. Recommended clinical interventions include addressing psychological distress, normalizing denial as an effective coping strategy, working with concerns about family disintegration, and helping families deal with stigmatization (Kaslow & Aronson, 2004). **EBN:** *Survivors of suicide may be reluctant to contact healthcare professionals, out of fear that they will be blamed or stigmatized. Group counseling addresses the blame, anger, guilt, shame, and search for a reason for the suicide that occurs in suicide survivors (Barlow & Morrison, 2002). Psychoeducational support group participants found relief in sharing a personal narrative of their suicide bereavement with others (Mitchell et al, 2003).*
- See the care plans for **Risk for self-directed Violence, Hopelessness,** and **Risk for Self-mutilation.** *Clients with suicidal ideation often are reacting to a feeling of hopelessness.*

 Pediatric

- The above interventions may be appropriate for pediatric clients.
- Use brief self-report measures to improve clinical management of at-risk cases. *The Risk of Suicide Questionnaire (RSQ) is available for children and adolescents (Horowitz et al, 2001).*
- Assess for both medical and psychiatric disturbances that may contribute to suicidality. *The process leading to suicide in young people often involves untreated depression (Houston, Hawton & Shepperd, 2001). Epilepsy has a fourfold risk increase of suicide, particularly documented in children and adolescents (Muzina, 2004).*
- Recognize that the developmental issues of childhood and adolescence may heighten suicide risks and involve different issues from those with adults. *Assessment of suicidality in children is difficult. Lethality of an action may be misperceived; motivation varies greatly among children. Reuniting with a lost loved one may be more dangerous than gaining attention or other motivations more common at an older age (Fritz, 2004). Physically aggressive behavior learned in early childhood may translate*

into suicide risk (Tremblay, 2004). The rates of attempted suicide are particularly higher during adolescence. Puberty, social, and cognitive changes can lead to greater unhappiness. Rage, hopelessness, despair, and guilt are common with suicide attempts, with greater variability of suicide timing, impulsivity, and mood (Spirito & Overholser, 2003).

- Assess specific stressors for the adolescent client. *Adolescents tend to experience concerns about personal issues, school pressures, and relationships. Poor familial communications and lack of a parental confidant may be present. Key interventions include improving family communications, addressing psychosocial issues, teaching problem-solving skills, and fostering decreased impulsivity (Webb, 2002).*

- Assess for exposure to suicide of a significant other. **EB:** *Among risk factors of previous psychiatric history, poor psychosocial function, dysphoric mood and psychomotor restlessness, suicide of a significant other was shown to create risk for adolescents diagnosed with Adjustment Disorder (Pelkonen et al, 2005).*

- Evaluate for the presence of self-mutilation and related risk factors. Refer to care plan for **Risk for Self-mutilation** for additional information. **EBN:** *Self-mutilation is common and suicide is possible for boys who have been sexually abused (Valente, 2005).*

- Be aware that complete overlap does not exist between suicidal behavior and self-mutilation. The motivation may be different (ending life rather than coping with difficult feelings), and the method is usually different. **EB:** *In one study, about half of the participants reported both attempted suicide and self-mutilation; in the other half there was no overlap in types of acts (Bolognini et al, 2003).*

- Assess for the presence of an eating disorder. *Suicidal behavior was shown to be more common among adolescents with dependence issues (drug abuse and eating disorders) (Bolognini et al, 2003). The thought processes of adolescents with an eating disorder were found to center on themes of feeling undeserving of receiving help, feeling helpless and hopeless in dealing with the eating disorder itself, difficulty with recognizing and expressing feelings, and ambivalence regarding treatment along with mistrust of healthcare providers (Manley & Leichner, 2003).*

- Involve the adolescent in multimodal treatment programs. **EB:** *Thorough assessment and multiple modes of treatment, including family sessions, were found to improve psychosocial functioning and self-image in a program for adolescent inpatients (Hintikka et al, 2006).*

- Before discharge from the hospital, ensure that the client's parent has a supply of ordered medications, has a plan for outpatient follow-up, has a caregiver who understands the plan or is able and willing to follow the plan, and has the ability to access outpatient treatment. *Lack of adequate follow-up has been associated with repeated suicide attempts among adolescents (Hulten et al, 2001).* **EB:** *A compliance enhancement intervention (including contracting interviews with parent and adolescent, and telephone contacts) improved attendance at follow-up appointments only when barriers to service were controlled (e.g., delays in getting appointments, placement on a waiting list, inability to switch therapists, problems with insurance coverage) (Spirito et al, 2002).*

- Parental education groups can influence suicide risk factors. **EB:** *A program of parent education groups focused on improved communication skills and relationships with adolescents. Students in the intervention group reported increased maternal care, decreased conflict with parents, decreased substance abuse, and decreased delinquency (Toumbourou & Gregg, 2002).*

- Support the implementation of school-based suicide prevention programs. *School nurses can be key to early intervention.* **EBN:** *An intervention study by school nurses on providing coping skills training and emotional support yielded a 55% decrease in suicidal ideation (Houck, Darnell & Lussman, 2002).* **EB:** *A test of the effectiveness of the Signs of Suicide (SOS) prevention program found that suicide attempts decreased, knowledge-based awareness increased, and adaptive attitudes toward depression and suicide were observed (Aseltine & DeMartino, 2004).*

- Encourage family meals. **EB:** *Frequency of family meals was inversely associated with tobacco, alcohol, and marijuana use; low grade point average; depressive symptoms; and suicide involvement (Eisenberg et al, 2004).*

Geriatric

- Evaluate the older client's mental and physical health status and financial stressors. *The possibility of reversible/medical causes of depression, including medical or neurological disorders, as well as psychomimetic reactions to medications, should inform nursing observations (Hall, Hall & Chapman, 2003).*

- Explore with client any concerns or pressures (physical and financial) regarding ability to secure support of medical care, especially perceived pressures about being a burden on family. **EB:** *The suicide notes of older adults were more likely than those of younger adults to contain the theme "burden to others" (Foster, 2003).*
- When assessing suicide risk factors, incorporate a higher degree of risk for older men and for some older adults who have lost a loved one in the previous year. **EB:** *Although mortality for oldest old adults (80+) has increased, the suicide mortality has not decreased. In one study, oldest old men had the highest increase in suicide risk after death of a partner (more so than oldest old women) and took a longer time to recover from the death of a spouse (Erlangsen et al, 2004). Suicide rate may be rising among men over age 65, and marriage may no longer be the protective factor it was once considered to be (Lamprecht et al, 2005).*
- Explore triggers of and barriers to suicidal behavior, with particular attention to real and perceived losses (e.g., professional role, health). **EB:** *For adults 75 years of age or older, predictors of suicide included family conflict, serious physical illness, and both major and minor depressions. For adults 65 to 74 years of age, but not for the older group, economic problems were predictive of suicide (Waern, Rubenowitz & Wilhelmson, 2003).* **EBN:** *A study of older Caucasian men revealed that losing connections initiated a process of loss and depression and triggered a decision point that could include suicidal ideation. Triggers included death of a spouse, emotional pain, health problems, and feelings of uselessness or hopelessness. A strong barrier was consequences to family members. Religion and social isolation were not relevant (Bell, 2000).*
- An older adult who shows self-destructive behaviors should be evaluated for dementia. **EB:** *In a study of nursing home residents, self-destructive behaviors were common; these behaviors were more likely related to dementia than to depression and were only weakly associated with suicidal intent (Draper et al, 2002).*
- Anticipate overall responsiveness to treatment, but monitor for early relapse. **EB:** *Older adults had high remission rates after antidepressant treatment, whether they had suicidal ideation or not. However, older adults with suicidal ideation had a higher relapse rate and a greater need for adjunctive psychotropic medications (Szanto et al, 2001).*
- ▲ Advocate for the older client with other professionals in securing treatment for suicidal states. Primary care physicians have been noted to underrecognize and undertreat older adult clients with depression. **EB:** *Older adults above age 75 with major or minor depression were less likely than those ages 65 to 74 to receive depression treatment (Waern et al, 2003).*
- Encourage physical activity in older adults. *Benefits to mood have been found with exercise. Activity therapy based on an ancient Chinese system of exercise (Qigong) has been proposed as a means of preventing disease, increasing strength, and resisting premature senility, as well as improving mood among depressed elders with chronic physical illnesses (Tsang, Cheung & Lak, 2002).* **EB:** *A study testing response to exercise, sertraline, or exercise plus sertraline found that the exercise-only group experienced the lowest depression levels, with the benefit of exercise continuing after the intervention period (Babyak et al, 2000).*
- Assist the older adult to identify protective factors that serve as resources to mitigate against suicidal ideation. *Internal and external factors that can serve as resources for the older adult include the ability to learn from experience and accept help, a sense of humor and interest in social concerns, a sense of purpose or meaning in life, a history of successful coping, caring and available family and a supportive community network, and membership in a religious community (Holkup, Tang & Titler, 2003).*
- Collaborative care management of older adults in primary care settings is a growing area for nursing intervention. **EB:** *A wide-scale study of individualized care provided by "depression care managers" (social workers, nurses, psychologists) in collaboration with physicians yielded a faster decline of suicidal ideation in the intervention group, along with a greater degree and speed of depression symptom reduction (Bruce et al, 2004).*
- Telephone contacts can serve as an effective intervention for suicidal older adults. **EBN:** *Nurse telehealth care, involving an average of 10 calls over 16 weeks to answer questions, offer support, and discuss overall health, reduced depressive symptoms more than did usual physician care (Hunkeler et al, 2000).* **EB:** *A protocol of twice-weekly support calls resulted in significantly fewer suicide deaths among women but not among men. The researchers concluded that outreach, continuity of care, and increased emotional support provided protection against suicide, at least for women (DeLeo, Della Buono & Dwyer, 2002).*

S

• = Independent;   ▲ = Collaborative;   EBN = Evidence-Based Nursing;   EB = Evidence-Based

Multicultural

- Assess for the influence of cultural beliefs, norms, and values on the individual's perceptions of suicide. **EBN:** *What the individual believes about suicide may be based on cultural perceptions (Leininger & McFarland, 2002). Among Hispanics, the largest proportion of suicides occurred among young persons; suicide rates were higher among males; and the most common method of suicide was by firearms (Centers for Disease Control and Prevention, 2004).*
- Identify and acknowledge the stresses unique to culturally diverse individuals. *Financial difficulties and maintaining cultural values are two of the most common family stressors cited by women of color (Majumdar & Ladak, 1998). Suicide rates among African-American male teenagers increased 105% from 1980 to 1986 (Surgeon General, 1999), with "suicide by cop" speculated to have increased these rates (Daugherty, 1999). A high rate of suicidal ideation has been reported as a result of the social discrimination experienced by gay and bisexual Latino men in the United States (Diaz et al, 2001). There may be a relationship between the possible relationship between rapid social change and the increasing rates of suicide among Alaska Natives (Richards, 2004).*
- Identify and acknowledge unique cultural responses to stressors in determining sensitive interventions to prevent suicide. **EBN:** *In a study of African-American, Hispanic/Latina, and Caucasian adolescent girls, the Hispanic/Latina girls had a significantly higher percentage of suicide attempts. Relationships were found between recent suicide attempts and family history of suicide attempts, friend's history of suicide attempt, history of physical or sexual abuse, and environmental stress. For all three groups, rate of recent suicide attempts was also associated with stress level, social connectedness, and religious influence (Rew et al, 2001). A recent study found African-American men committed suicide at rates much lower than those for Caucasians, but they do so at much younger ages (Garlow, Purselle & Heninger, 2005).*
- Encourage physical activity as intervention to decrease suicidal behavior. **EB:** *Increased physical activity was associated with lower suicidal feelings and suicidal behaviors in Hispanic and non-Hispanic boys (Brosnahan et al, 2004).*
- Encourage family members to demonstrate and offer caring and support to each other. **EB:** *The familial characteristics of care and support may be associated with fostering resilience in African-American families (Calvert, 1997). Family closeness is strong resiliency factor of suicidal behavior in African-American and Hispanic youths (O'Donnell et al, 2004).*
- Foster the client's use of available family and religious supports. **EB:** *Christian religious roots and family closeness, although eroding among many young African Americans, traditionally have worked against suicidal behavior among African Americans (Neeleman, Wessely & Lewis, 1998).*
- Validate the individual's feelings regarding concerns about the current crisis and family functioning. *Validation lets the client know that the nurse has heard and understood what was said, and it promotes the nurse-client relationship (Giger & Davidhizar, 2004).*

Home Care

- Communicate the degree of risk to family and caregivers; assess the family and caregiving situation for ability to protect the client and to understand the client's suicidal behavior. Provide the family and caregivers with guidelines on how to manage self-harm behaviors in the home environment. *Client safety between home visits is a nursing priority. Family and caregivers may become frightened by the client's suicidal ideation, may be angry at the client's perceived lack of self-control, or may feel as if they are walking on eggshells awaiting another suicide attempt.*
- ▲ If the client's suicidal ideation intensifies, or if a suicide plan with access to means becomes evident, institute an emergency plan for mental health intervention. *The degree of disturbance and the ability to manage care safely at home determines the level of services needed to protect the client. Approximately 25% of clients who are hospitalized after a suicide attempt kill themselves within 3 months after hospitalization (Appleby et al, 1999).*
- Counsel parents and homeowners to restrict unauthorized access to potentially lethal prescription drugs and firearms within the home. *Identifying teens at high risk of firearm suicide and limiting access to firearms are public health interventions likely to be successful in preventing firearm suicides (Shah et al, 2000).*
- Identify the client's concerns and implement interventions to address the consequences of dis-

---

• = Independent;   ▲ = Collaborative;   EBN = Evidence-Based Nursing;   EB = Evidence-Based

ability in a client with medical illness. **EB:** *In a study of cancer clients being cared for at home, primary factors influencing vulnerability to suicide were identified as real or feared loss of autonomy and independence, concerns about being a burden on others, hopelessness about the health condition, and fear of suffering (Filiberti et al, 2001). Hopelessness and demoralization in conjunction with dependence have been noted as precursors to suicidal ideation in palliative care clients (Kissane, Clarke & Street, 2001). Refer to the care plans for* **Hopelessness** *and* **Powerlessness.**

▲ Refer for homemaker or psychiatric home healthcare services for respite, client reassurance, and implementation of a therapeutic regimen. *Respite decreases the high degree of caregiver stress that goes with the responsibility of caring for a person at risk for suicide.* **EB:** *In a study of community-integrated home-based treatment for depression, depressive symptoms were significantly reduced in elderly participants, and improved health status was noted in chronically medically ill older adults with minor depression and dysthymia (Ciechanowski et al, 2004).*

▲ If the client is on psychotropic medications, assess the client's and family's knowledge of medication administration and side effects. Teach as necessary. *Knowledge of the medical regimen promotes compliance and promotes safe use of medications.*

▲ Evaluate the effectiveness and side effects of medications and adherence to the medication regimen. Review with the client and family all medications kept in the home; encourage discarding of old prescriptions. Monitor the amount of medications ordered/provided by the physician; limiting the amount of medications to which the client has access may be necessary. *Accurate clinical feedback improves the physician's ability to prescribe an effective medical regimen specific to the client's needs. At home, clients may have greater access to medications, including old prescriptions that may be used to overdose.*

Client/Family Teaching

• Establish a supportive relationship with family members. **EBN:** *When families with a suicidal member experienced mental healthcare personnel as reaching out to them, they reported an ability to trust the personnel, treatment, and care; a feeling of being trusted; and a sense of hope (Talseth, Gilje & Norberg, 2001).*

• Explain all relevant symptoms, procedures, treatments, and expected outcomes for suicidal ideation that is illness based (e.g., depression, bipolar disorder). *By increasing knowledge and adapting new behaviors, clients learn that they have some control over their health (Hennessy-Harstad, 1999).*

• Teach the family how to recognize that the client is at increased risk for suicide (changes in behavior and verbal and nonverbal communication, withdrawal, depression, or sudden lifting of depression). *A client may be at peace because a suicide plan has been made and the client has the energy to carry it out. Therefore when depression lifts, increased vigilance is necessary.*

• Provide written instructions for treatments and procedures for which the client will be responsible. *A written record provides a concrete reference so that the client and family can clarify any verbal information that was given.*

• Instruct the client in coping strategies (assertiveness training, impulse control training, deep breathing, progressive muscle relaxation). *Suicidal ideation may be triggered by stress and painful emotions. Once clients are able to identify these triggers, they need to learn how to respond to them more effectively through assertiveness, impulse control, or relaxation techniques, as appropriate.*

• Role play (e.g., say, "Tell me how you will respond if a friend asks why you were in the hospital"). *Role playing is the most commonly used technique in assertiveness training. It deconditions the anxiety that arises from interpersonal encounters by allowing the client to practice how he or she might respond in a given situation. Anxiety levels tend to be higher in situations that are unfamiliar.*

• Teach cognitive behavioral activities, such as active problem solving, reframing (reappraising the situation from a different perspective), or thought stopping (in response to a negative thought, picturing a large stop sign and replacing the image with a prearranged positive alternative). Teach the client to confront his or her own negative thought patterns (or cognitive distortions), such as catastrophizing (expecting the very worst), dichotomous thinking (perceiving events in only one of two opposite categories), or magnification (placing distorted emphasis on a single event). *Cognitive behavioral activities address clients' assumptions, beliefs, and attitudes about their situations and foster modification of these elements to be as realistic and optimistic as possible. Through*

• = Independent;   ▲ = Collaborative;   EBN = Evidence-Based Nursing;   EB = Evidence-Based

cognitive behavioral interventions, clients become more aware of their cognitive choices in adopting and maintaining their belief systems and thereby exercise greater control over their own reactions (Hagerty & Patusky, 2007).

- Provide the client and family with phone numbers of appropriate community agencies for therapy and counseling. *Continuous follow-up care should be implemented; therefore the method to access this care must be given to the client.*

evolve   See the EVOLVE website for World Wide Web resources for client education.

REFERENCES

American Psychiatric Association-Medical Specialty Society: *Practice guideline for the assessment and treatment of patients with suicidal behaviors.* Available www.ngc.gov/summary/summary.aspx?doc_id=45 29&nbr=3343&string=suicide, accessed January 10, 2005.

Appleby L, Shaw J, Amos T et al: Suicide within 12 months of contact with mental health services: national clinical survey, *BMJ* 318(7193):1235, 1999.

Apter A, Horesh N, Gothelf D et al: Relationship between self-disclosure and serious suicidal behavior, *Compr Psychiatry* 42(1):70, 2001.

Aseltine RH Jr, DeMartino R: An outcome evaluation of the SS suicide prevention program, *Am J Public Health* 94:446, 2004.

Babyak M, Blumenthal JA, Herman S et al: Exercise treatment for major depression: maintenance of therapeutic benefit at 10 months, *Psychosom Med* 62:633, 2000.

Barlow CA, Morrison H: Survivors of suicide. Emerging counseling strategies, *J Psychosoc Nurs Ment Health Serv* 40(1):28, 2002.

Befrienders International: *The warning signs of suicide,* available at http://befrienders.org/support/index.asp?PageURL=warningSigns. php. Accessed April 24, 2007.

Bell MA: *Losing connections: a process of decision-making in late-life suicidality,* doctoral dissertation, Tucson, Ariz, 2000, University of Arizona.

Bolognini M, Plancherel B, Laget J et al: Adolescents' self-mutilation: relationship with dependent behaviour, *Swiss J Psychol* 62(4):241, 2003.

Bowers L, Park A: Special observation in the care of psychiatric inpatients: a literature review, *Issues Ment Health Nurs* 22:769, 2001.

Brosnahan J, Steffen LM, Lytle L et al: The relation between physical activity and mental health among Hispanic and non-Hispanic white adolescents, *Arch Pediatr Adolesc Med* 158(8):818-823, 2004.

Brown GS, Jones ER, Betts E et al: Improving suicide risk assessment in a managed-care environment, *Crisis* 24(2):49, 2003.

Bruce ML, Ten Have TR, Reynolds CF III et al: Reducing suicidal ideation and depressive symptoms in depressed older primary care patients: a randomized controlled trial, *JAMA* 291:1081, 2004.

Burns J, Dudley M, Hazell P et al: Clinical management of deliberate self-harm in young people: the need for evidence-based approaches to reduce repetition, *Aus NZ J Psychiatry* 39:121, 2005.

Calvert WJ: Protective factors within the family, and their role in fostering resiliency in African American adolescents, *J Cult Divers* 4(4):110, 1997.

Centers for Disease Control and Prevention (CDC): Suicide among Hispanics—United States, 1997-2001, *MMWR Morb Mort Wkly Rep* 53(22):478-481, 2004.

Ciechanowski P, Wagner E, Schmaling K et al: Community-integrated home-based depression treatment in older adults: a randomized controlled trial, *JAMA* 291(13):1569, 2004.

Collins S, Cutcliffe JR: Addressing hopelessness in people with suicidal ideation: building upon the therapeutic relationship utilizing a cognitive behavioural approach, *J Psychiatr Ment Health Nurs* 10:175, 2003.

Cooper J, Kapur N, Webb R et al: Suicide after deliberate self-harm: a 4-year cohort study, *Am J Psychiatry* 162:297, 2005.

Cutcliffe JR, Barker P: The Nurses' Global Assessment of Suicide Risk (NGASR): developing a tool for clinical practice, *J Psychiatr Ment Health Nurs* 11(4):393, 2004.

Daugherty M: Suicide by cop, *J Calif Alliance Ment Ill* 10(2):79, 1999.

De Leo D, Della Buono M, Dwyer J: Suicide among the elderly: the long-term impact of a telephone support and assessment intervention in northern Italy, *Br J Psychiatr* 181:226, 2002.

Diaz RM, Ayala G, Bein E et al: The impact of homophobia, poverty, and racism on the mental health of gay and bisexual Latino men: findings from 3 US cities, *Am J Public Health* 91:927, 2001.

Draper B, Brodaty H, Low LF et al: Self-destructive behaviors in nursing home residents, *J Am Geriatr Soc* 50:354, 2002.

Drew BL: Self-harm behavior and no-suicide contracting in psychiatric inpatient settings, *Arch Psychiatr Nurs* 15:99, 2001.

Eisenberg ME, Olson RE, Neumark-Sztainer D et al: Correlations between family meals and psychosocial well-being among adolescents, *Arch Pediatr Adolesc Med* 158(8):792-796, 2004.

Ellis TE: Collaboration and a self-help orientation in therapy with suicidal clients, *J Contemp Psychother* 34(1):41, 2004.

Erlangsen A, Jeune B, Bille-Brahe U et al: Loss of partner and suicide risks among oldest old: a population-based register study, *Age Ageing* 33(4):378-383, 2004.

Farrow TL: "No suicide contracts" in community crisis situations: a conceptual analysis, *J Psychiatr Ment Health Nurs* 10:199, 2003.

Filiberti A, Ripamonti C, Totis A et al: Characteristics of terminal cancer patients who committed suicide during a home palliative care program, *J Pain Symptom Manage* 22:544, 2001.

Foster T: Suicide note themes and suicide prevention, *Int J Psychiatry Med* 33(4):323, 2003.

Francis E, Marchand W, Hart M et al: Utilization and outcome in an overnight psychiatric observation program at a Veterans Affairs medical center, *Psychiatr Serv* 51:92, 2000.

Franko DL, Keel PK, Dorer DJ et al: What predicts suicide attempts in women with eating disorders? *Psychol Med* 34:843, 2004.

Fritz GK: Suicide in young children (editorial), *Brown Univ Child Adolesc Behav Lett* 20(7):8, 2004.

Garlow SJ, Purselle D, Heninger M: Ethnic differences in patterns of suicide across the life cycle, *Am J Psychiatry* 162(2):319-323, 2005.

Giger, J, Davidhizar, R: *Transcultural nursing: assessment and intervention,* St Louis, 2004, Mosby.

Gonzalez-Pinto A, Aldama A, Gonzalez C et al: Predictors of suicide in first-episode affective and nonaffective psychotic inpatients: five-year follow-up of patients from a catchment area in Vitoria, Spain, *J Clin Psychiatry* 68:242, 2007.

Hagerty B, Patusky K: Mood disorders: depression and mania. In Fortinash KM, Holoday-Worret PA, editors: *Psychiatric mental health nursing,* ed 4, St Louis, 2007, Mosby.

Hall RCW, Hall RCW, Chapman MJ: Identifying geriatric patients at risk for suicide and depression, *Clin Geriatr* 11(10):36, 2003.

S

• = Independent;   ▲ = Collaborative;   EBN = Evidence-Based Nursing;   EB = Evidence-Based

Hennessy-Harstad EB: Empowering adolescents with asthma to take control through adaptation, *J Pediatr Health Care* 13:273, 1999.

Hintikka U, Marttunen M, Pelkonen M et al: Improvement in cognitive and psychosocial functioning and self-image among adolescent inpatient suicide attempters, *BMC Psychiatry* 6:58, 2006.

Holkup PA, Tang JH, Titler MG: Evidence-based protocol elderly suicide—secondary prevention, *J Gerontol Nurs* 29(6):6, 2003.

Horowitz LM, Wang PS, Koocher GP et al: Detecting suicide risk in a pediatric emergency department: development of a brief screening tool, *Pediatrics* 107:1133, 2001.

Houck GM, Darnell S, Lussman S: A support group intervention for at-risk female high school students, *J School Nurs* 18(4):212, 2002.

Houston K, Hawton K, Shepperd R: Suicide in young people aged 15-24: a psychological autopsy study, *J Affect Disord* 63(1-3):159, 2001.

Hulten A, Jiang GX, Wasserman D et al: Repetition of attempted suicide among teenagers in Europe: frequency, timing and risk factors, *Eur Child Adolesc Psychiatry* 10:161, 2001.

Hunkeler EM, Meresman JF, Hargreaves WA et al: Efficacy of nurse telehealth care and peer support in augmenting treatment of depression in primary care, *Arch Fam Med* 9:700, 2000.

Kaslow NJ, Aronson SG: Recommendations for family interventions following a suicide, *Prof Psychol Res Pract* 35(3):240, 2004.

Kissane DW, Clarke DM, Street AF: Demoralization syndrome-relevant psychiatric diagnosis for palliative care, *J Palliat Care* 17(1):12, 2001.

Lambert MT: Suicide risk assessment and management: focus on personality disorders, *Curr Opin Psychiatry* 16:71, 2003.

Lamprecht HC, Pakrasi S, Gash A et al: Deliberate self-harm in older people revisited, *Int J Geriatr Psychiatry* 20:1090, 2005.

Leininger MM, McFarland MR: *Transcultural nursing: concepts, theories, research and practices,* ed 3, New York, 2002, McGraw-Hill.

Lorig KR, Ritter P, Stewart AL et al: Chronic disease self-management program: 2-year health status and health care utilization outcomes, *Med Care* 39:1217, 2001.

Luoma JB, Martin CE, Pearson JL: Contact with mental health and primary care providers before suicide: a review of the evidence, *Am J Psychiatry* 159:909, 2002.

Majumdar B, Ladak S: Management of family and workplace stress experienced by women of color from various cultural backgrounds, *Can J Public Health* 89(1):48, 1998.

Malone KM, Oquendo MA, Haas GL et al: Protective factors against suicidal acts in major depression: reasons for living, *Am J Psychiatry* 157:1084, 2000.

Manley RS, Leichner P: Anguish and despair in adolescents with eating disorders: helping to manage suicidal ideation and impulses, *Crisis* 24(1):32, 2003.

McDermut W, Miller IW, Solomon D et al: Family functioning and suicidality in depressed adults, *Compr Psychiatry* 42:96, 2001.

Mitchell AM, Gale DD, Garand L et al: The use of narrative data to inform the psychotherapeutic group process with suicide survivors, *Issues Ment Health Nurs* 24:91, 2003.

Muzina DJ: What physicians can do to prevent suicide, *Cleveland Clinic J Med* 71(3):242, 2004.

Neeleman J, Wessely S, Lewis G: Suicide acceptability in African and white Americans: the role of religion, *J Nerv Ment Dis* 186:12, 1998.

O'Donnell L, O'Donnell C, Wardlaw DM et al: Risk and resiliency factors influencing suicidality among urban African American and Latino youth, *Am J Community Psychol* 33(1-2):37-49, 2004.

Pelkonen M, Marttunen M, Henriksson M et al: Suicidality in adjustment disorder: clinical characteristics of adolescent outpatients, *Eur Child Adolesc Psychiatry* 14:174, 2005.

Pies R: Bipolar disorder and suicide: an update, *Psychiatric Times Supplement, Bipolar Disorder and Impulsive Spectrum Letter* 21(2):1-4, 2004.

Pompili M, Mancinelli I, Girardi P et al: Suicide in anorexia nervosa: a meta-analysis, *Int J Eat Disord* 36:99, 2004.

Power PJR, Bell RJ, Mills R et al: Suicide prevention in first episode psychosis: the development of a randomized controlled trial of cognitive therapy for acutely suicidal patients with early psychosis, *Austr N Z J Psychiatry* 37:414, 2003.

Rew L, Thomas N, Horner SD et al: Correlates of recent suicide attempts in a triethnic group of adolescents, *J Nurs Scholarsh* 33:361, 2001.

Richards B: From respect to rights to entitlement, blocked aspirations and suicidal behavior, *Int J Circumpolar Health* (Suppl 1):19-24, 2004.

Rogers JR, Lewis MM, Subich LM: Validity of the Suicide Assessment Checklist in an emergency crisis center, *J Counsel Develop* 80:493, 2002.

Shah S, Hoffman RE, Wake L et al: Adolescent suicide and household access to firearms in Colorado: results of a case-control study, *J Adolesc Health* 26(3):157, 2000.

Sheehy N, O'Connor RC: Cognitive style and suicidal behaviour: implications for therapeutic intervention, research lacunae and priorities, *Br J Guidance Counsel* 30(4):353, 2002.

Sherbourne C, Schoenbaum M, Wells KB et al: Characteristics, treatment patterns, and outcomes of persistent depression despite treatment in primary care, *Gen Hosp Psychiatry* 26:106, 2004.

Skogman K, Ojehagen A: Motives for suicide attempts—the views of the patient, *Arch Suicide Res* 7:193, 2003a.

Skogman K, Ojehagen A: Problems of importance for suicide attempts—the patients' views, *Arch Suicide Res* 7:207, 2003b.

Spirito A, Boergers J, Donaldson D et al: An intervention trial to improve adherence to community treatment by adolescents after a suicide attempt, *J Am Acad Child Adolesc Psychiatry* 41(4):435, 2002.

Spirito A, Overholser J: The suicidal child: assessment and management of adolescents after a suicide attempt, *Child Adolesc Psychiatric Clin North Am* 12:649, 2003.

Surgeon General: *The Surgeon General's call to action to prevent suicide, 1999,* available at http://www.surgeongeneral.gov/library/calltoaction/default.htm. Accessed April 24, 2007.

Szanto K, Mulsant BH, Houck PR et al: Treatment outcome in suicidal vs. non-suicidal elderly patients, *Am J Geriatr Psychiatry* 9(3):261, 2001.

Talseth A, Gilje F, Norberg A: Being met—a passageway to hope for relatives of patients at risk of committing suicide: a phenomenological hermeneutic study, *Arch Psychiatr Nurs* 15:249, 2001.

Tang NK, Crane C: Suicidality in chronic pain: a review of the prevalence, risk factors, and psychological links, *Psychol Med* 36:575, 2006.

Torrey EF, Zdanowicz M: Outpatient commitment: what, why, and for whom, *Psychiatr Serv* 52(3):337, 2001.

Toumbourou JW, Gregg ME: Impact of an empowerment-based parent education program on the reduction of youth suicide risk factors, *J Adolesc Health* 31:277, 2002.

Tremblay RE: Physical aggression during early childhood: trajectories and predictors, *Pediatrics* 114(1):43, 2004.

Tsang HWH, Cheung L, Lak DCC: Qigong as a psychosocial intervention for depressed elderly with chronic physical illness, *Int J Geriatr Psychiatry* 17:1146, 2002.

Valente S, Saunders JM: Barriers to suicide risk management in clinical practice: a national survey of oncology nurses, *Issues Ment Health Nurs* 25:629, 2004.

Valente SM: Sexual abuse of boys, *JCAPN* 18:10, 2005.

Waern M, Rubenowitz E, Wilhelmson K: Predictors of suicide in the old elderly, *Gerontology* 49:328, 2003.

Webb L: Deliberate self-harm in adolescence: a systematic review of psychological and psychosocial factors, *J Adv Nurs* 38(3):235, 2002.

S

Delayed Surgical recovery   *Gail B. Ladwig, RN, MSN, CHTP*

NANDA   Definition

Extension of the number of postoperative days required to initiate and perform activities that maintain life, health, and well-being

Defining Characteristics

Difficulty in moving about; evidence of interrupted healing of surgical area (e.g., red, indurated draining, immobilized); fatigue; loss of appetite with or without nausea; perception that more time is needed to recover; postpones resumption of work/employment activities; requires help to complete self-care

Related Factors (r/t)

Extensive surgical procedure; obesity; pain; postoperative surgical site infection; preoperative expectations; prolonged surgical procedure

NOC   Outcomes (Nursing Outcomes Classification)

Suggested NOC Outcomes

Endurance, Infection Severity, Mobility, Pain Control, Self-Care: Activities of Daily Living (ADLs), Wound Healing: Primary Intention

Example NOC Outcome with Indicators
Wound Healing: Primary Intention as evidenced by the following indicators: Skin approximation/Scar formation (Rate the outcome and indicators of **Wound Healing as: Primary Intention:** 1 = none, 2 = limited, 3 = moderate, 4 = substantial, 5 = extensive [see Section I].)

Client Outcomes

Client Will (Specify Time Frame):

- Have surgical area that shows evidence of healing: no redness, induration, draining, or immobility
- State that appetite is regained
- State that no nausea is present
- Demonstrate ability to move about
- Demonstrate ability to complete self-care activities
- State that no fatigue is present
- State that pain is controlled or relieved after nursing interventions
- Resume employment activities/activities of daily living (ADLs)

NIC   Interventions (Nursing Interventions Classification)

Suggested NIC Interventions

Incision Site Care, Nutrition Management, Pain Management, Self-Care Assistance

Example NIC Activities—Incision Site Care
Teach the patient and/or the family how to care for the incision, including signs and symptoms of infection; Inspect the incision site for redness, swelling, or signs of dehiscence or evisceration

Nursing Interventions and *Rationales*

- Perform a thorough assessment of the client, including risk factors. Allow time to be with the client. **EBN:** *The perioperative dialogue allowed the clients time with the nurse and was experienced by them as having a positive effect on the healing process and recovery (Rudolffson et al, 2004). There*

S

• = Independent;   ▲ = Collaborative;   EBN = Evidence-Based Nursing;   EB = Evidence-Based

may not be a relationship between vital-signs collection and the occurrence or detection of complications (Zeitz & McCutcheon, 2006).

▲ Assess for the presence of medical conditions and treat appropriately before surgery. If the client is diabetic, maintain normal blood glucose levels before surgery. **EB:** *High blood glucose levels slow healing and increase risk of infection. The American Diabetes Association recommends that blood glucose should be less than 180 mg/dL for people in the hospital or having surgery. For some, the goal is less than 110 mg/dL (Anonymous, 2005).*

▲ Carefully assess client's use of dietary supplements such as feverfew, ginkgo biloba, garlic, ginseng, ginger, valerian, kava, St. John's wort, ephedra (Ma huang or metabo-lite), and echinacea. It is recommended that all clients be advised to stop all dietary supplements at least 1 week before major surgical or diagnostic procedures. *Certain dietary supplements can react or interact with frequently used surgical medications—including anesthesia—and may cause serious unforeseen consequences or complications. Arrhythmias, poor wound healing, bleeding, photosensitivity reaction, and prolonged sedation are among the serious reactions during and after surgical and diagnostic procedures that have been attributed to these products (Ciocon, Ciocon & Galindo, 2004).*

▲ Assess and treat for depression and anxiety in a client complaining of continuing fatigue after surgery. **EB:** *Fatigue is common after major surgery and delays recovery. The results of this study indicate that psychological processes may well be relevant in the etiology of postoperative fatigue (Rubin, Cleare & Hotopf, 2004).*

• Play music of the client's choice preoperatively, intraoperatively, and postoperatively. **EBN:** *In China it was demonstrated that the administration of self-selected music in the preprocedure period can be effective in the reduction of physiological parameters and anxiety (Lee, Henderson & Shum, 2004).* **EBN:** *Outpatient orthopedic clients indicate that participants overwhelmingly felt that music listening was a positive addition to traditional pain and anxiety management (Lukas, 2004).*

▲ Consider using healing touch in the perianesthesia setting and other mind-body-spirit interventions such as stress control and imagery. **EBN:** *Research showed that stress management, imagery, and touch therapy all produced reductions in reported worry, as compared with standard therapy (Seskevitch, Crater & Lane, 2004).*

• Use warmed cotton blankets to reduce heat loss during surgery. **EB:** *Warming helps a client maintain normothermia and appears to decrease client anxiety (Wagner, Byrne & Kolcaba, 2006). Normothermia is associated with low postoperative infection rates (Leaper, 2006).*

• Use careful aseptic technique when caring for wounds. **EBN:** *Client safety when performing aseptic technique is of the highest importance. There is a relationship between standards of aseptic technique and rise in hospital infection (Preston, 2005).*

• Suggest the use of a semipermeable dressing and suction drainage for selected orthopedic clients. **EB:** *This form of postoperative wound management appears to retain the nursing and hygiene advantages of suction drainage while preventing client discomfort and possibilities of wound infection associated with deep internal drainage (Panousis, Grigoris & Strover, 2004).*

• Clients should be allowed to shower after surgery to maintain cleanliness if not contra-indicated because of the presence of pacemaker wires. **EB:** *Clients undergoing open hernia repair who were allowed to shower showed no manifest infection and no difference in wound healing compared with those who were not allowed to shower (Riederer & Inderbitzi, 1997).*

• Promote early ambulation and deep breathing. Consider use of a transcutaneous electrical nerve stimulation (TENS) unit for pain relief. **EBN:** *TENS reduces pain intensity during walking and deep breathing and increases walking function postoperatively when used as a supplement to pharmacologic analgesia (Rakel & Franz, 2003). Early ambulation after hip fracture surgery accelerates functional recovery and is associated with more discharges directly home and less to high-level care (Oldmeadow et al, 2006).*

• The client should be provided with a complete, balanced therapeutic diet after the immediately postoperative period (24-48 hours). **EB:** *Improvement in nutritional status can improve outcomes of wound healing (Thomas, 2006).* **EBN:** *Good nutrition is important for effective wound healing (Anderson, 2005).*

• Provide 20-minute foot and hand massage (5 minutes to each extremity), 1 to 4 hours after a dose of pain medication. **EBN:** *The clients who had foot and hand massage experienced moderate*

S

• = Independent;   ▲ = Collaborative;   EBN = Evidence-Based Nursing;   EB = Evidence-Based

pain after they received pain medications. This pain was reduced by the intervention, thus supporting the effectiveness of foot and hand massage in postoperative pain management (Wang & Keck, 2004).

▲ Carefully consider the use of alternative therapy with a physician's order, such as application of aloe vera or aqueous cream to promote wound healing. **EBN:** *Aloe vera gel did not significantly reduce radiation-induced skin side effects in breast cancer clients. Aqueous cream was useful in reducing dry desquamation and pain related to radiation therapy (Heggie et al, 2002).*

▲ Consider the use of noetic therapies: stress management, imagery, and touch therapy. **EBN:** *The results of this study suggest that at least some noetic therapies may have beneficial effects on mood in the course of medical and surgical interventions (Seskevich, Crater & Lane, 2004).*

• Encourage the client to use prayer as a form of spiritual coping if this is comfortable for the client. **EB:** *This study demonstrated that greater internal control was positively associated with private prayer for coping in clients undergoing open-heart surgery (Ai et al, 2005).*

• See the care plans for **Anxiety, Acute Pain, Fatigue, Risk for deficient Fluid volume, Risk for perioperative positioning Injury, Impaired physical Mobility,** and **Nausea.**

Pediatric

• Support information the parents have gotten from the Internet regarding their child's condition. *The Internet is a useful educational tool in teaching parents about their child's condition. Parental use of the Internet is already widespread and may need to be specifically addressed during consultation and preoperative teaching (Sim, Kitteringham & Spitz, 2007).*

• Teach imagery and encourage distraction for children for postsurgical pain relief. **EBN:** *Distraction decreases pain in children undergoing painful procedures (Stubenrauch, 2007).* **EBN:** *Imagery using distraction was helpful in decreasing the use of analgesics for pain in a group of 7- to 12-year-olds who had had tonsillectomy and/or adenoidectomy (Huth, 2002).*

• Children who are at normal risk for aspiration/regurgitation should be allowed fluids prior to anesthesia. **EB:** *This study demonstrated that there is no evidence that children who are not permitted oral fluids for more than 6 hours preoperatively benefit in terms of intraoperative gastric volume and pH over children permitted unlimited fluids up to 2 hours preoperatively. Children permitted fluids have a more comfortable preoperative experience in terms of thirst and hunger (Brady et al, 2005).*

Geriatric

• Perform a thorough preoperative assessment, including a cardiac and social support assessment. **EB:** *Better preoperative risk assessment and preparation of the client have helped to improve outcomes in geriatric clients (Dharmarajan, Unnikrishnan & Dharmarajan, 2003).* **EBN:** *Older clients, those with preoperative comorbidities, and those without a caregiver at home experience delays in functional recovery and discharge. These findings support the addition of functional recovery and social support risk items to the preoperative cardiac surgery risk assessment (Anderson et al, 2006).*

• Assess for pain. **EBN:** *Often pain is undermanaged in older people. There is a need for individualized assessment (Brown, 2004).*

• Carefully evaluate the client's temperature. Know what is normal and abnormal for each client. Check baseline temperature and monitor trends. **EB:** *Older subjects have mean oral body temperatures lower than 98.6° F. Relatively few even achieve this temperature (Gomolin et al, 2005).*

• Teach guided imagery for pain relief. **EBN:** *Elderly clients with hip replacements demonstrated positive outcomes for pain relief, decreased anxiety, and decreased length of stay with guided imagery (Antall & Kresevec, 2004).*

• Offer spiritual support. **EB:** *In a qualitative study, religion and spirituality were found to help older adults maintain and recover both physical and mental health (Mackenzie et al, 2000).*

Home Care

• The above interventions may be adapted for the home setting.

• Provide supportive telephone calls from nurse to client as a means of decreasing anxiety and providing the psychosocial support necessary for recovery from surgery. **EB:** *Telephone calls are an effective method of providing supportive psychosocial care for individuals who may not be able to access this care because of geographic isolation, physical limitations, or discomfort with face-to-face interventions (Gotay & Bottomley, 1998).*

Client/Family Teaching

- Provide preoperative teaching by a nurse to decrease postoperative problems of anxiety, pain, nausea, and lack of independence. **EBN:** *Those clients awaiting coronary artery bypass grafting (CABG) who displayed high fear wanted informational support from nurses more often than clients who showed lower fear (Koivula et al, 2002).*
- Provide preoperative information in verbal and written form. **EB:** *Clients increasingly expect written information; however, amount, quality, and timeliness vary considerably. Combining commercially produced information with standard hospital information may be to the client's benefit (Sheard & Garrud, 2006).*
- Teach systematic muscle relaxation for pain relief. **EBN:** *Unrelieved pain after surgery can lead to complications, prolonged hospital stay, and delayed recovery. Substantial reductions in the sensation and distress of pain were found when postoperative clients used systematic relaxation (Roykulcharoen & Good, 2004).*
- Provide individualized teaching plans for the client with an ostomy. Consider basic needs: (1) maintenance of a pouching seal for a consistent, predictable wear time; (2) maintenance of peristomal skin integrity; and (3) social and professional support of the client. **EB:** *Guiding the client to the ostomy management system suited to his or her lifestyle can play a vital role toward achieving individual quality-of-life goals. Teaching plans should be individualized and customized to reflect and accommodate the phase of rehabilitation and client-defined quality-of-life goals at the time the nurse interacts with the client (Turnbull, Colwell & Erwin-Toth, 2004).*

evolve   See the EVOLVE website for World Wide Web resources for client education.

REFERENCES

Ai AL, Peterson C, Rodgers WL et al: Faith factors and internal health locus of control in patients prior to open-heart surgery, *J Health Psychol* 10(5):669-676, 2005.

Anderson B: Nutrition and wound healing: the necessity of assessment, *Br J Nurs* 14(19):S30, S32, S34, 2005.

Anderson JA, Petersen NJ, Kistner C et al: Determining predictors of delayed recovery and the need for transitional cardiac rehabilitation after cardiac surgery, *J Am Acad Nurse Pract* 18(8):386-392, 2006.

Anonymous: Diabetes in the hospital: taking charge, *Diabetes Spectrum* 18(1):49-50, 2005.

Antall GF, Kresevic D: The use of guided imagery to manage pain in an elderly orthopaedic population, *Orthop Nurs* 23(5):335-340, 2004.

Brady M, Kinn S, O'Rourke K et al: Preoperative fasting for preventing perioperative complications in children, *Cochrane Database Syst Rev* (2):CD005285, 2005.

Brown D: A literature review exploring how healthcare professionals contribute to the assessment and control of postoperative pain in older people, *J Clin Nurs* 13(6b):74-90, 2004.

Ciocon JO, Ciocon DG, Galindo DJ: Dietary supplements in primary care. Botanicals can affect surgical outcomes and follow-up, *Geriatrics* 59(9):20-24, 2004.

Dharmarajan TS, Unnikrishnan D, Dharmarajan L: Preparing the older adult for surgery, *Hosp Physician* 39(11):45-54, 2003.

Gomolin IH, Aung MM, Wolf-Klein G et al: Older is colder: temperature range and variation in older people, *J Am Geriatr Soc* 53(12):2170-2172, 2005.

Gotay CC, Bottomley A: Providing psychosocial support by telephone: what is its potential in cancer patients? *Eur J Cancer Care* 7(4):225-231, 1998.

Heggie S, Bryant GP, Tripcony L et al: A phase III study on the efficacy of topical aloe vera gel on irradiated breast tissue, *Cancer Nurs* 25(6):442-451, 2002.

Huth MM: *Imagery to reduce children's postoperative pain*, doctoral dissertation, Cleveland, Ohio, 2002, Case Western Reserve University.

Koivula M, Paunonen-Ilmonen M, Tarkka MT et al: Social support and its relation to fear and anxiety in patients awaiting coronary artery bypass grafting, *J Clin Nurs* 11(5):622-633, 2002.

Leaper D: Effects of local and systemic warming on postoperative infections, *Surg Infect (Larchmt)* (Suppl 2):S101-S103, 2006.

Lee D, Henderson A, Shum D: The effect of music on preprocedure anxiety in Hong Kong Chinese day patients, *J Clin Nurs* 13(3):297-303, 2004.

Lukas LK: Orthopedic outpatients' perception of perioperative music listening as therapy, *J Theory Construct Testing* 8(1):7-12, 2004.

Mackenzie ER, Rajagopal DE, Meibohm M et al: Spiritual support and psychological well-being: older adults' perceptions of the religion and health connection, *Altern Ther Health Med* 6(6):37-45, 2000.

Oldmeadow LB, Edwards ER, Kimmel LA et al: No rest for the wounded: early ambulation after hip surgery accelerates recovery, *ANZ J Surg* 76(7):607-611, 2006.

Panousis K, Grigoris P, Strover AE: Suction dressings in total knee arthroplasty—an alternative to deep suction drainage, *Acta Orthop Belg* 70(4):349-354, 2004.

Preston R: Aseptic technique: evidence-based approach for patient safety, *Br J Nurs* 14(10):540-544, 2005.

Rakel B, Frantz R: Effectiveness of transcutaneous electrical nerve stimulation on postoperative pain with movement, *J Pain* 4(8):455-464, 2003.

Riederer SR, Inderbitzi R: [Does a shower put postoperative wound healing at risk?] *Chirurg* 68(7):715-717, 1997 [article in German].

Roykulcharoen V, Good M: Systematic relaxation to relieve postoperative pain, *J Adv Nurs* 48(2):140-148, 2004.

Rubin GJ, Cleare A, Hotopf M: Psychological factors in postoperative fatigue, *Psychosom Med* 66(6):959-964, 2004.

Rudolffson G, Hallberg LRM, Ringsberg KC et al: The nurse has time for me: the perioperative dialogue from the perspective of patients, *J Adv Periop Care* 1(3):77-84, 2003.

Seskevich JE, Crater SW, Lane JD: Beneficial effects of noetic thera-

S

- = Independent;   ▲ = Collaborative;   EBN = Evidence-Based Nursing;   EB = Evidence-Based

pies on mood before percutaneous intervention for unstable coronary syndromes, *Nurs Res* 53(2):116-121, 2004.

Sheard C, Garrud P: Evaluation of generic patient information: effects on health outcomes, knowledge and satisfaction, *Patient Educ Couns* 61(1):43-47, 2006.

Sim NZ, Kitteringham L, Spitz L 2007: Information on the World Wide Web—how useful is it for parents? *J Pediatr Surg* 42(2):305-312, 2007.

Stubenrauch J: Striving for distraction, *AJN* 107(3):94-95, 2007.

Thomas DR: Prevention and treatment of pressure ulcers, *J Am Med Dir Assoc* 42(5):46-59, 2006.

Turnbull GB, Colwell J, Erwin-Toth P: Quality of life: pre, post, and beyond ostomy surgery: clinician strategies for helping people with a stoma lead healthy, productive lives, *Ostomy Wound Manage* 50(7): S2, 2004.

Wagner D, Byrne M, Kolcaba K: Effects of comfort warming on preoperative patients, *AORN J* 84(3):427-448, 2006.

Wang H, Keck JF: Foot and hand massage as an intervention for post-operative pain, *Pain Manage Nurs* 5(2):59-65, 2004.

Zeitz K, McCutcheon H: Observations and vital signs: ritual or vital for the monitoring of postoperative patients? *Appl Nurs Res* 19(4):204-211, 2006.

Impaired Swallowing   Betty J. Ackley, MSN, EdS, RN   *evolve*

NANDA   Definition

Abnormal functioning of the swallowing mechanism associated with deficits in oral, pharyngeal, or esophageal structure or function

Defining Characteristics

Esophageal phase impairment: Abnormality in esophageal phase by swallow study; acidic smelling breath; bruxism; complaints of "something stuck"; epigastric pain; food refusal; heartburn or epigastric pain; hematemesis; hyperextension of head (e.g., arching during or after meals); nighttime awakening; nighttime coughing; observed evidence of difficulty in swallowing (e.g., stasis of food in oral cavity, coughing/choking); odynophagia; regurgitation of gastric contents (wet burps); repetitive swallowing; unexplained irritability surrounding mealtime; volume limiting; vomiting; vomitus on pillow

Oral phase impairment: Abnormality in oral phase of swallow study; coughing, choking, or gagging before a swallow; falling of food from mouth; inability to clear oral cavity; incomplete lip closure; lack of chewing; lack of tongue action to form bolus; long meals with little consumption; nasal reflux; piecemeal deglutition; pooling in lateral sulci; premature entry of bolus; pushing of food out of mouth; sialorrhea or drooling; slow bolus formation; weak suck resulting in inefficient nippling

Pharyngeal phase impairment: Abnormality in pharyngeal phase by swallowing study; altered head position; choking, coughing, or gagging; delayed swallow; food refusal; gurgly voice quality; inadequate laryngeal elevation; multiple swallows; nasal reflux; recurrent pulmonary infections; unexplained fever

Related Factors (r/t)

Congenital Defects

Behavioral feeding problems; conditions with significant hypotonia; congenital heart disease; failure to thrive; history of tube feeding; mechanical obstruction (e.g., edema, tracheostomy tube, tumor); neuromuscular impairment (e.g., decreased or absent gag reflex, decreased strength or excursion of muscles involved in mastication, perceptual impairment, facial paralysis); protein energy malnutrition; respiratory disorders; self-injurious behavior; upper airway anomalies

Neurological Problems

Achalasia; acquired anatomic defects; cerebral palsy; cranial nerve involvement; developmental delay; esophageal defects; gastroesophageal reflux disease; laryngeal abnormalities; laryngeal defects; nasal defects; nasopharyngeal cavity defects; oropharynx abnormalities; prematurity; tracheal defects; traumas; traumatic head injury; upper airway anomalies

NOC   Outcomes (Nursing Outcomes Classification)

Suggested NOC Outcomes

Swallowing Status, Swallowing Status: Esophageal Phase, Oral Phase, Pharyngeal Phase

S

• = Independent;   ▲ = Collaborative;   EBN = Evidence-Based Nursing;   EB = Evidence-Based

Example NOC Outcome with Indicators
Swallowing Status as evidenced by the following indicators: Delivery of bolus to hypopharynx is timed with swallow reflex/Ability to clear oral cavity/Number of swallows appropriate for bolus size and texture/Voice quality/Choking, coughing, gagging not present/Normal swallow effort (Rate the outcome and indicators of **Swallowing Status:** 1 = severely compromised, 2 = substantially compromised, 3 = moderately compromised, 4 = mildly compromised, 5 = not compromised [see Section I].)

Client Outcomes

Client Will (Specify Time Frame):
- Demonstrate effective swallowing without choking or coughing
- Remain free from aspiration (e.g., lungs clear, temperature within normal range)

NIC   Interventions (Nursing Interventions Classification)

Suggested NIC Interventions
Aspiration Precautions, Swallowing Therapy

Example NIC Activities—Swallowing Therapy
Assist patient to sit in an erect position (as close to 90 degrees as possible) for feeding/exercise; Instruct patient not to talk during eating, if appropriate

Nursing Interventions and *Rationales*

- Determine the client's readiness to eat. The client needs to be alert, able to follow instructions, able to hold the head erect, able to swallow, and able to move the tongue in the mouth. *If one of these elements is missing, it may be advisable to withhold oral feeding and use enteral feeding for nourishment (Smith & Connolly, 2003).*
- ▲ If the swallowing impairment is of new onset, ensure that the client receives a diagnostic workup. *Swallowing impairment can have multiple causes, many of which are treatable (Smith & Connolly, 2003).* **EB:** *A referral for a formal swallowing evaluation is indicated in preventing aspiration pneumonia (Hammond & Goldstein, 2006).*
- Assess ability to swallow by positioning the thumb and index finger on the client's laryngeal protuberance. Ask the client to swallow; feel the larynx elevate. Ask the client to cough; test for a gag reflex on both sides of the posterior pharyngeal wall (lingual surface) with a tongue blade. Do not rely on the presence of a gag reflex to determine when to feed. *Normally the time required for the bolus to move from the point at which the reflex is triggered to the esophageal entry (pharyngeal transit time) is less than 1 second (Logemann, 1983). Clients can aspirate even if they have an intact gag reflex (Smith & Connolly, 2003).* **EB:** *CVA Clients who have experienced a cerebrovascular accident (CVA) and have prolonged pharyngeal transit times (prolonged swallowing) have an increased chance of developing aspiration pneumonia (Marik & Kaplan, 2003).*
- Consider the use of the Massey Bedside Swallowing Screen to screen for swallowing dysfunction. **EBN:** *The Massey Bedside Swallowing Screen demonstrated high sensitivity and specificity in predicting dysphagia, compared with assessment by experts in the field (Massey & Jedlicka, 2002).*
- Observe for signs associated with swallowing problems (e.g., coughing, choking, spitting of food, drooling, difficulty handling oral secretions, double swallowing or major delay in swallowing, watering eyes, nasal discharge, wet or gurgly voice, decreased ability to move the tongue and lips, decreased mastication of food, decreased ability to move food to the back of the pharynx, slow or scanning speech). **EB:** *A study demonstrated that voice analysis could accurately predict the clients with dysphagia by presence of perturbation, shimmer percentage, noise-to-harmonic ratio, and voice turbulence as tested by videofluoroscopic swallowing studies (Ryu, Park & Choi, 2004).*
- ▲ If the client has impaired swallowing, refer to a speech pathologist for bedside evaluation as soon as possible. Ensure that the client is seen by a speech pathologist within 48 hours after admis-

S

• = Independent;   ▲ = Collaborative;   EBN = Evidence-Based Nursing;   EB = Evidence-Based

sion if the client has had a CVA. **EBN:** *Early referral of CVA clients to a speech pathologist, along with early initiation of nutritional support, can result in decreased length of hospital stay, shortened recovery time, and reduced overall health costs (Runions, Rodrigue & White, 2004).*

▲ To manage impaired swallowing, use a dysphagia team composed of a rehabilitation nurse, speech pathologist, dietitian, physician, and radiologist who work together. *The dysphagia team can help the client learn to swallow safely and maintain a good nutritional status. Feeding a client who cannot adequately swallow results in aspiration and possibly death.* **EB:** *Enteral feedings via percutaneous endoscopic gastrostomy (PEG) tube are generally preferable to naso-gastric tube feedings, but further studies are needed (Bath, Bath-Hextall & Smithard, 2005).*

▲ If the client has impaired swallowing, do not feed until an appropriate diagnostic workup is completed. Ensure proper nutrition by consulting with a physician regarding enteral feedings, preferably using a PEG tube in most cases.

• If client is not eating sufficient amount of food, recognize that the immune system may be impaired with resultant increased risk of infection. **EB:** *A study comparing elderly clients with dysphagia who were tube fed versus others who were orally fed showed that the orally fed clients had much lower CD4 cell counts, as well as a low CD4/CD8 ratio (Leibovitz et al, 2004).*

• If the client has an intact swallowing reflex, attempt to feed. Observe the following feeding guidelines:
  ▪ Position the client upright at a 90-degree angle with the chin tucked forward at a 45-degree angle if this has been determined to be helpful (Metheny, 2007). *The chin tuck is protective for most people with dysphagia, because the epiglottis forms a protective shelf over the vocal folds as the client swallows (West & Redstone, 2004).*
  ▪ Ensure that the client is awake, alert, and able to follow sequenced directions before attempting to feed. *As the client becomes less alert, the swallowing response decreases, which increases the risk of aspiration.*
  ▪ Begin by feeding the client one third of a teaspoon of applesauce. Provide sufficient time to masticate and swallow.
  ▪ Place the food on the unaffected side of the tongue.
  ▪ During feeding, give the client specific directions (e.g., "Open your mouth, chew the food completely, and when you are ready, tuck your chin to your chest and swallow").
  ▪ Avoid rushing or forcing feeding.
  ▪ Ensure client is kept in an upright posture for an hour after eating. *An upright posture after eating has been associated with a decreased incidence of pneumonia in the elderly (Coleman, 2004; Metheny, 2007).*

▲ Watch for uncoordinated chewing or swallowing; coughing immediately after eating or delayed coughing, which may indicate silent aspiration; pocketing of food; wet-sounding voice; sneezing when eating; delay of more than 1 second in swallowing; or a change in respiratory patterns. If any of these signs is present, put on gloves, remove all food from the oral cavity, stop feedings, and consult with a speech and language pathologist and a dysphagia team. *These are signs of impaired swallowing and possible aspiration (Galvan, 2001).*

• If the client tolerates single-textured foods such as pudding, hot cereal, or strained baby food, advance to a soft diet with guidance from the dysphagia team. Avoid foods such as hamburgers, corn, and pastas that are difficult to chew. Also avoid sticky foods such as peanut butter and white bread. *The dysphagia team should determine the appropriate diet for the client based on progression in swallowing and needs to ensure that the client is nourished and hydrated.*

• Avoid providing liquids until the client is able to swallow effectively. Add a thickening agent to liquids to obtain a soft consistency that is similar to nectar, honey, or pudding, depending on the degree of swallowing problems. *Liquids can be easily aspirated; thickened liquids form a cohesive bolus that the client can swallow with increased efficiency (Langmore & Miller, 1994; Poertner & Coleman, 1998).*

• Thicken fluids as recommended from the swallowing evaluation. Preferably use prepackaged thickened liquids, or use a viscosimeter to ensure appropriate thickness. **EB:** *Using prepackaged thickened liquids or a viscosimeter to determine appropriate thickness can increase intake, which increases hydration and nutrition (Boczko, 2000; Goulding & Bakheit, 2000). The majority of clients*

S

with swallowing difficulties received liquids thickened to nectar-syrup consistency (60%), 33% received honey consistency, and only 6% received pudding consistency thickened fluids (Castellanos et al, 2004). NOTE: Several studies have shown that clients receiving thickened fluids do not meet daily fluid requirements (Finestone et al, 2001; Goulding & Bakheit, 2000).

▲ Work with the client on swallowing exercises prescribed by the dysphagia team (e.g., touching the palate with the tongue, stimulating the tonsillar arch and soft palate with a cold metal examination mirror [thermal stimulation], labial/lingual range-of-motion exercises). *Swallowing exercises, including both motor and sensory stimulation, can improve the client's ability to swallow (Hagg & Larsson, 2004). Exercises need to be done at intervals, which necessitates nursing involvement (Poertner & Coleman, 1998).* **EB:** *Clients who received a high-intensity swallowing intervention versus usual care or a low-intensity swallowing intervention were more likely to return to a normal diet and recover swallowing ability by 6 months (Carnaby, Hankey & Pizzi, 2006).*

▲ For many adult clients, avoid the use of straws if recommended by the speech pathologist. *Use of straws can increase the risk of aspiration, because straws can result in spilling of a bolus of fluid in the oral cavity, as well as decreased control of the posterior transit of fluid to the pharynx (Travers, 1999).* **EB:** *A reduction in airway protection with use of a straw was shown for drinking in the older men as compared with the younger men (Daniels et al, 2004).*

• Provide meals in a quiet environment away from excessive stimuli such as a community dining room. *A noisy environment can be an aversive stimulus and can decrease effective mastication and swallowing. Talking and laughing while eating increase the risk of aspiration (Galvan, 2001).*

• Ensure that there is adequate time for the client to eat. *Clients with swallowing impairments often take longer than others to eat, if they are being fed. Often, food is offered rapidly to speed up the task, and this can increase the chance of aspiration (Metheny, 2007).*

▲ Have suction equipment available during feeding. If choking occurs and suctioning is necessary, discontinue oral feeding until the client is safely assessed with a videofluoroscopic swallow study.

• Check the oral cavity for proper emptying after the client swallows and after the client finishes the meal. Provide oral care at the end of the meal. It may be necessary to manually remove food from the client's mouth. If this is the case, use gloves and keep the client's teeth apart with a padded tongue blade. *Food may become pocketed on the affected side and cause stomatitis, tooth decay, and possible later aspiration.*

• Praise the client for successfully following directions and swallowing appropriately. *Praise reinforces behavior and sets up a positive atmosphere in which learning takes place.*

• Keep the client in an upright position for 45 minutes to an hour after a meal. **EB:** *A study demonstrated that the number of elderly clients developing a fever was significantly reduced when clients were kept sitting upright after eating (Matsui et al, 2002).*

▲ Watch for signs of aspiration and pneumonia. Auscultate lung sounds after feeding. Note new crackles or wheezing, and note elevated temperature. Notify the physician as needed. *The presence of an increased respiratory rate, new crackles or wheezing, an elevated temperature or white blood cell count, a change in sputum, and also new onset of delirium could indicate aspiration of food or onset of pneumonia (Galvan, 2001; Metheny, 2007).* **EB:** *Bronchial auscultation of lung sounds was shown to be specific in identifying clients at risk for aspirating (Shaw et al, 2004).*

• Watch for signs of malnutrition and dehydration. Keep a record of food intake. *Malnutrition is common in dysphagic clients (Galvan, 2001). Clients with dysphagia are at serious risk for malnutrition and dehydration, which can lead to aspiration pneumonia resulting from depressed immune function and weakness, lethargy, and decreased cough (Langmore, 1999).*

▲ Weigh the client weekly to help evaluate nutritional status. Evaluate nutritional status daily. If the client is not adequately nourished, work with the dysphagia team to determine whether the client needs to avoid oral intake with therapeutic feeding only or needs enteral feedings until the client can swallow adequately. **EB:** *Dysphagic stroke clients who received thickened fluid dysphagia diets failed to meet their needs for fluids, whereas a group receiving enteral feeding and IV fluid did meet fluid requirements (Finestone et al, 2001).* **EBN:** *Four independent risk factors for dysphagia— hypoglossal nerve dysfunction, National Institutes of Health Stroke Scale score, incomplete oral labial closure, and wet voice after swallowing water—predicted the need for tube feedings in stroke clients with dysphagia (Wojner & Alexandrov, 2000).*

S

▲ If client has a tracheostomy, ask for referral to speech pathologist for swallowing studies before attempting to feed. After evaluation, decision should be made to have cuff either inflated or deflated when client eats. **EBN and EB:** *The presence of a tracheostomy tube increases the incidence of aspiration (Elpern, Jacobs & Bone, 1993). Clients who had aspiration after a tracheostomy had aspiration before the tracheostomy (Leder & Ross, 2000). For some clients, inflating the cuff may help decrease aspiration; for others, the inflated cuff will interfere with swallowing. This decision should be made after swallowing studies for the safety of the client's airway (Murray & Brzozowski, 1998).*

Pediatric

▲ Refer to a physician and a dietician a child who has difficulty swallowing and symptoms such as difficulty manipulating food, delayed swallow response, and pocketing of a bolus of food. **EB:** *Adequate nutrition is extremely important for children to ensure sufficient growth and development of all body systems (Morgan et al, 2004).*

• Provide oral motor stimulation that increases oral-sensory awareness by waking the mouth using exercises that focus on temperature, taste, and texture. *Many of these infants require supplemental tube feedings and special nipples or bottles to boost oral intake.*

• For infants with poor sucking and swallowing, do the following:
  ■ Support the cheeks and jaw to increase sucking skills.
  ■ Pace or rhythmically move the bottle, which encourages better suck-swallow-breath synchrony.

• Watch for indicators of aspiration: coughing, a change in web vocal quality while feeding, perspiration and color changes during feeding, sneezing, and increased heart rate and breathing.

• Watch for warning signs of reflux: sour-smelling breath after eating, sneezing, lack of interest in feeding, crying and fussing extraordinarily when feeding, pained expressions when feeding, and excessive chewing and swallowing after eating. *Many premature and medically fragile children experience growth deficits and respiratory problems from an underlying dysphagia. Some infants may need to work harder to breathe than others and, as a result, develop a decreased tolerance for food intake. They also demonstrate inconsistent arousal and poor/uncoordinated suck-swallow-breath synchrony. Many of these infants require supplemental tube feedings and the use of special nipples or bottles to boost oral intake.*

Geriatric

• Recognize that being elderly does not result in dysphagia, but having medical problems including such things as arthritis, hypertension, and other chronic medical problems can result in dysphagia. **EB:** *No delay in swallowing was found in elderly subjects, but clients with medical conditions did often have problems with dysphagia (Kendall, Leonard & McKenzie, 2004).*

▲ Evaluate medications the client is presently taking, especially if elderly. Consult with the pharmacist for assistance in monitoring for incorrect doses and drug interactions that could result in dysphagia. *Most elderly clients take numerous medications, which when taken individually can slow motor function, cause anxiety and depression, and reduce salivary flow. When taken together, these medications can interact, resulting in impaired swallowing function. Drugs that reduce muscle tone for swallowing and can cause reflux include calcium channel blockers and nitrates. Drugs that can reduce salivary flow include antidepressants, antiparkinsonism drugs, antihistamines, antispasmodics, antipsychotic agents or major tranquilizers, antiemetics, antihypertensives, and drugs for treating diarrhea and anxiety (Schechter, 1998).*

• Recognize that the elderly client with dementia needs a longer time to eat. *The dementia client has decreased cognition, distractibility, and decreased efficiency in chewing and is likely to have problems with swallowing (Granville, 2002).*

• Recognize that the loss of teeth can cause problems with chewing and swallowing. *Missing teeth and poorly fitting dentures predispose the client for aspiration, because of inadequate chewing and swallowing (Metheny, 2007).*

Home Care

▲ Refer to speech therapy. *Speech therapists can work with clients to enhance swallowing ability.*

• = Independent;   ▲ = Collaborative;   EBN = Evidence-Based Nursing;   EB = Evidence-Based

Client/Family Teaching

▲ Teach the client and family exercises prescribed by the dysphagia team.
- Teach the client a systematic method of swallowing effectively as prescribed by the dysphagia team.
- Educate the client, family, and all caregivers about rationales for food consistency and choices. *It is common for family members to disregard necessary dietary restrictions and give the client inappropriate foods that predispose to aspiration (Poertner & Coleman, 1998).*
- Teach the family how to monitor the client to prevent and detect aspiration during eating.

evolve See the EVOLVE website for World Wide Web resources for client education.

REFERENCES

Bath PM, Bath-Hextall FJ, Smithard EG: Interventions for dysphagia in acute stroke, *Cochrane Database Syst Rev* (2):CD000323, DJ9, 2005.

Boczko T: Increasing liquid consumption in patients with dysphagia, *Adv Speech Language Pathol Audiol* 10(45), 2000.

Carnaby G, Hankey G, Pizzi J: Behavioral intervention for dysphagia in acute stroke: a randomized controlled trial. *Lancet Neurol,* 5(1):31-37, 2006.

Castellanos VH, Butler E, Gluch L et al: Use of thickened liquids in skilled nursing facilities, *J ADA Assoc* 104(8):1222-1226, 2004.

Coleman PR: Pneumonia in the long-term care setting: etiology, management, and prevention, *J Gerontol Nurs* 30(4):14, 2004.

Daniels SK, Corey DM, Hadskey LD et al: Mechanism of sequential swallowing during straw drinking in healthy young and older adults, *J Speech Lang Hear Res* 47(1):33-45, 2004.

Elpern EH, Jacobs ER, Bone RC: Incidence of aspiration in tracheally intubated adults, *Heart Lung* 16:527, 1993.

Finestone HM, Foley NC, Woodbury MG et al: Quantifying fluid intake in dysphagic stroke patients: a preliminary comparison of oral and nonoral strategies, *Arch Phys Med Rehabil* 82(12):1744-1746, 2001.

Galvan TJ: Dysphagia: going down and staying down, *Am J Nurs* 101(1):37, 2001.

Goulding R, Bakheit A: Evaluation of the benefits of monitoring fluid thickness in the dietary management of dysphagic stroke patients, *Clin Rehabil* 14:119, 2000.

Granville L: *Introduction to comprehensive geriatric assessment.* Paper presented at the Florida Speech-Language Hearing Association Convention, Orlando, Fla, Sept 21-22, 2002.

Hagg, Larsson B: Effects of motor and sensory stimulation in stroke patients with long-lasting dysphagia, *Dysphagia* 19(4):219, 2004.

Hammond CA, Goldstein LB: Cough and aspiration of food and fluids due to oral-pharyngeal dysphagia: ACCP evidence-based clinical practice guidelines, *Chest* 129:154-168, 2006.

Kendall KA, Leonard RJ, McKenzie S: Common medical conditions in the elderly: impact on pharyngeal bolus transit, *Dysphagia* 19(2):71, 2004.

Langmore SE: Risk factors for aspiration pneumonia, *Nutr Clin Pract* 14(5):S41, 1999.

Langmore SE, Miller RM: Behavioral treatment for adults with oropharyngeal dysphagia, *Arch Phys Med Rehabil* 75:1154, 1994.

Leder SB, Ross DA: Investigation of the causal relationship between tracheostomy and aspiration in the acute care setting, *Laryngoscope* 100(4):641, 2000.

Leibovitz A, Sharon-Guidetti A, Segal R et al: CD4 lymphocyte count and CD4/CD8 ratio in elderly long-term care patients with oropharyngeal dysphagia: comparison between oral and tube enteral feedings, *Dysphagia* 19(2):83-86, 2004.

Logemann JA: *Evaluation and treatment of swallowing disorders*, San Diego, 1983, College Hill.

Marik PE, Kaplan D: Aspiration pneumonia and dysphagia in the elderly, *Chest* 124(1):328, 2003.

Massey R, Jedlicka D: The Massey Bedside Swallowing Screen, *J Neurosci Nurs* 34(5):252, 2002.

Matsui T, Yamaya M, Ohrui T et al: Sitting position to prevent aspiration in bed-bound patients, *Gerontology* 48(3):194-195, 2002.

Metheny NA: Preventing aspiration in older adults with dysphagia. Try This: Best practices in nursing care to older adults. *The Hartford Institute for Geriatric Nursing,* 20, 2007.

Morgan R et al: Challenges and strategies for proper pediatric nutrition and weight control, *N J Med* 101(5):33-36, 2004.

Murray KA, Brzozowski LA: Swallowing in patients with tracheotomies, *AACN Clin Issues* 9(3):416, 1998.

Poertner LC, Coleman RF: Swallowing therapy in adults, *Otolaryngol Clin North Am* 31(3):561, 1998.

Runions S, Rodrigue N, White C: Practice on an acute stroke until after implementation of a decision-making algorithm for dietary management of dysphagia, *J Neurosci Nurse* 36(4): 200, 2004.

Ryu JS, Park SR, Choi KH: Prediction of laryngeal aspiration using voice analysis, *Am J Phy Med Rehabil* 83(10):753, 2004.

Schechter GL: Systemic causes of dysphagia in adults, *Otolaryngol Clin North Am* 31(3):525, 1998.

Shaw JL, Sharpe S, Dyson SE et al: Bronchial auscultation: an effective adjunct to speech and language therapy bedside assessment when detecting dysphagia and aspiration? *Dysphagia* 19(4):211-218, 2004.

Smith HA, Connolly MJ: Evaluation and treatment of dysphagia following stroke, *Top Geriatr Rehabil* 19(1):43-60, 2003.

Travers P: Poststroke dysphagia: implications for nurses, *Rehabil Nurs* 24(2):69, 1999.

West JF, Redstone F: Feeding the adult with neurogenic disorders, *Top Geriatr Rehabil* 20(2):131-134, 2004.

Wojner AW, Alexandrov AV: Predictors of tube feeding in acute stroke patients with dysphagia, *AACN Clin Issues* 11(4):531, 2000.

S

Effective Therapeutic regimen management
Margaret Lunney, RN, PhD, and Dawn Fairlie, MS, ANP, FNP, GNP, CDE

NANDA   Definition

Pattern of regulating and integrating into daily living a program for treatment of illness and its sequelae that is satisfactory for meeting specific health goals

Defining Characteristics

Appropriate choices of daily activities for meeting the goals of a prevention program; appropriate choices of daily activities for meeting the goals of a treatment program; illness symptoms within a normal range of expectation; verbalizes desire to manage the treatment of illness; verbalizes desire to manage prevention of sequelae; verbalizes intent to reduce risk factors for progression of illness and sequelae

Related Factors (r/t)

To be developed.

NOC   Outcomes (Nursing Outcomes Classification)

Suggested NOC Outcomes

Knowledge: Treatment Regimen, Participation in Health Care Decisions, Risk Control

Example NOC Outcome with Indicators
Knowledge: Treatment Regimen as evidenced by the following indicator: Description of prescribed medication, activity, exercise, and specific disease process (Rate the outcome and indicators of **Knowledge: Treatment Regimen:** 1 = none, 2 = limited, 3 = moderate, 4 = substantial, 5 = extensive [see Section I].)

Client Outcomes

Client Will (Specify Time Frame):

*   Acknowledge appropriateness of choices for meeting goals of treatment or prevention programs
*   Agree to continue making appropriate choices
*   Verbalize intent to contact health provider(s) for additional information, support, or resources as needed

NIC   Interventions (Nursing Interventions Classification)

Suggested NIC Interventions

Health Education, Health System Guidance, Learning Facilitation, Learning Readiness Enhancement, Risk Identification

Example NIC Activities—Learning Facilitation
Present the information in a stimulating manner; Encourage the patient's active participation.

Nursing Interventions and *Rationales*

NOTE: Little or no research is being done to investigate interventions to maintain strengths. For many interventions, theoretical rationales are provided as evidence rather than research findings.
*   Review self-management strategies and related outcomes (e.g., changes in function and/or relief of symptoms such as pain). **EB:** *Self-management after client education is associated with positive outcomes (Holman & Lorig, 2004; Lorig et al, 2005; Lorig, Ritter & Jacquez, 2005; Lorig et al, 2006; Stanford University, 2007).*

• = Independent;   ▲ = Collaborative;   EBN = Evidence-Based Nursing;   EB = Evidence-Based

- Explore the meaning of the person's illness experience and identify uncertainties and needs through open-ended questions. **EB:** *This approach is necessary to know the person's perspective of self-management (Rogers et al, 2005).*
- Acknowledge the congruence of choices in activities of daily living (ADLs) with health-related goals. **EBN:** *Support from health provider(s) in efforts to self-manage therapeutic regimens motivates individuals to continue these efforts despite difficulties (Hibbard, 2004).*
- Support decisions regarding the person's methods of integrating therapeutic regimens into ADLs. **EBN:** *"A growing body of evidence shows that clients who are engaged, active participants in their own care have better health outcomes and measurable cost savings" (Hibbard, 2004).*
- Provide information on possible illness trajectories to allow planning for future management. **EBN:** *Knowledge and awareness of illness trajectories enables the person to plan for future management of therapeutic regimens (Lubkin & Larsen, 2006).*
- Help the person resolve ambivalent feelings about the illness and management of therapeutic regimens. **EBN:** *Wide variations may exist in attitudes and ambivalence toward illness and management of illness regimens. Ambivalence interferes with effective decision making regarding illness care (Pender, Murdaugh & Parsons, 2006).*
- Review methods of contacting health provider(s) for changes in therapeutic regimen and/or methods of incorporating therapeutic regimens into ADLs. **EBN:** *The partnership process includes continued contact as changes occur; people with chronic illnesses need to know how to obtain interventions that are needed in the future (Lubkin & Larsen, 2006).*
- Record the effectiveness of managing the therapeutic regimens. **EBN:** *For clients who are at risk of ineffective management of therapeutic regimens, health providers may continue to assess and diagnose this phenomenon unnecessarily. It saves the healthcare system time, effort, and money if the assessment and diagnosis of effective management is communicated to other health providers.*

Multicultural

- Assess health literacy in clients of diverse backgrounds. **EB:** *Individuals with marginal or inadequate functional health literacy have difficulty reading, understanding, and interpreting most written health texts and instructions. In addition, clients with marginal or inadequate health literacy scores are more likely to misunderstand directions for health care (Redman, 2007).*
- Assess cultural relevance of health information. **EB:** *A study of breast health information needs of women from minority ethnic groups found that healthcare professionals' lack of understanding about cultural beliefs, values, and knowledge, together with racial stereotyping and misconceptions about cancer in minority ethnic groups, posed challenges to information dissemination (Watts et al, 2004).*
- Refer to care plan **Ineffective Therapeutic regimen management.**

Client/Family Teaching

- Teach about the disease trajectory and ways to manage disease symptoms as the trajectory changes.

evolve   See the EVOLVE website for World Wide Web resources for client education.

REFERENCES

Hibbard JH: Moving toward a more patient-centered health care delivery system, *Health AFF (Millwood)*, Suppl Web Exclusives: VAR133-135, 2004.

Holman H, Lorig K: Patient self management: a key to effectiveness and efficiency in care of chronic disease, *Public Health Rep* 119:239-243, 2004.

Lorig KR, Hurwicz ML, Sobel D et al: A national dissemination of an evidenced-based self management program: a process evaluation study, *Patient Educ Couns* 59:69-79, 2005.

Lorig KR, Ritter PL, Jacquez A: Outcomes of border health Spanish/English chronic disease self management programs, *Diabetes Educ* 31:401-409, 2005.

Lorig KR, Ritter PL, Laurent DD et al: Internet-based chronic disease self management: a randomized trial, *Med Care* 44:964-971, 2006.

Lubkin IM, Larsen PD: *Chronic illness: impact and interventions,* ed 6, Boston, 2006, Jones and Bartlett.

Pender NJ, Murdaugh CL, Parsons MA: *Health promotion in nursing practice,* ed 5, Upper Saddle River, NJ, 2006, Prentice Hall.

Redman BK: *The practice of patient education: a case study approach,* ed 10, St Louis, 2007, Mosby.

Rogers A, Kennedy A, Nelson E et al: Uncovering the limits of patient centeredness. Implementing a self management trail for chronic illness, *Qual Health Res* 15(2):224-239, 2005.

Stanford University: *Educational materials,* available at http://patient-education.stanford.edu/internet/. Accessed April 25, 2007.

Watts T, Merrell J, Murphy F et al: Breast health information needs of women from minority ethnic groups, *J Adv Nurs* 47(5):526-535, 2004.

T

• = Independent;   ▲ = Collaborative;   EBN = Evidence-Based Nursing;   EB = Evidence-Based

Ineffective Therapeutic regimen management

Margaret Lunney, RN, PhD, and Dawn Fairlie, MS, ANP, FNP, GNP, CDE

NANDA   Definition

Pattern of regulating and integrating into daily living a program for treatment of illness and the sequelae of illness that is unsatisfactory for meeting specific health goals.

Defining Characteristics

Failure to include treatment regimens in daily routines; failure to take action to reduce risk factors; makes choices in daily living ineffective for meeting health goals; verbalizes desire to manage the illness; verbalizes difficulty with prescribed regimens

Related Factors (r/t)

Complexity of health care system; complexity of therapeutic regimen; decisional conflicts; economic difficulties; excessive demands made (e.g., individual, family); family conflict; family patterns of health care; inadequate number of cues to action; knowledge deficit; mistrust of healthcare personnel; mistrust of regimen; perceived barriers; powerlessness; perceived seriousness; perceived susceptibility; perceived benefits; social support deficit

NOC   Outcomes (Nursing Outcomes Classification)

Suggested NOC Outcomes

Decision Making, Knowledge: Disease Process, Knowledge: Treatment Regimen, Participation in Health Care Decisions

Example NOC Outcome with Indicators
Knowledge: Treatment Regimen as evidenced by the following indicator: Description of prescribed medication, activity, exercise, and specific disease process (Rate the outcome and indicators of **Knowledge: Treatment Regimen:** 1 = none, 2 = limited, 3 = moderate, 4 = substantial, 5 = extensive [see Section I].)

Client Outcomes

Client Will (Specify Time Frame):

- Describe daily food and fluid intake that meets therapeutic goals
- Describe activity/exercise patterns that meet therapeutic goals
- Describe scheduling of medications that meets therapeutic goals
- Verbalize ability to manage therapeutic regimens
- Collaborate with health providers to decide on a therapeutic regimen that is congruent with health goals and lifestyle

NIC   Interventions (Nursing Interventions Classification)

Suggested NIC Interventions

Health Education, Health Screening, Health System Guidance, Learning Facilitation, Learning Readiness Enhancement

Example NIC Activities—Learning Facilitation
Present the information in a stimulating manner; Encourage the patient's active participation

Nursing Interventions and *Rationales*

NOTE: This diagnosis does not have the same meaning as the diagnosis **Noncompliance.** This diagnosis is made with the client, so if the client does not agree with the diagnosis, it should not be

• = Independent;   ▲ = Collaborative;   EBN = Evidence-Based Nursing;   EB = Evidence-Based

made. The emphasis is on helping the client direct his or her own life and health, not on the client's compliance with the provider's instructions.

- Refer to the care plans for **Effective Therapeutic regimen management** and **Ineffective family Therapeutic regimen management.**
- Establish a collaborative partnership with the client for purposes of meeting health-related goals. **EBN:** *Nurse-client partnerships reflect nursing models for practice (Farrell, Wicks & Martin, 2004; Pellatt, 2004) and are consistent with national healthcare goals and objectives (U.S. Department of Health and Human Services, 2000). This approach differs from a traditional healthcare model in which the provider assumes authoritative and paternalistic approaches to care (Pellatt, 2004). At least one study (Pellatt, 2004) showed that the professionals' perceptions of partnership behaviors were actually paternalistic behaviors.*
- Listen to the person's story about his or her illness self management. **EB:** *In a study of the meaning of active participation in self-management from the perspective of 16 participants aged 30 to 81 years client participation was found to be more complex than expected (Haidet, Kroll & Sharf, 2006). Implications of the study were that physicians and other providers may be able to influence the person's illness story positively by recognizing their part in the illness story.*
- Explore the meaning of the person's illness experience and identify uncertainties and needs through open-ended questions. **EB:** *Even though providers agree that self-management is the ideal approach to client care, studies show significant discrepancies between providers' and clients' views. Providers talk about self-management but may still expect compliance (Rogers et al, 2005).*
- Help the client identify the "self" in self-management; show respect for the client's self-determination. **EBN:** *In a qualitative study with 24 older adults with asthma, three self-management models were developed that reflected data from the participants (Koch, Jenkin & Kralik, 2004). Even the participants interpreted self-management as medical management and were mainly talking about compliance and adherence. Self-management means that the person uses self-determination to adapt medical and nursing recommendations for their own lives and personal needs (Farrell, Wicks & Martin, 2004).*
- Help the client enhance self-efficacy or confidence in his or her own ability to mange the illness. **EBN:** *In a pilot study using a quasiexperimental pretest/posttest design with 48 persons recruited from two clinics, specific self-management strategies to improve self-efficacy were associated with significant improvements in self-efficacy and self-management behaviors (Farrell, Wicks & Martin, 2004). A review of the literature led Sol et al (2005) to conclude that enhancement of self-efficacy was important to achieve optimal self-management.*
- Involve family members in knowledge development, planning for self-management, and shared decision making. **EBN:** *Family support was one of two predictors of positive self-management strategies in a study of 53 women with type 2 diabetes (Whittemore, Melkus & Grey, 2005). In a review of research related to self-management, family management was found to be integral to self-management (Grey, Knafl & McCorkle, 2006).*
- Review factors of the Health Belief Model (individual perceptions of seriousness and susceptibility, demographic and other modifying factors, and perceived benefits and barriers) with the client. **EBN:** *Studies using the Health Belief Model support the view that individual perceptions and a variety of modifying factors affect the likelihood of changing health behaviors (Pender, Murdaugh & Parsons, 2006). In a study of 52 post–myocardial infarction clients, following a physical activity regimen was associated with health motivation, whereas following professional advice on smoking cessation was associated with self-efficacy (Leong, Molassiotis & Marsh, 2004).*
- Identify the reasons for actions that are not therapeutic and discuss alternatives. **EBN:** *Many possible reasons exist for actions that do not meet therapeutic goals. Fatigue and pain can have profound effects on the ability to perform therapeutic actions (Krein et al, 2005). Perceptions may differ according to diseases. In a longitudinal study of 7991 middle-age and older adults, those who did not take medications as prescribed because the medications were too costly were 50% more likely to have adverse events such as heart attacks (Heisler, 2004).*
- Use various formats to provide information about the therapeutic regimen, including group education, brochures, videotapes, written instructions, computer-based programs, and telephone contact. **EB and EBN:** *In a 5-year study at Stanford University of more than 1000 clients with chronic illnesses, self-management education was effective in achieving positive outcomes (Lorig et al, 2006; Stanford University, 2007). In a systematic review of controlled clinical trials of clients with diabetes, it was determined that group-based training for self-management had many positive effects*

T

• = Independent;   ▲ = Collaborative;   EBN = Evidence-Based Nursing;   EB = Evidence-Based

(Deakin et al, 2005). In a study of two groups of adults (n = 16) with dyspnea, the results of Internet-based support on outcomes were tested. Most subjects reported that the Internet-based program increased their access to information and resources for managing their dyspnea (Nguyen et al, 2005). A telephone survey with 781 persons was found to yield reliable and valid data on self-management and other variables (Baker et al, 2005).

- Help the client identify and modify barriers to effective self-management. *In a random sample of 446 people with diabetes and focus groups with subgroups of six to 12 persons, it was found that many barriers exist to self-management (Vijan et al, 2005). Cost was the most commonly identified barrier. Other barriers were moderation in diet, medication therapies, need for small portion sizes, difficulties communicating with providers, and staying on a rigid schedule. In a cross-sectional study of 993 diabetic clients in the Veterans Association system, pain was identified as a significant barrier to diabetes self-management (Krein et al, 2005). In a study of 24 adults diagnosed with diabetes, the respondents identified the barrier of lack of knowledge and understanding of the diet and its relation to the illness (Nagelkerk, Reick & Meengs, 2006).*

- Help the client self-manage his or her own health through teaching about strategies for changing habits such as overeating, sedentary lifestyle, and smoking. **EB:** *Self-management education helps achieve positive health outcomes such as reductions in glycosylated hemoglobin levels and systolic blood pressure as well as fewer asthmatic attacks (Warsi et al, 2004).*

- Develop a contract with the client to maintain motivation for changes in behavior. **EBN:** *The nursing intervention of client contracting provides a concrete means of keeping track of actions to meet health-related goals (Dochterman & Bulechek, 2004).*

- Help the client maintain consistency in therapeutic regimen management for optimal results. **EBN:** *With clients on hemodialysis, self-management activities varied tremendously (Curtin et al, 2004).*

- Review how to contact health providers as needed to address issues and concerns regarding self-management. **EBN:** *The partnership process includes continued contact as changes occur; people with chronic illnesses need to know how to obtain interventions that are needed in the future (Pellatt, 2004).*

- Implement organizational changes to facilitate shared decision making for self-management of chronic illnesses. **EB:** *With the goal of shared decision making and instructions on how to accomplish this goal, providers still approach client care as if compliance were the goal. Organizational structures and patterns were found to contribute to the difficulty of adopting a client-centered self-management approach (Rogers et al, 2005).*

- Use focus groups to evaluate the implementation of self-management programs. **EBN:** *The focus group format facilitated identification and understanding of themes that were important to self-management (Benavides-Vaello et al, 2004; Vijan et al, 2005). Themes identified were health maintenance, barriers to self-management, self-awareness, familial support, folk remedies, and confidence to manage diabetes (Benavides-Vaello et al, 2004). In a larger study with quantitative and qualitative components, cost, portion size, and family support were found to be major issues of concern (Vijan et al, 2005).*

Multicultural

- Conduct a self-assessment of the relation of culture to ethnically based care. **EBN:** *A tool was developed by the Midwest Bioethics Center Cultural Diversity Task Force (2001) to help providers conduct self-reflection and examination for ethnically based care.*

- Provide support for self-management throughout the process of care. **EB:** *In a survey of 956 people in 17 locations throughout the country, respondents perceptions of provider support for self-management were found to be significantly related to better self-management (Greene & Yedidia, 2005). African Americans constituted 34% of the sample; Hispanics constituted 14%.*

- Assess the influence of cultural beliefs, norms, and values on the individual's perceptions of the therapeutic regimen. **EBN:** *Cultural beliefs and values may be individual or group related. One study of 186 low-income African Americans (n = 100) and whites (n = 86) found no substantial differences in self-management between groups. Yet, in other studies, African Americans, Latinos born in the United States, and Latinos born in Mexico were less likely to follow dietary recommendations (Sharma et al, 2004). A recent study showed that Hispanic psychiatric outpatients experienced akathisia as an increase in nerviosismo. Addressing this issue, as well as using anxiolytics and low doses of antipsychotics when beginning treatment, led to an improvement in medication taking (Opler et al, 2004).*

• = Independent; ▲ = Collaborative; EBN = Evidence-Based Nursing; EB = Evidence-Based

- Discuss all strategies with the client in the context of the client's culture. **EBN:** *Research studies involving culture, health behaviors, and self-management show that culture significantly affects decision making for meeting therapeutic goals and is related to self-management strategies (Degazon, 2006; Grey, Knafl & McCorkle, 2006).*
- Provide health information that is consistent with the health literacy of clients. **EB:** *Individuals with marginal or inadequate functional health literacy have difficulty reading, understanding, and interpreting most written health texts and instructions. In addition, clients with marginal or inadequate health literacy scores are more likely to misunderstand directions for health care (Georges, Bolton & Bennett, 2004).*
- Determine that health information is culturally relevant. **EB:** *A study of breast health information needs of women from minority ethnic groups found that healthcare professionals' lack of understanding about cultural beliefs, values, and knowledge, together with racial stereotyping and misconceptions about cancer in minority ethnic groups, posed challenges to information dissemination (Watts et al, 2004).*
- Assess for barriers that may interfere with client follow-up of treatment recommendations. **EB:** *Optimal follow-up of treatment regimen is often compounded by variables such as cost, availability of services, and convenience of accessing care. Knowledge of barriers to seeking health care is important when developing interventions to address self-management of therapeutic regimens (Unzueta et al, 2004).*
- Discuss with the client his or her beliefs about medication and treatment to enhance self-management of medications and other treatments. **EB:** *A study of Hispanic and African-American women found that improved self-management was associated with recognition of the serious consequences of not following prescribed regimens, realization of the beneficial effects, and the belief that medicines are not harmful (Unson et al, 2003).*
- Use electronic monitoring to improve management of medications. **EB:** *A recent study showed that the use of electronic monitors had a positive effect on medication taking for minority women (Robbins et al, 2004).*
- Validate the client's feelings regarding the ability to manage his or her own care and the impact on current lifestyle. **EB:** *A recent study elicited the expectations of treatment in 93 hypertensive African-American clients (Ogedegbe, Mancuso & Allegrante, 2004). Client expectations of treatment could serve as the basis for client education and counseling about hypertension and its management in this client population.*

Home Care

- Prepare and instruct clients and family members in the use of a medication box. Set up an appropriate schedule for filling of the medication box, and post medication times and doses in an accessible area (e.g., attached by a magnet to the refrigerator). *Improved self-management of therapeutic regimen is increased through the use of cues and supports that help clients remember to take medications.*
- Monitor self-management of the medical regimen. **EBN:** *In elderly clients with diabetes mellitus living alone, home visits (both daily and weekly) were associated with reductions in fasting blood sugar, postmeal blood sugar, and hemoglobin A1c (Huang et al, 2004).*
- ▲ Consult physician and/or pharmacist as questions arise. **EBN:** *A study demonstrated that nurses monitoring medication regimen and appropriate referral for medication review helped increase clients' knowledge of medications and appropriate use of aids to self-management (Griffiths et al, 2004).*

Client/Family Teaching

- Identify what the client and/or family knows and adjust teaching accordingly. *Teach the client and family about all aspects of the therapeutic regimen, providing as much knowledge as the client and family will accept, in a culturally congruent manner.*
- Teach ways to adjust ADLs for inclusion of therapeutic regimens.
- Teach safety in taking medications.
- Teach the client to act as a self-advocate with health providers who prescribe therapeutic regimens.

evolve   See the EVOLVE website for World Wide Web resources for client education.

REFERENCES

Baker DW, Brown J, Chan KS et al: A telephone survey to measure communication, education, self-management, and health status for patients with heart failure: the improving chronic illness care evaluations (ICICE), *J Card Failure* 11(1):36-42, 2005.

Benavides-Vaello S, Garcia AA, Brown SA et al: Using focus group to plan and evaluate diabetes self-management interventions for Mexican Americans, *Diabetes Educ* 30(2):238-256, 2004.

Curtin RB, Sitter DCB, Schatell D et al: Self-management, knowledge, and functioning and well being of patients on hemodialysis, *Neph Nurs J* 31(4):378-386, 2004.

Deakin T, McShane CE, Cade JE et al: Group-based training for self management strategies in people with type 2 diabetes mellitus, *Cochrane Database Sys Rev* (2):CD003417, 2005.

Degazon C: Cultural influences in nursing in community health. In Stanhope M, Lancaster J: *Foundations of nursing in the community: community-oriented practice,* ed 2, St Louis, 2006, Mosby.

Dochterman JM, Bulechek GM: *Nursing interventions classification (NIC),* ed 4, St Louis, Mosby, 2004.

Farrell K, Wicks MN, Martin JC: Chronic disease self management improved with enhanced self efficacy, *Clin Nurs Res* 13(4):289-308, 2004.

Georges CA, Bolton LB, Bennett C: Functional health literacy: an issue in African-American and other ethnic and racial communities, *J Natl Black Nurses Assoc* 15(1):1-4, 2004.

Greene J, Yedidia MJ: Provider behaviors contributing to patient self-management of chronic illness among underserved populations, *J Health Care Poor Underserved* 16:808-824, 2005.

Grey M, Knafl K, McCorkle R: A framework for the study of self- and family management of chronic conditions, *Nurs Outlook* 54:278-286, 2006.

Griffiths R, Johnson M, Piper M et al: A nursing intervention for the quality use of medicines by elderly community clients, *Intl J Nurs Pract* 10(4):166, 2004.

Haidet P, Kroll TL, Sharf BF: The complexity of patient participation: lessons learned from patients' illness narratives, *Patient Educ Couns* 62:323-329, 2006.

Heisler M: The health effects of restricting prescription medication use because of cost, *Med Care* 42(7):626-634, 2004.

Huang CL, Wu SC, Jeng CY et al: The efficacy of a home-based nursing program in diabetic control of elderly people with diabetes mellitus living alone, *Publ Health Nurse* 21(1):49, 2004.

Koch T, Jenkin P, Kralik D: Chronic illness self management: locating the "self." *J Adv Nurs* 48:484-492, 2004.

Krein SL, Heisler M, Piette JD et al: The effect of chronic pain on diabetes patients' self-management, *Diabetes Care* 28(1):65-70, 2005.

Leong J, Molassiotis A, Marsh H: Adherence to health recommendations after a cardiac rehabilitation programme in post-myocardial infarction patients: the role of heath beliefs, locus of control and psychological status, *Clin Effectiveness Nurs* 8(1):26-38, 2004.

Lorig KR, Ritter PL, Laurent DD et al: Internet-based chronic disease self management: a randomized trial, *Med Care* 44:964-971, 2006.

Midwest Bioethics Center: Healthcare narratives from diverse communities—a self-assessment tool for health-care providers, *Bioethics Forum* 17(3-4):SS1, 2001.

Nagelkerk J, Reick K, Meengs L: Perceived barriers and effective strategies to diabetes self-management, *J Adv Nurs* 54:151-158, 2006.

Nguyen HQ, Carrieri-Kohlman V, Rankin SH et al: Is Internet-based support for dyspnea self-management in patients with chronic obstructive pulmonary disease possible? Results of a pilot study, *Heart Lung* 34(1):51-62, 2005.

Ogedegbe G, Mancuso CA, Allegrante JP: Expectations of blood pressure management in hypertensive African-American patients: a qualitative study, *J Natl Med Assoc* 96(4):442-449, 2004.

Opler LA, Ramirez PM, Dominguez LM et al: Rethinking medication prescribing practices in an inner-city Hispanic mental health clinic, *J Psychiatr Pract* 10(2):134-140, 2004.

Pellatt GC: Patient-professional partnership in spinal cord injury rehabilitation, *Br J Nurs* 13(16):948-953, 2004.

Pender NJ, Murdaugh CL, Parsons MA: *Health promotion in nursing practice,* ed 5, Upper Saddle River, NJ, 2006, Prentice Hall.

Robbins B, Rausch KJ, Garcia RI et al: Multicultural medication adherence: a comparative study, *J Gerontol Nurs* 30(7):25-32, 2004.

Rogers A, Kennedy A, Nelson E et al: Uncovering the limits of patient centeredness: implementing a self management trail for chronic illness, *Qual Health Res* 15(2):224-239, 2005.

Sharma S, Murphy SP, Wilkens LR et al: Adherence to the food guide pyramid recommendations among African Americans and Latinos: results from the Multiethnic Cohort, *J Am Diet Assoc* 104(12):1873-1877, 2004.

Sol BGM, Van Der Biji JJ, Banga JD et al: Vascular risk management through nurse-led self management programs, *J Vasc Nurs* 23(1):20-24, 2005.

Stanford University, Department of Medicine: *Educational materials,* available at http://patienteducation.stanford.edu/internet/. Accessed April 25, 2007.

Unson CG, Siccion E, Gaztambide J et al: Nonadherence and osteoporosis treatment preferences of older women: a qualitative study, *J Womens Health (Larchmt)* 12(10):1037-1045, 2003.

Unzueta M, Globe D, Wu J et al: Los Angeles Latino Eye Study Group. Compliance with recommendations for follow-up care in Latinos: the Los Angeles Latino Eye Study, *Ethn Dis* 14(2):285-291, 2004.

U.S. Department of Health and Human Services: *Healthy People 2010,* 2000, www.healthypeople.gov, accessed March 1, 2007.

Vijan S, Stuart, NS, Fitzgerald JT et al: Barriers to following dietary recommendations in type 2 diabetes, *Diabet Med* 22(1):32-38, 2005.

Warsi A, Wang PS, LaValley MP et al: Self management education programs in chronic disease, *Arch Intern Med* 164:1641-1649, 2004.

Watts T, Merrell J, Murphy F et al: Breast health information needs of women from minority ethnic groups, *J Adv Nurs* 47(5):526-535, 2004.

Whittemore R, Melkus GD, Grey M: Metabolic control, self management and psychosocial adjustment in women with type 2 diabetes, *J Clin Nurs* 14(2):195-204, 2005.

Ineffective community Therapeutic regimen management

Margaret Lunney, RN, PhD, and Dawn Fairlie, MS, ANP, FNP, GNP, CDE

NANDA   Definition

Pattern of regulating and integrating into community processes programs for treatment of illness and the sequelae of illness that are unsatisfactory for meeting health-related goals

• = Independent;   ▲ = Collaborative;   EBN = Evidence-Based Nursing;   EB = Evidence-Based

Defining Characteristics

Deficits in advocates for aggregates; deficits in community activities for prevention; illness symptoms above the norm expected for the population; insufficient healthcare resources (e.g., people, programs); unavailable healthcare resources for illness care; unexpected acceleration of illness

Related Factors (r/t)

To be developed.

NOC   Outcomes (Nursing Outcomes Classification)

Suggested NOC Outcomes

Community Competence, Community Health Status, Community Health Status: Immunity, Community Risk Control: Chronic Disease, Community Risk Control: Communicable Disease, Community Risk Control: Lead Exposure

Example NOC Outcome with Indicators
Community Health Status as evidenced by the following indicators: Participation rates in preventive health services/Prevalence of health protection and health promotion programs/Mortality rates/Morbidity rates/Mental health illness rates/Chronic disease rates/Low birth weight rates/Injury rates (Rate the outcome and indicators of **Community Health:** 1 = poor, 2 = fair, 3 = good, 4 = very good, 5 = excellent [see Section I].)

Community Outcomes

Community Members and Leaders Will (Specify Time Frame):

- Secure community members and/or health providers who will be accountable for illness care of specific groups.
- Remain involved in advocacy for illness care and prevention programs.
- Develop healthcare plans for effective prevention and treatment of illnesses.
- Make resources available for illness care and prevention.
- Initiate or improve strategies for prevention of the sequelae of illness.

NIC   Interventions (Nursing Interventions Classification)

Suggested NIC Interventions

Community Health Development, Case Management, Health Education, Environmental Management: Community, Health Policy Monitoring, Health Screening, Risk Identification
NOTE: NIC interventions that were developed for use with individuals can be adapted for use with communities.

Example NIC Activities—Community Health Development
Identify health concerns, strengths, and priorities with community partners; Facilitate implementation and revision of community plans

Nursing Interventions and *Rationales*

NOTE: Nursing interventions are conducted in collaboration with community leaders, community and public health nurses, and members of other disciplines (Anderson & McFarlane, 2006; Chinn, 2001).

- Implement strategies to engage community members to be team members for health assessments and development of community programs. **EB:** *In the conduct of community health assessments in 105 counties of Kansas, team building of health providers with community leaders was an important aspect of success (Curtis, 2002). The experiences of numerous other communities have shown that community participation is critical to the success of programs for illness prevention and control and reducing health disparities (e.g., Faust et al, 2005; Horowitz et al, 2004; Kieffer et al, 2004; Thacker, 2005).*

• = Independent;   ▲ = Collaborative;   EBN = Evidence-Based Nursing;   EB = Evidence-Based

▲ Request that a clinical nurse specialist in community health nursing work with coalitions of health providers and community leaders. **EBN:** *Community health nurses who are prepared as clinical nurse specialists have competencies in direct care of communities and community-based organizations and networks (Logan, 2005).*

▲ Recruit additional health providers as needed. **EB and EBN:** *Designing and implementing community-based programs requires the participation of providers from multiple disciplines working alongside community members (Anderson & McFarland, 2006; Chinn, 2001).*

• Establish special action groups for specific problems and/or localities to address health policies and practices. **EB:** *After 3 years, two special action groups in Arizona with a focus on diabetes prevention and control successfully documented changes in local policies and practices (Meister & Guernsey de Zapien, 2005).*

• Evaluate community infrastructures for adequacy in serving community illness-related needs. **EB:** *Community infrastructures are important aspects of self-management, including health policies, illness-focused education, availability of services and resources, and so forth (Chaffee & Arthur, 2002; Ingram, Gallegos & Elenes, 2005).*

• Advocate for and with the community in multiple arenas (e.g., newspapers, television, legislative bodies, community boards). **EBN:** *Many communities have benefited from the advocacy of nurses and other health providers whose opinions are respected (Anderson & McFarlane, 2006; Chinn 2001).*

• Provide information to public and private sources about community assessment, diagnosis, and plans of care. **EBN:** *The commitment needed for improvements in health services can be obtained only when community members have adequate information (Anderson & McFarland, 2006).*

• Mobilize support for the community to obtain the resources necessary for illness care and prevention. **EB:** *In a study of the Cardiovascular Health Network Project using focus groups with women participants, lack of community resources and support were identified as barriers for women from some communities to practice health-promoting activities such as physical exercise (Eyler et al, 2002).*

• Establish culturally sensitive community health programs for self-management. **EB:** *In New York City, between 2001 and 2004, emergency department and unscheduled physician office visits for asthma-related problems were reduced from 35% to 8% after 18 months of a culturally sensitive, community-based program (Centers for Disease Control and Prevention, 2005). Many other studies have shown that community-based programs for illness care and prevention have positive results (Garvin et al, 2004; Lee et al, 2004).*

• Provide coaching interventions in programs for chronic disease self-management. **EBN:** *The positive client outcomes of a community-based nursing program with a focus on coaching showed that nursing programs can successfully engage middle-age and older adults in health promotion and protection activities (Tidwell et al, 2004).*

• Integrate the Internet with community health programs. **EB:** *The Internet is widely used by consumers of all ages and ethnicities (e.g., in a study of 208 church-based African Americans, 47% used the Internet for health-related information) (Laken et al, 2004).*

• Determine the cultural appropriateness of all programs. **EBN:** *The cultural appropriateness of a program is an indicator of the potential success of the program (Leininger & McFarland, 2006).*

• Support the population of family caregivers through implementation of the National Family Support Program. **EB:** *A study of community leaders in 10 states showed that programs to support family caregivers are underway and are sorely needed to relieve the burden of family caregiving (Feinberg & Newman, 2004).*

• Write grant proposals for the funding of new programs or the expansion of existing programs (Coley & Scheinberg, 2007). **EB:** *Public and private sources of funds can often supply the financial bases of healthcare programs (Anderson & McFarlane, 2006).*

• Conduct research studies to convince others of the need to improve services or change policies. **EBN:** *Research findings may be needed to obtain broad support for needed changes (Anderson & McFarland, 2006). For example, in the last few decades nurses have conducted research studies on the topic of battered women who were successful in influencing legislators to change laws and public policies in ways that positively affected the prevention and treatment of violence against women. A recent example of this type of research showed a definite link between abuse during pregnancy and attempted and completed homicide of women (McFarlane et al, 2002).*

• = Independent;   ▲ = Collaborative;   EBN = Evidence-Based Nursing;   EB = Evidence-Based

- Avoid victim-blaming stances in efforts to promote community responsibility for health. **EB:** *Based on 40 years of work with multiple agencies, Green and Kreuter (2005) identified multiple determinants of health besides local community participation. Some of these determinants include national health policy, media, resources, and organizations.*

 Multicultural

- Refer to care plan **Ineffective community Coping.**
- Hire culturally diverse staff members for community agencies. **EB:** *In a study of 22 community agencies that provide end-of-life care in a southeastern state, the presence of more diverse staff members or volunteers was associated with more diverse clients. Culturally diverse services were more likely to be provided when directors provided leadership in welcoming diversity (Reese, Melton & Ciaravino, 2004).*
- Identify the health services and information resources currently available in the community. **EBN:** *This will help focus efforts and promote the wise use of valuable resources. Many communities of color lack access to culturally competent healthcare providers, pharmacies, and grocery stores (National Institutes of Health, 1998).*
- Identify cultural barriers such as acculturation issues, lack of community support, and lack of experience with a health behavior. **EBN:** *Cultural barriers to exercise regimens were identified in a series of focus groups with women in the Cardiovascular Health Network Project (Eyler et al, 2002).*
- Develop a health promotion directory that lists health resources for clients. **EB:** *A study that assessed utilization of a health promotion directory found that African-American group members were significantly more likely to contact one of the resources listed in the health directory (Haber & Looney, 2003).*

evolve See the EVOLVE website for World Wide Web resources for client education.

REFERENCES

Anderson ET, McFarlane J: *Community as partner: theory and practice in nursing,* ed 5, Philadelphia, 2006, Lippincott, Williams & Wilkins.

Centers for Disease Control and Prevention: Reducing childhood asthma through community-based service delivery, New York City, 2001-2004, *MMWR,* 54(1):11-14, 2005.

Chaffee MW, Arthur DC: Failure: lessons for health care leaders, *Nurs Econ* 20(5):225-228, 231, 2002.

Chinn PL: Making a difference in health care, *ANS Adv Nurs Sci* 24(1):v, 2001.

Coley SM, Scheinberg CA: *Proposal writing,* ed 3, Thousand Oaks, CA, 2007, Sage.

Curtis DC: Evaluation of community health assessment in Kansas, *J Public Manage Pract* 8(4):2-25, 2002.

Eyler AA, Matson-Koffman D, Vest JR et al: Environmental, policy, and cultural factors related to physical activity in a diverse sample of women: the Women's Cardiovascular Health Network Project—summary and discussion, *Women Health* 36(2):123, 2002.

Faust LA, Blanchard LW, Breyfogle DA et al: Discussion suppers as a means for community engagement, *J Rural Health* 21(1):92-95, 2005.

Feinberg LF, Newman SL: A study of 10 states since passage of the national family caregiver support program: policies, perceptions and program development, *Gerontologist* 44(6):760-769, 2004.

Garvin CC, Cheadle A, Chrisman N et al: A community-based approach to diabetes control in multiple cultural groups, *Ethn Dis* 14(3 suppl 1):S83-S92, 2004.

Green LW, Kreuter MW: *Health promotion planning: an education and ecological approach,* ed 4, New York, 2005, McGraw Hill.

Haber D, Looney C: Health promotion directory: development, distribution, and utilization, *Health Promotion Pract* 4(1):72-77, 2003.

Horowitz CR, Arniella A, James S et al: Using community-based participatory research to reduce health disparities in East and Central Harlem, *MT Sinai J Med* 71(6):368-374, 2004.

Ingram M, Gallegos G, Elenes J: Diabetes is a community issue: the

critical elements of a successful outreach and education model on the U.S.-Mexico Border, *Prev Chronic Dis* 2(1):A15, 2005.

Kieffer EC, Willis SK, Odoms-Young AM et al: Reducing disparities in diabetes among African American and Latino residents of Detroit: the essential role of community planning focus groups, *Ethn Dis* 14(3 suppl 1):S27-S37, 2004.

Laken MA, O'Rourke K, Duffy NG et al: Use of the Internet for health information by African Americans with modifiable risk factors for cardiovascular disease, *J E Health* 10(3):304-310, 2004.

Lee S, Naimark B, Porter MM et al: Effects of a long term, community-based cardiac rehabilitation program on middle aged and elderly cardiac patient, *Am J Geriatr Cardiol* 13(6):293-298, 2004.

Leininger MM, McFarland MR: *Cultural care diversity and universality: a worldwide nursing theory,* ed 2, Boston, 2006, Jones and Bartlett.

Logan L: The practice of certified community health CNSs, *Clin Nurse Spec* 19(1):43-48, 2005.

McFarlane J, Campbell JC, Sharps P et al: Abuse during pregnancy and femicide: urgent implications for women's health, *Obstet Gynecol* 100(1):27, 2002.

Meister JS, Guernsey de Zapien J: Bringing health policy issues front and center in the community: expanding the role of community health coalitions, *Prev Chronic Dis* 2(1):A16, 2005.

National Institutes of Health: *Salud para su corazo´n: bringing heart health to Latinos—a guide for building community programs,* DHHS Pub No. 98-3796, Washington, DC, 1998, U.S. Government Printing Office.

Reese DJ, Melton E, Ciaravino K: Programmatic barriers to providing culturally competent end-of-life care, *Am J Hosp Palliat Care* 21(5):357-364, 2004.

Thacker K: Academic-community partnerships: opening the doors to a nursing career, *J Transcult Nurs* 16(1):57-63, 2005.

Tidwell L, Holland SK, Greenberg J et al: Community-based nurse health coaching and its effect on fitness participation, *Lippincott Case Manag* 9(6):267-279, 2004.

T

• = Independent;   ▲ = Collaborative;   EBN = Evidence-Based Nursing;   EB = Evidence-Based

Ineffective family Therapeutic regimen management

Margaret Lunney, RN, PhD, and Dawn Fairlie, MS, ANP, FNP, GNP, CDE

NANDA   Definition

Pattern of regulating and integrating into family processes a program for treatment of illness and the sequelae of illness that is unsatisfactory for meeting specific health goals

Defining Characteristics

Acceleration of illness symptoms of a family member; failure to take actions to reduce risk factors; inappropriate family activities for meeting health goals; lack of attention to illness; verbalizes desire to manage the illness; verbalizes difficulty with therapeutic regimen

Related Factors (r/t)

Complexity of health care system; complexity of therapeutic regimen; decisional conflicts; economic difficulties; excessive demands; family conflict

NOC   Outcomes (Nursing Outcomes Classification)

Suggested NOC Outcomes

Health-Seeking Behavior, Knowledge: Treatment Regimen, Participation in Health Care Decisions

Example NOC Outcome with Indicators
Knowledge: Treatment Regimen as evidenced by the following indicator: Description of prescribed medication, activity, exercise, and specific disease process (Rate the outcome and indicators of **Knowledge: Treatment Regimen:** 1 = none, 2 = limited, 3 = moderate, 4 = substantial, 5 = extensive [see Section I].)

Family Outcomes

Family Will (Specify Time Frame):

- Make adjustments in usual activities (e.g., diet, activity, stress management) to incorporate therapeutic regimens of its members
- Reduce illness symptoms of family members
- Desire to manage therapeutic regimens of its members
- Describe a decrease in the difficulties of managing therapeutic regimens
- Describe actions to reduce risk factors

NIC   Interventions (Nursing Interventions Classification)

Suggested NIC Interventions

Family Involvement Promotion, Family Mobilization, Teaching: Disease Process

Example NIC Activities—Family Involvement Promotion
Identify and respect coping mechanisms used by family members; Provide crucial information to family members about the patient in accordance with client's preference

Nursing Interventions and *Rationales*

- Base family interventions on knowledge of the family, family context, and family function. **EBN:** *Family research has established that families differ widely from one another, even within cultures (Wright & Leahey, 2005). Family context includes all aspects of the larger societal systems. In a literature review, family functioning was shown to have positive effects on self-management (Grey, Knafl & McCorkle, 2006).*

• = Independent;   ▲ = Collaborative;   EBN = Evidence-Based Nursing;   EB = Evidence-Based

- Use a family approach when helping an individual with a health problem that requires therapeutic management. **EBN:** *In a family health model developed from three qualitative studies involving Appalachian families from Ohio, health habits were shown to be largely taught and defined within the family, so therapeutic regimens need to be addressed with the family (Denham, 2002). In studies of self-management, family support was found to be a predictor of positive self-management (Whittemore, Melkus & Grey, 2005; Leong, Molassiotis & Marsh, 2004).*
- Identify family interactions and their embedded contexts relative to specific health objectives. **EBN:** *Family-focused practice requires viewing each interaction to accomplish health objectives as an opportunity to address the household production of health or work toward health objectives (Denham, 2002).*
- Review with family members the congruence and incongruence of family behaviors and health-related goals. **EBN:** *To attain the motivation needed for changes in health habits, family members should understand the relation of daily habits to health-related goals (Wright & Leahey, 2005).*
- Help family members make decisions regarding ways to integrate therapeutic regimens into daily living. Provide advice or suggestions as solicited and accepted by the family. **EBN:** *Decisions made by the family rather than by health providers or others guide everyday actions (Denham, 2002).*
- Demonstrate respect for and trust in family decisions. **EBN:** *People make decisions that they believe are appropriate for them. Family members who are respected and trusted by health providers are more likely to collaborate effectively with them (Denham, 2002).*
- Acknowledge the challenge of integrating therapeutic regimens with family behaviors. **EBN:** *Therapeutic regimens require modifications of daily activities that have already been established based on family values and beliefs. Acknowledging the difficulty of changing family habits supports families through the process (Wright & Leahey, 2005).*
- Review the symptoms of specific illness(es) and work with the family toward development of greater self-efficacy in relation to these symptoms. **EBN:** *Knowledge of symptoms improves the ability of family members to adjust behaviors to prevent and manage symptoms (Lubkin & Larsen, 2006).*
- Support family decisions to adjust therapeutic regimens as indicated. **EBN:** *Sometimes families do not have access to health providers and should make independent decisions because of side effects or adverse effects of therapeutic regimens. Family members need to make informed decisions in their best interests (Wright & Leahey, 2005).*
- ▲ Advocate for the family in negotiating therapeutic regimens with health providers. **EB:** *Illness regimens generally are neither arbitrary nor absolute; therefore modifications can be discussed as needed to fit with the family lifestyle (Wright & Leahey, 2005).*
- Help the family mobilize social supports. **EBN:** *Increased social support helps families to meet health-related goals (Pender, Murdaugh & Parsons, 2006).*
- Help family members modify perceptions as indicated. **EBN:** *Individual perceptions of the seriousness of, susceptibility to, and threat of illness may be distorted or inaccurate and may be modified with new information (Pender, Murdaugh & Parsons, 2006).*
- Use one or more theories of family dynamics to describe, explain, or predict family behaviors (e.g., theories of Bowen, Satir, and Minuchin). **EBN:** *Family systems may not be understood by the nurse without adequate knowledge of family theory (Denham, 2002; Wright & Leahey, 2005).*
- ▲ Collaborate with expert nurses or other consultants regarding strategies for working with families. **EBN:** *Family systems are complex and challenging (Wright & Leahey, 2005); expert nurses can assist with problem solving and planning.*
- Promote and support public health programs to support families. **EB:** *Because the burden of family care is significant, a national effort is underway to support family caregivers, the National Family Caregiver Support Program. One study showed that 10 states have begun development of such programs (Feinberg & Newman, 2004).*
- Coaching methods can be used to help families improve their health. **EB:** *Coaching processes were shown to improve family outcomes related to improved nutrition and physical activity (Heimendinger et al, 2007).*

Multicultural

- Acknowledge racial and ethnic differences at the onset of care. **EBN:** *Acknowledgment of race and ethnicity issues enhances communication, establishes rapport, and promotes treatment outcomes (Leininger & McFarland, 2006).*

● = Independent;   ▲ = Collaborative;   EBN = Evidence-Based Nursing;   EB = Evidence-Based

- Ensure that all strategies for working with the family are congruent with the culture of the family. **EBN:** *Many nursing studies among people of a variety of cultures show that cultural variations exist in the management of therapeutic regimens, and these differences should be taken into account when working with families (Degazon, 2006; Leininger & McFarland, 2006).*
- Approach families of color with respect, warmth, and professional courtesy. **EBN:** *Instances of disrespect and lack of caring have special significance for families of color (Degazon, 2006).*
- Give a rationale when assessing African-American families about sensitive issues. **EBN:** *African Americans may expect white caregivers to hold negative and preconceived ideas about African Americans. Giving a rationale for questions asked may help reduce this perception.*
- Support religious beliefs and the comfort role of religion. **EBN:** *Studies have shown a strong relation between religion and subjective health and that subjective health is predictive of health outcomes (Harvey, 2006).*
- Use a family-centered approach when working with Latino, Asian, African-American, and Native-American clients. **EBN:** *Latinos may perceive the family as a source of support, solver of problems, and source of pride. Asian Americans may regard the family as the primary decision maker and influence on individual family members. Native-American families may have extended structures and exert powerful influences over functioning (Leininger & McFarland, 2006).*
- Facilitate modeling and role playing for the family regarding healthy ways to communicate and interact. **EBN:** *It is helpful for families and the client to practice communication skills in a safe environment before trying them in a real-life situation (Degazon, 2006; Wright & Leahey, 2005).*
- Use the nursing intervention of cultural brokerage to help families deal with the healthcare system. **EBN:** *Cultural brokerage helps individuals and families integrate their cultural values, beliefs, and traditions with health care decision making (Dagazon, 2006).*

Client/Family Teaching

- Teach about all aspects of therapeutic regimens. Provide as much knowledge as family members will accept, adjust instruction to account for what the family already knows, and provide information in a culturally congruent manner.
- Teach ways to adjust family behaviors to include therapeutic regimens.
- ▲ Teach safety in taking medications.
- ▲ Teach family members to act as self-advocates with health providers who prescribe therapeutic regimens.

evolve   See the EVOLVE website for World Wide Web resources for client education.

REFERENCES

Degazon C: Cultural influences in nursing in community health. In Stanhope M, Lancaster J, editors: *Foundations of nursing in the community: community-oriented practice*, ed 2, St Louis, 2006, Mosby.

Denham SA: Family routines: a structural perspective for viewing family health, *ANS Adv Nurs Sci* 24(4):60, 2002.

Feinberg LF, Newman SL: A study of 10 states since passage of the national family caregiver support program: policies, perceptions, and program development, *Gerontologist* 44:760-769, 2004.

Grey M, Knafl K, McCorkle R: A framework for the study of self- and family management of chronic conditions, *Nurs Outlook* 54:278-286, 2006.

Harvey IS: Self management of a chronic illness: an exploratory study on the role of spirituality among older African American women, *J Women Aging* 18(3):75-88, 2006.

Heimendinger J, Uyeki T, Andhara A et al: Coaching process outcomes of a family visit nutrition and physical activity intervention, *Health Educ Behav* 34:71-89, 2007.

Leininger MM, McFarland MR: *Culture care diversity and universality: a worldwide nursing theory*, ed 2, Boston, 2006, Jones & Bartlett.

Leong J, Molassiotis A, Marsh H: Adherence to health recommendations after a cardiac rehabilitation programme in post-myocardial infarction patients: the role of heath beliefs, locus of control and psychological status, *Clin Eff Nurs* 8(1):26-38, 2004.

Lubkin IM, Larsen PD: *Chronic illness: impact and interventions*, ed 6, Boston, 2006, Jones and Bartlett.

Pender NJ, Murdaugh CL, Parsons MA: *Health promotion in nursing practice*, ed 5, Upper Saddle River, NJ, 2006, Prentice Hall.

Whittemore R, Melkus GD, Grey M: Metabolic control, self management and psychosocial adjustment in women with type 2 diabetes, *J Clin Nurs* 14:195-204, 2005.

Wright LM, Leahey M: *Nurses and families: a guide to family assessment and intervention*, ed 4, Philadelphia, 2005, F.A. Davis.

T

• = Independent;   ▲ = Collaborative;   EBN = Evidence-Based Nursing;   EB = Evidence-Based

Readiness for enhanced Therapeutic regimen management

Margaret Lunney, RN, PhD, and Dawn Fairlie, MS, ANP, FNP, GNP, CDE

NANDA   Definition

Pattern of regulating and integrating into daily living a program for treatment of illness and its sequelae that is sufficient for meeting health-related goals and can be strengthened

Defining Characteristics

Choices of daily living are appropriate for meeting goals (e.g., treatment, prevention); describes reduction of risk factors; expresses desire to manage the illness (e.g., treatment, prevention of sequelae); expresses little difficulty with prescribed regimens; no unexpected acceleration of illness symptoms

NOC   Outcomes (Nursing Outcomes Classification)

Suggested NOC Outcomes

Health-Promoting Behavior, Health-Seeking Behavior, Knowledge: Health Behavior, Health Promotion, Health Resources, Illness Care, Medication, Prescribed Activity, Treatment Regimen

> #### Example NOC Outcome with Indicators
>
> **Health-Promoting Behavior** as evidenced by the following indicators: Monitors personal behavior for risks/ Seeks balance among exercise, work, leisure, rest, and nutrition/Performs healthy behaviors routinely/Uses financial and physical resources to promote health (Rate each indicator of **Health-Promoting Behavior:** 1 = never demonstrated, 2 = rarely demonstrated, 3 = sometimes demonstrated, 4 = often demonstrated, 5 = consistently demonstrated [see Section I].)

Client Outcomes

Client Will (Specify Time Frame):

- Describe integration of therapeutic regimen into daily living
- Demonstrate continued commitment to integration of therapeutic regimen into daily living routines

NIC   Interventions (Nursing Interventions Classification)

Suggested NIC Interventions

Anticipatory Guidance, Mutual Goal Setting, Patient Contracting, Self-Modification Assistance, Self-Responsibility Facilitation, Support System Enhancement, Teaching: Disease Process

> #### Example NIC Activities—Mutual Goal Setting
>
> Assist the patient in prioritizing (weighing) identified goals; Clarify with the patient roles of the healthcare provider and the patient, respectively

T

Nursing Interventions and *Rationales*

- Acknowledge the expertise that the client and family bring to self-management. **EBN:** *Older people diagnosed with asthma used three different models of self-management: a medical model, collaborative model, and self-agency model. To achieve optimal self-agency, it was recommended that healthcare professionals respect the expertise of clients (Koch, Jenkin & Kralik, 2004). The Patient Education Department of Stanford University, Department of Medicine, directed by Dr. Kate Lorig developed a client education program for self-management that is widely disseminated (Stanford University, 2007). Through 5 years of systematic research with more than 1000 clients, they established that client education in self-management is effective to improve health outcomes.*

• = Independent;   ▲ = Collaborative;   EBN = Evidence-Based Nursing;   EB = Evidence-Based

- Review factors that contribute to the likelihood of health promotion and health protection. Use Pender's Health Promotion Model and Becker's Health Belief Model to identify contributing factors (Pender, Murdaugh & Parsons, 2006). **EBN:** *Many studies using both the Health Promotion Model and the Health Belief Model support the view that individual perceptions and a variety of modifying factors affect the likelihood of improving health behaviors (Pender, Murdaugh & Parsons, 2006). In post–myocardial clients in the United Kingdom, adhering to physical activity was associated with health motivation, and adhering to smoking cessation was associated with self-efficacy (Leong et al, 2004). Adherence to healthy diet was accounted for by the extent that family members encouraged the client to follow the therapeutic regimen.*

- Assess for depression. **EB:** *In diabetic clients in a Korean clinic, depression was an explanatory factor for those reporting low adherence with self-care (Park et al, 2004). In post–myocardial clients in the United Kingdom, more than 19% had symptoms of depression, which were thought to contribute to low adherence (Leong et al, 2004).*

- Facilitate the client and family to obtain health insurance and drug payment plans whenever needed and possible. **EB:** *In African Americans, those who had health insurance reported the influence of health providers on self-care more frequently (Becker, Gates & Newsom, 2004). In older Americans, underuse of prescription medications because of cost was found to lead to adverse health effects (Heisler, 2004).*

- Further develop and reinforce contributing factors that might change with ongoing management of the therapeutic regimen (e.g., knowledge, self-efficacy, self-esteem, and perceived benefits). **EBN:** *Illness care is associated with ongoing changes and, over time, management of therapeutic regimens can become increasingly tedious and difficult (Lubkin & Larsen, 2006).*

- Support all efforts to self-manage therapeutic regimens. **EBN:** *Ongoing support and assistance from healthcare providers is needed to identify and enhance factors that contribute to the likelihood of taking action for health promotion and health protection (Pender, Murdaugh & Parsons, 2006). For adults with osteoarthritis, exercise was found to benefit the participants and increased attention by health providers to improving clients' self-efficacy and belief systems likely facilitated adherence (Belza et al, 2002).*

- Review the client's strengths in the management of the therapeutic regimen. **EBN:** *People who are doing the work of managing a therapeutic regimen may not even realize they are doing it well (Lubkin & Larsen, 2006).*

- Collaborate with the client to identify strategies to maintain strengths and develop additional strengths as indicated. **EBN:** *The client and provider working in partnership can facilitate, support, and reinforce the client's strengths (Bidmead & Cowley, 2005; Kettunen et al, 2006).*

- Identify contributing factors that may need to be improved now or in the future. **EBN:** *Health promotion and protection are complex behaviors that are difficult to implement on a daily basis. Based on the complexity of achieving these behaviors and the perceived barriers to implementation (e.g., time, energy, money), usually one or more contributing factors would benefit from increased focus and attention (Pender, Murdaugh & Parsons, 2006).*

- Provide knowledge as needed related to the pathophysiology of the disease or illness, prescribed activities, prescribed medications, and nutrition. **EBN:** *Knowledge is a factor that contributes significantly to the client's taking action for health promotion and protection (Pender, Murdaugh & Parsons, 2006). Remember, however, that knowledge is necessary but not sufficient to explain why people perform or do not perform actions for health promotion and protection (Pender, Murdaugh & Parsons, 2006).*

- Use coaching strategies such as educational reinforcement, psychosocial support, and motivational guidance. **EB:** *In a study involving individuals newly diagnosed with type 2 diabetes, nurse coaching yielded a modest increase in health-promoting behaviors and a decrease in fasting blood glucose level (Whittemore, Chase & Mandle, 2001).*

- Support positive health-promotion and health-protection behaviors. **EBN:** *Ongoing support may be needed to maintain these behaviors (Pender, Murdaugh & Parsons, 2006).*

- Help the client maintain existing support and seek additional supports as needed. **EBN:** *In numerous research studies, social support was shown to be a factor contributing to ongoing maintenance of positive health behaviors (Lubkin & Larsen, 2006; Pender, Murdaugh & Parsons, 2006). For example, in a study of long-term survivors of cancer, social support and self-esteem were two of the three variables that explained 53% of the variance in health-related quality of life (Pedro, 2001).*

Multicultural

- Manipulate community factors that may affect the management of the therapeutic regimen (e.g., barriers, supports, insurance, education about the illness, and provider-client relationships). **EBN:** *A study involving African-American clients with diabetes concluded that complex environmental factors can indirectly affect glycemic control and management of the therapeutic regimen (Brody et al, 2001).*
- Validate the client's feelings regarding the ability to manage his or her own care and the impact on current lifestyle. **EB:** *A recent study elicited the expectations of treatment in 93 hypertensive African-American clients. Client expectations of treatment could serve as the basis for client education and counseling about hypertension and its management in this client population (Ogedegbe, Mancuso & Allegrante, 2004).*
- Use electronic monitoring to improve medication adherence. **EB:** *A recent study showed that the use of electronic monitors had a positive effect on adherence for minority women (Robbins et al, 2004).*
- Discuss with clients their beliefs about medication and treatment to enhance medication and treatment adherence. **EB and EBN:** *Various cultures have different beliefs regarding medication and treatments (Leininger & McFarland, 2006). Fowles (2007) proposes that collaboration with underserved women is important to achieve health. In a study of Hispanic and African-American women, adherence was associated with recognition of the serious consequences of nonadherence, realization of the beneficial effects, and the belief that medicines are not harmful (Unson et al, 2003). In another study, the use of electronic monitors had a positive effect on adherence for minority women (Robbins et al, 2004).*

 Community Teaching

- Review therapeutic regimens and their optimal integration with daily living routines.
- Teach disease processes and therapeutic regimens for management of these disease processes.

evolve See the EVOLVE website for World Wide Web resources for client education.

REFERENCES

Becker G, Gates RJ, Newsom E: Self care among chronically ill African Americans: culture, health disparities, and health insurance status, *Am J Public Health* 94(12):2066-2073, 2004.

Belza B, Topolski T, Kinne S et al: Does adherence make a difference? Results from a community-based aquatic exercise program, *Nurs Res* 51(5):285, 2002.

Bidmead C, Cowley S: A concept analysis of partnership with clients, *Community Pract* 78:203-208, 2005.

Brody GH, Jack L Jr, Murry VM et al: Heuristic model linking contextual processes to self-management in African American adults with type 2 diabetes, *Diabetes Educ* 27(5):685, 2001.

Fowles ER: Collaborative methodologies for advancing the health of underserved women, *Fam Community Health* 30:S53-S63, 2007.

Heisler M: The health effects of restricting prescription medication use because of cost, *Med Care* 42(7):626-634, 2004.

Kettunen T, Liimatainen L, Villberg J et al: Developing empowering health counseling measurement. Preliminary results, *Patient Educ Couns* 64(1-3):159-166, 2006.

Koch T, Jenkin P, Kralik D: Chronic illness self management: locating the self, *J Adv Nurs* 48(5):484-492, 2004.

Leininger MM, McFarland MR: *Cultural care diversity and universality: a worldwide nursing theory*, ed 2, Boston, 2006, Jones and Bartlett.

Leong J, Molassiotis A, Marsh H: Adherence to health recommendations after a cardiac rehabilitation programme in post-myocardial infarction patients: the role of health beliefs, locus of control and psychological status, *Clin Effectiveness Nurs* 8(1):26-38, 2004.

Lubkin IM, Larsen PD: *Chronic illness: impact and interventions*, ed 6, Boston, 2006, Jones and Bartlett.

Ogedegbe G, Mancuso CA, Allegrante JP: Expectations of blood pressure management in hypertensive African-American patients: a qualitative study, *J Natl Med Assoc* 96(4):442-449, 2004.

Park H, Hong Y, Lee H et al: Individuals with type 2 diabetes and depressive symptoms exhibited low adherence with self care, *J Clin Epidemiol* 57:978-984, 2004.

Pedro LW: Quality of life for long-term survivors of cancer: influencing variables, *Cancer Nurs* 24(1):1-11, 2001.

Pender NJ, Murdaugh CL, Parsons MA: *Health promotion in nursing practice*, ed 5, Upper Saddle River, NJ, 2006, Prentice Hall.

Robbins B, Rausch KJ, Garcia RI et al: Multicultural medication adherence: a comparative study, *J Gerontol Nurs* 30(7):25-32, 2004.

Stanford University: *Patient education*, available at http://patient-education.stanford.edu/internet. Accessed April 25, 2007.

Unson CG, Siccion E, Gaztambide J et al: Nonadherence and osteoporosis treatment preferences of older women: a qualitative study, *J Womens Health* 12(10):1037-1045, 2003.

Whittemore R, Chase S, Mandle CL et al: The content, integrity and efficacy of a nurse coaching intervention in type 2 diabetes, *Diabetes Educ* 27(6):887, 2001.

T

• = Independent; ▲ = Collaborative; EBN = Evidence-Based Nursing; EB = Evidence-Based

Ineffective Thermoregulation *Betty J. Ackley, MSN, EdS, RN*

NANDA Definition

Temperature fluctuation between hypothermia and hyperthermia

Defining Characteristics

Cool skin; cyanotic nail beds; fluctuations in body temperature above and below the normal range; flushed skin; hypertension; increased respiratory rate; mild shivering; moderate pallor; piloerection; reduction in body temperature below normal range; seizures; slow capillary refill; tachycardia; warm to touch

Related Factors (r/t)

Aging; fluctuating environmental temperature; illness; immaturity; trauma

NOC Outcomes (Nursing Outcomes Classification)

Suggested NOC Outcomes

Thermoregulation, Thermoregulation: Newborn

Example NOC Outcome with Indicators
Thermoregulation as evidenced by the following indicators: Increased or decreased skin temperature/Hyper- or hypothermia/Skin color changes/Dehydration (Rate the outcome and indicators of **Thermoregulation:** 1 = severe, 2 = substantial, 3 = moderate, 4 = mild, 5 = none [see Section I].)

Client Outcomes

Client Will (Specify Time Frame):

- Maintain temperature within normal range
- Explain measures needed to maintain normal temperature
- Explain symptoms of hypothermia or hyperthermia

NIC Interventions (Nursing Interventions Classification)

Suggested NIC Interventions

Temperature Regulation, Temperature Regulation: Inoperative

Example NIC Activities—Temperature Regulation
Institute continuous core temperature monitoring device, as appropriate; Promote adequate fluid and nutritional intake

T

Nursing Interventions and *Rationales*

- Monitor temperature every 1 to 4 hours or use continuous temperature monitoring as appropriate. *Normal adult temperature is usually identified as 98.6° F (37° C), but in actuality the normal temperature fluctuates throughout the day. In the early morning it may be as low as 96.4° F (35.8° C) and in the late afternoon or evening as high as 99.1° F (37.3° C) (Bickley & Szilagyi, 2007). Disease, injury, and pharmacological agents may impair regulation of body temperature (Kasper et al, 2005).*
- Measure the temperature orally or rectally. Avoid using the axillary or tympanic site. **EBN:** *Oral temperature measurement provides a more accurate temperature than tympanic measurement (Fisk & Arcona, 2001; Giuliano et al, 2000). Axillary temperatures are often inaccurate. The oral temperature is usually accurate even in an intubated client (Fallis, 2000). The SolarTherm and DataTherm devices correlated strongly with core body temperatures obtained from a pulmonary artery catheter (Smith,*

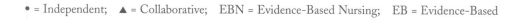

• = Independent;   ▲ = Collaborative;   EBN = Evidence-Based Nursing;   EB = Evidence-Based

2004). A study performed in Turkey found that axillary and tympanic temperatures were less accurate than oral temperatures (Devrim, 2007).

- Take vital signs every 1 to 4 hours, noting changes associated with hypothermia: first, increased blood pressure, pulse, and respirations; then decreased values as hypothermia progresses. *Mild hypothermia activates the sympathetic nervous system, which can increase the levels of vital signs; as hypothermia progresses, the heart becomes suppressed, with decreased cardiac output and lowering of vital sign readings (Ruffolo, 2002; Kasper et al, 2005).*

- Monitor the client for signs of hypothermia (e.g., shivering, cool skin, piloerection, pallor, slow capillary refill, cyanotic nail beds, decreased mentation, dysrhythmias) (Elliott, 2004).

- Note changes in vital signs associated with hyperthermia: rapid, bounding pulse; increased respiratory rate; and decreased blood pressure, accompanied by orthostatic hypotension (Worfolk, 2000). *Consistent monitoring promotes prevention and early intervention in clients with altered cardiopulmonary status associated with hypothermia or hyperthermia.*

- Monitor the client for signs of hyperthermia (e.g., headache, nausea and vomiting, weakness, absence of sweating, delirium, and coma) (Worfolk, 2000). *Monitoring for the defining characteristics of hypothermia and hyperthermia allows for prevention and/or early intervention.*

- Maintain a consistent room temperature (72° F [22.2° C]). *A consistent temperature limits environmental effects on thermoregulation.*

- Promote adequate nutrition and hydration. *These measures help maintain a normal body temperature.*

- Adjust clothing to facilitate passive warming or cooling as appropriate.

- See the Nursing Interventions and Rationales for **Hypothermia** or **Hyperthermia** as appropriate.

Pediatric

- Recognize that pediatric clients have a decreased ability to adapt to temperature extremes. Take the following actions to maintain body temperature in the infant or child:
  - Keep the head covered.
  - Use blankets to keep the client warm.
  - Keep the client covered during procedures, transport, and diagnostic testing.
  - Keep the room temperature at 72° F (22.2° C).

  The combination of a relatively larger body surface area, smaller body fluid volume, less well-developed temperature control mechanisms, and smaller amount of protective body fat limits the infant's and child's ability to maintain normal temperatures (Hockenberry, 2005).

- Recognize that the infant and small child are both vulnerable to heat stroke in hot weather and ensure they receive sufficient fluids and are protected from hot environments. *Infants and young children are at risk for heat stroke for many reasons, including a decreased thermoregulatory ability in the young body and the inability to obtain their own fluids (Carroll, 2002).*

Geriatric

- Do not allow an elderly client to become chilled or overheated. Keep the client covered when giving a bath and offer socks to wear in bed. Be aware of factors such as room temperature (heating/air conditioning), clothing (layered/loose), and fluid intake. *Older adults have a decreased ability to adapt to temperature extremes and need protection from extreme environmental temperatures. The response to cold environment is also compromised, with both the cutaneous vasoconstrictor response and the shivering process being less effective. Research indicates that this can be traced in part to medications used to treat chronic age-associated diseases. The rise in body temperature in response to pyrogens is blunted with increased aging. This deprives the elderly of the possible benefits of fever in coping with infections (Tallis, 2003).*

- Ensure that elderly clients receive sufficient fluids during hot days and stay out of the sun. *The elderly may have trouble walking independently to obtain fluids, have decreased thirst sensation, and have chronic illnesses that predispose to heat stroke (Carroll, 2002).*

- ▲ Assess the medication profile for the potential risk of drug-related altered body temperature. *Anesthetics, barbiturates, salicylates, nonsteroidal anti-inflammatory drugs, diuretics, antihistamines, anticholinergics, ß-blockers, and thyroid hormones have been linked to altered body temperature (Elliott, 2004).*

T

Home Care

- Prevent hypothermia in cold weather:
- Instruct the client to avoid prolonged exposure outdoors. When outdoors, the client should wear gloves and a cap on the head.
- Keep the room temperature at 68° to 72° F (20° to 22.2° C).
- ▲ Ensure an adequate source of heat. Refer to social services if the client/family has a low income and the heat could be turned off.
- Help the elderly client locate a warm environment to which the client can go for safety in cold weather if the home environment is no longer warm.
- Prevent hyperthermia in hot weather:
  - Encourage the client to wear lightweight cotton clothing. Help the elderly client remove the usual sweater.
  - Ensure that the client drinks adequate amounts of fluids (2000 mL/day).
  - Help the client obtain a fan or air conditioner to increase evaporation as needed.
  - Take the temperature of the elderly client in hot weather. *Elderly clients may not be able to tell that they are hot because of decreased sensation (Worfolk, 2000).*
  - Help the elderly client locate a cool environment to which the client can go for safety in hot weather.

Client/Family Teaching

- Teach the client and family the signs of hypothermia and hyperthermia and appropriate actions to take if either condition develops.
- Teach the client and family an age-appropriate method for taking the temperature.
- Teach the client to avoid alcohol and medications that depress cerebral function. *When the client is sedated or under the influence of alcohol, mentation is depressed, which results in decreased activities to maintain an adequate body temperature.*

evolve   See the EVOLVE website for World Wide Web resources for client education.

REFERENCES

Bickley LS, Szilagyj PJ: *Bates' guide to physical examination and history taking*, ed 9, Philadelphia, 2007, Lippincott.

Carroll P: The heat is on: protecting your patients from nature's silent killer, *Home Healthc Nurse* 20(6):376, 2002.

Devrim I, Kara A, Ceyhan M et al: Measurement accuracy of fever by tympanic and axillary thermometry, *Pediatr Emerg Care* 23(1):16-19, 2007.

Elliott F: You'd better watch out, *Occup Health Safety* 73(11):76, 2004.

Fallis WM: Oral measurement of temperature in orally intubated critical care patients: state-of-the-science review, *Am J Crit Care* 9(5):334, 2000.

Fisk J, Arcona S: Comparing tympanic membrane and pulmonary artery catheter temperatures, *Dimens Crit Care Nurs* 20(2):44, 2001.

Giuliano KK, Giuliano AJ, Scott SS et al: Temperature measurement in critically ill adults: a comparison of tympanic and oral methods, *Am J Crit Care* 9(4):254, 2000.

Hockenberry MJ: *Wong's essentials of pediatric nursing*, ed 7, St Louis, 2005, Mosby.

Kasper DL et al: *Harrison's principles of internal medicine*, ed 16, New York, 2005, McGraw Hill.

Ruffolo D: Hypothermia in trauma: the cold hard facts, *RN* 65(2), 2002.

Smith LS: Temperature measurement in critical care adults: a comparison of thermometry and measurement routes, *Biol Res Nurs* 6(2):117, 2004.

Tallis C: *Geriatric medicine and gerontology*, ed 6, Oxford, 2003, Churchill Livingstone.

Worfolk JB: Heat waves: their impact on the health of elders, *Geriatr Nurs* 21(2):70, 2000.

T

Disturbed Thought processes   *Judith R. Gentz, RN, CS, NP*

NANDA   ### Definition

Disruption in cognitive operations and activities

Defining Characteristics

Cognitive dissonance; distractibility; egocentricity; hypervigilance; hypovigilance; inaccurate interpretation of environment; inappropriate thinking; memory deficit

• = Independent;   ▲ = Collaborative;   EBN = Evidence-Based Nursing;   EB = Evidence-Based

Related Factors (r/t)

To be developed.

NOC   Outcomes (Nursing Outcomes Classification)

Suggested NOC Labels

Cognitive Ability, Cognitive Orientation, Concentration, Decision Making, Distorted Thought Self-Control, Identity, Information Processing, Memory, Neurological Status: Consciousness

Example NOC Outcome
Accomplishes **Distorted Thought Self-Control** as evidenced by the following indicators: Recognizes hallucinations or delusions are occurring/Refrains from attending to or responding to hallucinations or delusions/Exhibits reality-based thinking (Rate outcome and indicators of **Distorted Thought Self-Control:** 1 = never demonstrated, 2 = rarely demonstrated, 3 = sometimes demonstrated, 4 = often demonstrated, 5 = consistently demonstrated [see Section I].)

Client Outcomes

Client Will (Specify Time Frame):

- Remains oriented to time, place, person, and circumstance; demonstrates improved cognitive function
- Remains free from actual and potential harm by self or others
- Performs activities of daily living (ADLs) adequately and independently
- Identifies community resources for help after discharge
- Understands the actions and side effects of medications

NIC   Interventions (Nursing Interventions Classification)

Suggested NIC Labels

Delusion Management, Dementia Management

Example NIC Interventions—Delusion Management
Provide patient with opportunities to discuss delusions with caregivers; Focus discussion on the underlying feelings rather than the content of the delusion ("It appears as if you may be feeling frightened")

Nursing Interventions and *Rationales*

- Observe for causes of altered thought processes (see Related Factors). *In a descriptive study of older adults in an acute care setting, hypertension (21%) and cardiac dysrhythmias were the most common comorbidities (Park et al, 2004).*
- Monitor, record, and report changes in client's neurological status (level of consciousness, increased intracranial pressure), mental status (memory, cognition, judgment, and concentration), vital signs, laboratory results, and ability to follow commands. *Assessing cognitive, physical, and behavioral symptoms helps determine the relations among brain anatomy, neurochemical systems, and symptoms (Garand, Buckwater & Hall, 2000).*
- Obtain a medical history to rule out physical illness etiology for mental status changes. **EBN:** *Older adults are more likely to present with physical symptoms than mental health symptoms, so both must be closely assessed (Antai-Otong, 2003).*
- Complete a mental status examination of client, including a Mini Mental State Exam (MMSE). *A score of less than 24 on the MMSE may be considered cognitive impairment. (Joray, Wietlisbach & Büla, 2004).*
- Report any new onset or sudden increase in confusion. *Postoperative acute confusion is a significant problem among older surgical clients.*

T

• = Independent;   ▲ = Collaborative;   EBN = Evidence-Based Nursing;   EB = Evidence-Based

- Engage the client in conversation. **EBN:** *Socialization with the client helps the client maintain interpersonal relationship skills and social functioning (Washburn & Sands, 2006).*
- ▲ Assess pain and promptly provide comfort measures. **EBN:** *Confused clients cannot accurately report pain. Pain control reduces suffering and adverse health effects related to pain (Huffman & Kunik, 2000).*
- Identify and remove potentially dangerous items in the environment. **EBN:** *Interview clients in a private area while maintaining staff safety (Jensen, 2003).*
- Limit use of sedatives and drugs, which depress the central nervous system. *Confusion and/or disorientation are side effects of central nervous system depressants.*
- ▲ Use soft restraints with discretion and physician order. *Seclusion, restraint, and/or other behavioral management interventions must be used in accordance to the client's plan of care and regulatory guidelines (Health Care Financing Administration, 2000; Joint Commission on Accreditation of Healthcare Organizations, 2000).*
- Orient client, call client by name, and introduce self on each contact. Prominently display a clock and calendar that are easy to read in room and refer to them. **EB:** *External, written reminders are more effective than verbal reinforcement for memory aids (Day, Carreon & Stump, 2000).*
- Stay with clients if they are agitated and likely to be injured. *One-on-one contact from staff to client is the first step is successful de-escalation (Kozub & Skidmore, 2001).*
- Observe for therapeutic and side effects of psychotropic medications. *Side effects may mimic agitation, anxiety, and other primary symptoms and are usually remedied by altering the dosage or otherwise changing the medication schedule in consultation with the prescriber.*
- Develop a therapeutic alliance to increase trust with the client. **EBN:** *Approaching the client in a nonjudgmental manner, acknowledging the client's experience, and not challenging the client's reality help develop a therapeutic alliance (Jensen, 2003).*
- Assess client's assault potential and maintain staff safety. *Client resistance to staff direction requires immediate consideration of staff safety (Kozub & Skidmore, 2001).*
- Establish predictable care routines and maintain continuity of client's nursing staff. *Routines promote feelings of security.*
- Frequently check on client and have brief interactions to prevent sensory deprivation and/or overstimulation. **EB:** *Excessive environmental stimuli can adversely affect client's level of orientation and increase disorganization (Day, Carreon & Stump, 2000).*
- Evaluate the client's ability to safely engage in self-care activities. **EBN:** *Clients may minimize problems on self-reports and require staff observation for accurate assessment of self-care (Sousa & Frazier, 2004).*
- Observe for signs and symptoms of significant depression concomitant to altered thoughts. **EB:** *Severely depressed clients may also demonstrate declines in ADLs and cognitive functioning (McCall & Dunn, 2003).*
- Provide support and education to family during client's period of cognitive change. **EB:** *Integrating caregivers into the treatment process is key in treating elderly clients with cognitive changes (Miller & Reynolds, 2007).*
- ▲ Initiate a social service referral to find help for client after discharge. *Cognitive impairment in frail elderly is frequent, often undetected, and is associated with nursing home placement (Joray et al, 2004).*
- Observe for evidence of auditory and/or visual hallucination experiences. Teach management techniques. **EBN:** *Behavioral techniques taught to clients with auditory hallucinations were found to reduce negative characteristics of hallucinations (Buccheri et al, 2004).*
- Engage the psychotic client in simple, nonprobing conversation. **EBN:** *Psychosocial interventions are a recommended adjunct to psychopharmacotherapy (Isherwood, 2006).*
- Ask for clarification when necessary. **EB:** *There is a discrepancy between expression of emotion and experience of emotion in schizophrenia (Aghevli, Blanchard & Horan, 2003).*
- Help client state needs and ask for assistance. *Establish that staff should not automatically know the client's needs and wants and that it is acceptable to ask.*
- Assess need for referrals to other healthcare services, such as physical or occupational therapy. *Frail elderly engaged in strength training improved their MMSE (Mini Mental Status Exam) scores (Baum et al, 2003).*
- Refer to care plans for **Risk for self-** and **other-directed Violence** for further nursing interventions and rationales.

• = Independent;   ▲ = Collaborative;   EBN = Evidence-Based Nursing;   EB = Evidence-Based

Geriatric

- Monitor for dementia, as evidenced by gradual onset and a progressive deterioration, or for delirium, as evidenced by acute onset and generally reversible course. *Changes in behavior, cognitive functioning, and functional level occur with organic brain disease and other physiological changes in the body (Garand et al, 2000).*

Multicultural

- Assess the influence of cultural beliefs, norms, and values on the family's or caregiver's understanding of disturbed thought processes. **EBN:** *A recent study found that African-American families were unable to correctly identify early psychotic symptoms, which led to delays for treatment (Compton et al, 2004).*
- Inform the client's family or caregiver of the meaning of and reasons for common behaviors observed in the client with disturbed thought processes. *An understanding of behavior enables the client's family or caregiver to provide the client with a safe environment.*
- Validate the family members' feelings regarding the impact of the client's behavior on family lifestyle. **EBN:** *Validation is a therapeutic communication technique that lets the individual know that the nurse has heard and understood what was said, and it promotes the relationship between the nurse and the individual (Heineken, 1998).*

Home Care

- The interventions previously described may be adapted for home care use.
- ▲ Assess the client for the presence of a psychiatric disorder. Refer for mental health services as indicated. *Disturbed thought processes are part of several psychiatric disorders. Improvement in thought processes is unlikely unless the underlying disorder is treated.*
- Assess the family's knowledge of the disease process and plan of care; teach as necessary and encourage participation. *Illnesses associated with thought process disorders generally affect the family and family life as much as they do the client. Misinterpretation of the client's behavior is common, and instruction regarding the disease process is necessary to secure understanding of and cooperation with the treatment plan.*
- Identify the strengths of the caregiver and the caregiver's efforts to gain control of unpredictable situations. Help the caregiver to stay connected with a client who may be behaving differently than usual, to make life as routine as possible, to help the client set goals and sustain hope, and to allow the client space to experience progress. **EBN:** *Family members of persons with severe mental illness have found it helpful to work at staying connected to the person with mental illness, finding a role that they can feel comfortable with, and helping the relative move forward (Rose, 1998).*
- ▲ Assess the client's functional status as it relates to the ability for self-care; refer to a physician for evaluation of medication levels as indicated. *Negative symptoms, abnormal movements, and use of antiparkinsonism agents may increase the likelihood of functional impairment in older adults with schizophrenia (Cohen & Talavera, 2000).*
- Assess the home environment for the availability of distractions from hallucinations, such as playing music over headphones. **EB:** *Having schizophrenic clients listen to music produced beneficial effects (Glicksohn & Cohen, 2000).*
- ▲ If the client's condition deteriorates, seek acute medical or mental health intervention immediately, as appropriate. *Acute behavioral change could place the client or caregivers at risk; behavioral change often responds to sedation or an increase in medications.*
- ▲ Identify an emergency plan and discuss criteria for its use with the family or caregivers. *An appropriate level of clinical intervention supports client and family well-being.*
- ▲ Assess the client's ability to manage his or her own medications and make plans for assistance as needed to maintain safety of client. **EBN:** *Assistance, such as the use of a medication box or reminder telephone calls, may be sufficient to allow the client to perform care activities independently (Beebe, 2001).*
- Assess and modify environmental stimuli that could be misinterpreted (e.g., use a nightlight, evaluate placement of mirrors). *Nightlights help clients reorient themselves and decrease fear if clients awaken during the night.*

T

- Allow the client control over aspects of his or her environment, as he or she is able. *Control enhances self-esteem, although sometimes only for a short time. Refer to the care plan for* **Powerlessness.**
- Provide an opportunity for the client to pursue interests and use skills without taxing the client's judgment and cognitive ability. *Diversionary activities decrease anxiety and give meaning to life.*
- ▲ Refer the client and family to community support groups (e.g., psychosocial rehabilitation programs for the client, National Alliance for the Mentally Ill for the client and family). *Older adults may serve as a helpful resource to younger clients struggling with adjustment to their illness (Solano & Whitbourne, 2001).*
- ▲ In the presence of chronic thought process disorder, institute case management of frail elderly to support continued independent living. *Difficulties with thought disorder can lead to increasing needs for assistance in effectively using the healthcare system (Guttman, 1999).*
- ▲ When the client has a psychiatric disorder, pay special attention to the presence of comorbid medical conditions and the need for medical care. *Clients with schizophrenia have higher mortality rates and generally receive less-than-optimal health care (Folsom & Jeste, 2001).*
- ▲ When the client has a psychiatric disorder, refer for psychiatric home health care services for client reassurance and implementation of a therapeutic regimen. **EBN:** *Psychiatric home care nurses can address issues relating to the client's thought process disorder (Patusky, Rodning & Martinez-Kratz, 1996).*

Client/Family Teaching

- Teach family members reorientation techniques and about the need to repeat instructions frequently.
- Teach client distraction techniques to manage hallucinations.
- Teach family members ways to support client without supporting delusional beliefs.
- Help family identify coping skills, environmental supports, and community services for dealing with chronically mentally ill clients.
- Discuss caregiver's need for respite. Offer support, encouragement, and information for meeting those needs.

evolve See the EVOLVE web site for World Wide Web resources for client education.

REFERENCES

Aghevli, BH: The expression and experience of emotion in schizophrenia: a study of social interactions, *Psych Res,* 119(3):261, 2003.

Antai-Otong D: Managing geriatric psychiatric emergencies: delirium and dementia, *Nurs Clin North Am* 38(1):123, 2003.

Baum EE, Jarjoura D, Polen AE et al: Effectiveness of a group exercise program in a long-term care facility: a randomized pilot trial. *J Am Med Dir Assoc* 4(2):74, 2003.

Beebe LH: Community nursing support for clients with schizophrenia, *Arch Psychiatr Nurs* 15:214, 2001.

Buccheri R, Trygstad L, Dowling G et al: Long-term effects of teaching behavioral strategies for managing persistent auditory hallucinations in schizophrenia, *J Psychosoc Nurs Ment Health Serv* 42 (1):18, 2004.

Cohen CI, Talavera N: Functional impairment in older schizophrenic persons, *Am J Geriatr Psychiatry* 8:237, 2000.

Compton MT, Kaslow NJ, Walker EF: Observations on parent/family factors that may influence the duration of untreated psychosis among African American first-episode schizophrenia-spectrum patients, *Schizophr Res* 68(2-3):373-385, 2004.

Day K, Carreon D, Stump C: The therapeutic design of environments for people with dementia: a review of the empirical research, *Gerontologist* 40:4, 2000.

Folsom DP, Jeste DV: Medical comorbidity in patients with schizophrenia, *Home Health Consult* 8(9):17, 2001.

Garand L, Buckwater K, Hall G: The biological basis of behavioral symptoms in dementia, *Issues Ment Health Nurs* 21:21-107, 2000.

Glicksohn J, Cohen Y: Can music alleviate cognitive dysfunction in schizophrenia? *Psychopathology* 33(1):43, 2000.

Guttman R: Case management of the frail elderly in the community, *Clin Nurs Spec* 13(4):174, 1999.

Heineken J: Patient silence is not necessarily client satisfaction: communication in home care nursing, *Home Health Nurse* 16(2):115, 1998.

Huffman J, Kunik M: Assessment and understanding of pain in patients with dementia, *Gerontologist* 40:5, 2000.

Isherwood T: A qualitative analysis of the 'management of schizophrenia' within a medium-secure service for men with learning disabilities, *J Psych Ment Health Nurs,* 13(2):148, 2006.

Jensen LA: Managing acute psychotic disorder in an emergency department, *Nurs Clin North Am* 38(1):45, 2003.

Joray S, Wietlisbach V, Büla CJ: Cognitive impairment in elderly medical inpatients: detection and associated six-month outcomes, *Am J Ger Psych* 12(6):639, 2004.

Kozub M, Skidmore R: Least to most restrictive interventions, *J Psychos Nurs* 39:3, 2001.

McCall WV, Dunn AS: Cognitive deficits are associated with functional impairment in severely depressed patients, *Psychiatry Res* 121(2):179, 2003.

Miller MD, Reynolds CF 3d: Expanding the usefulness of interpersonal psychotherapy for depressed elders with co-morbid cognitive impairment, *Int J Geriatr Psych* 22(2):101-105, 2007.

Park M, Delaney C, Maas M et al: Using a nursing minimum data set

• = Independent;   ▲ = Collaborative;   EBN = Evidence-Based Nursing;   EB = Evidence-Based

with older patients with dementia in an acute care setting, *J Adv Nurs* 47:3, 2004.

Patusky KL, Rodning C, Martinez-Kratz M: Clinical lessons in psychiatric home care: a case study approach, *J Home Health Case Manag* 9:18, 1996.

Rose LE: Gaining control: family members relate to persons with severe mental illness, *Res Nurs Health* 21:363, 1998.

Solano NH, Whitbourne SK: Coping with schizophrenia: patterns in later adulthood, *Int J Aging Hum Dev* 53:1, 2001.

Sousa SA, Frazier R: A nursing tool for adherence and recovery in psychosis: a pilot study, *J Psychosoc Nurs Ment Health Serv* 42(3):28-36, 2004.

Washburn A, Sands L: Social cognition in nursing home residents with and without cognitive impairment, *J Gerontol B Psychol Sci Soc Sci* 61(3):P174-P179, 2006.

Impaired Tissue integrity   *Sharon Baranoski, MSN, DAPWCA, RN*

NANDA   Definition

Damage to mucous membrane, corneal, integumentary, or subcutaneous tissues

Defining Characteristics

Damaged tissue (e.g., cornea, mucous membrane, integumentary or subcutaneous tissue); destroyed tissue

Related Factors (r/t)

Altered circulation; chemical irritants; fluid deficit; fluid excess; impaired physical mobility; knowledge deficit; mechanical factors (e.g., pressure, shear, friction); nutritional factors (e.g., deficit or excess); radiation; temperature extremes

NOC   Outcomes (Nursing Outcomes Classification)

Suggested NOC Outcomes

Tissue Integrity: Skin & Mucous Membranes, Wound Healing: Primary Intention, Secondary Intention

Example NOC Outcome with Indicators
Intact **Tissue Integrity: Skin & Mucous Membranes** as evidenced by the following indicators: Skin intactness/Skin lesions absent/Tissue perfusion/Skin temperature (Rate the outcome and indicators of **Tissue Integrity: Skin & Mucous Membranes:** 1 = severely compromised, 2 = substantially compromised, 3 = moderately compromised, 4 = mildly compromised, 5 = not compromised [see Section I].)

Client Outcomes

Client Will (Specify Time Frame):

- Report any altered sensation or pain at site of tissue impairment
- Demonstrate understanding of plan to heal tissue and prevent injury
- Describe measures to protect and heal the tissue, including wound care
- Experience a wound that decreases in size and has increased granulation tissue

NIC   Interventions (Nursing Interventions Classification)

Suggested NIC Interventions

Incision Site Care, Pressure Ulcer Care, Skin Care: Topical Treatments, Skin Surveillance, Wound Care

Example NIC Activities—Pressure Ulcer Care
Monitor color, temperature, edema, moisture, and appearance of surrounding skin; Note characteristics of any drainage

● = Independent;   ▲ = Collaborative;   EBN = Evidence-Based Nursing;   EB = Evidence-Based

T

Nursing Interventions and *Rationales*

- Assess the site of impaired tissue integrity and determine the cause (e.g., acute or chronic wound, burn, dermatological lesion, pressure ulcer, leg ulcer, skin failure). **EB:** *The etiology or cause of the wound must be determined before appropriate interventions can be implemented. This provides the basis for additional testing and evaluation to start the assessment process (Baranoski & Ayello, 2003; Langemo, 2006).*
- Determine the size and depth of the wound (e.g., full-thickness wound, deep tissue injury, stage III or IV pressure ulcer). **EB:** *Serial wound assessments are more reliable when performed by the same caregiver, with the client in the same position, and using the same techniques (Ankrom et al, 2005; Black, 2005; Romero, Treston & O'Sullivan, 2006).*
- Classify pressure ulcers in the following manner (National Pressure Ulcer Advisory Panel, 2006; Black, 2005):
  - **Stage III:** Full-thickness skin loss involving damage to or necrosis of subcutaneous tissue that may extend down to but not through underlying fascia; ulcer appears as a deep crater with or without undermining of adjacent tissue.
  - **Stage IV:** Full-thickness skin loss with extensive destruction; tissue necrosis; or damage to muscle, bone, or supporting structures (e.g., tendons, joint capsules).
  - **Deep tissue injury:** A pressure-related injury to subcutaneous tissues under intact skin.
- Monitor the site of impaired tissue integrity at least once daily for color changes, redness, swelling, warmth, pain, or other signs of infection. Determine whether the client is experiencing changes in sensation or pain. Pay special attention to all high-risk areas such as bony prominences, skin folds, sacrum, and heels. *Systematic inspection can identify impending problems early.* **EBN:** *Pain secondary to dressing changes can be managed by interventions aimed at reducing trauma and other sources of wound pain (Rastinehad, 2006; Ayello & Braden, 2002; Moffatt, 2002; European Wound Management Association, 2001; Krasner 2001).*
- Monitor the status of the skin around the wound. Monitor the client's skin care practices, noting type of soap or other cleansing agents used, temperature of water, and frequency of skin cleansing. *Individualize the plan according to the client's skin condition, needs, and preferences. Avoid harsh cleansing agents, hot water, extreme friction or force, or too-frequent cleansing (Rodeheaver, 2001; Bergstrom et al, 1994).*
- Monitor the client's continence status and minimize exposure of the skin impairment site and other areas to moisture from urine or stool, perspiration, or wound drainage. *If the client is incontinent, implement an incontinence management plan to prevent exposure to chemicals in urine and stool that can strip or erode the skin. Refer to a continence care specialist, urologist, or gastroenterologist for incontinence assessment (Ratcliff, 2005; Wound, Ostomy, and Continence Nurses Society [WOCN], 2003).* **EB:** *Implementing an incontinence prevention plan with the use of a skin or cleanser protectant can significantly decrease skin breakdown and pressure ulcer formation (Clever et al, 2002; Warshaw et al, 2002).*
- Monitor for correct placement of tubes, catheters, and other devices. Assess the skin and tissue affected by the tape that secures these devices. *Mechanical damage to skin and tissues as a result of pressure, friction, or shear is often associated with external devices (Faller & Beitz, 2001).*
- In an orthopedic client, check every 2 hours for correct placement of foot boards, restraints, traction, casts, or other devices, and assess skin and tissue integrity. Be alert for symptoms of compartment syndrome (refer to the care plan for **Risk for Peripheral neurovascular dysfunction**). *Mechanical damage to skin and tissues (pressure, friction, or shear) is often associated with external devices.*
- For a client with limited mobility, use a risk assessment tool to assess immobility-related risk factors systematically. **EBN and EB:** *A validated risk assessment tool such as the Norton or Braden scale should be used to identify clients at risk for immobility-related skin breakdown (Ayello & Braden, 2002). Targeting variables (e.g., age and Braden Scale risk category) can focus assessment on particular risk factors (e.g., pressure) and help guide the plan of prevention and care (WOCN, 2003; Young et al, 2002; Ratcliff, 2005).*
- Implement a written treatment plan for the topical treatment of the skin impairment site. *A written treatment plan ensures consistency in care and documentation (Baranoski & Ayello, 2003; Maklebust & Sieggreen, 2001).*

T

▲ Identify a plan for debridement if necrotic tissue (eschar or slough) is present and if consistent with overall client management goals. *Healing does not occur in the presence of necrotic tissue (Bergstrom et al, 1994; WOCN, 2003).*

• Select a topical treatment that maintains a moist wound-healing environment and also allows absorption of exudate and filling of dead space. *No single wound care product provides the optimal environment for healing all wounds.* **EBN:** *Choose dressings that provide a moist environment, keep periwound skin dry, and control exudate and eliminate dead space (Ayello, 2006; Brett, 2006; WOCN, 2003; Bergstrom et al, 1994; Panel for the Prediction and Prevention of Pressure Ulcers in Adults, 1992).*

• Do not position the client on the site of impaired tissue integrity. *If it is consistent with overall client management goals, turn and position the client at least every 2 hours and transfer the client carefully to avoid adverse effects of external mechanical forces (pressure, friction, and shear) (WOCN, 2003).*

• Evaluate for the use of specialty mattresses, beds, or devices as appropriate (Fleck, 2001; Geyer, 2001).

• If the goal of care is to keep the client comfortable (e.g., for a terminally ill client), turning and repositioning may not be appropriate. *Maintain the head of the bed at the lowest degree of elevation possible to reduce shear and friction and use lift devices, pillows, foam wedges, and pressure-reducing devices in the bed (WOCN, 2003; Krasner, Rodeheaver & Sibbald, 2001).*

• Avoid massaging around the site of impaired tissue integrity and over bony prominences. **EB:** *A study demonstrated that massage over an immobile client's bony prominences with skin discoloration resulted in a lower skin blood flow than before massage (Ek, Gustavsson & Lewis, 1985). In a descriptive study, postmortem biopsies documented macerated, degenerated tissue in areas exposed to massage that were not documented on nonmassaged individuals (Dyson, 1978).* **EB:** *A review of the literature found no evidence that massage was appropriate for pressure ulcers in at-risk individuals (Buss, Halfens & Abu-Saad, 1997). Massage may lead to deep tissue trauma.*

• Assess the client's nutritional status; refer for a nutritional consultation and/or institute use of dietary supplements. **EB:** *The benefit of nutritional evaluation and intensive nutritional support in clients at risk for and with pressure ulcers is not supported by rigorous clinical trials. Despite this lack of evidence, the National Pressure Ulcer Advisory Panel endorses the application of reasonable nutritional assessment and treatment for clients at risk for and with pressure ulcers (available at www.npuap.org).*

▲ A comprehensive plan of care includes a thorough wound assessment, treatment interventions, support surfaces, nutritional products, adjunctive therapies, and evaluation of the outcome of care. *Documentation of these essential elements is paramount to establishing a framework for quality care (Baranoski, 2006).*

 Home Care

• Some of the interventions previously described may be adapted for home care use.

▲ Assess the client's current phase of wound healing (inflammation, proliferation, maturation) and stage of injury; initiate appropriate wound management. **EB:** *Accurate understanding of tissue status combined with knowledge of underlying diagnoses and product validity provide a basis for determining appropriate treatment objectives (Ovington, 1999).*

• Instruct and assist the client and caregivers in understanding how to change dressings and the importance of maintaining a clean environment. Provide written instructions and observe them completing the dressing change (Ovington & Schaum, 2001).

▲ Initiate a consultation in a case assignment with a wound specialist or wound, ostomy, and continence nurse to establish a comprehensive plan as soon as possible. Plan case conferencing to promote optimal wound care. *Case conferencing ensures that cases are regularly reviewed to discuss and implement the most effective wound care management to meet client needs (Biala, 2002).*

▲ Consultation with other healthcare disciplines provides a thorough, comprehensive assessment. *Consider referring to the dietitian, physical therapist, occupational therapist, and social worker as needed.*

 Client/Family Teaching

• Teach skin and wound assessment and ways to monitor for signs and symptoms of infection, complications, and healing. *Early assessment and intervention help prevent serious problems from developing.*

T

- Teach the client why a topical treatment has been selected. Explain wound bed changes that the caregiver can expect to see. Instruct on when the dressing needs to be changed. **EBN:** *The type of wound dressing needed may change over time as the wound heals and/or deteriorates (WOCN, 2003; Brett, 2006).*
- ▲ If it is consistent with overall client management goals, teach how to turn and reposition the client at least every 2 hours. **EB:** *If the goal of care is to keep the client comfortable (e.g., for a terminally ill client), turning and repositioning may not be appropriate (Krasner, Rodeheaver & Sibbald, 2001).*
- Teach the use of pillows, foam wedges, and pressure-reducing devices to prevent pressure injury. *The use of effective pressure-reducing seat cushions for elderly wheelchair users significantly prevented sitting-acquired pressure ulcers (Geyer et al, 2001).*

evolve See the EVOLVE website for World Wide Web resources for client education.

REFERENCES

Ankrom MA, Bennett RG, Sprigle S et al: Pressure related deep tissue injury under intact skin and the current pressure ulcer staging system, *Adv Skin Wound Care* 18(1):35-42, 2005.

Ayello EA: New evidence for an enduring wound-healing concept: moisture control. *J Wound Ostomy Continence Nurs* 33(6S):S1-S2, 2006.

Ayello EA, Braden B: How and why to do pressure ulcer risk assessment, *Adv Skin Wound Care* 15(3):125, 2002.

Baranoski S: Pressure ulcers: a renewed awareness, *Nursing* 36(8):36-41, 2006.

Baranoski S, Ayello EA, editors: *Wound care essentials: practice principles,* Springhouse, PA, 2003, Lippincott Williams & Wilkins.

Bergstrom N et al: *Treatment of pressure ulcers: clinical practice guideline no. 15,* Rockville, MD, 1994, U.S. Department of Health and Human Services.

Biala KY: Case conferencing for wound care patients, *Home Healthc Nurs* 20(2):120, 2002.

Black JM, National Pressure Ulcer Advisory Panel: Moving toward a consensus on deep tissue injury and pressure ulcer staging, *Adv Skin Wound Care* 18(8):415-421, 2005.

Brett DW: A review of moisture-control dressings in wound care, *J Wound Ostomy Continence Nurse* 33(6S):S3-S7, 2006.

Buss IC, Halfens RJ, Abu-Saad HH: The effectiveness of massage in preventing pressure sores: a literature review, *Rehabil Nurs* 22(5):229-234, 242, 1997.

Clever K, Smith G, Bowser C et al: Evaluating the efficacy of a uniquely delivered skin protectant and its effect on the formation of sacral/buttock pressure ulcers, *Ostomy Wound Manage* 48(12):60-67, 2002.

Dyson R: Bed sores—the injuries hospital staff inflict on patients, *Nurs Mirror* 146(24):30-32, 1978.

Ek AC, Gustavsson G, Lewis DH: The local skin blood flow in areas at risk for pressure sores treated with massage, *Scand J Rehabil Med* 17(2):81-86, 1985.

European Wound Management Association: *Pain at wound dressing changes, position document,* London, 2001, Medical Education Partnership.

Faller N, Beitz J: When a wound isn't a wound: tubes, drains, fistulas and draining wounds. In Krasner D, Rodeheaver G, Sibbald RG, editors: *Chronic wound care: a clinical source book for healthcare professionals,* ed 3, Wayne, PA, 2001, HMP Communications.

Fleck D: Support surfaces: criteria and selection. In Krasner D, Rodeheaver G, Sibbald RG, editors: *Chronic wound care: a clinical source book for healthcare professionals,* ed 3, Wayne, PA, 2001, HMP Communications.

Geyer MJ, Brienza DM, Karg P et al: A randomized control trial to evaluate pressure-reducing seating cushions for elderly wheelchair users, *Adv Skin Wound Care* 14(3):120-129, 2001.

Krasner D: Caring for the person experiencing chronic wound pain. In Krasner D, Rodeheaver G, Sibbald RG, editors: *Chronic wound care: a clinical source book for healthcare professionals,* ed 3, Wayne, PA, 2001, HMP Communications.

Krasner D, Rodeheaver G, Sibbald RG, editors: *Chronic wound care: a clinical source book for healthcare professionals,* ed 3, Wayne, PA, 2001, HMP Communications.

Langemo DK, Brown G: Skin fails too: acute, chronic and end-stage skin failure. *Adv Skin Wound Care* 19(4)206-211, 2006.

Maklebust J, Sieggreen M: *Pressure ulcers: guidelines for prevention and nursing management,* ed 3, Springhouse, PA, 2001, Springhouse.

Moffatt CJ et al: *Understanding wound pain and trauma: an international perspective, European Wound Management Association (EWMA) position document: pain at wound dressing changes 2-7,* 2002, available at http://www.tendra.com/item.asp?id=1321&si=3. Accessed April 27, 2007.

Ovington L: Dressings and adjunctive therapies: AHCPR guidelines revisited, *Ostomy Wound Manage* 45(suppl 1A):94S-106S, 1999.

Ovington LG, Schaum KD: Wound care products: how to choose, *Home Healthc Nurs* 19(4):224, 2001.

Panel for the Prediction and Prevention of Pressure Ulcers in Adults: *Pressure ulcers in adults: prediction and prevention, clinical practice guideline no 3,* Rockville, MD, 1992, US Department of Health and Human Services.

Rastinehad D: Pressure ulcer pain, *J Wound Ostomy Continence Nurs* 33(3):252-257, 2006.

Ratcliff CR: WOCN's evidence-based pressure ulcer guideline, *Adv Skin Wound Care* 18(4):204-208, 2005.

Rodeheaver GT: Wound cleansing, wound irrigation wound disinfection. In Krasner D, Rodeheaver G, Sibbald RG, editors: *Chronic wound care: a clinical source book for healthcare professionals,* ed 3, Wayne, PA, 2001, HMP Communications.

Romero DV, Treston J, O'Sullivan AL: Raising awareness of pressure ulcer prevention and treatment, *Adv Skin Wound Care* 19(7):398-404, 2006.

Sussman C, Bates-Jensen BM: *Wound care: a collaborative practice manual for physical therapists and nurses,* Gaithersburg, MD, 1998, Aspen.

van Rijswijk L: Wound assessment and documentation. In Krasner D, Rodeheaver G, Sibbald RG: *Chronic wound care: a clinical source book for healthcare professionals,* ed 3, Wayne, PA, 2001, HMP Communications.

Warshaw E, Nix D, Kula J et al: Clinical and cost effectiveness of a cleanser protectant lotion for treatment of perineal skin breakdown

● = Independent;   ▲ = Collaborative;   EBN = Evidence-Based Nursing;   EB = Evidence-Based

in low-risk patients with incontinence, *Ostomy Wound Manage* 48(6):44-51, 2002.

Wound, Ostomy, and Continence Nurses Society: *Guideline for prevention and management of pressure ulcers, WOCN Clinical Practice Guideline Series 2,* Glenview, IL, 2003, Wound, Ostomy, and Continence Nurses Society.

Young J, Nikoletti S, McCaul K, et al: Risk factors associated with pressure ulcer development at a major Western Australia teaching hospital from 1998 to 2000. secondary data analysis, *J Wound Ostomy Continence Nurs* 29(5):234-241, 2002.

Ineffective Tissue perfusion (specify type: renal, cerebral, cardiopulmonary, gastrointestinal, peripheral)

Marian Crowther, MSN, RN, APNC, CCRN, and Betty J. Ackley, MSN, EdS, RN

NANDA   Definition

Decrease in oxygen resulting in failure to nourish tissues at capillary level

Defining Characteristics

Cardiopulmonary

Abnormal arterial blood gasses; altered respiratory rate outside of acceptable parameters; arrhythmias; bronchospasm; capillary refill >3 seconds; chest pain; chest retraction; dyspnea; nasal flaring; sense of "impending doom"; use of accessory muscles

Cerebral

Altered mental status; behavior changes; changes in motor response; changes in papillary reactions; difficulty in swallowing; extremity weakness; paralysis; speech abnormalities

Gastrointestinal

Abdominal distention; abdominal pain or tenderness; absent bowel sounds; hypoactive bowel sounds; nausea

Peripheral Arterial

Altered sensation; altered skin characteristics (hair, moisture) or nails; cold extremities; diminished arterial pulses; intermittent claudication (Gengo de Silva et al, 2006); pale skin upon elevation of leg, with color not returning upon lowering of leg; pallor; shiny, waxy skin; skin temperature changes; slow healing of lesions; weak or absent pulses

Peripheral Venous

Edema; brawny hemosideric skin discoloration; dependent blue or purple skin color; positive Homan's sign; slow healing of lesions

Renal

Altered blood pressure outside of acceptable parameters; anuria; elevation in blood urea nitrogen/creatinine ratio; hematuria; oliguria

Related Factors (r/t)

Altered affinity of hemoglobin for oxygen; decreased hemoglobin concentration in blood; enzyme poisoning; exchange problems; hypoventilation; hypovolemia; hypervolemia; impaired transport of oxygen; interruption of blood flow; mismatch of ventilation with blood flow

NOC   Outcomes (Nursing Outcomes Classification)

Suggested NOC Outcomes

Cardiac Pump Effectiveness, Circulation Status, Fluid Balance, Hydration, Tissue Perfusion: Cardiac, Cerebral, Peripheral, Urinary Elimination

T

• = Independent;   ▲ = Collaborative;   EBN = Evidence-Based Nursing;   EB = Evidence-Based

Client Outcomes

Client Will (Specify Time Frame):

- Demonstrate adequate tissue perfusion as evidenced by palpable peripheral pulses, warm and dry skin, adequate urinary output, and absence of respiratory distress
- Verbalize knowledge of treatment regimen, including appropriate exercise and medications and their actions and possible side effects
- Identify changes in lifestyle needed to increase tissue perfusion

NIC   Intervention (Nursing Interventions Classification)

Suggested NIC Intervention

Circulatory Care: Arterial Insufficiency

Example NIC Activities—Circulatory Care: Arterial Insufficiency

Evaluate peripheral edema and pulses; inspect skin for arterial ulcers and tissue breakdown

Nursing Interventions and *Rationales*

Cerebral Perfusion

▲ If the client has a period of syncope or other signs of a possible transient ischemic attack, assist the client to a resting position, perform a neurological assessment, and report to the physician. *Syncope may be caused by dysrhythmias, hypotension caused by decreased tone or volume, cerebrovascular disease, or anxiety. Unexplained recurrent syncope, especially if associated with structural heart disease, is associated with a high risk of death (Kasper et al, 2005).*

- If the client experiences dizziness because of postural hypotension when getting up, teach methods to decrease dizziness, such as remaining seated for several minutes before standing, flexing feet upward several times while seated, rising slowly, sitting down immediately if feeling dizzy, and trying to have someone present when standing. *Postural hypotension can be detected in up to 30% of elderly clients. These methods can help prevent falls (Tinetti, 2003).*

▲ If symptoms of a new cerebrovascular accident occur (e.g., slurred speech, change in vision, hemiparesis, hemiplegia, or dysphasia), notify a physician immediately. **EB:** *New onset of these neurological symptoms can signify a stroke. If the stroke is caused by a thrombus and the client receives thrombolytic treatment within 3 hours, effects can often be reversed and function improved, although there is an increased risk of intracranial hemorrhage (Wardlaw et al, 2003).*

- If symptoms of a stroke are present, use the National Institute of Health Stroke Scale to evaluate the condition of the client. *The neglect subscale of the NIHSS includes extinction and inattention. Information on the scale is available at www.ninds.nih.gov/doctors/NIH_Stroke_Scale.pdf.*

▲ If an ischemic stroke has occurred, determine the position of the head of the bed after consulting the physician. In some situations it is appropriate to raise the head of the bed 30 degrees to lower intracranial pressure. Other times it is appropriate to keep the client mostly flat to increase cerebral perfusion. **EBN:** *An examination of the velocity of blood flow in the middle cerebral artery demonstrated increased flow when the head was lower than 30 degrees or flat (Wojner, El-Mitwalli & Alexandrov, 2002). A systematic review demonstrated that cerebral perfusion pressure showed no statistical significance in the magnitude of change from a flat position to 30-degree elevation (Fan, 2004).* **EB:** *Middle cerebral artery stroke clients demonstrated that cerebral perfusion pressure was highest at 0*

T

degrees compared with 15 degrees and 30 degrees during periods of normal intracranial pressure (Schwarz et al, 2002).

- See the care plans for **Decreased Intracranial adaptive capacity, Risk for Injury,** and **Acute Confusion.**

Renal Perfusion

- Be aware that renal blood flow and glomerular filtration rate may decrease in response to exercise and with a variety of medications. **EB:** *A study assessing renal integrity during exercise after administration of COX-2 inhibitors found that renal blood flow and glomerular filtration rate fell by 40% in response to exercise and COX-2 inhibitors, which significantly reduce free water clearance compared with placebo during exercise recovery (Baker et al, 2005; Neumayr et al, 2005).*

Peripheral Perfusion

- ▲ Check the brachial, radial, dorsalis pedis, posterior tibial, and popliteal pulses bilaterally. If unable to find them, use a Doppler stethoscope and notify the physician immediately if new onset of pulses is not present. *Diminished or absent peripheral pulses indicate arterial insufficiency with resultant ischemia (Kasirajan & Ouriel, 2002).*
- Note skin color and feel the temperature of the skin. *Skin pallor or mottling, cool or cold skin temperature, or an absent pulse can signal arterial obstruction, which is an emergency that requires immediate intervention (Dillon, 2003). Rubor (reddish-blue color accompanied by dependency) indicates dilated or damaged vessels. Brownish discoloration of the skin on the anterior tibia indicates chronic venous insufficiency (Simon, Dix & McCollum, 2004; Bickley & Szilagyi, 2007).*
- Check capillary refill. *Nail beds usually return to a pinkish color within 2 to 3 seconds after compression (Dillon, 2003).*
- Note skin texture and the presence of hair, ulcers, or gangrenous areas on the legs or feet. *Thin, shiny, dry skin with hair loss; brittle nails; and gangrene or ulcerations on toes and anterior surfaces of the feet are seen in clients with arterial insufficiency. If ulcerations are on the side of the leg, they are usually associated with venous insufficiency (Bickley & Szilagyi, 2007).*
- Note the presence of edema in the extremities and rate severity on a four-point scale. Measure the circumference of the ankle and calf at the same time each day in the early morning.
- Assess for pain in the extremities, noting severity, quality, timing, and exacerbating and alleviating factors. Differentiate venous from arterial disease. *In clients with venous insufficiency the pain lessens with elevation of the legs and exercise. In clients with arterial insufficiency the pain increases with elevation of the legs and exercise (Kasper et al, 2005). Some clients have both arterial and venous insufficiency. Arterial insufficiency is associated with pain when walking (claudication) that is relieved by rest. Clients with severe arterial disease have foot pain while at rest, which keeps them awake at night. Venous insufficiency is associated with aching, cramping, and discomfort (Kasper et al, 2005).*

Arterial Insufficiency

- ▲ Monitor peripheral pulses. If there is new onset of loss of pulses with bluish, purple, or black areas and extreme pain, notify the physician immediately. *These are symptoms of arterial obstruction that can result in loss of a limb if not immediately reversed.*
- Do not elevate the legs above the level of the heart. *With arterial insufficiency, leg elevation decreases arterial blood supply to the legs.*
- ▲ For early arterial insufficiency, encourage exercise such as walking or riding an exercise bicycle from 30 to 60 minutes per day as ordered by the physician. *Exercise therapy should be the initial intervention in nondisabling claudication (Zafar, Farkouh & Chesebro, 2000; Treat-Jacobson & Walsh, 2003).* **EB:** *Participation in an exercise program was shown to increase walking times more effectively than angioplasty and antiplatelet therapy (Leng et al, 2004).*
- Keep the client warm and have the client wear socks and shoes or sheepskin-lined slippers when mobile. Do not apply heat. *Clients with arterial insufficiency report being constantly cold; keep extremities warm to maintain vasodilation and blood supply. Heat application can easily damage ischemic tissues.*
- Use a variety of leg positions after surgical intervention for peripheral arterial disease (either supine with legs extended, sitting with legs extended, or supine with legs elevated 20 degrees)

T

• = Independent;   ▲ = Collaborative;   EBN = Evidence-Based Nursing;   EB = Evidence-Based

when getting this population out of bed. **EBN:** *There were no significant changes in transcutaneous oxygen measurements between positions used (Rich, 2004).*

▲ Pay meticulous attention to foot care. Refer to a podiatrist if the client has a foot or nail abnormality. *Ischemic feet are vulnerable to injury; meticulous foot care can prevent further injury.*

• If the client has ischemic arterial ulcers, refer to the care plan for **Impaired Tissue integrity.**

▲ If client smokes, aggressively counsel the client to stop smoking and refer to the physician for medications to support nicotine withdrawal and a smoking withdrawal program. **EB:** *A combination of psychosocial and pharmacological interventions was more effective than either intervention alone to stop smoking behavior (van der Meer, Wagena & Ostelo, 2003).* **EB:** *There is 45% smaller hyperemic vascular responsive in smokers than nonsmokers, indicating that pressure ulcers are more likely to occur in even light smokers (Noble, Voegeli & Clough, 2003).*

Venous Insufficiency

• Elevate edematous legs as ordered and ensure no pressure under the knee. *Elevation increases venous return, helps decrease edema, and can help heal venous leg ulcers (Simon, Dix & McCollum, 2004). Pressure under the knee decreases venous circulation.*

• Apply graduated compression stockings as ordered. Ensure proper fit by measuring accurately. Remove the stocking at least twice a day, in the morning with the bath and in the evening, to assess the condition of the extremity, then reapply. **EBN and EB:** *The use of graduated compression stockings reduced the incidence of deep vein thrombosis in a high-risk orthopedic surgical population. Implementation of additional antithrombotic measures along with stocking use decreased the incidence even further (Joanna Briggs Institute, 2001). Graduated compression stockings, alone or used in conjunction with other prevention modalities, help prevent deep vein thrombosis in hospitalized clients (Amarigiri & Lees, 2005).*

• Encourage the client to walk with compression stockings on and perform toe-up and point-flex exercises. *Exercise helps increase venous return, builds up collateral circulation, and strengthens the calf muscle pumps (Simon, Dix & McCollum, 2004).*

• If the client is overweight, encourage weight loss to decrease venous disease. *Obesity is a risk factor for development of chronic venous disease (Kunimoto et al, 2001).*

• If the client has venous leg ulcers, encourage the client to avoid prolonged sitting, standing, and elevation of the involved leg. **EBN:** *Wound perfusion was lower when the client with venous leg ulcers was sitting, standing, or elevating the involved leg than when the client was lying supine (Wipke-Tevis et al, 2001).*

• Discuss lifestyle with the client to determine if the client's occupation requires prolonged standing or sitting, which can result in chronic venous disease (Kunimoto et al, 2001).

▲ If the client is mostly immobile, consult with the physician regarding use of a calf-high pneumatic compression device for prevention of deep vein thrombosis. *Pneumatic compression devices can be effective in preventing deep vein thrombosis in the immobile client (Roman, 2005; Van Gerpen & Mast, 2004).*

• Observe for signs of deep vein thrombosis, including pain, tenderness, swelling in the calf and thigh, and redness in the involved extremity. Take serial leg measurements of the thigh and calf circumferences. In some clients a tender venous cord can be felt in the popliteal fossa. Do not rely on Homans' sign. *Thrombosis with clot formation is usually first detected as swelling of the involved leg and then as pain. Homans' sign is not reliable (Kasper et al, 2005). Symptoms of existing deep vein thrombosis are not found in 25% to 50% of client examinations, even when a thrombus is present (Launius & Graham, 1998).*

▲ Note the results of a D-dimer test and ultrasounds. *High levels of D-dimer, a fibrin degradation fragment, are found in deep vein thrombosis and pulmonary embolism (Sadovsky, 2005), but results should be confirmed with a duplex venous ultrasonogram (Kasper et al, 2005).*

▲ If deep vein thrombosis is present, observe for symptoms of a pulmonary embolism, including dyspnea, tachypnea, and tachycardia, especially with a history of trauma. **EB:** *Fatal pulmonary embolisms are reported in one third of trauma clients (Agency for Healthcare Research and Quality, 2000).*

• If client is receiving heparin subcutaneously, do not change the needle after drawing up the dose. **EBN:** *Changing the subcutaneous needle after withdrawing heparin from a vial did not reduce the size of ecchymoses at the injection site of study subjects (Klingman, 2000).*

T

• = Independent;   ▲ = Collaborative;   EBN = Evidence-Based Nursing;   EB = Evidence-Based

- If client develops deep vein thrombosis, after treatment and hospital discharge recommend client wear below-the-knee elastic compression stockings during the day on the involved extremity. **EB:** *Clients who wore compression stockings had a 50% less likely incidence of developing postthrombotic syndrome than did clients who did not wear the stockings (Shaughnessy, 2005). There is substantial evidence that compression stockings reduce the occurrence of postthrombotic syndrome after deep vein thrombosis (Kolbach et al, 2004).*

Geriatric

- Change the client's position slowly when getting the client out of bed. *Postural hypotension can be detected in up to 30% of elderly clients (Tinetti, 2003).*
- Recognize that the elderly have an increased risk of developing pulmonary embolism; if it is present, the symptoms are nonspecific and often mimic those of heart failure or pneumonia (Berman, 2001).

Home Care

- The interventions previously described may be adapted for home care use.
- Differentiate between arterial and venous insufficiency. *Accurate diagnostic information directs nursing care.*
- If arterial disease is present and the client smokes, aggressively encourage smoking cessation. See the care plan for **Health-seeking behaviors.**
- Examine the feet carefully at frequent intervals for changes and new ulcerations. *Lower Extremity Amputation Prevention Program (LEAP) documentation forms are available at www.hrsa.gov/leap (Feldman, 1998).*
- ▲ Assess the client's nutritional status, paying special attention to obesity, hyperlipidemia, and malnutrition. Refer to a dietitian if appropriate. *Malnutrition contributes to anemia, which further compounds the lack of oxygenation to tissues. Obese clients have poor circulation in adipose tissue, which can create increased hypoxia in the tissues.*
- Monitor for development of gangrene, venous ulceration, and symptoms of cellulitis (redness, pain, and increased swelling in an extremity). *Cellulitis often accompanies peripheral vascular disease.*

Client/Family Teaching

- ▲ Explain the importance of good foot care. Teach the client and family to wash and inspect the feet daily. Recommend that the diabetic client wear padded socks, special insoles, and jogging shoes. *Use of cushioned footwear can decrease pressure on the feet, decrease callus formation, and help save the feet.*
- ▲ Teach the diabetic client that he or she should have a comprehensive foot examination at least annually, including assessment of sensation using the Semmes-Weinstein monofilaments. If good sensation is not present, refer to a footwear professional for fitting of therapeutic shoes and inserts, the cost of which is covered by Medicare. **EB:** *Testing with Semmes-Weinstein monofilaments is effectively diagnostic of impaired sensation, especially when combined with clinical examination (Pham et al, 2000).*
- For arterial disease, stress the importance of not smoking, following a weight loss program (if the client is obese), carefully controlling a diabetic condition, controlling hyperlipidemia and hypertension, maintaining intake of antiplatelet therapy, and reducing stress. *All these risk factors for atherosclerosis can be modified (Treat-Jacobson, 2003).*
- Teach the client to avoid exposure to cold; limit exposure to brief periods if going out in cold weather and wear warm clothing.
- For venous disease, teach the importance of wearing compression stockings as ordered, elevating the legs at intervals, and watching for skin breakdown on the legs (Shaughnessy, 2005).
- Teach the client to recognize the signs and symptoms that should be reported to a physician (e.g., change in skin temperature, color, or sensation or the presence of a new lesion on the foot).
- NOTE: If the client is receiving anticoagulant therapy, see the care plan for **Ineffective Protection.**

 See the EVOLVE website for World Wide Web resources for client education.

• = Independent;   ▲ = Collaborative;   EBN = Evidence-Based Nursing;   EB = Evidence-Based

REFERENCES

Agency for Healthcare Research and Quality: *Prevention of venous thromboembolism after injury,* www.ahrq.gov/clinic/epcsums/vt-summ.htm, accessed March 11, 2005.

Amarigiri SV, Lees TA: Elastic compression stockings for prevention of deep vein thrombosis, *Cochrane Database Syst Rev* (3): CD001484, 2005.

Baker J, Cotter JD, Gerrard DF et al: Effects of indomethacin and celecoxib on renal function in athletes, *Med Sci Sports Exerc* 37(5):712-717, 2005.

Berman AR: Pulmonary embolism in the elderly, *Clin Geriatr Med* 17(1):107, 2001.

Bickley LS, Szilagyi PG, *Bates guide to physical examination and history taking,* ed 9, Philadelphia, 2007, Lippincott.

Dillon PM: *Nursing health assessment,* Philadelphia, 2003, F.A. Davis.

Fan J: Effect of backrest position on intracranial pressure and cerebral perfusion pressure in individuals with brain injury: a systematic review, *J Neurosci Nurs* 36(5):278-288, 2004.

Feldman CB: Caring for feet: patients and nurse practitioners working together, *Nurse Pract Forum* 9(2):87, 1998.

Gengo de Silva R, Monteiro da Cruz D, Bortolotto LA et al: Ineffective peripheral tissue perfusion: clinical validation in patients with hypertensive cardiomyopathy, *Int J Nurs Terminol Classif* 17(2):97-107, 2006.

Joanna Briggs Institute: Best practice: graduated compression stockings for the prevention of post-operative venous thromboembolism, *Evidence based practice information sheets for health professions,* available at http://www.joannabriggs.edu.au/pubs/best_practice.php?pageNum_rsBestPractice=/&totalRows_ersBestPractice=47, *Australia* 5:2, 2001. Accessed April 27, 2007.

Kasirajan K, Ouriel K: Current options in the diagnosis and management of acute limb ischemia, *Prog Cardiovasc Nurs* 17(1):26, 2002.

Kasper DL et al: *Harrison's principles of internal medicine,* ed 16, New York, 2005, McGraw-Hill.

Klingman L: Effects of changing needles prior to administering heparin subcutaneously, *Heart Lung* 29(1):70, 2000.

Kolbach DN, Sandbrink MW, Hamulyak K et al: Non-pharmaceutical measures for prevention of post-thrombotic syndrome, *Cochrane Database Syst Rev* (1):CD004174, 2004.

Kunimoto B, Cooling M, Gulliver W et al: Best practices for the prevention and treatment of venous leg ulcers, *Ostomy Wound Manage* 47(2):34, 2001.

Launius BK, Graham BD: Understanding and preventing deep vein thrombosis and pulmonary embolism, *AACN Clin Issues* 9(1):91-99, 1998.

Leng GC, Fowler B, Ernst E: Exercise for intermittent claudication, *Cochrane Database Syst Rev* (2):CD000990, 2004.

Neumayr G, Pfister R, Hoertnagl H et al: Renal function and plasma volume following ultramarathon cycling, *Int J Sports Med* 26(1):2-8, 2005.

Noble M, Voegeli D, Clough GF: A comparison of cutaneous vascular responses to transient pressure loading in smokers and nonsmokers, *J Rehabil Res Dev* 40(3):283-288, 2003.

Pham H, Armstrong DG, Harvey C et al: Screening techniques to identify people at high risk for diabetic foot ulceration: a prospective multicenter trial, *Diabetes Care* 23(5):606, 2000.

Rich KA: *The effects of leg/body position on transcutaneous oxygen measurements in age-matched healthy subjects and PAD subjects after lower extremity arterial revascularization* [thesis], Chicago, 2004, Rush University College of Nursing.

Roman M: Deep vein thrombosis: an overview, *Med-Surg Matters* 14(1), 2005.

Sadovsky R: D-Dimer assays for prediction of venous thromboembolism, *Am Fam Physician* 71(4):775-806, 2005.

Schwarz S, Georgiadis D, Aschoff A et al: Effects of body position on intracranial pressure and cerebral perfusion in patients with large hemispheric stroke, *Stroke* 33:497-501, 2002.

Shaughnessy AF: Compression stockings and post-thrombotic syndrome, *Am Fam Physician* 71(1):139-188, 2005.

Simon DA, Dix FP, McCollum CN: Management of venous leg ulcers, *BMJ* 328(7452):1358, 2004.

Tinetti ME: Preventing falls in elderly persons, *N Engl J Med* 348(1):421, 2003.

Treat-Jacobson D, Walsh ME: Treating patients with peripheral arterial disease and claudication, *J Vasc Nurs* 21(1):5, 2003.

van der Meer RM, Wagena EJ, Ostelo RW et al: Smoking cessation for chronic obstructive pulmonary disease, *Cochrane Database Syst Rev* (2):CD002999, 2003.

Van Gerpen RV, Mast ME: Thromboembolic disorders in cancer, *Clin J Oncol Nurs* 8(3):289, 2004.

Wardlaw JM, Zoppo G, Yamaguchi T et al: Thrombolysis for acute ischaemic stroke, *Cochrane Database Syst Rev* (3):CD000213, 2003.

Wipke-Tevis DD, Stotts NA, Williams DA et al: Tissue oxygenation, perfusion, and position in patients with venous leg ulcers, *Nurs Res* 50(1):24, 2001.

Wojner AW, El-Mitwalli A, Alexandrov AV: Effect of head positioning on intracranial blood flow velocities in acute ischemic stroke: a pilot study, *Crit Care Nurs Q* 24(4):57, 2002.

Zafar MU, Farkouh ME, Chesebro JH: A practical approach to lower-extremity arterial disease, *Patient Care* 30:96, 2000.

T | Impaired Transfer ability   *Brenda Emick-Herring, RN, MSN, CRRN*

NANDA   Definition

Limitation of independent movement between two nearby surfaces

Defining Characteristics

Inability to transfer: between uneven levels; from bed to chair; from chair to bed; on or off a toilet; on or off a commode; in or out of tub; in or out of shower; from chair to car; from car to chair; from chair to floor; from floor to chair; from standing to floor; from floor to standing; from bed to standing; from standing to bed; from chair to standing; from standing to chair

Related Factors (r/t)

Cognitive impairment; insufficient muscle strength; musculoskeletal impairment (e.g., contractures); neuromuscular impairment; obesity; pain

• = Independent;   ▲ = Collaborative;   EBN = Evidence-Based Nursing;   EB = Evidence-Based

Suggested functional level classifications include the following:

0—Completely independent

1—Requires use of equipment or device

2—Requires help from another person for assistance, supervision, or teaching

3—Requires help from another person and equipment or device

4—Dependent; does not participate in activity

NOC   Outcomes (Nursing Outcomes Classification)

Suggested NOC Outcomes

Balance, Body Positioning: Self-Initiated, Transfer Performance

Example NOC Outcome with Indicators
Transfer Performance as evidenced by the following indicators: Transfers from bed to chair and back/Transfers from wheelchair to toilet and back/Transfers from wheelchair to vehicle and back (Rate the outcome and indicators of **Transfer Performance:** 1 = severely compromised, 2 = substantially compromised, 3 = moderately compromised, 4 = mildly compromised, 5 = not compromised [see Section I].)

Client Outcomes

Client Will (Specify Time Frame):

- Transfer from bed to chair and back successfully
- Transfer from chair to chair successfully
- Transfer from wheelchair to toilet and back successfully
- Transfer from wheelchair to car and back successfully

NIC   Interventions (Nursing Interventions Classification)

Suggested NIC Interventions

Exercise Promotion: Strength Training, Exercise Therapy: Muscle Control

Example NIC Activities—Exercise Promotion: Strength Training
Obtain medical clearance for initiating a strength-training program, as appropriate; Assist to set realistic short- and long-term goals and to take ownership of the exercise plan

Nursing Interventions and *Rationales*

- ▲ Request consult for a physical and/or occupational therapist (PT and OT) to develop exercise and strengthening program early in the client's recovery. *Leg and trunk strength are key for doing partial or full weight-bearing transfers; arm and trunk strength are key for slide-board transfers.*
- ▲ Obtain a consult for a PT, OT, or orthotist to evaluate and fit clients with proper orthoses, braces, collars, and walking aids before helping them stand. *Equipment must be individualized to help clients move and function safely, comfortably, and independently (Hoeman, 2002).*
- • Help client don/doff collars, prostheses, antiembolism stockings, and abdominal binders while in bed. *Devices stabilize and align body parts during motion. Antiembolism stockings and abdominal binders help prevent postural hypotension; the binder must be put on and taken off in bed to ensure hemodynamic stability.*
- ▲ Ergonomically assess clients' dependence, weight, strength, balance, tolerance to position change, cooperation, and cognition plus available equipment and staff ratio and experience to decide whether to do a manual or device-assisted transfer. **EBN:** *A wheelchair ramp and hoist scale to weigh clients reduced stress on employees' shoulders and backs, reducing compressive and shear forces at L5-S1 (Owen & Garg, 1994). Staff reported work fatigue, demands, and back and shoulder pain decreased, and safety increased after education on "safe" and "no strenuous" lifting; musculoskeletal injuries did not change (Yassi et al, 2001). A trained nursing lift team successfully transferred*

• = Independent;   ▲ = Collaborative;   EBN = Evidence-Based Nursing;   EB = Evidence-Based

maximal assist clients and prevented injury, and the system was positively received (Caska, Patnode & Clickner, 1998).

▲ Collaborate with PT and use algorithms to identify technological aids to handle and transfer dependent clients safely (VISN 8, 2006; U.S. Department of Labor, 2006). *Powered stand-assist devices, sling and support lifts, stretchers to chairs, and friction-reducing devices prevent work-related musculoskeletal injuries of staff (Baptiste et al, 2002).*

• Do not use the under-axilla method or manual handling to transfer dependent clients; rather, use mechanical handling equipment such as powered mechanical lifts and stand-assist lifts. (U.S. Department of Labor, 2005). *Axilla lifts triggers shoulder injury and pain in clients and staff injury.* **EBN:** *Under-axilla lifts can cause overexertion back injuries to staff; clients seemed to be more physically and psychologically comfortable when lifted with mechanical devices (Owen, Welden & Kane, 1999).*

• Apply a gait belt to client's low back or under the axilla before transfers; keep the belt and client close to you during the transfer. *If used incorrectly, such as at arm's length, it prevents support of client and places staff at risk for back and arm injury (Minor & Minor, 1999).* **EBN:** *Use of a gait belt decreased staff exertion, back stress, and compressive force at L5-S1 (Owen & Garg, 1993). Garg et al (1991) concluded that the use of two staff using a walking belt and a rocking motion followed by a pulling motion was preferred by staff over four other transfer methods.*

▲ Remind clients to comply with weight-bearing restrictions ordered by the physician. *Weight bearing may retard healing in fractured bones.*

• Adjust transfer surfaces so they are similar in height. For example, lower a hospital bed to equal commode height. **EB:** *Equal heights between seat surfaces require much less upper extremity muscular effort during transfers (Wang et al, 1994).*

• Help clients don shoes and socks with nonskid soles, and educate diabetics to wear shoes before transfers. *Wearing shoes helps prevent slips and falls. Diabetics' feet heal poorly if injured (Yetzer, 2002).*

• Nursing staff should wear positive-grip shoe covers or nonslip shoes when transferring clients off shower chairs on tile floors. **ENB:** *Results from a small quality improvement study indicated nurses did not slip or fall when wearing such shoe products (Staal, White & Brasser, 2004).*

• Remove or swivel wheelchair armrests, leg rests, and footplates to the side, especially with squat or slide board transfers. *This gives clients and nurses feet space to maneuver in and provides fewer obstacles to trip over (Minor & Minor, 1999).*

• Place wheelchair and commode at a slight angle toward the surface to which client will transfer onto. *The two surfaces are close together yet allow room for the caregiver to adjust the client's movements during the transfer (Hoeman, 2002).*

• Teach client to consistently lock brakes on wheelchair/commode/shower chair before transferring. *Wheels will roll if not locked, thus creating risk for falls. Pneumatic wheelchair tires must be adequately inflated for brakes to lock effectively (Minor & Minor, 1999).*

• Position walking aids logistically so client can grasp and use them once he or she is standing. *These aids help provide support, balance, and stability to help client stand and step safely (Bohannon, 1997).* **EB:** *Elders with peripheral neuropathy had less risk of losing balance while standing on an unstable (tilting) surface in normal and low light when using a cane in the nondominant hand (Ashton-Miller et al, 1996).*

• Reinforce that clients are to place one hand on walker and push with opposite hand against chair arm or surface from which they are rising. *Placing both hands on the walker may cause it to tip and the client to lose balance and fall.*

• Give clear, simple cues and instructions, allow client time to process information, and let him or her do as much of the transfer as possible. *Overassistance by staff and family may decrease client learning and self-esteem.* **EBN:** *The ability to perform bed transfers was shown to be the most important factor in enabling frail elderly clients to live independently (Seidenfeld, Eberle & Potter, 2000).*

▲ Implement and document type of transfer (slide board, pivot, etc.), weight-bearing status (non-weight-bearing, partial, etc.), equipment (walker, sling lift, etc.), and level of assistance (standby, moderate, etc.) on care plan. *Team consistency is critical for clients' motor (re)learning, progress, and staff safety. (Rehabilitation Nursing Standards Task Force, 2000; APTA, ARN, VHA Task Force, 2005).* **EBN:** *Kjellberg, Lagerstrom & Hagberg (2004) found a positive relation between nurses' skill*

• = Independent;   ▲ = Collaborative;   EBN = Evidence-Based Nursing;   EB = Evidence-Based

in performing client transfers, and quality of care (clients' feeling of safety and comfort during lifts and transfers).

• Place client in set position before standing him or her; for example, sitting on edge of surface with bilateral weight bearing on buttocks and hips, with knees flexed, balls of feet aligned under knees, and head in midline. *This position prepares individuals for bearing weight and permits shifting of weight from pelvis to feet as the center of gravity changes while rising (Kumagai, 1998).*

• Support and stabilize clients weak knee(s) by placing one or both of your knees next to or encircling client's knee(s), rather than blocking them. *This allows client to flex his or her knee(s) and lean forward to stand and transfer. (See Gee and Passarella, 1985; Ossman and Campbell, 1990; Kumagai, 1998; and Minor and Minor, 1999 for instructions and pictures of additional transfers.)*

  ▪ Squat transfer: client leans well forward, slightly raises flexed hips off the surface, pivots, and sits down on new surface. *This is beneficial for clients with slight weight-bearing ability.*

  ▪ Standing pivot transfer: client leans forward with hips flexed and pushes up with hands from seat surface (or arms of chair), then stands erect, pivots, and sits down on new surface. *This is beneficial for clients who have partial weight-bearing ability.*

  ▪ Slide board transfer: client should have on pants or have a pillowcase over the board. Remove arm and leg rest from wheelchair and slightly angle it toward new surface. Help client lean sideways, thus shifting his or her weight so transfer board can be placed well under the upper thigh of the leg next to new surface. Make sure board is safely angled across both surfaces. Help client return to neutral alignment and place one hand on board and the other hand on seat surface. Remind and help client perform a series of pushups with arms while leaning slightly forward and lifting (not sliding) hips in small increments across board with each pushup. *This benefits clients with little to no weight-bearing ability (Hoeman, 2002; Minor & Minor, 1999).*

▲ Use extra staff to transfer debilitated bariatric (extremely obese) clients and place their beds against a corner wall. Help them into the set position, with both knees level with thighs (a footstool may be needed). Help clients lean well forward. *The wall helps prevent bed movement. Level knees prevent feet (and weight) from drifting downward. Clients should lean forward; staff use this momentum to help transfer them (Daus, 2001).*

▲ Use bariatric moving devices, including mattress overlay, transfer sheet, sliding or roller board, 60-inch long gait belt or two regular gait belts buckled together, standing-lift device, overhead ceiling-mounted or A-frame lifts (Dionne, 2000, 2002), and chairs/commodes (1000-pound limit) (Daus 2001, 2003).

• Perform initial and subsequent fall risk assessment. *Fall assessment tools help quickly identify persons at risk so prevention and protection measures can be implemented (Morse, 2006).* **EBN:** *The Morse Fall Scale was tested in three clinical areas; it effectively identified clients prone to falling and was quick and easy for nursing staff to use (Morse et al, 1989).*

▲ Collaborate with PT, OT, and pharmacy for early individualized preventative fall/recurrent fall plan, for example, scheduled toileting, balance and strength training, removal of hazards, chair alarms, call system in reach, and review of medications (Browne et al, 2004; Resnick & Junlapeeya, 2004*). **EBN:** *Clients on digoxin, class 1A antiarrhythmics, and diuretics fell slightly more; persons taking three or more medications had more recurrent falls (Leipzig, Cumming & Tinetti, 1999).*

 Home Care

▲ Obtain referral for occupational therapy and physical therapy to teach home exercises and balance as well as fall prevention and recovery and evaluate for modifications such as ramps, wide doorways, floor surfaces, lighting, grab bars, tub and toilet seats, and clutter elimination. *Access and safety promote independence.* **EB:** *Finlayson & Havixbeck (1992) concluded that nonuse of prescribed equipment could be prevented with therapist home visits, but tub transfers were frightening or difficult even after inpatient training. Allen (2001) found canes and crutches reduced the number of hours of care a person needed with ADLs, and walkers and wheelchairs supplemented human aid.*

▲ Assess for optimal furniture placement for function, maneuverability, and stability for those using assistive devices at home. For example, fitted bedspreads help prevent tripping. *Home evaluations promote safety; steady furniture can be used to pull oneself up if a fall occurs (Aiello et al, 2001).*

T

▲ Involve social worker or case manager to educate clients about potential assistive technology, financial cost and benefits, regulations of payers, and local resources. *Information helps clients understand options and cost of services and aids (Berry & Ignash, 2003).*

• Implement ergonomic approaches for home care staff and family to safely handle and transfer clients. *Risk of injury is high because people often work alone, without mechanical aids or adjustable beds and in crowded spaces while giving care (Galinsky, Waters & Malit, 2001).*

• For further information, refer to care plans for **Impaired physical Mobility** and **Impaired Walking.**

Client/Family Teaching

• Assess for readiness to learn and use teaching modalities conducive to personal learning styles. *Learning varies but may be enhanced with visual, auditory, tactile, and cognitive stimulus (Allen, 2002).*

• Supervise practice sessions in which client and family apply gait belt, brace, or orthoses; check skin once aids are removed; and perform recommended transfer or lift ergonomically. *Repetition reinforces learning; correct techniques and mechanical devices help prevent caregiver injury.*

• Teach and monitor client and family for consistent use of safety precautions for transfers, including nonskid shoes, correctly placed equipment and chairs, locked brakes, leg rests swiveled away, and so forth. *Such actions help prevent falls and injury to clients and caregivers.*

▲ Teach client and family how to check brakes on chairs to ensure they engage and how to check tires for adequate air pressure; advise routine inspection and annual tune-up of devices. *Long-term use may loosen brakes or cause them to slip; brakes work only if they make sound contact with tire or wheel. Thus pneumatic tires must be adequately inflated (Minor & Minor, 1999).*

▲ Offer information on safe use of shower and commode chairs to prevent discomfort, pressure, and falls during transfer, transport, care, and hygiene. **EBN:** *Three shower/bowel chairs were evaluated by clients or caregivers for comfort, safety, transportability, bowel accessibility, and repeated shower use; once unsafe features were identified (Malassigne et al, 1993), the research team designed and tested a new chair to minimize risks and client error in use (Nelson et al, 2000).*

• For further information, refer to the care plans for **Impaired physical Mobility, Impaired Walking,** and **Impaired wheelchair Mobility.**

evolve See the EVOLVE website for World Wide Web resources for client education.

REFERENCES

Aiello DD, Cole M, Ryan L et al: Safety in the home, *Rehabil Manag* 14(5):54, 2001.

Allen JC: Outcome-directed client and family education. In Hoeman SP, editor: *Rehabilitation nursing: process, application, and outcomes,* ed 3, St Louis, 2002, Mosby.

Allen SM: Canes, crutches and home care services: the interplay of human and technological assistance, *Cent Home Care Policy Res Policy Briefs* (4)1:1-6, 2001.

American Physical Therapy Association, Association of Rehabilitation Nurses and Veterans Health Administration Task Force: Strategies to improve patient and healthcare provider safety in patient handling and movement tasks, *Rehabil Nurs* 30(3):80-83, 2005.

Ashton-Miller JA, Yeh MW, Richardson JK et al: A cane reduces loss of balance in patients with peripheral neuropathy: results from a challenging unipedal balance test, *Arch Phys Med Rehabil* 77(5):446-452, 1996.

Baptiste A, Tiesman H, Nelson A et al: Technology to reduce nurses' back injuries, *Rehabil Nurs* 27(2):43, 2002.

Berry BE, Ignash S: Assistive technology: providing independence for individuals with disabilities, *Rehab Nurs* 28(1):6, 2003.

Bohannon RW: Gait performance with wheeled and standard walkers, *Percept Mot Skills* 85:1185, 1997.

Browne JA, Covington BG, Davila Y et al: Using information technology to assist in redesign of a fall prevention program, *J Nurs Care Qual* 19(3):218, 2004.

Caska BA, Patnode RE, Clickner D: Feasibility of a nurse staffed lift team, *AAOHN J* 46(6):283, 1998.

Daus C: Rehab and the bariatric patient, *Rehabil Manag* 14(9):42, 2001.

Daus C: The right fit, *Rehabil Manag* 16(7):32, 2003.

Dionne M: Maximizing efficiency with minimum effort: transferring the bariatric patient, *Rehab Manag* 13(6):64, 2000.

Dionne M: Ten tips for safe mobility in the bariatric population, *Rehabil Manag* 15(8):28, 2002.

Finlayson M, Havixbeck K: A post-discharge study on the use of assistive devices, *Can J Occup Ther* 59(4):201, 1992.

Galinsky T, Waters T, Malit B: Overexertion injuries in home health care workers and the need for ergonomics, *Home Health Care Serv Q* 20(3):57, 2001.

Garg A, Owen B, Beller D et al: A biomechanical and ergonomic evaluation of patient transferring tasks: wheelchair to shower chair and shower chair to wheelchair, *Ergonomics* 34(4):407-419, 1991.

Gee AL, Passarella PM: *Nursing care of the stroke patient: a therapeutic approach,* Pittsburgh, 1985, Harmarville Rehabilitation Center.

Hoeman SP: Movement, functional mobility, and activities of daily living. In Hoeman SP, editor: *Rehabilitation nursing: process, application, and outcomes,* ed 3, St Louis, 2002, Mosby.

T

Kjellberg K, Lagerstrom M, Hagberg M: Patient safety and comfort during transfers in relation to nurses' work technique, *J Adv Nurs* 47(3):251, 2004.

Kumagai KAS: Physical management of the neurologically involved client: techniques for bed mobility and transfers. In Chin PA, Finocchiaro D, Rosebrough A, editors: *Rehabilitation nursing practice,* New York, 1998, McGraw-Hill.

Leipzig RM, Cumming RG, Tinetti ME: Drugs and falls in older people: a systematic review and meta-analysis: II. Cardiac and analgesic drugs, *J Am Geriatr Soc* 47(1):40, 1999.

Malassigne P, Nelson A, Amerson T et al: Toward the design of a new bowel care chair for the spinal cord injured: a pilot study, *SCI Nurs* 10(3):84-90, 1993.

Minor MAD, Minor SD: *Patient care skills,* ed 4, Stamford, CT, 1999, Appleton and Lange.

Morse JM: The safety of safety research: the case of patient fall research, *Can J Nurs Res* 38(2):74, 2006.

Morse JM, Black C, Oberle K et al: A prospective study to identify the fall-prone patient, *Soc Sci Med* 28(1):81, 1989.

Nelson A, Malassigne P, Cors MW et al: Promoting safe use of equipment for neurogenic bowel management, *SCI Nurs* 17(3):119-124, 2000.

Ossman NJH, Campbell M: *Adult positions, transitions, and transfers: reproducible instruction cards for caregivers,* Tucson, AZ, 1990, Therapy Skill Builders.

Owen BD, Garg A: Back stress isn't part of the job, *Am J Nurs* 93(2):48, 1993.

Owen BD, Garg A: Reducing back stress through an ergonomic approach: weighing a patient, *Int J Nurs Stud* 31(6):511, 1994.

Owen BD, Welden N, Kane J: What are we teaching about lifting and transferring patients? *Res Nurs Health* 22(1):3, 1999.

Rehabilitation Nursing Standards Task Force: *Standards and scope of rehabilitation nursing practice,* ed 2, Glenview, IL, 2000, Association of Rehabilitation Nurses.

Resnick B, Junlapeeya P: Falls in a community of older adults: findings and implications for practice, *Appl Nurs Res* 17(2):81, 2004.

Seidenfeld SE, Eberle CM, Potter JF: Functional abilities of frail elderly that enable return to the community, *Home Health Care Consult* 7(8):29, 2000.

Staal C, White B, Brasser B: Reducing employee slips, trips, and falls during employee-assisted patient activities, *Rehabil Nurs* 29(6):211, 2004.

U.S. Department of Labor, Occupational Safety and Health Administration: *Ergonomics: guidelines for nursing homes,* 2005, available at http://www.osha.gov/ergonomics/guidelines/nursinghome/index.html. Accessed April 27, 2007.

Wang YT, Kim CK, Ford HT 3d et al: Reaction force and EMG analyses of wheelchair transfers, *Percep Mot Skills* 79:763-766, 1994.

Yassi A, Cooper JE, Tate RB et al: A randomized controlled trial to prevent patient lift and transfer injuries of health care workers, *Spine* 26(16):1739-1746, 2001.

Yetzer EA: Causes and prevention of diabetic foot skin breakdown, *Rehabil Nurs* 27(2):52, 2002.

Risk for Trauma   *Michele Walters, RN, MSN, ARNP*

NANDA   Definition

Accentuated risk of accidental tissue injury (e.g., wound, burn, fracture)

Risk Factors

External

Accessibility of guns; bathing in very hot water (e.g., unsupervised bathing of young children); bathtub without antislip equipment; children playing with dangerous objects; children playing without gates at top of stairs; children riding in the front seat in car; contact with corrosives; contact with intense cold; contact with rapidly moving machinery; defective appliances; delayed lighting of gas appliances; driving a mechanically unsafe vehicle; driving at excessive speeds; driving while intoxicated; driving without necessary visual aids; entering unlighted rooms; experimenting with chemicals; exposure to dangerous machinery; faulty electrical plugs; flammable children's clothing; flammable children's toys; frayed wires; grease waste collected on stoves; high beds; high-crime neighborhood; inappropriate call-for-aid mechanisms for bed-resting client; inadequate stair rails; inadequately stored combustibles (e.g., matches, oily rags); inadequately stored corrosives (e.g., lye); knives stored uncovered; lack of protection from heat source; large icicles hanging from the roof; misuse of necessary headgear; misuse of seat restraints; nonuse of seat restraints; obstructed passageways; overexposure to radiation; overloaded electrical outlets; overloaded fuse boxes; physical proximity to vehicle pathways (e.g., driveways, lanes, railroad tracks); playing with explosives; pot handles facing toward front of stove; potential ignition of gas leaks; slippery floors (e.g., wet or highly waxed); smoking in bed; smoking near oxygen; struggling with restraints; unanchored electric wires; unanchored rugs; unsafe road; unsafe walkways; unsafe window protection in homes with children; use of cracked dishware; use of unsteady chairs; use of unsteady ladders; wearing flowing clothes around open flame

T

• = Independent;   ▲ = Collaborative;   EBN = Evidence-Based Nursing;   EB = Evidence-Based

Internal

Balancing difficulties; cognitive difficulties; emotional difficulties; history of previous trauma; insufficient finances; lack of safety education; lack of safety precautions; poor vision; reduced muscle coordination; reduced sensation; weakness

Related Factors (r/t)

See Risk Factors.

NOC   Outcomes (Nursing Outcomes Classification)

Suggested NOC Outcomes

Risk Control, Fall Prevention Behavior

Example NOC Outcome with Indicators
Accomplishes **Risk Control** as evidenced by the following indicators: Monitors environmental risk factors/Develops effective risk control strategies/Modifies lifestyle to reduce risk (Rate the outcome and indicators of **Risk Control:** 1 = never demonstrated, 2 = rarely demonstrated, 3 = sometimes demonstrated, 4 = often demonstrated, 5 = consistently demonstrated [see Section I].)

Client Outcomes

Client Will (Specify Time Frame):

* Remain free from trauma
* Explain actions that can be taken to prevent trauma

NIC   Interventions (Nursing Interventions Classification)

Suggested NIC Interventions

Environmental Management: Safety, Skin Surveillance

Example NIC Activities—Environmental Management
Provide family/significant other with information about making home environment safe for patient; Remove harmful objects from the environment

Nursing Interventions and *Rationales*

* Screen clients with a fall risk factor assessment tool to identify those at risk for falls. **EBN:** *This may reduce the incidence of client falls and provides an opportunity to offer health education to high-risk clients (Hsu et al, 2004).*
* Provide vision aids for visually impaired clients. *A client with a sensory loss must be protected from injury; therefore the visually impaired client must use vision aids (Potter & Perry, 2003).*
* Help the client with ambulation. Allow the client to use assistive devices in ADLs as needed. *Assistive devices can augment the client's ability to perform ADLs (Potter & Perry, 2003).*
* Have a family member evaluate water temperature for the client. *A client with a tactile sensory impairment resulting from age or psychological or physiological factors must be protected from burns (Potter & Perry, 2003).*
* Assess the client for causes of impaired cognition. **EB:** *Clients with dementia have a higher rate of injurious falls than those without dementia (Doorn et al, 2003).* **EB:** *Fall prevention programs will be more beneficial to clients with a higher level cognition by decreasing the number of falls (Jensen et al, 2003).*
* Provide assistive devices in bathrooms (e.g., hand rails, nonslip decals on the floor of the shower and bathtub). **EB:** *Home hazard assessment and modification are personal safety measures to prevent falls (Gillespie et al, 2003).*

T

- Ensure that call light systems are functioning and that the client is able to use them in conjunction with the nurse making hourly rounds. **EBN:** *The preliminary results of a study conducted by the Alliance for Health Care Research concludes that hourly checks ensure availability of the call light while saving nursing time and energy by reducing call light use (Trinsey, 2006).*
- Use a nightlight after dark to assist in orientation and improve visual acuity.
- Teach the client to observe safety precautions in high-crime neighborhoods (e.g., lock doors, do not leave home at night without a companion, keep entryways well lighted). *Adequate lighting helps protect the home and its inhabitants from crime (Potter & Perry, 2003).*
- ▲ Instruct the client not to drive under the influence of alcohol or drugs. Assess for a substance abuse problem and refer to appropriate resources for drug and alcohol education. **EB:** *The use of alcohol or drugs (e.g., benzodiazepines, cocaine, opiates) is related to increased risk for motor vehicle accidents. Alcohol and drug combinations were the highest risk of experiencing injurious road accidents (Movig et al, 2004).*
- ▲ Review drug profile for potential side effects that may inhibit performance of ADLs. **EB:** *Benzodiazepines have a fivefold increase injury risk for drivers (Movig et al, 2004). A significant increase in traumatic occupational injury risk occurs with sedating antihistamines (Hanrahan & Paramore, 2003).*
- See Nursing Interventions and Rationales in the care plans for **Risk for Aspiration, Impaired Home maintenance, Risk for Injury, Risk for Poisoning,** and **Risk for Suffocation.**

Pediatric

- Assess the client's socioeconomic status. **EB:** *Pediatric clients living in poverty are at higher risk for injury (Shenassa, Stubbendick & Brown, 2004).*
- Assess family interests in safety topics to identify priority areas for counseling. **EB:** *Soliciting parents' interest before counseling may help identify priority areas for counseling as well as dispel myths and unfounded fears regarding childhood injury risk (McDonald et al, 2006).*
- Never leave young children unsupervised around water or cooking areas. *Young children are at risk for drowning even in small amounts of water. Heat and fire from cooking are a hazard to young children (Potter & Perry, 2003).*
- Keep flammable and potentially flammable articles out of the reach of young children.
- Lock up harmful objects such as guns. *Increased access to guns and limited parental supervision significantly increase the risk of youths' exposure to gun violence (Slovak, 2002).*

Geriatric

- Assess the geriatric client's cognitive level of functioning both at admission and periodically. **EB:** *Delirium after day 7 of inpatient care, sleeping disturbances, and male sex were associated with inpatient falls. Intervention programs should include prevention and treatment of delirium and sleep disturbances as well as increased supervision of male clients (Stenvall et al, 2006).*
- Assess for routine eye examinations and use of appropriate prescription glasses. *Poor vision reduces postural stability and significantly increases the risk of fall and fractures in older people (Lord, 2006).*
- Perform a home safety assessment and recommend the following preventive measures: keep electrical cords out of the flow of traffic; remove small rugs or make sure they are slip resistant; increase lighting in hallways and other dark areas; place a light in the bathroom; keep towels, curtains, and other items that might catch fire away from the stove; store harmful products away from food products; provide at least one grab bar in tubs and showers; check prescribed medications for appropriate labels; store medications in original containers or in a dispenser of some type (e.g., egg carton, 7-day plastic dispenser); if the client cannot administer medications according to directions, secure someone to administer medications. **EB:** *Home hazard assessment and modification are personal safety measures to prevent falls (Gillespie et al, 2003). Identifying risks and implementing changes decrease risk of injury (National Center for Disease Control and Prevention, 2006).*
- Mark stove knobs with bright colors (yellow or red) and outline the borders of steps. *Easily visible markings are helpful for clients with decreased depth perception (Potter & Perry, 2003).*
- Discourage driving at night. *A decline in depth perception and night blindness are common in the elderly, making night driving a difficult and unsafe task.*

T

• = Independent;   ▲ = Collaborative;   EBN = Evidence-Based Nursing;   EB = Evidence-Based

- Encourage the client to participate in resistance and impact exercise programs as tolerated. **EB:** *Muscle strengthening and balance retraining are beneficial in preventing falls (Gillespie et al, 2003). Structured, group-based exercise programs offered by community organizations can successfully increase balancing ability among community-dwelling older adults concerned about falls (Robitaille et al, 2005).*
- Implement fall and injury prevention strategies in residential care facilities. **EB:** *An interdisciplinary and multifactorial prevention program targeting residents, staff, and the environment may reduce falls and femoral fractures (Jensen et al, 2002).*
- Attend a fall prevention screening clinic. **EB:** *Clients who attended a fall prevention screening clinic demonstrated improved confidence during ADLs and reduced falls (Perell et al, 2006).*

Client/Family Teaching

- Educate the family regarding age-appropriate child safety precautions, environmental safety precautions, and intervention in an emergency. **EB:** *Infants and toddlers are more likely to be injured than are older children, regardless of setting (Waibel & Ranjita, 2003).*
- Teach the family to assess the childcare provider's knowledge regarding child safety, environmental safety precautions, and assistance of a child in an emergency. **EB:** *Infants and toddlers are more likely to be injured than are older children, regardless of setting (Waibel & Ranjita, 2003).*
- Educate the client and family regarding helmet use during recreation and sports activities. *Each year 1.5 million people sustain traumatic brain injuries, which account for one third of all injury deaths (National Center for Injury Prevention and Control, 2002).*
- Encourage the use of proper car seats and safety belts. *Every state requires that children ride buckled up; using a car safety seat or belt correctly can prevent injuries to children (American Academy of Pediatrics, 2002).*
- Teach parents to restrict nighttime driving after 10 PM for young drivers. **EB:** *The injury crash rate for drivers aged 16 or 17 years increases during nighttime hours and in the absence of adult supervision, with or without other passengers (Rice, Peek-Asa & Kraus, 2003).*
- Teach how to plan safe prom and graduation parties. *Guests can have fun and live to tell about it (Mothers Against Drunk Driving, 1994).*
- Teach parents the importance of monitoring youths after school. *Firearm injuries increase after school, and violent crimes by youths peak between 3 PM and 4 pm (Slovak, 2002).*
- Teach firearm safety. Encourage the family to keep firearms and ammunition in locked storage. **EB:** *Behavioral skills training programs are effective for teaching children to perform gun safety skills during supervised role play, but the skills were not used when the children were assessed by real-life assessments. More research is needed to determine the most effective way to promote the use of the skills outside the training sessions (Himle et al, 2004).*
- ▲ Educate that the use of psychotropic medications may increase the risk of falls and that withdrawal of psychotropic medications should be considered. **EB:** *Withdrawal of psychotropic medication decreased risk of falls in the elderly (Gillespie et al, 2003).*
- For further information, refer to care plans for **Risk for Aspiration, Impaired Home maintenance, Risk for Injury, Risk for Poisoning,** and **Risk for Suffocation.**

evolve See the EVOLVE website for World Wide Web resources for client education.

REFERENCES

American Academy of Pediatrics: *Car safety seats: a guide for families,* 2007, available at www.aap.org/family/carseatguide.htm. Accessed April 25, 2007.

Doorn C, Gruber-Baldini A, Zimmerman S et al: Dementia as a risk factor for falls and fall injuries among nursing home residents, *J Am Geriatr Soc* 51:1213-1218, 2003.

Gillespie LD, Gillespie WJ, Robertson MC et al: Interventions for preventing falls in elderly people *Cochrane Database Syst Rev* (4): CD000340, 2003.

Hanrahan LP, Paramore LC: Aeroallergens, allergic rhinitis, and sedating antihistamines: risk factors for traumatic occupational injury and economic impact, *Am J Ind Med* 44(4):438-446, 2003.

Himle M, Miltenberger R, Gatheridge B et al: An evaluation of two procedures for training skills to prevent gun play in children, *Pediatrics* 113(1):70-77, 2004.

Hsu S, Lee C, Wang S et al: Fall risk factors assessment tool: enhancing effectiveness in falls screening, *J Nurs Res* 12(3):169-178, 2004.

Jensen J, Lundin-Olsson L, Nyberg L et al: Fall and injury prevention in older people living in residential care facilities, *Ann Intern Med* 136(10):733, 2002.

Jensen J, Nyberg L, Gustafson Y et al: Fall and injury prevention in residential care: effects in residents with higher and lower levels of cognition, *J Am Geriatr Soc* 51:627-635, 2003.

• = Independent;   ▲ = Collaborative;   EBN = Evidence-Based Nursing;   EB = Evidence-Based

Lord SR: Visual risk factors for falls in older people, *Age Ageing* 35(2):1142-1145, 2006.

McDonald EM, Solomon BS, Shields WC et al: Do urban parents' interests in safety topics match their children's injury risks? *Health Promot Pract* 7(4):388-395, 2006.

Movig K, Mathijssen M, Nagel P et al: Psychoactive substance use and the risk of motor vehicle accidents, *Accid Anal Prev* 36:631-636, 2004.

Mothers Against Drunk Driving: *A parent's guide to sober teen celebration,* 1994, available at http:www.madd.org/under21/2710. Accessed April 25, 2007.

National Center for Injury Prevention and Control: *Traumatic brain injury,* 2002, www.cdc.gov/ncipc/factsheets/tbi.htm, accessed January 11, 2003.

National Center for Disease Control and Prevention: Injury Center: Preventing falls among older adults, 2006, available at http://www.cdc.gov/ncipc/preventadultfalls.htm. Accessed April 25, 2007.

Perell KL, Manzano ML, Weaver R et al: Outcomes of a consult fall prevention screening clinic, *Am J Phys Med Rehabil* 85(11):882-888, 2006.

Potter P, Perry A: *Basic nursing: essentials for practice,* St Louis, 2003, Mosby.

Rice TM, Peek-Asa C, Kraus JF: Nighttime driving, passenger transport, and injury crash rates of young drivers, *Inj Prev* 9(3):245-250, 2003.

Robitaille Y, Laforest S, Fournier M et al: Moving forward in fall prevention: an intervention to improve balance among older adults in real-world settings, *Am J Public Health* 95(11):2049-2056, 2005.

Shenassa E, Stubbendick A, Brown M: Social disparities in housing and related pediatric injury: a multilevel study, *Am J Pub Health* 94(4):633-640, 2004.

Slovak K: Gun violence and children: factors related to exposure and trauma, *Health Soc Work* 27(2):104, 2002.

Stenvall M, Olofsson B, Lundstrom M et al: Inpatient falls and injuries in older patients treated for femoral neck fracture, *Arch Gerontol Geriatr* 43(3):389-399, 2006.

Trinsey M: Hourly rounds keep call lights quiet, *Nursing* 36(2):33, 2006.

Waibel R, Ranjita M: Injuries to preschool children and infection control practices in childcare programs, *J School Health* 73(4):167-172, 2003.

Impaired Urinary elimination   *Mikel Gray, PhD, RN*

NANDA   Definition

Disturbance in urine elimination

NOTE: This broad diagnosis may be used to describe many dysfunctional voiding conditions. Refer to **Functional urinary Incontinence, Reflex urinary Incontinence, Stress urinary Incontinence, Total urinary Incontinence, Urge urinary Incontinence,** and **Urinary retention** for information on these more specific diagnoses.

Defining Characteristics

The term *lower urinary tract symptoms* (LUTS) is now used to describe the variety of complaints associated with disorders of bladder filling/storage or altered patterns of urine elimination (Abrams et al, 2002). Bothersome bladder filling/storage symptoms include diurnal frequency (voiding more than every 2 hours), infrequent urination (voiding less then every 6 hours), and nocturia (arising from sleep more than twice to urinate). Our understanding of the physiologic desire is incomplete, but the term *urgency* has been defined as "a sudden and strong desire to urinate that is not easily deferred" (Abrams et al, 2002). Lower urinary tract pain may present as dysuria (pain associated with micturition), burning, pressure, or cramping discomfort during bladder filling and storage. Voiding symptoms may include reduced force of the urinary stream, intermittency, hesitancy, and the need to strain to evacuate the bladder. Other voiding symptoms are postvoid dribbling, feelings of incomplete bladder emptying, or the total inability to urinate (acute urinary retention).

Urinary incontinence is the uncontrolled loss of urine of sufficient magnitude to constitute a problem for the client, family, or caregivers (Abrams et al, 2002). Stress urinary incontinence is the loss of urine with physical exertion. Urge urinary incontinence is the loss of urine associated with overactive detrusor contractions and a precipitous desire to urinate. It is part of a larger symptom syndrome called *overactive bladder*. The overactive bladder is characterized by bothersome urgency and typically associated with frequent daytime voiding and nocturia. Approximately 37% of patients with overactive bladder dysfunction experience urge urinary incontinence (Stewart et al, 2003).

Reflex urinary incontinence is urine loss associated with neurogenic detrusor overactivity, diminished or absent sensations of bladder filling, and dyssynergia between the detrusor and striated urethral sphincter muscles. Functional urinary incontinence is urine loss associated with deficits of mobility, dexterity, cognition, or environmental barriers to timely toileting. Urine loss from an extraurethral source can be defined as total incontinence, and urinary retention is the condition where the client is unable to completely evacuate urine from the bladder despite micturition. Chronic urinary retention is defined as the inability to completely evacuate urine from the bladder after voiding, and acute urinary retention is the inability to urinate (Gray, 2000).

U

• = Independent;   ▲ = Collaborative;   EBN = Evidence-Based Nursing;   EB = Evidence-Based

Related Factors (r/t)

Bothersome LUTS (urological disorders, neurological lesions, gynecological conditions, dysfunction of bowel elimination); incontinence (refer to specific diagnosis); urinary retention (refer to specific diagnosis); acute urinary retention (refer to **Urinary retention**)

NOC Outcomes (Nursing Outcomes Classification)

Suggested NOC Outcomes

Urinary Continence, Urinary Elimination

Example NOC Outcome with Indicators
Urinary Continence as evidenced by the following indicators: Has no urine loss leakage with increased abdominal pressure (e.g., sneezing, laughing, lifting)/Voids in appropriate receptacle/Gets to toilet between urge and passage of urine/Keeps underclothing dry during day/Keeps underclothing or bedding dry during night (Rate the outcome and indicators of **Urinary Continence**: 1 = never demonstrated, 2 = rarely demonstrated, 3 = sometimes demonstrated, 4 = often demonstrated, 5 = consistently demonstrated [see Section I].)

Client Outcomes

Client Will (Specify Time Frame):

- Demonstrate diurnal frequency no more than every 2 hours
- Demonstrate nocturia two times or less per night
- Be able to postpone voiding until toileting facility is accessed and clothing is removed
- Be able to perceive and recognize cues for toileting, move to toilet or use urinal or portable toileting apparatus, and remove clothing as necessary for toileting
- Demonstrate postvoiding residual volumes less than 150 mL to 200 mL or 25% of total bladder capacity
- State absence of pain or excessive urgency during bladder storage or during urination

NIC Interventions (Nursing Interventions Classification)

Suggested NIC Intervention

Urinary Elimination Management

Example NIC Activities—Urinary Elimination Management
Monitor urinary elimination, including frequency, consistency, odor, volume, and color, as appropriate; Teach patient signs and symptoms of urinary tract infection

Nursing Interventions and Rationales

- Routinely screen all adult women and aging men for urinary incontinence or LUTS including bothersome urgency. *Urinary incontinence and overactive bladder dysfunction are prevalent problems, particularly among women and aging males in the sixth decade of life or older (Hunskaar et al, 2005). Routine screening is justified because urinary incontinence is prevalent, negatively affects physical health and psychosocial function, and is amenable to treatment (Gray, 2003).*
- ▲ Assess bladder function using the following techniques:
  - ■ Take a focused history including duration of bothersome LUTS, characteristics of symptoms, patterns of diurnal and nocturnal urination, frequency and volume of urine loss, alleviating and aggravating factors, and exploration of possible causative factors.
  - ■ In close consultation with a physician or advanced practice nurse, administer a validated questionnaire querying lower urinary symptoms, associated bowel elimination symptoms, and symptoms of pelvic organ prolapse in women.
  - ■ Perform a focused physical assessment of perineal skin integrity, evaluation of the vaginal

• = Independent;   ▲ = Collaborative;   EBN = Evidence-Based Nursing;   EB = Evidence-Based

vault, evaluation of urethral hypermobility, and neurological evaluation including bulbocavernosus reflex and perineal sensations.

- Review results of urinalysis for the presence of urinary infection, polyuria, hematuria, proteinuria, and other abnormalities, or obtain urine for analysis.

A focused history and physical examination are essential elements of the initial evaluation of impaired urine elimination (Staskin et al, 2005). **EBN:** *There is limited evidence to support the diagnostic value of the physical examination in the diagnosis of urinary incontinence and differential diagnosis of stress versus urge incontinence in elderly women (van Gerwen & Largo-Janssen, 2006). There are 23 validated tools for the evaluation of lower urinary tract symptoms, bowel elimination symptoms, and symptoms associated with pelvic organ prolapse in women. These instruments can assist the clinician to differentiate the primary type of incontinence, distinguish urgency form pelvic pain, and identify associated bowel elimination disorders and pelvic organ prolapse (Avery et al, 2007).*

- Complete a more detailed assessment on selected clients including a bladder log and functional/cognitive assessment. (Refer to **Functional urinary Incontinence, Reflex urinary Incontinence, Stress urinary Incontinence, Total urinary Incontinence,** and **Urge urinary Incontinence.**)
- Assess the client for urinary retention. (Refer to **Urinary retention.**)
- Teach the client general guidelines for bladder health:
  - Clients should avoid dehydration and its irritative effects on the bladder; fluid consumption for the ambulatory, normally active adult should be approximately 30 mL/kg of body weight (0.5 oz per pound per day).
  - Clients with storage LUTS, overactive bladder dysfunction, or urinary incontinence should reduce or cease caffeine intake (Gray, 2001).
  - Clients with lower urinary tract pain or interstitial cystitis should be encouraged to eliminate potential bladder irritants: caffeine, alcohol, aspartame, carbonated beverages, alcohol, citrus juices, chocolate, vinegar, and highly spiced foods such as those flavored with curries or peppers (Bade, Peeters & Mensink, 1997; Interstitial Cystitis Association, 1999). These foods should be reintroduced singly to the diet to determine their effect (if any) on bothersome LUTS.
  - All clients should be counseled about measures to alleviate or prevent constipation including adequate consumption of dietary fluids, dietary fiber, exercise, and regular bowel elimination patterns.
  - All clients should be strongly advised to stop smoking; it is associated with an increased risk of bladder cancer (Bjerregaard et al, 2006), urinary incontinence (Danforth et al, 2006), and bothersome lower urinary tract symptoms in men (Haidenger et al, 2000).

Dehydration increases irritating voiding symptoms and may enhance the risk of urinary infection. Constipation predisposes the individual to urinary retention, and it increases the risk of urinary infection. Smoking may increase the severity and risk of stress incontinence, and it is clearly linked with an increased risk for bladder cancer (Tampakoudis et al, 1995). **EBN:** *Client education, alteration of fluid volume intake, reduction of caffeine consumption, and bladder training and pelvic floor muscle training administered by generic and advanced practice nurses reduce the frequency of urinary incontinence, pad use, and perceived severity of bothersome LUTS (Borrie et al, 2002; Dougherty et al, 2002; Dowd, Kolcaba & Steiner, 2000; Sampselle et al, 2000).*

- ▲ Consult the physician for culture and sensitivity testing and antibiotic treatment in the individual with evidence of a urinary infection. *UTI is a transient, reversible condition that is associated with urge urinary incontinence and overactive bladder syndrome (Brown et al, 2001). Although the precise nature of this relationship remains unclear, it is known that eradication of UTI will alleviate or reverse LUTS including suprapubic pressure and discomfort, bothersome urgency, daytime voiding frequency, and dysuria (Malterud & Baerheim, 1999).*
- ▲ Refer the individual with chronic lower urinary tract pain to a urologist or specialist in the management of pelvic pain. *Bladder pain and storage symptoms, in the absence of an acute urinary infection, may indicate the presence of interstitial cystitis, a chronic condition requiring ongoing treatment (Gray, Hufstuttler & Albo, 2002).*
- ▲ Teach the client to recognize symptoms of UTI (dysuria that crescendos as the bladder nears complete evacuation; urgency to urinate followed by micturition of only a few drops; suprapubic aching discomfort; malaise; voiding frequency; sudden exacerbation of urinary incontinence with

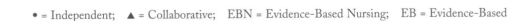

• = Independent;   ▲ = Collaborative;   EBN = Evidence-Based Nursing;   EB = Evidence-Based

or without fever, chills, and flank pain). *There are a variety of typical and unexpected symptoms in women with a history of recurring UTI (Malterud & Baerheim, 1999).*

▲ Teach colleagues that a cloudy or malodorous urine, in the absence of other lower urinary tract symptoms, does not indicate the presence of a urinary tract infection and that asymptomatic bacteriuria, in the elderly, does not justify the need for a course of antibiotics. *Nurses are more likely than physicians to interpret presence of cloudy urine as indicating the presence of a UTI in the frail elder. Asymptomatic bacteriuria may be associated with cloudy or malodorous urine, but these signs alone do not justify antimicrobial therapy when balanced against the potential adverse effects of treatment including adverse side effects of the various antibiotics and encouragement of colonization of the urine with antibiotic-resistant bacterial strains (Midthun et al, 2005).*

• Teach the client to recognize hematuria and to seek help promptly if hematuria occurs. *Hematuria in the presence of irritative voiding symptoms typically indicates urinary infection; however, gross or microscopic, in the absence of an existing UTI it raises the risk for urinary system tumor and requires further investigation (Kincaid-Smith & Fairley, 2005).*

• Assist the individual with urinary leakage to select a product that adequately contains urine, avoids soiling clothing, is not apparent when worn under clothing, and protects the underlying skin. (See the care plan for **Total urinary Incontinence.**)

• Teach perineal care including judicious use of soaps and use of vaginal douches only under special circumstances. (See the care plan for **Total urinary Incontinence.**)

Geriatric

• Provide an environment that encourages toileting for the elderly client cared for in the home or in acute care, long-term care, or critical care units. *Insufficient toileting opportunities, medications, acute or chronic illnesses, and environmental factors may contribute to functional incontinence or exacerbate other forms of urinary leakage in the elderly client (Gray & Burns, 1996; Jirovec & Wells, 1990; Morris, Browne & Saltmarche, 1992).*

• Perform urinalysis in all elderly persons who experience a sudden change in urine elimination patterns, lower abdominal discomfort, acute confusion, or a fever of unclear origin. *Elderly persons, particularly adults aged 80 years and older, often experience atypical symptoms with a UTI or pyelonephritis (Bostwick, 2000; Suchinski et al, 1999).*

• Encourage elderly women to drink at least 10 oz of cranberry juice daily, regularly consume one to two servings of fresh blueberries, or supplement the diet with cranberry concentrate capsules (usually taken in 500 mg doses with each meal). **EBN:** *Systematic literature review reveals that consumption of 400 mg of cranberry tablets, 8 to 10 oz of cranberry juice, or an equivocal portion of foods containing whole cranberries or blueberries exerts a bacteriostatic effect on* Escherichia coli, *the most common pathogen associated with urinary infection among community-dwelling adult women. Mixed evidence tends to support a reduction in UTI risk among community-dwelling women, although no beneficial effect has been found in clients with neurogenic bladder dysfunction who are managed by intermittent or indwelling catheters (Gray, 2002).*

Client/Family Teaching

• Provide all clients with the basic principles for optimal bladder function.
• Teach the community and healthcare providers that urinary incontinence is not a normal part of aging and that incontinence can be corrected or managed with proper evaluation and care.
• Provide information to healthcare providers and the community about the signs, symptoms, and management of UTIs and interstitial cystitis.
• Teach all persons the signs and symptoms of UTI and its management.
• Teach all persons to recognize hematuria and to promptly seek care if this symptom occurs.

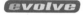 See the EVOLVE website for World Wide Web resources for client education.

• = Independent;   ▲ = Collaborative;   EBN = Evidence-Based Nursing;   EB = Evidence-Based

REFERENCES

Abrams P, Cardozo L, Fall M et al: The standardization of terminology of lower urinary tract function: report from the Standardization Subcommittee of the International Continence Society, *Am J Obstet Gynecol* 187(1):116-126, 2002.

Avery KN, Bosch JL, Gotoh M et al: Questionnaires to assess urinary and anal incontinence: review and recommendations, *J Urol* 177(1):39-49, 2007.

Bade JJ, Peeters JM, Mensink HJ: Is the diet of patients with interstitial cystitis related to their disease? *Eur Urol* 32(2):179-183, 1997.

Bjerregaard BK, Raaschou-Nielsen O, Sorensen M et al: Tobacco smoke and bladder cancer-in the European Prospective Investigation into Cancer and Nutrition, *Int J Cancer* 119(10):2412-2416, 2006.

Borrie MJ, Bawden M, Speechley M et al: Interventions led by nurse continence advisers in the management of urinary incontinence: a randomized controlled trial, *Can Med Assoc J* 166(10):1267-1273, 2002.

Bostwick JM: The many faces of confusion. Timing and collateral history often hold the key to diagnosis, *Postgrad Med* 108(6):60-62, 65-66, 71-72, 2000.

Brown JS, Vittinghoff E, Kanaya AM et al: Urinary tract infections in postmenopausal women: effect of hormone therapy and risk factors, *Obstet Gynecol* 98(6):1045-1052, 2001.

Danforth KN, Townsend MK, Lifford K et al: Risk factors for urinary incontinence among middle-aged women, *Am J Obst Gynecol* 194(2):339-345, 2006.

Dougherty MC, Dwyer JW, Pendergast JF et al: A randomized trial of behavioral management for continence with older rural women, *Res Nurs Health* 25:3-13, 2002.

Dowd T, Kolcaba K, Steiner R: Using cognitive strategies to enhance bladder control and comfort, *Holist Nurs Pract* 14(2):91-103, 2000.

Gray M: Are cranberry juice or cranberry products effective in the prevention or management of urinary tract infection? *J Wound Ostomy Continence Nurs* 29:122-126, 2002.

Gray M: Caffeine and urinary incontinence, *J Wound Ostomy Continence Nurs* 28:66-69, 2001.

Gray M: The importance of screening, assessing and managing urinary incontinence in primary care, *J Am Acad Nurse Practitioners* 15(3):102, 2003.

Gray M: Urinary retention. Management in the acute care setting. Part 1, *Am J Nurs* 100(7):40-47, 2000.

Gray M, Hufstuttler S, Albo M: Interstitial cystitis: a guide to recognition, evaluation and management for the nurse practitioner, *J Wound Ostomy Continence Nurs* 29:93-102, 2002.

Gray ML, Burns SB: Continence management, *Crit Care Clin North Am* 8:29, 1996.

Hunskaar S et al: Epidemiology of urinary (UI) and fecal incontinence (FI) and pelvic organ prolapse (POP). In Abrams P, Cardozo L, Khoury S et al, editors: *3rd International consultation on incontinence,* ed 3, Plymouth, UK, 2005, Plymbridge, Health Publications.

Interstitial Cystitis Association: *Interstitial cystitis and diet,* Rockville, Md, 1999, The Association.

Jirovec MM, Wells TJ: Urinary incontinence in nursing home residents with dementia: the mobility-cognition paradigm, *Appl Nurs Res* 3:112-117, 1990.

Kincaid-Smith P, Fairley K: The investigation of hematuria, *Semin Nephrol* 25(3):127-135, 2005.

Malterud K, Baerheim A: Peeing barbed wire. Symptom experiences in women with lower urinary tract infection, *Scand J Prim Health Care* 17(1):49-53, 1999.

Midthun S, Paur R, Bruce AW et al: Urinary tract infections in the elderly: a survey of physicians and nurses, *Geriatr Nurs* 26(4):245-251, 2005.

Morris A, Browne G, Saltmarche A: Urinary incontinence: correlates among cognitively impaired elderly veterans, *J Gerontol Nurs* 18(10):33-40, 1992.

Sampselle CM, Wyman JF, Thomas KK et al: Continence for women: evaluation of AWHONN's third research utilization project. Association of Women's Health Obstetric and Neonatal Nurses, *J Obstet Gynecol Neonatal Nurs* 29(1):9-17, 2000.

Staskin D et al: Initial assessment of incontinence. In Abrams P, Cardozo, L, Khoury S et al, editors: *Incontinence: 3rd international consultation on incontinence,* ed 3, Plymouth, UK, 2005, Plymbridge, Health Publications.

Stewart WF, Van Rooyen JB, Cundiff GW et al: Prevalence and burden of overactive bladder in the United States, *World J Urol* 20(6):327-336, 2003.

Suchinski GA, Piano MR, Rosenberg N et al: Treating urinary tract infections in the elderly, *Dimens Crit Care Nurs* 18(1):21-27, 1999.

Tampakoudis P, Tantanassis T, Grimbizis G et al: Cigarette smoking and urinary incontinence in women—a new calculative method of estimating the exposure to smoke, *Eur J Obstet Gynecol Reprod Biol* 63(1):27-30, 1995.

van Gerwen M, Lagro-Janssen AL: [Diagnostic value of patient history and physical examination in elderly patients with urinary incontinence; a literature review] [article in Dutch], *Ned Tijdschr Geneeskd* 150(32):1771-1775, 2006.

U

Readiness for enhanced Urinary elimination   *Mikel Gray, PhD, RN*

NANDA   **Definition**

A pattern of urinary functions that is sufficient for meeting eliminatory needs and can be strengthened

Defining Characteristics

Amount of output is within normal limits; expresses willingness to enhance urinary elimination; fluid intake is adequate for daily needs; positions self for emptying of bladder; specific gravity is within normal limits; urine is odorless; urine is straw colored

• = Independent;   ▲ = Collaborative;   EBN = Evidence-Based Nursing;   EB = Evidence-Based

NOC   Outcomes (Nursing Outcomes Classification)

Suggested NOC Outcomes

Urinary Continence, Urinary Elimination

Example NOC Outcome with Indicators
Urinary Continence as evidenced by the following indicators: Voids >150 mL each time/Empties bladder completely/Absence of postvoid residual/Postvoid residual <100 to 200 mL (Rate the outcome and indicators of **Urinary Continence:** 1 = never demonstrated, 2 = rarely demonstrated, 3 = sometimes demonstrated, 4 = often demonstrated, 5 = consistently demonstrated [see Section I].)

Client Outcomes

Client Will (Specify Time Frame):

- Eliminate or reduce incontinent episodes
- Recognize sensory stimulus indicating readiness for urine elimination
- Respond to prompts for toileting

NIC   Interventions (Nursing Interventions Classification)

Suggested NIC Intervention

Urinary Elimination Management

Example NIC Activities—Urinary Elimination Management
Monitor urinary elimination, including frequency, consistency, odor, volume, and color, as appropriate; Teach patient signs and symptoms of urinary tract infection

Nursing Interventions and *Rationales*

- Assess the client for readiness for improving urine elimination patterns, focusing on need for physical assistance to access toilet, cognitive awareness of sensations indicating readiness for urine elimination, and current continence status (bladder management strategy, frequency of incontinent episodes). *Definitions of urinary continence and incontinence applied to ambulatory adults must be modified for the frail, elder client who is homebound or who resides in a long-term care setting (Palmer et al, 1997).*
- Using information from the Minimum Data Set (MDS), evaluate the client for potentially reversible or modifiable factors contributing to urinary incontinence. **EBN:** *A review of the MDS often reveals reversible or modifiable causes of urinary incontinence that lie outside of the urinary tract such as administration of specific drugs, acute delirium, bed-rails, trunk restraints, chair restraints, or impaired mobility that may be alleviated or modified, reducing or ablating urinary incontinence (Brandeis et al, 1997).*
- Complete a bladder diary of diurnal and nocturnal urine elimination patterns and patterns of urinary leakage. *A bladder diary provides a more objective verification of urine elimination patterns than a history (Resnick et al, 1994).* **EBN:** *A bladder diary is an integral portion of the evaluation of urinary incontinence in the client who is homebound or residing in a long-term setting, and it provides a baseline against which outcomes of treatment can be evaluated (Pfister, 1999).*
- Begin a scheduled toileting program (usually every 2 to 3 hours) for the client who has mild to moderately impaired cognition and who requires some physical assistance to access the toilet. **EBN:** *Elders with no to moderate cognitive impairment, who are able to cooperate with toileting, and who have adequate mobility to toilet with minimal or moderate assistance are ideal candidates for scheduled toileting (Jirovec & Templin, 2001).*
- Remove environmental barriers to toilet access.
- Provide a urinal or bedside toilet as indicated.

• = Independent;   ▲ = Collaborative;   EBN = Evidence-Based Nursing;   EB = Evidence-Based

- Assist client to remove clothing, transfer to the toilet, cleanse the perineal skin, and redress as indicated.
- Ensure that toileting opportunities are offered both during daytime hours and during hours of sleep. *Certain clients who are homebound or reside in a long-term care facility have the potential for continence but experience urine loss because they lack adequate physical assistance needed to access the toilet, remove clothing, and redress after toileting is finished. The level of assistance varies significantly and depends on the client's mobility and dexterity, as well as the availability of bedside toileting aids (Palmer et al, 1997).*
- For the client experiencing urinary incontinence who has mild cognitive deficits, begin a prompted voiding program or patterned urge response toileting program. Begin a prompted toileting program based on the results of bladder log over a period of 2 to 3 days, using a check and change system as indicated.
    - Approach the client and briefly explain that it is time to toilet.
    - Assist the client to the toilet, provide assistance removing clothing and urine-containment devices (pads, adult urine-containment briefs), and check for urinary leakage since the last scheduled toileting.
    - Praise the client when toileting occurs with prompting.
    - If the client does not toilet or has evidence of an incontinence episode, refrain from praise, gently inform the client of the urine loss, remove and replace the soiled containment device, and assist the client to redress and rejoin activities or return to bed.

    EBN: *There is weak evidence that prompted voiding increases successful, self-initiated voiding episodes and diminishes incontinent episodes (Eustice, Roe & Paterson, 2000).*
- Institute regular use of incontinence-containment devices combined with a structured perineal skin care program for the client with severe cognitive impairment, significant functional impairment, or no reduction in urinary incontinence frequency or severity with a scheduled or prompted toileting program. (Refer to **Total urinary Incontinence**.) *Urine-containment products include a variety of absorptive pads, incontinent briefs, under-pads for bedding, absorptive inserts that fit into specially designed undergarments, and condom catheters. Careful selection of an absorptive device and education concerning its use maximizes its effectiveness in controlling urine loss in a particular individual (Dunn et al, 2002).*

evolve   See the EVOLVE website for World Wide Web resources for client education.

REFERENCES

Brandeis GH, Baumann MM, Hossain M et al: The prevalence of potentially remediable urinary incontinence in frail older people: a study using the Minimum Data Set, *J Geriatr Soc* 45(2):179-184, 1997.

Dunn S, Kowanko I, Paterson J et al: Systematic review of the effectiveness of urinary continence products, *J Wound Ostomy Continence Nurs* 29(3):129-142, 2002.

Eustice S, Roe B, Paterson J: Prompted voiding for the management of urinary incontinence in adults, *Cochrane Database Syst Rev* (2): CD002113, 2000.

Jirovec MM, Templin T: Predicting success using individualized scheduled toileting for memory-impaired elders at home, *Res Nurs Health* 24(1):1-8, 2001.

Palmer MH, Czarapata BJ, Wells TJ et al: Urinary outcomes in older adults: research and clinical perspective, *Urol Nurs* 17(1):2-9, 1997.

Pfister SM: Bladder diaries and voiding patterns in older adults, *J Gerontol Nurs* 25(3):36-41, 1999.

Resnick NM, Beckett LA, Branch LG et al: Short term variability of self-report of incontinence in older persons, *J Am Geriatr Soc* 42:202-207, 1994.

U

Urinary retention   *Mikel Gray, PhD, RN*   **evolve**

NANDA   **Definition**

Incomplete emptying of the bladder

Defining Characteristics

Measured urinary residual greater than 200 to 250 mL or 25% of total bladder capacity; voiding and postmicturition LUTS (slow stream, intermittency of stream, hesitancy of urination, postvoid dribbling, feelings of incomplete bladder emptying); often accompanied by storage LUTS

• = Independent;   ▲ = Collaborative;   EBN = Evidence-Based Nursing;   EB = Evidence-Based

(urgency, day and nighttime voiding frequency); occasionally accompanied by overflow incontinence (dribbling urine loss caused when intravesical pressure overwhelms the sphincter mechanism)

Related Factors (r/t)

Bladder outlet obstruction (benign prostatic hyperplasia [BPH], prostate cancer, prostatitis, acute prostatic congestion and inflammation after implantation of irradiated seeds, urethral stricture, bladder neck dyssynergia, bladder neck contracture, detrusor striated sphincter dyssynergia, high tone pelvic floor muscle dysfunction, obstructing cystocele, urethral tumor, urethral polyp, posterior urethral valves, postoperative complication)

Deficient detrusor contraction strength (sacral level spinal lesions, cauda equina syndrome, peripheral polyneuropathies, herpes zoster or simplex affecting sacral nerve roots, injury or extensive surgery causing denervation of pelvic plexus, medication side effect, complication of illicit drug use, impaction of stool)

Defining characteristics and related factors adapted from the work of NANDA.

NOC   Outcomes (Nursing Outcomes Classification)

Suggested NOC Outcomes

Urinary Continence, Urinary Elimination

Example NOC Outcome with Indicators
Urinary Continence as evidenced by the following indicators: Absence of urinary leakage between catheterizations or containment of micturition by condom catheter and drainage bag/Absence of UTI (negative leukocytes and bacterial growth negative or <100,000 CFU/mL)/Underclothing dry during day/Underclothing or bedding dry during night (Rate the outcome and indicators of **Urinary Continence:** 1 = never demonstrated, 2 = rarely demonstrated, 3 = sometimes demonstrated, 4 = often demonstrated, 5 = consistently demonstrated [see Section I].)

CFU, Colony-forming units; *UTI,* urinary tract infection.

Client Outcomes

Client Will (Specify Time Frame):

- Demonstrate consistent ability to urinate when desire to void is perceived or via timed schedule; measured urinary residual volume is <200 to 250 mL or 25% of total bladder capacity (voided volume plus urinary residual volume)
- Experience correction or relief from voiding and postvoid LUTS
- Experience correction or alleviation of storage LUTS
- Be free of upper urinary tract distress (renal function remains sufficient; febrile urinary infections are absent)

NIC   Interventions (Nursing Interventions Classification)

Suggested NIC Interventions

Urinary Catheterization, Urinary Retention Care

Example NIC Activities—Urinary Retention Care
Perform a comprehensive urinary assessment focusing on incontinence (e.g., urinary output, urinary voiding pattern, cognitive function, and preexistent urinary problems); Use the power of suggestion by running water, or flushing toilet; Provide enough time for bladder emptying/Use double voiding technique

Nursing Interventions and *Rationales*

- Obtain a focused urinary history emphasizing the character and duration of lower urinary tract symptoms. Query the client about episodes of acute urinary retention (complete inability to void) or chronic retention (documented elevated postvoid residual volumes). *Although the presence of obstructive or irritative voiding symptoms is not diagnostic of urinary retention (Roehrborn et al, 2002), a focused nursing history can provide clues to the likely cause of retention and its management (Gray, 2000a).*
- Question the client concerning specific risk factors for urinary retention including:
  - Disorders affecting the sacral spinal cord such as spinal cord injuries of vertebral levels T12-L2, disk problems, cauda equina syndrome, tabes dorsalis
  - Acute neurological injury causing sudden loss of mobility such as spinal shock or ischemic stroke
  - Metabolic disorders such as diabetes mellitus, chronic alcoholism, and related conditions associated with polyuria and peripheral polyneuropathies
  - Herpetic infection involving the sacral skin and underlying spinal dermatomes
  - Heavy-metal poisoning (lead, mercury) causing peripheral polyneuropathies
  - Advanced stage human immunodeficiency virus (HIV)
  - Medications including antispasmodics/parasympatholytics, alpha-adrenergic agonists, antidepressants, sedatives, narcotics, psychotropic medications, illicit drugs
  - Recent surgery requiring general or spinal anesthesia
  - Bowel elimination patterns, history of fecal impaction, encopresis
  - Recent surgical procedures
  - Recent prostatic biopsy or brachytherapy therapy

  Urinary retention is related to multiple factors affecting either detrusor contraction strength or urethral resistance to urinary outflow (Acheson & Mudd, 2004; Darabi et al, 2004; Gray, 2000a; Kong & Young, 2000; Gehrich et al, 2005; Thomas et al, 2005; Ohashi et al, 2006). **EBN:** *Multiple factors in the surgical client are associated with an increased risk of postoperative urinary retention including preoperative voiding difficulty, advanced age, total amount of fluid replacement during a 24-hour postoperative period, type of anesthesia, pain management medications, and route and length of medication administration (Wynd et al, 1996).*
- ▲ Perform a focused physical assessment or review results of a recent physical including perineal skin integrity; inspection, percussion, and palpation of the lower abdomen for obvious bladder distention; a neurological examination including perineal skin sensation and the bulbocavernosus reflex; and vaginal vault examination in women and digital rectal examination in men. *The physical assessment provides clues to the likely cause of urinary retention and its management.*
- ▲ Determine the urinary residual volume by catheterizing the client immediately after urination or by obtaining a bladder ultrasound after micturition. *Although catheterization provides the most accurate method to determine urinary residual volume, it is invasive, produces discomfort, and carries a risk of infection (Gray, 2000b).* **EBN:** *Postvoid bladder ultrasound performed by registered nurses provided reasonable estimates of postvoid residual bladder volumes in clients treated in acute care and geriatric rehabilitation units (Borrie et al, 2001; O'Farrell et al, 2001). The results of the ultrasonic measurement changed nursing practice by 51% of instances, reducing unneeded catheterizations by 32% (O'Farrell et al, 2001).*
- Complete a bladder log including patterns of urine elimination, urine loss (if present), nocturia, and volume and type of fluids consumed for a period of 3 to 7 days. *The bladder log provides an objective verification of urine elimination patterns and allows comparison of fluids consumed versus urinary output during a 24-hour period (Nygaard & Holcomb, 2000).*
- ▲ Consult with the physician concerning eliminating or altering medications suspected of producing or exacerbating urinary retention. *Medication side effects may cause or greatly exacerbate urinary retention in susceptible individuals (Gray, 2000a,b).*
- Teach the client with mild to moderate obstructive symptoms to double void by urinating, resting in the bathroom for 3 to 5 minutes, and then trying again to urinate. *Double voiding promotes more efficient bladder evacuation by allowing the detrusor to contract initially and then rest and contract again (Gray, 2000b).*

- Teach the client with urinary retention and infrequent voiding to urinate by the clock. *Timed or scheduled voiding may reduce urinary retention by preventing bladder overdistention (Gray, 2000b).*
- Advise the male client with urinary retention related to BPH to avoid risk factors associated with acute urinary retention as follows:
  - Avoid over-the-counter cold remedies containing a decongestant (alpha-adrenergic agonist).
  - Avoid taking over-the-counter dietary medications (frequently contain alpha-adrenergic agonists).
  - Discuss voiding problems with a healthcare provider before beginning new prescription medications.
  - After prolonged exposure to cool weather, warm the body before attempting to urinate.
  - Avoid overfilling the bladder by regular urination patterns and refrain from excessive intake of alcohol.

  These modifiable factors predispose the client to acute urinary retention by overdistending the bladder and compromising detrusor contraction strength or by increasing outlet resistance (Gray, 2000b). **EB:** *Medications with alpha-adrenergic agonistic effects increased the risk for acute urinary retention in elder men with prostatic enlargement (Meigs et al, 1999).*

- ▲ Teach the elderly male client with BPH to self-administer a 5 alpha-reductase inhibitor, such as *finasteride* or *dutasteride*, or an alpha-adrenergic–blocking agent, such as *tamsulosin, alfuzosin,* doxazosin, or terazosin, as directed. Provide careful instruction concerning the dose, administration schedule, and side effects of these drugs, including possible adverse side effects (postural hypotension) when multiple doses are inadvertently missed. *Finasteride is a 5-alpha-reductase inhibitor that reduces the risk of acute urinary retention when taken by men with BPH over a prolonged period (McConnell et al, 1998). The magnitude of obstruction associated with BPH is also reduced by routine administration of alpha-adrenergic–blocking agents including alfuzosin, tamsulosin, terazosin, or doxazosin. Terazosin and doxazosin must be taken regularly to reduce the risk of side effects including postural hypotension (Narayan & Tewari, 1998; Lepor et al, 1997, 1998). Some agents must be titrated, and a risk for postural hypotension increases if doses are missed; other agents do not require titration and are associated with a reduced risk of postural hypotension (Schulman, 2003).*

- ▲ Teach the client who is unable to void specific strategies to manage this potential medical emergency as follows:
  - Attempt urination in complete privacy.
  - Place the feet solidly on the floor.
  - If unable to void using these strategies, take a warm sitz bath or shower and void (if possible) while still in the tub or shower.
  - Drink a warm cup of caffeinated coffee or tea to stimulate the bladder, which may promote voiding.
  - If unable to void within 6 hours or if bladder distention is producing significant pain, seek urgent or emergency care.

  Attempting urination in complete privacy and placing the feet solidly on the floor help relax the pelvic muscles and may encourage voiding. Warm water also stimulates the bladder and may produce voiding; the cooling experienced by leaving the tub or shower may again inhibit the bladder (Gray, 2000b).

- ▲ Remove the indwelling urethral catheter at midnight in the hospitalized client to reduce the risk of acute urinary retention. **EBN:** *Removal of indwelling catheters in clients undergoing urologic surgery at midnight offers several advantages to "morning removal," including a larger initial voided volume and earlier hospital discharge with no increased risk for readmission compared with those undergoing morning removal (Griffiths, Fernandez & Murie, 2004).*

- ▲ Consult the physician about bladder stimulation in the client with urinary retention caused by deficient detrusor contraction strength. **EBN:** *High-frequency transvaginal electrical stimulation of the bladder neck has been shown to be beneficial in a small case series involving women with chronic urinary retention owing to deficient detrusor contraction strength (Bernier & Davila, 2000).*

- ▲ Perform sterile or clean intermittent catheterization as directed for clients with urinary retention. **EBN:** *Intermittent catheterization using clean technique had no more symptomatic UTI than those managed by intermittent catheterization using sterile technique (Moore, Burt & Volklander, 2006).*

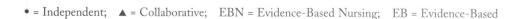

▲ Teach the client with significant urinary retention to perform clean, self-intermittent catheterization as directed. **EBN:** *Intermittent catheterization allows regular, complete bladder evacuation without serious complications (Horsley, Crane & Reynolds, 1982; Robinson, 2006).*

• Advise clients who undergo intermittent catheterization that bacteria are likely to colonize the urine but that this condition does not indicate a clinically significant urinary tract infection. *Bacteriuria frequently occurs in the client undergoing intermittent catheterization; only symptoms producing infections warrant treatment (Wyndaele, 2002).*

• Insert an indwelling catheter for the individual with urinary retention who is not a suitable candidate for intermittent catheterization. *An indwelling catheter provides continuous drainage of urine; however, the risks of serious urinary complications with prolonged use are significant (Weld et al, 2000).*

• Advise clients with indwelling catheters that bacteria in the urine is an almost universal finding after the catheter has remained in place for a period of 30 days or longer and that only symptomatic infections warrant treatment. *The long-term indwelling catheter is inevitably associated with bacterial colonization. Most bacteriuria does not produce significant infection, and attempts to eradicate bacteriuria often produce subsequent morbidity because resistant bacteria are encouraged to reproduce while more easily managed strains are eradicated (Gray, 2004). Intermittent catheterization was preferred in a rehabilitation setting because it improves client quality of life and diminishes the time required to recover spontaneous voiding with a postvoid residual volume <150ml (Tang et al, 2006).*

• Use the following strategies to reduce the risk for catheter associated UTI whenever feasible:
  ▪ Insert a silver impregnated catheter for short-term indwelling catheterization (<14 days).
  ▪ Maintain a closed drainage system whenever feasible.
  ▪ Change the catheter every 4 weeks whenever possible; more frequent catheter changes should be reserved for clients who experience catheter encrustation and blockage.
  ▪ Place clients managed in an acute or long-term care facility with a catheter-associated UTI in a separate room from others managed by an indwelling catheter to reduce the risk of spreading the offending pathogen.
  ▪ Educate staff about the risks of catheter-associated UTI and specific strategies to reduce this risk.

  EBN: *These strategies are supported by sufficient evidence to recommend routine use. Strategies that lack sufficient evidence to support routine use include (1) aseptic technique when replacing a long-term indwelling catheter, (2) routine meatal care, (3) application of antimicrobial ointments or creams to the urethral meatus, (4) adding hydrogen peroxide or silver sulfadiazine or slow-releasing silver ions to the catheter drainage bag, (5) frequent drainage bag changes, or (6) one-way catheter valves (Gray, 2004).*

 Geriatric

• Aggressively assess elderly clients, particularly those with dribbling urinary incontinence, UTI, and related conditions for urinary retention. *Elderly women (and men) may experience urinary retention of 1500 mL or more with few or no apparent symptoms; a urinary residual volume and related assessments are necessary to determine the presence of retention in this population (Williams, Wallhagen & Dowling, 1993).*

• Assess elderly clients for impaction when urinary retention is documented or suspected. *Fecal impaction and urinary retention frequently coexist in elderly clients and, unless reversed, may lead to acute delirium, UTI, or renal insufficiency (Waale, Bruijns & Dautzenberg, 2001).*

• Assess elderly male clients for retention related to prostatic enlargement (BPH or prostate cancer). *Prostate enlargement in elderly men increases the risk of acute and chronic urinary retention (Loh & Chin, 2002; McNeill & Hargreave, 2000).*

 Home Care

• The interventions listed previously may be adapted for home care use.

• Encourage the client to report any inability to void. *Pathophysiological factors of urinary retention require follow-up.*

▲ Maintain an up-to-date medication list; evaluate side effect profiles for risk of urinary retention. *New medications or changes in dose may cause urinary retention.*

▲ Refer the client for physician evaluation if urinary retention occurs. *Identification of cause is important. Left untreated, urinary retention may lead to UTI or kidney failure.*

U

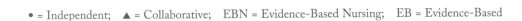
• = Independent;   ▲ = Collaborative;   EBN = Evidence-Based Nursing;   EB = Evidence-Based

Client/Family Teaching

- Teach techniques for intermittent catheterization including use of clean rather than sterile technique, washing using soap and water or a microwave technique, and reuse of the catheter.
- Teach the client with an indwelling catheter to assess the tube for patency, maintain the drainage system below the level of the symphysis pubis, and routinely cleanse the bedside bag.
- Teach the client with an indwelling catheter or undergoing intermittent catheterization the symptoms of a significant urinary infection including hematuria, acute-onset incontinence, dysuria, flank pain, or fever.

evolve See the EVOLVE website for World Wide Web resources for client education.

REFERENCES

Acheson J, Mudd D: Acute urinary retention attributable to sacral herpes zoster, *Emerg Med J* 21(6):752-753, 2004.

Bernier F, Davila GW: The treatment of nonobstructive urinary retention with high-frequency transvaginal electrical stimulation, *Urol Nurs* 20(4):261-264, 2000.

Borrie MJ, Campbell K, Arcese ZA et al: Urinary retention in patients in a geriatric rehabilitation unit: prevalence, risk factors, and validity of bladder scan evaluation, *Rehab Nurs* 26(5):187-191, 2001.

Darabi K, Segal AM, Torres G: Herpes zoster infection: a rare cause of urinary retention, *Can J Urol* 11(4):2314, 2004.

Gehrich AP, Aseff JN, Iglesia CB et al: Chronic urinary retention and pelvic floor hypertonicity after surgery for endometriosis: a case series, *Am J Obst Gynecol* 193(6):2133-2137, 2005.

Gray M: Urinary retention. Management in the acute care setting. Part 1, *Am J Nurs* 100(7):40-47, 2000a.

Gray M: Urinary retention. Management in the acute care setting. II. *Am J Nurs* 100(8):36-43, 2000b.

Gray M: What nursing interventions reduce the risk of symptomatic urinary tract infection in the patient with an indwelling catheter? *J Wound Ostomy Continence Nurs* 31(1):3-13, 2004.

Griffiths RD, Fernandez RS, Murie P: Removal of short-term indwelling urethral catheters: the evidence, *J Wound, Ostomy Continence Nurs* 31(5):299-308, 2004.

Horsley JA, Crane J, Reynolds MA: *Clean intermittent catheterization: conduct and utilization of research in nursing project*, New York, 1982, Grune & Stratton.

Kong K, Young S: Incidence and outcome of poststroke urinary retention: a prospective study, *Arch Phys Med Rehabil* 81(11):1464-1467, 2000.

Lepor H, Kaplan SA, Klimberg I et al: Doxazosin for benign prostatic hyperplasia: long-term efficacy and safety in hypertensive and normotensive patients, *J Urol* 157:525-530, 1997.

Lepor H, Williford WO, Barry MJ et al: The impact of medical therapy due to symptoms, quality of life and global outcome, and factors predicting response, *J Urol* 160:1358-1367, 1998.

Loh SY, Chin CM: A demographic profile of patients undergoing transurethral resection of the prostate for benign prostate hyperplasia and presenting in acute urinary retention, *Br J Urol Int* 89(6):531-533, 2002.

McConnell JD, Bruskewitz R, Walsh P et al: The effect of finasteride on the risk of acute urinary retention and the need for surgical treatment among men with benign prostatic hyperplasia. Finasteride Long-Term Efficacy and Safety Study Group, *N Engl J Med* 338(9):557-563, 1998.

McNeill SA, Hargreave TB: Efficacy of PSA in the detection of carcinoma of the prostate in patients presenting with acute urinary retention, *J R Coll Surg Edinb* 45(4):227-230, 2000.

Meigs JB, Barry MJ, Giovannucci E et al: Incidence rates and risk factors for acute urinary retention: the health professionals follow-up study, *J Urol* 162(2):376-382, 1999.

Moore KN, Burt J, Voaklander DC: Intermittent catheterization in the rehabilitation setting: a comparison of clean and sterile technique, *Clin Rehabil* 20(6):461-468, 2006.

Narayan P, Tewari A: A second phase III multicenter placebo study of 2 dosages of modified release tamsulosin in patients with symptoms of benign prostatic hyperplasia. United States 93-01 study group, *J Urol* 160:1701-1706, 1998.

Nygaard I, Holcomb R: Reproducibility of the seven day voiding diary in women with stress urinary incontinence, *Int Urogynecol J Pelvic Floor Dysfunct* 11:15-17, 2000.

O'Farrell B, Vandervoort MK, Bisnaire D et al: Evaluation of portable bladder ultrasound: accuracy and effect on nursing practice in an acute neuroscience unit, *J Neurosci Nurs* 33(6):301-309, 2001.

Ohashi T, Yorozu A, Toya K et al: Predictive factors of acute urinary retention requiring catheterization following 125I prostate brachytherapy, *Jpn J Clin Oncol* 36(5):285-289, 2006.

Robinson J: Intermittent self-catheterization: principles and practice, *Br J Community Nurs* 11(4):144, 146, 148 passim, 2006.

Roehrborn CG, McConnell JD, Saltzman B et al: Storage (irritative) and voiding (obstructive) symptoms as predictors of benign prostatic hyperplasia progression and related outcomes, *Eur Urol* 42(1):1-6, 2002.

Schulman CC: Lower urinary tract symptoms/benign prostatic hyperplasia: minimizing morbidity caused by treatment, *Urology* 62(3 Suppl 1):24-33, 2003.

Tang MW, Kwok TC, Hui E et al: Intermittent versus indwelling urinary catheterization in older female patients, *Maturitas* 53(3):274-281, 2006.

Thomas AW, Cannon A, Bartlett E et al: The natural history of lower urinary tract dysfunction in men: minimum 10-year urodynamic follow-up of untreated bladder outlet obstruction, *BJU Int* 96(9):1301-1306, 2005.

Waale WH, Bruijns E, Dautzenberg PJ: Delirium due to urinary retention: confusing for both the patient and the doctor, *Tijdschr Gerontol Geriatr* 32(3):100-103, 2001.

Weld KJ, Wall BM, Mangold TA et al: Influences on renal function in chronic spinal cord injured patients, *J Urol* 164(5):1490-1493, 2000.

Williams MP, Wallhagen M, Dowling G: Urinary retention in elderly hospitalized women, *J Gerontol Nurs* 19:7-14, 1993.

Wynd CA, Wallace M, Smith KM et al: Factors influencing postoperative urinary retention following orthopaedic surgical procedures, *Orthop Nurs* 15(1):43-50, 1996.

Wyndaele JJ: Complications of intermittent catheterization: their prevention and treatment, *Spinal Cord* 40(10):536, 2002.

Impaired spontaneous Ventilation   *Elizabeth A. Henneman, PhD, RN*

NANDA   Definition

Decreased energy reserves result in an individual's inability to maintain breathing adequate to support life

Defining Characteristics

Apprehension; decreased cooperation; decreased Po_2; decreased SaO_2; decreased tidal volume; dyspnea; increased heart rate; increased metabolic rate; increased Pco_2; increased restlessness; increased use of accessory muscles

Related Factors (r/t)

Metabolic factors; respiratory muscle fatigue

NOC   Outcomes (Nursing Outcomes Classification)

Suggested NOC Outcomes

Neurological Status: Central Motor Control, Respiratory Status: Gas Exchange, Ventilation

Example NOC Outcome with Indicators
Achieves appropriate **Respiratory Status: Ventilation** as evidenced by the following indicators: Respiratory rate/Respiratory rhythm/Depth of inspiration/Symmetrical chest expansion/Ease of breathing/Moves sputum out of airway/Accessory muscle use not present/Adventitious breath sounds not present/Chest retraction not present/ Auscultated breath sounds/Tidal volume/Vital capacity (Rate the outcome and indicators of **Respiratory Status: Ventilation:** 1 = severely compromised, 2 = substantially compromised, 3 = moderately compromised, 4 = mildly compromised, 5 = not compromised [see Section I].)

Client Outcomes

Client Will (Specify Time Frame):

- Maintain arterial blood gases within safe parameters
- Remain free of dyspnea or restlessness
- Effectively maintain airway
- Effectively mobilize secretions

NIC   Interventions (Nursing Interventions Classification)

Suggested NIC Interventions

Artificial Airway Management, Mechanical Ventilation: Invasive, Respiratory Monitoring, Resuscitation: Neonate, Ventilation Assistance, Mechanical Ventilation Management: Noninvasive

Example NIC Activities—Mechanical Ventilation Management: Invasive
Monitor for conditions indicating a need for ventilation support (e.g., respiratory muscle fatigue, neurological dysfunction second to trauma, anesthesia, drug overdose, refractory respiratory acidosis); Consult with other healthcare personnel in selection of a ventilator mode

Nursing Interventions and *Rationales*

▲ Collaborate with the client, family, and physician regarding possible intubation and ventilation. Ask whether the client has advanced directives and, if so, integrate them into the plan of care with clinical data regarding overall health and reversibility of the medical condition. **EB:** *Client preferences must be acknowledged when planning care. Advanced directives protect client autonomy and help to ensure that the client's wishes are respected (Garas & Pantilat, 2001).*

• = Independent;   ▲ = Collaborative;   EBN = Evidence-Based Nursing;   EB = Evidence-Based

- Assess and respond to changes in the client's respiratory status. Monitor the client for dyspnea, increase in respiratory rate, use of accessory muscles, retraction of intercostal muscles, flaring of nostrils, decrease in O_2 saturation, and subjective complaints (Schultz, 2005). **EBN:** *It is essential to monitor for these signs of impending respiratory failure or inability to tolerate mechanical ventilation/weaning (Earven et al, 2004).*
- Have the client use a numerical scale (0-10) to rate dyspnea before and after interventions. **EBN:** *The numerical rating scale is a valid measure of dyspnea and has been found to be easiest for clients to use. This allows measurement of the intensity, progression, and resolution of dyspnea (Gift & Narsavage, 1998; Powers & Bennett, 1999).*
- Assess for history of chronic respiratory disorders when administering oxygen. *With chronic obstructive pulmonary disease (COPD) the respiratory drive is primarily in response to hypoxia, not hypercarbia; oxygenating too aggressively can result in respiratory depression. When managing acute respiratory failure in clients with COPD, use caution in administering oxygen because hyperoxygenation can lead to respiratory depression.*
- ▲ Collaborate with the physician and respiratory therapists in determining the appropriateness of noninvasive positive pressure ventilation (NPPV) for the decompensated client with COPD.
- ▲ Assist with implementation, client support, and monitoring if NPPV is used. **EB:** *In a client with exacerbation of COPD, NPPV can be as effective as intubation with use of a ventilator. It can also be used if the client has other complications, such as hypotension or severely impaired mental status (Perkins & Shortall, 2000; Pierson, 2002). The use of continuous positive airway pressure (CPAP) and bi-level positive airway pressure (bi-PAP) has been shown to improve oxygenation and decrease the rate of endotracheal intubation in clients with acute pulmonary edema (Park et al, 2004).*
- If the client has apnea, pH <7.25, $PaCO_2$ >50 mm Hg, PaO_2 <50 mm Hg, respiratory muscle fatigue, or somnolence, prepare the client for intubation and placement on a ventilator. **EBN:** *These indicators are predictive of the need for invasive mechanical ventilation (Burns, 2005; Pierson, 2002).*

Ventilator Support

- ▲ Explain the intubation intervention to the client and family as appropriate, and during the procedure, administer sedation for client comfort according to the physician's orders. **EBN:** *Explanation of the procedure decreases anxiety and reinforces information; premedication allows for a more controlled intubation with decreased incidence of insertion problems (Burns, 2005).*
- Secure the endotracheal tube in place using either tape or a device, auscultate bilateral breath sounds, use a CO_2 detector, and obtain a chest radiograph to confirm endotracheal tube placement. **EBN:** *Secure taping is needed to prevent inadvertent extubation. Nursing studies have shown conflicting results regarding the preferable way to secure the endotracheal tube (Barnason et al, 1998; Clarke et al, 1998; Kaplow & Bookbinder, 1994).* **EB:** *Auscultation alone is an unreliable method for checking endotracheal tube placement (Takeda, 2003). A CO_2 detector can be used to confirm tube placement in the trachea (Takeda et al, 2003); however, correct position of the endotracheal tube in the trachea (3-5 cm above the carina) must be confirmed by chest radiograph (Burns, 2005; Henneman, Ellstrom & St. John, 1998).*
- Ensure that ventilator settings are appropriate to meet the client's minute ventilation requirements. *Pay careful attention to the tidal volume and respiratory rate settings to prevent hyperventilation or hypoventilation. Tidal volume VT should be 8-12 ml/kg and respiratory rate ≤20 breaths/minute (Burns, 2005).*
- Suction as needed, and hyperoxygenate and hyperventilate according to policy. Refer to the care plan **Ineffective Airway clearance** for further information on suctioning.
- Ensure activation of all monitor alarms each shift. *This action helps ensure client safety (Burns, 2005).*
- Respond to ventilator alarms promptly. If unable to rapidly locate the source of the alarm, use a manual self-inflating resuscitation bag to ventilate the client while waiting for assistance. *Common causes of a high-pressure alarm include secretions, condensation in the tubing, biting of the endotracheal tube, decreased compliance of the lungs, and compression of the tubing. Common causes of a low-pressure alarm are ventilator disconnection, leaks in the circuit, and changing compliance and increased resistance (e.g., due to bronchospasm). Using a manual self-inflating resuscitation bag with supplemental oxygen, the nurse can provide immediate ventilation and oxygenation as needed (Burns, 2005).*

- Prevent unplanned extubation by maintaining stability of endotracheal tube and using soft wrist restraints on the client if needed and ordered. *Use only when other methods are ineffective, such as orienting client and allowing family at bedside.*
- Drain collected fluid from condensation out of ventilator tubing as needed. *This action reduces the risk of infection by decreasing inhalation of contaminated water droplets (Burns, 2005).*
- Note ventilator settings of flow of inspired oxygen, peak inspiratory pressure, tidal volume, and alarm activation at intervals and when removing the client from the ventilator for any reason. *Checking the settings ensures that safety measures are taken and that the client is not left on 100% oxygen after suctioning (Burns, 2005).*
- ▲ Administer analgesics and sedatives as needed with a defined protocol to facilitate client comfort and rest. Use pain and sedation scales to provide a consistent way of monitoring sedation levels and ensuring that therapeutic outcomes are being met (Consensus Conference on Sedation Assessment, 2004). **EBN:** *A study demonstrated that a nurse-implemented sedation protocol decreased the number of days of intubation, the need for a tracheotomy, and the length of hospital stay (Brook et al, 1999).* **EB:** *Avoid oversedation; use of continuous IV sedative infusions is associated with longer duration of mechanical ventilation compared with bolus sedation (Kress et al, 2000; Kollef et al, 1998; Brook et al, 1999). Clients receiving continuous sedative infusions should undergo once daily interruptions of the medication to assess the client's level of anxiety and need for medication (Kress et al, 2000). Oral intubation and inadequate sedation have been noted to be indicators for unplanned extubation (Chevron et al, 1998).*
- Assess level of sedation with such tools as the Riker Sedation-Agitation Scale, the Motor Activity Assessment Scale, or the Richmond Agitation-Sedation Scale. **EB:** *Each of these instruments has established reliability and validity and can be used to monitor the effect of sedative therapy (Jacobi et al, 2003; Ely et al, 2003).*
- To decrease anxiety, use music therapy with selections of the client's choice played on headphones at intervals. **EBN:** *Music therapy has been reported to decrease anxiety and reduced heart and respiratory rate in critically ill and intubated clients (Chlan, 1998; White, 2000).*
- Analyze and respond to arterial blood gas results, end-tidal CO_2 levels, and pulse oximetry values. *Ventilatory support must be closely monitored to ensure adequate oxygenation and acid-base balance.* **EBN:** *End-tidal CO_2 monitoring is best used as an adjunct to direct client observation and is used to monitor a client's ventilatory status and pulmonary blood flow (Good, 2005; St John, 2003).*
- Use an effective means of verbal and nonverbal communication with the client. A variety of communication devices are available, including electronic voice output communication aids, alphabet boards, picture boards, computers, and writing slate. Ask the client for input into care as able. Ensure client's human rights are met. **EBN:** *Inability to communicate can lead to client frustration, insecurity, and sometimes panic (Happ, 2001). Clients have reported a high level frustration in communicating their needs while being mechanically ventilated (Patak et al, 2004) and believe the use of a communication board would have decreased this frustration (Patak et al, 2006).* **EB:** *Use of a voice-output communication device was shown to be effective in a group of intubated surgery clients (Costello, 2000).* **EBN:** *Practitioner behaviors reported to facilitate communication include being kind, informative, and physically present at the bedside (Patak et al, 2004).*
- Move the endotracheal tube from side to side every 24 hours, and tape it or secure it with a device. Assess and document client's skin condition, and ensure correct tube placement at lip line. *These steps help prevent skin breakdown at the lip line resulting from endotracheal tube pressure (Scott & Vollman, 2005).*
- ▲ Implement steps to prevent ventilator associated pneumonia (VAP), including continuous removal of subglottic secretions, elevation of the head of bed to 30-45 degrees unless medically contraindicated, change of the ventilator circuit no more than every 48 hours, and hand washing before and after contact with each client (Tablan et al, 2004). See details in the sections that follow.
- Use endotracheal tubes that allow for the continuous aspiration of subglottic secretions (CASS) (if available). **EB:** *The accumulation of contaminated oropharyngeal secretions above the endotracheal tube may contribute to the risk of aspiration. Two studies have suggested a decrease in the rate of VAP in clients requiring mechanical ventilation for >3 days when CASS was used (Mahul et al, 1992; Valles*

et al, 1995). This practice is recommended by the Centers for Disease Control and Prevention (Tablan et al, 2004).

• Position the client in a semirecumbent position with the head of the bed at a 30- to 45-degree angle to decrease the aspiration of gastric secretions. **EB:** *Studies have shown that mechanically ventilated clients have a decreased incidence of pneumonia if the client is placed in a 30- to 45-degree semirecumbent position as opposed to a supine position (Collard, Saint & Matthay, 2003; Drakulovic et al, 1999; Torres et al, 1992).*

• Perform hand washing using either soap and water (if hands are visibly soiled) or alcohol based solution before and after all client contact (Tablan et al, 2004). **EB:** *Hand washing with an alcohol-based solution decreases bacterial counts (Girou et al, 2002; Lucet et al, 2002; Trick et al, 2003).*

• Provide routine oral care using toothbrushing and/or oral rinsing with an antimicrobial agent. **EB:** *Most episodes of VAP are thought to result from aspiration of oropharyngeal secretions containing potentially pathogenic organisms (Collard et al, 2003). Tooth brushing is recommended (versus use of sponge toothettes) to remove plaque (Munro & Grap, 2004). The use of an oral rinse of chlorhexidine is effective in preventing nosocomial pneumonia in clients after cardiac surgery (Houston et al, 2002).*

• Turn the client from side to side every 2 hours or as indicated. Use rotational bed therapy in clients for whom side-to-side turning is contraindicated or difficult. **EBN:** *Changing position frequently decreases the incidence of atelectasis, pooling of secretions, and resultant pneumonia (Burns, 2005).* **EB:** *Continuous, lateral rotational therapy has been shown to improve oxygenation and decrease the incidence of VAP (Wang et al, 2003).*

• Assess bilateral anterior and posterior breath sounds every 2-4 hours and PRN; respond to any relevant changes.

• Assess responsiveness to ventilator support; monitor for subjective complaints and sensation of dyspnea (Burns, 2005).

▲ Collaborate with the interdisciplinary team in treating clients with acute respiratory failure. **EB:** *A collaborative approach to caring for mechanically ventilated clients has been demonstrated to reduce length of time on the ventilator and length of stay in the ICU (Henneman et al, 2001, 2002). The mechanical ventilator is usually a temporary support until the underlying pathology can be effectively resolved.*

Geriatric

• Recognize that older adults have a high rate of morbidity when mechanically ventilated. *Implement such interventions as positioning and nutrition maintenance early to prevent decline (Phelan, Cooper & Sangkachand, 2002).*

Home Care

▲ Some of the interventions listed previously may be adapted for home care use. Begin discharge planning as soon as possible with the case manager or social worker to assess the need for home support systems, assistive devices, and community or home health services.

▲ With help from a medical social worker, assist the client and family to determine the fiscal affect of care in the home vs. an extended care facility.

• Assess the home setting during the discharge process to ensure the home can safely accommodate ventilator support (e.g., adequate space and electricity).

• Have the family contact the electric company and place the client residence on a high-risk list in case of a power outage. *Some home-based care requires special conditions for safe home administration.*

• Assess the caregivers for commitment to supporting a ventilator-dependent client in the home. *Commitment to care and valuing home as a healing place provides meaning for participating in caregiving and decrease caregiver role strain (Boland & Sims, 1996).*

• Be sure that the client and family or caregivers are familiar with operation of all ventilation devices, know how to suction secretions if needed, are competent in doing tracheostomy care, and know schedules for cleaning equipment. Have the designated caregiver or caregivers demonstrate care before discharge. *Some home-based care involves specialized technology and requires specific skills for safe and appropriate care.*

• Assess client and caregiver knowledge of the disease, client needs, and medications to be administered via ventilation-assistive devices. Avoid analgesics. Assess knowledge of how to use equipment. Teach as necessary. *A client receiving ventilation support may not be able to articulate needs. Respiratory medications can have side effects that change the client's respiration or level of consciousness.*

- Establish an emergency plan and criteria for use. Identify emergency procedures to be used until medical assistance arrives. Teach and role play emergency care. *A prepared emergency plan reassures the client and family and ensures client safety.*
- ▲ Institute case management of frail elderly clients to support continued independent living. *Respiratory difficulties represent and can lead to increasing need for assistance in using the healthcare system effectively.*

 Client/Family Teaching

- Explain to the client the potential sensations that will be experienced, including relief of dyspnea, the feeling of lung inflations, the noise of the ventilator, and the reality of alarms. **EBN:** *Knowledge of potential sensations and experiences before they are encountered can decrease anxiety. Administration of sedatives or narcotics may be needed to provide adequate oxygenation and ventilation in some clients (Burns, 2005).*
- Explain to the client and family about being unable to speak, and work out an alternative system of communication. See previously mentioned interventions.
- Demonstrate to the family how to perform simple procedures, such as suctioning secretions in the mouth with a tonsil-tip catheter, providing range-of-motion exercises, and reconnecting the ventilator immediately if it becomes disconnected. *Families often need to be part of the client's care, may be present at the bedside for prolonged periods of time, and need information about the plan of care (Burns, 2005; Henneman & Cardin, 2002).*
- Offer both the client and family explanations of how the ventilator works and answer any questions. *Having questions answered is often cited as an important need of clients and families when a client is on a ventilator (Burns, 2005).*

evolve See the EVOLVE website for World Wide Web resources for client education.

REFERENCES

Barnason S, Graham J, Wild MC et al: Comparison of two endotracheal tube securement techniques on unplanned extubation, oral mucosa, and facial skin integrity, *Heart Lung* 27(6):409, 1998.

Boland D, Sims S: Family care giving at home as a solitary journey, *Image* 28:1, 1996.

Brook AD, Ahrens TS, Schaiff R et al: Effect of a nursing-implemented sedation protocol on the duration of mechanical ventilation, *Crit Care Med* 27(12):2609, 1999.

Burns SM: Ventilatory management—volume and pressure modes. In Lynn-McHale DJ, Carlson KK, editors: *AACN procedure manual for critical care*, ed 4, Philadelphia, 2005, WB Saunders.

Chevron V, Menard JF, Richard JC et al: Unplanned extubation risk factors of development and predictive criteria for reintubation, *Crit Care Med* 26(6):1049, 1998.

Chlan L: Effectiveness of a music therapy intervention on relaxation and anxiety for patients receiving ventilatory assistance, *Heart Lung* 27(3):169, 1998.

Clarke T, Evans S, Way P et al: A comparison of two methods of securing an endotracheal tube, *Aust Crit Care* 11(2):45, 1998.

Collard HR, Saint S, Matthay MA: Prevention of ventilator-associated pneumonia: an evidence-based systemic review, *Ann Intern Med* 138(6):494, 2003.

Consensus conference on sedation assessment. Abbott Laboratories, American Association of Critical Care Nurses, St. Thomas Health System, *Crit Care Nurse* 24:33, 2004.

Costello JM: AAC intervention in the intensive care unit: the Children's Hospital Boston model, *Augment Altern Commun* 16, 2000.

Drakulovic MB, Torres A, Bauer TT et al: Supine body position as a risk factor for nosocomial pneumonia in mechanically ventilated patients: a randomized trial, *Lancet* 354(9193):1851, 1999.

Earven S, Fisher C, Lewis R et al: The experience of four outcomes managers: an institutional approach to weaning patients from long-term mechanical ventilation, *Crit Care Nurs Clin North Am* 16:395, 2004.

Ely EW, Truman B, Shintani A et al. Monitoring sedation status over time in ICU patients: reliability and validity of the Richmond Agitation-Sedation Scale (RASS), *JAMA* 289(22):2983-2991, 2003.

Garas N, Pantilat SZ: Advance planning for end-of-life care. In Shojania KG, Duncan BW, McDonald KM et al, editors: *Making healthcare safer: a critical analysis of patient safety practices. Evidence report/technology assessment No. 43*, AHRQ Publication No. 01-E058, Rockville, Md, July 2001, Agency for Healthcare Research and Quality, p 561.

Gift A, Narsavage G: Validity of the numeric rating scale as a measure of dyspnea, *Am J Crit Care* 7(3):200, 1998.

Girou E, Loyeau S, Legrand P et al: Efficacy of hand rubbing with alcohol based solution versus standard handwashing with antiseptic soap: randomized, clinical trial, *BMJ* 325:362, 2002.

Good VS: Continuous end-tidal carbon-dioxide monitoring. In Lynn-McHale DJ, Carlson KK, editors: *AACN procedure manual for critical care*, ed 4, Philadelphia, 2005, WB Saunders, pp 87-93.

Happ MB: Communicating with mechanically ventilated patients: state of the science, *AACN Clin Issues* 12(2):247, 2001.

Henneman EA, Cardin C: Family centered critical care: a practical approach to making it happen, *Crit Care Nurse* 22(6):12-19, 2002.

Henneman EA, Dracup K, Ganz T et al: Effect of a collaborative weaning plan on patient outcome in the critical care setting, *Crit Care Med* 29:297, 2001.

Henneman EA, Dracup K, Ganz T et al: Using a collaborative weaning plan to decrease duration of mechanical ventilation and length of stay in the intensive care unit for patients receiving long-term ventilation, *Am J Crit Care* 11:132, 2002.

Henneman EA, Ellstrom KE, St. John RE: *Airway management. AACN practice protocol.* Aliso Viejo, Calif, 1998, American Association of Critical Care Nursing.

Houston S, Hougland P, Anderson JJ et al: Effectiveness of 0.12% chlorhexidine gluconate oral rinse in reducing prevalence of nosocomial pneumonia in patients undergoing heart surgery, *Am J Crit Care* 11(6):567-570, 2002.

Jacobi J, Fraser GL, Coursin DB et al: Clinical practice guidelines for the sustained use of sedatives and analgesics in the critically ill adult, *Crit Care Med* 30 (1):119-141, 2003.

Kaplow R, Bookbinder M: A comparison of four endotracheal tube holders, *Heart Lung* 23:59, 1994.

Kollef MH, Levy NT, Ahrens TS et al: The use of continuous IV sedation is associated with prolongation of mechanical ventilation, *Chest* 114(2):541, 1998.

Kress JP, Pohlman AS, O'Connor MF et al: Daily interruption of sedative infusions in critically ill patients undergoing mechanical ventilation, *N Eng J Med* 342:1471, 2000.

Lucet JC, Rigaud MP, Menter F et al: Hand contamination before and after different hygiene techniques: a randomized clinical trial, *J Hosp Infect* 50:276-280, 2002.

Mahul P, Auboyer C, Jospe R et al: Prevention of nosocomial pneumonia in intubated patients: respective role of mechanical sub-glottic secretions drainage and stress ulcer prophylaxis, *Intensive Care Med* 18:20, 1992.

Munro CL, Grap MJ: Oral health and care in the intensive care unit: state of the science, *Am J Crit Care* 13(1):25-33, 2004.

Park M, Sangean MC, Volpe MS et al: Randomized, prospective trial of oxygen, continuous positive airway pressure and bilevel positive airway pressure by face mask in acute cardiogenic pulmonary edema, *Crit Care Med* 32:2407, 2004.

Patak L, Gawlinski A, Fung NI et al: Patient's reports of healthcare practitioner interventions that are related to communication during mechanical ventilation, *Heart Lung* 33:308, 2004.

Patak L, Gawlinski A, Fung NI et al: Communication boards in critical care: patient's views. *Appl Nurs Res* 19:182-190, 2006.

Perkins LA, Shortall SP: Ventilation without intubation, *RN* 63(1):34, 2000.

Phelan BA, Cooper DA, Sangkachand P: Prolonged mechanical ventilation and tracheostomy in the elderly, *AACN Clin Issues* 13:1, 2002.

Pierson DJ: Indications for mechanical ventilation in adults with acute respiratory failure, *Respir Care* 47:3, 2002.

Powers J, Bennett SJ: Measurement of dyspnea in patients treated with mechanical ventilation, *Am J Crit Care* 8(4):254-261, 1999.

Schultz SL: Oxygen saturation monitoring by pulse oximetry. In Lynn-McHale DJ, Carlson KK, editors: *AACN procedure manual for critical care,* ed 4, Philadelphia, 2005, WB Saunders, pp 101-107.

Scott JM, Vollman KM: Endotracheal tube and oral care. In Wiegand DJL, Carlson KK, editors: *AACN procedure manual for critical care,* ed 5, St Louis, 2005, Saunders, pp 28-33.

St John RE: End-tidal carbon dioxide monitoring, *Crit Care Nurse* 23:83, 2003.

Tablan O, Anderson L, Besser R et al: Guidelines for preventing health-care—associated pneumonia, 2003. recommendations of CDC and the Healthcare Infection Control Practices Advisory Committee, *MMWR Recomm Rep* 53(RR-3):1-36, 2004.

Takeda T, Tanigawa K, Tanaka H et al: The assessment of three methods to verify tracheal tube placement in the emergency setting, *Resuscitation* 56(2):153-157, 2003.

Torres A, Serra-Batlles J, Ros E et al: Pulmonary aspiration of gastric contents in patients receiving mechanical ventilation: the effect of body position, *Ann Intern Med* 116:540, 1992.

Trick W, Vernon M, Hayes R et al: Impact of ring wearing on hand contamination and comparison of hand hygiene agents in a hospital, *Clin Infect Dis* 36:1383-1390, 2003.

Valles J, Artigas A, Rello J et al: Continuous aspiration of subglottic secretions in preventing ventilator-associated pneumonia, *Ann Intern Med.* 122:179, 1995.

Wang JY, Chuang PY, Lin CJ et al: Continuous lateral rotational therapy in the medical intensive care unit, *J Formos Med Association* 102:788, 2003.

White JM: State of the science of music interventions: critical care and perioperative practice, *Crit Care Nurs Clin North Am* 12(2):219-225, 2000.

Dysfunctional Ventilatory weaning response   *Elizabeth A. Henneman, PhD, RN*

NANDA   Definition

Inability to adjust to lowered levels of mechanical ventilator support that interrupts and prolongs the weaning process

Defining Characteristics

Mild

Breathing discomfort; expressed feelings of increased need for oxygen; fatigue; increased concentration on breathing; queries about possible machine malfunction; restlessness; slight increase of respiratory rate from baseline; warmth

Moderate

Slight increase from baseline blood pressure (<20 mm Hg); baseline increase in respiratory rate (<5 breaths/min); slight increase from baseline heart rate (<20 beats/min); pale, slight cyanosis; slight respiratory accessory muscle use; inability to respond to coaching; inability to cooperate;

• = Independent;   ▲ = Collaborative;   EBN = Evidence-Based Nursing;   EB = Evidence-Based

apprehension; color changes; decreased air entry on auscultation; diaphoresis; eye widening, wide-eyed look; hypervigilance to activities

Severe

Deterioration in arterial blood gases from current baseline; respiratory rate increases significantly from baseline; increase from baseline blood pressure (20 mm Hg); agitation; increase from baseline heart rate (20 beats/min); paradoxical abdominal breathing; adventitious breath sounds, audible airway secretions; cyanosis; decreased level of consciousness; full respiratory accessory muscle use; shallow, gasping breaths; profuse diaphoresis; breathing uncoordinated with the ventilator

Related Factors (r/t)

Physiological

Ineffective airway clearance; sleep pattern disturbance; inadequate nutrition; uncontrolled pain or discomfort

Psychological

Knowledge deficit of the weaning process and client role; perceived inefficacy about the ability to wean; decreased motivation; decreased self-esteem; moderate or severe anxiety or fear; hopelessness; powerlessness; insufficient trust in nurse

Situational

Uncontrolled episodic energy demands or problems; inappropriate pacing of diminished ventilator support; inadequate social support; adverse environment (e.g., noise, activity, negative events in the room); low nurse-client ratio; extended nurse absence from bedside; unfamiliar nursing staff; history of ventilator dependence for >4 days to 1 week; history of multiple unsuccessful weaning attempts

NOC   Outcomes (Nursing Outcomes Classification)

Suggested NOC Outcomes

Respiratory Status: Gas Exchange, Ventilation

Example NOC Outcome with Indicators
Respiratory Status: Ventilation as evidenced by the following indicators: Respiratory rate/Respiratory rhythm/Depth of inspiration/Chest expansion symmetrical/Ease of breathing/Moves sputum out of airways/Accessory muscle use not present/Adventitious breath sounds not present/Chest retraction not present/Auscultated breath sounds/Tidal volume/Vital capacity (Rate the outcome and indicators of **Respiratory Status: Ventilation:** 1 = extremely compromised, 2 = substantially compromised, 3 = moderately compromised, 4 = mildly compromised, 5 = not compromised [see Section I].)

Client Outcomes

Client Will (Specify Time Frame):

- Wean from ventilator with adequate arterial blood gases
- Remain free of unresolved dyspnea or restlessness
- Effectively clear secretions

NIC   Interventions (Nursing Interventions Classification)

Suggested NIC Interventions

Mechanical Ventilation Management: Invasive, Mechanical Ventilatory Weaning

Example NIC Activities—Mechanical Ventilatory Weaning
Monitor for optimal fluid and electrolyte status; Monitor to assure patient is free of significant infection prior to weaning

• = Independent;   ▲ = Collaborative;   EBN = Evidence-Based Nursing;   EB = Evidence-Based

Nursing Interventions and *Rationales*

- Assess client's readiness for weaning as evidenced by the following:
  - Physiological readiness: (Brochard et al, 1994; Dries, 1997; Esteban et al, 1995; Lessard & Brochard, 1996; Mancebo, 1996)
    - ❑ Resolution of initial medical problem that led to ventilator dependence
    - ❑ Hemodynamic stability
    - ❑ Normal hemoglobin levels
    - ❑ Absence of fever
    - ❑ Normal state of consciousness
    - ❑ Metabolic, fluid, and electrolyte balance
    - ❑ Adequate nutritional status with serum albumin levels >2.5 g/dL
    - ❑ Adequate sleep

    EB: *Adequate respiratory parameters include the following: adequate gas exchange (PaO_2/FiO_2 ratio >200), respiratory rate ≤35 breaths/min, a negative inspiratory pressure <−20 cm, positive expiratory pressure >30 cm H_2O, spontaneous tidal volume >5 mL/kg, vital capacity >10-15 mL/kg.* **EBN:** *These respiratory predictors of weaning success have limited value in the management of clients receiving long-term mechanical ventilation (Burns, 2004).*
  - Psychological readiness: There has been little research devoted to the study of psychological readiness to wean. **EBN:** *An in-depth qualitative nursing research study has provided new insight into the weaning process and suggests that three key criteria give an indication of a client's psychological readiness: (1) being orientated, (2) mental ease, and (3) a positive attitude (Logan & Jenny, 1997).*
- For best results ensure that the client is in an optimal physiological and psychological state before introducing the stress of weaning (Burns, 2004; Earven et al, 2004; MacIntyre, 2004; Martensson & Fridlund, 2002; Blackwood, 2000). *For more information on weaning assessment, please refer to the Burns Weaning Assessment Program (Burns, 2005).*
- Involve family as appropriate to help the client provide a maximal effort during weaning readiness measurements (Burns, 2005).
- Provide adequate nutrition to ventilated clients, using enteral feeding when possible. **EB:** *Protein malnutrition results in decreased muscle strength, which will impair the weaning process. Enteral nutrition is preferred to total parenteral nutrition because it provides an equal number of calories at lower cost and with fewer complications, while preserving gut integrity (Parrish & McCray 1999; Romand & Sutter, 2000). The use of a nutrition management program has been shown to decrease the number of days on a ventilator (Barr et al, 2004).*
- Use evidence-based weaning protocols as appropriate. **EB:** *Protocol-directed weaning has been demonstrated to be safe and effective but not superior to other weaning methods that used structured rounds and other processes that allow for timely and ongoing clinical decision-making by expert nurses and physicians (Crocker, 2002; Kress et al, 2000; Brook et al, 1999; Kollef et al, 1997; Ely et al, 1996; Grap et al, 2003; Krishnan et al, 2004; Keogh Courtney & Coyer, 2003). Two large randomized studies have demonstrated that no one method or mode of mechanical ventilation has been demonstrated to be superior in weaning clients (Esteban et al, 1995; Brochard et al, 1994).*
- Identify reasons for previous unsuccessful weaning attempts, and include that information in development of the weaning plan. **EBN:** *Analyzing client responses after each weaning attempt prevents repeated unsuccessful weaning trials (Burns, 2004; Henneman et al, 2002; Henneman et al, 2001; Henneman, 2001).*
- ▲ Collaborate with an interdisciplinary team (physician, nurse, respiratory therapist, physical therapist, and dietician) to develop a weaning plan with a time line and goals; revise this plan throughout the weaning period. Use a communication device, such as a weaning board or flow sheet. **EBN:** *Effective interdisciplinary collaboration can positively affect client outcomes (Baggs et al, 1992; Grap et al, 2003). Collaborative weaning plans using dry-erase boards and flow sheets have been demonstrated to decrease the number of days on a ventilator and length of stay in the intensive care unit (Henneman et al, 2002; Henneman et al, 2001). Decisions related to weaning trials should be made in conjunction with members of the interdisciplinary team (Burns, 2005).*
- Assist client to identify personal strategies that result in relaxation and comfort (e.g., music, visualization, relaxation techniques, reading, television, family visits). Support implementation of these strategies. **EBN:** *Personal strategies for relaxation are effective (Gift, Moore & Soeken, 1992).*

• = Independent;   ▲ = Collaborative;   EBN = Evidence-Based Nursing;   EB = Evidence-Based

A study demonstrated that playing relaxing music decreased anxiety and increased relaxation, as shown by reduced heart and respiratory rates in intubated adults (Chlan, 1998).

- Provide a safe and comfortable environment. Stay with the client during weaning if possible. If unable to stay, make the call light button readily available and assure the client that needs will be met responsively. **EBN:** *A client who feels safe and trusts the healthcare providers can focus on the immediate work of weaning; support from the nurse helps decrease anxiety (Blackwood, 2000; Burns, 2005).*

▲ Coordinate pain and sedation medications to minimize sedative effects. **EB:** *Appropriate use of sedation is key to successful weaning. Use of continuous IV sedation is associated with longer duration of mechanical ventilation compared with bolus sedation (Brook et al, 1999; Kress et al, 2000).*

- Schedule weaning periods for the time of day when the client is most rested. Cluster care activities to promote successful weaning. Avoid other procedures during weaning: keep the environment quiet and promote restful activities between weaning periods. *It is important that the client receive adequate rest between weaning periods. Control of external noises and stimuli can promote restful periods (Cropp et al, 1994).*

- Promote a normal sleep-wake cycle, allowing uninterrupted periods of nighttime sleep (Higgins, 1998). *Limit visitors during weaning to close and supportive persons; ask visitors to leave if they are negatively affecting the weaning process.*

- During weaning, monitor the client's physiological and psychological responses; acknowledge and respond to fears and subjective complaints. Validate the client's efforts during the weaning process. **EBN:** *Weaning is a stressful experience that requires active participation by the client. The client's work needs to be understood and supported by clinicians to facilitate recovery from mechanical ventilation and weaning (Blackwood, 2000; Burns, 2005).*

- Monitor subjective and objective data (breath sounds, respiratory pattern, respiratory effort, heart rate, blood pressure, oxygen saturation per oximetry, amount and type of secretions, anxiety, and energy level) throughout weaning to determine client tolerance and responses (Burns, 2005).

- Involve the client and family in the weaning plan. Alert them as to possible client responses to weaning (e.g., potential feelings of dyspnea) (Burns, 2005).

- Coach the client through episodes of increased anxiety. Remain with the client or place a supportive and calm significant other in this role. Give positive reinforcement, and with permission use touch to communicate support and concern. *It is not unusual for a client with lung disease to experience self-limiting episodes of increased shortness of breath. Supporting and coaching a client through such episodes allows weaning to continue.*

- Terminate weaning when the client demonstrates predetermined criteria or when the following signs of weaning intolerance occur:
  - Tachypnea, dyspnea, or chest and abdominal asynchrony
  - Agitation or mental status changes
  - Decreased oxygen saturation: SaO_2 <90%
  - Change in pulse rate or blood pressure or onset of new dysrhythmias
  Discontinue weaning trial when client intolerance leads to fatigue and possible cardiovascular failure (Burns, 2005).

▲ If the dysfunctional weaning response is severe, consider slowing weaning to brief periods (e.g., 5 minutes). Continue to collaborate with the team to determine whether an untreated physiological cause for the dysfunctional weaning pattern remains. Consider an alternative care setting (subacute, rehabilitation facility, home) for clients with prolonged ventilator dependence as a strategy that can positively affect outcomes. **EB:** *One study indicated that half of the clients admitted to a rehabilitation facility were weaned from the ventilator (Modawal et al, 2002).*

Geriatric

- Recognize that older clients may require longer periods to wean. **EBN:** *A study demonstrated that older clients required a longer period to wean, especially if they were older than 80 years (Epstein, El-Modadem & Peerless, 2002).*

Home Care

NOTE: Weaning from a ventilator at home should be based on client stability and comfort of the client and caregivers under an intermittent care plan. The client and/or family may be more comfortable having the client hospitalized for the process.

• = Independent;   ▲ = Collaborative;   EBN = Evidence-Based Nursing;   EB = Evidence-Based

- Assess comfort and coping ability of the client and/or family to wean at home, fiscal implications, and home care coverage. *Compromises in respiratory function are frightening for clients and family who perceive the availability of a high-technology, structured environment as a more appropriate environment for weaning (Sevick & Bradham, 1997).*
- Establish an emergency plan and methods of implementation. Include emergency aeration and reestablishment of the ventilation assistive device. *Having a prepared emergency plan reassures the client and family and provides for client safety.*
- ▲ Obtain orders for alternative routes of medication administration when medications have been administered via a ventilation device. Instruct the client and family about these changes.

evolve   See the EVOLVE website for World Wide Web resources for client education.

REFERENCES

Baggs JG, Ryan SA, Phelps CE et al: The association between interdisciplinary collaboration and patient outcomes in a medical intensive care unit, *Heart Lung* 21(1):18, 1992.

Barr J, Hecht M, Flavin KE et al: Outcomes in critically ill patients before and after the implementation of an evidence-based nutritional management protocol, *Chest* 125(4):1446-1457, 2004.

Blackwood B: The art and science of predicting patient readiness for weaning from mechanical ventilation, *Int J Nurs Stud* 37:145, 2000.

Brochard L, Rauss A, Benito S et al: Comparison of three methods of gradual withdrawal from ventilatory support during weaning from mechanical ventilation, *Am J Respir Crit Care Med* 150:896, 1994.

Brook AD, Ahrens TS, Schaiff R et al: Effect of a nursing-implemented sedation protocol on the duration of mechanical ventilation, *Crit Care Med* 27:2609, 1999.

Burns SM: The science of weaning: when and how? *Crit Care Nurs Clin North Am* 16:379, 2004.

Burns SM: Weaning process. In Lynn-McHale DJ, Carlson KK, editors: *AACN procedure manual for critical care*, ed 4, Philadelphia, 2005, WB Saunders.

Chlan L: Effectiveness of a music therapy intervention on relaxation and anxiety for patients receiving ventilatory assistance, *Heart Lung* 27(3):169, 1998.

Crocker C: Nurse-led weaning from ventilatory and respiratory support, *Intensive Crit Care Nurs* 18:272, 2002.

Cropp AJ, Woods LA, Raney D et al: Name that tone: the proliferation of noise in the intensive care unit, *Chest* 105:1217, 1994.

Dries DJ: Weaning from mechanical ventilation, *J Trauma* 43:372, 1997.

Earven S, Fisher C, Lewis R et al: The experience of four outcomes managers: an institutional approach to weaning patients from long-term mechanical ventilation, *Crit Care Nurs Clin North Am* 16:395, 2004.

Ely EW, Baker AM, Dunagan DP et al: Effect on the duration of mechanical ventilation of identifying patients capable of breathing spontaneously, *N Engl J Med* 335:1864, 1996.

Epstein CD, El-Modadem N, Peerless JR: Weaning older patients from long-term mechanical ventilation: a pilot study, *Am J Crit Care* 11:4, 2002.

Esteban A, Frutos F, Tobin MJ et al: A comparison of four methods of weaning patients from mechanical ventilation, *N Eng J Med* 332:345, 1995.

Gift AG, Moore T, Soeken K: Relaxation to reduce dyspnea and anxiety in COPD patients, *Nurs Res* 41(4):242-246, 1992.

Grap MJ, Strickland D, Tormey L et al: Collaborative practice: development, implementation, and evaluation of a weaning protocol for patients receiving mechanical ventilation, *Am J Crit Care* 12(5):454-460, 2003.

Henneman EA: Liberating patients from mechanical ventilation, a team approach, *Crit Care Nurs* 21(3):25, 2001.

Henneman EA, Dracup K, Ganz T et al: Effect of a collaborative weaning plan on patient outcome in the critical care setting, *Crit Care Med* 29:297, 2001.

Henneman EA, Dracup K, Ganz T et al: Using a collaborative weaning plan to decrease duration of mechanical ventilation and length of stay in the intensive care unit for patients receiving long-term ventilation, *Am J Crit Care* 11:132, 2002.

Higgins P: Patient perception of fatigue while undergoing long term mechanical ventilation: incidence and associated factors, *Heart Lung* 27:177, 1998.

Keogh S, Courtney M, Coyer F: Weaning from ventilation in paediatric intensive care: an intervention study, *Intensive Crit Care Nurs* 19(4):186-197, 2003.

Kollef MH, Shapiro SD, Silver P et al: A randomized controlled trial of protocol-directed versus physician-directed weaning from mechanical ventilation, *Crit Care Med* 25(4):567, 1997.

Kress JP, Pohlman AS, O'Connor MF et al: Daily interruption of sedative infusions in critically ill patients undergoing mechanical ventilation, *N Engl J Med* 342:1471, 2000.

Krishnan JA, Moore D, Robeson C et al: A prospective, controlled trial of a protocol-based strategy to discontinue mechanical ventilation, *Am J Respir Crit Care Med* 169(6):673-678, 2004.

Lessard MR, Brochard LJ: Weaning from mechanical support, *Clin Chest Med* 17:475, 1996.

Logan J, Jenny J: Qualitative analysis of patients' weaning work during mechanical ventilation and weaning, *Heart Lung* 26:140, 1997.

MacIntyre NR: Evidence-based guidelines for weaning and discontinuing ventilatory support, *Respir Care* 47(1):69, 2004.

Mancebo J: Weaning from mechanical ventilation, *Eur Respir J* 9:1923, 1996.

Martensson IE, Fridlund B: Factors influencing the patient during weaning from mechanical ventilation: a national survey, *Intensive Crit Care Nurs* 18:223, 2002.

Modawal A, Candadai NP, Mandell KM et al: Weaning success among ventilator-dependent patients in a rehabilitation facility, *Arch Phys Med Rehabil* 83(2):154, 2002.

Parrish CR, McCray SF: Nutrition support for the mechanically ventilated patient, *Crit Care Nurse* 19(1):91-94, 1999.

Romand JA, Sutter PM: Enteral nutrition: the right stuff at the right time in the right place, *Crit Care Med* 28(7):2671-2672, 2000.

Sevick MA, Bradham DD: Economic value of caregiver effort in maintaining long term ventilatory assisted individuals, *Heart Lung* 26(2):148, 1997.

V

• = Independent;   ▲ = Collaborative;   EBN = Evidence-Based Nursing;   EB = Evidence-Based

Risk for other-directed Violence   *Kathleen L. Patusky, PhD, APRN-BC*

NANDA   Definition

At risk for behaviors in which an individual demonstrates that he or she can be physically, emotionally, and/or sexually harmful to others

Risk Factors

Body language: rigid posture, clenching of fists and jaw, hyperactivity, pacing, breathlessness, threatening stances; history of violence against others (e.g., hitting someone, kicking someone, spitting at someone, scratching someone, throwing objects at someone, biting someone, attempted rape, rape, sexual molestation, urinating/defecating on someone); history of threats of violence (e.g., verbal threats against property, verbal threats against person, social threats, cursing, threatening notes/letters, threatening gestures, sexual threats); history of violent antisocial behavior (e.g., stealing, insistent borrowing, insistent demanding of privileges, insistent interrupting of meetings, refusing to eat, refusing to take medication, ignoring instructions); history of violence, indirect (e.g., tearing off clothes, ripping objects off walls, writing on walls, urinating on floor, defecating on floor, stamping feet, displaying temper tantrum, running in corridors, yelling, throwing objects, breaking a window, slamming doors, making sexual advances); neurological impairment (e.g., positive EEG, CAT, or MRI; head trauma; positive neurological findings; seizure disorders); cognitive impairment (e.g., learning disabilities, attention deficit disorder, decreased intellectual functioning); history of childhood abuse; history of witnessing family violence; cruelty to animals; fire setting; prenatal/perinatal complications or abnormalities; history of drug or alcohol abuse; pathological intoxication; psychotic symptomatology (e.g., auditory, visual, command hallucinations; paranoid delusions; loose, rambling, or illogical thought processes); motor vehicle offenses (e.g., frequent traffic violations, use of a motor vehicle to release anger); suicidal behavior; impulsivity; availability/possession of weapon(s)

NOC   Outcomes (Nursing Outcomes Classification)

Suggested NOC Outcomes

Abuse Cessation, Abusive Behavior Self-Restraint, Aggression Self-Control, Distorted Thought Self-Control, Impulse Self-Control, Parenting: Psychosocial Safety, Risk Detection

Example NOC Outcome with Indicators
Aggression Self-Control as evidenced by the following indicators: Refrains from harming others/Communicates needs and feelings appropriately/Identifies when angry (Rate the outcome and indicators of **Aggression Self-Control:** 1 = never demonstrated, 2 = rarely demonstrated, 3 = sometimes demonstrated, 4 = often demonstrated, 5 = consistently demonstrated [see Section I].)

The Broset Violence Checklist (BVC) has been developed for short-term prediction of violence in psychiatric inpatients. Some false-positive cases were met with preventive measures, which may have avoided violence (Abderhalden et al, 2004).

The Alert Assessment Form may be used to identify potentially aggressive clients with moderate (71%) sensitivity and high (94%) specificity (Kling, et al, 2006).

The Caregiver Psychological Elder Abuse Behavior Scale may be used to identify elder abuse behavior (Wang, 2005).

Client Outcomes

Client Will (Specify Time Frame):

- Stop all forms of abuse (physical, emotional, sexual; neglect; financial exploitation)
- Have cessation of abuse reported by victim
- Display no aggressive activity
- Refrain from verbal outbursts
- Refrain from violating others' personal space

• = Independent;   ▲ = Collaborative;   EBN = Evidence-Based Nursing;   EB = Evidence-Based

- Refrain from antisocial behaviors
- Maintain relaxed body language and decreased motor activity
- Identify factors contributing to abusive/aggressive behavior
- Demonstrate impulse control or state feelings of control
- Identify impulsive behaviors
- Identify feelings/behaviors that lead to impulsive actions
- Identify consequences of impulsive actions to self or others
- Avoid high-risk environments and situations
- Identify and talk about feelings; express anger appropriately
- Express decreased anxiety and control of hallucinations as applicable
- Displace anger to meaningful activities
- Communicate needs appropriately
- Identify responsibility to maintain control
- Express empathy for victim
- Obtain no access or yield access to harmful objects
- Use alternative coping mechanisms for stress
- Obtain and follow through with counseling
- Demonstrate knowledge of correct role behaviors

Victim (and Children If Applicable) Will (Specify Time Frame):

- Have safe plan for leaving situation or avoiding abuse
- Resolve depression or traumatic response

Parent Will (Specify Time Frame):

- Monitor social/play contacts
- Provide supervision and nurturing environment
- Intervene to prevent high-risk social behaviors

NIC   Interventions (Nursing Interventions Classification)

Suggested NIC Interventions

Abuse Protection Support, Anger Control Assistance, Behavior Management, Calming Technique, Coping Enhancement, Crisis Intervention, Delusion Management, Dementia Management, Distraction, Environmental Management: Violence Prevention, Mood Management, Physical Restraint, Seclusion, Substance Use Prevention

Example NIC Intervention—Environmental Management: Violence Prevention

Remove other individuals from the vicinity of a violent or potentially violent patient; Provide ongoing surveillance of all patient access areas to maintain patient safety and therapeutically intervene as needed

Nursing Interventions and *Rationales*
Client Violence

- ▲ Monitor the environment, evaluate situations that could become violent, and intervene early to de-escalate the situation. Consider that family members or other staff may initiate violence. Enlist support from other staff rather than attempting to handle the situation alone. **EBN:** *One study suggested that systematic risk assessment, aggression management training, and decreasing nurses' coercive responses to clients could reduce coercion and client violence (Needham et al, 2004).*
- ▲ Know and follow institution's policies and procedures concerning violence. *Being familiar with and following policies and procedures of the department prevents violence. Policies should be developed, and training programs should be provided in proper use and application of restraints. All nursing units should develop a proactive plan for dealing with violent situations.*
- Initiate client assessment by distinguishing the broadest categories of causes of aggression: social versus biological. *A nursing concept analysis of aggression examined the causes of aggression, identify-*

• = Independent;   ▲ = Collaborative;   EBN = Evidence-Based Nursing;   EB = Evidence-Based

ing social causes (learned behavior, frustration) and biological causes (brain dysfunction, high levels of testosterone, low levels of serotonin, birth complications, nutrition deficiency). Knowledge of the source of aggression is important in applying and developing the most appropriate interventions (Liu, 2004). **EBN:** *Knowing the client, having experience with similar clients, paying attention, and planning interventions are expert practices used by nurses to predict and respond to aggressive behavior effectively (Pryor, 2006).*

▲ Assess the client for risk factors of violence, including those in the following categories: psychiatric disorders (particularly paranoid or bipolar disorders, substance abuse), neurological disorders (e.g., head injury, temporal lobe epilepsy), psychological precursors (e.g., low tolerance for stress, impulsivity), coping difficulties (e.g., inability to plan solutions or see long-term consequences of behavior), and personal history (e.g., past violent behavior). *All of these risk factors have been implicated in aggressive, agitated, or violent behavior.*

▲ Assess for potential indicators of impending violence against others: frequent medication change, high use of sedative drugs, past violent behavior, a *Diagnostic and Statistical Manual of Mental Health IV* diagnosis of antisocial personality or borderline personality disorder, and long hospitalization. Other indicators include hypervigilance, hostility, substance use, and lack of adherence to medication regimen. *Knowing, recognizing, and promptly intervening in early precipitating factors prevents violence.*

• Assess the client with a history of previous assaults. Listen to and acknowledge feelings of anger, observe for increased motor activity, and prepare to intervene if the client becomes aggressive. **EBN:** *Assaultive clients had significantly more previous assaults, had more difficulty appropriately verbalizing angry feelings, and before the assault, were more verbally hostile with more increased motor activity than control subjects (Lanza et al, 1996).*

• Assess the client for physiological signs and external signs of anger. *Internal signs of anger include increased pulse rate, respiration rate, and blood pressure; chills; prickly sensations; numbness; choking sensation; nausea; and vertigo. External signs include increased muscle tone, changes in body posture (clenched fists, set jaw), eye changes (eyebrows lower and drawn together, eyelids tense, eyes assuming a "hard" appearance), lips pressed together, flushing or pallor, goose bumps, twitching, and sweating (Harper-Jacques & Reimer, 2002).*

• Assess for the presence of hallucinations. *Command hallucinations may direct the client to behave violently (McNeil, Eisner & Binder, 2000).*

• Determine the presence and degree of homicidal or suicidal risk. A number of questions will elicit the necessary information. "Have you been thinking about harming someone? If yes, who? How often do you have these thoughts, and how long do they last? Do you have a plan? What is it? Do you have access to the means to carry out that plan? What has kept you from hurting the person until now?" Refer to the care plan for **Suicide Risk.** *Psychotherapists are required to report harm or threats of harm to another person, referred to as the duty to warn. State laws and mental health codes should be checked to determine local mandates for threat reporting by specific healthcare professionals.*

• Take action to minimize personal risk: Use nonthreatening body language. Respect personal space and boundaries. Maintain at least an arm's length distance from the client; do not touch the client without permission (unless physical restraint is the goal). Do not allow the client to block access to an exit. If speaking with the client alone, keep the door to the room open. Be aware of where other staff is at all times. Notify other staff of where you are at all times. Take verbal threats seriously and notify other staff. Wear clothing and accessories that are not restricting and that will not be dangerous (e.g., sandals or shoes with heels can lead to twisted ankles; necklaces or dangling earrings could be grabbed). **EBN:** *Programs for violence prevention have been implemented that reduce workplace violence. For OSHA guidelines, visit www.osha.gov/SLTC/ workplaceviolence/index.html (Lipscomb et al, 2006).*

• Remove potential weapons from the environment. Be prepared to remove obstructions to staff response from the environment. Search the client and his or her belongings for weapons or potential weapons on admission to the hospital as appropriate. *Clients prone to violence may use available weapons opportunistically. If client restraint becomes necessary, environmental hazards (e.g., chairs, wastebaskets) should be moved out of the way to prevent injuries.*

• Inform the client of unit expectations for appropriate behavior and the consequences of not meeting these expectations. Emphasize that the client must comply with the rules of the unit. Give positive reinforcement for compliance. *Clients benefit from clear guidance and positive reinforcement regarding behavioral expectations and consequences, providing much-needed structure and emphasizing client responsibility for his or her own behavior. The unit serves as a microcosm of the client's outside world, so adherence to social norms while on the unit models adherence upon discharge and provides the client with staff support to learn appropriate coping skills and alternative behaviors.*

- Increase surveillance of the hospitalized client at smoking, meal, and medication times. **EBN:** *Physical control use (mechanical restraint and locked seclusion) at a state psychiatric hospital increased at clients' smoking, meal, and medication times. Increased demands on clients, difficulty adjusting to shifts in activity, close proximity to other clients, or denial of privileges (e.g., smoking) may have accounted for the increases (Vittengl, 2002).*

- Assign a single room to the client with a potential for violence toward others. *The client will be able to take time away from unit stimulation to calm self as needed. Another client will not be placed at risk as a roommate.* **EBN:** *Research suggests lack of single-bed rooms may reduce rest and privacy and increase the risk of overstimulation (Stolker, Nijman & Zwanikken, 2006).*

- Maintain a secluded area for the client to be placed when violent. Ensure that staff are continuously present and available to client during seclusion. **EBN:** *Clients perceived seclusion to be punishment; however, the main negative effect reported by clients was that seclusion intensified preexisting feelings of exclusion, rejection, abandonment, and isolation. Staff presence is necessary to prevent the harmful effects of social isolation and to honor clients' motivation to connect with staff (Holmes, Kennedy & Perron, 2004).*

- Maintain a calm attitude in response to the client. Provide a low level of stimulation in the client's environment; place the client in a safe, quiet place, and speak slowly and quietly. *Anxiety is contagious.*

- Redirect possible violent behaviors into physical activities (e.g., walking, jogging) if the client is physically able. *Using a punching bag or hitting a pillow may not be indicated, because they are not calming activities and they continue patterning violent behavior. However, activities that distract while draining excess energy help to build a repertoire of alternative behaviors for stress reduction.*

- Provide sufficient staff if a show of force is necessary to demonstrate control to the client. *When staff responds to an escalating or violent situation, it can reassure clients that they will not be allowed to lose control. On the other hand, leave immediately if the client becomes violent and you are not trained to handle it.*

- Protect other clients in the environment from harm. Remove other individuals from the vicinity of a violent or potentially violent client. Follow safety protocols of the department. *Proper preparation, training, and implementation of strict protocols can save nurses' and others' lives when violence occurs. Others can be injured during a violent outburst; therefore their safety must be considered. The risk of a violent client to others in the area (other clients, visitors) should be anticipated, even as efforts proceed to de-escalate the situation with the client.*

- ▲ Use chemical restraints as ordered. Obtain an order for medication and administer it immediately. *Medications should be offered before physical restraints or seclusion is considered.*

- ▲ Use mechanical restraints if ordered and as necessary. *Physical restraint can be therapeutic to keep the client and others safe.* **EBN:** *Restraint skill training, audits of adverse events, and examination of the safe use of restraints and medications are important to safe restraint practices (Ryan & Bowers, 2006).*

- Follow the institution's protocol for releasing restraints. Observe the client closely, remain calm, and provide positive feedback as the client's behavior becomes controlled. *The period during which restraints are removed can be dangerous for staff if they do not recognize that the client may choose to reinitiate violence. Protocols will specify safe procedures for removing restraints.*

- If restraints are necessary, provide the client with musical tapes and a headset. *Music can provide a distraction from negative thoughts or auditory hallucinations.*

- Encourage clients to eat a balanced diet instead of junk food. *In clients with a poor dietary history, particularly indigent clients or clients with alcoholism, deficiencies of thiamine and niacin may lead to irritability, disorientation, and paranoia (Harper-Jacques & Reimer, 2002).*

- Form a therapeutic alliance with the client, identifying the source of anger as external to both nurse and client. *The development of a therapeutic relationship before aggressive behavior occurs pro-*

V

• = Independent;   ▲ = Collaborative;   EBN = Evidence-Based Nursing;   EB = Evidence-Based

vides an alternative for working through anger and frustration. Assisting the client to identify a source of anger or frustration that is external to both the nurse and client prevents the need for defensiveness by both and directs energy at solving an external problem.

- Allow, encourage, and assist the client to verbalize feelings appropriately either one-on-one or in a group setting. Actively listen to the client; explore the source of the client's anger, and negotiate resolution when possible. *When clients' feelings are not addressed, when an individual feels threatened, or when gratification is delayed or denied, violence may be used as a manifestation of the internal feeling state.*

- Teach healthy ways to express feelings/anger, appropriate gender roles, and how to communicate needs appropriately. *Clients may become violent if their perceived needs are thwarted. Instruction that prepares them to express their needs appropriately, while recognizing that others are under no obligation to meet their needs, prepares them to defuse this anger trigger.*

- Have the client keep an anger diary and discuss alternative responses together. Teach cognitive-behavioral techniques. *Clients with anger management difficulties may not be alert to physiological changes or cues that they are becoming angry. They may not be aware of any time delay between the stimulus and their angry response. Instruction in cognitive-behavioral techniques and review of the diary with staff assists the clients in identifying thought processes leading to anger and the space between stimulus and response.*

- Identify stimuli that initiate violence and the means of dealing with the stimuli. *Assisting the client to identify situations and people that upset him or her provides information needed for problem solving. The client may then identify alternative responses (e.g., leaving the stimulus; using relaxation techniques, such as deep breathing; initiating thought stopping; initiating a distracting activity; responding assertively rather than aggressively).*

- Emphasize that the client is responsible for his or her choices and behavior. Introduce descriptions of possible effects of a client's aggressive/violent behavior on others. *In most cases clients are capable of learning to control angry impulses. In many cases clients operate from a worldview that perceives others as instruments of the clients' gratification. A difficult but important insight that clients must gain is that they are dealing with other human beings who experience pain. Clients' behaviors influence how others respond to them.*

- ▲ Always follow up a violent episode with a debriefing of clients and staff. *Allowing discussion of a violent episode, either individually or in a group, among other clients present reveals clients' responses to the event and provides the opportunity for staff to offer reassurance and support. Clients may have concerns that staff will attempt to restrain them without reason or may feel uncertain whether staff can keep them safe.* **EBN:** *Staff report a range of feelings in response to adverse incidents. Consequences include increased containment, increased focus on risk assessment, and an ignoring of client responses (Bowers et al, 2006).*

Domestic Violence

NOTE: Before implementation of interventions in the face of domestic violence, nurses should examine their own emotional responses to abuse, their knowledge base about abuse, and systemic elements within the emergency department (ED) to ensure that interventions will be compassionate and appropriate. **EBN:** *Barriers to domestic violence screening in the ED include lack of education and instruction about how to ask about abuse, the nurse's personal or family history of abuse, and lack of a sense of self-efficacy (Hollingsworth & Ford-Gilboe, 2006; Yonaka et al, 2007). The ability of nurses to provide effective care was found to be compromised by a lack of knowledge about the influence of domestic abuse on the mental health of children and adolescents (De Wit & Davis, 2004).*

- Screen for possible abuse in women or children with a pattern of multiple injuries, particularly if any suspicion exists that the physical findings are inconsistent with the explanation of how the injuries were incurred. **EBN:** *Although 86% of women approaching the justice system for domestic violence actions (filing charges, restraining orders) reported healthcare visits in the previous year, only 24% had been assessed for interpersonal violence. Universal screening for interpersonal violence was urged (Willson et al, 2001).*

- ▲ Report suspected child abuse to Child Protective Services. Refer women suspected of being in a spouse abuse situation to an area crisis center and provide phone number of area crisis hotline. *Rapid screening tools are helpful to identify intimate partner violence. All nurses are required by law to report suspected child abuse.* **EB:** *A study found that hotline, advocacy, counseling, and shelter services for domestic violence were effective in achieving positive outcomes (Bennett et al, 2004). If a child has been mistreated, there is a likelihood that spousal violence also exists (Appel & Kim-Appel, 2006).*

- With women who repeatedly experience injuries from domestic violence, maintain a nonjudgmental approach and continue to offer resources/referrals. If the woman voices a willingness to leave her situation, assist with developing an emergency plan that will consider all contingencies possible (e.g., safe location, financial resources, care of children, when to leave safely) (Amar & Cox, 2006). *A women in a domestic violence situation may change her mind several times before actually leaving. Proactive organization of an emergency plan helps to increase the possibility that women will be able to leave safely. The most dangerous time of a domestic violence situation is when the spouse tries to leave.* **EB:** *Forgiveness of the partner for abusive behavior and willingness to let go of anger has been found to be a more reliable predictor of intention to return to the relationship than severity of violence, attributions regarding violence, or psychological constraints or investments (Gordon, Burton & Porter, 2004).*

▲ In dealing with abused wives, maintain a nonjudgmental response when clients return to husbands or refuse to leave them. *Reasons for remaining in or returning to the relationship include economic concerns (especially with children), socialization about the women's role, political or legal obstacles, traumatic bonding that leaves the woman feeling powerless, and realistic fear of retaliation or death (Boyd & Mackey, 2000; Wallace, 1999).* **EB:** *A study found that interventions with victims of domestic violence that focus on dysphoria, hopelessness, or self-esteem are unlikely to be effective unless issues of perceived control and coping are also addressed (Clements, Sabourin & Spiby, 2004). Refer to the care plan for* **Powerlessness.** **EBN:** *Experienced nurses working with abused women came to redefine success as client personal growth over time, rather than leaving the relationship (Webster et al, 2006).*

- Particular attention should be paid to the potential for domestic violence during pregnancy. **EBN:** *Pregnant women will remain in an abusive relationship if they perceive it to be in the best interest of the child, part of a process of "double-binding" with child and abusive spouse (Libbus et al, 2006; Lutz et al, 2006). Choking is a danger that should be added to routine screening (Bullock et al, 2006).*

- Women with physical or mental disabilities require extended assessment if abuse is suspected or present, to determine unique ways in which they may experience abuse. In addition to an assessment of the usual power and control concerns, a comprehensive functional assessment should be conducted along with attention to cultural issues, the nature of the disability, and needed resources. **EB:** *A study of services used by disabled women in abusive situations noted the need for collaboration to ensure that the women's unique needs are met (Chang et al, 2003).*

▲ Women with disabilities may experience abuse from multiple sources, and particular attention should be paid to the additional emotional stresses for these women. **EBN:** *The limitations of disabilities can mean that women cannot leave the home situation without much difficulty; shelters may not be prepared to accommodate the disabilities; and nursing home placement may be an undesirable option (Curry, Hassouneh-Phillips & Johnston-Silverberg, 2001). Women with disabilities may be vulnerable to abuse from any caregiver, including personal-assistance providers. Themes expressed by women with disabilities included (1) confusion of social and personal boundaries (e.g., intrusiveness into client's personal business), (2) challenging power dynamics (e.g., client as employer but dependent upon assistance), (3) additional forms of abuse (e.g., financial, neglectful), and (4) inability of client to confront abusive behavior (fear of retaliation, potential loss of care provider) (Saxton et al, 2001). Women with schizophrenia are especially vulnerable and have complex needs (Bengtsson-Tops & Tops, 2007; Rice, 2006).*

▲ In cases where spouse or child abuse accompanies substance abuse, refer the abusive client to a substance abuse treatment program. Refer the spouse receiving abuse to Al-Anon and the children to Alateen. *Use of drugs or alcohol decreases impulse control and aggravates abusive behavior.* **EB:** *A study found that marital violence decreased significantly after the husband received substance abuse treatment (Stuart et al, 2003).*

▲ In cases where an adult reveals a history of unresolved/untreated sexual abuse as a child, referral to a local Adults Molested as Children (AMAC) group may be helpful. **EB:** *Childhood sexual* *abuse has been associated with adult depression, attempted suicide, self-harm, and higher risk for later interpersonal violence (Gladstone et al, 2004). Interventions tailored to the AMAC experience may be helpful.* Refer to the care plans for **Risk for Suicide, Self-mutilation,** and **Risk for Self-mutilation.**

▲ Intervention may include referral to a number of programs available, including parenting classes or a parental counseling support group. **EBN:** *Theraplay (Bennett, Shiner & Ryan, 2006) and INSIGHT (Zust, 2006) address domestic violence issues.*

Social Violence

• Assess for acute stress disorder (ASD) and posttraumatic stress disorder (PTSD) among victims of violence. **EB:** *In the acute phase following an assault, women reported high rates of ASD symptoms. Four months after an attack, dissatisfaction with previous life, prior mental health problems, recent life events, and earlier abuse were risk factors for PTSD (Renck, 2006).*

▲ Assess the support network of women who become victims of violent crime and refer for appropriate levels of assistance. **EB:** *In a national study of female crime victims, three help-seeking strategies were identified: (1) minimal or no help seeking, (2) family and friend help seeking, and (3) substantial help seeking (from family, friends, psychiatrists, social service providers, and police) (Kaukinen, 2004). Of particular concern would be women who do not have family or friends to provide support or who have difficulty accessing other types of assistance.*

• Be aware that hate crime is increasing, particularly toward transgendered individuals, and it requires support and advocacy for victims. *The growth of hate crimes toward transgendered individuals has been noted, and more research is needed to understand the influence of hate crimes on gay males (Thomas, 2004; Willis, 2004).*

▲ Victims of violence seen in the ED should receive an assessment for needed services and assignment to case management. *Establishment of linkages with social service agencies can provide important services for referral.* **EB:** *An ED study provided linkages with internal services, such as primary care, gang-related tattoo removal, psychiatric services, substance abuse treatment, and dental care; and with a social service agency providing such services as programs in personal development and education, comprehensive employment preparation, computer skills, and others. Outside agencies were also used for legal assistance, spiritual counseling, GED classes, and financial assistance. With case management initiated in the ED as the key element, the number of resources used by young victims of interpersonal violence as compared with controls was significantly increased (Zun, Downey & Rosen, 2003).*

Pediatric

• Be alert for both shaken baby syndrome and exposure of children to violence. *Nurse practitioners can play an important role in identifying shaken baby syndrome and educating others about prevention (Walls, 2006). Approaches for addressing children exposed to family violence include the Ploeger Model of enhanced maternal and child health (Edgecombe & Ploeger, 2006) and the Health Promotion Model for Violence Prevention (Skybo & Polivka, 2007).*

• Assess for dating violence among adolescent girls. Additional assessments may be required for sexually transmitted diseases and pregnancy. **EB:** *Adolescent girls who have been intentionally hurt by a date in the previous year were found to be more likely to experience sexual health risks and pregnancy (Silverman, Raj & Clements, 2004). A high rate of dating violence by both male and female university students has been found worldwide (Straus, 2004).*

• Pregnant teens should be assessed for abuse, particularly if they are with an older partner. **EBN:** *In a study of predominantly African-American pregnant teens, 13% reported domestic violence during pregnancy. Teens with adult partners (4 or more years older) were twice as likely to report abuse as teens with similar age partners (Harner, 2004).*

▲ When physical abuse by parents is present, parent-child interaction therapy (PCIT) may be helpful. **EB:** *PCIT is an empirically supported treatment that has been shown to reduce abuse (Chaffin et al, 2004; Chambless & Ollendick, 2000).*

▲ In the case of child abuse or neglect, refer for early childhood home visitation. **EB:** *Home visits during a child's first 2 years of life have been found to be effective in preventing child abuse and neglect (Hahn et al, 2003).*

Geriatric

- Be alert to the potential for elder abuse in clients, including the possibility of psychological abuse. *Abuse may occur along a continuum, from neglect to physical or sexual abuse. Family and strangers may commit financial exploitation. Look for signs of bruising, malnutrition, and fearful responses to or around caregivers.* **EBN:** *Female caregivers, those with more education, and those with greater burdens showed more severe psychologically abusive behavior (Wang, Lin & Lee, 2006).*
- Assess for changes in physiological functions (e.g., constipation, dehydration) or impairment of the ability to meet basic needs (e.g., inadequate toileting, decreased mobility). Observe for signs of fear, anxiety, anger, and agitation, and intervene immediately. *In older adults subtle physiological changes, interruptions of or changes in routine, or fears about medical disorders or potential loss of independence can be transformed into anger, irritability, or agitation.* **EB:** *Agitation in nursing home clients was predicted independently by cognitive impairment, vision and hearing impairment, and gender. Individuals with significant hearing impairment were more likely to become agitated than less impaired individuals (Vance et al, 2003).*
- Observe for dementia and delirium. *Clients with dementia or delirium may strike out if they are frustrated or if they have the sense that their personal space is being violated. However, this may not occur within a cognitive capacity that permits discussion of the behavior.*
- Assess sensory impairments and the influence they may have on the client's behavior. *Agitation and striking out may be precipitated in older adults who are experiencing either sensory impairment or difficulty communicating (Allen, 1999).*
- Be alert for the potential of sexual abuse of elders. *Nurses are in the position not only to provide acute care intervention, but also to collect forensic evidence and report suspected cases to the authorities (Burgess et al, 2006).* **EB:** *Sensitive assessment and intervention is called for, to overcome the marginalization of elders who may experience inadequate response to issues of violence and power (Burgess & Clements, 2006; Jones & Powell, 2006). Refer to care plan for* **Rape-trauma syndrome.**
- ▲ Monitor for paradoxical drug reactions, and report any to the physician. *Violent behavior can be stimulated by a medication intended to calm the client.*
- ▲ Assess for brain insults, such as recent falls or injuries, strokes, or transient ischemic attacks. *Clients with brain injuries may respond to stimulus control, problem solving, social skills training, relaxation training, and anger management to reduce aggressive behaviors. Brain injuries, lowered impulse control, and reduced coping can cause violent reactions to self or others. Brain injury symptoms may be mistaken for mental illness.*
- Decrease environmental stimuli if violence is directed at others. *Removal of the client to a quiet area can reduce violent impulses. Use a calm voice to "talk down" the client.*
- Provide hand or back rubs and calming music when an elderly client experiences agitation. **EBN:** *In a study of older adults in nursing homes, calming music and hand massage were found to soothe agitation for up to 1 hour. No additional benefit was found from combining the two interventions (Remington, 2002).*
- ▲ If abuse or neglect of an elderly client is suspected, report the suspicion to an adult protective services agency with jurisdiction over the geographical area where the client lives.

Multicultural

- Exercise cultural competence when dealing with domestic violence. *Within the demands and difficulties of an increasingly diverse healthcare environment, increased need exists for awareness, education, cultural sensitivity, and action in responding to multicultural issues of family violence (Anderson & Aviles, 2006; Hindin, 2006; Sumter, 2006).* **EBN:** *Battered Latina women voiced equal fear of the abuser and of disclosing the abuse to healthcare professionals, based on the consequences, but wanted to be asked about abuse and receive help (Kelly, 2006).*

Home Care

- Be alert to the potential for violent behavior in the home setting. Respond to verbal aggression with interventions to de-escalate negative emotional states. *Violence is a process that can be recognized early. De-escalation involves reducing client stressors, responding to the client with respect, acknowledging the client's feeling state, and assisting the client to regain control. If de-escalation does not*

V

work, the nurse should leave the home (Distasio, 2000). **EB:** *Verbal aggression was shown to be a predictor of negative psychological outcomes (Bussing & Hoge, 2004).*

- Assess family members or caregivers for their ability to protect the client and themselves. *The safety of the client between home visits is a nursing priority. Caregivers often need assistance with recognizing or admitting fear of or danger from a loved one.*
- Include an initial and ongoing assessment and evaluation of potential abuse and neglect. Photograph evidence of abuse or neglect when possible. *Victims of abuse perceive themselves to be powerless to change the situation. Indeed, the abuser fosters this perception and may threaten violence or death if the victim attempts to leave. Chronic abuse and neglect by a spouse or other family among the elderly is often hidden until home care is actively involved. Refer to the care plan for* **Powerlessness.**
- ▲ If neglect or abuse is suspected, identify an emergency plan that addresses the problem immediately, ensures client safety, and includes a report to the appropriate authorities. Discuss when to use hotlines and 911. Role play access to emergency resources with the client and caregivers. *Client safety is a nursing priority. An emergency plan should address either immediate removal to a safe environment or identification of appropriate steps to take in the event of abuse and the securing of resources for the anticipated action (e.g., available phone, packed bag, alternative living arrangements). Reporting is a legal requirement of healthcare workers.*
- Encourage appropriate safety behaviors in abused women; call the client at intervals during a 6-month period to determine whether safety behaviors are being carried out. **EBN:** *A study of telephone contacts to women who sought help through the district attorney's office demonstrated that safety behaviors increased dramatically. Safety behaviors included hiding money; hiding an extra set of house and car keys; establishing a code for abuse occurrence with family or friends; asking neighbors to call police if violence occurred; removing weapons; keeping available family social security numbers, rent and utility receipts, family birth certificates, identification or drivers licenses, bank account numbers, insurance policies and numbers, marriage license, valuable jewelry, important phone numbers, and a hidden bag with extra clothing (McFarlane et al, 2002).*
- Assess the home environment for harmful objects. Have the family remove or lock objects as able. *The safety of the client and caregivers is a nursing priority.*
- ▲ Refer for homemaker or psychiatric home healthcare services for respite, client reassurance, and implementation of a therapeutic regimen. *Responsibility for a person who may become violent provides high caregiver stress. Respite decreases caregiver stress. The presence of caring individuals is reassuring to both the client and caregivers, especially during periods of client anxiety. Individuals exhibiting violent behaviors can respond to the interventions described previously, modified for the home setting.*
- ▲ If the client is taking psychotropic medications, assess client and family knowledge of medication and its administration and side effects. Teach as necessary. *Knowledge of the medical regimen supports compliance.*
- ▲ Evaluate effectiveness and side effects of medications. *Accurate clinical feedback improves the physician's ability to prescribe an effective medical regimen specific to a client needs.*
- If client displays mildly intensifying aggressive behavior, attempt to diffuse anger or violence (e.g., ask for a glass of water to distract client). Later in the visit explain that aggressive behavior is not acceptable and present consequences of continued aggressive behavior (i.e., right of agency to discontinue services). *Mild aggression can be diffused safely. Confronting the client before severe aggression is evident places responsibility on the client and family for respectful partnership in care.*
- Document all acts or verbalizations of aggression. *Safety of the staff is a primary responsibility of home health agencies. Law enforcement intervention may be necessary.*
- ▲ If client verbalizes or displays threatening behavior, notify your supervisor and plan to make joint visits with another staff person or a security escort. *Having a second person at the visit is a show of power and control used to subdue aggressive behavior.*
- If the client's behavior is not overtly threatening but makes the nurse uncomfortable, a meeting may be held outside the home in sight of others (e.g., front porch). *The nurse should trust a "gut" reaction that prompts concern regarding the client's potential for aggressive or violent behavior. Such intuitive reactions are often the result of subliminal cues that are not readily voiced.*

• = Independent;   ▲ = Collaborative;   EBN = Evidence-Based Nursing;   EB = Evidence-Based

- Never enter a home or remain in a home if aggression threatens your well-being.
▲ Never challenge a show of force, such as a gun threat. Leave and notify your supervisor and the appropriate authorities. Document the incident. *Safety of the staff is a primary responsibility of home health agencies. Law enforcement intervention may be necessary.*
▲ If client behaviors intensify, refer for immediate mental health intervention. *The degree of disturbance and ability to manage care safely at home determines the level of services needed to protect the client.*

Client/Family Teaching

- Teach relaxation and exercise as ways to release anger.
- Teach cognitive-behavioral activities, such as active problem solving, reframing (reappraising the situation from a different perspective), or thought stopping (in response to a negative thought, picture a large stop sign and replace the image with a prearranged positive alternative). Teach the client to confront his or her own negative thought patterns (or cognitive distortions), such as catastrophizing (expecting the very worst), dichotomous thinking (perceiving events in only one of two opposite categories), magnification (placing distorted emphasis on a single event), or unrealistic expectations (e.g., "I should get what I want when I want it."). *Cognitive-behavioral activities address clients' assumptions, beliefs, and attitudes about their situations, fostering modification of these elements to be as realistic as possible. Through cognitive-behavioral interventions, clients become more aware of their cognitive choices in adopting and maintaining their belief systems, thereby exercising greater control over their own reactions (Hagerty & Patusky, 2007; Sinclair et al, 1998).*
- For religious couples, encourage the use of prayer. *Prayer appears to be a significant "softening" event for religious couples, facilitating reconciliation and problem solving. It de-escalates hostile emotions and reduces emotional reactivity (Butler, Gardner & Bird, 1998).*
▲ Refer to individual or group therapy.
- Teach the adolescent client violence prevention, and encourage him or her to become involved in community service activities. *School programs that couple community service with classroom health instruction can have a measurable effect on violent behaviors of young adolescents at high risk for being both the perpetrators and victims of peer violence. Community service programs may be a valuable part of multicomponent violence-prevention programs (O'Donnell et al, 1999).*
▲ Teach the use of appropriate community resources in emergency situations (e.g., hotline, community mental health agency, ED, 911 in most places in the United States, the toll-free National Domestic Violence Hotline [1-800-799-SAFE]). *Internet resources are increasing and should be made available to clients (Hopkins et al, 2003). It is necessary to get immediate help when violence occurs.*
▲ Encourage the use of self-help groups in nonemergency situations.
▲ Inform the client and family about medication actions, side effects, target symptoms, and toxic reactions.

evolve   See the EVOLVE website for World Wide Web resources for client education.

REFERENCES

Abderhalden C, Needham I, Miserez B et al: Predicting inpatient violence in acute psychiatric wards using the Broset violence checklist: a multicenter prospective cohort study, *J Psychiatr Ment Health Nurs* 11(4):422, 2004.

Allen LA: Treating agitation without drugs, *Am J Nurs* 99(4):36, 1999.

Amar AF, Cox CW: Intimate partner violence: implications for critical care nursing, *Crit Care Nurs Clin North Am* 18:287, 2006.

Anderson TR, Aviles AM: Diverse faces of domestic violence, *ABNF J* 17:129, 2006.

Appel JK, Kim-Appel D: Child maltreatment and domestic violence: human services issues, *J Health Hum Serv Adm* 29:228, 2006.

Bengtsson-Tops A, Tops D: Self-reported consequences and needs for support associated with abuse in female users of psychiatric care, *Int J Ment Health Nurs* 16:35, 2007.

Bennett L, Riger S, Schewe P et al: Effectiveness of hotline, advocacy, counseling, and shelter services for victims of domestic violence, *J Interpers Violence* 19(7):815, 2004.

Bennett LR, Shiner SK, Ryan S: Using Theraplay in shelter settings with mothers & children who have experienced violence in the home, *J Psychosoc Nurs Ment Health Serv* 44:38, 2006.

Bowers L, Simpson A, Eyres S et al: Serious untoward incidents and their aftermath in acute inpatient psychiatry: the Tompkins Acute Ward study, *Int J Ment Health Nurs* 15:226, 2006.

Boyd MR, Mackey M: Alienation from self and others: the psychosocial problem of rural alcoholic women, *Arch Psychiatr Nurs* 14:134, 2000.

Bullock L, Bloom T, Davis J et al: Abuse disclosure in privately and Medicaid-funded pregnant women, *J Midwifery Womens Health* 51:361, 2006.

Burgess AW, Clements PT: Information processing of sexual abuse in elders, *J Forensic Nurs* 2:113, 2006.

V

• = Independent;   ▲ = Collaborative;   EBN = Evidence-Based Nursing;   EB = Evidence-Based

Burgess AW, Watt ME, Brown KM et al: Management of elder sexual abuse cases in critical care settings, *Crit Care Nurs Clin North Am* 18:313, 2006.

Bussing A, Hoge T: Aggression and violence against home care workers, *J Occup Health Psychol* 9(3):206, 2004.

Butler MH, Gardner BC, Bird MH: Not just a time-out: change dynamics of prayer for religious couples in conflict situations, *Fam Process* 37(4):451, 1998.

Chaffin M, Silovsky JF, Funderburk B et al: Parent-child interaction therapy with physically abusive parents: efficacy for reducing future abuse reports, *J Consult Clin Psychol* 72(3):500, 2004.

Chambless DL, Ollendick TH: Empirically supported psychological interventions: controversies and evidence, *Annu Rev Psychol* 52:685, 2000.

Chang JC, Martin SL, Moracco KE et al: Helping women with disabilities and domestic violence: strategies, limitations, and challenges of domestic violence programs and services, *J Womens Health* 12(7):699, 2003.

Clements CM, Sabourin CM, Spiby L: Dysphoria and hopelessness following battering: the role of perceived control, coping, and self-esteem, *J Fam Violence* 19(1):25, 2004.

Curry MA, Hassouneh-Phillips D, Johnston-Silverberg A: Abuse of women with disabilities: an ecological model and review, *Violence Against Women* 7(1):60, 2001.

De Wit K, Davis K: Nurses' knowledge and learning experiences in relation to the effects of domestic abuse on the mental health of children and adolescents, *Contemp Nurse* 16(3):214, 2004.

Distasio CA: Violence against home care providers. Stop it before it starts, *Caring* 19(10):14, 2000.

Edgecombe G, Ploeger H: Working with families experiencing violence: the Ploeger Model of enhanced maternal and child health nursing practice, *Contemp Nurse* 21:287, 2006.

Gladstone GL, Parker GB, Mitchell PB et al: Implications of childhood trauma for depressed women: an analysis of pathways from childhood sexual abuse to deliberate self-harm and revictimization, *Am J Psychiatry* 161(8):1417, 2004.

Gordon KC, Burton S, Porter L: Predicting the intentions of women in domestic violence shelters to return to partners: does forgiveness play a role? *J Fam Psychol* 18(2):331, 2004.

Hagerty B, Patusky K: Mood disorders: depression and mania. In Fortinash KM, Holoday-Worret PA, editors: *Psychiatric mental health nursing,* ed 4, St Louis, 2007, Mosby.

Hahn RA, Bilukha OO, Crosby A et al: First reports evaluating the effectiveness of strategies for preventing violence: early childhood home visitation, *MMWR Recomm Rep* 52(RR-14):1, 2003.

Harner HM: Domestic violence and trauma care in teenage pregnancy: does paternal age make a difference? *J Obstet Gynecol Neonatal Nurs* 33(3):312, 2004.

Harper-Jacques S, Reimer M: Management of aggression. In Boyd MA, editor: *Psychiatric nursing. Contemporary practice,* ed 2, Philadelphia, 2002, Lippincott Williams & Wilkins.

Hindin PK: Intimate partner violence screening practices of certified nurse-midwives, *J Midwifery Womens Health* 51:216, 2006.

Hollingsworth E, Ford-Gilboe M: Registered nurses' self-efficacy for assessing and responding to woman abuse in emergency department settings, *Can J Nurs Res* 38:54, 2006.

Holmes D, Kennedy SL, Perron A: The mentally ill and social exclusion: a critical examination of the use of seclusion from the patient's perspective, *Issues Ment Health Nurs* 25:559, 2004.

Hopkins K, Sleet DA, Mickalide A et al: Internet resources for injury and violence prevention, *Am J Health Educ Supplement* 34(5): S-62, 2003.

Jones H, Powell JL: Old age, vulnerability and sexual violence: implications for knowledge and practice, *Int Nurs Rev* 53:211, 2006.

Kaukinen C: The help-seeking strategies of female violent crime victims, *J Interpers Violence* 19(9):967, 2004.

Kelly U: "What will happen if I tell you?" Battered Latina women's experiences of health care, *Can J Nurs Res* 38:78, 2006.

Kling R, Corbiere M, Milord R et al: Use of a violence risk assessment tool in an acute care hospital: effectiveness in identifying violent patients, *AAOHN J* 54:481, 2006.

Lanza ML, Kayne HL, Pattison I et al: The relationship of behavioral cues to assaultive behavior, *Clin Nurs Res* 5(1):6, 1996.

Libbus MK, Bullock LF, Neltson T et al: Abuse during pregnancy: current theory and new contextual understandings, *Issues Ment Health Nurs* 27:927, 2006.

Lipscomb J, McPhaul K, Rosen J et al: Violence prevention in the mental health setting: the New York state experience, *Can J Nurs Res* 38:96, 2006.

Liu J: Concept analysis: aggression, *Issues Ment Health Nurs* 25:693, 2004.

Lutz KE, Curry MA Robrecht LC et al: Double binding, abusive intimate partner relationships, and pregnancy, *Can J Nurs Res* 38(4):118-134, 2006.

McFarlane J, Malecha A, Gist J et al: An intervention to increase safety behaviors of abused women: results of a randomized clinical trial, *Nurs Res* 51:347, 2002.

McNeil DE, Eisner JP, Binder RL: The relationship between command hallucinations and violence, *Psychiatr Serv* 51(10):1288, 2000.

Needham I, Abderhalden C, Meer R et al: The effectiveness of two interventions in the management of patient violence in acute mental inpatient settings: report on a pilot study, *J Psychiatr Ment Health Nurs* 11(5):595, 2004.

O'Donnell L, Stueve A, San Doval A et al: Violence prevention and young adolescents' participation in community youth service, *J Adolesc Health* 24(1):28, 1999.

Pryor J: What do nurses do in response to their predictions of aggression? *J Neurosci Nurs* 38:177, 2006.

Remington R: Calming music and hand massage with agitated elderly, *Nurs Res* 51:317, 2002.

Renck B: Psychological stress reactions of women in Sweden who have been assaulted: acute response and four-month follow-up, *Nurs Outlook* 54:312, 2006.

Rice E: Schizophrenia and violence: the perspective of women, *Issues Ment Health Nurs* 27:961, 2006.

Ryan CJ, Bowers L: An analysis of Nurses' post-incident manual restraint reports, *J Psychiatr Ment Health Nurs* 13:527, 2006.

Saxton M, Curry MA, Powers L et al: "Bring my scooter so I can leave you": a study of disabled women handling abuse by personal assistance providers, *Violence Against Women* 7(4):393, 2001.

Silverman JG, Raj A, Clements K: Dating violence and associated sexual risk and pregnancy among adolescent girls in the United States, *Pediatrics* 114(2):220, 2004.

Sinclair VG, Wallston KA, Dwyer KA et al: Effects of a cognitive-behavioral intervention for women with rheumatoid arthritis, *Res Nurs Health* 21:315, 1998.

Skybo T, Polivka B: Health promotion model for violence prevention and exposure, *J Clin Nurs* 16:38, 2007.

Stolker JJ, Nijman HL, Zwanikken PH: Are patients' views on seclusion associated with lack of privacy in the ward? *Arch Psychiatr Nurs* 20:282, 2006.

Straus MA: Prevalence of violence against dating partners by male and female university students worldwide, *Violence Against Women* 10(7):790, 2004.

Stuart GL, Ramsey SE, Moore TM et al: Reductions in marital violence following treatment for alcohol dependence, *J Interpers Violence* 18(10):1113, 2003.

• = Independent;   ▲ = Collaborative;   EBN = Evidence-Based Nursing;   EB = Evidence-Based

Sumter M: Domestic violence and diversity: a call for multicultural services, *J Health Hum Serv Adm* 29:173, 2006.

Thomas SP: Rising violence against transgendered individuals (editorial), *Issues Ment Health Nurs* 25:557, 2004.

Vance DE, Burgio LD, Roth DL et al: Predictors of agitation in nursing home residents, *J Gerontol* 58B(2):P129, 2003.

Vittengl JR: Temporal regularities in physical control at a state psychiatric hospital, *Arch Psychiatr Nurs* 16:80, 2002.

Wallace H: *Family violence: legal, medical, and social perspectives,* ed 2, Boston, 1999, Allyn & Bacon.

Walls C: Shaken baby syndrome education: a role for nurse practitioners working with families of small children, *J Pediatr Health Care* 20:304, 2006.

Wang JJ: Psychological abuse behavior exhibited by caregivers in the care of the elderly and correlated factors in long-term care facilities in Taiwan, *Nurs Res* 13:271, 2005.

Wang JJ, Lin JN, Lee FP: Psychologically abusive behavior by those caring for the elderly in a domestic context, *Geriatr Nurs* 27:284, 2006.

Webster F, Bouck MS, Wright BL et al: Nursing the social wound: public health nurses' experience of screening for woman abuse, *Can J Nurs Res* 38:136, 2006.

Willis D: Hate crimes against gay males: an overview, *Issues Ment Health Nurs* 25:115, 2004.

Willson P, Cesario S, Fredland N et al: Primary healthcare provider's lost opportunity to help abused women, *J Am Acad Nurse Pract* 13(12):565, 2001.

Yonaka L, Yoder MK, Darrow JB et al: Barriers to screening for domestic violence in the emergency department, *J Contin Educ Nurs* 38:37, 2007.

Zun LS, Downey LV, Rosen J: Violence prevention in the ED: linkage of the ED to a social service agency, *Am J Emerg Med* 21(6):454, 2003.

Zust BL: Meaning of INSIGHT participation among women who have experienced intimate partner violence, *Issues Ment Health Nurs* 27:775, 2006.

Risk for self-directed Violence   *Kathleen L. Patusky, PhD, APRN-BC*

NANDA   Definition

At risk for behaviors in which an individual demonstrates that he/she can be physically, emotionally and/or sexually harmful to self

Risk Factors

Age 15-19; age over 45; behavioral clues (e.g., writing forlorn love notes, directing angry messages at a significant other who has rejected the person, giving away personal items, taking out a large life insurance policy); conflictual interpersonal relationships; emotional problems (e.g., hopelessness, despair, increased anxiety, panic, anger, hostility); employment problems (e.g., unemployed, recent job loss/failure); engagement in autoerotic sexual acts; family background (e.g., chaotic or conflictual, history of suicide); history of multiple suicide attempts; lack of personal resources (e.g., poor achievement, poor insight, affect unavailable and poorly controlled); lack of social resources (e.g., poor rapport, socially isolated, unresponsive family); physical health problems (e.g., hypochondriasis, chronic or terminal illness); marital status (single, widowed, divorced); mental health problems (e.g., severe depression, psychosis, severe personality disorder, alcoholism, or drug abuse); occupation (executive, administrator/owner of business, professional, semiskilled worker); sexual orientation (bisexual [active], homosexual [inactive]); suicidal ideation; suicidal plan; verbal clues (e.g., talking about death, "better off without me," asking questions about lethal dosages of drugs)

NOC   Outcomes (Nursing Outcomes Classification)

Suggested NOC Outcomes

Depression Self-Control, Distorted Thought Self-Control, Impulse Self-Control, Loneliness Severity, Mood Equilibrium, Risk Detection, Self-Mutilation Restraint, Suicide Self-Restraint

Example NOC Outcome with Indicators
Suicide Self-Restraint as evidenced by the following indicators: Expresses feelings and seeks help when feeling self-destructive/Verbalizes and controls suicidal ideas and impulses (Rate the outcome and indicators of **Suicide Self-Restraint:** I = never demonstrated, 2 = rarely demonstrated, 3 = sometimes demonstrated, 4 = often demonstrated, 5 = consistently demonstrated [see Section I].)

● = Independent;   ▲ = Collaborative;   EBN = Evidence-Based Nursing;   EB = Evidence-Based

Client Outcomes

Client Will (Specify Time Frame):

- Refrain from self-injury
- State appropriate ways to cope with increased psychological or physiological tension
- Talk about feelings; express anger appropriately
- Seek help when feeling self-destructive or having urges to self-mutilate
- Maintain self-control without supervision
- Use appropriate community agencies when caregivers are unable to attend to emotional needs
- Maintain connectedness in relationships
- Express decreased anxiety and control of impulses
- Refrain from using mood-altering substances
- Obtain no access to harmful objects
- Yield access to harmful objects
- Maintain self-control without supervision

NIC   Interventions (Nursing Interventions Classification)

Suggested NIC Interventions

Anger Control Assistance, Anxiety Reduction, Behavior Management: Self-Harm, Calming Technique, Coping Enhancement, Crisis Intervention, Mood Management, Substance Use Prevention, Suicide Prevention, Surveillance

Example NIC Activities—Suicide Prevention

Determine presence and degree of suicidal risk; Encourage patient to seek out care providers to talk as urge to harm self occurs

Nursing Interventions and *Rationales*

Refer to care plans for **Risk for Suicide**, **Self-mutilation**, and **Risk for Self-mutilation.**

Impaired Walking   *Brenda Emick-Herring, RN, MSN, CRRN*

NANDA   Definition

Limitation of independent movement within the environment on foot (or artificial limb)

Defining Characteristics

Impaired ability to: climb stairs, walk on uneven surface, walk required distances, walk on even surfaces, walk on an incline or decline, navigate curbs

Related Factors (r/t)

Cognitive impairment; deconditioning; depressed mood; environmental constraints (e.g., stairs, inclines, uneven surfaces, unsafe obstacles, distances, lack of assistive devices or person, restraints); fear of falling; impaired balance; impaired vision; insufficient muscle strength; lack of knowledge; limited endurance; musculoskeletal impairment (e.g., contractures); neuromuscular impairment; obesity; pain

NOTE: These are the same as the etiologies for **Impaired physical Mobility** with the addition of lower extremity amputation.

Suggested functional level classifications follow:
0—Completely independent
1—Requires use of equipment or device
2—Requires help from another person for assistance, supervision, or teaching
3—Requires help from another person and equipment device
4—Dependent (does not participate in activity)

• = Independent;   ▲ = Collaborative;   EBN = Evidence-Based Nursing;   EB = Evidence-Based

Suggested NOC Outcomes

Ambulation, Mobility

Example NOC Outcome with Indicators

Ambulation as evidenced by the following indicators: Walks with effective gait/Walks at moderate pace/Walks up and down steps/Walks moderate distance (Rate the outcome and indicators of **Ambulation:** 1 = severely compromised, 2 = substantially compromised, 3 = moderately compromised, 4 = mildly compromised, 5 = not compromised [see Section I].)

Client Outcomes/Goals

Client Will (Specify Time Frame):

- Demonstrate optimal independence and safety in walking
- Demonstrate the ability to direct others on how to assist with walking
- Demonstrate the ability to properly and safely use and care for assistive walking devices

Suggested NIC Intervention

Exercise Therapy: Ambulation

Example NIC Activities—Exercise Therapy: Ambulation

Assist patient to use footwear that facilitates walking and prevents injury; Encourage to sit in bed, on side of bed ("dangle"), or in chair, as tolerated

Nursing Interventions and *Rationales*

- ▲ Reinforce "bridging" (lifting hips up while supine); have client use it to move to side of bed and raise buttocks off bed. *This prepares clients for walking, because it involves hip extension with simultaneous weight bearing through foot/leg, especially in hemiplegics (Bobath, 1978; Gee & Passarella, 1985).*
- ▲ Progressively mobilize clients (gradual elevation of head of bed, sitting in reclined chair, standing, etc.). *Helps clients adapt to and tolerate upright position changes/postures.*
- • Assist clients to apply orthoses, immobilizers, splints, and braces before walking. *Maintain joint stability, immobilization, and alignment during motion (Hoeman, 2002).*
- • Apply thromboembolic deterrent stockings (TEDs), elastic wraps, abdominal binders; raise head of bed in small increments; have clients move feet up/down, sit up/stand slowly, and avoid prolonged standing for orthostatic hypotension. *Enhances circulatory redistribution so blood doesn't pool in legs/feet (Sclater & Alagiakrishnan, 2006).*
- ▲ Compare morning and lying/sitting/standing blood pressures. If systolic pressure falls 20 mm Hg or diastolic pressure falls 10 mm Hg from lying to standing within 3 minutes, and/or if light-headedness, dizziness, syncope, or unexplained falls occur, consult a physician (Bradley & Davis, 2003; Irvin & White, 2004). *Detection of orthostatic hypotension is key to fall prevention; medication or fluid adjustment may be needed.* **EB:** *Persons with orthostatic hypotension are often symptomatic and have postprandial (after meal) hypotension/heart rate variability (Ejaz et al, 2004).*
- ▲ Give hydration and prescribed medications to treat orthostatic hypotension. *Water has a pressor effect in those with autonomic orthostatic hypotension (Shannon et al, 2002).* **EB:** *A small group of seated persons with severe orthostatic postprandial hypotension had elevated blood pressures after rapid ingestion of 500 ml of water (Shannon et al, 2002).*
- • Screen for and vigilantly apply compression stockings/intermittent pneumatic compression devices; exercise feet and ankles and give prophylactic anticoagulants as ordered to persons at

• = Independent;   ▲ = Collaborative;   EBN = Evidence-Based Nursing;   EB = Evidence-Based

risk for deep vein thrombosis (DVT). Refer to the care plan for **Ineffective Tissue perfusion.** *Screening for risk, using mechanical devices to prevent stasis, and treating with anticoagulants prevent blood clots (Kehl-Pruett, 2006; Van Wicklin, Ward & Cantrell, 2006).*

▲ Assist persons with DVT to walk, because early ambulation may be ordered. *A literature review suggested ambulation 24-48 hours after anticoagulation treatment started was safe in those with ". . . adequate cardiopulmonary reserve and no evidence of pulmonary embolism" (Aldrich & Hunt, 2004).*

▲ Cue clients regarding weight-bearing restrictions and how to correctly use prescribed devices. *Full weight bearing may retard bone healing in fractured limbs. Standard walkers are commonly used by clients with full weight-bearing restrictions and wheeled walkers are often used by clients with partial weight-bearing restrictions and low endurance (Kreger, 2006).*

• As weight bearing resumes after prolonged bed rest, teach clients to ingest protein but avoid nonsteroidal antiinflammatory drugs (NSAIDs); be alert for depression. *Protein helps muscle repair, whereas NSAIDs may delay muscle recovery; muscle soreness physiology may contribute to depression (St. Pierre & Flaskerud, 1995).* **EBN:** *Animal studies showed muscle fiber damage occurred with non–weight bearing for 7 days (St. Pierre & Tidball, 1994).*

• Encourage clients to stand and walk frequently. *Skeletal muscle contraction stimulates bone growth and calcium resorption (International Food Information Council Foundation, 2002; Sims & Olson, 2002).* **EB:** *Risk of hip fracture was reduced 20%-40% in active elders (Gregg, Pereira & Casperson, 2000).*

• Teach clients with leg amputations to correctly don sheath, stump socks, liner, and prosthesis before walking. *A thin nylon sheath prevents the limb from turning in the socket of the prosthesis. A stump sock establishes proper fit between limb and socket. The liner helps prevent pressure ulcers (Kipnis, 1993; Yeltzer, 1998).*

▲ Use a snug gait belt and assistive devices while walking clients, as recommended by the physical therapist (PT). *Belts help staff steady the clients; devices give clients support and help compensate for poor balance and endurance (Kreger, 2006).* **EBN:** *Use of a gait belt decreased staff exertion, back stress, and compressive force from L5-S1 (Owen & Garg, 1993).* **EB:** *Older adults living in a residential facility who were physically active and used walking aids had fewer falls (Graafmans et al, 2003). Use of two-wheeled walkers allowed persons with leg amputations and prosthetics to walk faster and halt less often than when four-footed walkers were used (Tsai et al, 2003).*

• Walk clients with an appropriate number of people; have one team member state short simple motor instructions. *This helps prevent falls, fear, and mixed messages, because walking requires concentration and visualization, especially if the client is learning new information.* **EB:** *Stroke survivors engaging in a verbal task while walking had poorer balance and gait velocity (Bowen et al, 2001). Older adults lost their balance and swayed while standing when an auditory task was introduced (Shumway-Cook & Woollacott, 2000).*

• Document the number of helpers, level of assistance (maximum, standby, etc.), type of assistance, and devices needed on the care plan. *Communication, repetition, and practice promote motor (re)learning.*

• Collect baseline pulse rate/rhythm before walking clients, and reassess after 5 minutes of walking. If either are abnormal, have the client sit for 5 minutes then retake pulse rate. If it is still abnormal, walk clients more slowly and with more help, or for a shorter time. *Pulse rate indicates cardiac tolerance; if it rises too high after a few walking trials, the physician should be notified (Radwanski & Hoeman, 1996).*

▲ Monitor the client's tolerance for walking. Initiate a 5-minute rest period if shortness of breath, use of accessory muscles, chest pain, nausea, sweating, pale/flushed skin, dizziness, syncope, or mental confusion occurs. If signs persist, notify the physician. Refer to the care plan for **Activity intolerance.**

▲ Perform initial and subsequent screening for risk of falling. *Fall assessment tools help identify persons at risk so prevention and protection measures can be implemented (Morse, 2006).*

• Individualize interventions to prevent falls and overuse of restraints. Interventions include scheduled toileting, balance/strength training, sleep hygiene, education on risk of medication/alcohol use, and removal of hazards (Browne et al, 2004; Resnick & Junlapeeya, 2004). **EBN:** *Assessment and root cause analysis indicated that inpatients who fell had gait problems, were confused, and were self-toileting; individualizing preventions decreased fall rates (Gowdy & Godfrey, 2003).*

• = Independent;   ▲ = Collaborative;   EBN = Evidence-Based Nursing;   EB = Evidence-Based

Balance and fear of falling improved in older adults in nursing homes after ankle strengthening and walking programs were begun (Schoenfelder & Rubenstein, 2004). Retrospective analysis of inpatients indicated that the number of falls that occurred when bed rails were up was equal to or higher than when they were not up; one death occurred from falling over the bed rails (van Leeuwen et al, 2001).

Geriatric

- Monitor pulse, respirations, and blood pressure before and 5 minutes after the client has started a new upright activity; stop if resting heart rate >100 beats/min, exercise heart rate is 35% greater than resting rate, systolic blood pressure is 25-35 mm Hg above resting pressure, or decrease in systolic blood pressure >20 mm Hg (Radwanski & Hoeman, 1996). *Activity may be too physically strenuous for older clients.*

▲ Collaborate with PT to obtain the correct walking device for the client's endurance and balance abilities; recognize that devices increase energy and may raise pulse rate/blood pressure. *Wheeled walkers help clients walk more easily but may not offer enough support physically or psychologically (Kreger, 2006).*

- Encourage walking and recognize that older adults often walk slowly. *Slow gait may be related to fear of falling; decreased strength in hip extensors, hip abductors, or plantar flexor muscles; reduced balance or visual acuity; knee flexion contractures; and foot pain (Jones, 2001; Sims & Olson, 2002).*

▲ Assess risk then implement fall precautions, such as using a visual identifier to indicate clients at risk, placing a call system within reach, recommending an exercise/education program, clearing obstacles, and reviewing medication. *Previous fall, physiological changes, and adverse effects from multiple medications puts older adults at risk for falls (Alexander, 1994; Ulfarsson & Robinson, 1997).* **EB:** *After falling, older clients who received education about fall prevention, home safety, and environmental modification had fewer recurrent falls than members of a control group (Close et al, 1999).*

- Assess for swaying, poor balance, and short first step length during standing and walking. **EB:** *Researchers found that older adults who were prone to falling had a shorter first step as they began to walk; this may be a factor to help identify postural problems (Mbourou, Lajoie & Teasdale, 2003). Leg weakness and poor tandem walking ability were predictive of older adult inpatients who later fell (Chu et al, 1999).*

▲ Encourage participation in therapeutic exercise programs. **EB:** *A randomized controlled trial of older adults living at home and attending a rehabilitation exercise program had fewer falls and injuries than control subjects attending health classes (Means et al, 2005). A randomized controlled trial in a subacute care hospital indicated 30% fewer falls in subjects enrolled in an exercise/education program (Haines et al, 2004).*

- Emphasize the importance of wearing firm, low-heeled shoes with nonskid and nonfriction soles and seeking medical care for foot pain, foot problems, and diabetes. **EB:** *Older women had more foot problems than older men; subjects with foot pain did worse with leaning, going up and down stairs, alternate step up, and timed 6-meter walk testing (Menz & Lord, 2001).*

- Introduce and reinforce positive perceptions of old age. **EB:** *Older adults exposed to positive and negative stereotypes of aging reported significant improvements in gait with positive images (Hausdorff, Levy & Wei, 1999). A positive association was found between two variables—living alone and belief in self—and walking, even if clients had physical difficulties (Simonsick, Guralnik & Fried, 1999).*

Home Care

- Establish a support system for emergency and contingency care (e.g., Lifeline). *Impaired walking may pose a life threat during a crisis (e.g., fall, fire, orthostatic episode).*

- Teach compensatory strategies mentioned previously for orthostatic hypotension. *Older adults develop arterial stiffness and reduced autonomic nervous system functioning. Their baroreceptors respond slowly so they are less able to maintain blood pressure when standing (Sclater & Alagiakrishnan, 2006). Retrospective chart review identified concurrent medications that contributed to orthostatic hypotension in older adults (Poon & Braun, 2005).*

- Assess for and modify any barriers to walking in the home environment. **EB:** *In a randomized controlled trial, occupational therapists (OTs) made home visits to advise clients on removing fall hazards. These clients fell less often than those in the control group; it's unclear if elimination of hazards or changes in client behavior reduced falls (Cumming et al, 1999).*

• = Independent;   ▲ = Collaborative;   EBN = Evidence-Based Nursing;   EB = Evidence-Based

- Stress the importance of adequate lighting, tacking down carpet edges, removing throw rugs, using nonskid backings with throw rugs, applying nonskid wax to floors, and removing clutter. *Prophylaxis and removal of hazards may prevent falls (Ulfarsson & Robinson, 1997).*
▲ Obtain referral for PT home visits for individualized strength, balance retraining, and a walking plan. *Diseases, medications, and a history of falls place clients at risk for falling (Hertel & Trahiotis, 2001; Sloan, Haslam & Foret, 2001).* **EB:** *Older women with individually tailored exercise programs had fewer falls and injuries from falls during the 2-year study (Campbell et al, 1999).*
▲ Make referrals for home health aide services for assistance with activities of daily living (ADLs). *Walking impairment may serve as a barrier to self-care, including eating and drinking.*
▲ Listen to and support client/caregivers; refer to case manager, social services, or support groups. *Immobility may necessitate role changes and create anger and frustration; supportive services as needed promote validation of feelings and alternative methods of problem solving.*

Client/Family Teaching

- Teach the client to routinely check walking devices, such as removing dirt from and replacing rubber tips of walkers and canes; checking push button locks on walkers with telescoping legs (Minor & Minor, 1999); and inspecting prostheses for cracks, rough spots inside the socket, and odd noises and movement at joints or the foot (Yeltzer, 1998). *Routine checks keep devices in safe working order, and sound tips grip the floor.*
▲ Instruct men and women at risk for osteoporosis or hip fractures to bear weight, walk, take calcium and vitamin D supplements, drink milk, stop smoking, and consult a physician for estrogen replacement and antiresorptive therapy (Franzen-Korzendorfer, 2002). **EB:** *In 50 of 52 studies, high calcium intake increased accumulation of bone, prevented bone loss, and decreased risk of fractures in older adults (Heaney, 2000). Older men surviving hip fractures rarely received antiresorptive therapy, or calcium or vitamin D supplements (Kiebzak et al, 2002).*
- For more information, please refer to the care plans for **Impaired Transfer ability** and **Impaired wheelchair Mobility.**

 See the EVOLVE website for World Wide Web resources for client education.

REFERENCES

Aldrich D, Hunt DP: When can the patient with deep venous thrombosis begin to ambulate? *Phys Ther* 84(3):268, 2004.

Alexander NB: Postural control in older adults, *J Am Geriatr Soc* 42(1):93, 1994.

Bobath B: *Adult hemiplegia: evaluation and treatment,* London, 1978, William Heinemann.

Bowen A, Wenman R, Mickelborough J et al: Dual-task effects of talking while walking on velocity and balance following stroke, *Age Ageing* 30(4):319, 2001.

Bradley JG, Davis KA: Orthostatic hypotension, *Am Fam Physician* 68(12):2393, 2003.

Browne JA, Covington BG, Davila Y et al: Using information technology to assist in redesign of a fall prevention program, *J Nurs Care Qual* 19(3):218, 2004.

Campbell AJ, Robertson MC, Gardner MM, et al: Falls prevention over 2 years: a randomized controlled trial in women 80 years and older, *Age Ageing* 28:513, 1999.

Chu LW, Pei CK, Chiu A et al: Risk factors for falls in hospitalized older medical patients, *J Gerontol* 54(1):M38, 1999.

Close J, Ellis M, Hooper R et al: Prevention of falls in the elderly trial (PROFET): a randomised controlled trial, *Lancet* 353(9147):93, 1999.

Cumming RG, Thoomas M, Szonyi G et al: Home visits by an occupational therapist for assessment and modification of environmental hazards: a randomized trial of falls prevention, *J Am Geriatr Soc* 47:1397, 1999.

Ejaz AA, Haley WE, Wasiluk A et al: Characteristics of 100 consecutive patients presenting with orthostatic hypotension, *Mayo Clin Proc* 79(7):890, 2004.

Franzen-Korzendorfer H: The silent disease, *Rehab Manag* 15(8):30, 2002.

Gee ZL, Passarella PM: *Nursing care of the stroke patient: a therapeutic approach,* Pittsburgh, 1985, AREN.

Gowdy M, Godfrey S: Using tools to assess and prevent inpatient falls, *Jt Comm J Qual Saf* 29(7):363, 2003.

Graafmans WC, Lips P, Wijlhuizen GJ et al: Daily physical activity and the use of a walking aid in relation to falls in elderly people in a residential care setting, *Z Gerontol Geriatr* 36(1):23, 2003.

Gregg EW, Pereira MA, Casperson CJ: Physical activity, falls, and fractures among older adults: a review of the epidemiologic evidence, *J Am Geriatr Soc* 48:883, 2000.

Haines TP, Benell KL, Osborne RH et al: Effectiveness of targeted falls prevention programme in subacute hospital setting: randomized controlled trial, *BMJ* 328:676, 2004.

Hausdorff JM, Levy BR, Wei JY: The power of ageism on physical function of older persons: reversibility of age-related gait changes, *J Am Geriatr Soc* 47:1346, 1999.

Heaney RP: Calcium, dairy products and osteoporosis, *J Am Coll Nutr* 19:835, 2000.

Hertel KL, Trahiotis MG: Exercise in the prevention and treatment of osteoporosis, *Nurs Clin North Am* 36(3):441, 2001.

Hoeman SP: Movement, functional mobility, and activities of daily living. In Hoeman SP, editor: *Rehabilitation nursing: process, application, and outcomes,* ed 3, St Louis, 2002, Mosby.

International Food Information Council Foundation (IFIC): *IFIC review: physical activity, nutrition and bone health.* Available at http://ific.org/healthybones, accessed on April 27, 2002.

Irvin DJ, White M: The importance of accurately assessing orthostatic hypotension, *Geriatr Nurs* 25(2):99, 2004.

Jones DA: Successful aging: maintaining mobility in a geriatric patient population, *Rehab Manag* 14(9):46, 2001.

Kehl-Pruett, W: Deep vein thrombosis in hospitalized patients: a review of evidence based guidelines for prevention, *Dimens Crit Care Nurs* 25(2):53, 2006.

Kiebzak GM, Beinart GA, Perser K et al: Undertreatment of osteoporosis in men with hip fracture, *Arch Intern Med* 162(19):2217, 2002.

Kipnis ND: Musculoskeletal/orthopedic disorders. In McCourt A, editor: *The specialty practice of rehabilitation nursing: a core curriculum,* ed 3, Skokie, Ill, 1993, Rehabilitation Foundation.

Kreger A: Choosing mobility, *Rehab Manag* 19(3):34, 2006.

Mbourou GA, Lajoie Y, Teasdale N: Step length variability at gait initiation in elderly fallers and anon-fallers, and young adults, *Gerontology* 49(1):21, 2003.

Means KM, Rodell DE, O'Sullivan PS et al: Balance, mobility, and falls among community-dwelling elderly persons: effects of a rehabilitation exercise program, *Am J Phys Med Rehabil* 84(4):238, 2005.

Menz HB, Lord SR: Foot pain impairs balance and functional ability in community-dwelling older people, *J Am Podiatr Med Assoc* 91(5):222, 2001.

Minor MAD, Minor SD: *Patient care skills,* ed 4, Stamford, Conn, 1999, Appleton & Lange.

Morse JM: The safety of safety research: the case of patient fall research, *Can J Nurs Res* 38(2):74, 2006.

Owen BD, Garg A: Back stress isn't part of the job, *Am J Nurs* 93(2):48, 1993.

Poon IO, Braun U: High prevalence of orthostatic hypotension and its correlation with potentially causative medications among elderly veterans. *J Clin Pharm Ther* 30(2):173, 2005.

Radwanski MB, Hoeman SP: Geriatric rehabilitation nursing. In Hoeman SP, editor: *Rehabilitation nursing: process and application,* ed 2, St Louis, 1996, Mosby.

Resnick B, Junlapeeya P: Falls in a community of older adults: findings and implications for practice, *Appl Nurs Res* 17(2):81, 2004.

Schoenfelder DP, Rubenstein LM: An exercise program to improve fall-related outcomes in elderly nursing home residents, *Appl Nurs Res* 17(1):21, 2004.

Sclater A, Alagiakrishnan K: Orthostatic hypotension: a primary care primer for assessment and treatment, *Geriatrics* 59(8):22, 2006.

Shannon JR, Diedrich A, Biaggioni I et al: Water drinking as a treatment for orthostatic syndromes, *Am J Med* 112(5):355, 2002.

Shumway-Cook A, Woollacott M: Attention demands and postural control: the effect of sensory context, *J Gerontol A Biol Sci Med Sci* 55(1):M10, 2000.

Simonsick EM, Guralnik JM, Fried LP: Who walks? Factors associated with walking behavior in disabled older women with and without self-reported walking difficulty, *J Am Geriatr Soc* 47(6):672, 1999.

Sims GL, Olson RS: Muscle and skeletal function. In Hoeman SP, editor, *Rehabilitation nursing: process, application, and outcomes,* ed 3, St Louis, 2002, Mosby.

Sloan HL, Haslam K, Foret CM: Teaching the use of walkers and canes, *Home Health Nurs* 19:241, 2001.

St. Pierre BA, Flaskerud JH: Clinical nursing implications for the recovery of atrophied skeletal muscle following bed rest, *Rehabil Nurs* 20(6):314, 1995.

St. Pierre BA, Tidball JG: Differential response of macrophage subpopulations to soleus muscle reloading after rat hindlimb suspension, *J Appl Physiol* 77:290, 1994.

Tsai HA, Kirby RL, MacLeod DA et al: Aided gait of people with lower-limb amputations: comparisons of 4-footed and 2-wheeled walkers, *Arch Phys Med Rehabil* 84(4):584, 2003.

Ulfarsson J, Robinson BE: Falls and falling. In Ham RJ, Sloane PD, editors: *Primary care geriatrics: a case-based approach,* ed 3, St Louis, 1997, Mosby.

van Leeuwen M, Bennett L, West S et al: Patient falls from bed and the role of bedrails in the acute care setting, *Aust J Adv Nurs* 19(2):8, 2001.

Van Wicklin, SA, Ward KS, Cantrell SW: Implementing a research utilization plan for prevention of deep vein thrombosis, *AORN J* 83(6):1353, 2006.

Yeltzer EA: Care of the client with an amputation. In Chin PA, Finocchiaro D, Rosebrough A, editors: *Rehabilitation nursing practice,* New York, 1998, McGraw-Hill.

Wandering   *Donna Algase, PhD, RN, FAAN*

NANDA   Definition

Meandering; aimless or repetitive locomotion that exposes the individual to harm; frequently incongruent with boundaries, limits, or obstacles

Defining Characteristics

Frequent or continuous movement from place to place, often revisiting the same destinations; persistent locomotion in search of "missing" or unattainable people or places; haphazard locomotion; locomotion in unauthorized or private spaces; locomotion resulting in unintended leaving of a premise; long periods of locomotion without an apparent destination; fretful locomotion or pacing; inability to locate significant landmarks in a familiar setting; locomotion that cannot be easily dissuaded or redirected; following behind or shadowing a caregiver's locomotion; trespassing; hyperactivity; scanning, seeking, or searching behaviors; periods of locomotion interspersed with periods of nonlocomotion (e.g., sitting, standing, sleeping); getting lost

• = Independent;   ▲ = Collaborative;   EBN = Evidence-Based Nursing;   EB = Evidence-Based

Related Factors (r/t)

Cognitive impairment, specifically memory and recall deficits, disorientation, poor visuoconstructive (or visuospatial) ability, and language (primarily expressive) defects; cortical atrophy; premorbid behavior (e.g., outgoing, sociable personality); separation from familiar people and places; sedation; emotional state, especially fear, anxiety, boredom, or depression (agitation); overstimulating/understimulating social or physical environment; physiological state or need (e.g., hunger/thirst, pain, urination, constipation); time of day

NOC   Outcomes (Nursing Outcomes Classification)

Suggested NOC Outcomes

Caregiver Home Care Readiness, Fall Prevention Behavior, Falls Occurrence

Example NOC Outcome with Indicators
Caregiver Home Care Readiness as evidenced by the following indicators: Knowledge of recommended treatment regimen/Knowledge of prescribed activity/Knowledge of emergency care/Confidence in ability to manage care at home (Rate the outcome and indicators of **Caregiver Home Care Readiness:** 1 = not adequate, 2 = slightly adequate, 3 = moderately adequate, 4 = substantially adequate, 5 = totally adequate [see Section I].)

Client Outcomes

Client Will (Specify Time Frame):

- Decrease incidence of falls (preferably free of falls)
- Decrease incidence of elopements
- Maintain appropriate body weight

Caregiver Will (Specify Time Frame):

- Be able to explain interventions he or she can use to provide a safe environment for a care receiver who displays wandering behavior

NIC   Interventions (Nursing Interventions Classification)

Suggested NIC Intervention

Dementia Management

Example NIC Activities—Dementia Management
Place identification bracelet on the patient; Provide space for safe pacing and wandering

Nursing Interventions and *Rationales*

- Assess and document the amount (frequency and duration), pattern (random, lapping, or pacing), and 24-hour distribution of wandering behavior over 3 days. **EBN:** *Assessment over time provides a baseline against which behavior change can be evaluated (Algase et al, 1997). Such assessment can also reveal the time of day when wandering is greatest and when surveillance or other precautionary measures are most necessary.*
- Document particular aspects of wandering that are troubling. **EBN:** *Such instruments as the Algase Wandering Scale (Version 2 or Community Version) (Algase et al, 2001, 2004a) can indicate whether the behavior is persistent, spatially disordered, or prone to elopement. The Everyday Spatial Questionnaire (Chiu et al, 2005) or the Wayfinding Effectiveness Scale (Algase et al, in press) can be used to assess the nature of navigational deficits. Information from such instruments can direct caregivers toward more appropriate intervention strategies.*
- Obtain a history of personality characteristics and behavioral responses to stress. **EBN and EB:** *Information about long-standing behavioral tendencies may reveal circumstances under which wander-*

ing will occur and can aid in interpreting both positive and negative meanings of wandering behavior of the client (Kolanowski, Strand & Whall, 1997; Thomas, 1997).

- Evaluate for neurocognitive strengths and limitations, particularly language, attention, visuospatial skills, and perseveration. **EBN:** *Wanderers may have expressive language deficits that hamper their ability to communicate needs (Algase, 1992; Dawson & Reid, 1987).* **EBN and EB:** *Knowledge of attentional and visuospatial deficits, which may account for certain patterns of wandering or wayfinding deficits, can lead to identification of appropriate environmental modifications that could enhance functional ambulation, such as elimination of distractions and enhancement of cues marking desired destinations (Algase et al, 2004b; Chiu et al, 2004; Fischer, Marterer & Danielczyk, 1990; Henderson, Mack & Williams, 1989; Kavcic & Duffy, 2003; Monacelli et al, 2003, Mapstone, Steffenella & Duffy, 2003; Passini et al, 1995, 2000).* **EB:** *The presence of perseveration may indicate that the wanderer is unable to voluntarily stop his or her behavior (Passini et al, 1995; Ryan et al, 1995), thus calling for nursing judgment as to when wandering should be interrupted to enhance the wanderer's safety, comfort, or well-being.*

- Assess for physical distress or needs, such as hunger, thirst, pain, discomfort, or elimination. **EBN:** *Although physical needs have not been documented in relation to wandering, the Need-Driven Dementia-Compromised Model hypothesizes this relationship (Algase et al, 1996).*

- Assess for emotional or psychological distress, such as anxiety, fear, or feeling lost. **EB:** *Anxiety and depression frequently accompany wandering (Teri et al, 1999).*

- Observe wandering episodes for antecedents and consequences. **EBN and EB:** *People, events, or circumstances surrounding the onset or conclusion of wandering may provide cues about triggers or rewards that are stimulating or reinforcing wandering behavior (Heard & Watson, 1999; Hirst & Metcalf, 1989; Hussian, 1981, 1982).*

- Apply observed consequences of wandering, such as personal attention, food, and so forth, at times when the person is not wandering, and withhold them while the person is wandering. **EB:** *Differential reinforcement of other behavior (nonwandering) can reduce wandering episodes by 50% to 80% (Heard & Watson, 1999).*

- Assess regularly for the presence of or potential for negative outcomes of wandering, such as declining social skills, falls, elopement, and getting lost. **EB:** *Wanderers are at greater risk for falls than other cognitively impaired persons (Kippenbrock & Soja, 1993; Morse, Tylko & Dixon, 1987; Rowe & Bennet, 2003; Rowe, Feinglass & Wiss, 2004). Wanderers have also shown greater loss in social skills over time than nonwandering counterparts (Cornbleth, 1977).*

- Weigh the client at defined intervals to detect onset of weight loss, and watch for symptoms associated with inadequate food intake, including constipation, dehydration, muscle wasting, and starvation. *Wandering behavior can affect the client's ability to eat, when the client is unable to sit at a table for the time needed to eat a meal (Beattie & Algase, 2002).*

- For the client who displays wandering behavior during mealtimes, use behavioral interventions to shape behavior, including verbal statements, nonverbal social behavior, and systematic extinguishing of undesirable client behavior. **EBN:** *Results of a study using behavior interventions demonstrated that they were effective in increasing the time the client sat at the table, and the amount of food the client ate (Beattie, Algase & Song, 2004).*

- Provide for safe ambulation with comfortable and well-fitting clothes, shoes with nonskid soles and foot support, and any necessary walking aids (e.g., a cane, walker, or Merry Walker). **EB:** *For persons with advanced dementia who had previously led active lives, falls are often related to a decline in vigor (Brody et al, 1984). Wanderers are at increased risk for falls (Katz et al, 2004).*

- Provide safe and secure surroundings that deter accidental elopements, using perimeter control devices, camouflage, or electronic tracking systems. **EBN:** *Eloping can have hazardous outcomes, including death (Rowe & Glover, 2001).* **EB:** *Perimeter control devices can effectively reduce or prevent exiting behavior (Negley, Molla & Obenchain, 1990).* **EBN and EB:** *However, under some circumstances, these devices are viewed as unnecessarily restrictive, and more passive means, such as camouflage, have been substituted. Camouflage techniques, such as masking the doorknob or creating striped floor patterns in front of exits, have been used with success (Namazi, Rosner & Calkins, 1989; Hussian & Brown, 1987), particularly in subjects with Alzheimer's disease (Hewewasam, 1996), but the effectiveness may be mitigated by other architectural features of the setting (Hamilton, 1993; Chafetz, 1990). A Cochrane review found that no randomized controlled trials have been done to validate the effectiveness*

of subjective barriers to prevent wandering in cognitively impaired clients (Price, Hermans & Grimley-Evans, 2000). Newer electronic monitoring and tracking systems are highly effective and reduce care-giver burden (Altus et al, 2000; Nelson et al, 2004; Siders et al, 2004).

- During periods of inactivity, position the wanderer so that desirable destinations (e.g., bathroom) are within the client's line of vision and undesirable destinations (e.g., exits or stairwells) are out of sight. **EBN and EB:** *Functional, nonwandering ambulation is possible even into late-stage dementia and may be facilitated by keeping appropriate visual cues accessible (Passini et al, 2000; Algase, 1999).*

- If wandering takes a random or haphazard route, reduce environmental distractions and increase relevant environmental cues. Note and eliminate stimuli that distract the wanderer while in route. Provide afternoon rest periods if assessment reveals that random-pattern wandering worsens as the day progresses. **EBN:** *Random-pattern wandering may be affected by environmental stimuli (Algase, 1999). The proportion of wandering that is random increases as the day progresses (Algase et al, 1997; Algase, 1999) and may indicate fatigue.*

- Enhance institutional settings with areas that provide interesting views and opportunities to sit. **EB:** *Enhanced environments can improve mood, and they encourage wanderers to linger or sit more than purely institutional surroundings do (Cohen-Mansfield & Werner, 1998).*

- Engage wanderers in social interaction and structured activity, especially when wanderers appear distressed or otherwise uncomfortable, or their wandering presents a challenge to others in the setting. **EBN and EB:** *Wandering and social interaction are inversely related. Wanderers often have an outgoing or sociable personality and also have deficits in expressive language skills. Thus although they may prefer social interaction, their ability to initiate it may be compromised (Algase, 1992; Thomas, 1997).*

- If wandering has a pacing quality, attempt to identify and address any underlying problems or concerns. Offer stress-reducing approaches, such as music, massage, or rocking. Attempts to distract or redirect the pacing wanderer may worsen wandering. **EBN:** *Pacing, as a wandering pattern, is not associated with level of cognitive impairment and may reflect anxiety, agitation, pain, or another internal process (Algase, Beattie & Therrien, 2001; Gerdner, 2000; Snyder & Olson, 1996).*

- If wandering is a recently acquired behavior or if it increases in intensity over previous levels, evaluate for constipation, pneumonia, or acute physical problems. **EBN and EB:** *Persons who first exhibit wandering within 3 months after admission to a nursing home are more likely than others to have developed physical problems that stimulate wandering (Keily, Morris & Algase, 2000).*

- If wandering has a lapping or circuitous pattern, signs or labels may be effective. Substitute another repetitive activity, such as folding or rocking, if lapping becomes problematic or excessive. **EBN:** *Not all wanderers display lapping-pattern wandering, and when it does occur, it tends to occur early in the day or to follow rest periods. Thus it may be a more functional pattern than random wandering and may indicate a slightly better level of cognitive function for the individual, even if transient. Thus wanderers who lap may be better able to use information in the environment (Algase, Beattie & Therrien, 2001).* **EB:** *However, this pattern of wandering may also be a form of perseveration, and therefore the person may be unable to disengage voluntarily (Passini et al, 1995; Ryan et al, 1995).*

- Provide a regularly scheduled and supervised exercise or walking program, particularly if wandering occurs excessively during the night or at times that are inconvenient in the setting. **EBN and EB:** *Although exercise or walking programs do not reduce daytime wandering, they have been shown to reduce or eliminate nighttime wandering (Carillon Nursing and Rehabilitation Center, 2000; Robb, 1987) and to decrease general agitation levels (Holmberg, 1997).*

- Use slow-stroke, hand, or foot massage before the times of day or events that induce wandering. **EBN and EB:** *Various massage techniques have been shown to reduce wandering and diffuse agitation in persons with dementia (Kilstoff & Chenoweth, 1998; Malaquin-Pavan, 1997; Rowe & Alfred, 1999; Snyder, Egan & Burns, 1995; Sutherland, Reakes & Bridges, 1999).*

Multicultural

- Assess for the influence of cultural beliefs, norms, and values on the family's understanding of wandering behavior. **EBN:** *Latina caregivers of people with dementia delay institutionalization significantly longer than female Caucasian caregivers. In addition, Latino cultural values and positive*

• = Independent;   ▲ = Collaborative;   EBN = Evidence-Based Nursing;   EB = Evidence-Based

views of the caregiving role are important factors that may significantly influence their decision to institutionalize loved ones with dementia (Mausbach et al, 2004). Another study found that black and Latino community-dwelling clients with moderate to severe dementia have a higher prevalence of wandering and other dementia-related behaviors (Sink et al, 2004).

▲ Refer the family to social services or other supportive services to assist with the impact of caregiving for the wandering client. **EBN:** *African-American caregivers of dementia clients may evidence less desire than other caregivers to institutionalize their family members and are more likely to report unmet service needs (Hinrichsen & Ramirez, 1992). African-American and white families of clients with dementia may report restricted social activity (Haley et al, 1995).*

• Encourage the family to use support groups or other service programs. **EBN:** *Studies indicate that minority families of clients with dementia use few support programs, even though these programs could have a positive impact on caregiver well-being (Cox, 1999).*

• Validate the family's feelings regarding the impact of client wandering on family lifestyle. **EBN:** *Validation is a therapeutic communication technique that lets the client know that the nurse has heard and understands what was said (Heineken, 1998).*

 ### Home Care

• Help the caregiver set up a plan to deal with wandering behavior using the interventions mentioned in Nursing Interventions and Rationales.

• Assess the home environment for modifications that will protect the client and prevent elopement. *Security devices are available to notify the caregiver of the client's movements (e.g., alarms at doors, bed alarms).*

• Assist the family to set up a plan of exercise for the client, including safe walking. *Walking is a valuable source of exercise, even for clients with dementia (Oddy, 2004).*

• Enroll wanderers in the Safe Return Program of the Alzheimer's Association, and help the caregiver develop a plan of action to use if the client elopes. **EBN:** *The Safe Return Program has assisted in locating numerous persons who have eloped from their homes or other residential care settings. Mortality rates are high if there is failure to locate elopers within the first 24 hours (Rowe & Glover, 2001).*

• Help the caregiver develop a plan of action to use if the client elopes.

▲ Institute case management of frail elderly clients to support continued independent living. *Wandering behavior represents and can lead to increasing needs for assistance in using the healthcare system effectively. Case management combines nursing activities of client and family assessment, planning and coordination of care among all healthcare providers, delivery of direct nursing care, and monitoring of care and outcomes. These activities are able to address continuity of care, mutual goal setting, behavior management, and prevention of worsening health problems (Guttman, 1999).*

▲ Refer for homemaker or psychiatric home healthcare services for respite, client reassurance, and implementation of a therapeutic regimen. Refer to the care plan for **Caregiver role strain.** *Responsibility for a person at high risk for wandering provides high caregiver stress. Respite care decreases caregiver stress. The presence of caring individuals is reassuring to both the client and caregivers, especially during periods of client anxiety. Wandering behavior can make use of the interventions described previously, modified for the home setting.*

 ### Client/Family Teaching

• Inform the client and family of the meaning of and reasons for wandering behavior. *An understanding of wandering behavior will enable the client and family to provide the client with a safe environment.*

• Teach the caregiver/family methods to deal with wandering behavior using the interventions mentioned in Nursing Interventions and Rationales.

W

 See the EVOLVE website for World Wide Web resources for client education.

REFERENCES

Algase DL: Cognitive discriminants of wandering among nursing home residents, *Nurs Res* 41(2):78, 1992.

Algase DL: Wandering: a dementia-compromised behavior, *J Gerontol Nurs* 25(9):10, 1999.

Algase DL, Beattie ER, Song JA et al: Validation of the Algase Wandering Scale: version 2 in a cross cultural sample, *Aging Ment Health* 8(2):133-142, 2004a.

Algase DL, Beattie ERA, Therrien B: Impact of cognitive impairment on wandering behavior, *West J Nurs Res* 23:283, 2001.

Algase DL, Beattie ER, Bogue EL et al: The Algase Wandering Scale: initial psychometrics of a new caregiver reporting tool, *Am J Alzheimers Dis Other Demen* 16(3):141-152, 2001.

Algase DL, Beck C, Kolanowski A et al: Need-driven dementia-compromised behavior: an alternative view of disruptive behavior, *Am J Alzheimers Dis Other Demen* 11(6):10-19, 1996.

Algase DL, Kupferschmid B, Beel-Bates CA et al: Estimates of stability of daily wandering behavior among cognitively impaired long-term care residents, *Nurs Res* 46(3):172-178, 1997.

Algase DL, Son GR, Beattie E et al: The interrelatedness of wandering and wayfinding in a community sample of persons with dementia, *Dement Geriatr Cogn Disord* 17(3):231-239, 2004b.

Algase DL et al: Initial psychometric evaluation of the wayfinding effectiveness scale, *West J Nurs Res*, in press.

Altus DE, Mathews RM, Xaverius PK et al: Evaluating an electronic monitoring system for people who wander, *Am J Alzheimers Dis* 15(2):121-125, 2000.

Beattie ERA, Algase DL: Improving table-sitting behavior of wanderers via theoretic substruction, *J Gerontol Nurs* 28(10):6, 2002.

Beattie ERA, Algase DL, Song J: Keeping wandering nursing home residents at the table: improving food intake using a behavior communication intervention, *Aging Ment Health* 8(2):109, 2004.

Brody EM, Kleban MH, Moss MS et al: Predictors of falls among institutionalized females with Alzheimer's disease, *J Am Geriatr Soc* 32(12):877-882, 1984.

Carillon Nursing and Rehabilitation Center: Nature walk: from aimless wandering to purposeful walking, *Nurs Homes Long Term Care Manage* 49(11):50, 2000.

Chafetz PK: Two dimensional grid is ineffective against demented patients' exiting through glass doors, *Psychol Aging* 5:146, 1990.

Chiu Y, Algase D, Whall A et al: Getting lost: directed attention and executive function in early Alzheimer's disease patients, *Dement Geriatr Cogn Disord* 17(3):174-180, 2004.

Chiu YC, Algase D, Liang J et al: Conceptualization and measurement of getting lost behavior in persons with early dementia, *Int J Geriatr Psychiatry* 20(8):760-768, 2005.

Cohen-Mansfield J, Werner P: The effects of an enhanced environment on nursing home residents who pace, *Gerontologist* 38(2):199, 1998.

Cornbleth T: Effects of a protected hospital ward area on wandering and non-wandering geriatric patients, *J Gerontol* 32:573, 1977.

Cox C: Race and caregiving: patterns of service use by African American and white caregivers of persons with Alzheimer's, *J Gerontol Soc Work* 32(2):5, 1999.

Dawson P, Reid DW: Behavioral dimensions of patients at risk for wandering, *Gerontologist* 27:104, 1987.

Fischer P, Marterer A, Danielczyk W: Right-left disorientation in dementia of the Alzheimer's type, *Neurology* 40:1619, 1990.

Gerdner LA: Effects of individualized versus classical "relaxation" music on the frequency of agitation in elderly persons with Alzheimer's disease and related disorders, *Int Psychogeriatr* 12(1):49, 2000.

Guttman R: Case management of the frail elderly in the community, *Clin Nurse Spec* 13(4):174, 1999.

Haley WE, West CA, Wadley VG et al: Psychological, social, and health impact of caregiving: a comparison of black and white dementia family caregivers and noncaregivers, *Psychol Aging* 10(4):540-552, 1995.

Hamilton C: *The use of tape patterns as an alternative method for controlling wanderers' exiting behavior in a dementia care unit* (unpublished master's thesis), Blacksburg, Va, 1993, Virginia Polytechnic Institute and State University.

Heard K, Watson TS: Reducing wandering by persons with dementia using differential reinforcement, *J Appl Behav Anal* 32(9): 381, 1999.

Heineken J: Patient silence is not necessarily client satisfaction: communication in home care nursing, *Home Healthc Nurse* 16(2):115, 1998.

Henderson V, Mack W, Williams BW: Spatial disorientation in Alzheimer's disease, *Arch Neurol* 46:391, 1989.

Hewewasam L: Floor patterns limit wandering of people with Alzheimer's, *Nurs Times* 92:41, 1996.

Hinrichsen GA, Ramirez M: Black and white dementia caregivers: a comparison of their adaptation, *Gerontologist* 32(3):375, 1992.

Hirst ST, Metcalf BJ: Whys and whats of wandering, *Geriatr Nurs* 10(5):237, 1989.

Holmberg SK: Evaluation of a clinical intervention for wanderers on a geriatric nursing unit, *Arch Psychiatr Nurs* 11:21, 1997.

Hussian RA: Psychotherapeutic intervention: organic mental disorders In Hussian RA: *Geriatric psychology: a behavioural perspective,* New York, 1981, Van Nostrand Reinhold.

Hussian RA: Stimulus control in the modification of problematic behavior in elderly institutionalized patients, *Int J Behav Geriatr* 1:33, 1982.

Hussian RA, Brown DC: Use of two dimensional grid patterns to limit hazardous ambulation in demented patients, *J Gerontol* 42: 558, 1987.

Katz IR, Rupnow M, Kozma C et al: Risperidone and falls in ambulatory nursing home residents with dementia and psychosis or agitation: secondary analysis of a double-blind, placebo-controlled trial, *Am J Geriatr Psychiatry* 12(5):499-508, 2004.

Kavcic V, Duffy CJ: Attentional dynamics and visual perception: mechanisms of spatial disorientation in Alzheimer's disease, *Brain* 126(pt 5):1173-1181, 2003.

Keily DK, Morris JN, Algase DL: Resident characteristics associated with wandering in nursing homes, *Int J Geriatr Psychiatry* 15:1013, 2000.

Kilstoff K, Chenoweth L: New approaches to health and well-being for dementia day-care clients, family carers and day care staff, *Int J Nurs Pract* 4(2):72, 1998.

Kippenbrock T, Soja M: Preventing falls in the elderly: interviewing patients who have fallen, *Geriatr Nurs* 14:205, 1993.

Kolanowski AM, Strand G, Whall A: A pilot study of the relation in premorbid characteristics to behavior in dementia, *J Gerontol Nurs* 23:21, 1997.

Malaquin-Pavan E: Therapeutic benefit of touch-massage in the overall management of demented elderly, *Rech Soins Infirm* 49:11, 1997.

Mapstone M, Steffenella TM, Duffy CJ: A visuospatial variant of mild cognitive impairment: getting lost between aging and AD, *Neurology* 60(5):802-808, 2003.

Mausbach BT, Coon DW, Depp C et al: Ethnicity and time to institutionalization of dementia patients: a comparison of Latina and Caucasian female family caregivers, *J Am Geriatr Soc* 52(7):1077-1084, 2004.

Monacelli AM, Cushman LA, Kavcic V: Spatial disorientation in Alzheimer's disease: the remembrance of things passed, *Neurology* 61(11):1491-1497, 2003.

Morse J, Tylko S, Dixon H: Characteristics of the fall-prone patient, *Gerontologist* 27:516, 1987.

Namazi KH, Rosner TT, Calkins MP: Visual barriers to prevent ambulatory Alzheimer's patients from exiting through an emergency door, *Gerontologist* 29:699, 1989.

Negley E, Molla PM, Obenchain J: No exit: the effects of an electronic security system on confused patients, *J Gerontol Nurs* 16: 21, 1990.

Nelson A, Powell-Cope G, Gavin-Dreschnack D et al: Technology to promote safe mobility in the elderly, *Nurs Clin North Am* 39(3):649-671, 2004.

Oddy R: Walk this way: assisted exercise for all people with dementia, *J Dement Care* 12(1):21, 2004.

Passini R, Pigot H, Rainville C et al: Wayfinding in a nursing home for advanced dementia of the Alzheimer's type, *Environ Behav* 32(5):684-710, 2000.

Passini R, Rainville C, Marchand N et al: Wayfinding in dementia of the Alzheimer's type: planning abilities, *J Clin Exp Neuropsychol* 17(6):820-832, 1995.

Price JC, Hermans DG, Grimley Evans J: Subjective barriers to prevent wandering of cognitively impaired people, *Cochrane Database Syst Rev* (4):CD001932, 2000.

Robb SS: Exercise treatment for wandering. In Altman HJ, editor: *Alzheimer's disease: problems, prospects, and perspectives*, New York, 1987, Plenum.

Rowe M, Alfred D: The effectiveness of slow stroke massage in diffusing agitated behaviors in individuals with Alzheimer's disease, *J Gerontol Nurs* 25(6):22, 1999.

Rowe MA, Bennett V: A look at deaths occurring in persons with dementia lost in the community, *Am J Alzheimers Dis Other Demen* 18(6):343-348, 2003.

Rowe MA, Feinglass NG, Wiss ME: Persons with dementia who become lost in the community: a case study, current research, and recommendations, *Mayo Clin Proc* 79(11):1417-1422, 2004.

Rowe MA, Glover JC: Antecedents, descriptions and consequences of wandering in cognitively-impaired adults and the Safe Return (SR) program, *Am J Alzheimers Dis* 16(6):344, 2001.

Ryan JP, McGowan J, McCaffrey N et al: Graphomotor perseveration and wandering in Alzheimer's disease, *J Geriatr Psychiatry Neurol* 8(4):209-212, 1995.

Siders C, Nelson A, Brown LM et al: Evidence for implementing nonpharmacological interventions for wandering, *Rehabil Nurs* 29(6):195-206, 2004.

Sink KM, Covinsky KE, Newcomer R et al: Ethnic differences in the prevalence and pattern of dementia-related behaviors, *J Am Geriatr Soc* 52(8):1277-1283, 2004.

Snyder M, Egan E, Burns K: Interventions for decreasing agitation behaviors in persons with dementia, *J Gerontol Nurs* 21(7):34, 1995.

Snyder M, Olson J: Music and hand massage interventions to produce relaxation and reduce aggressive behaviors in cognitively impaired elders: a pilot study, *Clin Gerontol* 17(1):64, 1996.

Sutherland JA, Reakes J, Bridges C: Foot acupressure and massage for patients with Alzheimer's disease and related dementias, *J Nurs Sch* 31(4):34, 1999.

Teri L, Ferretti LE, Gibbons LE et al: Anxiety of Alzheimer's disease: prevalence and comorbidity, *J Gerontol A Biol Sci Med Sci* 54(7): M348-M342, 1999.

Thomas DW: Understanding the wandering patient: a continuity of personality perspective, *J Gerontol Nurs* 23(1):16, 1997.

Nursing Diagnoses Arranged by Maslow's Hierarchy of Needs

Because human beings adapt in many ways to establish and maintain the self, health problems are much more than simple physical matters. Maslow's Hierarchy of Needs (see diagram below) is a system of classifying human needs. Maslow's hierarchy is based on the idea that lower-level physiological needs must be met before higher-level, abstract needs can be met.

For nurses, Maslow's hierarchy has special significance in decision making and planning for care. By considering need categories as you identify client problems, you will be able to provide more holistic care. For example, a client who demands frequent attention for a seemingly trivial matter

may require help with self-esteem needs. Need levels vary from client to client. If a client is short of breath, the client is probably not interested in or capable of discussing spirituality. In addition, a client's need level may change throughout planning and intervention, so you will need to be vigilant in your assessment.

Read the descriptions of each category in the diagram and see how you would relate them to nursing diagnoses. Compare your evaluation with how the authors categorized the nursing diagnoses according to this hierarchy. Be sure to assess clients for potential problems at all levels of the pyramid, regardless of their initial symptom.

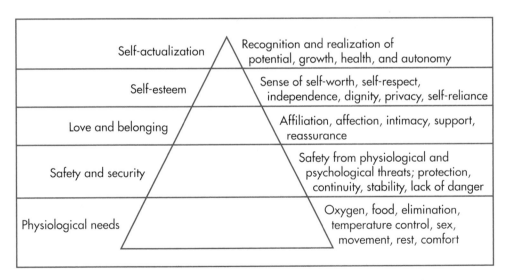

- Self-actualization — Recognition and realization of potential, growth, health, and autonomy
- Self-esteem — Sense of self-worth, self-respect, independence, dignity, privacy, self-reliance
- Love and belonging — Affiliation, affection, intimacy, support, reassurance
- Safety and security — Safety from physiological and psychological threats; protection, continuity, stability, lack of danger
- Physiological needs — Oxygen, food, elimination, temperature control, sex, movement, rest, comfort

PHYSIOLOGICAL NEEDS

Activity intolerance
Activity intolerance, risk for
Airway clearance, ineffective
Allergy response, latex
Aspiration, risk for
Body temperature, risk for imbalanced
Bowel incontinence
Breastfeeding, effective
Breastfeeding, ineffective
Breastfeeding, interrupted
Breathing pattern, ineffective
Cardiac output, decreased
Comfort, readiness for enhanced
Constipation
Constipation, perceived
Constipation, risk for
Dentition, impaired
Diarrhea
Fatigue
Fluid balance, readiness for enhanced
Fluid volume, deficient
Fluid volume, excess
Fluid volume, risk for deficient
Fluid volume, risk for imbalanced
Gas exchange, impaired
Glucose level, risk for unstable
Hyperthermia
Hypothermia
Immunization status, readiness for enhanced
Incontinence, functional urinary
Incontinence, overflow
Incontinence, reflex urinary
Incontinence, risk for urge urinary
Incontinence, stress urinary
Incontinence, total urinary
Incontinence, urge urinary
Infant behavior, disorganized
Infant behavior, readiness for enhanced organized
Infant behavior, risk for disorganized
Infant feeding pattern, ineffective
Insomnia
Intracranial adaptive capacity, decreased
Liver function, risk for impaired
Mobility, impaired bed
Mobility, impaired physical
Mobility, impaired wheelchair
Nausea
Nutrition, imbalanced: less than body requirements
Nutrition, imbalanced: more than body requirements
Nutrition, imbalanced: risk for more than body requirements
Oral mucous membrane, impaired
Pain, acute
Pain, chronic

Protection, ineffective
Self-care deficit, bathing/hygiene
Self-care deficit, dressing/grooming
Self-care deficit, feeding
Self-care deficit, toileting
Sensory perception, disturbed (specify): visual, auditory, kinesthetic, gustatory, tactile, olfactory
Sexual dysfunction
Sexuality patterns, ineffective
Skin integrity, impaired
Skin integrity, risk for impaired
Sleep deprivation
Sleep, readiness for enhanced
Surgical recovery, delayed
Swallowing, impaired
Thermoregulation, ineffective
Thought processes, disturbed
Tissue integrity, impaired
Tissue perfusion, ineffective (specify type): cerebral, renal, cardiopulmonary, gastrointestinal, peripheral
Transfer ability, impaired
Urinary elimination, readiness for enhanced
Urinary elimination, impaired
Urinary retention
Ventilation, impaired spontaneous
Ventilatory weaning response, dysfunctional
Walking, impaired

SAFETY AND SECURITY NEEDS

Allergy response, risk for latex
Anxiety
Anxiety, death
Autonomic dysreflexia
Autonomic dysreflexia, risk for
Communication, readiness for enhanced
Communication, impaired verbal
Confusion, acute
Confusion, risk for acute
Confusion, chronic
Contamination
Contamination, risk for
Death syndrome, risk for sudden infant
Disuse syndrome, risk for
Environmental interpretation syndrome, impaired
Falls, risk for
Family role performance, supportive
Family processes, dysfunctional: alcoholism
Fear
Grieving
Grieving, complicated
Grieving, risk for complicated
Growth, risk for disproportionate
Health maintenance, ineffective
Home maintenance, impaired

Infection, risk for
Injury, risk for
Perioperative-positioning injury, risk for
Knowledge, deficient
Knowledge of (specify), readiness for enhanced
Memory, impaired
Neglect, unilateral
Peripheral neurovascular dysfunction, risk for
Poisoning, risk for
Religiosity impaired
Religiosity, risk for impaired
Sorrow, chronic
Suffocation, risk for
Therapeutic regimen management, ineffective
Therapeutic regimen management, ineffective community
Therapeutic regimen management, ineffective family
Therapeutic regimen management, readiness for enhanced
Trauma, risk for
Wandering

LOVE AND BELONGING NEEDS

Anxiety
Attachment, risk for impaired parent/infant/child
Caregiver role strain
Caregiver role strain, risk for
Conflict, parental role
Coping, compromised family
Coping, disabled family
Coping, readiness for enhanced
Coping, readiness for enhanced family
Failure to thrive, adult
Family processes, interrupted
Family processes, readiness for enhanced
Grieving Loneliness, risk for
Parenting, impaired
Parenting, readiness for enhanced
Parenting, risk for impaired
Relocation stress syndrome
Relocation stress syndrome, risk for
Social interaction, impaired
Social isolation

SELF-ESTEEM NEEDS

Body image, disturbed
Conflict, decisional
Coping, defensive
Coping, ineffective
Coping, ineffective community
Coping, readiness for enhanced community
Decision Making, readiness for enhanced
Denial, ineffective
Dignity, risk for compromised human
Diversional activity, deficient
Health behavior, risk prone
Hope, readiness for enhanced
Hopelessness
Identity, disturbed personal
Noncompliance
Post-trauma syndrome
Post-trauma syndrome, risk for
Power, readiness for enhanced
Powerlessness
Powerlessness, risk for
Rape-trauma syndrome
Rape-trauma syndrome: compound reaction
Rape-trauma syndrome: silent reaction
Role performance, ineffective
Self-esteem, chronic low
Self-esteem, situational low
Self-esteem, risk for situational low
Self-mutilation
Self-mutilation, risk for
Suicide, risk for
Violence, risk for other-directed
Violence, risk for self-directed
Self-Actualization Needs
Development, risk for delayed
Energy field, disturbed
Growth and development, delayed
Health-seeking behaviors
Nutrition, readiness for enhanced
Religiosity readiness for enhanced
Sedentary lifestyle
Self-Care, readiness for enhanced
Self-concept, readiness for enhanced
Spiritual distress
Spiritual distress, risk for
Spiritual well-being, readiness for enhanced
Therapeutic regimen management, effective

Nursing Diagnoses Arranged by Gordon's Functional Health Patterns[1]

Diagnoses currently accepted by NANDA International (North American Nursing Diagnosis Association, new/revised diagnoses are indicated by *). Italicized diagnoses were developed by Marjory Gordon, not yet reviewed by NANDA-I, but are found to be useful in clinical practice.

HEALTH-PERCEPTION-HEALTH-MANAGEMENT PATTERN

Health-seeking behaviors (specify)
Ineffective Health maintenance (specify)
Ineffective Therapeutic regimen management (specify area)
Risk for ineffective Therapeutic regimen management (specify area)
Readiness for enhanced Therapeutic regimen management
Effective Therapeutic regimen management (specify area)
Health-Management Deficit (specify area)
Risk for Health-Management Deficit (specify area)
Noncompliance (specify area)
Risk for Noncompliance (specify area)
Risk for Infection (specify type and area)
Risk for Injury (trauma)
Risk for Falls
Risk for perioperative-positioning Injury
Risk for Poisoning
Risk for Suffocation
Ineffective Protection (specify)
Disturbed Energy field
Contamination*
Risk for Contamination*
Readiness for enhanced Immunization status*

NUTRITIONAL-METABOLIC PATTERN

Adult Failure to thrive
Imbalanced Nutrition: more than body requirements or *Exogenous Obesity*
Risk for imbalanced Nutrition: more than body requirements or *Risk for Obesity*
Imbalanced Nutrition: less than body requirements or *Nutritional Deficit (specify type)*
Readiness for enhanced Nutrition
Interrupted Breastfeeding
Ineffective Breastfeeding
Effective Breastfeeding
Ineffective Infant feeding pattern

Impaired Swallowing (uncompensated)
Nausea
Risk for Aspiration
Impaired Oral mucous membrane (specify impairment)
Impaired Dentition
Risk for imbalanced Fluid volume
Excess Fluid volume
Deficient Fluid volume
Risk for deficient Fluid volume
Readiness for enhanced Fluid balance
Impaired Skin integrity
Risk for impaired Skin integrity or *Risk for Skin Breakdown*
Impaired Tissue integrity (specify type)
Pressure Ulcer (specify type)
Latex Allergy response
Ineffective Thermoregulation
Hypothermia
Risk for imbalanced Body temperature
Risk for unstable blood Glucose*
Risk for Impaired Liver function*

ELIMINATION PATTERN

Constipation
Perceived Constipation
Intermittent Constipation Pattern
Risk for Constipation
Diarrhea
Bowel Incontinence
Reflex urinary Incontinence
Stress urinary Incontinence
Urge urinary Incontinence
Risk for Urge urinary Incontinence
Total urinary Incontinence
Urinary Retention
Readiness for enhanced Urinary elimination
Overflow urinary Incontinence*

ACTIVITY-EXERCISE PATTERN

Activity intolerance (specify level)
Risk for Activity intolerance
Sedentary lifestyle
Fatigue
Deficient Diversional activity
Impaired physical Mobility (specify level)
Impaired Walking (specify level)
Impaired wheelchair Mobility
Impaired bed Mobility (specify level)
Impaired Transfer ability (specify level)

From Gordon M: *Manual of nursing diagnosis*, ed 11, Sudbury Mass, 2007, Jones & Bartlett.
[1]As updated by Gail Ladwig to incorporate the 2007-2008 NANDA-I Nursing Diagnoses.

Wandering
 Risk for Disuse syndrome
Risk for Joint Contractures
Total Self-care deficit (specify level)
Bathing/hygiene Self-care deficit (specify level)
Dressing/grooming Self-care deficit (specify level)
Feeding Self-care deficit (specify level)
Toileting Self-care deficit (specify level)
Developmental Delay: Self-care Skills (specify level)
Delayed Surgical recovery
Delayed Growth and development
Risk for delayed Development
Risk for disproportionate Growth
Impaired Home maintenance
Dysfunctional Ventilatory weaning response
Impaired spontaneous Ventilation
Ineffective Airway clearance
Ineffective Breathing pattern
Impaired Gas exchange
Decreased Cardiac output
Ineffective Tissue perfusion (specify Type)
Autonomic dysreflexia
Risk for Autonomic dysreflexia
Risk for sudden infant Death syndrome
Disorganized Infant behavior
Risk for disorganized Infant behavior
Readiness for enhanced organized Infant behavior
Risk for peripheral Neurovascular dysfunction
Decreased Intracranial adaptive capacity
Readiness for enhanced Self-Care*

SLEEP-REST PATTERN

Insomnia*
Sleep deprivation
Delayed Sleep Onset
Sleep Pattern Reversal
Readiness for enhanced Sleep

COGNITIVE-PERCEPTUAL PATTERN

Acute Pain (specify location)
Chronic Pain (specify location)
Chronic Pain Self-Management Deficit
Uncompensated Sensory Loss (specify type/degree)
Sensory Overload
Sensory Deprivation
Unilateral Neglect
Deficient Knowledge
Readiness for enhanced Knowledge
Disturbed Thought processes
Attention-Concentration Deficit
Acute Confusion

Chronic Confusion
Impaired Environmental interpretation syndrome
Uncompensated Memory Loss
Impaired Memory
Risk for Cognitive Impairment
Decisional Conflict (specify)
Risk for Acute Confusion*
Readiness for enhanced Decision making*
Readiness for enhanced Comfort*

SELF-PERCEPTION-SELF-CONCEPT PATTERN

Fear (specify focus)
Anxiety
Mild Anxiety
Moderate Anxiety
Severe Anxiety (panic)
Anticipatory Anxiety (mild, moderate, severe)
Death Anxiety
Reactive Depression (specify focus)
Risk for Loneliness
Hopelessness
Powerlessness (severe, moderate, low)
Risk for Powerlessness
Chronic low Self-esteem
Situational low Self-esteem
Risk for situational low Self-esteem
Disturbed Body image
Disturbed personal Identity
Readiness for enhanced Self-concept
Risk for self-directed Violence
Readiness for enhanced Hope*
Readiness for enhanced Power*

ROLE-RELATIONSHIP PATTERN

Grieving*
Complicated Grieving*
Risk for Complicated Grieving*
Chronic Sorrow
Ineffective Role Performance (specify)
Unresolved Independence-Dependence Conflict
Social isolation or *Social rejection*
Social isolation
Impaired Social interaction
Developmental Delay: Social Skills (specify)
Relocation stress syndrome
Risk for Relocation stress syndrome
Interrupted Family Processes (specify)
Dysfunctional Family processes: alcoholism
Readiness for enhanced Family processes
Impaired Parenting (specify Impairment)
Risk for impaired Parenting (specify)

Weak Parent-Infant Attachment
Risk for impaired parent/infant/child Attachment
Parent-Infant Separation
Readiness for enhanced Parenting
Caregiver role strain
Impaired verbal Communication
Readiness for enhanced Communication
Developmental Delay: Communication Skills (specify type)
Risk for other-directed Violence

SEXUALITY-REPRODUCTIVE PATTERN

Ineffective Sexuality patterns
Sexual dysfunction
Rape trauma syndrome
Rape trauma syndrome: compound reaction
Rape trauma syndrome: silent reaction

COPING-STRESS-TOLERANCE PATTERN

Ineffective Coping (specify)
Readiness for enhanced Coping
Avoidance Coping

Defensive Coping
Ineffective Denial or *Denial*
Risk for Suicide
Compromised family Coping
Disabled family Coping
Readiness for enhanced family Coping
Ineffective community Coping
Readiness for enhanced community Coping
Support System Deficit
Risk-prone Health Behavior*
Post-trauma syndrome
Risk for Post-trauma syndrome
Self-mutilation
Risk for Self-mutilation
Stress overload*
Risk for Compromised Human Dignity*
Moral Distress*

VALUE-BELIEF PATTERN

Spiritual distress
Risk for Spiritual distress
Readiness for enhanced Spiritual well-being
Impaired religiosity
Risk for impaired Religiosity
Readiness for enhanced Religiosity

Wellness-Oriented Diagnostic Categories

This is a list of NANDA-I diagnoses in a wellness format. When available, readiness diagnoses are listed first in each category. Risk diagnoses are listed next. The goal is to support wellness, prevent illness, and intervene when illness is present.

Diagnoses are arranged first by priority according to the ABCs (airway, breathing, circulation). They are then arranged according to possible priority physiological needs and then psychosocial needs. Diagnoses dealing with family, infant, and child are grouped together. It is the responsibility of the nurse to individualize and reorder based on the patient's assessment data.

Adult: (asterisked diagnoses have pediatric interventions in care plans**)

PHYSIOLOGICAL

Airway/Breathing

- Risk for Aspiration
- Risk for Suffocation
- Impaired Swallowing
- Ineffective Airway clearance
- Ineffective Breathing pattern
- Impaired Gas exchange
- Impaired spontaneous Ventilation
- Dysfunctional Ventilatory weaning response

Circulation

- Risk for **Peripheral** neurovascular dysfunction
- Decreased **Cardiac** output
- Ineffective **Tissue** perfusion

Cognition/Sensory Perception

- Risk for acute **Confusion**
- Risk **Autonomic** dysreflexia
- **Autonomic** dysreflexia
- Decreased **Intracranial** adaptive capacity
- Disturbed **Sensory** perception
- Acute **Confusion**
- Chronic **Confusion**
- Impaired **Environmental** interpretation syndrome
- Impaired **Memory**
- Disturbed **Thought** processes

Injury: Falls/Infection/Poisoning/Trauma

- Readiness for Enhanced **Immunization** Status**
- Risk for **Contamination**
- Risk for **Falls**
- Risk for **Injury****

- Risk for Infection**
- Risk for latex Allergy response
- Risk for perioperative positioning Injury
- Risk for Poisoning**
- Risk for Trauma
- Acute Pain** (psychosocial)
- Chronic Pain** (psychosocial)
- Contamination
- Delayed Surgical recovery
- Ineffective Protection
- Latex Allergy response
- Rape-trauma syndrome
- Rape-trauma syndrome: silent reaction
- Rape-trauma syndrome: compound reaction

Homeostasis

- Risk for impaired **Liver** function
- Risk for unstable **Blood** sugar
- Risk for imbalanced **Body** temperature**
- Adult **Failure** to thrive
- Disturbed **Energy** field**
- **Hyperthermia**
- **Hypothermia****
- Ineffective **Thermoregulation**

Fluid/Nutrition/Oral/Dental Management

- Readiness for enhanced **Fluid** balance
- Readiness for enhanced **Nutrition**
- Risk for imbalanced **Nutrition:** more than body requirements
- Risk for imbalanced **Fluid** volume
- Risk for deficient **Fluid** volume
- **Nausea**
- Imbalanced **Nutrition:** more than body requirements
- Imbalanced **Nutrition:** less than body requirements
- Deficient **Fluid** volume**
- Excess **Fluid** volume
- Impaired **Oral** mucous membrane
- Impaired **Dentition**

Elimination
Urinary Elimination

- Readiness for enhanced **Urinary** elimination
- Impaired **Urinary** elimination
- **Urinary** retention

Incontinence, Bowel

- **Bowel** incontinence

Incontinence, Bladder

- Risk for urge urinary **Incontinence**
- Functional urinary **Incontinence**
- Overflow urinary **Incontinence**
- Reflex urinary **Incontinence**
- Stress urinary **Incontinence**
- Urge urinary **Incontinence**

Bowel Elimination
Constipation

- Risk for Constipation
- Perceived Constipation
- Constipation

Diarrhea

- Diarrhea**

Activity/Movement/Self-Care

- Readiness for enhanced **Self-Care**
- Risk for **Activity** intolerance
- Risk for **Disuse** syndrome
- Sedentary **Lifestyle****
- Deficient **Diversional** activity**
- **Activity** intolerance
- **Fatigue**
- Impaired physical **Mobility**
- Bathing/hygiene **Self-care** deficit
- Dressing/grooming **Self-care** deficit
- Feeding **Self-care** deficit
- Toileting **Self-care** deficit
- Impaired **Walking**
- Impaired **Transfer** ability
- Impaired bed **Mobility**
- Impaired wheelchair **Mobility**
- Unilateral **Neglect** syndrome
- **Wandering**

Skin/Tissue

- Risk for impaired **Skin** integrity
- Impaired **Skin** integrity
- Impaired **Tissue** integrity

Sleep

- Readiness for enhanced **Sleep**
- **Insomnia**
- **Sleep** deprivation

PSYCHOSOCIAL

Comfort

- Readiness for enhanced **Comfort**
- Impaired **Comfort**
- Acute **Pain** (Physiological)**
- Chronic **Pain** (Physiological)**

Communication/Healthy Behaviors/Therapeutic Regimen/Knowledge
Individual

- Readiness for enhanced **Communication****
- Readiness for enhanced Therapeutic regimen management
- Readiness for enhanced Knowledge**
- Risk-prone health Behavior
- Effective Therapeutic regimen management
- Health-seeking behaviors**
- Impaired verbal **Communication****
- Ineffective Therapeutic regimen management
- Deficient Knowledge**
- Ineffective Health maintenance

Community

- Ineffective community **Therapeutic** regimen management

Family

- Ineffective family **Therapeutic** regimen management

Spirituality/Religious Beliefs

- Readiness for enhanced **Spiritual** well-being
- Readiness for enhanced **Religiosity****
- Readiness for enhanced **Hope**
- Risk for **Spiritual** distress
- Risk for impaired **Religiosity**
- Impaired **Religiosity**
- **Spiritual** distress
- Impaired **Religiosity**
- **Hopelessness**

Harm: Self and Others

- Risk for **Suicide**
- Risk for **Self-mutilation**
- Risk for other-directed **Violence**
- Risk for self-directed **Violence**
- **Self-mutilation**

Anxiety/Stress

- Readiness for enhanced **Decision** making
- Risk for **Relocation stress syndrome**
- Risk for compromised human **Dignity**
- **Anxiety**
- Death **Anxiety**
- Ineffective **Denial**
- Decisional **Conflict**
- Dysfunctional **Family** processes: alcoholism**
- **Fear****
- **Noncompliance**
- **Relocation** stress syndrome**
- **Stress** overload

Coping
Individual

- Readiness for enhanced **Coping****
- Readiness for enhanced **Power**
- Risk for **Caregiver** role strain
- Risk for **Powerlessness**
- Risk for **Loneliness****
- Risk for **Post-trauma** syndrome**
- **Social** isolation
- Defensive **Coping**
- Deficient health **Behavior**
- Ineffective **Coping**
- **Caregiver** role strain
- Impaired **Social** interaction
- **Post-trauma** syndrome
- **Powerlessness**
- Ineffective **Role** performance**

Community

- Readiness for enhanced community **Coping**
- Compromised family **Coping**
- Ineffective community **Coping**

Sexuality/Body Image

- Disturbed **Body** image
- **Sexual** dysfunction
- Ineffective **Sexuality** patterns**

Grief/Sorrow

- Risk for complicated Grieving**
- Grieving**
- Complicated Grieving**
- Chronic Sorrow

Self-concept/Self-esteem/Personal Identity

- Readiness for enhanced **Self-concept****
- Risk for situational low **Self-esteem**
- Situational low **Self-esteem**
- Chronic low **Self-esteem**

FAMILY/INFANT/CHILD

Sudden Infant Death

- Risk for sudden infant **Death** syndrome

Development/Growth

- Risk for delayed **Development**
- Risk for disproportionate **Growth**
- Delayed **Growth** and development

Infant Care

- Readiness for enhanced organized **Infant** behavior
- Readiness for enhanced **Immunization** status
- Risk for disorganized **Infant** behavior
- Risk for impaired parent/child **Attachment**
- Disorganized **Infant** behavior
- Ineffective **Infant** feeding pattern

Parenting

- Readiness for enhanced **Parenting**
- Risk for impaired **Parenting**
- Impaired **Parenting**
- Parental role **Conflict**

Breastfeeding

- Effective Breastfeeding
- Interrupted Breastfeeding
- Ineffective Breastfeeding

Coping/Family

- Readiness for enhanced family **Coping**
- Compromised family **Coping**
- Disabled family **Coping**
- Ineffective family **Therapeutic** regimen management

Family Processes

- Readiness for enhanced **Family** processes
- Interrupted **Family** processes
- Dysfunctional **Family** processes: alcoholism

A Guide to Using Equianalgesic Charts

- Equianalgesic means approximately the same pain relief.
- The equianalgesic chart is a guideline. Doses and intervals between doses are titrated according to the individual's response.
- The equianalgesic chart is helpful when switching from one drug to another or switching from one route of administration to another. (Exception: see comments for methadone.)
- Dosages in the equianalgesic chart for moderate to severe pain are not necessarily starting doses. The doses suggest a ratio for comparing the analgesia of one drug to another.
- For elders, initially reduce the recommended adult opioid dose for moderate to severe pain by 25% to 50%.
- The longer the client has been receiving opioids, the more conservative the starting doses of a *new* opioid.

Equianalgesic Chart: Approximate Equivalent Doses of Opioids for Moderate to Severe Pain

Analgesic	Parenteral (IM, SC, IV) Route (mg)*†	PO Route* (mg)	Comments
mu-Opioid Agonists			
Morphine	10	30	Standard for comparison Multiple routes of administration Available in immediate-release and controlled-release formulations Active metabolic M6G can accumulate with repeated dosing in renal failure
Codeine	130	200 NR	IM has unpredictable absorption and high side effect profile Used PO for mild to moderate pain Usually compounded with nonopioid (e.g., Tylenol 3).
Fentanyl	100 micrograms/h parenterally and transdermally ≅4 mg/h morphine parenterally; 1 microgram/h transdermally ≅2 mg/24 h morphine PO	—	Short half-life, but at a steady state slow elimination from tissues can lead to a prolonged half-life (up to 12 h) Start opioid-naive clients on no more than 12 to 25 micrograms/h transdermally Transdermal fentanyl NR for acute pain management Available by oral transmucosal route
Hydrocodone (Vicodin, Lortab)		30? (NR)	Equianalgesic information lacking
Hydromorphone (Dilaudid)	1.5	7.5	Useful alternative to morphine with shorter duration than morphine Available in high-potency parenteral formulation (10 mg/mL) useful for SC infusion; 3 mg rectal ≅650 mg aspirin PO. With repeated dosing (e.g., client-controlled analgesia), it is more likely that 2 to 3 mg parenteral hydromorphone = 10 mg parenteral morphine.
Levorphanol (Levo-Dromoran)	2	4	Longer acting than morphine when given repeatedly Long half-life can lead to accumulation within 2 to 3 days of repeated dosing
Meperidine	75	300 NR	Not a first-line opioid for the management of acute or chronic pain because of potential toxicity from accumulation of metabolite normeperidine Normeperidine has 15- to 20-h half-life and is not reversed by naloxone NR in elderly or clients with impaired renal function NR by continuous IV infusion

Analgesic	Parenteral (IM, SC, IV) Route (mg)*†	PO Route* (mg)	Comments
mu-Opioid Agonists (cont'd)			
Methadone (Dolophine)	—	—	Longer acting than morphine when given repeatedly Long half-life can lead to delayed toxicity from accumulation within 3 to 5 days Equianalgesic dosing is controversial and use of an equianalgesic chart is usually not recommended when switching to methadone. Instead, many clinicians use a ratio approach such as the following (Miaskowski et al, 2005): 1. Stop morphine or other opioid. 2. Give methadone at fixed intervals, q 8 h. 3. If the total daily PO morphine dose is: • Less than 90 mg/day, use morphine: methadone ratio of 4:1 • 90 to 300 mg/day, use ratio of 8:1 • Greater than 300 mg/day, use ratio of 12:1 4. Breakthrough dose of short-acting opioid should be 10% of total daily methadone dose. Start PO dosing on PRN schedule In opioid-tolerant clients converted to methadone, start with 10% to 25% of equianalgesic dose
Oxycodone	—	20	Used for moderate pain when combined with a nonopioid (e.g., Percocet, Tylox) Available as a single entity in immediate-release and controlled-release formulations (e.g., OxyContin) Can be used like PO morphine for severe pain
Oxymorphone (Numorphan)	1	10	Used for moderate to severe pain Oral extended-release formulation available for twice-daily dosing
Agonist-Antagonist Opioids			
Not recommended for severe, escalating pain. If used in combination with μ-agonists, may reverse analgesia and precipitate withdrawal in opioid-dependent clients.			
Buprenorphine (Buprenex)	0.4	—	Not readily reversed by naloxone NR for laboring clients
Butorphanol (Stadol)	2	—	Available in nasal spray
Dezocine (Dalgan)	10	—	
Nalbuphine (Nubain)	10	—	
Pentazocine (Talwin)	60	180	

*Duration of analgesia is dose dependent; the higher the dose, usually the longer the duration.

†IV boluses may be used to produce analgesia that lasts approximately as long as IM or SC doses. However, of all routes of administration, IV produces the highest peak concentration of the drug, and the peak concentration is associated with the highest level of toxicity, e.g., sedation. To decrease the peak effect and lower the level of toxicity, IV boluses may be administered more slowly (e.g., 10 mg of morphine over a 15-minute period) or smaller doses may be administered more often (e.g., 5 mg of morphine every 1 to 1.5 hours).

IM, Intramuscular; *SC,* subcutaneous; *IV,* intravenous; *PO,* by mouth; *NR,* not recommended; *PRN,* as needed.

Adapted from McCaffery M, Pasero C: *Pain: clinical manual,* St Louis, 1999, Mosby, based on the recommendations from the American Pain Society: *Principles of analgesic use in the treatment of acute pain and cancer pain,* ed 5, Glenview, IL, 2003, The Society, and Miaskowski C, Cleary J, Burney R et al: *Guideline for the management of cancer pain in adults and children,* Glenview, Ill, 2005, American Pain Society.